D1232038

Molecular Genetic Testing in Surgical Pathology

Molecular Genetic Testing in Surgical Pathology

■ JOHN D. PFEIFER, M.D., Ph.D.

Associate Professor
Department of Pathology and Immunology
Washington University School of Medicine
St. Louis, Missouri

with contributions by
DANIEL A. ARBER, M.D.
CHRISTINE E. FULLER, M.D.
M. RAJAN MARIAPPAN, M.D., Ph.D.
ARIE PERRY, M.D.
PANG-HSIEN TU, M.D., Ph.D.
MARK A. WATSON, M.D., Ph.D.
and
BARBARA A. ZEHNBAUER, Ph.D.

 Lippincott Williams & Wilkins
a Wolters Kluwer business
Philadelphia · Baltimore · New York · London
Buenos Aires · Hong Kong · Sydney · Tokyo

Acquisitions Editor: Jonathan W. Pine, Jr.
Managing Editor: Anne E. Jacobs
Project Manager: Alicia Jackson
Senior Manufacturing Manager: Benjamin Rivera
Marketing Manager: Angela Panetta
Cover Designer: Joseph DePinho
Production Service: GGS Book Services
Printer: Edwards Brothers

© 2006 by LIPPINCOTT WILLIAMS & WILKINS
530 Walnut Street
Philadelphia, PA 19106 USA
LWW.com

Library of Congress Cataloging-in-Publication Data
Molecular genetic testing in surgical pathology/editor, John D. Pfeifer; with contributions by Daniel A. Arber . . . [et al.].
p.   ; cm.
Includes index.
ISBN 13: 978-0-7817-4748-6
ISBN 10: 0-7817-4748-1
1. Pathology, Surgical—Technique.   2. Human molecular genetics.
3. Tumors—Genetic aspects. I. Pfeifer, John D.
[DNLM: 1. Neoplasms—pathology.   2. Pathology, surgical.
3. Molecular Diagnostic Techniques—methods.   4.Neoplasms—genetics.
WO 142 M718 2006]
RD57 .M595 2006
617′ .07—dc22   2005027606

Care has been taken to confirm the accuracy of the information presented and to describe generally accepted practices. However, the authors, editors, and publisher are not responsible for errors or omissions or for any consequences from application of the information in this book and make no warranty, expressed or implied, with respect to the currency, completeness, or accuracy of the contents of the publication. Application of the information in a particular situation remains the professional responsibility of the practitioner.

The authors, editors, and publisher have exerted every effort to ensure that drug selection and dosage set forth in this text are in accordance with current recommendations and practice at the time of publication. However, in view of ongoing research, changes in government regulations, and the constant flow of information relating to drug therapy and drug reactions, the reader is urged to check the package insert for each drug for any change in indications and dosage and for added warnings and precautions. This is particularly important when the recommended agent is a new or infrequently employed drug.

Some drugs and medical devices presented in the publication have Food and Drug Administration (FDA) clearance for limited use in restricted research settings. It is the responsibility of the health care provider to ascertain the FDA status of each drug or device planned for use in their clinical practice.

To purchase additional copies of this book, call our customer service department at (800) 638-3030 or fax orders to (301) 223-2320. International customers should call (301) 223-2300.

Visit Lippincott Williams & Wilkins on the Internet: at LWW.com. Lippincott Williams & Wilkins customer service representatives are available from 8:30 am to 6 pm, EST.

10 9 8 7 6 5 4 3

This book is dedicated to the patients behind the tissue specimens, with the hope that molecular genetic testing will increase diagnostic accuracy, provide reliable prognostic information, and identify effective treatment regimens to help ease the physical and psychological burden of their disease.

Contents

Contributing Authors

DANIEL A. ARBER, M.D., Professor, Department of Pathology, Stanford University, Stanford, California; Director, Clinical Hematology Laboratory, and Associate Director, Molecular Pathology, Department of Pathology, Stanford University Hospital and Lucile Packard Children's Hospital, Stanford, California

CHRISTINE E. FULLER, M.D., Assistant Member, Department of Pathology, St. Jude Children's Research Hospital, Memphis, Tennessee

M. RAJAN MARIAPPAN, M.D., PH.D., Clinical Fellow, Hematopathology and Molecular Genetic Pathology, Department of Pathology, Stanford University Medical Center, Stanford, California

ARIE PERRY, M.D., Associate Professor, Department of Pathology and Immunology, Division of Neuropathology, Washington University School of Medicine, St. Louis, Missouri.

PANG-HSIEN TU, M.D., PH.D., Instructor, Department of Pathology and Immunology, Division of Neuropathology, Washington University School of Medicine, St. Louis, Missouri.

MARK A. WATSON, M.D., PH.D., Associate Professor, Department of Pathology and Immunology, Washington University School of Medicine, St. Louis, Missouri

BARBARA A. ZEHNBAUER, PH.D., Professor, Department of Pathology and Immunology and Department of Pediatrics, Washington University School of Medicine, St. Louis, Missouri

Preface

Molecular genetic testing has been an ancillary method in surgical pathology for only about 10 years, but has already had a profound impact on the discipline. Pathologists' interest in structured information about emerging molecular methods is apparent in the high attendance at courses focused on molecular pathology offered at national meetings, and by pathologists' enthusiastic reception of several monographs on the subject. However, my interactions with the residents and fellows in the Department of Pathology at Washington University School of Medicine, as well as my contact with pathologists who send cases to us in consultation, have made it clear that much of the information on molecular analysis is disconnected from the issues that affect the utility of testing in routine practice. There is a need for a practice-based guide to the application of molecular genetic testing in surgical pathology, and this book is intended to serve that function.

This book addresses the various molecular genetic techniques that can be used to provide ancillary information on tissue or cytology samples; the advantages, disadvantages, capabilities, and limitations of the different techniques; and the settings in surgical pathology in which the techniques provide results that are of diagnostic, prognostic, or therapeutic utility. Because the book is intended as a practical guide, it presents the testing approaches for individual tumor types organ system by organ system, and discusses the diagnostic issues that can complicate interpretation of test results, as, for example, when more than one tumor type harbors the same aberration, when more than one mutation is characteristic of a specific tumor type, and so on.

The book is intended to stand on its own, but there is no doubt that space constraints limited the amount of background material that could be included to place molecular genetic testing in the broader context of tumor biology and oncology. Readers are therefore strongly encouraged to consult a text devoted to human molecular biology for more detail on gene structure and function and a text dedicated to oncogenic mechanisms for more detailed descriptions of the aberrations in cellular pathways that are responsible for tumor development.

Acknowledgments

I have had the extreme good fortune to have Drs. John Kissane, Peter Humphrey, and Pepper Dehner as mentors, colleagues, and friends. They have provided a model of diagnostic excellence, academic productivity, and commitment to resident and fellow education. I also want to acknowledge Dr. Emil Unanue, Chairman of the Department of Pathology and Immunology, for providing an environment in which academic surgical pathology can flourish.

I especially recognize the contributions of my colleagues who so willingly contributed their time and expertise to write chapters for the book, including Dr. Barbara A. Zehnbauer, Dr. Mark A. Watson, Dr. Arie Perry, Dr. Pang-hsien Tu, Dr. Christine E. Fuller, Dr. M. Rajan Mariappan, and Dr. Daniel A. Arber. I also thank my colleagues who generously helped me with illustrations of specific diseases, including Dr. Diane Arthur, Dr. Helen Liapis, Dr. Phyllis Huettner, Dr. Ashley Hill, Dr. Jon Ritter, and Dr. Richard Burack. I would be remiss if I did not acknowledge a number of other people who also provided considerable assistance, including my secretary, Sherry Ellis, who typed virtually the entire book; Marcy Hartstein, who drew the figures; Walter Clermont, who helped with photography; and Sherry Cannon, who spent endless hours tracking down references.

I have also been fortunate to have the opportunity to interact with a wonderful group of people at Lippincott, Williams & Wilkins. Ruth Weinberg, Senior Acquisitions Editor, was receptive to my idea for the book. Jonathan Pine, Senior Executive Editor, provided the steady and patient direction needed to ensure the book's completion. Anne Jacobs, Managing Editor, provided encouragement and sage advice when needed most (although it is customary for an author to recognize his Managing Editor as a most helpful, supportive, and understanding person, in my case it also happens to be true).

Finally, and most importantly, I want to thank my kids, Claire and Ethan, and my wife, Andrea, for their patience, good humor, and support over the past 2 1/2 years, when I did little else besides sit in the sun porch and write.

John D. Pfeifer

Molecular Genetic Testing in Surgical Pathology

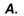

A.

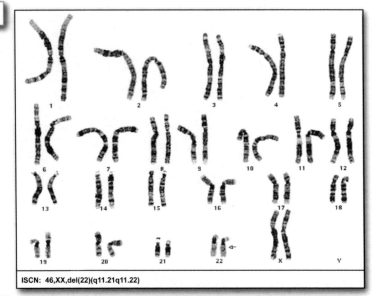

ISCN: 46,XX,del(22)(q11.21q11.22)

B.

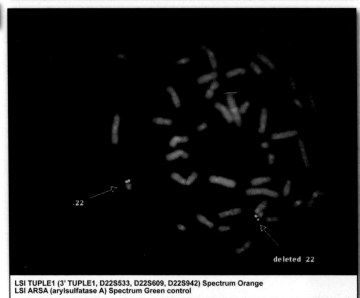

.22

deleted 22

LSI TUPLE1 (3' TUPLE1, D22S533, D22S609, D22S942) Spectrum Orange
LSI ARSA (arylsulfatase A) Spectrum Green control

Figure 3.4 Example of metaphase FISH using a unique sequence probe. **A**, High resolution G-banded karyotype (from peripheral blood lymphocytes) showing a microdeletion of the proximal long arm of one chromosome 22 (arrow). Panel B: Metaphase FISH with the LSI TUPLE1 SpectrumOrange/LSI ARSA SpectrumGreen probe mixture (Vysis, Inc.) confirms deletion of the DiGeorge/velocardiofacial syndrome region (TUPLE1) of one chromosome 22. (Courtesy Dr. Diane Arthur, Head, Clinical Cytogenetics Section, U.S. National Institutes of Health.)

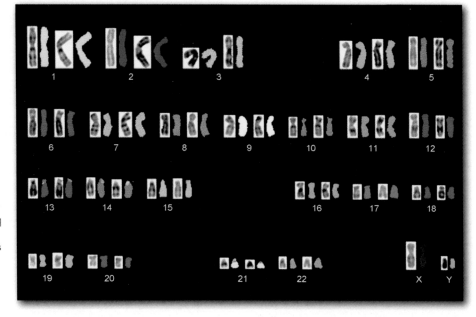

Figure 3.5 Spectral karyotype (SKY, Applied Spectral Imaging, Inc., Vista, CA) of peripheral blood lymphocytes from a normal 46,XY male. For each chromosome pair, black and white DAPI-banded chromosomes are shown on the *left*, and SKY painted chromosomes are shown on the *right*. (Courtesy Dr. Diane Arthur, Head, Clinical Cytogenetics Section, U.S. National Institutes of Health.)

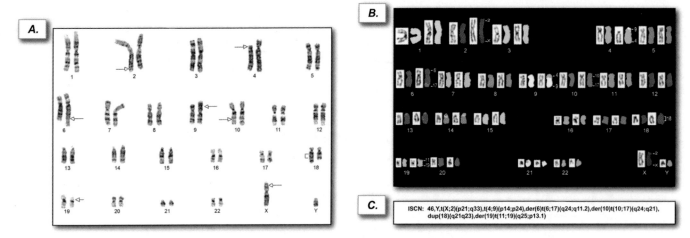

A.

B.

C. ISCN: 46,Y,t(X;2)(p21;q33),t(4;9)(p14;p24),der(6)t(6;17)(q24;q11.2),der(10)t(10;17)(q24;q21),
dup(18)(q21q23),der(19)t(11;19)(q25;p13.1)

Figure 3.6 Example of SKY to establish the origin of rearrangements that cannot be defined based on routine cytogenetic analysis. **A**, G-banded karyotype from bone marrow of a patient with relapsed diffuse large B-cell non-Hodgkin's lymphoma showing a pseudodiploid male karyotype with complex structural rearrangements involving chromosomes X, 2, 4, 6, 9, 10, 18, and 19 (*arrows*). **B**, Spectral karyotyping is necessary to completely define the complex rearrangements noted with G-banding. **C**, Final karyotype. (Courtesy Dr. Diane Arthur, Head, Clinical Cytogenetics Section, U.S. National Institutes of Health.)

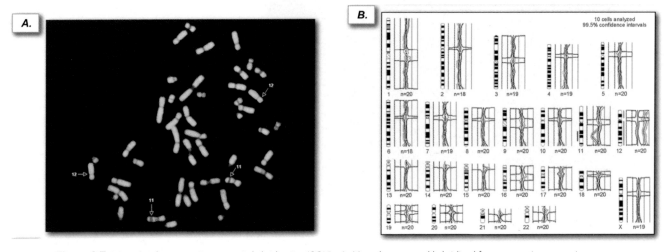

A.

B.

Figure 3.7 Example of comparative genomic hybridization (CGH). **A**, Metaphase spread hybridized for comparative genomic hybridization (GCH, Applied Imagining Corporation, San Jose, CA) showing interstitial deletion of part of the long arm of chromosome 11 and gain of chromosome 12 in a patient with chronic lymphocytic leukemia. **B**, CGH software analysis confirms 11q deletion and trisomy 12. (Courtesy Dr. Diane Arthur, Head, Clinical Cytogenetics Section, U.S. National Institutes of Health.)

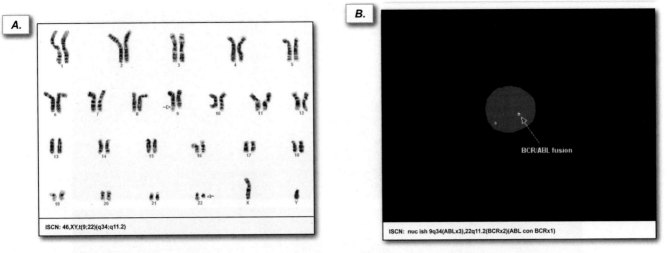

A.

ISCN: 46,XY,t(9;22)(q34;q11.2)

B.

BCR/ABL fusion

ISCN: nuc ish 9q34(ABLx3),22q11.2(BCRx2)(ABL con BCRx1)

Figure 3.8 Example of interphase FISH using the probe fusion approach. **A**, G-banded karyotype from bone marrow showing a single Philadelphia chromosome (Ph) arising from the common t(9;22) translocation (*arrows*) in a patient with chronic myelogenous leukemia in chronic phase. **B**, Interphase FISH with the LSI BCR/ABL ES Dual Color Translocation Probe (Vysis, Inc.) showing the Ph BCR/ABL fusion. (Courtesy Dr. Diane Arthur, Head, Clinical Cytogenetics Section, U.S. National Institutes of Health.)

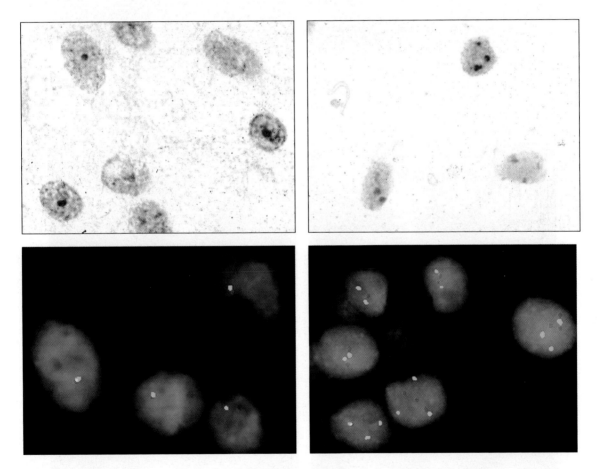

Figure 4.1 Examples of aneusomies using CISH (**A,B**) and FISH (**C,D**). CISH utilizing CEP probes in a glioblastoma with monosomy 10 (**A**, only one brown signal per nucleus) and trisomy 7; **B**, up to 3 brown intranuclear signals). Monosomy 10 (or 10q deletion) is similarly seen with FISH utilizing locus-specific probes against *PTEN* on 10q23 (green) and *DMBT1* on 10q25-q26 (red) (**C**, one green and one red signal per nucleus). Trisomy 17 is seen in a subset of breast cancer cells with 3 CEP 17 (green) and 3 *HER-2/neu* (red) signals (**D**).

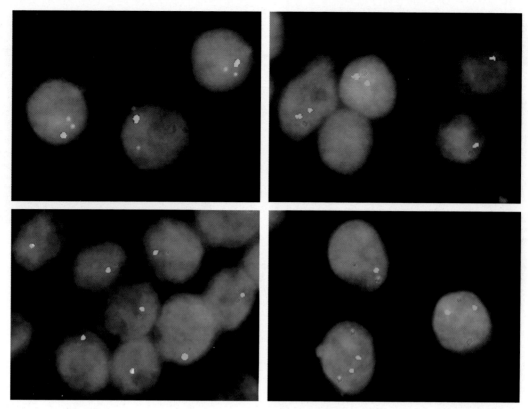

Figure 4.2 Examples of deletions detected by FISH, including an oligodendroglioma with 1p (**A**, one green 1p32 and two red 1q42 signals per nucleus) and 19q deletions (**B**, one red 19q13 and two green 19p13 signals), and an atypical teratoid/rhabdoid tumor (**C**, one green *BCR* and one red *NF2* signal). A glioma with normal complements of chromosome 1 (two green and two red signals in most nuclei) is shown for comparison (**D**).

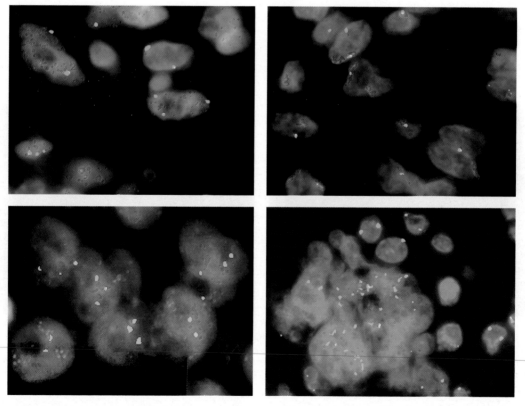

Figure 4.3 Examples of gene amplification, including glioblastomas with EGFR amplification (**A**, "double minute" pattern with small individual red signals; **B**, "homogenously staining region" pattern with large, coalescent red signals; CEP7 in green) and *HER-2/neu* amplification with numerous red gene signals and considerably fewer green CEP17 signals (**C**, *HER-2/neu* to CEP17 signal ratio >2.0). A dramatic example of polysomy 7 is shown for comparison with a multinucleated giant cell containing numerous copies of both the p16 gene on 9p21 in red and the CEP9 reference in green (**D**). In contrast to true gene amplification, the p16 to CEP9 signal ratio was close to 1.0 and several smaller, near diploid cells are seen nearby with two green and two red signals.

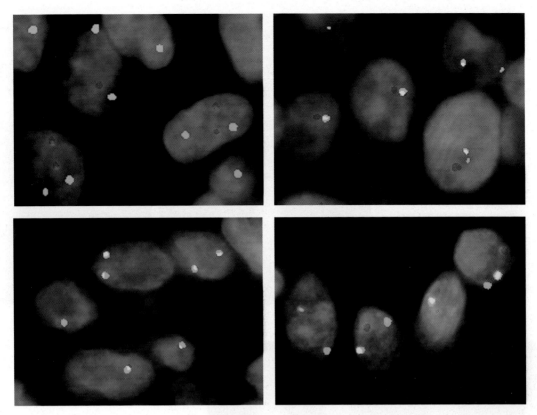

Figure 4.4 Examples of common FISH assays for translocation, including FISH-F negative (**A**, green and red signals split) and FISH-F positive cases (**B**, one yellow fusion signal and one pair of split red and green signals in most nuclei) tested with probes against *EWS* on 22q12 (red) and *FLI1* on 11q24 (green). The FISH-BA strategy for *SYT* is similarly illustrated with negative (**C**, only fused signals) and positive (**D**, one fusion signal and one pair of split red and green signals) cases.

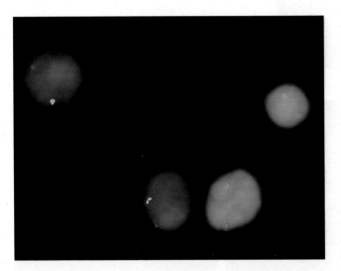

Figure 4.5 Chimeric bone marrow in patient with sex-mismatched transplant showing a mixture of donor and recipient, male (*left*) and female (*right*) cells (CEPX in red, CEPY in green).

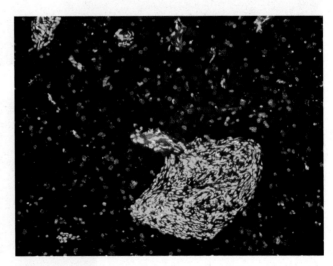

Figure 4.6 Low-magnification (100X) FISH image of a heterogeneous brain tissue sample involved by meningioangiomatosis. Because the morphology is retained, it is relatively simple to distinguish the perivascular spindled cells of interest (*lower center*) from the surrounding neocortex without the need for microdissection.

Figure 4.7 Relative 1p deletion within near-tetraploid cells of an oligodendroglioma with enlarged nuclei containing four copies of the red 1q32 reference probe signals and two copies of the green 1p32 test probe signals (**A**). A near-diploid tumor cell with one green and two red signals is also seen on the right. A homozygous deletion of the p16 gene on 9p21 is shown, wherein the majority of cells have retained green CEP9 signals, but no red p16 signals (**B**). A normal pattern of two paired red and green signals is seen in the lower right, likely representing an entrapped non-neoplastic cell.

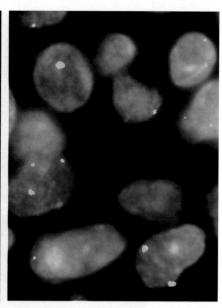

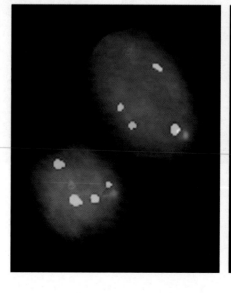

Figure 4.8 Interphase FISH study to verify the appropriate cytogenetic localization for a homemade DNA probe against the 4.1G gene on 6q23 (4.1G in red, CEP6 in green).

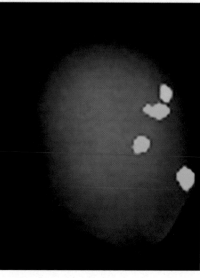

Figure 4.9 Three-color aneusomy/deletion FISH cocktail for CLL in negative (**A**, two green CEP12, two red 13q14.3, and two aqua 13q34 signals) and positive (**B**, three green, one red, one aqua) examples.

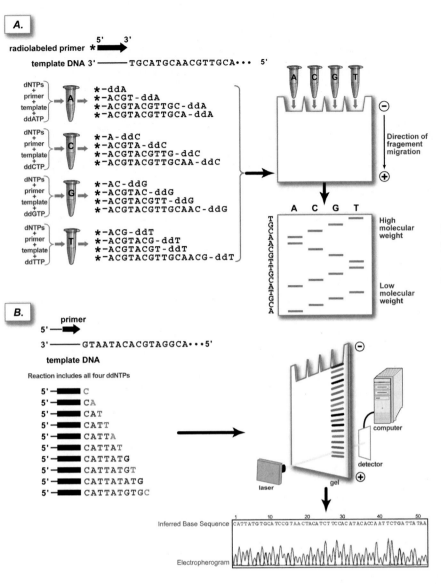

A.

radiolabeled primer *→ 5'   3'

template DNA 3' ———TGCATGCAACGTTGCA••• 5'

dNTPs + primer + template + ddATP	→ A	*-ddA *-ACGT-ddA *-ACGTACGTTGC-ddA *-ACGTACGTTGCA-ddA
dNTPs + primer + template + ddCTP	→ C	*-A-ddC *-ACGTA-ddC *-ACGTACGTTG-ddC *-ACGTACGTTGCAA-ddC
dNTPs + primer + template + ddGTP	→ G	*-AC-ddG *-ACGTAC-ddG *-ACGTACGTT-ddG *-ACGTACGTTGCAAC-ddG
dNTPs + primer + template + ddTTP	→ T	*-ACG-ddT *-ACGTACG-ddT *-ACGTACGT-ddT *-ACGTACGTTGCAACG-ddT

Direction of fragment migration

A C G T

High molecular weight

Low molecular weight

TGCAACGTTGCATGCA

B.

primer
5' →
3' ———GTAATACACGTAGGCA•••5'

template DNA

Reaction includes all four ddNTPs

5'—■ C
5'—■ CA
5'—■ CAT
5'—■ CATT
5'—■ CATTA
5'—■ CATTAT
5'—■ CATTATG
5'—■ CATTATGT
5'—■ CATTATATG
5'—■ CATTATGTGC

computer

detector

laser   gel

Inferred Base Sequence
1   10   20   30   40   50
CATTATGTGCA TCCG TAA CTACA TCT TCCAC ATACACCA AT TCTGA TTA TAA

Electropherogram

Figure 7.2 Schematic diagram of enzymatic DNA sequencing by the chain termination method. **A**, Traditional method. Four parallel base-specific reactions are performed, each with the same primer and all four dNTPs; each reaction is radiolabeled either by use of a labeled primer (illustrated here by asterisks) or much more commonly by use of labeled dNTPs. Each reaction also includes a low concentration of one ddNTP. Competition for incorporation into the growing DNA strand between the ddNTP and its conventional dNTP analog results in infrequent but specific chain termination at the position where the ddNTP is incorporated, generating a population of DNA strands of assorted lengths that all have the same 5' end defined by the sequencing primer. The four separate enzymatic reactions are size-fractioned in parallel lanes in a denaturing polyacrylimide gel. The pattern of bands produced by autoradiography of the gel (read from smallest to largest) yields the sequence of the complementary strand. **B**, Automated method. In the dye terminator method (illustrated), all four base-specific reactions are performed simultaneously in a single tube in which each ddNTP is labeled with a different fluorescent dye. The reaction products are size-fractionated in a single lane, and a laser beam focused at a constant position on the gel causes the dyes to fluoresce as they migrate past. The fluorescence emissions are recorded, and computer analysis converts the electropherogram into an inferred base sequence. The illustrated sequence is from human papilloma virus type 6.

Figure 7.3 Errors in automated sequence analysis. **A**, Photomicrograph of a gastric gastrointestinal stromal tumor (GIST), a tumor type that often harbors mutations in exon 11 of the *c-kit* gene (Chapter 15). **B**, Exon 11 was amplified by PCR and subjected to automated sequence analysis. A homology search of the computer-generated inferred base sequence search identified a putative single base pair insertion. Inspection of the actual electropherogram demonstrates that the putative mutation is a base-calling error (*arrow, bottom*). **C**, Automated sequence analysis of the total DNA product from PCR amplification of exon 11 from another GIST. Visual inspection of the electropherogram (*top*) shows a complicated pattern of overlapping peaks that calls into question the validity of the inferred base sequence. Sequence analysis of the cloned PCR products shows that some of the DNA molecules have a wild-type sequence (*middle*) while others have a mutant sequence containing a 6-bp deletion involving codons 562-564 (*bottom*). This result indicates that the tumor is actually heterozygous for an exon 11 deletion.

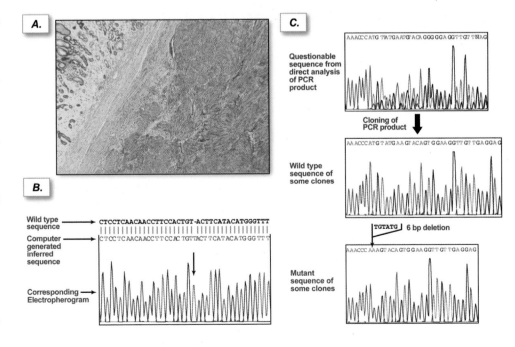

A.

B.

Wild type sequence → CTCCTCAACAACCTTCCACTGT-ACTTCATACATGGGTTT

Computer generated inferred sequence → CTCCTCAACAACCTTCCAC TGTTACT TCATACA TGGG TTT

Corresponding Electropherogram →

C.

Questionable sequence from direct analysis of PCR product

AAACCCATG TATGAATGTACA GGG GGA GGTTGT TNAG

Cloning of PCR product

Wild type sequence of some clones

AA ACCCATGT ATGAAGT ACAGT GGAA GGTT GT TGAGGA G

TGTATG 6 bp deletion

AAACCC AAAGT ACA GT GGAA GGTT GT TGA GGAG

Mutant sequence of some clones

Figure 7.10 Partial output of a nucleotide similarity search using the NCBI Basic Local Alignment Search Tool (BLAST) at www.ncbi.nlm.nih.gov/BLAST for the query sequence of exon 11 of the *c-kit* gene illustrated in the lower panel of Figure 7.3C. The upper region of the output graphically summarizes the BLAST alignment results; each horizontal bar (#1) indicates the region of the query sequence that is homologous to individual sequences in the Entrez Nucleotides database; the bar's color indicates the degree of homology (#2). Mouse-over of a bar (#3) displays the name of the matching sequence in the textbox (#4). The middle region of the output provides a brief description of sequences with significant homology. The output includes the identifier for the database sequence linked to the GenBank entry (#5), the bit score measure of the homology in the alignment that is higher the better the alignment (#6), and an E value that provides a statistical measure of the significance of the alignment (#7). The output also provides links, where applicable, to curated sequence and descriptive information about genetic loci at NCBI LocusLink (#8), non-redundant gene-oriented clusters at UniGene (#9), and expression and hybridization array data at the Gene Expression Omnibus GEO (#10). The lower region of the output shows the actual alignments for the sequences with significant homology. For simplicity, the only alignment shown is the one that corresponds to the moused-over sequence at #3 and #4 and highlighted at #5. In addition to the identifier and brief description, the output includes a link to the full homologous subject sequence in the database (#11), and indicates the position of the nucleotides in the query and subject sequences that delineate the region of homology (#12). The horizontal dashes indicate the site of the 6 bp deletion. The boundaries of exon 11 have been added for clarity.

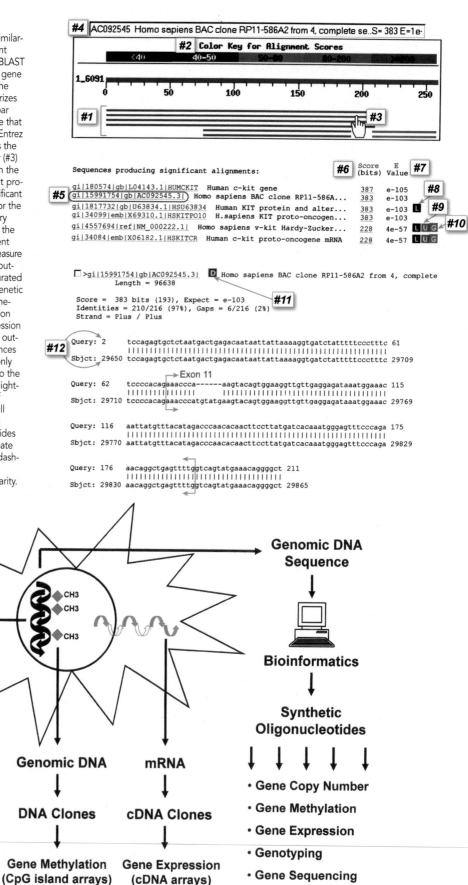

Figure 9.2 Approaches to nucleic acid microarray fabrication. Molecular constituents of a cell (genomic DNA or mRNA) may be isolated and cloned (bacterial artificial chromosome [BAC] clones, DNA clones, cDNA clones). Libraries of clones are then spotted as probes onto the microarray surface to be used for genome copy number assessment (array comparative genetic hybridization [CGH]), DNA methylation analysis (CpG island arrays), or gene expression profiling (cDNA arrays). Alternatively, genome sequence information may be used with bioinformatics algorithms to design and synthesis oligonucleotides that may be spotted or synthesized directly on the array surface. Oligonucleotide probes may be used to perform a wide variety of microarray-based genomic assays.

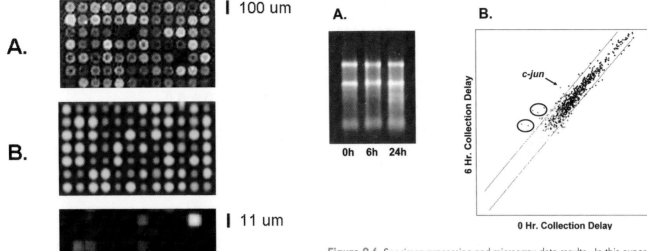

A.

B.

C.

D.

A. | 100 um

| 11 um

Figure 9.3 Microarray morphology. Representative images of scanned nucleic acid gene expression microarrays are shown. **A**, Image from two-color spotted microarray. Independent red and green signals reflect the hybridization intensities of the two different target samples. Note the extensive non-uniformity (doughnut holes) associated with the pin-based spotting process. **B**, Image from two-color Agilent ink-jet array, demonstrating greater uniformity of hybridization intensity across each feature. **C**, Image from Affymetrix single-color GeneChip microarray. Note the regular, grid-shaped hybridization feature pattern that reflects the mask-based in situ synthesis of oligonucleotides using photolithography. (D) In the GeneChip® technology platform, 11 pairs of features that are randomly distributed across the array are electronically aggregated. The composite single of 11 probes and 11 negative control (mismatch) probes are utilized to generate a single intensity value for a transcript.

A.

0h 6h 24h

B.

6 Hr. Collection Delay

c-jun

0 Hr. Collection Delay

Figure 9.6 Specimen processing and microarray data results. In this experiment, three biopsies from non-malignant splenic tissue were either snap-frozen immediately after surgical removal (0 h) or stored in normal saline solution for 6 hours (6 h) or 24 hours (24 h) prior to freezing. RNA was isolated from each of the three specimens and analyzed by conventional agarose gel electrophoresis (**A**) and ethidium bromide staining. Based on ribosomal RNA band intensity, RNA derived from snap-frozen tissue or tissue maintained at room temperature for 24 hours appear equally intact, while tissue maintained at room temperature for 24 hours shows evidence of slight RNA degradation. RNAs from 0 hour and 6 hour time points were then subjected to gene expression profiling using Affymetrix GeneChip microarrays. Expression values of ~1500 transcripts are represented as a scatter plot (**B**), where level of transcript expression in the snap-frozen sample is plotted on the x-axis and corresponding transcript levels in the 6 hour sample are plotted on the y-axis. Note that blue diagonal lines denote the limits of ± two-fold change between samples. Grey points represent transcripts that were undetected in either sample. Black points correspond to transcripts that were detected in both samples; red points denote transcripts whose expression was detected in one sample but not the other. Although the majority of gene transcript levels remained unchanged between the 0 hour and 6 hour samples, several transcripts (e.g. *c-jun*) demonstrate greater than two-fold differences in expression between tissue specimens that have been frozen after differing warm ischemia times.

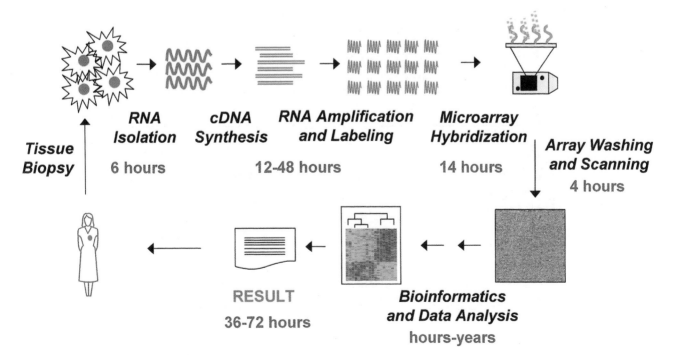

Tissue Biopsy

RNA Isolation
6 hours

cDNA Synthesis
12-48 hours

RNA Amplification and Labeling

Microarray Hybridization
14 hours

Array Washing and Scanning
4 hours

RESULT
36-72 hours

Bioinformatics and Data Analysis
hours-years

Figure 9.7 Outline of a gene expression microarray experiment. The experimental steps involved in performing a gene expression profiling experiment are outlined along with estimates of time required for each step in the process, from patient biopsy to end results. If a pre-validated microarray-based assay is being used for clinical diagnostics, data analysis may require only several minutes to one hour to complete. Otherwise, as described in the text, data analysis of research studies for biomarker discover may require months or years to complete and validate.

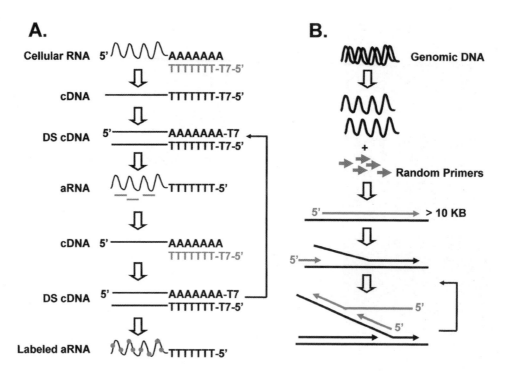

Figure 9.8 Nucleic acid amplification strategies for microarray analysis. In amplifying small quantities of mRNA for gene expression microarray analysis (**A**), cellular RNA is converted into first-strand cDNA using an oligo-dT/T7 RNA polymerase promoter primer and double-stranded (DS) cDNA is then made using a standard Gubler-Hoffman synthesis protocol. The resulting cDNA template is used for in vitro transcription to generate cRNA. Amplified cRNA is converted back into first-strand cDNA using random primers and then into double-stranded DNA using the dT/T7 primer. The amplified cDNA can be used again for in vitro transcription to generate labeled cRNA target for microarray hybridization. Alternatively, another round of transcript amplification may be performed. For whole genome amplification (WGA) using strand-displacing Phi29 DNA polymerase (**B**), genomic DNA is denatured and annealed to random primers. In the presence of Phi29 polymerase and dNTPs, primers are extended along the denatured, single-stranded DNA template for at least 10 kb. Subsequent primers can bind again to single-stranded DNA, displace the first synthesized strand, and generate additional single-stranded DNA copies. In the meantime, single-stranded DNA copies that are generated from template genomic DNA can themselves serve as templates for additional priming and polymerization in the opposite direction. This process continues in a linear and isothermal manner until reagents (primers, dNTPs, enzyme activity) are exhausted or the reaction is halted. Amplified, single-stranded genomic fragments can then be labeled for microarray hybridization using a wide variety of techniques.

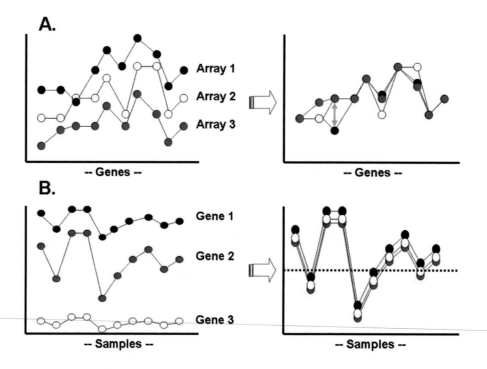

Figure 9.9 Microarray data normalization. (**A**) In order to compare patterns of gene expression (or gene copy number) across multiple microarrays, each associated with differing overall intensity as a result of technical variability, data may be normalized across arrays (samples). The effect of the inter-array normalization process (*arrow*) is to make all data sets comparable so that true biologic changes in gene expression between samples (*green arrow*) can be appreciated. (**B**) To compare patterns of gene expression between different genes, where the absolute level of gene expression may be quite different, data for a given gene may be normalized across samples. The effect of the intergene normalization process (*arrow*) is to make all genes comparable by transforming their expression level relative to a mean (*dotted line*), so that similar patterns of gene expression can be identified across samples, irrespective of absolute hybridization signal.

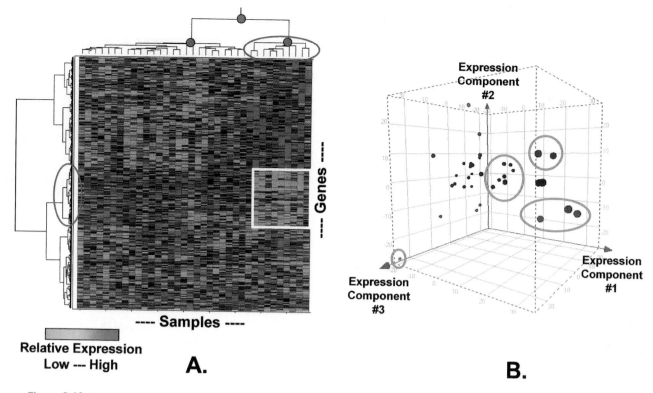

Figure 9.10 Microarray data visualization. When using hierarchical clustering and heat-map representation of gene expression microarray data (**A**), samples (represented as 36 columns in this data set) are organized based on similarity of gene expression while genes (represented by approximately 9000 rows) are simultaneously organized based on similarity of expression across all samples. In the heat-map image, *green lines* represent transcripts that are relatively less expressed in a sample while *red lines* represent transcripts that are relatively overexpressed in a sample. The tree (dendrogram) at top quantifies the relative similarity between samples. Each blue node is associated with a correlation coefficient that describes the relatedness of samples among the two subsequent branches of the dendrogram. Samples with higher similarity to each other based on gene expression are depicted as lower 'branches' on the tree (horizontal ellipse). Similarly, the tree on the left quantifies the relative similarity between gene expression patterns. Genes that show similar patterns of expression across all samples are depicted as smaller branches on the tree (*vertical ellipse*). Note subgroups of genes that demonstrate identical patterns of expression in subgroups of samples (*white box*). In principle components analysis (B), gene expression values may be condensed into two or three principle components that represent the majority of variation in gene expression across all samples. Each sample is plotted in two- or three-dimensional space (as shown here) based upon the value of its principle expression components. Each point may be further color-coded base on other features of the sample (e.g. tumor grade, patient age, etc). In this view, it is easy to demonstrate clusters of samples (*green ellipses*) that are very distinct in their gene expression profiles. (Visualizations generated using DecisionSite for Functional Genomics software, Spotfire, Inc., Somerville, MA.)

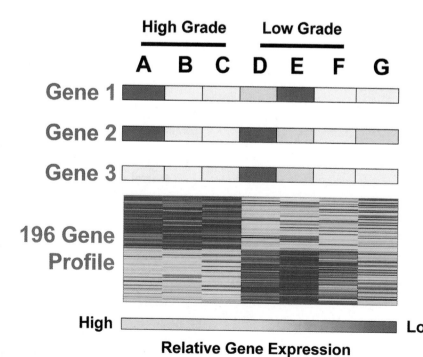

Figure 9.11 Synergism of gene expression signatures. In this study, seven oligodendroglioma tumors of low **A** to **C**, high **D** to **F**, and intermediate (**G**) histological grade were analyzed on a gene expression microarray representing approximately 1500 transcripts. Note that when examined individually, the expression of three different genes appears to have little correlation with tumor grade. However, when the same three genes are examined in the context of 193 other genes, the composite gene expression signature clearly delimits a molecular difference between tumor grades.

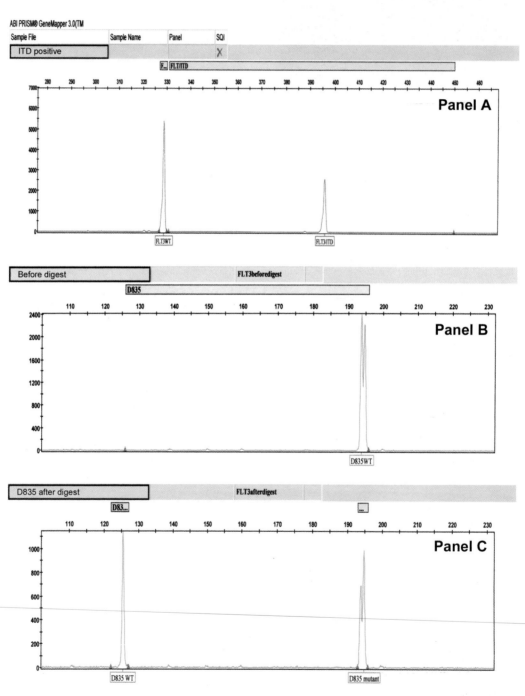

Figure 12.4 Example of *MYCN* amplification in neuroblastoma. **A**, A poorly differentiated neuroblastoma from a 4-year-old girl who presented with an adrenal mass. The tumor had a high mitosis-karyorrhexis index. **B**, FISH analysis using a probe for *MYCN* demonstrates high-level amplification of the gene. (Courtesy Drs. Ashley Hill and Arie Perry, Washington University School of Medicine, St. Louis, MO.)

Figure 13.6 A shows the *FLT3* – ITD. The patient sample with internal tandem duplication in one allele (*FLT3*/ITD-peak at 395 base pairs [BP]) is 66 bp larger than the wild-type (*FLT3*/WT-peak at 329 bp). **B** and **C** show the D835 mutation. The mutation is resistant to restriction enzyme digestion by EcoRV (Panel C – D835 mutant), whereas the normal allele is digested to a smaller fragment (D835WT).

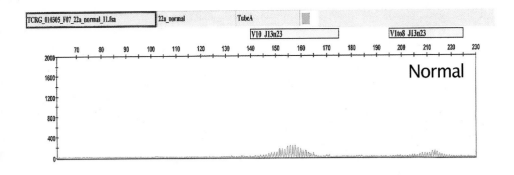

Normal

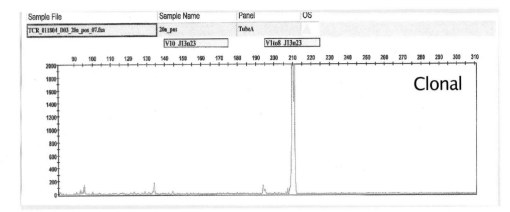

Clonal

Figure 13.8 Electropherogram of *TCRγ* rearrangement. **A**, The products of amplification by the primers targeting *V10-J13* (BIOMED-2) show a Gaussian distribution, confirming that the rearrangements were random. **B** shows one dominant peak, revealing that the amplification product was of one size, which could originate only in the presence of a clonal rearrangement.

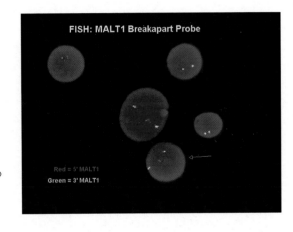

Figure 13.9 Break-apart FISH targeting 3' and 5' regions of *MALT1* shows a fusion of red and green (*yellow signal*) in the normal allele. In the presence of a translocation (indicated by the *arrow*), the targets are spliced apart, resulting in two different signals (*red* and *green*). The nucleus also shows one normal allele. (Courtesy Mr. Charles Dana Bangs, Cytogenetics Laboratory, Stanford University Medical Center.)

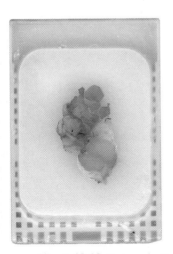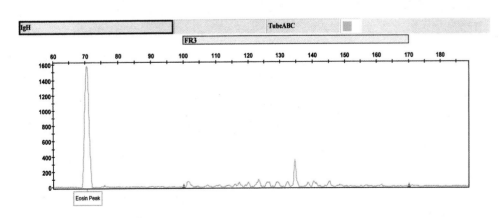

Figure 13.10 Eosin peak. Tissue marked with eosin (paraffin block) for visibility during processing, retain minute amounts of eosin during DNA extraction. Electropherogram tracings in the 71 base pair (bp) region shows a very bright signal, resulting from autofluorescence of eosin. In this particular specimen, which was tested for *IGH* rearrangements, this eosin peak did not fall within the clonal region. A clonal peak about 133 bp is also seen in this patient with a B-cell non-Hodgkin lymphoma.

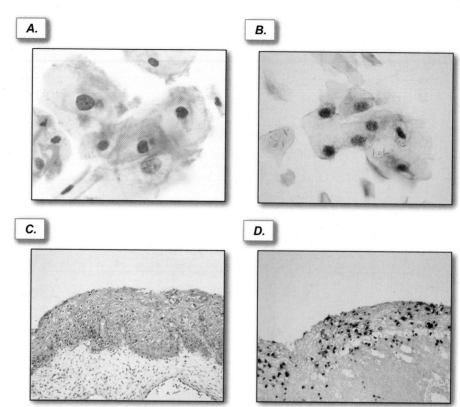

Figure 16.2 Chromogenic in situ hybridization (CISH) of cytology and biopsy specimens. **A**, A conventional PAP smear from a woman less than 30 years old shows ASCUS. **B**, Strong staining by CISH demonstrates the presence of high-risk human papilloma virus (HPV) infection. **C**, A cervical biopsy showing koilocytosis. **D**, Strong staining by CISH demonstrates the presence of high-risk HPV infection.

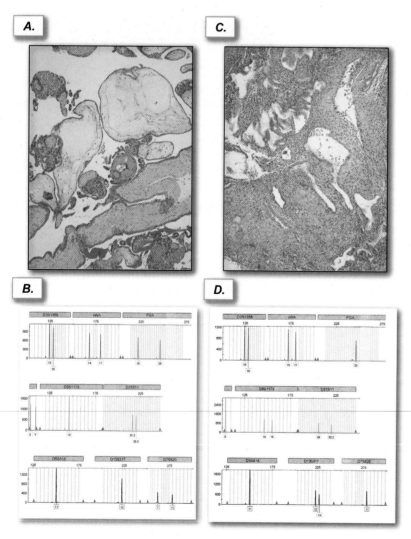

Figure 16.6 Use of STR to evaluate products of conception suspicious for a molar pregnancy. **A**, The histologic features of the villi make it difficult to distinguish between an early molar pregnancy and hydropic change in a nonmolar pregnancy. **B**, DNA typing using a subset of the *CODIS* loci (Table 23.3) on villi microdissected from the tissue block shows a diploid gestation. Parallel analysis on maternal tissue (endometrium microdissected from the tissue block) (**C**) shows the maternal genotype (**D**), and demonstrates that products of conception contain a maternal allele at each locus. Taken together, the findings exclude a complete or partial molar gestation.

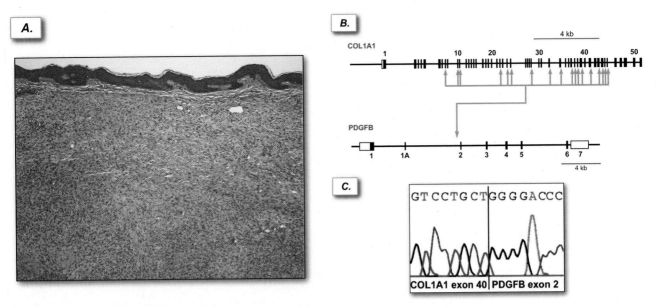

Figure 18.5 The *COLIA1-PDGFB* gene fusion is characteristic of dermatofibrosarcoma protuberans (DFSP). **A**, DFSP arising in the skin of the groin; the photomicrograph illustrates the tumor's storiform pattern, and growth immediately beneath a thinned epidermis. **B**, The translocation breakpoint that produces the *COLIA1-PDGFB* fusion can occur in wide region of the *COLIA1* gene, but almost always occurs in intron 1 of *PDGFB*. **C**, Multiplex RT-PCR analysis of the groin neoplasm shows an in-frame fusion between *COL1A1* exon 40 and *PDGFB* exon 2, consistent with the diagnosis of DFSP.

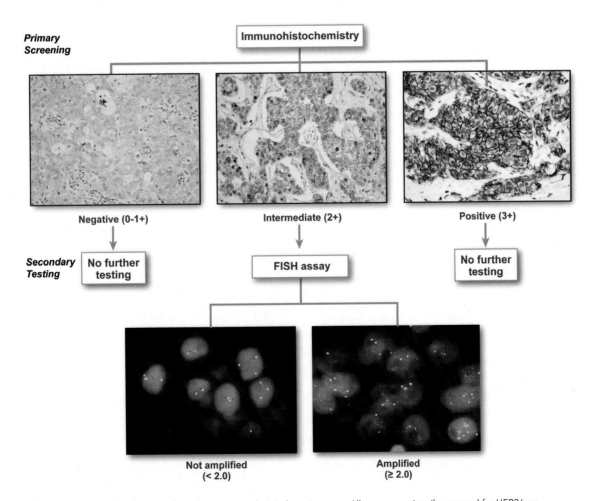

Figure 20.4 Testing algorithm for tissue-based *HER2/neu* analysis in breast cancer. All cases are primarily screened for HER2/neu overexpression by immunohistochemistry. Secondary testing by FISH analysis is only performed on cases with an intermediate (2+) level of immunohistochemical staining. In this illustration, primary screening was performed by HerceptTest immunohistochemical staining; 0 indicates no membrane staining, 1+ indicates partial membrane staining in more than 10% of cells without circumferential staining, 2+ indicates thin circumferential membrane staining in more than 10% of cells, and 3+ indicates thick circumferential membrane staining in more than 10% of cells. Secondary screening was performed by the PathVysion FISH assay, where *HER2* amplification is indicated by a ratio of *HER2* (red signals) to chromosome 17 (green signals) that is 2.0 or greater.

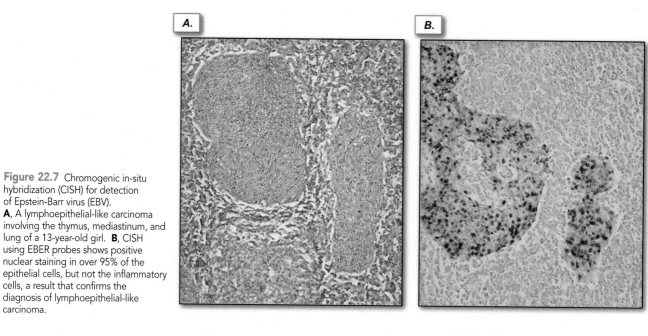

Figure 22.7 Chromogenic in-situ hybridization (CISH) for detection of Epstein-Barr virus (EBV). **A**, A lymphoepithelial-like carcinoma involving the thymus, mediastinum, and lung of a 13-year-old girl. **B**, CISH using EBER probes shows positive nuclear staining in over 95% of the epithelial cells, but not the inflammatory cells, a result that confirms the diagnosis of lymphoepithelial-like carcinoma.

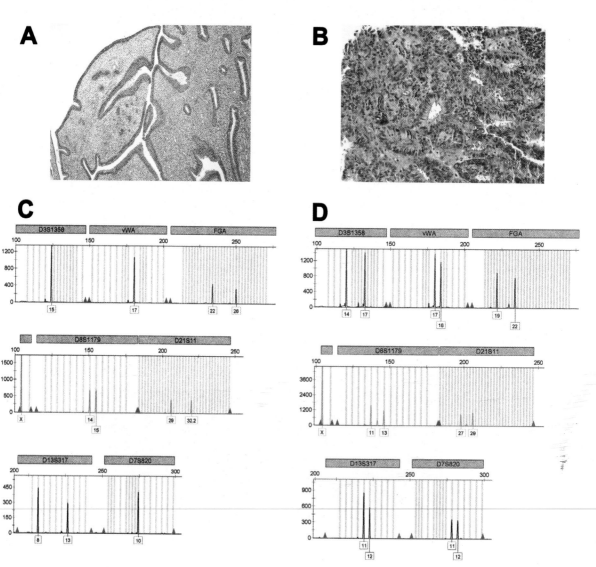

Figure 23.1 Example of the use of STR loci to resolve a specimen identity issue. Sections of the uterine cervix of a 40-year-old woman with persistently abnormal pap smears showed unremarkable cervical mucosa (**A**, magnification 40x), but a detached fragment of an atypical glandular proliferation was also present (**B**, magnification 400x). DNA typing using a subset of the CODIS loci (see Table 23.3) showed that the cervical mucosa (**C**) and atypical glandular fragment (**D**) had different genotypes, identifying the fragment as a contaminant.

Structure and Function of DNA and RNA

This chapter is intended as a general review of the details of gene structure and function that are of importance in the context of the types of molecular genetic tests performed on tissue samples. More detailed information can be found in general molecular biology texts (1,2) or texts that specifically focus on human molecular biology (3,4).

DNA STRUCTURE

Deoxyribonucleic acid (DNA) is a double-stranded antiparallel helix composed of deoxyribonucleotides (Table 1.1 and Fig. 1.1) linked together in a linear polymer by phosphodiester bonds between neighboring sugar residues (Fig. 1.2). The strands are held together by hydrogen bonds between laterally opposed base pairs in which adenine shares two hydrogen bonds with thymidine (A:T pairing) and guanine shares three hydrogen bonds with cytosine (G:C pairing). As a result, the nucleotide sequence of one DNA strand is complementary to the nucleotide sequence of the other DNA strand (5).

Because the phosphodiester bonds that form the linear backbone of the nucleic acid molecule link the 3′ carbon atom of the sugar residue to the 5′ carbon atom of the

TABLE 1.1

BASES IN DNA AND RNA WITH CORRESPONDING NUCLEOSIDES AND NUCLEOTIDES[a]

Base	Purines		Pyrimidines		
	Adenine (A)	Guanine (G)	Cytosine (C)	Thymine (T)	Uracil (U)
Nucleoside = Base + Sugar					
Base + ribose	Adenosine	Guanosine	Cytidine	—[b]	Uridine
Base + deoxyribose	2′-Deoxyadenosine	2′-Deoxyguanosine	2′-Deoxycytidine	2′-Deoxythymidine	—
Nucleotide = Nucleoside + Phosphate[c]					
In RNA	Adenosine 5′-triphosphate (ATP)	Guanosine 5′-triphosphate (GTP)	Cytidine 5′-triphosphate (CTP)	—	Uridine 5′-triphosphate (UTP)
In DNA	2′-Deoxyadenosine 5′-triphosphate (dATP)	2′-Deoxyguanosine 5′-triphosphate (dGTP)	2′-Deoxycytidine 5′-triphosphate (dCTP)	2′-Deoxythymidine 5′-triphosphate (dTTP)	—

[a]Only the common bases are shown; rare bases, such as xanthine and hypoxanthine, that result from spontaneous chemical changes are not included (Chapter 2). Similarly, rare bases found in tRNA such as pseudouridine are not included.
[b]Not normally found.
[c]Nucleotides can be monophosphates, diphosphates, or triphosphates; for simplicity, only the nucleotide triphosphates are presented, followed by their abbreviation in parentheses.

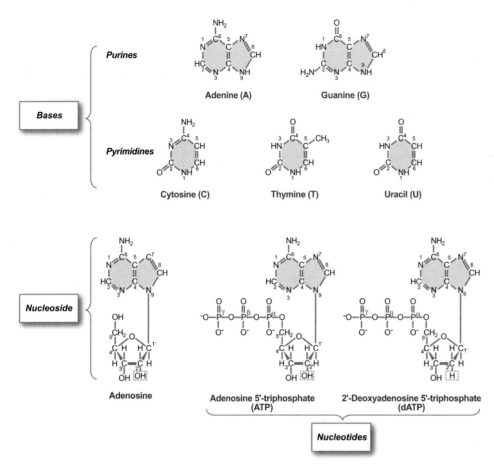

Figure 1.1 Structure of bases, nucleosides, and nucleotides. Numbering of the sugars ribose and dioxyribose is confined to the five carbon atoms (numbers 1′ to 5′); numbering of the bases includes both carbon and nitrogen atoms in the heterocyclic rings; phosphate groups are sequentially denoted as α, β, and δ according to their proximity to the sugar ring. Note that purines are connected to the sugar group by the nitrogen at position 9 and pyrimidines by the nitrogen at position 1. The boxed hydroxyl and hydrogen atoms connected to the 2′ carbon of the sugars are the essential difference between ribose and dioxyribose, respectively.

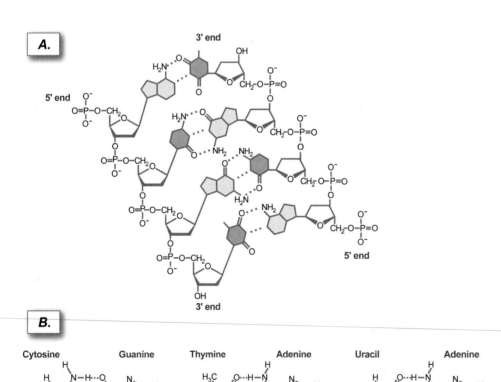

Figure 1.2 The double-stranded, antiparallel DNA helix. **A** emphasizes that the two strands are antiparallel because of the opposite orientation of the 3′ carbon to 5′ carbon phosphate linkages between adjacent sugar residues. The double helix is stabilized by hydrogen bonds between opposed bases, illustrated schematically in **A** and shown in more detail in **B**. **B** also shows the hydrogen bonding between adenine and uracil. By convention, DNA and RNA sequences are always given in the 5′ to 3′ direction, and so the sequence of the left hand strand in **A** is ACGT.

adjacent sugar residue, the molecule has a chemical polarity. By definition, the nucleotide whose 5′ carbon atom is not linked to an adjacent sugar residue is the 5′ end and the opposite end of the nucleic acid molecule is the 3′ end. This chemical polarity is the basis of the antiparallel orientation of the two strands of a DNA molecule. In a similar way, a strand of DNA and a strand of ribonucleic acid (RNA) in a DNA-RNA heteroduplex will also have an antiparallel orientation. In a single nucleic acid strand, regions of complementarity stabilized by intramolecular hydrogen bonds also have an antiparallel orientation. By convention, DNA and RNA sequences are always indicated in the 5′ to 3′ direction.

The hydrogen bonds between complementary base pairs not only maintain the structure of DNA but also underlie DNA replication and RNA transcription, processing, and translation. Intramolecular base pairing is also responsible for the secondary structure that is integral to the function of messenger RNA (mRNA), transfer RNA (tRNA), and ribosomal RNA (rRNA). And, because hydrogen bonds can be readily disrupted and reformed, complementary nucleic strands can be easily separated (denatured) or reannealed (renatured), reversible processes that are exploited in vitro in many molecular genetic tests.

The right-handed double helix originally posed by Watson and Crick on the basis of x-ray crystallography data has ten base pairs (bp) per turn and is termed B-DNA. It is the structural form that predominates in vivo. However, DNA can also adopt two other helical configurations. A-DNA is also a right-handed helix, but it has 11 bp per turn. A-DNA may participate in RNA-DNA binding. Z-DNA forms a left-handed helix with 12 bp per turn. Although the in vivo role of Z-DNA remains uncertain, the Z-DNA configuration can be induced by stretches of alternating purines and pyrimidines. This fact raises the possibility that Z-DNA affects the efficiency of gene transcription because alternating GC-rich sequences are often present upstream of genes (6–8).

HISTONES AND NUCLEOSOMES

Multiple hierarchies of DNA organization are required to produce chromosomes (Fig. 1.3). The fundamental unit of organization is the nucleosome, which consists of a stretch of 146 bp of double-stranded DNA wrapped around a central core of eight histone proteins (9). Nucleosomes are connected by short spacer segments of DNA that range from 20 to 70 bp long, yielding an arrangement that classically is said to resemble "beads on a string." The nucleosomes are in turn coiled into a 30-mm-diameter chromatin fiber that constitutes the next level of chromatin organization. During cell division, DNA becomes even more compact; loops of the chromatin fiber (20 to 100 kb of DNA per loop) are attached to a central protein scaffold, and in metaphase chromosomes the loop–scaffold complex is still further condensed by coiling. Although euchromatin, which constitutes most of the chromatin, is dispersed throughout the nucleus in an extended state during interphase, the regions of DNA that

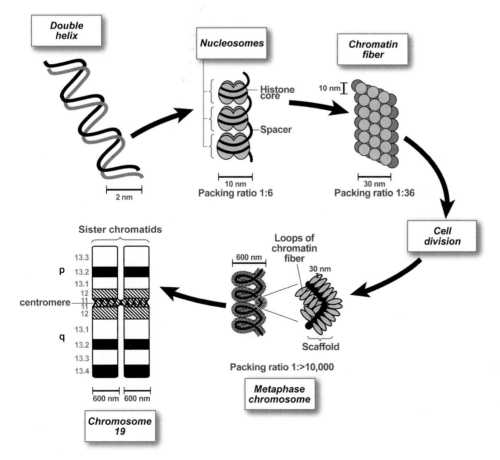

Figure 1.3 DNA packing. The nucleosome has a packing ratio (degree of compaction of the linear DNA molecule) of 1:6. Coiling of the nucleosomes into the chromatin fiber achieves a packing ratio of 1:36. Further compaction occurs during cell division; 20- to 100-kb loops of the chromatin fiber are attached to a central scaffold, and coiling of the loop–scaffold complex itself achieves a final packing ratio of about 1:10,000. The relationship between a fully compacted DNA molecule and a standard G-band ideogram is shown for human chromosome 19.

form heterochromatin are highly condensed throughout the cell cycle. Genes within the euchromatin may or may not be expressed depending on the individual cell type and its metabolic requirements, but genes within the heterochromatin are expressed only rarely, if ever.

Nucleosomes are not static structures that simply compact the huge amount of DNA in a cell's nucleus. Instead, nucleosomal structure is continuously modified by two major classes of protein complexes, adenosine triphosphate (ATP)-dependent complexes that remodel chromatin and complexes that covalently modify the histone proteins themselves (10). These protein complexes control the accessibility of DNA to the binding factors that are required for a range of genetic processes, including DNA replication, recombination, and repair; maintenance of transcriptionally active and inactive chromatin; regulation of gene expression; and even regulation of telomere length (11–20).

Covalent Modifications

Histones can be covalently but reversibly modified at a number of different sites by a diverse group of enzymatic reactions that includes acetylation, phosphorylation, methylation, ubiquitination, and poly-(ADP-ribosyl)ation.

Acetylation

In the absence of acetylation, lysine residues close to the N-termini of histone subunit proteins are positively charged and therefore exhibit strong ionic affinity for the negatively charged phosphate backbone of nucleosomal DNA. This strong affinity leads to a highly condensed chromatin confirmation, particularly prominent in heterochromatin. In the opposite way, acetylation of the lysine residues of the histone proteins decreases the net positive charge of histones, which results in reduced affinity of

TABLE 1.2

DISEASES ASSOCIATED WITH HISTONE ACETYLTRANSFERASE AND DEACETYLASE MUTATIONS

Altered Activity	Mutation	Resulting Disease
Histone acetyltransferase activity		
CREBBP	Point mutations, deletions, translocations, inversions	Rubinstein-Taybi syndrome
	HRX-CREBBP chimeric protein caused by t(11;16)(q23;p13)	Acute myeloid leukemia; treatment-related hematologic disorders
EP300	Missense mutations in Cys/His-rich regions	Colorectal and gastric disorders
	HRX-EP300 chimeric protein caused by t(11;22)(q23;q13)	Acute myeloid leukemia
MOZ, CREBBP	MOZ-CREBBP chimeric protein caused by t(8;16)(p11;p13)	Acute myeloid leukemia M4/M5
MOZ, TIF2	MOZ-TIF2 chimeric protein caused by inv(8)(p11q13)	Acute mixed lineage leukemia
Histone deacetyltransferase activity		
HDAC1, 2, and 3	Papilloma virus protein E7 causes release of HDAC1 from retinoblastoma tumor suppressor protein RB1	Induction of warts or carcinoma
	Pharmacologic doses of retinoids overcome the association of the histone deacetylase complex with the PML-RARα chimeric protein formed by t(15;17)(q21;q21) in one type of promyelocytic AML	Remission of APML harboring PML-RARα fusions
	Pharmacologic doses of retinoids do not overcome the association of the histone deacetylase complex with the PLZF-RARα chimeric protein formed by t(11;17)(q23;q21) in one type of promyelocytic AML	Lack of sensitivity to retinoid therapy of APML harboring PLZF-RARα fusions
MECP2	Loss-of-function mutations cause defective gene silencing through decreased histone recruitment	Rett syndrome

binding between histones and DNA, allowing a more open and extended chromatin structure.

In general, histone acetylation is associated with gene expression, presumably because binding sites for the proteins required to initiate transcription are more accessible when DNA has a more open chromatin structure (14,15, 21,22). The relationships between histone acetylation and gene expression are emphasized by the observations that known activators of gene transcription have histone acetyltransferase (HAT) activity (23) and that proteins with HAT activity are also involved in the control of cell proliferation and differentiation (24). Conversely, histone deacetylation, which is coupled to DNA methylation, is associated with repression of gene transcription (14,15,23,25,26). The importance of the links between histone acetylation, gene expression, chromatin structure, and epigenetic modifications of DNA (23,27,28) are emphasized by the features of diseases caused by alterations in histone acetyltransferase or deacetylase activity (Table 1.2).

Poly-(ADP-Ribosyl)ation

This modification involves the addition of long, branched sugar chains to histones at glutamic acid or aspartic amino acid residues, a modification that is thought to create an anionic matrix that results in reduced affinity of binding between histones and DNA, promoting chromatin decondensation (29,30).

Other Modifications

Other important covalent modifications of histones include reversible methylation of lysine residues and phosphorylation of serine residues. These types of alterations may not have a direct effect on chromatin–DNA interactions, but instead mediate changes in nucleosomal structure by functioning as binding sites that recruit other proteins or RNA to the nucleosome (16,31,32).

Noncovalent Modifications

The ATP-dependent protein complexes that remodel nucleosomes can be grouped into three general families based on the identity of their catalytic subunit, although the biochemical features of the different families are quite involved (10). The complexes remodel chromatin by two general mechanisms, either catalysis of conformational changes (which alter the accessibility of DNA on the surface of the histone octamer) or shifts in the position of the nucleosome along DNA (which expose or occlude different DNA sequences) (10,33–35). ATP-dependent remodelers are thought to have an especially important role in the regulation of transcription, where there is strong evidence that they act in concert with the enzymes that covalently modify histones.

DNA METHYLATION

DNA methylation is an indirect, non–sequence-based (or epigenetic) modification of DNA (28). At least three different DNA methyltransferases are capable of performing

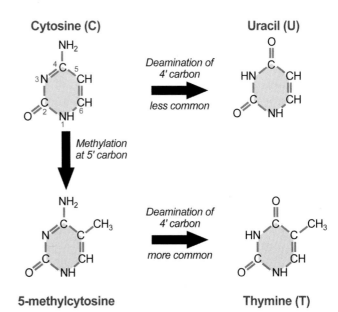

Figure 1.4 DNA methylation. Cytosines occurring in the sequence 5'-CpG-3' (and a smaller percentage of cytosines in the sequence 5'-CpNpG-3') are a target for methylation at the 5' carbon. 5-Methylcytosine is chemically unstable and prone to deamination that forms thymine, and the resulting T:G mismatch is subject to inefficient DNA repair. Together, these facts account for the underrepresentation of the CpG dinucleotide in DNA.

the enzymatic reaction in which a methyl group from *S*-adenosyl methionine is transferred to a cytosine, converting it to 5-methylcytosine (Fig. 1.4). Most methylated cytosines are found in the CpG dinucleotide (the nomenclature used to indicate a 5'-CG-3' DNA sequence), although a small percentage of methylated cytosines also occur in the sequence CpNpG, where N is any base. Cytosine methyltransferases preferentially recognize hemimethylated DNA (DNA methylated on one strand only), and so a cell's methylation pattern is heritable; the dyad symmetry intrinsic to CpG sequences ensures that following replication, the newly synthesized DNA strands will have the same CpG methylation pattern as the parental DNA strands. Although only about 3% of cytosines in human DNA are methylated, methylation is important for X chromosome inactivation and genomic imprinting (25, 36–38), and, because the pattern changes by developmental stage and cell type, methylation also is an important mechanism for developmentally regulated and tissue-specific gene regulation (39–41).

The methylated CpG dinucleotide is chemically unstable and is prone to deamination followed by ineffective DNA repair (Chapter 2), consistent with the observation that the CpG dinucleotide is underrepresented in human DNA. Regions of DNA that are comparatively GC rich are typically 50 to 2000 bp long and are termed GC islands. GC islands are usually found in the 5' region of genes that are widely expressed, often in the promoter region; however, for genes that show restricted expression patterns, GC islands are often located a distance downstream from the transcription initiation site. In general, GC islands associated with the transcription start site of tissue-specific genes tend to be methylated in tissues where the gene is not expressed. However, the relationships between the location of a GC island, its methylation status, and the level of expression of the related gene are quite complex. It is often difficult to know in advance how an altered level of DNA methylation will affect expression of a particular gene. The mechanisms by which changes in methylation affect gene activation are not entirely clear, although it is likely that the methylation state of specific sequence elements regulates transcription factor binding and is responsible for structural changes in chromatin necessary to permit transcription itself to proceed (42).

The pattern of DNA methylation is significantly altered in neoplastic cells, which in general show an overall decrease in genome methylation (25,43,44). The lower level of methylation likely results in unregulated expression of many genes (45,46) and may also be responsible for the genomic instability that is a hallmark of malignancy because unmethylated interspersed repetitive DNA sequences (see below) are more likely to undergo recombination (46–48). However, it has recently become clear that increased methylation of CpG islands, with resultant transcriptional silencing, is also a characteristic feature of some tumors (28,49). The significance of this observation lies in the identity of the repressed genes, some of which encode proteins that are important for the control of DNA repair, such as O^6-methyguanine methyltransferase and hMLH1, and others of which are tumor suppressor genes such as *BRCA1* (22,50) (Chapter 2).

It is important to emphasize that abnormalities in DNA methylation are associated with benign disease, as well as malignancies. Mutations in genes that are involved directly or indirectly in DNA methylation have been correlated with several genetic disorders, including Rett syndrome, the ICF immunodeficiency syndrome, and X-linked α-thalassemia/mental retardation syndrome (51–54). Similarly, defects in imprinted genes are responsible for a number of disorders characterized by parental-origin inheritance effects (28,55–57), including disease syndromes such as Beckwith-Wiedemann syndrome and Prader-Willi/Angelman syndromes (36–41), as well as specific neoplasms, including neuroblastoma, Wilms tumor, acute myeloblastic leukemia, rhabdomyosarcoma, sporadic osteosarcoma, and glomus tumor (36,58). A number of DNA methyltransferase inhibitors that have potential use as chemotherapeutic drugs are under development (59).

THE CENTROMERE

The centromere is the region of a normal chromosome that is responsible for chromosomal segregation during mitotic and meiotic cell division. Structurally, centromeres consist of repetitive DNA composed of various families of tandomly repeated sequences termed satellite DNA (Fig. 1.5 and Table 1.3) (60,61). Human centromeres primarily contain alphoid satellite DNA that consists of 171-bp-long repeating units organized into higher order repeats that share 95% to 99% sequence homology (62–67). The nucleotide sequence of the alphoid DNA and its precise organization into higher order repeats varies on different chromosomes, as does the length of the overall centromeric array, ranging from 0.2 to 5 Mb in length (65–67). Pericentromeric regions contain more degenerate repeats and also appear to be frequent sites of intrachromosomal segmental duplications (62,68,69).

In humans, some evidence suggests that an internal 17-bp degenerate sequence must be present in the alphoid DNA in order to produce a functional centromere (70–73). However, other evidence indicates that human centromeres can function without alphoid DNA altogether (74–76), suggesting epigenetic mechanisms are also involved in centromere organization (72,77–81).

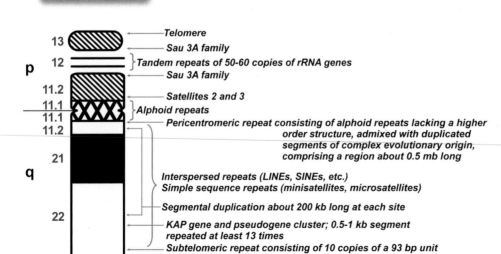

Figure 1.5 As an example of the distribution of repetitive sequence elements in a human chromosome, the repetitive elements of chromosome 21 are schematically diagrammed as they relate to the chromosome's standard G-band ideogram (compiled from references 60 and 82).

TABLE 1.3

MAJOR CLASSES OF REPETITIVE HUMAN DNA

Class	Size of Repeat Unit	Number of Copies and Location
Tandemly repeated DNA		
Megasatellite DNA	Greater than 1 kb	Blocks up to hundreds of kb long
RS447	4.7 kb	Approximately 50–70 copies (chromosomes 4p15 and 8p); contains the deubiquitinating enzyme gene USP17
rRNA transcription unit	13 kb with an adjacent 27-kb spacer	A 2-Mb-long cluster of about 50–60 tandem repeats is present on 13p, 14p, 15p, 21p and 22p
Satellite DNA	5–171 bp	Blocks from hundreds of kb to several Mb long, often forming centromeric heterochromatin
Alphoid DNA	171 bp	Centromeric heterochromatin of all chromosomes
Sau3A family	68 bp	Centromeric heterochromatin of 1, 9, 13, 14, 15, 21, 22, Y
Satellite 1	25–48 bp	Centromeric and other heterochromatin
Satellites 2 and 3	5 bp	Most chromosomes
Minisatellite DNA	14–500 bp	Simple sequence repeats interspersed throughout all chromosomes; blocks from 0.1 to 20 kb long; often referred to as variable number of tandem repeats (VNTR)
Telomeric family	6 bp	Telomeres of all chromosomes
Hypervariable family	9–64 bp	All chromosomes, often near telomeres
Microsatellite DNA	1–13 bp	Simple sequence repeats dispersed throughout all chromosomes; often occur in coding sequences; often referred to as short tandem repeats (STR)
Repetitive interspersed DNA		
LINEs	6–8 kb	Interspersed throughout all chromosomes (21% of genome)
LINE1		516,000
LINE2		315,000
LINE3		37,000
SINEs	80–300 bp	Interspersed throughout all chromosomes (13% of genome)
Alu		1,090,000
MIR		393,000
MIR3		75,000
LTR elements	1.5–11 kb	Interspersed throughout all chromosomes (8% of genome)
ERV—Class I		112,000
ERV(k)—Class II		8,000
ERV(c)—Class II		83,000
MaLR		240,000
DNA elements	80–3,000 bp	Interspersed throughout all chromosomes (3% of genome)
hAT group		195,000
Tc-1 group		75,000
PiggyBac-like		2,000
Unclassified		22,000

THE TELOMERE

The other specialized component that is an essential element of every chromosome is the telomere. Evidence for the role of the telomere in maintaining the integrity of the chromosome end is provided by the observation that chromosomes lacking a telomere are unstable and tend to fuse with the ends of other broken chromosomes, undergo recombination, or be degraded (83).

The unique structure of the telomere provides the mechanism for maintenance of the integrity of the chromosome's end. Telomeres are several kilobases long and are composed of a tandomly repeated hexamer sequence, which in humans is 5′-TTAGGG-3′. Telomeres end with a 3′ single-stranded overhang of the repeated hexamer sequence that is 200 to 600 nucleotides long. The stability of the end of the chromosome is due to the formation of a loop that results when this 3′ overhang displaces a series of TTAGGG repeats in a more proximal region of the telomere, converting a double-stranded region of the DNA into a structure resembling a t-loop (Fig. 1.6). This looping reaction is catalyzed by a specific enzyme, and the entire t-loop structure is stabilized by a complex of telomere-specific proteins (84).

Because synthesis of the lagging strand during DNA replication is discontinuous (as discussed below), a mechanism is required to replicate the region of the telomere that is at the extreme end of the chromosome. In the absence of this mechanism, incomplete replication would lead to a progressive shortening of the telomere, and subsequently the chromosome, with each cell division. The enzyme telomerase, a large ribonucleoprotein, catalyzes the unique reaction by which telomeres are synthesized. Telomerase has three main structural components, an RNA component, the telomerase-associated protein TEP1, and a reverse transcriptase domain (83). Although telomerase synthesizes the

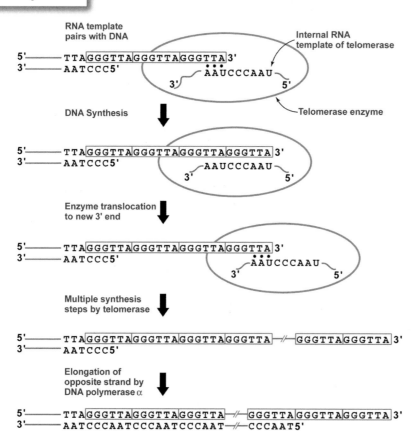

A. Telomere Synthesis

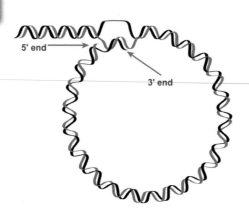

B. Telomere t-loop

Figure 1.6 Telomere synthesis and structure. Telomerase positions itself through base pairing between the internal RNA template and the protruding single-stranded DNA and then adds the complementary bases one at a time (**A**). The t-loop at the end of human chromosomes forms when the 3′ single-stranded end of the telomere displaces homologous repeats from duplex DNA (**B**). Although diagrammed as only 12 bp long, the 3′ single-stranded end involved in t-loop formation is actually several hundred nucleotides long.

individual repeats that are added to the chromosomal end, it does not itself control the number of repeats. Instead, telomerase activity is tightly regulated through a variety of processes (17,83,85–87), although the details of the different mechanisms are not fully understood.

Methods for molecular genetic analysis of telomerase activity (Chapter 5) have been widely employed in surgical pathology because abnormalities in telomere length have been associated with many neoplasms (88–95).

DNA REPLICATION

The process of DNA synthesis generates two daughter DNA duplexes that are each identical to the parent molecule (96). In humans, DNA replication is initiated at 10^4 to 10^5 different origins, each serving up to a 300-kb region of DNA, and replication from different origins is initiated at different times during S-phase of the cell cycle (97).

Control of chromosome replication is achieved via regulation of assembly of a prereplication protein complex at replication origins, with subsequent regulation of the activation of the complex (97–99). The overall process, known as replication licensing, not only coordinates DNA replication from the thousands of origins but also ensures that DNA replicates only once during each cell cycle (97,100,101). The DNA sequence that defines an origin of replication in humans has recently been defined for some sites (100), but specification of other replication origins may involve epigenetic mechanisms (102–104).

After initiation at a specific origin, replication advances by way of the replication fork, the point at which the parental DNA duplex bifurcates into the two daughter DNA duplexes (Fig. 1.7). However, the antiparallel structure of the two parental DNA strands, coupled with the fundamental biochemical fact that nucleic acids are synthesized only from the 5' end toward the 3' end, results in asymmetry

in DNA replication. On the leading strand, DNA synthesis can proceed continuously in the 5' to 3' direction as the parental duplex is unwound. In contrast, the lagging strand can only be synthesized as a series of short strands that are each polymerized in the 5' to 3' direction. Termed Okazaki fragments after their discoverer, these segments are typically 100 to 1,000 nucleotides long and are eventually joined (ligated) to create an intact lagging strand.

The polymerases that are responsible for nuclear DNA replication in humans are pol α, pol δ, and pol ε (although several other DNA polymerases exist, they are primarily involved in DNA repair [Chapter 2]). Pol γ replicates mitochondrial DNA. The activity of the individual DNA polymerases is controlled by a number of regulatory proteins, all of which are ultimately governed by the cell cycle (105). Additional enzymes are also required to unwind or relax the DNA as replication proceeds, including helicases and topoisomerases.

REPETITIVE DNA

When classified on the basis of the number of copies of a specific sequence present in the genome, DNA can be categorized into single-copy sequences, moderately repetitive sequences, and highly repetitive sequences. Single-copy DNA sequences are present in single or low copy number, as exemplified by the coding and intronic sequences of most structural genes. Moderately repetitive sequences are present at 10 to 10^5 copies per genome and are found throughout the euchromatin. Moderately repetitive sequences include some multiple-copy genes, such as the 250 to 1,000 copies of the immunoglobulin heavy-chain variable region genes at 14q32, but primarily consist of tandemly repeated or interspersed noncoding DNA. Highly repetitive DNA sequences are present at greater than 10^5 copies per genome, are noncoding, and are usually located in the heterochromatic regions of the centromere or telomere as tandemly repeated arrays. Websites devoted to repeated sequences (106,107) have greatly simplified analysis of repetitive elements.

Only a small percentage of the DNA within a human cell is ever transcribed, and, even though different cells transcribe the different segments of DNA that correspond with their physiologic function, the great majority of DNA is never transcribed in any cell. In fact, less than 5% of human DNA encodes a functional product, whether a protein, rRNA, tRNA, small nuclear RNA (snRNA), and so on (62). Nonetheless, many regions of noncoding repetitive DNA do have important functions, as is the case with centromeres, telomeres, origins of replication, and regulatory elements that control gene expression. However, the largest percentage of noncoding genetic material is so-called junk DNA, which separates functional genes. Although there is at present no known role for the vast majority of these stretches of DNA, they may actually serve structural or organizational functions that have yet to be appreciated. For example, it has recently been suggested that a significant fraction of conserved noncoding DNA may mediate attachment of chromatin loops to the nuclear matrix, a structural role that may also influence regulation of transcription activation (108).

In any event, the more than 50% of human DNA that consists of multiple copies of noncoding repetitive DNA

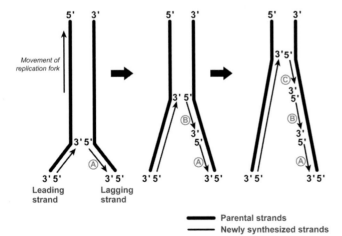

Figure 1.7 Schematic diagram of DNA replication. Because DNA polymerization occurs in the 5' to 3' direction, synthesis of the leading strand is continuous and in the same direction as the movement of the replication fork. However, the lagging strand can be synthesized only as a series of short Okazaki fragments (first A, then B, then C in the diagram) that are subsequently linked together. In eukaryotic cells the leading and lagging strands are synthesized by DNA polymerases δ and α, respectively.

has two major types of organization, tandemly repeated and interspersed.

Tandemly Repeated DNA

Tandemly repeated DNA can be grouped into four classes: megasatellite, satellite, minisatellite, and microsatellite. Each class is defined by blocks of repeated sequence that occur at only a few or at many different chromosomal locations (Table 1.3).

Megasatellite DNA is characterized by tandemly repeated DNA in which the repeated unit itself is several kilobases long. Depending on the family of megasatellite DNA, the unit is repeated approximately 50 to 400 times, producing blocks that can be hundreds of kilobases long (109). Some megasatellites are composed of coding repeats, for example, rRNA genes, and the deubiquitinating enzyme gene USP17.

Satellite DNA consists of very large arrays of tandemly repeated DNA sequences in which the repeat unit ranges from 5 to over 170 bp in length. Individual blocks of satellite DNA can range from 100 kb to several megabases (Mb) long. Satellite DNA is not transcribed, accounts for about 15% of human DNA, forms the bulk of the heterochromatic regions of the genome, and is prominent in the vicinity of the centromeres (70).

Minisatellite DNA is the class of simple sequence repeats comprising tandemly repeated DNA sequences in which the size of the repeat unit is approximately 14 to 500 bp. The repeats comprise blocks that are usually 0.1 to 20 kb long. Minisatellites, sometimes referred to as variable number of tandem repeats (VNTRs), are dispersed over most portions of the genome, although the family that forms telomeres provides an example of minisatellite DNA that has a very restricted distribution. Some hypervariable minisatellites encode proteins that are characteristically highly polymorphic as a result of variation in the exact number of minisatellite-encoded repeats (110).

Microsatellite DNA is the class of sequence that is composed of tandemly repeated sequences in which the repeat unit is 1 to 13 bp long (62,111). Microsatellite DNA forms blocks that are often less than 150 bp long, sometimes referred to as short tandem repeats (STRs). Microsatellites are interspersed throughout the genome and are generally intergenic, although they also occur within introns or coding sequences. Microsatellites are thought to arise as a result of template slippage during DNA replication (Chapter 2). Even in the absence of any physiologic function, microsatellite DNA has great utility in identity determination (Chapter 23).

Interspersed Repetitive DNA

There are four major classes of human interspersed repetitive DNA (Table 1.3). Even though the individual units of interspersed repetitive noncoding DNA are not clustered, taken together they account for approximately 45% of the human genome (62,112–114).

The most abundant class is the long interspersed nuclear elements (LINEs), which together make up 21% of the human genome. The most abundant LINE family is the LINE1 repeat, which is the most abundant sequence in the human genome and alone accounts for over 20% of

human DNA (62). Despite its abundance, the LINE1 repeat has no known function.

Short interspersed nuclear elements (SINEs) are the other major class of human interspersed repetitive DNA and account for almost 11% of the human genome (62). It has been suggested that SINE RNAs promote protein translation under stress (115), especially *Alu* elements, although this hypothesis remains controversial.

LINEs, SINEs, and LTR elements are retroposons, defined as transposons mobilized via RNA, reverse-transcribed into DNA, and then inserted at a new site in the genome (116,117). The *Alu* repeat is thought to have originated through retrotransposition of the 7SL RNA gene, and ongoing transposition of *Alu* sequences (118) and LINE family members (116,119) has been documented. This mobility provides LINEs and *Alu* repeats with the capability to cause genetic disease by insertional mutagenesis (117,120–122), although the most common mechanism by which they cause mutations is via homologous unequal recombination (Chapter 2). Although the repeats are a source of genetic disease, they are apparently also responsible for important functional contributions to the genome, including regulatory elements and even new genes. In fact, it has been estimated that the human genome has at least 47 genes derived from transposons (62).

RNA TRANSCRIPTION

In a typical human cell, the most abundant types of RNA are those types that are functional end molecules (62); approximately 70% to 75% of RNA is rRNA, 10% to 15% is tRNA, and 10% is heterogeneous nuclear RNA (hnRNA), itself composed of several RNA types, including snRNA, small nucleolar RNA (snoRNA), and the short RNA molecules responsible for RNA interference (see below). Even though mRNA constitutes less than 5% of the RNA within a human cell, because it is the intermediate required to produce polypeptide chains, it is the most complex type of RNA and is virtually the only type of RNA currently analyzed in the molecular genetic evaluation of human disease.

mRNA, like all nucleic acid molecules, is synthesized in the 5′ to 3′ direction. Because the transcript is complementary to the DNA template strand directing its polymerization, the mRNA has the same 5′ to 3′ the base sequence as the opposite nontemplate strand, except that the base uracil replaces thymine. By convention, the nontemplate strand of DNA is therefore referred to as the sense strand and gene sequences are indicated as the sequence of the sense strand in the direction of RNA transcription. Thus, the 5′ end of a gene refers to sequences at the 5′ end of the DNA sense strand, and upstream sequences are those sequences flanking the gene at its 5′ end. Similarly, the 3′ end of the gene refers to the sequences at the 3′ end of the DNA sense strand and downstream sequences are those flanking the 3′ end of the sense strand. By definition, a transcriptional unit encompasses not only the DNA sequence encoding the polypeptide but upstream regulatory sequences as well as downstream terminator signals.

As shown in Figure 1.8, the transcription start site for RNA polymerase II (the polymerase used to transcribe genes encoding proteins) is located approximately 25

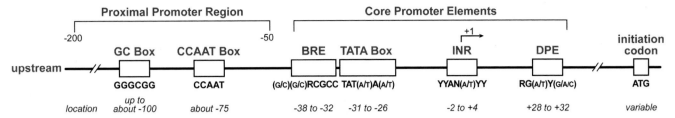

Figure 1.8 Schematic diagram of conserved promoter elements bound by ubiquitous transcription factors. The core promoter of individual genes does not necessarily contain all of the core promoter elements illustrated. The proximal promoter region and the further upstream region harbors the sequence elements that are recognized by transcription factors that regulate tissue, cell, and developmental–stage specific gene expression (not shown). Y, C or T; R, A or G; N, any nucleotide; +1 indicates the transcription start site.

nucleotides downstream of the TATA box, although many genes contain alternative transcription start sites. The mRNA translation start site of the gene, which lies 3′ to the transcriptional start site, is encoded by an ATG on the DNA sense strand (corresponding to an AUG codon in mRNA) and marks the beginning of the amino acid coding region, or open reading frame, of the gene. Both the region of the RNA transcript between the transcription start site and the translation start site, the 5′ untranslated region (UTR), and the region 3′ to the translation stop site and the end of the transcript, the 3′ UTR, assist in binding and stabilizing mRNA on ribosomes and have important regulatory functions discussed more fully below.

RNA polymerase II cannot initiate transcription by itself, so the transcription of genes that encode polypeptides is absolutely dependent on upstream *cis*-acting DNA sequence elements to recruit *trans*-acting proteins that are required to initiate transcription (Tables 1.4 and 1.5). Regulation of transcription is achieved through the presence of different combinations of the *cis*-acting regulatory elements and through either ubiquitous or tissue-specific expression of the *trans*-acting factors that bind to them. The short *cis*-acting transcription elements clustered upstream of the transcription start site collectively constitute the promoter. The core promoter contains the components that direct the basal transcription complex to initiate transcription (Fig. 1.8). The core promoter elements are usually located in the region that extends from about 45 bp upstream to about 40 bp downstream from the transcription start site. These promoter elements include the TATA box, the BRE (TFIIB recognition element) immediately upstream from the TATA box (123), the Inr (initiator) sequence (124), and the DPE (downstream promoter element), which is located about 30 bp downstream from the site of initiation of transcription (125). The proximal promoter region, which extends for about 200 bp upstream from the core promoter, contains several other sequence elements that are also recognized by ubiquitous transcription factors, including the CCAAT box (about 75 bp upstream from the transcription start site) and the GC box sequence (about 100 bp upstream from the transcription start site). Multiple regulatory DNA sequence elements are located still further upstream from the transcription start; these distal promoter elements also consist of short DNA sequences that are recognized by sequence-specific transcription factors.

It is the core promoter, however, that is the site of the assembly of the basal transcription apparatus that is necessary to initiate transcription. At promoters that contain a TATA box, assembly of the basal transcription apparatus requires recognition of the TATA sequence by TATA-binding protein (TBP), binding of TBP by 8 to 12 additional TBP-associated factors (TAFs) to form the evolutionary conserved *trans*-acting apparatus TFIID, and recruitment of additional auxiliary transcription factors as well as RNA polymerase II (126). Although the details of assembly of the basal transcription apparatus are quite complex (127), two features of the process are important. First, many other general transcription complexes (named TFIIA, TFIIB, etc.) can also prime transcription by RNA polymerase II, so that neither TBP nor TFIID are indispensable for transcription initiation. Second, although every gene is constitutively expressed at a minimum rate determined by its core promoter, the rate of transcription can be markedly increased or decreased, or even virtually shut off, by additional positive or negative regulatory elements that may be located within, or some distance away from, the promoter. Regulatory sequence elements, response elements, enhancers, silencers, and boundary elements are among the more or less remote *cis*-acting sequence elements required to achieve the sophisticated level of control characteristic of the developmentally regulated or tissue-restricted transcription pattern of many genes.

Regulatory Sequence Elements

Regulatory sequence elements are *cis*-acting short DNA motifs that are found in the promoter or enhancer region of a gene that, together with developmentally controlled or tissue-restricted *trans*-acting transcription factors that recognize and bind to them, provide a mechanism for regulation of gene expression (Table 1.4). X-ray crystallography and protein microarrays have been used to study the structure of several different DNA-transcription factor complexes to define the molecular basis for the specificity that is ultimately responsible for control of gene expression (128–130). These studies have demonstrated that binding between transcription factors, and between transcription factors and precise DNA sequence motifs, is stabilized by a small number of hydrogen bonds, ionic bonds, or hydrophobic interactions between individual amino acids and nucleotides. When all the weak interactions are taken together, they produce interactions that are both strong and specific.

Transcription factors classically have two distinct functional domains, a DNA binding domain and an activation (or repressor) domain. The DNA binding domain is the

TABLE 1.4
EXAMPLES OF *cis* REGULATORY SEQUENCE ELEMENTS

cis Sequence Element	Consensus Binding Sequence	Position[a]	Transcription Factors That Recognize the Element	Transcription Factor Expression Pattern
Core promoter elements				
TATA box	TAT(A/T)A(A/T) surrounded by GC rich sequences	About −25 bp	TATA-box binding protein (a subunit of TFIID)	Ubiquitous
BRE element	(G/C)(G/C)RCGCC[b]	Immediately upstream of the TATA box	TFIIB	Ubiquitous
Inr (initiator) sequence	YYA^{+1}N(T/A)YY[c]	At the start site	TFII-I	Ubiquitous
DPE	RG(A/T)Y(G/A/C)	+30 bp		Ubiquitous
Proximal promoter region elements				
GC boxes (Sp1 boxes)	GGGCGG	Within −100 bp	Sp1	Ubiquitous
CCAAT box	GGCCAATCT	−75 bp	CTF/NF-1 and CBF/NF-Y	Ubiquitous
GATA site	(A/T)GATA(A/G)	Proximal promoter region	GATA-1, GATA-2, etc.; Myb	Erythroid cells, megakaryocytes, spermatogonia
HNF-5 motif	T(G/A)TTTG(C/T)	Proximal promoter region	HNF-5	Liver
Ker1 motif	GCCTGCAGGC	Proximal promoter region	Ker1	Keratinocytes
E box	CANNTG	Proximal promoter region	MyoD; myogenin; C-Myc family proteins	Myoblasts and myotubes
TCF-1 motif	(C/A)A(C/A)AG	Proximal promoter region	TCF-1	T cells
AP1 motif	TGAGTCA	Proximal promoter region	JUN/FOS heterodimer	
NFκB motif	GGGACTTTCC	Proximal promoter region	NFκB	Present in promoters and enhancers of lymphoid and nonlymphoid cells
Response elements for inducible gene expression				
CRE (cAMP response element)	GTGACGT(A/C)A(A/G)	Within −1 kb	CREB family	Ubiquitous
PE element	GTTAATNATTAAC	Within −1 kb	Hnf-1	Differentiated cells of liver, kidney, GI tract, spleen
Heat shock response element	CTNGAATNTTCTAGA	Within −1 kb	Heat shock proteins, including HSP70	
GAS elements	TTNCNNNAAA	Within −1 kb	Stat family	Macrophages, lymphocytes
Steroid receptor response elements	AGAACANNNTGTTCT	Within −1 kb	Glucocorticoid receptor	
	AGGTGANNNTGACCT	Within −1 kb	Estrogen receptor	
	AGGGTCANNNNNAGACCA	Within −1 kb	Retinoid acid receptor	
	AGGTCATGACCT	Within −1 kb	Thyroxine receptor	
	AGGTCANNNAGGTCA	Within −1 kb	Vitamin D receptor	

[a]Relative to the site of transcription initiation.
[b]Y, C or T; R, A or G; N any nucleotide.
[c]The A^{+1} is the transcription initiation site.
GI, gastrointestinal.

region of the protein that is responsible for specific binding to the defined DNA sequence element. A relatively small number of conserved structural motifs, including the leucine zipper, helix-loop-helix, zinc finger, helix-turn-helix, and bZIP motifs (Table 1.5) are shared by many different transcription factors (131–134) and provide the general structure for binding DNA. Within a given motif, differences in the amino acid sequence of the individual transcription factors provide the basis for recognition of specific DNA sequence elements. After a transcription factor has bound to its target sequence, its activation (or repressor) domain interacts with other transcription

TABLE 1.5

EXAMPLES OF RECURRING MOTIFS IN *trans*-ACTING TRANSCRIPTION FACTORS[a]

Transcription Factor Domain	Motif Structure	Binding Targets	Binding Mechanism	Examples
Helix-loop-helix	Two α-helices connected by a flexible loop	E box	Dimers bind major groove of DNA	MyoD, myogenin, Myc family
Helix-turn-helix	Two short α-helices separated by a short amino acid sequence that induces a turn	RY(A/C)AAYA[b]	Dimers bind major groove of DNA	Forkhead transcription factors, POU-domain proteins, Myb factors
Zinc finger	Zinc ion bound by a loop (finger)		α-Helix binds to major groove of DNA	
	Two conserved cysteine and two conserved histidine amino acids form loop	GC box, (T/A)GATAR sites		General transcription factors including Sp1, GATA-1, WT1
	Four conserved cysteine amino acids form loop	Steroid hormone response elements		Steroid hormone receptors
bZIP	Helix-loop-helix domain mediates DNA binding; adjacent leucine zipper domain mediates oligomerization		Y-shaped dimer grips DNA double helix like a clothes peg grips a clothesline	
	Homodimerizing	ATTACGTAAT TGACGY(C/A)R		PAR family CREB family
	Homodimerizing and hetero-dimerizing	ATTGCGCAAT TGA(C/G)T(C/A)A		C/EBP family JUN family
	Heterodimerizing	Various		FOS, CNC, and L-MAF families

[a]Compiled from references 131–135.
[b]The core binding sequence of the majority of forkhead proteins; Y, C or T; R, A or G.

factors to assist (or inhibit) assembly of the basal transcription apparatus (132). Although some transcription factors bind DNA as monomers (134), those that can only bind DNA as dimers usually also have a third functional domain that regulates their pairing. Although many transcription factors form homodimers, some dimerization motifs such as the leucine zipper and the helix-loop-helix motifs also permit heterodimerization (130–132).

Given that transcription factors have a central role in controlling gene expression, it is not surprising that the activity of transcription factors themselves is tightly regulated by several different mechanisms. First, the activity of a transcription factor can be regulated based on the level of its own synthesis. Expression of a transcription factor in only one cell type provides an obvious and direct mechanism for tissue-specific gene regulation. Second, the activity of dimeric transcription factors can vary depending on which partners are involved. Third, the activity of a transcription factor can be controlled by covalent modifications such as phosphorylation or by cleavage. Fourth, although a transcription factor may be constitutively expressed, its availability, and hence its activity, can vary because of sequestration or binding by other proteins. Fifth, the activity of a transcription factor can be regulated by ligand binding. Mutations in a number of different transcription factors that interfere with their normal activity have been described, and are responsible for a variety of abnormalities (Table 1.6).

Response Elements

Response elements are short consensus DNA sequences (Table 1.4) that modulate transcription in response to external stimuli. The modulation is achieved via

TABLE 1.6
EXAMPLES OF TRANSCRIPTION FACTORS RESPONSIBLE FOR HUMAN DISEASE

Transcription Factor	Disease	Mutation and Mechanism of Action
Developmental abnormalities		
WT1	Renal neoplasia or embryonic malformation; Denys-Drash syndrome; WAGR syndrome	Germline mutations abolish DNA binding that normally inhibits expression of insulin-like growth factor-2
Endocrinopathies		
Vitamin D receptor	Hereditary vitamin D-resistant rickets	Point mutation causes abnormal dimerization (analogous disorders involve the antigen receptor and thyroxin receptor)
Hairless (GATA-like gene product)	Alopecia universalis	Deletion
Tbx1	diGeorge syndrome	Haploinsufficiency resulting from heterozygous deletion of chromosome 22q11.2
GATA-3	Hypoparathyroidism, deafness, and renal anomalies resembling diGeorge syndrome	Haploinsufficiency
Viral infections		
Tax	Transcription factor encoded by HTLV1	Stimulation of HIV transcription and viral replication requires binding to bZIP domain of CREB
Hepatitis B virus X protein		Binds to bZIP domain of CREB and interacts with TATA-box binding protein
Neoplasms		
WT1	Desmoplastic small round cell tumor	t(11;22) produces *EWS-WT1* oncogenic chimeric gene
PAX3 and PAX7	Alveolar rhabdomyosarcoma	t(2;13) and t(1;13) produce oncogenic *PAX3-FKHR* and *PAX7-FKHR* chimeric genes, respectively
PAX8	Follicular thyroid carcinoma	t(2;3) produces oncogenic *PAX8-PPARγ1* chimeric gene
ETV6	Congenital fibrosarcoma, congenital mesoblastic nephroma, secretory breast carcinoma	t(12;15) produces oncogenic *ETV6-NTRK3* chimeric gene
ATF1	Clear cell sarcoma	t(12;22) produces oncogenic *EWS-ATF1* chimeric gene
CHOP	Myxoid liposarcoma	t(11;16) produces oncogenic *TLS-CHOP* chimeric gene
TFE3	Alveolar soft part sarcoma; Xp11.1-associated renal carcinomas	Translocations involving Xp11.1 and a number of different partner loci produce oncogenic chimeric genes

HIV, human immunodeficiency virus.

transcription factors that, following activation by hormones or intracellular second messengers (135), bind to the response elements. Response elements are usually located within several hundred bp upstream of a promoter, although they have also been described in enhancers.

Enhancers

Enhancers provide for upregulation of gene expression. They usually contain, within a span of only several hundred bp, *cis*-acting DNA sequence elements that are recognized by ubiquitous transcription factors as well as sequence elements recognized by tissue-specific transcription factors. In aggregate, the clustered sequence elements increase the basal level of transcription initiated through the gene's core promoter elements (136). Functionally, enhancers are also the likely initial sites of binding of histone acetyltransferases that, through an ordered process of histone acetyltransferation and other covalent histone modifications, assist in recruiting transcriptional complexes to adjacent promoter sequences (32).

However, enhancers differ from promoters in several important ways. First, enhancers are not essential for transcription initiation, although enhancer elements may be an internal component of a promoter. Second, enhancers can be located over 10 to 15 kb from the gene promoter they regulate. Third, although they are usually situated 5' to the transcription start site, they can also be located within introns, within the open reading of the gene, or even 3' to the gene. Fourth, the function of the enhancer, unlike that of the core promoter, is independent of orientation.

Silencers

Two classes of silencers have been distinguished, both of which diminish a gene's expression level. The first class is composed of position-independent elements that direct an active repression mechanism, although the functional basis for the repression by most members of this class remains uncharacterized. The second class is composed of negative regulatory elements (NREs) that are position-dependent sequences with a passive repression mechanism that seems to be demarcated by changes in histone acetylation (137). Repression is thought to result from physical inhibition of the interaction of transcription factors with other DNA sequence motifs by specific silencer-bound proteins (137–139). Silencer elements have been identified in a variety of positions in human genes, both near the promoter and within introns, exons, or flanking sequences. In some mammalian systems, silencers located within an exon have been shown to function at the level of DNA for regulation of gene transcription and also at the level of RNA for control of translation through interference with normal RNA processing or trafficking (137).

Boundary Elements

Boundary elements, also known as insulator elements, are regions of DNA from 0.5 to 3 kb long that demarcate the 5' and 3' margins of a gene (140). From the perspective of gene regulation, the capability of enhancers to exert an upregulatory effect on regions of DNA that are many kb long requires a mechanism to prevent inappropriate activation of neighboring genes, and boundary elements perform this task. Boundary elements likely function by establishing an intricate three-dimensional chromatin structure (that is probably important for DNA replication and RNA processing, not just regulation of transcription) (140,141). Boundary elements also block the inappropriate repression of transcription caused by local silencers.

RNA Interference

Several classes of short double-stranded or single-stranded RNA molecules have recently been shown to have a role in regulation of gene expression (142–144). Often referred to as RNA interference (RNAi), RNA-mediated control of gene expression constitutes an entirely new pathway of gene regulation and occurs through several different mechanisms.

As an aside, it is worth noting that the discovery of RNAi has suggested novel strategies for treating a wide variety of illness, ranging from cancer to infectious diseases (145). Although delivery of short RNA molecules remains an obstacle to the development of RNAi-based therapies (145), several model systems have been developed that demonstrate the potential of RNAi-based approaches. For example, injection of siRNA has been used to protect mice from viral hepatitis (146), and nasally administered siRNA has been used to protect mice from respiratory virus infection (147,148).

Short Interfering RNA

RNAi through short interfering RNA (siRNA) is thought to have initially developed as a mechanism to silence the expression of genes encoded by repetitive sequence elements. siRNAs are double-stranded RNA molecules that are 21 to 22 nucleotides long. They are produced from long double-stranded RNA molecules that are cut into shorter fragments by an enzyme named Dicer. An RNA-induced silencing complex (RISC) removes the sense strand (via a process that is not yet fully characterized), leaving the antisense strand to guide the RISC to mRNAs produced from the target gene. Through repeated cycles of degradation of the target mRNAs, the RISC prevents production of the encoded protein, effectively silencing the gene from which the mRNA is produced.

siRNAs also are capable of directly inhibiting gene expression by transcriptional silencing. Although the details of the process are unknown, transcriptional silencing involves DNA methylation as well as chromatin remodeling through histone methylation (142,149,150).

Micro RNA

Micro RNAs (miRNAs) are short single-stranded molecules that are 19 to 25 nucleotides long. They are evolutionarily conserved and have roles in gene regulation and development (151). In humans, there are approximately 200 to 255 genes encoding miRNAs (152,153).

Functionally, miRNAs are thought not to inhibit transcription but rather to inhibit translation of mRNA by binding to partially complementary sequences in the 3' untranslated region of mRNA. A typical mRNA contains many miRNA binding sites in its 3' untranslated region, and because binding is by only partially complementary sequences, several miMRA can bind to each transcript, and each miMRA can bind to mRNA transcripts from several hundred different genes.

Other Short RNAs

Several potential new classes of short RNAs have recently been described, including small modulatory RNA (smRNA). smRNAs are short double-stranded RNA molecules that are 20 to 23 nucleotides long and, like miRNAs, are evolutionarily conserved. Although the details are again unknown, smRNAs apparently exert control over gene expression via interaction with specific regulatory proteins (154).

TRANSCRIPT ELONGATION

It turns out that the activity of RNA polymerase II is regulated at additional steps beside just the initiation of transcription. During transcript elongation, the enzyme pauses at various sites in a gene's sequence, and the frequency and duration of the pauses is under control of several cellular proteins (155–157). The significance of the control these proteins exert on the process of elongation is shown by their role in a diverse collection of human diseases, including HIV-1 infection, acute myeloid leukemia, and von Hippel-Lindau disease (155,158–160).

RNA PROCESSING

The initial RNA transcript is subjected to two immediate processing events. The first reaction is RNA capping, in which 7-methylguanosine is linked to the initial 5′ nucleotide of the RNA transcript co-transcriptionally. RNA capping protects the nascent transcript from 5′ to 3′ exonuclease attack (161), facilitates RNA splicing and transport from the nucleus to the cytoplasm, and is integral for attachment of the 40S subunit of cytoplasmic ribosomes to mRNA. The second initial processing event is polyadenylation, in which approximately 200 adenylate (AMP) residues are added to the 3′ end of the transcript by the enzyme poly(A) polymerase to form the poly(A) tail. Two or more polyadenylation signals are found in the 3′ UTR of many human genes, and different types of polydenylation sites have been described (162). Transcripts polyadenylated at an alternative site can show a different pattern of tissue specificity or an alternative pattern of RNA splicing (162,163). Regardless of the site of polyadenylation, the poly(A) tail is thought to facilitate transfer of the RNA transcript to the cytoplasm, stabilize the transcript, and enhance translation by facilitating recognition of the mRNA by the ribosomal machinery.

RNA Splicing

The coding sequence of the vast majority of human genes is split into segments (exons), which are separated by noncoding intervening sequences (introns). The few human genes not interrupted by introns tend to be very small and include the genes for histones, small functional RNA molecules, most tRNAs, various neurotransmitter and hormone receptors, and cytokines such as alpha interferon.

RNA splicing is the processing by which introns are excised from the primary full-length RNA transcript. Splicing is mediated by the spliceosome, a large RNA–protein complex that contains five types of snRNA and at least 50 proteins. The mechanism by which the spliceosome catalyzes endonucleolytic cleavage and excision of intronic RNA segments, with subsequent ligation of the adjacent exonic RNA segments, is known in some detail (Fig. 1.9) and provides the explanation for why 5′-GU and

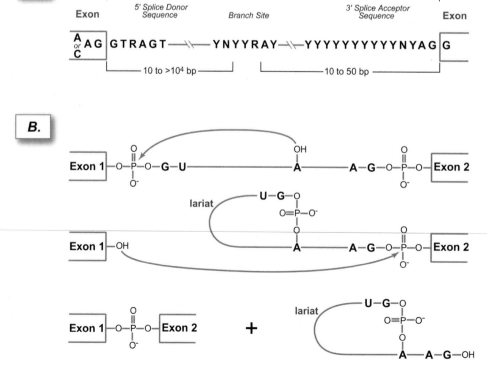

Figure 1.9 RNA splicing. **A,** Consensus sequence (at the DNA level) for the 5′ splice donor, 3′ splice acceptor, and branch point. R, purine (A or G); Y, pyrimidine (C or T); N, any base. **B,** Schematic diagram of the mechanism of RNA splicing. Splicing occurs by two sequential transesterification reactions involving nucleophilic attack of a phosphodiester bond by a free OH end. Note that the first transesterification reaction involves the 2′-hydroxyl group of the ribose (Fig. 1.1) attached to the conserved adenine at the branch site.

AG-3' dinucleotide pairs at the exon–intron boundaries (known as the splice junctions) are critical to splicing. However, it is important to recognize that the mere presence of 5'-GU and AG-3' dinucleotide pairs in an RNA transcript is not sufficient to specify the presence of an intron; highly conserved sequences must also be present in the sequences adjacent to the dinucleotide pairs, and a branch site must be located within 40 nucleotides of the AG-3' dinucleotide. The vast majority of introns follow the GU-AG rule, but a much rarer class of introns also exists in which the conserved GU and AG dinucleotides are replaced by AU and AC, respectively. Introns that belong to the AU-AC class are processed by a spliceosome that has a slightly different component of snRNAs.

The order in which intronic sequences are excised is not governed by their linear order in the initial RNA transcript. Instead, the accessibility of splice sites is thought to be determined by the conformation of the RNA transcript. As initially accessible introns are removed, the RNA conformation changes, new pairs of splice sites become available, and splicing continues. In addition, it has recently become clear that exonic splicing enhancers (ESEs) and exonic splicing silencers (ESSs) affect exon skipping or inclusion (164–166). ESEs are discrete but degenerate sequence motifs roughly 6 to 18 nucleotides long that enhance the use of weak splice sites; they can be located within exons or introns (167–171). ESSs, for which a consensus sequence has yet to be determined, inhibit the use of splice sites and so promote exon skipping (172).

The mechanism of RNA splicing explains why mutations of splice site consensus sequences, even those that are intronic and therefore outside the region of the gene that encodes the amino acid sequence of polypeptide, can nonetheless have a profound effect on protein function and cause disease (173–176). In addition, ESEs and ESSs provide the means for missense or even silent mutations within exons to influence protein structure independent of an effect on the protein's amino acid sequence (164,165,174,177,178). In fact, nearly 15% of point mutations known to cause human genetic disease and result in defective splicing are located in exons, distinct from splice junctions and not associated with cryptic splice sites (164).

Alternative Splicing

The majority of human genes are transcribed into an RNA molecule that gives rise to a single type of mRNA after splicing. However, for some genes, the process of alternative splicing produces mature mRNA molecules that have different exon combinations (179–181). For some genes, alternative splicing is regulated so that only one mRNA occurs under a given set of circumstances, whereas for other genes, alternative splicing produces different mRNAs encoding different isoforms of the same protein in the same cell at the same time (179,181–183).

Several mechanisms direct the pattern of alternative splicing (180,184,185). First, use of different promoters can change the transcriptional start site, which then alters the number of exons in the initial RNA transcript, which then affects the pattern of splicing (181,186). Second, use of different 3' polyadenylation signals can change the length of the initial transcript and alter the pattern of RNA splicing

(181). Third, specific proteins (including some encoded by viruses) can exert control over the pattern of splicing (180). Fourth, alternative splicing may be governed by ESEs and ESSs (164). For many genes, however, the mechanisms that control alternative splicing are unknown.

The functional significance of alternative splicing lies in the fact that it provides a means to produce, from the same gene, different protein isoforms that have different functions (187). Alternative splicing can produce tissue-specific isoforms of a protein; for example, calcitonin and calcitonin gene-related peptide result from alternative splicing of the calcitonin gene in thyroid and brain, respectively. Alternative splicing can change the ligand binding affinity of a growth factor receptor or lead to production of a protein isoform that is soluble rather than membrane bound (188). Alternative splicing can even generate protein isoforms with opposed functions. For example, alternative splicing of transcripts from the same gene gives rise to the transcriptional activators NFI-B1 and NFI-B2, as well as the transcriptional repressor NFI-B3 (189). Similarly, alternative splicing of transcripts from the same gene underlies production of bcl-X_L and bcl-X_S, which are positive and negative regulators of programmed cell death, respectively (190). As could be expected, mutations that affect the pattern of alternative splicing are responsible for a number of hereditary diseases (191).

RNA Editing

RNA editing is a rare form of post-translation processing. Although insertion/deletion editing has been described in kinetoplastid protoza and slime molds (192), RNA editing in humans is restricted to base-specific changes that are introduced at the pre-mRNA level by deamination reactions catalyzed by specific enzymes (193–197). The base change that results from RNA editing often alters the sequence of the encoded protein, but some evidence suggests that the most commons sites of editing are within noncoding sequences where the effect of the base change is unknown (197). Although it is very rare, the significance of RNA editing lies in the fact that it represents a process whereby the informational content of a transcript can be changed at the level of the mRNA itself, essentially diversifying the information encoded in the genome.

Editing of the pre-mRNA of several different human proteins has been documented (Table 1.7) at sites that include coding sequences, introns, and 5' and 3' untranslated regions (194,195,197,200). In the first described example, a cytidine deaminase acting on RNA from the *ApoB* gene converts C to U in enterocytes of the small intestine, a change that generates a stop codon, leading to the production of a truncated ApoB48 protein involved in chylomicron metabolism; hepatocytes do not edit *ApoB* RNA and instead produce the full-length ApoB100 gene product that is a component of lipoproteins (201). In another well-characterized example, adenosine deaminases acting on RNA edit the transcripts of ligand-gated ion channels in a process that apparently helps modulate the myriad of protein–protein interactions that regulate cell signaling (193). Although these two examples illustrate situations in which RNA editing is a component of normal physiologic processes, editing also plays a role in the pathogenesis of

TABLE 1.7

HUMAN RNA EDITING ENZYMES

Enzyme	Base Change	Examples
Cytidine deaminases acting on RNA (CDAR)		
APOBEC-1[a]	Site specific C→U in pre-mRNA	ApoB editing in small intestine; editing of neurofibromin tumor suppressor protein in NF-1
CEM15 (APOBEC3G)	C→U in specific sequence contexts	Anti-retroviral defense
Adenosine deaminases acting on RNA (ADAR)		
ADAR1, ADAR2, ADAR3 (RED2)	Promiscuous or site-specific A→I[b] in dsRNA and pre-mRNA	Coding sequence: all five glutamate receptor subunits; serotonin receptor; HDV antigenome; measles virus, parainfluenza virus, RSV, VSV, polyoma virus Noncoding sequence: NADH-dehydrogenase; proteosome subunit HsC7-I
Adenosine deamination in tRNA		
ADAT1	A→I in tRNA	Performs A→I reaction immediately adjacent to the anticodon
ADAT2/ADAT3 heterodimer	A→I in tRNA	Performs A→I reaction that generates the I present at the first (wobble) anticodon position in eight tRNAs
Enzymatic addition of amine group		
Unknown	U→C	Converts a leucine to a proline in the Wilms tumor gene (WT1) mRNA; the two forms of the protein have slightly different levels of activity as transcriptional regulators
Nucleotide replacement rather than covalent modification[c]		
Unknown	U→A	A-galactosidase mRNA

[a]APOBEC-1 is the catalytic subunit of a multisubunit complex required for editing.
[b]Inosine, read as a G during translation.
[c]There is controversy as to whether this form of editing exists (198,199).
HDV, hepatitis D virus; RSV, respiratory syncytial virus; VSV, vesicular stromatitis virus.

several diseases. Editing of endothelin B receptor transcripts may be involved in the development of some cases of Hirschsprung disease (202), of *NF1* gene transcripts may play a role in the pathogenesis and progression of neoplasms associated with neurofibromatosis type 1 (203,204), and of *WT1* transcripts may be responsible for some renal tumors and developmental abnormalities (205,206). Editing even plays a role in host defense to retroviral infection (207,208).

PROTEIN SYNTHESIS

mRNA transcribed from genes in nuclear DNA is transported to the cytoplasm, where it directs the synthesis of polypeptides on ribosomes (209–211). In humans, these large protein–RNA complexes are composed of a large subunit (the 60S subunit, which itself is composed of three rRNA species and 49 proteins) and a small subunit (the 40S subunit composed of one rRNA and 33 proteins). Ribosomes have several active centers that direct the assembly of the

polypeptide chain via the base pairing interaction of mRNA codons and the complementary anti-codons of tRNA. The active centers of ribosomes are not discrete small regions similar to the active centers of enzymes, but instead are relatively large and, when taken together, comprise about two thirds of ribosomal structure. Active centers include the P and A sites (the sites occupied by the peptidyl-tRNA that carries the growing polypeptide chain, and the site that exposes the codon representing the next amino acid to be added, respectively); an exit channel (where the polypeptide chain emerges from the ribosome, and which can associate with a cell membrane); elongation factor binding sites; the peptidyltransferase center; and so on. Protein synthesis on the ribosome can be divided into three general stages, initiation, elongation, and termination.

Initiation

The initiation step includes all the reactions that precede formation of the peptide bond between the first two amino acids of the nascent polypeptide chain. Initiation requires ribosomal binding to mRNA, a slow process that usually determines the rate at which an mRNA molecule is translated.

According to the scanning model of initiation, the 40S ribosomal subunit initially recognizes the 5' cap of the mRNA and then migrates linearly along the mRNA until it encounters an AUG initiation codon. The first AUG codon usually, though not always, initiates translation (212), but the trinucleotide by itself is not sufficient to stop migration of the 40S subunit. The AUG is only recognized as an initiation codon in the context of the sequence GCCRC-CAUGG, where R indicates a purine. The 60S subunit joins the 40S subunit at the initiation site, forming an intact ribosome.

The overwhelming majority of initiation events involve scanning from the 5' cap, but it is worth noting that an alternative initiation mechanism exists that involves direct association of the 40S subunit with an internal mRNA sequence termed an IRES site. An increasing number of cellular genes have been shown to harbor an IRES, which either has a role in the control of translation or functions primarily when cap-dependent translation is physiologically impaired, such as during mitosis, quiescence, stress, and apoptosis (213,214). IRES are also important for initiation of translation of many viral proteins (214–217), especially those encoded by picornavirus, because during infection picornavirus specifically destroys cap structures in order to inhibit host protein synthesis (218).

Elongation

The growth of the polypeptide chain occurs through a cycle of reactions that repeats with the addition of each amino acid: an aminoacyl-tRNA enters the A site of a ribosome whose P site is occupied by the peptidyl-RNA; a peptide bond is formed as the polypeptide chain is transferred to the aminoacyl-tRNA in the A site; the ribosome translocates three nucleotides along the mRNA, which expels the now uncharged tRNA from the P site and simultaneously vacates the A site by shifting the peptidyl-RNA to the P site (219). Although each tRNA has a specific trinucleotide sequence that provides the specificity required to interpret the nucleotide sequence of the mRNA molecule, translational accuracy is also dependent on the aminoacyl-tRNA synthetase enzymes (220). The fidelity of aminoacyl-tRNA synthetases and aminoacyl-tRNA binding at the A site of the ribosome, together with proofreading processes at each of these two steps, result in the remarkable overall accuracy of translation, in which errors occur at a rate of only about 1 per 10^5 amino acid residues synthesized.

Termination

The termination step of translation requires several specific reactions to release the completed polypeptide chain and disassociate the ribosomal complex from the mRNA. Each of the three termination, or stop, codons is necessary and sufficient to end protein synthesis. Because none of the termination codons is represented by a tRNA, the termination reaction does not depend on codon–anticodon recognition. Instead, the termination codons are recognized directly by protein factors that catalyze three reactions that direct termination of transcription, specifically release of the completed polypeptide chain, expulsion of the last tRNA from the ribosome, and disassociation of the ribosome from the mRNA.

THE GENETIC CODE

Each codon consists of a nucleotide triplet, and thus there are 64 total codons. Although 20 amino acids have classically been ascribed to humans, it has recently become clear that the amino acid selenocysteine can be inserted into protein via its own tRNA, establishing selenocysteine as the 21st amino acid in mammals, including humans (62,221,222). In the revised genetic code that incorporates selenocysteine (Appendix 1), 61 codons represent amino acids and two codons terminate protein synthesis, but one codon that usually terminates protein synthesis can also represent selenocysteine. Because there are only 21 amino acids, most amino acids are therefore represented by more than one codon. Similarly, because there are only 38 unique types of cytoplasmic tRNA (62), the rules that govern codon–anticodon recognition on the ribosome during protein synthesis must allow for some lack of stringency in base pairing. The decreased stringency is summarized by the wobble hypothesis, which states that conventional base paring rules are followed for the first two base positions in a codon, but that there is reduced specificity at the third position. Appendix 2 presents the biochemical features of the 21 amino acids specified by the genetic code.

POST-TRANSCRIPTIONAL CONTROL OF GENE EXPRESSION

Regulation of the level of expression of most protein-encoding genes is primarily achieved by controlling the level of transcription; however, gene expression can also be controlled post-transcriptionally through a variety of mechanisms, including regulation of mRNA stability, mRNA localization, translation initiation, or RNA interference (142,211,223–225).

Translational Control

The level of gene expression can be controlled by the efficiency of translation of mRNA in the absence of corresponding changes in the level of mRNA production or in the absence of changes in the steady-state level of the mRNA. Translational control of gene expression is important because it provides a mechanism for cells to respond to external stimuli more rapidly than is possible by activation of transcription. Control can be exerted via the 5' UTR, the 3' UTR, or even the coding region of the gene itself (163,226–231). Mechanistically, control is usually exerted through cis-acting sequence elements of the mRNA that are recognized by trans-acting RNA-binding proteins that either cause alterations of mRNA secondary structure or target mRNA to specific intracellular locations (163,226,227,229,232–236). And, as discussed above, RNA translation also can be inhibited by miRNAs that bind to partially complementary sequences in the 3' untranslated region of mRNA (142).

Translational control has long been known to play a critical role during development, when the embryologic events involved in pattern formation, germ cell specification, cell fate, and cell division are programmed by sequence-specific translational activation of stored maternal mRNA (237). Recently, translational control has been shown to play a role in drug metabolism, in which some of the same RNA-binding proteins may also interact with specific sequence elements of mRNAs for proteins involved in cell cycle control (238). These observations have important clinical ramifications because they suggest that mutations that disrupt translational regulation may provide a novel mechanism for malignant transformation that is linked to the emergence of drug resistance in neoplastic cells.

Control of mRNA Stability

Regulation of cytoplasmic mRNA degradation has emerged as a particularly important mechanism of post-transcriptional control of protein expression (224,239). The 3' UTR is a region that harbors many determinates involved in the control of mRNA decay (226,228,229), and A+U-rich elements (AREs) have been demonstrated to be particularly potent destabilizing elements in a wide variety of mRNAs (163,229). AREs usually contain a variable number of overlapping AUUUA pentamers, and accelerated mRNA decay is mediated by a diverse set of RNA-binding proteins, some of which have RNA-binding domains that show structural homology with functional motifs of DNA-binding proteins (229,235). Most ARE-binding proteins have a destabilizing function and therefore increase the rate of mRNA decay, although some lead to increased message stability. The iron response element (IRE) is an interesting example of an mRNA sequence motif that can have opposite effects on mRNA stability; multiple IREs located in the 3' UTR of transferrin receptor mRNA are recognized by IRE-binding proteins that stabilize the message, while a single IRE present in the 5' UTR of ferritin mRNA causes transcription repression when bound by IRE-binding proteins (240).

RNA interference is another mechanism that regulates cytoplasmic mRNA degradation. As noted above, in addition to their role in transcriptional silencing, siRNAs guide the catalytic destruction of target mRNAs by the RISC enzymatic complex (142). Even though the details of the process by which siRNAs guide the RISC are unknown, the mechanism can effectively silence any gene as long as the complementary short double-stranded is present.

POST-TRANSLATIONAL MODIFICATION OF PROTEINS

Over 100 different post-translational modifications of proteins have been described. Some of the chemical modifications (Table 1.8) involve the attachment of simple structural groups to single amino acids, such as phosphorylation, hydroxylation, methylation, and acetylation. Other proteins undergo more extensive modifications that involve attachment of complex molecules, often at several sites (241,242). The modifications are often required for correct protein folding (especially true for carbohydrate modifications), proper intracellular trafficking, or protein function. Consequently, even conservative missense mutations, mutations that result in the substitution of one amino acid by another that is chemically similar, can still have a profound affect on a protein's function if they alter its post-translational processing.

Glycosylation

The few proteins in the cytosol that are glycosylated have a single N-acetylglucosamine sugar residue attached to either serine or threonine. By contrast, proteins that are secreted or exported to lysosomes, the Golgi apparatus, or the cell membrane undergo several classes of glycosylation reactions in which oligosaccharides that are largely preformed are added en bloc. N-Glycosylation involves transfer of an oligosaccharide to the amino group of the asparagine side chain. The reaction occurs within the endoplasmic reticulum, with subsequent modification of the common oligosaccharide in the Golgi. O-Glycosylation is less frequent and involves linkage of a core oligosaccharide to serine, threonine, or hydroxylysine. Proteoglycans are proteins in which the attached sugars are glycosaminoglycans that usually consist of repeating disaccharide units containing glucosamine or galactosamine.

Addition of Lipid Groups

The lipid groups that are attached to proteins typically function as membrane anchors. The myristoyl group is added to a glycine amino acid at the N-terminus of a protein. Prenyl groups are attached to proteins via a thioester linkage to cysteine residues near the C-terminus of a protein, and palmitoyl fatty acyl groups are linked through a sulfide bound to a cysteine residue close to either the N- or C-terminus of the protein. Glycosylphosphatidyl inositol (GPI) is a complex glycolipid that is attached to proteins by a C-terminal aspartate residue and is used to anchor proteins to the outer layer of the cell membrane.

Post-translational Cleavage

For many proteins, the primary translated polypeptide undergoes internal cleavage to generate the mature protein product. The proteolytic reactions include excision of the initial methionine residue, excision of the signal sequence, and even production of multiple functional polypeptide chains from the single precursor protein encoded by the mRNA.

INTRACELLULAR PROTEIN TRAFFICKING

Protein trafficking is accomplished by specific localization signals embedded in the structure of the protein, signals that usually take the form of short polypeptide sequences (Table 1.9). Some localization signals determine whether nasciently synthesized proteins will be secreted or will be exported to specific intracellular organelles such as the nucleus, mitochondria, or peroxisome (242–245). Other

TABLE 1.8
POST-TRANSLATIONAL MODIFICATION OF PROTEINS

Type of Modification	Target	Comments
Addition of small chemical groups		
Phosphorylation (PO_4^-)	Tyrosine, serine, threonine	Reversible; kinases add phosphate groups, phosphatases remove them
Methylation (CH_3)	Lysine	Reversible; methylases add methyl groups, demethylases remove them
Hydroxylation (OH)	Aspartic acid, lysine, proline	Particularly common modification of collagen; a deficiency in the required co-factor vitamin C causes scurvy
Acetylation (CH_3CO)	Lysine	Reversible; acetylases add acetyl groups, deacetylases remove them
Carboxylation (COOH)	Glutamic acid	The γ-carboxylation of blood clotting factors requires vitamin K as a co-factor
Sulfation (SO_4^-)	Tyrosine	Occurs in the *trans*-Golgi network
Glycosylation reactions		
N-Glycosylation (addition of complex carbohydrates)	Asparagine, usually in the N-Z[a]-S/T consensus sequence	Occurs in the endoplasmic reticulum
O-Glycosylation (addition of complex carbohydrates)	Serine, threonine, hydroxylysine	Occurs in the Golgi apparatus
N-Acetylglucosamine addition	Serine, threonine	Modification of cytosolic proteins rather than surface proteins or exported proteins
Addition of fatty residues		
Glypiation (addition of glycosylphosphatidyl inositiol group, GPI)	Aspartic acid at C-terminus	Anchors protein to outer layer of plasma membrane
Myristoylation (C_{14} fatty acyl group)	Glycine at N-terminus in M-G-Z-Z-Z-S/T	Terminal methionene is removed to make glycine available; membrane anchor
Palmitoylation (C_{16} fatty acyl group)	Cysteine near C-terminus, or rarely N-terminus	Membrane anchor via *S*-palmitoyl link
Farnesylation (C_{15} isoprenoid group)	Cysteine at C-terminus in Cys-Ali[b]-Ali-Met/Ser	Terminal tripeptide is removed to make cysteine available; membrane anchor
Geranylgeranylation (C_{20} isoprenoid group)	Cysteine at C-terminus in Cys-Ali-Ali-Leu	Terminal tripeptide is removed to make cysteine available; membrane anchor
Ribosylation		
ADP-ribosylation	Arginine, cysteine, acetyllysine	Occurs in both cytoplasmic and nuclear proteins
Poly(ADP-ribosyl)ation	Glutamic acid, aspartic acid	Poly(ADP-ribosyl)ation of DNA-binding proteins within the nucleus appears to play a protective role in the DNA damage response
Ubiquitinylation	Lysine; phosphorylated P-E-S-T	The 76 amino acid protein ubiquitin marks proteins for proteosomal destruction

[a]Z represents multiple possible amino acids.
[b]Ali represents aliphatic amino acid.

short peptide sequences function as sorting signals to specify the ultimate destination of proteins that are part of the soluble component of the cytosol (246,247) or act to control functional protein trafficking, such as internalization of membrane receptors after ligand binding (248).

Mutations in sequences that control polypeptide trafficking can have a profound effect on protein function, even if they occur in a region that is not present in the mature protein. For example, the signal sequence (or leader sequence) consists of the first 10 to 25 amino acids

TABLE 1.9

EXAMPLES OF PROTEIN TRAFFICKING SIGNALS

Routing	Signal
Proteins synthesized by ER-associated ribosomes	
Endoplasmic reticulum followed by secretion from the cell	Hydrophobic leader sequences consisting of an N-terminal sequence of 10–25 very hydrophobic amino acids
Retention in endoplasmic reticulum	C-terminal salvage signal K-D-G-L in addition to hydrophobic leader sequence
Proteins required for lysosomal structure and function	Addition of mannose-6-phosphate
Proteins synthesized by non-ER-associated ribosomes	
To mitochondria	N-terminal amphipathic α-helix with positively charged residues on one face and hydrophobic residues on the other
To peroxisome	S-K-L tripeptide at C-terminus
To nucleus	Stretch of 4–8 positiviely charged amino acids with neighboring prolines; a split (bipartite) distribution of the signal, separated by about 10 amino acids, is often present
Functional trafficking	
Lysosomal import of cytosolic proteins fated for lysosomal destruction	K-F-E-R-Q pentapeptide
Internalization of membrane receptors	Tetrapeptide N-P-Z[a]-Y in the cytoplasmic domain (LDL receptor); tetrapeptide Y-Z-R-F in the cytoplasmic domain (transferrin receptor)

[a]Z represents multiple possible amino acids
LDL, low-density lipoprotein.

at the N-terminal end of proteins destined to be secreted from the cell, but after the signal sequence guides translocation of the nascent protein into the lumen of the RER, it is cleaved from the protein.

MITOCHONDRIAL GENES

Mitochondria apparently originated as the result of an endosymbiotic event between a precursor to the eukaryotic cell and an ancient eubacterium. Although it is likely that the proto-organelle initially retained all the genes necessary for independent function, with time, most of its genes were either lost or transferred to the cell nucleus (249). The evolutionary history of mitochondria explains many of their unique genetic characteristics.

The human mitochondrial genome is only 16.6 kb long, and its organization is extremely compact (250). The genome includes only 22 tRNA genes, 2 rRNA genes, and 13 protein encoding genes, all of which encode components of oxidative phosphorylation. Mitochondrial genes lack introns and are closely opposed, and the coding sequences of some genes overlap. Because each mitochondrion has from 2 to 10 copies of the genome, and because human cells contain hundreds to thousands of mitochondria, mitochondrial DNA nonetheless accounts for up to 0.5% of the DNA in a somatic cell.

The mitochondrial genome encodes the large subunit of the mitochondrial ribosome (the 23S rRNA) and the small subunit of the mitochondrial ribosome (the 16S rRNA), as well as the different types of tRNA that are required for synthesizing the 13 encoded polypeptides on mitochondrial ribosomes. However, all the other components of the translational machinery (e.g., the protein components of mitochondrial ribosomes, aminoacyl tRNA synthetases, etc.), as well as all other structural and enzymatic proteins of the mitochondria, are encoded by nuclear genes and must be translated on cytoplasmic ribosomes before being imported into the mitochondria. The human mitochondrial genetic code itself differs slightly from the nuclear genetic code, as indicated in Appendix 1.

Mitochondrial DNA evolves at a different rate from nuclear DNA for two reasons. First, mitochondrial DNA (mtDNA) has a higher intrinsic rate of mutation that is a result of, among other factors, a high rate of oxidative damage resulting from the production of reactive oxygen intermediates by the respiratory chain and the lack of some DNA repair systems. Second, the unique pattern of mitochondrial inheritance results in a very high rate of fixation of mtDNA mutations. Although a sperm contributes half of the zygote's nuclear genome, it contributes none of the zygote's mtDNA, and so the mitochondrial genome is maternally inherited (although a recent report of paternal transmission of mtDNA in skeletal muscle in a patient with a mitochondrial myopathy [251] serves as a warning that maternal inheritance of mtDNA is not absolute). This pattern of inheritance of mtDNA not only helps explain the high rate of mtDNA evolution but also

TABLE 1.10

EXAMPLES OF MITOCHONDRIAL DISEASES[a]

Mutated Gene	Gene Location	Altered Product(s)	Disease
Mitochondrial respiratory-chain genes			
ND1, ND2, ND3, ND4, ND4L, ND5, ND6	mtDNA	Structural components of complex I of respiratory chain	LHON, MELAS, LHON and dystonia, sporadic myopathy
Cytb	mtDNA	Structural components of complex III of respiratory chain	Sporadic myopathy, encephalomyopathy, septo-optic dysplasia, cardiomyopathy
COXI, COXII, COXIII	mtDNA	Structural components of complex IV of respiratory chain	Sporadic anemia, sporadic myopathy, encelphalomyopathy, ALS-like syndrome
ATPase 6	mtDNA	Structural components of complex V of respiratory chain	NARP, MILS, FBSN
Mitochondrial tRNA genes			
tRNA$^{Leu (UUR)}$	mtDNA	Mitochondrial leucine tRNA	MELAS
tRNA^{Lys}	mtDNA	Mitochondrial lysine tRNA	MERRF
tRNA^{Ile}	mtDNA	Mitochondrial isoleucine tDNA	Hypertension, hypercholesterolemia, and hypomagnesemia
Nuclear respiratory-chain genes			
SDHC, SDHD	nDNA	Structural components of complexes I and II of respiratory chain	Leigh's syndrome, leukodystrophy, paraganglioma, pheochromocytoma
BCS1L	nDNA	Ancillary protein required for assembly of complex III of respiratory chain	Leigh's syndrome, GRACILE syndrome
SCO1, SCO2, COX10, COX15, SURF1	nDNA	Ancillary proteins required for assembly or insertion of cofactors of complex IV of respiratory chain	Leigh's syndrome, hepatopathy, cardioencephalomyopathy, leukodystrophy and tubulopathy
Defects in membrane lipid milieu			
G4.5	nDNA	Acyl-coenzyme A synthase with likely role in cardiolipin synthesis	Barth syndrome
Defects of mitochondrial protein importation			
TIMM8A	nDNA	Encodes the protein DDP1, a component of the mitochondrial protein-import machinery in the intramembranous space	Mohr-Tranebjaerg syndrome
Defects in mitochondrial response to oxidant stress			
FRDA	nDNA	Encodes frataxin, loss of which is associated with mitochondrial iron accumulation, deficiency in iron-sulfer proteins, and increased oxidant stress	Friedreich ataxia
OGG1	nDNA	DNA glycosylase required for repair of oxidative base damage	Age-dependent decrease in import
Defects in mitochondrial motility			
OPA1	nDNA	Encodes dynamin-related guanosine triphophatase required for mitochondrial movement along cytoskeleton microtubules	Optic atrophy

[a]The MITOMAP database of mitochondrial mutations (http://infinity.gen.emory.edu/mitomap.html) summarizes all the information on genotypes and phenotypes.
LHON, Leber's hereditary optic myopathy; MELAS, mitochondrial encephalomyopathy, lactic acidosis; nDNA, nuclear DNA. GRACILE, growth retardation, aminoaciduria, lactic acidosis, and early death; ALS, amyotrophic lateral sclerosis; NARP, neuropathy, ataxia, and retinitis pigmentosa; MILS, maternally inherited Leigh's syndrome; FBSN, familial bilateral striatal necrosis; MERRF, myoclonus epilepsy with ragged-red fibers

TABLE 1.11
SELECTED EXAMPLES OF COMPLEXITY IN THE ONE GENE/ONE ENZYME HYPOTHESIS

Concept	Example	Disease Caused by Genetic Defect
One gene/one enzyme	Glucose-6-phophatase	Hypoglycemia; hepatomegaly
One gene/one nonenzymatic protein	Fibrillin FBN1	Marfan syndrome
One gene/one RNA product	Mitochondrial tRNA	Maternally inherited myopathy and hypertrophic cardiomyopathy
One functional enzyme requires multiple subunits from separate genes	Hexosaminidase	Tay-Sachs disease
One polypeptide has multiple enzymatic activities	Orotate phosphoribosyl transferase and orotidine-5'-phosphate decarboxylase	Orotic aciduria
One polypeptide is a component of multiple enzymes	β-Subunit of hexosaminidase A and B	Sandoff disease
One polypeptide is a component of multiple nonenzymatic proteins	γ-Chain of IL-2, IL-4, IL-7, IL-11, IL-15 receptors	X-linked severe combined immunodeficiency syndrome
Deficiency of one enzyme causes multiple secondary enzyme deficiencies	UDP-N-acetylglucosamine (GlcNAc)-1- phosphotransferase	Mucolipidosis II (I-cell disease)
One transcript encoding a single polypeptide produces multiple protein products via post-translational cleavage	ACTH (adrenocorticotrophic hormone) and endorphins	
One multigenic transcript is subsequently cleaved to give rise to mature mRNAs encoding different proteins	Mitochondrial P_H and P_L transcripts	
One transcript encodes multiple RNA products	18S, 5.8S, and 28S rRNA	
One transcript undergoes alternative splicing to produce different isoforms of the same protein	Production of both IgM and IgD by immature B cells	
One transcript undergoes alternative splicing to produce two unrelated mature proteins	Calcitonin gene alternatively spliced to produce calcitonin in the thyroid, CGRP in neural tissue	
Alternative promoters used for transcription of the same gene	Dystrophin	Duchenne muscular dystrophy
Alternative polyadenylation sites for the same transcript	Cyclin D1	
Post-transcriptional editing of mRNA	Apolipoproteins B100 and B48	Hypobetalipoproteinemia
DNA rearrangements before transcription	Immunoglobulins, T-cell receptors	Agammaglobulinemia combined immunodeficiency
Overlapping genes	Mitochondrial genes for ATPase subunits 6 and 8 (translated in different reading frames)	
Same disease caused by mutations in different genes (locus heterogeneity)	RET, NTRK1, and BRAF	Papillary thyroid carcinoma
Different mutations in the same gene result in a spectrum		
Of disease severity	CFTR	Ranging from classic cystic fibrosis, to sinusitis with congenital absence of the vas deferens, to normal females
Of related diseases	COL2A1	Stickler syndrome/Kniest dysplasia/spondyloepiphyseal dysplasia
Of different diseases	RET	MEN2A/MEN2B/Hirschsprung disease
Mutations leading to the deficiency of a protein are not in the structural gene-encoding the protein	Tyrosine kinase Btk	X-linked (Bruton) hypogammaglobulinemia

provides the reason for the nonmendelian pattern of inheritance that is a feature of diseases resulting from mitochondria mutations.

The high rate of mtDNA mutation, coupled with the presence of thousands of mtDNA molecules in each cell, means that cells and tissues generally harbor both wild-type and mutant genomes, known as heteroplasmy (note that heteroplasmy can also exist at the organellar level when a single mitochondrion harbors both wild-type and mutant mtDNA molecules). Because a minimal number of mutant mtDNAs must be present before a level of organellar dysfunction occurs that causes clinical disease, a threshold effect characterizes many mitochondrial diseases, especially respiratory chain disorders; the threshold is lower in tissues highly dependent on oxidative metabolism, such as brain, heart, skeletal muscle, renal tubules, retina, and endocrine glands (252). Random distribution of mitochondria during cell division can change the proportion of wild-type and mutant mtDNA within the daughter cells, and so the pathogenic threshold in a previously unaffected tissue can potentially be surpassed with time. This mechanism explains the tissue-related and age-related variability that are also characteristic clinical features of mtDNA-related diseases (252). Taken together, the unique features of the molecular biology of mitochondria help explain why there are so many human diseases with such protean features resulting from mutations in mtDNA (Table 1.10), and why it can be so difficult to characterize pathogenic mtDNA mutations (253).

CONCLUSION

As shown in Table 1.11, a more detailed understanding of gene structure, regulation of gene activation and transcription, RNA processing, post-translation protein modifications, and protein trafficking has challenged the classical one gene–one enzyme hypothesis and required modification of the classical definition of a gene. The significance of this complexity, from the perspective of human disease, is that the relationship between the DNA sequence of a gene and the structure of the encoded mature protein is often quite complicated, and the relationship between a specific mutation (genotype) and the manifestation of the genetic abnormality (phenotype) is often far from obvious. Consequently, the clinical features of a disease may provide little insight into the underlying genetic mechanism and, conversely, the mechanism by which a mutation causes a specific disease may not be intuitively obvious. Application of molecular genetic testing to the study of human disease in clinical practice therefore requires a broad perspective and an open mind if specific genetic defects are to be correctly correlated with individual diseases.

REFERENCES

1. Watson JD, Baker TA, Bell SP, et al. eds. *Molecular Biology of the Gene*, 5th ed. Redwood City, CA: Benjamin Cummings Publishing Co., Inc., 2003.
2. Lewin B, ed. *Genes VIII*. Oxford, UK: Oxford University Press, 2003.
3. Strachan T, Read AP, eds. *Human Molecular Genetics*, 3rd ed. London: Garland Science Publishers, 2004.
4. Epstein RJ, ed. *An Introduction to the Molecular Basis of Health and Disease*. Cambridge, UK: Cambridge University Press, 2003.
5. Watson JD, Crick FH. Molecular structure of nucleic acids: a structure for deoxyribose nucleic acid. *Nature* 1953;171:737–738.
6. Herbert A, Rich A. The biology of left-handed Z-DNA. *J Biol Chem* 1996; 271:11595–11598.
7. Rothenburg S, Koch-Nolte F, Haag F. DNA methylation and Z-DNA formatin as mediators of quantitative differences in the expression of alleles. *Immunol Rev* 2001; 184:286–298.
8. Gagna CE, Kuo H, Lambert WC. Terminal differentiation and left-handed ZDNA: a review. *Cell Biol Int* 1999;23:1–5.
9. Richmond TJ, Davey CA. The structure of DNA in the nucleosome core. *Nature* 2003;423:145–150.
10. Narlikar GJ, Fan HY, Kingston RE. Cooperation between complexes that regulate chromatin structure and transcription. *Cell* 2002;108:475–487.
11. Grewal SI, Elgin SC. Heterochromatin: new possibilities for the inheritance of structure. *Curr Opin Genet Dev* 2002;12:178–187.
12. Berger SL. Histone modifications in transcriptional regulation: histone modifications in transcriptional regulation. *Curr Opin Genet Dev* 2002;12:142–148.
13. Plath K, Fang J, Mlynarczyk-Evans SK, et al. Role of histone H3 lysine 27 methylation in X inactivation. *Science* 2003;300:131–135.
14. Ng HH, Bird A. DNA methylation and chromatin modification. *Curr Opin Genet Dev* 1999;9:158–163.
15. Jones PL, Wolffe AP. Relationships between chromatin organization and DNA methylation in determining gene expression. *Cancer Biol* 1999;9:339–347.
16. Berger SL. Histone modifications in transcriptional regulation. *Curr Opin Genet Dev* 2002;12:142–148.
17. Garcia-Cao M, O'Sullivan R, Peters AH, et al. Epigenetic regulation of telomere length in mammalian cells by the Suv39h1 and Suv39h2 histone methyltransferases. *Nat Genet* 2004;36:94–99.
18. Maile T, Kwoczynski S, Katzenberger RJ, et al. TAF1 activates transcription by phosphorylation of serine 33 in histone H2B. *Science* 2004;304:1010–1014.
19. Downs JA, Jackson SP. Cancer: protective packaging for DNA. *Nature* 2003; 424:732–734.
20. Milne TA, Briggs SD, Brock HW, et al. MLL targets SET domain methyltransferase activity to *Hox* gene promoters. *Mol Cell* 2002;10:1107–1117.
21. Fu XH, Liu DP, Liang CC. Chromatin structure and transcriptional regulation of the beta-globin locus. *Exper Cell Res* 2002;278:1–11.
22. Kouzarides T. Histone methylation in transcriptional control. *Curr Opin Genet Dev* 2002;12:198–209.
23. Roux-Rouquie M, Chauvet ML, Munnich A, et al. Human genes involved in chromatin remodeling in transcription initiation, and associated diseases: an overview using the GENATLAS database. *Mol Genet Metab* 1999;67:261–277.
24. Lehrmann H, Pritchard LL, Harel-Bellan A. Histone acetyltransferases and deacetylases in the control of cell proliferation and differentiation. *Adv Cancer Res* 2002;86:41–65.
25. Jaenisch R, Bird A. Epigenetic regulation of gene expression: how the genome integrates intrinsic and environmental signals. *Nat Genet* 2003;33:245–254.
26. Geiman TM, Robertson KD. Chromatin remodeling, histone modifications, and DNA methylation: how does it all fit together? *J Cell Biochem* 2002;87:117–125.
27. Balmer D, Arredondo J, Samaco RC, et al. MECP2 mutations in Rett syndrome adversely affect lymphocyte growth, but do not affect imprinted gene expression in blood or brain. *Hum Genet* 2002;110:545–552.
28. Feinberg AP, Tycko B. The history of cancer epigenetics. *Nat Rev Cancer* 2004; 4:143–153.
29. Tong WM, Cortes U, Wang ZQ. Poly(ADP-ribose) polymerase: a guardian angel protecting the genome and suppressing tumorigenesis. *Biochim Biophys Acta* 2001;1552:27–37.
30. Kraus WL, Lis JT. PARP goes transcription. *Cell* 2003;113:677–683.
31. Wang Y, Wysocka J, Sayegh J, et al. Human PAD4 regulates histone arginine methylation levels via demethylimination. *Science* 2004;306:279–283.
32. Agalioti T, Chen G, Thanos D. Deciphering the transcriptional histone acetylation code for a human gene. *Cell* 2002;111:381–392.
33. Lomvardas S, Thanos D. Nucleosome sliding via TBP DNA binding in vivo. *Cell* 2001;106:685–696.
34. Svejstrup JQ. Transcription: histones face the FACT. *Science* 2003;301:1053–1055.
35. Owen-Hughes T, Bruno M. Molecular biology: breaking the silence. *Science* 2004;303:324–325.
36. Falls JG, Pulford DJ, Wylie AA. Genomic imprinting: implications for human disease. *Am J Pathol* 1999;154:635–647.
37. Kono T, Obata Y, Wu Q, et al. Birth of parthenogenetic mice that can develop to adulthood. *Nature* 2004;428:860–864.
38. Kaneda M, Okano M, Hata K, et al. Essential role for de novo DNA methyltransferase Dnmt3a in paternal and maternal imprinting. *Nature* 2004;429:900–903.
39. Paulsen M, Ferguson-Smith AC. DNA methylation in genomic imprinting, development, and disease. *J Pathol* 2001;195:97–110.
40. Park KY, Pfeifer K. Epigenetic interplay. *Nat Genet* 2003;34:126–128.
41. Paulsen M, Ferguson-Smith AC. DNA methylation in genomic imprinting, development, and disease. *Pathology* 2001;195:97–110.
42. Boyes J, Bird A. DNA methylation inhibits transcription indirectly via a methyl-CpG binding protein. *Cell* 1991;64:1123–1134.
43. Widschwendter M, Jones PA. The potential prognostic, predictive, and therapeutic values of DNA methylation in cancer. *Clin Cancer Res* 2002;8:17–21.
44. Kwong J, Lo KW, To KF, et al. Promoter hypermethylation of multiple genes in nasopharyngeal carcinoma. *Clin Cancer Res* 2002;8:131–137.
45. Gaudet F, Hodgson JG, Eden A, et al. Induction of tumors in mice by genomic hypomethylation. *Science* 2003;300:489–492.
46. Lengauer C. Cancer: an unstable liaison. *Science* 2003;300:442–443.
47. Hanahan D, Weinberg RA. The hallmarks of cancer. *Cell* 2000;7:57–70.
48. Eden A, Gaudet F, Waghmare A, et al. Chromosomal instability and tumors promoted by DNA hypomethylation. *Science* 2003;300:455.
49. Herman JG, Baylin SB. Gene silencing in cancer in association with promoter hypermethylation. *N Engl J Med* 2003;349:2042–2054.

50. Esteller M, Garcia-Foncillas J, Andion E, et al. Inactivation of the DNA-repair gene MGMT and the clinical response of gliomas to alkylating agents. *Engl J Med* 2000; 343:1350–1354.

51. Hansen RS, Wijmenga C, Luo P, et al. The DNMT3B DNA methyltransferase gene is mutated in the ICF immunodeficiency syndrome. *Proc Natl Acad Sci USA* 1999; 96:14412–14417.

52. Bienvenu T, Carrie A, de Roux N, et al. MECP2 mutations account for most cases of typical forms of Rett syndrome. *Hum Mol Genet* 2000;9:1377–1384.

53. Amir RE, Van den Veyver IB, Wan M, et al. Rett syndrome is caused by mutations in X-linked MECP2, encoding methyl-CpG-binding protein 2. *Nat Genet* 1999;23:185–188.

54. Gibbons RJ, McDowell TL, Raman S, et al. Mutations in changes in the pattern of DNA methylation. *Nature Genet* 2000;24:368–371.

55. Morison IM, Reeve AE. A catalogue of imprinted genes and parent-of-origin effects in humans and animals. *Hum Mol Genet* 1998;7:1599–1609.

56. http://www.geneimprint.com.

57. http://www.cancer.otago.ac.nz/IGC/Web/home.html.

58. Falls JG, Pulford DJ, Wylie AA, et al. Genomic imprinting: implications for human disease. *Am J Pathol* 1999;154:635–647.

59. Goffin J, Eisenhauer E. DNA methyltransferase inhibitors-state of the art. *Ann Oncol* 2002;13:1699–1716.

60. Tyler-Smith C, Willard HF. Mammalian chromosome structure. *Curr Opin Genet Dev* 1993;3:390–397.

61. Lee C, Wevrick R, Fisher RM, et al. Human centromeric DNAs. *Hum Genet* 1997;100:291–304.

62. Lander ES, Linton LM, Birren B, et al. Initial sequencing and analysis of the human genome. *Nature* 2001;409:860–921.

63. Eichler EE, Archidiacono N, Rocchi M. CAGGG repeats and the pericentromeric duplication of the hominoid genome. *Genome Res* 1999;9:1048–1058.

64. Horvath JE, Schwartz S, Eichler EE. The mosaic structure of human pericentromeric DNA: a strategy for characterizing complex regions of the human genome. *Genome Res* 2000;10:839–852.

65. Horvath JE, Viggiano L, Loftus BJ, et al. Molecular structure and evolution of an alpha satellite/non-alpha satellite junction at 16p11. *Hum Mol Genet* 2000;9:113–123.

66. Schueler MG, Higgins AW, Rudd MK, et al. Genomic and genetic definition of a functional human centromere. *Science* 2001;294:109–115.

67. Ugarkovic D, Plohl M. Variation in satellite DNA profiles: causes and effects. *EMBO J* 2002;21:5955–5959.

68. International Human Genome Sequencing Consortium. Finishing the euchromatic sequence of the human genome. *Nature* 2004;431:931–945.

69. Martin J, Han C, Gordon LA, et al. The sequence and analysis of duplication-rich human chromosome 16. *Nature* 2004;432:988–994.

70. Larin Z, Mejia JE. Advances in human artificial chromosome technology. *Trends Genet* 2002;18:313–319.

71. Grimes B, Cooke H. Engineering mammalian chromosomes. *Hum Mol Genet* 1998;7:1635–1640.

72. Kouprina N, Ebersole T, Koriabine M, et al. Cloning of human centromeres by transformation-associated recombination in yeast and generation of functional human artificial chromosomes. *Nucleic Acids Res* 2003;31:922–934.

73. Koch J. Neocentromeres and alpha satellite: a proposed structural code for functional human centromere DNA. *Hum Mol Genet* 2000;9:149–154.

74. Lamb JC, Birchler JA. The role of DNA sequence in centromere formation. *Genome Biol* 2003;4:214.

75. Lo AW, Craig JM, Saffery R, et al. A 330 kb CENP-A binding domain and altered replication timing at a human neocentromere. *EMBO J* 2001;20:2087–2096.

76. Lo AW, Magliano DJ, Sibson MC, et al. A novel chromatin immunoprecipitation and array (CIA) analysis identifies a 460-kb CENP-A-binding neocentromere DNA. *Genome Res* 2001;11:448–457.

77. Sullivan BA, Blower MD, Karpen GH. Determining centromere identity: cyclical stories and forking paths. *Nat Rev Genet* 2001;2:584–596.

78. Warburton PE, Dolled M, Mahmood R, et al. Molecular cytogenetic analysis of eight inversion duplications of human chromosome 13q that each contain a neocentromere. *Am J Hum Gen* 2000;66:1794–1806.

79. Willard HF. Centromeres: the missing link in the development of human artificial chromosomes. *Curr Opin Genet Dev* 1998;8:219–225.

80. Murphy TD, Karpen GH. Centromeres take flight: alpha satellite and the quest for the human centromere. *Cell* 1998;93:317–320.

81. Amor DJ, Choo KHA. Neocentromeres: role in human disease, evolution, and centromere study. *Am J Hum Pathol* 2002;71:695–714.

82. Hattori M, Fujiyama A, Taylor TD. The DNA sequence of human chromosome 21. *Nature* 2000;405:311–319.

83. Cong Y, Wright WE, Shay JW. Human telomerase and its regulation. *Microbiol Mol Biol Rev* 2002;66:407–425.

84. Griffith JD, Comeau L, Rosenfield S, et al. Mammalian telomeres end in a large duplex loop. *Cell* 1999;97:503–514.

85. Aisner DL, Wright WE, Shay JW. Telomerase regulation: not just flipping the switch. *Curr Opin Genet Dev* 2002;12:80–85.

86. Loayza D, de Lange T. POT1 as a terminal transducer of TRF1 telomere length control. *Nature* 2003;424:1013–1018.

87. Colgin LM, Baran K, Baumann P, et al. Human POT1 facilitates telomere elongation by telomerase. *Curr Biol* 2003;13:942–946.

88. Tang SJ, Dumot JA, Wang L, et al. Telomerase activity in pancreatic endocrine tumors. *Am J Gastroenterol* 2002;4:1022–1030.

89. Artandi SE, Depinho RA. Mice without telomerase: what can they teach us about human cancer? *Nat Med* 2000;6:852–855.

90. Soria JC, Viehl P, El-Naggar A. Telomerase activity in cancer: a magic bullet or a mirage? *Adv Anat Pathol* 1998;5:86–94.

91. Lee BK, Diebel E, Neukam FW, et al. Diagnostic and prognostic relevance of expression of human telomerase subunits in oral cancer. *Int J Oncol* 2001;19:1063–1068.

92. Kumaki F, Kawai T, Hiroi S, et al. Telomerase activity and expression of human telomerase RNA component and human telomerase reverse transcriptase in lung carcinomas. *Hum Pathol* 2001;32:188–195.

93. Niiyama H, Mizumoto K, Sato N, et al. Quantitative analysis of hTERT mRNA expression in colorectal cancer. *Am J Gastroenterol* 2001;96:1896–1900.

94. Shay JW, Wright WE. Telomerase activity in human cancer. *Curr Opin Oncol* 1996;8:66–71.

95. Ince TA, Crum CP. Telomerase: promise and challenge. *Hum Pathol* 2004;35:393–395.

96. Alberts B. DNA replication and recombination. *Nature* 2003;421:431–435.

97. Lei M, Tye BK. Initiating DNA synthesis: from recruiting to activating the MCM complex. *J Cell Sci* 2001;114:1447–1454.

98. Takisawa H, Mimura S, Kubota Y. Eukaryotic DNA replication: from pre-replication complex to initiation complex. *Curr Opin Cell Biol* 2000;12:690–696.

99. Li X, Rosenfeld MG. Transcription: origins of licensing control. *Nature* 2004; 427:687–688.

100. Bielinsky AK, Gerbi SA. Where it all starts: eukaryotic origins of DNA replication. *J Cell Sci* 2001;114:643–651.

101. Blow JJ, Hodgson B. Replication licensing: defining the proliferative state? *Trends Cell Biol* 2002;12:72–78.

102. Mechali M. *DNA replication origins: from sequence specificity to epigenetics*. Macmillan Magazines, Ltd. 2001.

103. Gilbert DM. Making sense of eukaryotic DNA replication origins. *Science* 2001;294:96–100.

104. Gerbi SA, Bielinsky AK. DNA replication and chromatin. *Curr Opin Genet Dev* 2002;12:243–248.

105. Hobscher U, Maga G, Spadari S. Eukaryotic DNA polymerases. *Annu Rev Biochem* 2002;71:133–163.

106. http://www.hgmp.mrc.ac.uk/GenomeWeb/nuc-repeats.html.

107. http://www.girinst.org.

108. Glazko GV, Koonin EV, Rogozin IB, et al. A significant fraction of conserved noncoding DNA in human and mouse consists of predicted matrix attachment regions. *Trends Genet* 2003;19:119–124.

109. Gondo Y, Okada T, Matsuyama N, et al. Human megasatellite DNA RS447: copy-number polymorphisms and interspecies conservation. *Genomics* 1998;54:39–49.

110. Swallow DM, Gendler S, Griffiths B, et al. The human tumour-associated epithelial mucins are coded by an expressed hypervariable gene locus PUM. *Nature* 1987;328:82–84.

111. Li YC, Korol AB, Fahima, et al. Microsatellites: genomic distribution, putative functions and mutational mechanisms—a review. *Mol Ecol* 2002;11:2453–2465.

112. Smit AFA. The origin of interspersed repeats in the human genome. *Curr Opin Genet Dev* 1996;6:743–748.

113. Smit A, Riggs AD. *Tiggers* and other DNA transposon fossils in the human genome. *Proc Natl Acad Sci USA* 1993;93:1443–1448.

114. Rowold DJ, Herrera RJ. *Alu* elements and the human genome. *Genetica* 2000; 108:57–72.

115. Weiner AM. SINEs and LINEs: the art of biting the hand that feeds you. *Curr Opin Cell Biol* 2002;14:343–350.

116. Sassaman DM, Dombroski BA, Moran JV, et al. Many human L1 elements are capable of retrotransposition. *Nat Genet* 1997;16:37–43.

117. Kazazian HH, Moran JV. The impact of L1 retrotransposons on the human genome. *Nat Genet* 1998;19:19–24.

118. Dewannieux M, Esnault C, Heidmann T. LINE-mediated retrotransposition of marked Alu sequences. *Nat Genet* 2003;35:41–48.

119. Meischl BB, Ostertag C, deBoer E, et al. Evidence consistent with human L1 retrotransposition in maternal meiosis I. *Am J Hum Gen* 2002;71:327–336.

120. Van de Water N, Williams R, Ockelford P, et al. A 20.7 kb deletion within the factor VIII gene associated with LINE-1 element insertion. *Thromb Haemost* 1998;79:938–942.

121. Li X Scaringe WA, Hill KA, Roberts S, et al. Frequency of recent retrotransposition events in the human factor IX gene. *Hum Mutat* 2001;175:511–519.

122. Ostertag EM, Kazazian HH Jr. Biology of mammalian L1 retrotransposons. *Annu Rev Genet* 2001;35:501–538.

123. Lagrange T, Kapanidis AN, Tang H, et al. New core promoter element in RNA polymerase II-dependent transcription: sequence-specific DNA binding by transcription factor IIB. *Genes Dev* 1998;12:34–44.

124. Javahery R, Khachi A, Lo K, et al. DNA sequence requirements for transcriptional initiator activity in mammalian cells. *Mol Cell Biol* 1994;14:116–127.

125. Burke TW, Kadonaga JT. The downstream core promoter element, DPE, is conserved from *Drosophila* to humans and is recognized by TAFII60 of *Drosophila. Genes Dev* 1997;11:3020–3031.

126. Nikolov DB, Burley SK. RNA polymerase II transcription initiation: a structural view. *Proc Natl Acad Sci USA* 1997;94:15–22.

127. Cosma MP. Ordered recruitment: gene-specific mechanism of transcription activation. *Mol Cell* 2002;10:227–236.

128. Ellenberger T, Fass MA, Harrison S. Crystal structure of transcription factor E47: e-box recognition by a basic regin helix-loop-helix dimmer. *Genes Dev* 1994;8:970–980.

129. Clark KL, Halay ED, Lei E, et al. Co-crystal structure of the HNF-3/fork head DNA-recognition motif resembles histone H5. *Nature* 1993;364:412–420.

130. Newman JR, Keating AE. Comprehensive identification of human bZIP interactions with coiled-coil arrays. *Science* 2003;300:2097–2101.

131. Vinson C, Myakishev M, Acharya A, et al. Classification of human B-ZIP proteins based on dimerization properties. *Mol Cell Biol* 2002;22:6321–6335.

132. Massari ME, Murre C. Helix-loop-helix proteins: regulators of transcription in eucaryotic organisms. *Mol Cell Biol* 2000;20:429–440.

133. Carlsson P, Mahlapuu M. Forkhead transcription factors: key players in development and metabolism. *Dev Biol* 2002;250:1–23.

134. Warren AJ. Eukaryotic transcription factors. *Curr Opin Struct Biol* 2002;12:107–114.

135. Klinge CM. Estrogen receptor interaction with estrogen response elements. *Nucleic Acids Res* 2001;29:2905–2919.

136. Merika M, Thanos D. Enhanceosomes. *Curr Opin Genet Dev* 2001;11:205–208.

137. Dhillon N, Kamakaka RT. Breaking through to the other side: silencers and barriers. *Curr Opin Genet Dev* 2002;13:188–192.

138. Frenkel S, Mijnes J, Aronow MA, et al. Position and orientation-slective silencer in protein-coding sequences of the rat osteocalcin gene. *Biochemistry* 1993;32:13636–13643.

139. Ogbourne S, Antalis TM. Transcriptional control and the role of silencers in transcriptional regulation in eukaryotes. *Biochem J* 1998;3331:1–14.

140. Geyer PK. The role of insulator elements in defining domains of gene expression. *Curr Opin Genet Dev* 1997;7:242–248.
141. Labrador M, Corces VG. Setting the boundaries of chromatin domains and nuclear organizaton. *Cell* 2002;111:151–154.
142. Novina CD, Sharp PA. The RNAi revolution. *Nature* 2004;430:161–164.
143. Tijsterman M, Ketting RF, Plasterk RH. The genetics of RNA silencing. *Annu Rev Genet* 2002;36:489–519.
144. Bartel DP. MicroRNAs: genomics, biogenesis, mechanism, and function. *Cell* 2004;116:281–297.
145. Stevenson M. Therapeutic potential of RNA interference. *N Engl J Med* 2004; 351:1772–1777.
146. Song E, Lee SK, Wang J, et al. RNA interference targeting Fas protects mice from fulminant hepatitis. *Nat Med* 2003;9:347–351.
147. Zhang W, Yang H, Kong X, et al. Inhibition of respiratory syncytial virus infection with intranasal siRNA nanoparticles targeting the viral NS1 gene. *Nat Med* 2005;11:56–62.
148. Bitko V, Musityenko A, Shulyayeva O, et al. Inhibition of respiratory viruses by nasally administered siRNA. *Nat Med* 2005;11:50–55.
149. Morris KV, Chan SW, Jacobsen SE, et al. Small interfering RNA-induced transcriptional gene silencing in human cells. *Science* 2004;305:1289–1292.
150. Kawasaki H, Taira K. Induction of DNA methylation and gene silencing by short interfering RNAs in human cells. *Nature* 2004;431:211–217.
151. Chen CZ, Li L, Lodish HF, et al. MicroRNAs modulate hematopoietic lineage differentiation. *Science* 2004;303:83–86.
152. Lim LP, Glasner ME, Yekta S, et al. Vertebrate microRNA genes. *Science* 2003;299:1540.
153. Griffiths-Jones S. The microRNA Registry. *Nucleic Acids Res* 2004;32:D109–D111.
154. Kuwabara T, Hsieh J, Nakashima K, et al. A small modulatory dsRNA specifies the fate of adult neural stem cells. *Cell* 2004;116:779–793.
155. Conaway JW, Conaway RC. Transcription elongation and human disease. *Annu Rev Biochem* 1999;68:301–319.
156. Taube R, Lin X, Irwin D, et al. Interaction between P-TEFb and the C-Terminal domian of RNA polymerase II activates transcriptional elongation from sites upstream or downstream of target genes. *Mol Cell Biol* 2002;22:321–331.
157. Shilatifard A. Factors regulating the transcriptional elongation activity of RNA polymerase II. *FASEB* J. 1998;12:1437–1446.
158. Garber ME, Jones KA. HIV-1 Tat: coping with negative elongation factors. *Curr Opin Immunol* 1999;11:460–465.
159. Kamura T, Brower CS, Conaway RC. A molecular basis for stablization of the von Hippel-Landau (VHL) tumor suppressor protein by components of the VHL ubiquitin ligase. *J Biol Chem* 2002;277:30388–30393.
160. Latif F, Tory K, Gnarra J, et al. Identification of the von Hippel-Lindau disease tumor suppressor gene. *Science* 1993;260:1317–1320.
161. Sheth U, Parker R. Decapping and decay of messenger RNA occur in cytoplasmic processing bodies. *Science* 2003;300:805–808.
162. Edwalds-Gilbert G, Veraldi KL, Milcarek C. Alternative poly(A) site selection in complex transcription units: means to an end? *Nucleic Acids Res* 1997;25:2547–2561.
163. Conne B, Stutz A, Vassali J. The 3' untranslated region of messenger RNA: a molecular 'hotspot' for pathology? *Nat Med* 2000;6:637–641.
164. Maquat LE. The power of point mutations. *Nat Genet* 2001;27:5–6.
165. Liu HX, Cartegni L, Zhang MQ, et al. A mechanism for exon skipping caused by nonsense or missense mutations in *BRCA1* and other genes. *Nat Genet* 2001;27:55–58.
166. Fairbrother WG, Chasin LA. Human genomic sequences that inhibit splicing. *Mol Cell Biol* 2000;20:6816–6825.
167. Guil S, Darzynkiewicz E, Bach-Elias M. Study of the 2719 mutant of the c-H-*ras* oncogene in a bi-intronic alternative splicing system. *Oncogene* 2002;21:5649–5653.
168. Fairbrother WG, Yeh RF, Sharp PA, et al. Predicitive identification of exonic splicing enhancers in human genes. *Science* 2002;297:1007–1013.
169. Smith PJ, Spurrell EL, Coakley J, et al. An exonic splicing enhancer in human IGF-I pre-mRNA mediates recognition of alternative exon 5 by the serine-arginine protein splicing factor-2/alternative splicing factor. *Endocrinology* 2002;143:146–154.
170. Woerfel G, Bindereif A. *In vitro* selection of exonic splicing enhancer sequences: identification of novel CD44 enhancers. *Nucleic Acids Res* 2001;29:3204–3211.
171. Hastings ML, Ingle HA, Lazar MA, et al. Post-transcriptional regulation of thyroid hormone receptor expression by cis-acting sequences and a naturally occurring antisense RNA. *J Biol Chem* 2000;275:11507–11513.
172. Kan JL, Green MR. Pre-mRNA splicing of IgM exons M1 and M2 is directed by a juxtaposed splicing enhancer and inhibitor. *Genes Dev* 1999;13:462–471.
173. Krawczak M, Reiss J, Cooper D. The mutational spectrum of single base-pair substitutions in mRNA splice junctions of human genes: causes and consequences. *Hum Genet* 1992;90:41–54.
174. Liu HX, Cartegni L, Zhang MQ, et al. A mechanism for exon skipping caused by nonsense of missense mutations in *BRCA1* and other genes. *Nat Genet* 2001;27:55–58.
175. Mendell JT, Dietz HC. When the message goes awry: disease-producing mutations that influence mRNA content and performance. *Cell* 2001;107:411–414.
176. Cartegni L, Chew SL, Krainer AR. Listening to silence and understanding nonsense: exonic mutatins that affect splicing. *Nat Rev Genet* 2002;3:285–298.
177. Carteni L, Krainer AR. Disruption of an SF2/ASF-dependent exonic splicing enhancer in SMN2 causes spinal muscular atrophy in the absence of SMN1. *Nat Genet* 2002;30:377–384.
178. Kashima T, Manley JL. A negative element in SMN2 exon 7 inhibits splicing in spinal muscular atrophy. *Nat Genet* 2003;34:460–463.
179. Ladd AN, Cooper TA. Finding signals that regulate alternative splicing in the post-genomic era. *Genome Biol* 2002;3:0008.1–0008.4.
180. Cáceres JF, Kornblihtt AR. Alternative splicing: multiple control mechanisms and involvement in human disease. *Trends Genet* 2002;18:186–193.
181. Yudt MR, Cidlowski JA. The glucocorticoid receptor: coding a diversity of proteins and responses through a single gene. *Mol Endocrinol* 2002;16:1719–1726.
182. Jensen K, Shiels C, Freemont PS. PML protein isoforms and the RBCC/TRIM motif. *Oncogene* 2001;20:7223–7233.
183. Kuo BA, Uporova TM, Liang H, et al. Alternative splicing during chondrogenesis: modulation of fibronectin exon EIIIA splicing by SR proteins. *J Cell Biochem* 2002;86:45–55.
184. Lopez AJ. Alternative splicing of PRE-mRNA: developmental consequences and mechanisms of regulation. *Annu Rev Genet* 1998;32:279–305.
185. Cooper TA, Mattox W. The regulation of splice-site section, and its role in human disease. *Am J Hum Gen* 1997;61:259–266.
186. Pekhletsky RI, Chernov BK, Rubtsov PM. Variants of the 5'-untranslated sequence of human growth hormone receptor mRNA. *Mol Cell Endocrinol* 1992;90:103–109.
187. Zhu J, Shendure J, Mitra RD, et al. Single molecule profiling of alternative pre-mRNA splicing. *Science* 2003;301:836–838.
188. Matsumoto S, Katoh M, Saito S, et al. Identification of solumble type of membrane-type matrix metalloproteinase-3 formed by alternatively spliced mRNA. *Biochim Biophys Acta* 1997;1354:159–170.
189. Liu Y, Bernard HU, Apt D. NFI-B3, a novel transcriptional repressor of the nuclear factor I family, is generated by alternative RNA processing. *J Biol Chem* 1997; 272:10739–10745.
190. Boise LH, Gonzalez-Garcia M, Posterma CE, et al. bcl-x, a bcl-2-related gene that functions as a dominant regulator of apoptotic cell death. *Cell* 1993;74:597–608.
191. Caceres JF, Kornblihtt AR. Alternative splicing: multiple control mechanisms and involvement in human disease. *Trends Genet* 2002;18:186–193.
192. Simpson L, Thiemann OH. Sense from nonsense: RNA editing in mitochondria of kinetoplastid protozoa and slime molds. *Cell* 1995;81:837–840.
193. Higuchi M, Maas S, Single FN, et al. Point mutation in an AMPA receptor gene rescues leathality in mice deficient in the RNA-editing enzyme ADAR2. *Nature* 2000;406:78–81.
194. Gerber AP, Keller W. RNA editing by base deamination: more enzymes, more targets, new mysteries. *Trends Biochem Sci* 2001;26:376–384.
195. Scott J. A place in the world for RNA editing. *Cell* 1995;81:833–836.
196. Melcher T, Maas S, Herb A, et al. A mammalian RNA editing enzyme. *Nature* 1996;379:460–464.
197. Bass BL. RNA editing by adenosine deaminases that act on RNA. *Annu Rev Biochem* 2002;71:817–846.
198. Novo FJ, Kruszewski A, MacDermot KD, et al. Editing of human alpha-galactosidase RNA resulting in a pyrimidine to purine conversion. *Nucleic Acids Res* 1995;23:2636–2640.
199. Blom D, Speijer D, Linthorst GE, et al. Recombinant enzyme therapy for Fabry disease: absence of editing of human alpha-galactosidase A mRNA. *Am J Hum Genet* 2003;72:23–31.
200. Hoopengardner B, Bhalla T, Staber C, et al. Nervous system targets of RNA editing identified by comparative genomics. *Science* 2003;301:832–836.
201. Skuse GR, Cappione AJ, Sowden M, et al. The neurofibromatosis type I messenger RNA undergoes base-modification RNA edition. *Nucleic Acids Res* 1996;24:478–486.
202. Tanoue A, Koshimizu T, Tsuchiya M, et al. Two novel transcripts for human endothelin B receptor produced by RNA editing/alternative splicing from a single gene. *J Biol Chem* 2002;277:33205–33212.
203. Powell LM, Wallis SC, Pease RJ, et al. A novel form of tissue-specific RNA processing produces apolipoprotein-B48 in intestine. *Cell* 1987:50:831–84.
204. Cappione AJ, French BL, Skuse GR. A potential role for NF1 mRNA editing in the pathogenesis of NF1 tumors. *Am J Hum Genet* 1997;60:305–312.
205. Mrowka C, Schedl A. Wilms' tumor suppressor gene WT1: from structure to renal pathophysiologic features. *J Am Soc Nephrol* 2000;11:S106–S115.
206. Sharma PM, Bowman M, Madden SL, et al. RNA editing in the Wilms' tumor susceptibility gene, WT1. *Genes Dev* 1994;8:720–731.
207. Mangeat B, Turelli P, Caron G, et al. Broad antiretroviral defence by human APOBEC3G through lethal editing of nascent reverse transcripts. *Nature* 2003;424:99–103.
208. Zhang H, Yan B, Pomerantz RJ, et al. The cytidine deaminase CEM15 induces hypermutation in newly synthesized HIV-1 DNA. *Nature* 2003;424:94–98.
209. Dreyfuss G, Kim VN, Kataoka N. Messenger-RNA-binding proteins and the messages they carry. *Nat Rev Mol Cell Biol* 2002;3:195–205.
210. Reed R, Hurt E. A conserved mRNA export machinery coupled to pre-mRNA splicing. *Cell* 2002;108:523–531.
211. Derrigo M, Cestelli A, Savettierei G, et al. RNA-protein interactions in the control of stability and localization of messenger RNA. *Int J Mol Med* 2000;5:111–123.
212. Kozak M. An analysis of vertebrate mRNA sequences: intimations of translational control. *J Cell Biol* 1991;115:887–903.
213. Vagner S, Galy B, Pyronnet S. Irresistible IRES. *EMBO Rep* 2001;2:893–898.
214. Pestova TV, Kolupaeva VG, Lomakin IB, et al. Molecular mechanisms of translation initiation in eukaryotes. *Proc Natl Acad Sci USA* 2001;98:7029–7036.
215. Jang SK, Krausslich HG, Nicklin MJ, et al. A segment of the 5'-nontranslated regin of encephalomyocarditis vius RNA directs internal entry of ribosomes during *in vitro* translation. *J Virol* 1988;62:2636–2643.
216. Pelletier J, Sonenberg N. Internal initiation of translation of eukaryotic mRNA directed by a sequence derived from poliovirus RNA. *Nature* 1988;334:320–325.
217. Jubin R. Hepatitis C IRES: translating translation into a therapeutic target. *Curr Opin Mol Ther* 2001;3:278–287.
218. Lamphear BJ, Kirchweger R, Skern T, et al. Mapping of functional domains in eukaryotic protein synthesis initiation factor 4G (eIF4G) with picornaviral proteases: implications for cap-dependent and cap-independent translational initiation. *J Biol Chem* 1995;270:21975–21983.
219. Fredrick K, Noller HF. Catalysis of ribosomal translocation by sparsomycin. *Science* 2003;300:1159–1162.
220. Francklyn C, Perona JJ, Puetz J, et al. Aminoacyl-tRNA synthetases: versatile players in the changing theater of translation. *RNA* 2002;8:1363–1372.
221. Hatfield DL, Gladyshev VN. How selenium has altered our understanding of the genetic code. *Mol Cell Biol* 2002;22:3565–2576.
222. Kryukov GV, Castellano S, Novoselov SV, et al. Characterization of mammalian selenoproteomes. *Science* 2003;300:1439–1443.
223. Hazelrigg T. The destinies and destinations of RNAs. *Cell* 1998;95:451–460.
224. Dodson RE, Shapiro DJ. Regulation of pathways of mRNA destabilization and stabilization. *Prog Nucleic Acid Res Mol Biol* 2002;72:129:129–164.
225. Clark A. Post-transcriptional regulation of pro-inflammatory gene expression. *Arthr Res* 2000;2:172–174.
226. Wickens M, Bernstein DS, Kimble J, et al. A PUF family portrait: 3'UTR regulation as a way of life. *Trends Genet* 2002;18:150–157.

227. Kwon S, Barbarese E, Carson JH. The cis-acting RNA trafficking signal from myelin basic protein mRNA and its cognate trans-acting ligand hnRNP A2 enhance cap-dependent translation. *J Cell Biol* 1999;175:247–256.

228. Makeyev AV, Liebhaber SA. The poly(C)-binding proteins: a multiplicity of functions and a search for mechanisms. *RNA* 2002;8:265–278.

229. Wilusz CJ, Wormington M, Peltz SW. The cap-to-tail guide to mRNA turnover. *Nat Rev Mol Cell Biol* 2001;2:237–248.

230. Wickens M, Anderson P, Jackson RJ. Life and death in the cytoplasm: messages from the 3' end. *Curr Opin Genet Dev* 1997;7:220–232.

231. Vivinus S, Baulande S, Zanten M, et al. An element within the 5' untranslated region of human *Hsp70* mRNA translation. *Eur J Biochem* 2001;268:1908–1917.

232. Carson JH, Cui H, Barbarese E. The balance of power in RNA trafficking. *Curr Opin Neurobiol* 2001;11:558–563.

233. Ma ASW, Moran-Jones K, Shan J, et al. Heterogeneous nuclear ribonucleoprotein A3, a novel RNA trafficking response element-binding protein. *J Biol Chem* 2002;277:18010–18020.

234. Veyrune JL, Carillo S, Vie A, et al. c-fos mRNA instability determinants present within both the coding and the 3' non coding region link the degradation of this mRNA to its translation. *Oncogene* 1995;11:2127–2134.

235. Siomi H, Dreyfuss G. RNA-binding proteins as regulators of gene expression. *Curr Opin Genet Dev* 1997;7:345–353.

236. Mouland AJ, Xu H, Cui H, et al. RNA trafficking signals in human immunodeficiency virus type I. *Mol Cell Bio* 2001;21:2133–2143.

237. Stebbins-Boaz B, Richter, JD. Translational control during early development. *Crit Rev Eukaryot Gene Expr* 1997;7:73–94.

238. Schmitz JC, Liu J, Lin X, et al. Translational regulation as a novel mechanism for the development of cellular drug resistance. *Cancer Metastasis Rev* 2001;20:33–41.

239. Guhaniyogi J, Brewer G. Regulation of mRNA stability in mammalian cells. *Gene* 2001;265:11–23.

240. Klausner RD, Rouault TA, Harford JB. Regulating the fate of mRNA: the control of cellular iron metabolism. *Cell* 1993;72:19–28.

241. Wells L, Whelan SA, Hart GW. O-GlcNAc: a regulatory post-translational modification. *Biochem Biophys Res Commun* 2003;302:435–441.

242. Corda D, Di Girolamo M. Functional aspects of protein mono-ADP-ribosylation. *EMBO J* 2003;22:1953–1958.

243. Sato TK, Overduin M, Emr SD. Location, location, location: membrane targeting directed by PX domains. *Science* 2001;294:1881–1885.

244. Tekirian TL. The central role of the trans-Golgi network as a gateway of the early secretory pathoway: physiologic vs nonphysiologic protein transit. *Exper Cell Res* 2002;281:9–18.

245. Lalioti V, Vergarajauregui S, Sandoval IV. Targeting motifs in GLUT4. *Mol Membr Biol* 2001;18:257–264.

246. Hung AY, Sheng M. PDZ domains: structural modules for protein complex assembly. *J Biol Chem* 2002;277:5699–5702.

247. Kirchhausen T. Clathrin adaptors really adapt. *Cell* 2002;109:413–416.

248. Collawn JF, Stangel M, Kuhn LA, et al. Transferrin receptor internalization sequence YXRF implicates a tight turn as the structural recognition motif for endocytosis. *Cell* 1990;63:1061–1072.

249. Gabaldon T, Huynen MA. Reconstruction of the proto-mitochondrial metabolism. *Science* 2003;301:609.

250. Graff C, Clayton DA, Larsson NG. Mitochondrial medicine: recent advances. *J Intern Med* 1999;246:11–23.

251. Schwartz M, Vissing J. Paternal inheritance of mitochondrial DNA. *N Engl J Med* 2002;347:576–580.

252. DiMauro S, Schon EA. Mitochondrial respiratory-chain diseases. *N Engl J Med* 2003;348:2656–2668.

253. Moraes CT, Atencio DP, Oca-Cossio J, et al. Techniques and pitfalls in the detection of pathogenic mitochondrial DNA mutations. *J Mol Diagn* 2003;5:197–208.

DNA Damage, Mutations, and Repair

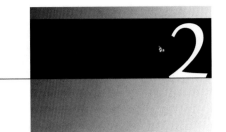

Constant and unavoidable sources of deoxyribonucleic acid (DNA) damage include spontaneous chemical changes, reactive oxygen species and other endogenous reactive metabolites, ionizing radiation, ultraviolet (UV) light, and genotoxic chemicals present in air and in food. Together, these agents cause a variety of DNA lesions ranging from abasic sites, to base adducts, to DNA strand breaks and crosslinks (1), and cells consequently contain a number of repair systems that correct these types of lesions to minimize the likelihood that the damage will cause a mutation.

However, some types of DNA alterations, such as insertions and deletions, duplications, inversions, and translocations are not the result of DNA damage but are instead the result of DNA polymerase errors, illegitimate recombination events, and unstable repeat sequences. These types of DNA alterations are directly mutagenic and are not targeted by cellular DNA repair pathways.

DNA DAMAGE

Endogenous Sources of Damage

The sources of background DNA damage are summarized in Table 2.1.

Reactive Oxygen Species

Reactive oxygen species (ROS) include ·OH, NO·, and peroxides. ROS are produced as a result of normal cellular metabolism, as well as by ionizing radiation, infection, and reperfusion of ischemic tissue. The DNA damage produced by ROS is collectively referred to as oxidative damage and includes sugar and base modifications, DNA–DNA and DNA–protein crosslinks, and DNA strand breaks (2–8), examples of which are shown in Fig. 2.1. Among the oxidative lesions of DNA, 8-oxodeoxyguanosine is a major cause of mutagenesis during replication because it can pair with adenine almost as efficiently as with cytosine, causing G:C to T:A transversion mutations; similarly, misincorporation of 8-oxodeoxyguanosine formed in the nucleotide pool of the cell can cause A:T to C:G transversions.

Spontaneous Chemical Reactions

Most spontaneous chemical changes that alter the structure of nucleotides are deamination and depurination reactions, but spontaneous hydrolysis, alkylation, and adduction reactions also occur (9). The mutagenic potential of the different types of spontaneous reactions vary.

For example, the deamination of cytosine that produces uracil (Fig. 2.2) creates a mismatched U:G pair. Normally, this mutation is efficiently repaired by the enzyme uracil-DNA glycosylase, and so the substitution infrequently results in a permanent mutation. The deamination of 5-methylcytosine produces thymine and creates a mismatched T:G pair, but because thymine is a normal component of DNA, this mismatch is subject to less efficient DNA repair, leading to an T:A substitution after DNA replication. Similarly, adenine can undergo deamination to form hypoxanthine, creating a mismatched H:T pair, but because hypoxanthine pairs with cytosine instead of thymine, the adenine deamination reaction leads to substitution of cytosine in the complementary strand after DNA replication.

TABLE 2.1
BACKGROUND SOURCES OF DNA DAMAGE

Type	Sources	Examples	Estimated Damage Level in DNA (lesions per genome unless otherwise indicated)[a]
Reactive oxygen species (ROS)	**Endogenous:** Products of cell metabolism; metal catalyzed generation, ionizing radiation; infection; tissue reperfusion	·OH, NO·, peroxides	26,000[b]
Depurination reactions	**Endogenous:** Spontaneous chemical reactions	Loss of adenine or guanine from DNA	35,000
Deamination reactions	**Endogenous:** Spontaneous chemical reactions	Conversion of cytosine to uracil, adenine to hypoxanthine, guanine to xanthine, 5-methycytosine to thymine	23,000
Alkylation	**Endogenous:** Spontaneous chemical reactions **Exogenous:** therapeutic drugs	**Endogenous:** Formation of 6-methylguanine **Exogenous:** Cytotoxic alkylating agents, including nitrogen mustard, nitrosurea, cyclophosphamide	2,600; higher with drug therapy
Adduct formation	**Exogenous:** Carcinogens in ambient air; smoking and passive smoking; natural dietary toxins	Polycyclic aromatic hydrocarbons, aflatoxin B1	1,000–17,000; highest in smokers
Photoproducts	**Exogenous:** Ultraviolet radiation	Pyrimidine dimer; 6-4 pyrimidine-pyrimidone photoproduct	Exposure dependent
DNA–DNA and DNA–protein crosslinks	**Endogenous:** ROS **Exogenous:** Therapeutic drugs; ionizing radiation	**Endogenous:** ·OH, NO·, and peroxides **Exogenous:** Cytotoxic alkylating agents, high and low LET radiation	Exposure dependent[c]
DNA single-strand and double-strand breaks	**Endogenous:** ROS **Exogenous:** Ionizing radiation; therapeutic drugs	**Endogenous:** ·OH, NO·, peroxides **Exogenous:** Cytotoxic alkylating agents, low and high LET radiation	Exposure dependent

[a]Conservative estimates were taken from reference 1 and references therein. A discussion of possible methodologic factors that have potentially influenced damage level measurements is also contained in reference 1.
[b]Including 8-oxodeoxyguanosine and other hydroxylated nucleotides; does not include sugar modifications, DNA–DNA and DNA–protein crosslinks, or DNA strand breaks caused by ROS.
[c]The estimated damage due to DNA–protein crosslinks alone is about 2,000 lesions per genome.
Compiled from Tables 1 and 2 in reference 1.
LET, linear energy transfer.

Depurination is another spontaneous chemical reaction that damages DNA, resulting in the loss of adenine and guanine from DNA. However, depurination reactions do not result in single base pair (bp) substitutions. Instead, if not corrected before the next cycle of DNA replication, the depurination often results in a single bp deletion.

Metal Ions

Although the evidence for DNA damage by endogenous metals is especially strong for iron and copper, the metals nickel, chromium, magnesium, and cadmium are well-established human carcinogens (2,5,10). Oxidative damage via metal-catalyzed ROS generation is by far the most important mechanism of DNA damage (2,10,11). However, metals also act as catalytic centers for reactions that produce a wide spectrum of oxygen-, carbon-, or sulfur-centered radicals from lipids, polypeptide chains, and the ligands of the metal itself.

Endogenous metals also mediate DNA damage caused by a variety of organic compounds, including mono-

nuclear and polynuclear aromatic hydrocarbons (2). The damage is caused by an indirect route; metal-catalyzed reactions either generate ROS from the organic compounds or produce metabolites that form DNA adducts (Fig. 2.3).

Finally, metals such as arsenic, cadmium, nickel, and lead directly inhibit DNA repair and thus augment the mutagenic potential of the DNA damage they cause (5,12–16).

Exogenous Sources of DNA Damage

Chemical Mutagens

Although a virtually infinite number of chemicals can damage DNA, a few families of environmental and therapeutic compounds illustrate the general mechanisms involved.

With the exception of the 5' methylation of cytosine involved in gene regulation (Chapter 1), addition of a methyl or ethyl groups to DNA bases (known as alkylation)

A.

8-oxodeoxyguanosine

B.

thymidine glycol

C.

2,5-dideoxypentose-4-ulose

D.

DNA-protein crosslink

Figure 2.1 DNA damage caused by reactive oxygen species (ROS). 8-Oxodeoxyguanosine (**A**) and thymidine glycol (**B**) are examples of damage to nucleotides caused by hydroxyl radical adds; compare with Figure 1.1. 2,5-Dideoxypentose-4-ulose is an example of ROS damage to a sugar moiety that leads to an abasic site (*open arrow*) as well as a DNA strand break (*closed arrow*) (**C**). The thymidine–tyrosine crosslink between DNA and histone proteins is an example of a DNA–protein crosslink induced by hydroxyl radicals (**D**).

A.

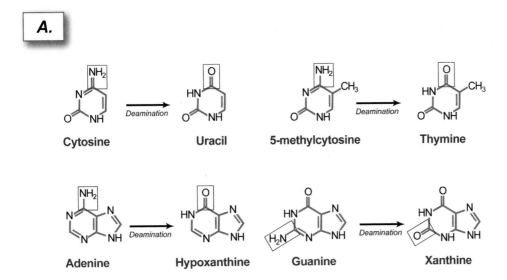

Cytosine → Uracil   5-methylcytosine → Thymine

Adenine → Hypoxanthine   Guanine → Xanthine

B.

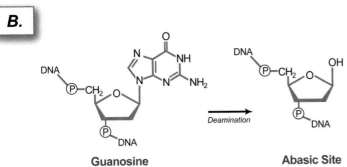

Guanosine → Abasic Site

Figure 2.2 Spontaneous deamination and depurination reactions of the bases in DNA. **A,** Deamination of cytosine to uracil (U pairs with A), 5-methycytosine to thymine, adenine to hypoxanthine (H pairs with C), and guanine to xanthine (X pairs with C). **B,** Depurination of the nucleotide guanosine.

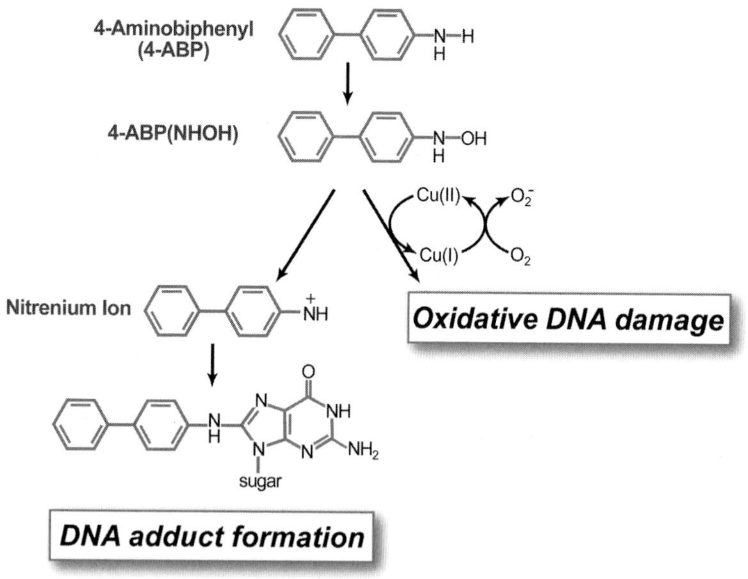

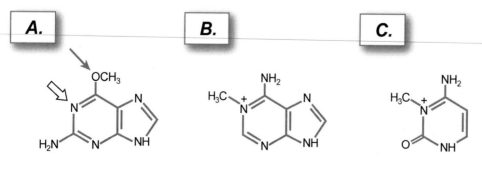

4-Aminobiphenyl
(4-ABP)

4-ABP(NHOH)

Nitrenium Ion

Oxidative DNA damage

DNA adduct formation

sugar

Figure 2.3 Example of a proposed mechanism for DNA damage mediated by metals. 4-Aminobiphenyl (4-ABP) is a binuclear aromatic amine present in tobacco smoke. In the liver, 4-ABP is oxidized to 4-ABP(NHOH), leading to the production of nitrenium ions that cause DNA adduct formation. However, copper-mediated autoxidation of 4-ABP(NHOH) also occurs, resulting in oxidative DNA damage.

can be a direct cause of single bp substitutions. For example, the alkylation reaction that produces O6-methylguanine (Fig. 2.4) results in a base that pairs with thymine, which, if not corrected, leads to a G:C to A:T mutation during the next round of DNA replication.

Polycyclic aromatic hydrocarbons and related compounds do not cause significant direct DNA damage. Instead, this class of molecules is converted into reactive intermediate metabolites by the normal physiologic action of cytochrome P450, a process termed metabolic activation. It is the metabolites that mediate DNA damage through the formation of DNA adducts (2,17–19). Cigarette smoke is a particularly rich source of compounds that mediate DNA damage through the formation of DNA adducts (Fig. 2.3 and 2.5B), although both the vapor phase and particulate phase of cigarette smoke also contain numerous free radicals that cause oxidative DNA damage (19,20,21). Given the tremendous variety of exogenous compounds that are metabolized by cytochrome P450 and related pathways, the spectrum of DNA damage caused by the adducts is almost limitless. Because DNA adducts are a such a significant DNA lesion, variation in the balance between metabolic activation and detoxification among individuals influences cancer rates, providing a rationale for pharmacogenomic analysis of the relevent enzymatic pathways in individual patients (18,22).

Some antineoplastic agents, such as cisplatin, act primarily by causing intrastrand and interstrand crosslinks (Fig. 2.5D). However, cytotoxic alkylating agents used for the treatment of neoplasms, such as cyclophosphamide, busulfan, nitrogen mustard, nitrosourea, and thiotepa, damage DNA through the formation of covalent linkages that produce alkylated nucleotides, DNA–DNA crosslinks (Fig. 2.5A), DNA–protein crosslinks, and DNA strand breaks (23,24). The reactivity and selectivity of alkylating agents is influenced by their chemical structure (mono-, bi, or tri-functional), their pattern of metabolic activation, and the physiology of their target tissue (23). The significance of the genetic damage that accompanies treatment with cytotoxic alkylating agents is indicated by the increased occurrence of secondary malignancies following their therapeutic use.

Radiation

Radiation-induced DNA damage can be classified in two general categories, damage caused by ultraviolet radiation (UV light) and damage caused by ionizing radiation.

UVB radiation from sunlight (wavelength of 280 to 315 nm) induces covalent bonds between adjacent thymine bases in the same strand of DNA (Fig. 2.6A), producing bulky intrastrand TT cyclobutane pyrimidine dimers. UVB radiation also generates 6-4 pyrimidine-pyrimidone photoproducts from TC or CC dimers in the same strand of DNA (Fig. 2.6B). If unrepaired, all these lesions not only inter-

A.

OCH₃

H₂N

B.

NH₂

H₃C

C.

NH₂

H₃C

Figure 2.4 Examples of DNA bases damaged by alkylation reactions. **A,** O6-methylguanine; methylation at the O6 position of guanine (*closed arrow*) results in deprotonation of the adjacent N1 nitrogen (*open arrow*), giving the base ambiguous base-pairing properties. **B,** 1-Methyladenine. **C,** 3-Methylcytosine. Compare with Figure 1.1.

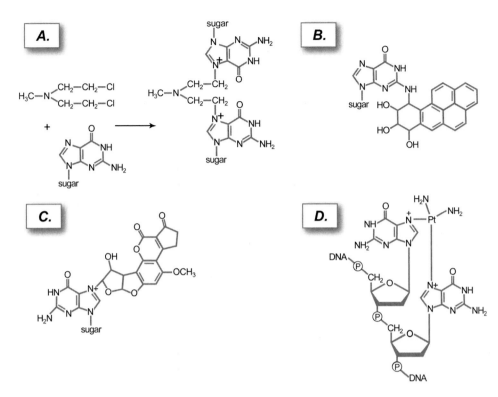

Figure 2.5 Examples of damaged DNA bases caused by exogenous compounds. **A,** DNA–DNA crosslink caused by the bifunctional alkylating agent nitrogen mustard. **B,** Guanosine adduct formed by benz[a]pyrene, a common polycyclic hydrocarbon in cigarette smoke. **C,** Guanosine adduct formed from aflatoxin B1, a dietary toxin (a metabolite produced by mold that grows on peanuts) and a potent hepatocarcinogen. **D,** An intrastrand DNA–DNA crosslink produced by the drug cisplatin.

fere with transcription, but also promote error-prone translesion DNA synthesis. Compared with UVB, DNA damage caused by UVA radiation (wavelength 315 to 400 nm) is more likely to be due to ROS-mediated mechanisms (25).

Ionizing radiation causes a broad spectrum of DNA damage, including individual base lesions, crosslinks, and single- and double-strand breaks (4,26,27). Ionizing radiation characteristically causes clusters of DNA lesions called multiple damaged sites (MDS) that typically span less than 20 bp, and when an MDS contains two single-strand breaks on opposite DNA strands, a double-strand break is created, a principal lesion responsible for both the chromosomal abnormalities and mutations caused by ionizing radiation (28–30).

Even though there appears to be no site specificity for radiation-induced point mutations or DNA break points on a genomewide basis, the organization of chromatin results in a nonrandom distribution of damage on smaller scales. For example, for low linear energy transfer (LET) radiation (x-rays, γ-rays, electrons, and β particles that have a typical LET less than 10 keV/μm), the initial group of ·OH radicals produced by the radioactive particle, coupled with the diffusion distance of the radicals, produces a pattern of damage that reflects the periodicity of DNA wrapped around histones in the nucleosome core (30,31). However, when high LET radiation (protons and neutrons have a typical LET of 10 to 100 keV/μm, while α-particles have an LET greater than 175 keV/μm) traverses the 30-nm chromatin fiber, a stretch of DNA about 2 kb long is heavily damaged. For example, a single 100-keV/μm particle would have enough energy to produce a double-strand break and roughly 100 additional lesions in the surrounding DNA, ranging from individual damaged bases to single-strand breaks (30).

Nucleosomal Influence on the Pattern of DNA Damage

As discussed in Chapter 1, the fundamental unit of DNA packaging is the nucleosome, which consists of 146 bp of DNA wrapped around a central core of eight histone proteins and a 20 to 70-bp long spacer region. The structure of the nucleosome helps protect DNA from attack by many classes of reactive compounds. Regions of DNA that face the histone surfaces are relatively protected, but DNA wound around the nucleosomal core has an underlying 10- to 11-bp periodicity of sites where the DNA backbone faces away from the histone octamer, which correlates with the 10 to 11-bp periodicity of DNA damage caused by singlet oxygen and the hydroxyl radical (32). The DNA damage induced by UV light also apparently occurs primarily at DNA sites facing away from the histone surface.

However, many classes of compounds cause DNA damage that does not demonstrate the anticipated 10 to 11 bp periodicity but instead shows a difference between the core and linker regions of the nucleosome (32). Though modest, this site selectivity has traditionally been attributed to a relative inability of bulky molecules to interact with DNA wrapped around the histones in the core region of the nucleosome. For example, many compounds that produce DNA damage through the formation of adducts or strand breaks show about a 5-fold preference for sites in the linker region relative to core DNA, and compounds that damage DNA through crosslinks or alkylation reactions cause a 2- to 5-fold increase in damage outside the nucleosomal core (32). Active chromatin seems to be more vulnerable to damage, indicating that the unwinding of DNA from nucleosomes that is necessary to provide access to regulatory proteins must expose DNA to reactive metabolites that can cause damage.

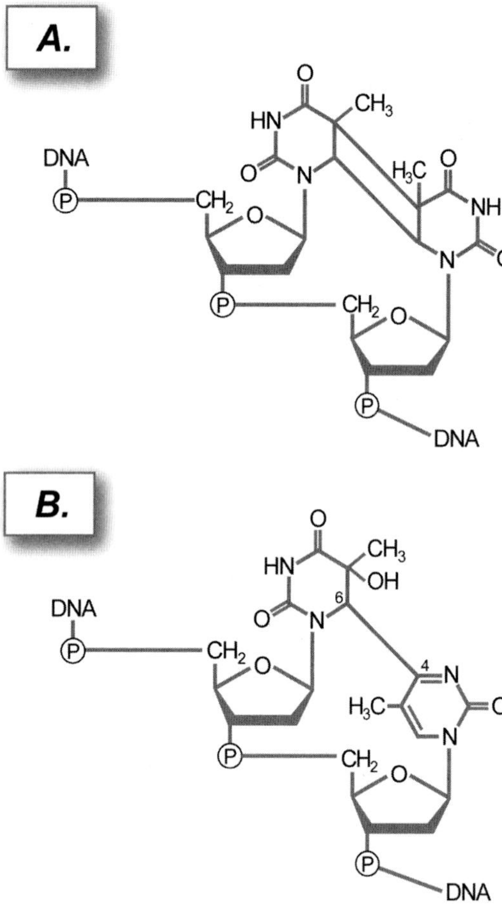

Figure 2.6 UV-induced base damage. **A,** The most abundant type of damage, the TT cyclobutane pyrimidine dimer. **B,** The T(6-4)T photoproduct, an example of the less common 6-4 pyrimidine-pyrimidone photoproduct induced by UV light.

DNA MUTATIONS

The main classes of DNA mutations are listed in Table 2.2. Appendix 3 summarizes the recommended nomenclature for describing sequence mutations, and Chapter 3 summarizes the nomenclature used to describe larger chromosomal structural abnormalities.

Single Base Pair Substitutions

Single bp substitutions are among the most common mutations. Because most mechanisms produce single bp substitutions that are distributed randomly throughout the genome, coding and noncoding regions are about equally susceptible to this type of mutation (33). However, selection pressure reduces the overall frequency of surviving mutations in coding DNA and in associated regulatory sequences, with the result that the overall substitution rate in coding DNA is much less than that of noncoding DNA.

TABLE 2.2

MAIN CLASSES OF DNA MUTATIONS

Single base substitutions (transversions and transitions)
    Coding region
      Synonymous substitutions
      Nonsynonymous substitutions
       Missense mutations
       Nonsense mutations
    Noncoding region
      Substitutions in regulatory regions
      Substitutions that effect RNA processing

Deletions
    Single base pair (bp) deletions to gross structural
    abnormalities
Insertions
    Single bp insertions to gross structural abnormalities
    Trinucleotide repeat expansions
    Retrotransposition of repetitive sequence elements

Gene conversion

Duplications
    Short duplications to gross structural abnormalities

Inversions
    Short sequences to gross structural abnormalities

Gross chromosomal structural abnormalities
    Translocations, ring chromosomes, marker chromosomes, etc.

Numerical chromosomal abnormalities
    Monosomy, trisomy, aneuploidy, etc.

Transitions and Transversions

Transitions are substitutions of a purine by a purine, or a pyrimidine by a pyrimidine; transversions are substitutions of a purine by a pyrimidine, or a pyrimidine by a purine (Fig. 2.7). Despite the expectation that the transversion rate would be higher (because when one base is substituted by another, there is only one choice for a transition but two choices for a transversion), in the human genome the transition rate is actually higher. At least three factors account for this unexpectedly high transition rate. First, because the cytosine in CpG dinucleotides is often methylated (Chapter 1), there is a comparatively high frequency of C to T transitions as a result of the susceptibility of 5-methylcytosine to spontaneous deamination. In fact, the CpG dinucleotide is a hot spot for mutation, with a rate over eight times higher than that of dinucleotides in general (34). Second, at least in coding sequences, transitions usually result in a more conserved polypeptide sequence (and are thus less likely to have a significant functional effect). The genetic code appears to have evolved so as to minimize the effect of nucleotide substitution by specifying chemically related amino acids by codons that have related trinucleotide sequences. Third, the sequence-dependent proofreading activities of the four primary nuclear replicative DNA polymerases may not repair all mispaired bases with equal efficiency, with the net result that transitions over transversions are favored (35,36).

Whether transversions or transitions, single bp substitutions are the end result of a number of different processes,

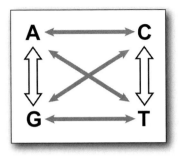

Figure 2.7 Transversions (*closed arrows*) and transitions (*open arrows*). Note that transversions are theoretically twice as frequent as transitions.

including errors in DNA replication, spontaneous chemical reactions, oxidant damage caused by reactive oxygen species, chemical mutagens, and ionizing radiation.

Errors in DNA Replication

The final accuracy of DNA replication depends on the fidelity of the enzymes that polymerize the new DNA strands and on the efficiency of subsequent error-correction mechanisms (35,36). In human cells, replicative DNA polymerases have an error rate that is approximately 10^{-6} to 10^{-7} errors per bp, but mismatch repair lowers the net rate to approximately 10^{-10} errors per residue. However, even this level of DNA replication fidelity results in a high number of mutations over the lifetime of every person. Just considering the coding region of genes, and assuming in very general terms that the coding region of an average human gene is about 2 kb long, coding mutations resulting from misincorporation during DNA replication will therefore occur spontaneously with an average frequency of about 2×10^{-7} per gene per cell division. Given that during an average human lifetime there are an estimated 10^{16} cell divisions (about 10^{14} divisions are required to generate the approximately 10^{14} cells in the adult, with additional mitoses required for cell renewal), each gene will consequently be the site of about 10^{9} mutations. Although only a tiny fraction of cells will carry a mutation for any one gene, and although for many somatic cells the mutation will be inconsequential because it either has no deleterious effect or is lethal for that particular cell type, DNA replication errors nonetheless provide a large reservoir of mutations (34).

Consequences of Single Base Pair Mutations in Coding DNA

A single bp substitution in the coding sequence of a protein can cause a significant change in the encoded amino acid, but will not cause a shift in the translational reading frame. Single bp substitutions in coding DNA are classified into synonymous (silent) mutations and nonsynonymous mutations of which there are two types, missense mutations and nonsense mutations.

Synonymous Mutations

This type of single bp substitution results in a different codon that still specifies the same amino acid. Although synonymous mutations usually occur at the third base position of a codon because of third base wobble, base substitutions at the first position of a codon can also give rise to synonymous substitutions (see Appendix 1). They are the most frequently observed coding mutations and have traditionally been thought to provide no advantage or disadvantage to the cell in which they arise and therefore are often referred to as neutral mutations. However, there are situations in which synonymous substitutions can have a profound effect on the encoded polypeptide. For example, a synonymous substitution within the coding region can cause defective gene expression by activating a cryptic splice site within an exon (37), or a synonymous mutation in an exonic splicing enhancer or exonic splicing silencer can produce an altered pattern of exon skipping or inclusion that causes disease (38,39).

Missense Mutations

Missense mutations are nonsynonymous substitutions in which the mutated codon specifies a different amino acid. A conservative substitution results in the replacement of one amino acid by another that is chemically similar. The effect of conservative substitutions on protein function is usually minimal. A nonconservative substitution results in replacement of one amino acid by another that is chemically dissimilar, typically in charge or hydrophobicity. Functionally, most nonsynonymous mutations have a deleterious effect on gene expression.

Nonsense Mutations

Nonsense mutations are nonsynonymous substitutions in which a codon specifying an amino acid is replaced by a stop codon. Although single bp substitutions that produce nonsense mutations are a direct mechanism for substituting a normal codon with a stop codon, a variety of splice site mutations can also introduce a premature termination codon if the altered pattern of exon joining results in a change in the codon reading frame. The level of function of a truncated protein is usually difficult to predict, because it depends on both on the extent of the truncation and the stability of the truncated polypeptide, but it is usually reduced. Consequently, nonsense mutations are invariably subject to selection pressure and are therefore relatively rare.

Consequences of Single Base Pair Substitutions on RNA Processing

A summary of effects that single BP substitutions can have on gene function is presented in Table 2.3.

Altered RNA Splicing

Single bp substitutions that cause a defect in messenger ribonucleic acid (mRNA) splicing appear to represent about 15% of all point mutations that cause human disease

(33,34,37,40) and fall into four main categories. First, mutations within 5' or 3' consensus splice sites result in the production of mature mRNAs that either lack part of the coding sequence or that contain extra sequences of intronic origin (41). However, mutations that influence a 5' or 3' splice site do not always result in a lack of protein function, as is the case with a single bp substitution in a 5' splice site of the *ras* gene that results in production of a protein with an enhanced level of activity (42). Second, as alluded to above, mutations within an intron or exon can activate cryptic splice sites or create novel splice sites (41,43). Third, also alluded to above, mutations in exonic splicing enhancers or exonic splicing silencers can change the pattern of RNA splicing (38,39,44). An excellent example of this category of mutations is provided by disease-associated point mutations in exonic splicing enhancers of the *BRCA1* gene, many of which are silent at the amino acid sequence level (38,39). In fact, almost 15% of point mutations known to cause human genetic diseases by defective splicing are apparently due to mutations in exonic splicing enhancers or exonic splicing silencers (39,44). Fourth, single bp substitutions at the branch site

sequence required for lariat formation can interfere with normal RNA splicing. Such mutations have been reported, albeit rarely, in association with congenital anomalies (45) and a number of specific diseases (37,46–51).

Pathogenic single bp substitutions have been described that affect RNA processing at stages other than RNA splicing (33,52). Single bp mutations at the CAP site result in either incomplete or unstable transcripts (53). Mutations in the 5' UTR region have been described that appear to exert their affect at the transcriptional level or at the translational level through the creation of new AUG initiation codons (53). Pathogenic single bp substitutions also occur in the 3' UTR; for example, single bp substitutions at the cleavage/polyadenylation signal sequences of α_2- and β-globin genes are the cause of relatively mild forms of thalassemia (53,54).

Production of Premature Termination Codons

Although the most obvious deleterious effect of a nonsense mutation is the production of a truncated polypeptide, premature termination codons also have a significant

TABLE 2.3

EXAMPLES OF WAYS BY WHICH SINGLE BASE PAIR MUTATIONS ALTER THE FUNCTION OF A GENE PRODUCT

Single BP Change	Effect
Single bp substitution	
Synonymous mutation in coding region	Activation of a cryptic splice site in an exon; alteration of an exonic splicing enhancer or exonic splicing silencer
Missense mutation in coding region	Replacement of an essential amino acid; prevention of post-transcriptional processing; prevention of correct cellular localization of product; disruption of RNA editing[a]
Nonsense mutation in coding region	Production of a truncated protein; increased nonsense-mediated RNA decay
In the upstream regulatory region	Decreased or increased gene expression
At a splice site	Inactivation of donor or acceptor splice site; activation of cryptic splice site
In an intron	Alteration of branch site sequence required for lariat formation during splicing; disruption of RNA editing[a]
At the CAP site	Incomplete or unstable RNA transcripts
In the 5' UTR	Mutation of the initiation codon; creation of a new initiation codon; disruption of RNA editing
In the 3' UTR	Polyadenylation/cleavage signal mutations
Single bp additions	
In coding region	Frame shift
In noncoding regions	Additions in regulatory sequences, splice sites, introns, 5' and 3' UTRs, etc., can potentially alter gene function through the same mechanisms listed above for single bp substitutions
Single bp deletions	
In coding regions	Frame shift
In noncoding regions	Deletions in regulatory sequences, splice sites, introns, 5' and 3' UTRs, etc., can potentially alter gene function through the same mechanisms listed above for single bp substitutions

[a]Mutations in noncoding regions that are far removed from the editing site itself can also effect editing.

effect on mRNA stability. mRNAs carrying a premature codon are usually rapidly degraded in vivo by a form of RNA surveillance known as nonsense-mediated mRNA decay (55–58). The mechanism of RNA surveillance is not yet well characterized, but some estimates suggest that perhaps a quarter of all known mutations cause nonsense-mediated mRNA decay (55).

Single Base Pair Substitutions in Regulatory Regions

Most single bp substitutions responsible for genetic disease lie within gene coding regions, but some lie in the 5′ flanking sequences that contain constitutive promoter elements, enhancers, repressors, and other gene regulatory elements. For example, mutations in the TATA box of the core promoter and of the CACCC motif in the proximal promoter region of the β-globin gene are associated with mild β-thalassemia, whereas some mutations in the binding site of *cis*-acting regulatory proteins of γ-globin genes result in increased gene expression (52,59,60).

GROSS GENE DELETIONS

There are two types of recombination events that give rise to gross gene deletions. Homologous unequal recombination is mediated by either related gene sequences or repetitive sequence elements and involves the cleavage and rejoining of homologous but nonallelic DNA sequences. In contrast, nonhomologous recombination (or illegitimate recombination) occurs between DNA loci that have minimal or no sequence homology.

Homologous Recombination

Homologous equal recombination (crossover) occurs between identical or very similar DNA sequences during meiosis or less often during mitosis. Homologous equal recombination involves breakage of a pair of alleles with rejoining of the fragments to generate new recombinant strands; the process does not cause insertions or deletions, although intragenic equal crossover between two alleles can result in a fusion or hybrid gene (Fig. 2.8). In contrast, unequal recombination (unequal crossover) occurs at homologous but nonallelic DNA sequences. One result of unequal recombination is creation of gene fusions that encode abnormal hybrid molecules, for example, between the δ-globin and β-globin genes, leading to hemoglobin Lepore (61); between the α and β-myosin heavy-chain genes, leading to familial hypertrophic cardiomyopathy (62); and between the genes encoding the red and green visual pigments, leading to visual dichromacy (red-green color blindness) (63). However, homologous unequal recombination can also result in a deletion of one of the participating DNA strands (Fig. 2.8).

Because the sites at which homologous unequal recombination occurs show considerable sequence homology, which presumably stabilizes the mispairing of the DNA strands required for recombination, repetitive DNA sequences are especially prone to unequal crossovers and are the site of many large-scale deletions, as well as insertions, duplications, inversions, and translocations (Table 2.4). As noted in Chapter 1, the most abundant repetitive element in the human genome is the interspersed repetitive *Alu* repeat, each copy of which is from 70% to over 95% homologous to the *Alu* consensus sequence. There are about 10^6 copies of the *Alu* repeat in the human genome (64,65), and the observation that *Alu* repetitive sequences flank deletion break points responsible for a considerable number of human genetic diseases has suggested a general role for *Alu* sequences in promoting recombination events (66). In the usual model, recombination between chromosomes misaligned at highly homologous *Alu* sequences with the same orientation generates deletions and concomitant insertions, while *Alu* sequences in opposite orientations mediate crossovers that cause deletions or inversions. One example of the role of recombination at *Alu* sequences in oncogenesis is provided by *Alu*-mediated *BRCA1* deletions that have been implicated as founder mutations in breast cancer patients (67).

Other types of repetitive sequence elements can also mediate homologous unequal recombination. Examples

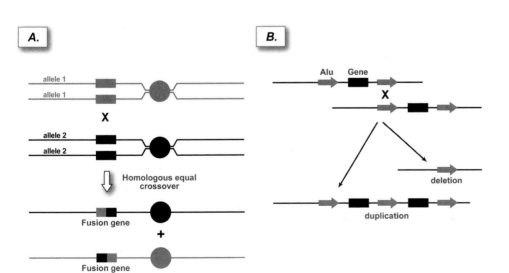

Figure 2.8 Homologous recombination. **A,** Homologous equal recombination that occurs between alleles can generate a novel fusion gene composed of segments of the two alleles (note that a similar exchange between sister chromatids does not result in a novel allele because the sequences on sister chromatids are identical). **B,** Homologous unequal recombination results from pairing of similar but nonallelic sequences of nonsister chromatids or sister chromatids (in this example, *Alu* repetitive sequences). The exchange is unequal in that one DNA strand loses a stretch of DNA (a deletion) while the other strand gains a stretch of DNA (an insertion).

TABLE 2.4

EXAMPLES OF MUTATIONS CAUSED BY REPETITIVE DNA SEQUENCES

Type of Repeat	Type of Mutation	Mechanism
Tandem repeats		
Very short repeats (ranging from several to dozens of base pairs [bp] long)	Short deletions, frame shift mutations	Slipped strand mispairing (Figs. 2.10 and 2.13)
	Short insertions, frame shift mutations	Slipped strand mispairing (Fig. 2.10)
	Trinucleotide expansion	Precise mechanism unknown (Table 2.6)
Larger size repeats (hundreds to thousands of bp long)	Alteration of gene sequences	Unequal crossover; unequal sister chromatid exchange (Fig. 2.8); gene conversion (Fig. 2.9)
	Fusion genes	Unequal crossover; unequal sister chromatid exchange
	Partial or total gene deletion	Unequal crossover; unequal sister chromatid exchange
	Partial or total gene duplication	Unequal crossover; unequal sister chromatid exchange
Palindromes	Short gene deletions, frame shift mutations	Intrastrand formation of hairpin loop (Fig. 2.11)
Interspersed repeats		
Interspersed repeat elements (*Alu* and LINE elements)	Deletions	Unequal crossover; unequal sister chromatid exchange (Fig 2.8)
	Duplications	Unequal crossover; unequal sister chromatid exchange (Fig. 2.8)
	Inversions	Unequal crossover; unequal sister chromatid exchange; intrachromatid exchange (Fig. 2.8)
	Complicated rearrangements	Unequal crossover; unequal sister chromatid exchange; intrachromatid exchange
Active transposable elements (*Alu* and LINE elements)	Insertion	Retrotransposition

include LINE elements (68,69), S232-type low-copy repetitive-sequence repeats that may be responsible for the high frequency of deletions at the steroid sulfatase locus that are characteristic of ichthyosis (70,71), a THE-1 family transposonlike element involved in deletions of the dystrophin gene in Duchenne muscular dystrophy patients (72), and so-called low-copy repeats that mediate constitutional rearrangements of chromosome 22 (73). The segmental aneusomy syndromes (Table 2.5) are genetic disorders that result from inappropriate dosages of genes in a genomic segment, apparently as the result of aberrant recombination at sites of segmental duplications that are 1 to 400 kb long (74).

Nonhomologous recombination

Nonhomologous or illegitimate recombination occurs between two sites that show minimal DNA sequence homology. This type of event is proposed to explain DNA rearrangements such as translocations that show no sequence homology at the break points, or at most very limited sequence homology over a region of only a few nucleotides (75). The observation that translocation-prone gene loci, specifically those that are the site of disease-specific chromosomal rearrangements, are preferentially positioned in close spatial proximity as a consequence of high-order gene structure suggests that the spatial proximity of two genetic loci may contribute to the likelihood of rearrangements via nonhomologous recombination (76–78).

Gene Conversion

Gene conversion is a nonreciprocal transfer of sequence information between a pair of loci. One of the pair of interacting sequences (the donor or source) remains unchanged, whereas the other sequence (the target or acceptor) is altered by partial or total replacement by a sequence copied from the donor sequence. Consequently, only the acceptor sequence is modified and the sequence exchange is therefore directional (Fig. 2.9). A likely mechanism for gene conversion involves homologous recombination in which, following heteroduplex formation,

TABLE 2.5

GENOMIC DISORDERS MEDIATED BY SEGMENTAL DUPLICATIONS

Genomic Disorder	Chromosomal Rearrangement	Chromosomal Location	Rearrangement Size (Mb)
Charcot-Marie-Tooth disease type 1A	Interstitial duplication	17p12	1.5
Hereditary neuropathy with pressure palsies	Deletion	17p12	1.5
Smith-Magenis syndrome	Deletion	17p11.2	5
Duplication 17p11.2	Interstitial duplication	17p11.2	5
Neurofibromatosis type1	Deletion	17q11.2	1.5
Prader-Willi syndrome	Deletion	15q11-15q13	4
Angelman syndrome	Deletion	15q11-15q13	4
Inverted duplication 15	Supernumerary marker chromosome	15q11-15q14	4
Williams-Beuren syndrome	Deletion	7q11.23	1.6
DiGeorge and velocardiofacial syndromes	Deletion	22q11.2	3
Cat eye syndrome	Supernumerary marker chromosome	22q11.2	3
X-linked ichthyosis	Deletion	Xp22	1.9
Hemophilia A	Inversion	Xq28	0.5

Reprinted from Zucman-Rossi J, Legoix P, Victor JM, et al. Chromosome translocation based on illegitimate recombination of human tumors. *Proc Natl Acad Sci USA* 1998;95: 11786–11791; used with permission.

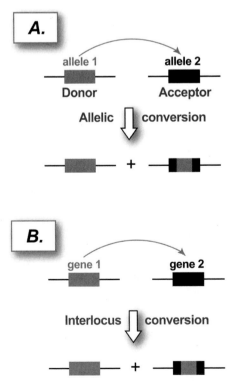

Figure 2.9 Gene conversion. Allelic gene conversion (**A**) and interlocus (nonallelic) conversion (**B**). Note that there is a nonreciprocal sequence exchange in both cases; the acceptor sequence is altered by incorporating a sequence copied from the donor sequence, which remains unchanged.

conversion of the acceptor gene segment occurs via DNA mismatch repair. In this model, DNA repair enzymes recognize the lack of complete complementarity between the two strands of the heteroduplex and "correct" the DNA sequence of the acceptor strand.

Tandemly repeated and clustered gene families seem to be prone to gene conversion, and interlocus sequence exchanges between functional genes and nonfunctional but closely related pseudogenes have been clearly associated with gene conversion events. The classic example of disease pathogenesis resulting from gene–pseudogene exchanges is steroid 21-hydroxylase deficiency, in which over 95% of pathogenic mutations result from sequence exchanges between the functional gene and a very closely related pseudogene on a tandemly repeated DNA segment (79,80).

SHORT GENE DELETIONS

Although variable, the germline mutation rate at some microsatellites (short tandem repeats [STRs]) is remarkably high. Because new mutant alleles have been observed to differ from the parental allele by a single repeat unit, without exchange of flanking markers, the proposed mechanisms for the generation of short gene deletions involve the misalignment of the short direct repeats. Most replication-based models are adaptations of the slipped mispairing hypothesis, also referred to as replication slippage or polymerase slippage (Fig. 2.10). Slipped mispairing can also

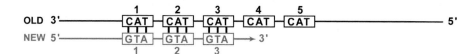

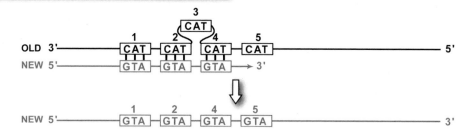

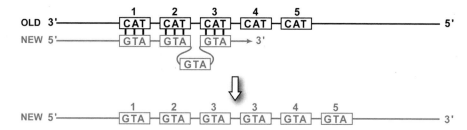

Figure 2.10 Slipped strand mispairing of short tandem repeats. During replication, backward slippage causes an insertion in the newly synthesized DNA strand, while forward slippage causes a deletion in the newly synthesized DNA strand.

provide the mechanism for large deletions (and duplications) through mispairing between noncontinuous repeats (81) and for the production of frame shift errors by misalignment that occurs within a run of identical bases (35,82). However, microsatellite variation does not depend on replication slippage alone but is also influenced by other factors, including repeat number, repeat type, flanking sequences, and the efficiency of mismatch repair (83,84).

Even short direct repeats that do not represent a type of repetitive DNA sequence can apparently cause deletions through a replication slippage mechanism. One well-documented example is the deletion of intervening

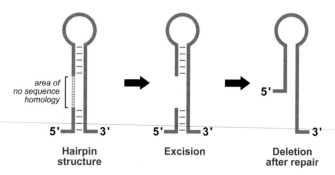

Figure 2.11 Proposed mechanism for deletions mediated by palindromic or quasipalindromic sequences. A hairpin or cruciform secondary structure is produced when a single DNA strand folds back upon itself at the self-complementary palindromic sequences. These misaligned secondary structures provide templates for frameshifts and short deletions by DNA repair mechanisms.

sequences between two perfect 13-bp repeats in Kearns-Sayer syndrome, one of a number of pathogenic deletions in the mitochondrial genome that are bounded by short direct repeats (85). In these diseases, the evidence that the deletions result from a replication slippage mechanism is provided by the fact that the mitochondrial genome is recombination-deficient.

Inverted Repeats

Two types of inverted repeats, palindromes and quasi-palindromes, are frequently observed in the vicinity of short gene deletions. The finding has led to the proposal (86) that the inverted repeats are responsible for frame shifts and short deletions through intrastrand formation of hairpin or cruciform secondary structures in which unpaired bases are deleted through DNA repair mechanisms (Fig. 2.11). Sequence motifs that possess an axis of internal symmetry have also been shown to be overrepresented in the vicinity of short human gene deletions, although the role of these types of sequences in mediating DNA mutation remains uncertain (53).

INSERTIONS

Slipped mispairing of microsatellite loci at the replication fork can, in theory, account for short insertions just as it can for short deletions (35,82–84) (Fig. 2.10). Replication

TABLE 2.6

EXAMPLES OF DISEASES CAUSED BY EXPANSION OF UNSTABLE REPEAT SEQUENCES

Disease	Pattern of Inheritance[a]	Gene	Repeat	Stable Repeat Number (Normal)	Unstable Repeat Number (Mutant)	Repeat Location
Expansion of repeats outside coding sequence						
Fragile-X site A	XLD	FMR1	CGG	6–52	6–200 premutation/ 230–1,000 full mutation	5′ UTR
Fragile-XE site E	XLD	FMR2	GCC	7–35	130–150 premutation/ 230–750 full mutation	5′ UTR
Friedreich ataxia	AR	X25	GAA	6–34	80 premutation/112–1,700 full mutation	Intron
Myotonic dystrophy (DM1)	AD	DMPK	CTG	5–37	50–3,000	3′ UTR
Mytonic dystrophy (DM2)	AD	ZFP9	CCTG	12	75 to >10,000	Intron
Spinocerebellar ataxia type 8	AD	SCA8	CTG	16–37	110 to >500	3′ UTR
Spinocerebellar ataxia type 12	AR	SCA12	CAG	7–25	66–78	5′ UTR
Progressive myoclonus epilepsy	AR	CSTB	CCCCGCCCCGCG	2–3	35–80	Promoter
Spinocerebellar ataxia type 10	AD	SCA10	ATTCT	10–22	280 to >4,500	Intron
Expansion of CAG repeats within coding sequence (expanded glutamine tracts)						
Huntington disease	AD	HD	CAG	6–39	36–121	Coding
Spinobulbar muscular atrophy (Kennedy disease)	XLR	AR	CAG	11–33	38–66	Coding
Spinocerebellar ataxia type 1	AD	SCA1	CAG	6–39[b]	41–81	Coding
Spinocerebellar ataxia type 2	AD	SCA2	CAG	14–31	35–64	Coding
Spinocerebellar ataxia type 3 (Machado-Joseph disease)	AD	SCA3 MJD1	CAG	12–41	40–84	Coding
Spinocerebellar ataxia type 6 (Episodic atypia type 2)	AD	SCA6	CAG	7–18	20–27	Coding
Spinocerebellar ataxia type 7	AD	SCA7	CAG	7–17	38–130	Coding
Dentatorubral-pallidoluysian atrophy	AD	DRPLA	CAG	6–35	51–88	Coding
Spinocerebellar ataxia type 17	AD	SCA17[c]	CAG	25–42	46–63	Coding
Expansion of other repeats within coding sequences						
Synpolydactyly	AD	HOXD13	(GCG)n(GCT)n (GCA)n	15	22–29	Coding
Oculopharynegeal muscular dystrophy	AD	PABP2	GCG	6	7–13	Coding

[a]XLD, X-linked dominant; XLR, X-linked recessive; AD, autosomal dominant; AR, autosomal recessive.
[b]Alleles with 21 or more repeats are interrupted by 1 to 3 CAT trinucleotides; disease alleles consist of only CAG repeats.
[c]Encodes transcription initiation factor TFIID.

slippage also provides a mechanism to generate large duplications by mispairing between noncontiguous repeats.

Homologous unequal recombination between repetitive sequence elements provides another mechanism for the generation of larger insertions, as noted above. However, repetitive DNA elements can also mediate larger insertions through active transposition (87). It turns out that short interspersed nuclear elements (SINEs, of which the *Alu* repeat is the most prominent number) and long interspersed nuclear elements (LINEs) are retrotransposons, a class of transposons that are mobilized via RNA, reverse-transcribed into DNA, and then inserted at a new site in the genome. Although *Alu* and LINE elements are typically found in intergenic noncoding sequences and are conspicuously absent from most coding regions of DNA, there are nonetheless established examples of insertional mutagenesis that result from the retrotransposition of these elements. For example, retrotransposition events have been shown to be responsible for some cases of breast cancer (88), hemophilia A and B (89,90), Duchenne muscular dystrophy (91), neurofibromatosis type 1 (92), chronic granulomatous disease (93), and others (94,95).

Expansion of Unstable Repeat Sequences

A small subset of the tandem trinucleotide repeats in the human genome, as well as a very limited number of longer repeats, show anomalous behavior that causes abnormal gene expression (96–98). At these loci, repeats below a certain length are stable in mitosis and meiosis while repeats above a certain threshold length become extremely unstable. The unstable repeats are virtually never transmitted unchanged from parent to child, and although expansions and contractions occur, there is a bias toward expansion. The increasing size of the trinucleotide repeats between generations accounts for the nonmendelian phenomenon of anticipation that is characteristic of these diseases, a pattern of inheritance in which the disease becomes more severe with successive generations (96). Several mechanisms have been proposed for the repeat instability and associated expansion, including replication slippage, misalignment during excision repair, and unequal recombination.

Genes containing unstable expanding trinucleotide repeats can be grouped into two major classes (99). The first class includes genes that show very large expansions of repeats outside coding sequences. As is shown in Table 2.6, the repeats can be in the promoter, the 5′ untranslated region, introns, or in the 3′ untranslated region of the affected gene. Regardless of their location, the stable and nonpathologic alleles typically have from about 5 to 50 repeats while the unstable alleles that cause disease have several hundreds or thousands of repeats. The second class consists of genes that show modest expansion of repeats within coding sequences. Most, though not all (100), involve CAG repeats for which the stable and nonpathologic alleles typically have about 10 to 40 repeats while the unstable pathologic alleles have expansions in the range of 40 to 200 repeats. The expanded number of trinucleotide repeats does not affect transcription and translation of the abnormal genes. Instead, the long polyglutamine tract encoded by the CAG repeat causes the mutant protein to aggregate, which results in cell death, and the different clinical features of the individual diseases reflect differences in the particular cell populations involved.

Molecular genetic methods, including PCR amplification and Southern blot analysis, have traditionally been employed for laboratory diagnosis of the diseases caused by unstable repeat sequences (96–98,101). However, immunohistochemical evaluation of the level of expression of the associated proteins can provide a simpler method of analysis (102,103).

DUPLICATIONS

Depending on the exact region of DNA involved, unequal crossing over caused by homologous recombination between repetitive sequence elements can cause insertions that are actually gene duplications (Fig. 2.8). The fact that exons duplicated in the *C1I* and *COL2A1* genes, responsible for a type of hereditary angioedema and spondyloepiphyseal dysplasia, respectively, are deleted in other patients with disease due to deficiencies of these proteins demonstrates the capability of unequal recombination to cause disease via duplications as well as deletions (104–106). However, for many duplications there is little or no homology at the duplication break point junctions. Topoisomerase activity has been proposed as one possible alternative mechanism in this setting, a suggestion based on the finding of potential sites for topoisomerases I and II interaction with DNA that are coincident with the break points in some duplications (107–109).

INVERSIONS

A high degree of sequence similarity between repeats on the same chromosome may predispose to either deletions or inversions by a mechanism that involves the chromatid bending back upon itself. Although repetitive DNA sequences such as the *Alu* element have been associated with some inversions (110), other pathogenic inversions are not associated with repetitive DNA sequence elements (74,111–113). Inversions that disrupt the factor VIII gene and cause severe hemophilia A are a classic example of the latter. These inversions have been shown to be due to homologous intrachromosomal recombination that results from mispairing between the *F8A* gene (located within intron 22 of the factor VIII gene) and two closely related sequences oriented in the opposite direction (located approximately 500 kb upstream of the factor VIII gene) (114,115).

Other inversions are not associated with significant sequence homology and are apparently the result of nonhomologous recombination events. A paracentric inversion on chromosome 2 that is responsible for hereditary nonpolyposis colorectal cancer in one kindred is an example of such an inversion (112).

ILLEGITIMATE RECOMBINATION

The enzyme RAG that is responsible for the double-stranded DNA breaks that underlie the V(D)J recombination of antigen receptor genes also occasionally cuts DNA at unrelated loci that have complementary recombination signals, producing a translocation (116). When these fortuitous, cryptic signals are present near a protooncogene, the resulting translocation can be oncogenic, as is the case with follicular lymphomas. The pseudo-signals that induce cleavage by RAG apparently cause DNA to assume a non–B-form structure, producing short stretches of single-stranded DNA that are prone to RAG cleavage (117).

MITOCHONDRIAL DNA DAMAGE AND MUTATIONS

Although mitochondrial DNA (mtDNA) is damaged by all the same processes that damage nuclear DNA, ROS are an especially important source of mtDNA damage (118). The proximity of mtDNA to the reactive intermediates produced by electron transport/oxidative phosphorylation of the respiratory chain likely contributes to the increased susceptibility of mtDNA to ROS damage, as does the fact that mtDNA is not bound by histones. In addition, there appears to be an increased production of ROS as a by-product of aging-associated respiratory function decline, and oxidative damage of mtDNA has been shown to increase with age in various human tissues (119).

The types of mtDNA mutations are also similar to those of nuclear DNA and include single bp substitutions, deletions, duplications, and inversions (120–124). However, there are some unique features to the spectrum of mtDNA mutations. First, large-scale deletions and duplications of mtDNA apparently increase with age (119). Second, even if mtDNA does undergo recombination at a low rate (125–127), because the mitochondrial genome is recombination deficient, deletions are thought to arise primarily by a replication slippage mechanism similar to that occurring at STRs, rather than through homologous equal or unequal recombination events (85). Third, the ends of duplicated or deleted sequences are often marked by short direct repeats, a finding that suggests the underlying mechanisms are related to homologous recombination, although they remain largely uncharacterized (128).

Although mtDNA is subject to the same types of damage and mutation as nuclear DNA, the unique features of mitochondrial genetics (Chapter 1) result in an entirely different pattern of phenotype–genotype correlations. The maternal inheritance of mitochondria (and therefore mtDNA), the presence of homoplasmy (every mtDNA molecule harbors the causative mutation) or heteroplasmy (a cell or a tissue harbors a mixed population of both normal and mutant mtDNA), the threshold effect, and mitotic segregation all lead to a situation in which the proportion of mutant mtDNA within a cell or tissue can change with time. Consequently, the same mutation can be associated with age-related and tissue-related variability of clinical features within individual patients, or even different syndromes in different patients.

DNA REPAIR

Cells have different DNA repair mechanisms to correct the different types of DNA damage. Repair only rarely involves simple chemical reversal of the damage, but instead usually

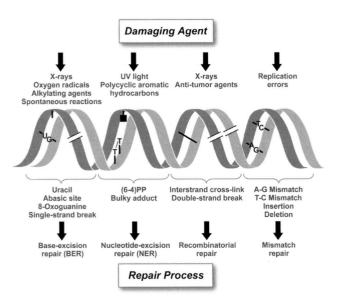

Figure 2.12   DNA damage and repair mechanisms. The top of the diagram lists common agents that damage DNA, the middle shows examples of the resulting DNA lesions, and the bottom indicates the associated DNA repair mechanism. (Reprinted from Hoeijmakers JH. Genome maintenance mechanisms for preventing cancer. *Nature* 2001; 411: 366–374; with permission.)

entails excision of the stretch of DNA containing the altered nucleotides, followed by resynthesis of DNA to fill the gap. The partially overlapping DNA damage repair pathways in human cells are direct repair, base excision repair (BER), nucleotide excision repair (NER), transcription coupled repair, mismatch repair (MMR), and recombinatorial repair (129–133). Figure 2.12 provides a diagrammatic summary of the different DNA repair processes.

DIRECT REPAIR

Human cells produce only a few enzymes that directly reverse DNA damage. One of the few is O6-methylguanine methyltransferase, an enzyme that removes the nonnative methyl group from O6-methylguanine (Fig. 2.4); this dealkylation reaction is quite important because the altered base pairs with either C or T, and hence is highly mutagenic (134). Another set of recently discovered enzymes catalyze oxidative demethylation of 1-methyladenine and 3-methylcytosine (Fig. 2.4); remarkably, these enzymes can apparently repair alkylation damage of both DNA and RNA (135,136). However, human cells lack many other direct repair enzymes that have been described in prokaryotes. For example, bacteria can repair pyrimidine dimers caused by UV light through a single-step photoreactivation process catalyzed by a photolyase enzyme (137); although mammals possess enzymes with homology to photolyases, they are not used for DNA repair but instead appear to be essential components involved in maintenance of circadian rhythms (138).

BASE EXCISION REPAIR

The DNA damage repaired by BER usually is due to small chemical alterations. For example, BER is responsible for repair of oxidized bases (e.g., 8-oxoguanine), alkylated bases, and spontaneously formed bases (e.g., hypoxanthine) and is also responsible for repair of spontaneous depurination events, single strand breaks, and some mismatched bases (139). Because the lesions repaired by BER are the most common types of DNA damage, do not typically impede transcription or DNA replication, and are therefore prone to produce mutations, BER is especially relevant for maintaining the integrity of the genome. Many of the lesions repaired by BER are also substrates for repair by NER, but there is a fundamental difference between the two types of repair. BER employs a number of different damage-recognition proteins that are each specific for a limited set of DNA lesions, whereas NER employs a smaller number of enzymes to recognize many different types of DNA damage (as discussed below).

The first step of BER consists of removal of the damaged base by a DNA glycosylase. Several glycosylases have been identified in humans, each of which excises an overlapping subset of spontaneously formed oxidized, alkylated, or mismatched bases (140). The abasic site is recognized by an apurinic/apyrimidinic endonuclease that cuts the phosphodiester bond of the sugar–phosphate backbone of the DNA strand, leaving behind a single strand break with a normal 3'-hydroxyl group and an abnormal 5'-abasic terminus. The abasic residue is replaced via the lyase and polymerase activities of DNA polβ, and DNA ligase then completes the repair by sealing the remaining nick. A minor pathway, long-patch BER, involves repair synthesis of 2 to 10 bases through a homologous mechanism (129,141).

Defective Base Excision Repair

Demonstration that germline mutations in the gene *MYH*, a glycosylase that removes adenines mispaired with 8-oxoguanine or guanine, are associated with recessive inheritance of multiple colorectal adenomas provides an example of a human disease caused by defective BER (142,143). However, no other human diseases caused by mutations in the core BER pathway have been described, a fact that suggests defective BER is lethal, which is not unexpected given that BER is responsible for repair of the most common types of DNA damage.

NUCLEOTIDE EXCISION REPAIR

NER is the most flexible of the DNA repair pathways and is responsible for correction of various structurally unrelated lesions (129,145). The common denominator of the different types of damage repaired by NER seems to be significant helix distortion with interference of normal base pairing. For example, NER corrects damage caused by bulky base adducts, as well as lesions caused by UV light such as TT cyclobutane pyrimidine dimers.

Biochemically, NER is quite complicated, involving as many as 30 separate proteins. Briefly, the first step in NER is recognition of a DNA lesion that causes disrupted base pairing by the XPC/HHR23B protein complex. Next, the XPB and XPD helicases of the multisubunit repair factor TFIIH open about 30 bp of DNA around the lesion, an intermediate that is stabilized by the factor XPA. Replication protein-A also stabilizes the open intermediate by binding to the undamaged DNA strand. The endonucleases XPG and XPF/ERCC1 then cleave the 3' and 5' borders of the unwound stretch of the damaged strand, defining the margins of a roughly 30-bp region that contains the site of damage. Components of the conventional DNA replication machinery, specifically DNA polδ and polε, then degrade the damaged strand via their 5'$\rightarrow$3' endonuclease activity and fill in the gap. The repair is completed when the remaining nicks are sealed by DNA ligase (129,146).

Defective Nucleotide Excision Repair

Inborn defects in NER are associated with the autosomal recessive photosensitivity syndrome xeroderma pigmentosum and the photosensitive form of the brittle hair disorder trichothiodystrophy (129,130,145) (Table 2.7).

Xeroderma pigmentosum patients are exquisitely sensitive to UV light, and the sun-exposed skin of these patients shows a marked propensity to develop actinic keratosis, as well as malignant neoplasms, including basal cell carcinomas, squamous cell carcinomas, and melanomas. Some patients also develop progressive neurologic degeneration

(151,152). Cell fusion complementation analysis has demonstrated that the mutations causing xeroderma pigmentosum cluster into seven groups, designated XPA through XPG. The XPB and XPD groups are due to mutations in the *XPB* and *XPD* genes, which, as discussed above, encode the helicases that are subunits of the transcription factor TFIIH required for NER (153,154). The XPG and XPF groups are due to mutations in the *XPG* and *XPF* genes that encode endonucleases involved in NER, as also discussed above.

A small number of patients have been identified with a clinical disorder that combines features of both xeroderma pigmentosum and Cockayne syndrome. Specifically, these patients demonstrate a pattern of UV hypersensitivity characteristic of xeroderma pigmentosum together with neurologic and somatic abnormalities characteristic of Cockayne syndrome. Cell fusion complementation analysis has demonstrated that the mutations causing combined xeroderma pigmentosum/Cockayne syndrome fall into the XPB, XPD, and XPG groups defined by complementation analysis of conventional xeroderma pigmentosum. However, different specific mutations in the *XPB*, *XPD*, and *XPG* genes are apparently responsible for the different pattern of clinical manifestations that characterize xeroderma pigmentosum or combined xeroderma pigmentosum/Cockayne syndrome.

Trichothiodystrophy consists of a group of several diseases that exhibit common features, including sparse, dry hair that is easily broken; ichthyosis; sensitivity to UV light; impaired intelligence; and neurologic disfunction (152,155). Cell fusion experiments have identified three complementation groups in the subset of trichothiodystrophy patients who are hypersensitive to UV light. Two of the complementation groups correspond to the XPB and XPD groups of xeroderma pigmentosum, although a different group of mutations is again responsible for the different pattern of clinical disease.

TRANSCRIPTION COUPLED REPAIR

Damage to the nontranscribed strand of active genes and to regions of the genome that are transcriptionally silent is efficiently repaired by NER and BER, often referred to as global genome repair. However, NER and BER inefficiently repair damage to the transcribed DNA strand in regions of the genome that are actively expressed, because RNA polymerase II stalls at the site of the damage on the transcribed strand and sterically inhibits NER and BER. Transcription coupled repair is the system responsible for displacing the stalled RNA polymerase and for repairing the damage that led to the block. Because the stalled RNA polymerase II effectively inactivates the gene, independent of whether or not the DNA damage would result in a mutation effecting gene function, transcription coupled repair in essence not only fixes the DNA damage but also restores gene expression (156).

The initial step in transcription coupled repair requires at least two specific factors, CSA and CSB, which displace the stalled RNA polymerase and make the site of damage accessible for repair. The subsequent stages of transcription coupled repair are thought to be identical to those of BER or NER, depending on the lesion (156–159).

TABLE 2.7

DISEASES WITH DEFECTIVE GENOME MAINTENANCE

Disease	Mutated Gene	Affected Maintenance Mechanism	Pattern of Inheritance	Predominant Type of Genomic Instability	Major Cancer Predisposition
Xeroderma pigmentosum (XP)	XPA through XPG	NER (±TCR)	AR	Point mutations	UV-induced skin cancer (basal cell carcinoma, squamous cell carcinoma, melanoma)
XP variant	Polη	TLS	AR	Point mutations	UV-induced skin cancer
Cockayne syndrome	CSA, CSB	TCR	AR	Point mutations	None
Trichothiodystrophy[a]	XPB, XPD, TTD-A	NER and TCR	AR	Point mutations	None
Ataxia telangiectasia	ATM	DSB	AR	Chromosome aberrations	Acute lymphocytic leukemia, T-cell prolymphocytic leukemia[b]
Ataxia telangiectasia–like disorder	hMRE11	DSB	AR	Chromosome aberrations	Lymphomas
Nijmegen breakage syndrome	NBS1	DSB	AR	Chromosome aberrations	Lymphomas
Familial breast cancer syndrome	BRCA1, BCRA2	HR/DSB	AD	Chromosome aberrations	Breast cancer and ovarian cancer[c]
Werner syndrome	WRN[d]	DSB?	AR	Chromosome aberrations	Sarcomas[c]
Bloom syndrome	BLM[d]	HR	AR	Chromosome aberrations	Leukemias and lymphomas, skin cancer[c]
Rothmund-Thomson syndrome	RECQL4[d]	DSB?HR?	AR	Chromosome aberrations	Osteosarcoma
Hereditary nonpolyposis colorectoral cancer (HNPCC)	hMHL1, hMSH2, hPMS1, hPMS2, hMSH6	MMR	AD	Point mutations	Colorectal cancer[c]
Fanconi anemia	FANCA, FANCB, FANCC, FANCDI, FANCD2/BRCA2, FANCE-FANCL	NER? DSB?	AR (XL for FANCB)	Defective crosslink repair	Acute myelogenous leukemia[c]
Muir-Torre syndrome[e]	hMSH2, hMLH1	MMR	AD	Point mutations	Colorectal cancer plus basal cell carcinoma, squamous cell carcinoma, and sebaceous gland tumors
Multiple colorectal adenomas	MYH	BER	AR	Point mutations	
Mosaic variegated aneuploidy	BUB1B	Checkpoint control	AR	Aneuploidy	Childhood malignancies including Wilms tumor, rhabdomyosarcoma, leukemia

NER, nucleotide excision repair; AR, autosomal recessive; BER, base excision repair; TLS, translesion synthesis; TCR, transcription-coupled repair; DSB, double-strand break response and repair; HR, homologous recombination; MMR, mismatch repair; AD, autosomal dominant; XL, X-linked.
[a]Mechanism for different pattern of disease, despite mutations at some of the same loci as XP, remains unknown.
[b]Heterozygotes also show an increased risk of breast cancer.
[c]Only the predominant type of malignancy is listed; the disease also carries an increased risk of numerous other malignancies.
[d]All are homologues of a DNA helicase that unwinds double-stranded DNA into single-stranded DNA, but their precise role in the different DNA maintenance pathways is uncertain.
[e]Mechanism for different pattern of disease, despite mutations at some of the same loci as HNPCC, remains unknown.
Compiled from references 129, 147–150.

Defective Transcription Coupled Repair

Inborn defects in transcription coupled repair are associated with Cockayne syndrome, a rare pleiotrophic disorder with extensive variation in symptoms and disease severity (152). Common symptoms include photosensitivity, somatic abnormalities often associated with growth failure, progressive ocular abnormalities, hearing loss, and neurodevelopmental dysfunction (151,152). The mutations causing Cockayne syndrome have been shown by complementation analysis to fall into two groups, designated

CSA and CSB. As discussed above, the corresponding CSA and CSB proteins are responsible for displacement of stalled RNA polymerase during the initial steps of transcription coupled repair. Nevertheless, the mechanisms by which mutations that disrupt the general pathway of transcription coupled repair produce disease with the specific features of Cockayne syndrome are unclear.

MISMATCH REPAIR

The mismatch repair system removes nucleotides that are mispaired by DNA polymerases. The repair system also removes insertion/deletion loops ranging from 1 to over 10 bp long that result from polymerase slippage during replication of repetitive sequences or during recombination (160–162). Cells that are defective in the mismatch repair pathway have mutation rates up to a thousand times higher than the rates of normal cells, with a particular tendency for replication slippage at STRs or homopolymeric stretches. One particular mechanism by which defective mismatch repair facilitates malignant transformation is by producing mutations in genes that harbor microsatellites in their coding regions, some of which have critical roles in the regulation of cell growth and apoptosis (163,164).

Mechanistically, mismatch repair can be divided into several steps (129,160,162). The first step is mismatch recognition; hMSH2/6 heterodimers recognize mismatches as single base loops, whereas hMSH2/3 heterodimers recognize larger insertion and deletion loops. During the second step, additional mismatch repair factors are recruited, including heterodimeric complexes of hMLH1/hPMS2 and hMLH1/hPMS1. The third step involves differentiation of the new mutant DNA strand from the old correct strand. Strand discrimination in bacteria relies on the absence of DNA methylation in the newly synthesized strand; however, the mechanism of discrimination in mammals is as yet unclear, although it may be based on the pattern of contact with nearby replication machinery. The fourth step entails degradation of the incorrect strand past the mismatch with subsequent DNA resynthesis, a step that requires a host of ancillary proteins, as well as DNA polδ and polε. Recent experimental evidence suggests that a number of additional proteins are also involved in mismatch repair, although their precise role has yet to be characterized (165).

Defective Mismatch Repair

Mutations in *hMLH1* and *hMSH2* account for 40% to 50% of all patients with hereditary nonpolyposis colorectal cancer (HNPCC); mutations in *hPMS1* and *hPMS2* have been associated with a much smaller subset of cases of HNPCC (129,160,166). Defects in *hMSH6* are responsible for late-onset atypical HNPCC (161,162).

Defects in some mismatch repair genes, *hMLH1*, for example, are associated with an increased incidence of carcinomas of the colon, endometrium, and ovary without a similarly increased incidence of carcinomas at other epithelial sites. In contrast, patients who have mutations in *hMSH2* also suffer from a higher rate of epithelial malignancies of the renal pelvis, ureter, and stomach. The reasons for the differences are as yet unexplained (161).

It is important to recognize that although the microsatellite instability phenotype can be demonstrated in a variety of malignancies, in most cases the phenotype is due to somatic rather than germline mutations at mismatch repair loci. For example, microsatellite instability is present in 12% to 28% of sporadic colorectal adenocarcinomas, although HNPCC accounts for less than 5% of colorectal adenocarcinomas (164,166).

TRANSLESION SYNTHESIS

The polymerases in humans that are primarily responsible for replication of nuclear DNA, specifically polymerases α, δ, and ε, are specialized enzymes that replicate templates containing the four normal nucleotides at high speed with high fidelity (146,168,169). However, replication is hampered when these polymerases encounter a chemically altered base because they inefficiently add a nucleotide opposite the damaged base in the template DNA strand. Furthermore, when extension does occur, the resulting distorted terminus triggers the 3′→5′ exonuclease proofreading activity of the polymerase, triggering futile addition–excision cycles (Fig. 2.13). Translesion synthesis is the mechanism by which cells manage to replicate damaged nuclear DNA templates despite the almost limitless diversity of DNA lesions encountered by DNA polymerases.

Given the variety of chemical modifications that alter DNA nucleotides, it is not surprising that translesion synthesis is error prone. Chemical damage itself is responsible for some errors; if a chemical modification has destroyed the coding properties of the preexisting base, insertion of a

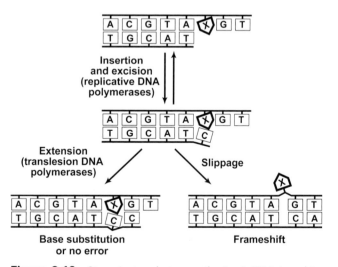

Figure 2.13 Steps in translesion synthesis. A DNA template lesion (X) distorts the DNA backbone. Because none of the dNTPs can pair with X, addition of even the "best" nucleotide will still distort the terminus, precluding further extension. In addition, the 3′→5′ exonuclease proofreading activity of replicative DNA polymerases will excise the newly incorporated nucleotide, initiating futile addition–excision cycles. Translesion synthesis is frequently mutagenic, inducing base substitutions or frameshift mutations (especially when the nucleotide inserted across the lesion is complementary to the next base of the template). (Modified from Pages, V and Fuchs, RPP, How DNA lesions are turned into mutations within cells. *Oncogene* 2001;21:8957–8966; with permission from Nature Publishing Group. http://www.nature.com/.)

nucleotide opposite the damaged base is essentially random, producing a base substitution 75% of the time. However, other errors are a direct consequence of the enzymatic properties of the specific DNA polymerases involved in translesion synthesis.

In general terms, the mechanism of translesion synthesis involves transient replacement of the conventional DNA polymerase in the vicinity of the DNA lesion by one (or several) of a group of specialized polymerases that have the ability to replicate damaged DNA (168,170,171). The specialized polymerases have several properties that make them enzymatically distinct from the conventional replicative DNA polymerases. As a group, translesion synthesis polymerases display low fidelity replication of nondamaged templates, have a slow rate of polymerization and little processivity, have a propensity to use mismatched termini for extension, lack a proofreading function, and have flexible (and even alternative) base-pairing properties (146,168,171–174). Although each polymerase seems to exhibit maximum activity for a particular type of DNA damage (175), the polymerase involved in the bypass of a lesion also apparently depends on the local sequence context within which the lesion is located. As would be expected from the diversity of DNA modifications that

must be bypassed, the number of polymerases that favor damaged templates far exceeds the number of polymerases that replicate undamaged DNA (Table 2.8).

Although the flexible base-pairing properties of translesion polymerases provide cells with the capability to replicate damaged DNA at sites where conventional replicative DNA polymerases are blocked (Fig. 2.14), the capability comes at the expense of a high error rate. [In the final analysis, DNA damage produced by many mutagens is nothing more than a stable chemical modification of an individual DNA base, and translesion synthesis is a mechanism by which the inert chemical alteration becomes permanently fixed in the genome as a mutation.] Translesion synthesis is also prone to generate frame shift mutations, a tendency that is apparently the result of primer-template misalignment or slippage that occurs when the nucleotide added across from the damaged DNA base is complementary to the next base in the template DNA strand.

Defective Translesion Synthesis

About 20% of xeroderma pigmentosum patients are classified as xeroderma pigmentosum variants. Affected individuals often cannot be clinically distinguished from patients

TABLE 2.8
DNA POLYMERASES

Polymerase	Base Substitution Error Rate[a]	Associated Activities[b]	Proposed Functions[c]
Classical DNA polymerases			
α	10^{-4}	Primase	Chromosomal replication; DSB repair
β	10^{-3} to 10^{-4}	dRP lyase	BER; SSB repair
γ	10^{-5} to 10^{-6}	$3' \rightarrow 5'$ exonuclease; dRP lyase	Mitochondrial replication; mitochondial BER
δ	10^{-6} to 10^{-7}	$3' \rightarrow 5'$ exonuclease	Chromosomal replication; NER; BER; MMR; DSB repair
ε	10^{-6} to 10^{-7}	$3' \rightarrow 5'$ exonuclease	Chromosomal replication; NER; BER; MMR; DSB repair
Error-prone repair DNA polymerases			
ζ	10^{-4} to 10^{-5}		TLS; DSB repair; SHM; ICL repair?
η	10^{-1} to 10^{-3}		TLS; SHM
θ			ICL repair?
ι	10^{-2} to 10^{-4}	dRP lyase	SHM; TLS? BER?
κ	10^{-3} to 10^{-4}		TLS
λ		dRP lyase	DSB repair; BER?
μ	NA	TdT	DSB repair
σ			Sister chromatid cohesion
REV1	NA	TdT for dCTP	TLS

[a]In regions without DNA damage. Does not include frame shift errors. Error rates vary by base and local sequence environment from the representative values given. For polymerases γ, δ, and ε, mismatch repair following DNA polymerization is responsible for an overall mutation rate of $<10^{-10}$ misincorporations per base pair.
[b]dRP, 5'-deoxyribose phosphate; TdT, terminal deoxynucleotidyl transferase
[c]BER, base excision repair; DSB, double-strand break; SSB, single-strand break; NER, nucleotide excision repair; MMR, mismatch repair; TLS, translesion synthesis; ICL, intrastrand crosslink; SHM, somatic hypermutation; NA, not applicable.
Modified from reference 146 (with permission), and references 40 and 167.

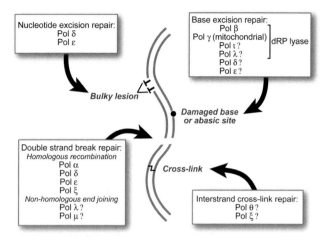

Figure 2.14 DNA polymerases involved in DNA damage repair. (Reprinted from Shcherbakova PV, Bebenck K, Kunkel TA. Functions of eukaryotic DNA polymerases. Science's Sage KE; http://sageke.sciencemag.org/cgi/content/full/sageke; 2003/8/re3; with permission.)

with conventional xeroderma pigmentosum, but cell culture studies have shown that the variant form of the disease has a different genetic cause; as discussed above, most patients with xeroderma pigmentosum harbor defects in NER, but patients with xeroderma pigmentosum variant exhibit defective replication of damaged DNA resulting from inherited mutations in *Polη* (176,177). In fact, xeroderma pigmentosum variant is the first example of a human disorder caused by a deficiency in the translesion synthesis pathway. It is interesting to note that Polη has an intrinsically high capacity to accurately replicate through TT cyclobutane dimers, where it preferentially inserts an AA dinucleotide opposite the lesion (170). Polη therefore seems to have been evolutionarily selected to prevent mutations caused by TT cyclobutane dimers, the most abundant UV light–induced lesion (171).

RECOMBINATORIAL REPAIR

Repair of Double-Strand Breaks

Double-strand breaks can lead to mutagenic rearrangements such as translocations, inversions, and deletions. Because they create a substrate for both single and double strand exonucleases, double-strand breaks can also lead to the loss of genetic information even in the absence of rearrangements. The two main double-strand break repair mechanisms are homologous recombination and nonhomologous end joining (148). Both activate a cascade of kinase reactions, which not only recruit repair factors to the site of the break but also delay or stop the cell cycle in a process known as DNA damage cell cycle checkpoint control (150,178–182). The identity of the sensor proteins that detect the double-strand break, as well as the biochemical basis of the recognition event, remain unknown (183,184). Models have been proposed in which the critical structure may be a complex formed by replication protein-A (also involved in NER, as noted previously) or p53 binding protein (185,186), or in which changes in

chromatin structure induced by the double-strand break may expose covalent histone modifications that recruit specific proteins that initiate checkpoint control (187). A third minor pathway of double-strand break repair, single-strand annealing, has also been described but is best considered as a subpathway of the homologous recombination mechanism (188).

Homologous Recombination

For homologous recombination, an intact DNA duplex of identical or near identical sequence is used to repair the broken DNA molecule. The repair process conceptually consists of three stages (148). During first stage, known as presynapsis, the 5' and 3' ends of the broken DNA duplex are processed by the MRE11/RAD50/NBS1 protein complex and then coated with additional proteins required for the repair process. In the second stage, synapsis, homologous regions between the broken and intact DNA strands anneal, forming a D-loop. The group of proteins that catalyze this step includes the recombinase RAD51 that initiates strand exchange between the paired DNA molecules, an activity that is regulated by BRCA2 (189,190). In the final stage, postsynapsis, the D-loop matures into a Holliday junction, the intact double-stranded DNA duplex is used as a template to fill in the gaps of the broken duplex, and the Holliday junction is resolved.

Nonhomologous End Joining

Most double-strand breaks are repaired by the nonhomologous end joining pathway, a process by which broken DNA ends are joined regardless of sequence similarity. Although nonhomologous end joining is intrinsically error prone and therefore highly mutagenic, it nonetheless provides a mechanism to join breaks that may have noncomplimentary overhanging ends, limiting the additional loss of genetic information that would result from degradation of the exposed DNA ends by nucleases. Nonhomologous end joining is also the pathway used to process the site-specific DNA double-strand breaks introduced during V(D)J recombination of antigen receptor gene loci.

Mechanistically, the end joining pathway simply links the ends of two double strand breaks together without use of an intervening template. The pathway involves a Ku70–Ku80 heterodimer that binds the DNA ends and activates the catalytic subunit of DNA dependent protein kinase DNA-PK, and rejoining is completed by a DNA ligase/Xrcc4 heterodimer (188). End joining is sometimes associated with the loss or gain of a few nucleotides if internal microhomologies are used for alignment before repair, a finding that implies that DNA polymerases may also be involved at some point in the process.

Repair of DNA Crosslinks

The mechanism of crosslink repair in human cells remains unknown (146,191). One recent model suggests that crosslink repair involves components of NER, as well as double-strand break repair through the homologous recombination pathway (191–196).

Defective Double-strand Break and Crosslink Repair

Some human diseases have been associated with mutations in the proteins involved in double strand-break repair by homologous recombination, and, not unexpectedly, the diseases share radiosensitivity, genome instability, cancer susceptibility, and immunodeficiency as prominent clinical features (129,147,197).

Ataxia telangiectasia, an autosomal recessive disease characterized by progressive cerebellar degeneration, conjunctival telangiectasias, extreme radiation sensitivity, and an increased incidence of malignancies, is due to germline mutations in the *ATM* gene (198,199). ATM is a protein kinase that is one of the early initiators of DNA damage cell cycle checkpoint control, which, as noted above, is responsible for delaying or stopping the cell cycle when double-strand breaks occur (181,200–202). It is noteworthy that somatic mutations in *ATM* also cause disease. For example, *ATM* is mutated in most, if not all, patients with sporadic T-cell prolymphocytic leukemia, a malignancy with phenotypic similarities to one of the leukemias characteristic of ataxia telangiectasia (203,204).

Germ line mutations in *MRE11* give rise to the disease ataxia telangiectasia–like disorder, and mutations in NBS1 are characteristic of the Nijmegen breakage syndrome (205,206). As noted above, both MRE11 and NBS1 are involved in the presynapsis stage of double-strand break repair by the homologous recombination pathway, and it is therefore not surprising that hypersensitivity to ionizing radiation, chromosomal instability, defects in cell cycle checkpoint control, and a predisposition to malignancies are characteristic of both disorders.

Fanconi anemia is an autosomal or X-linked disease characterized by diverse congenital abnormalities, a predisposition to bone marrow failure and malignancy, and cellular sensitivity to DNA crosslinking agents (191,207). Cell fusion experiments have demonstrated that the responsible germ line mutations involve at least 11 separate genes (208,209). One of the genes, FANCD2, encodes a multifunctional protein that interacts with MRE11/ RAD50/NBS1 in the repair of DNA crosslinks and is phosphorylated by ATM as part of cell cycle checkpoint control. Somatic defects in the activation of FANCD2 are a feature of several sporadic malignancies, providing a possible explanation for the chromosomal instability that is characteristic of some tumors (191). At least five of the other genes responsible for Fanconi anemia encode proteins that regulate activation of FANCD2, and the *FANCD1* gene turns out to be *BRCA2*.

Inherited mutations in *BRCA1* or *BRCA2* are the cause of familial breast and ovarian cancer syndromes. Both genes encode proteins that are apparently involved in a multitude of different pathways, including DNA repair and recombination, cell cycle control, and gene transcription (190,210–213). BRCA1 participates in protein complexes that regulate MRE11 and has been implicated in cell cycle checkpoint control events including sequence-specific transcriptional regulation of genes whose expression affects downstream checkpoint enforcement (190,212, 213). Disordered regulation of RAD51 may be the most important mechanism by which mutant *BRCA2* contributes to oncogenesis in familial cancer syndromes (189,212, 213); however, as yet there is no explanation for the fact that cancer predisposition associated with *BRCA2* mutations is limited to particular epithelial tissues (190). The proposed overlaps between double-strand break repair and DNA crosslink repair likely explain the sensitivity of cells harboring mutations in *BRCA1* or *BRCA2* to DNA crosslinking agents (191).

Werner, Bloom, and Rothmund-Thomson syndromes are all associated with a high degree of genomic instability and a predisposition to cancer, but they are not due to mutations in genes directly responsible for DNA repair (214–218). Instead, the syndromes are due to mutations in members of the RecQ family of helicases, proteins that unwind the complementary strands of the DNA duplex and appear to maintain genomic stability by functioning at the interface between DNA replication and DNA repair (214,215,219,220). For example, the *WRN* gene, mutated in Werner syndrome, encodes a protein that interacts with DNA polδ, as well as the replication protein-A complex (215,219,221,222), and the *BLM* gene product, mutated in Bloom syndrome, has been shown to interact with ATM, RAD51, and replication protein-A (219). The *WRN* gene product has also been shown to have a pivotal role in telomere lagging strand synthesis, which provides a link between the genetic instability and the premature aging that is characteristic of Werner syndrome (223).

MITOCHONDRIAL DNA REPAIR

As discussed in more detail in Chapter 1, human mtDNA contains only 37 genes, which encode just 2 rRNAs, 22 tRNAs, and 13 subunits of the respiratory chain. Consequently, all the proteins needed for mtDNA repair are encoded by nuclear DNA and must be imported into the organelle, and it is through this route that mitochondria acquire the basic enzymes required for the BER pathway of DNA repair, including several DNA glycosylases, an apurinic/apyrimidinic endonuclease, and a DNA ligase (123,224). The repair polymerase in the mitochondrial BER pathway is apparently the mtDNA replicative polymerase polγ, and consequently it is not surprising that mutations in the enzyme's proofreading domain that underlie the rare inherited disease progressive external ophthalmoplegia cause accumulation of mitochondrial mutations (225,226). It is interesting to note that some of the aging-associated increases in oxidative damage seen in mtDNA may also result from mutations in *polγ* (227), as well as from deficiencies in the import of the glycosylases required for the mitochondrial BER pathway (228).

Mismatch repair activity has also been demonstrated in mammalian mitochondria (229). Although the repair pathway has not been well characterized, the mitochondrial pathway exhibits several important differences from the nuclear pathway, including an apparent lack of involvement by hMSH2 and a lack of strand bias (229).

The nuclear NER pathway does not operate in mammalian mitochondria (229,230). However, helix-distorting DNA lesions are nonetheless removed from mtDNA, although no details of the process have been described

(231). Similarly, even though the mitochondrial genome is recombination deficient, complex lesions such as cisplatin-induced crosslinks are removed, athough the mechanism for the repair process is unknown (232).

HEREDITARY CANCER SYNDROMES

Some of the most striking examples of hereditary cancer syndromes are due to mutations affecting genes involved in repair of DNA damage (Table 2.9). However, not all familial cancer syndromes are caused by defects in DNA repair. Germline mutations in other tumor suppressor genes besides those encoding DNA repair enzymes also cause hereditary cancer syndromes, as do germline mutations in oncogenes. To help put the syndromes caused by defects in DNA repair into perspective, the other causes of familial cancer syndromes are briefly reviewed here.

Tumor Suppressor Genes

The proteins encoded by tumor suppressor genes are involved in a wide range of cell processes, including cell cycle control, differentiation, and apoptosis, as well as maintenance of genome integrity. Over 20 tumor suppressor genes have been identified, and at least 10 other candidates have been described (233,234). As far as conceptualizing their roles in familial cancer syndromes is concerned, tumor suppressor genes have been broadly divided into two classes, gatekeepers and caretakers (147,235).

Gatekeepers

The products of gatekeeper genes directly regulate cell growth by either inhibiting cellular proliferation or promoting apoptosis (235,236). Because the functions of these genes are rate limiting for tumor growth, both maternal and paternal copies must be inactivated for a tumor to develop. In accordance with Knudson's hypothesis (237–239), individuals with an autosomal dominant cancer susceptibility inherit one damaged copy of this type of gene and as a result require only one additional somatic mutation to inactivate the remaining wild-type allele and initiate tumor formation. However, mutation of both alleles of a gatekeeper gene is usually insufficient for acquisition of a fully transformed phenotype. Additional mutations, often in other tumor suppressor genes or oncogenes, are required for a cell to express a malignant phenotype (233,240–246).

Gatekeepers vary with tissue type, so inactivation of a particular gatekeeper gene leads to specific forms of cancer predisposition. For example, inherited mutations of *WT1* predispose to Wilms tumor and inherited mutations of *VHL* predispose to clear cell renal cell carcinoma, and, although both neoplasms involve the kidney, they are clinicopathologically different diseases; in contrast, inherited mutations *APC* predispose to colonic adenocarcinoma but not tumors of the kidney. And, just as germline mutations that inactivate gatekeepers underlie familial cancer syndromes, somatic inactivating mutations are frequently found in sporadic malignancies (233,245). Sporadic tumors are particularly likely to harbor somatic mutations in the genes that are responsible for syndromic neoplasms of the same histologic type.

Caretakers

The proteins encoded by caretaker genes do not directly promote cell growth (235). Instead, inactivation of a caretaker gene leads to genetic instability that indirectly promotes proliferation by causing an increased rate of mutation. Cells with defective caretaker genes accumulate mutations in other tumor suppressor genes and oncogenes, apparently via random chance rather than a direct targeting mechanism (233,240–246). The genes that encode proteins involved in DNA repair are classic examples of caretaker genes.

Somatic mutations of caretaker genes are rarely the initiating events in nonfamilial or sporadic neoplasms, presumably because an extended length of time is required for random inactivation of both alleles of a caretaker gene and subsequent mutation of several additional loci.

Oncogenes

Proto-oncogenes encode proteins that regulate the events that control cell growth and differentiation (234,240). More than 75 proto-oncogenes have been identified, and their products include extracellular cytokines and growth factors, transmembrane growth factor receptors, cytoplasmic proteins that transmit intracellular biochemical signals to the nucleus, transcription factors, and nuclear proteins involved in the control of DNA replication.

Oncogenes are mutated forms of proto-oncogenes that cause neoplastic transformation by interfering with normal cell growth or differentiation, often by disrupting control of the cell cycle. Accumulated evidence from human malignancies, as well as transgenic animal models, indicates that mutation of a single oncogene is insufficient for acquisition of a fully transformed malignant phenotype. Instead, additional mutations that activate other oncogenes or inactivate tumor-suppressor genes are necessary (240–244). Admittedly, it is sometimes uncertain as to whether a gene is best classified as an oncogene or as a gatekeeper tumor suppressor gene.

Oncogenes also can be divided into two general groups based on the mechanism of their action. Oncogenes in the first group induce continuous or unregulated cell proliferation by inactivation of growth inhibitory signals, or by activation of growth-promoting genes, growth factors, receptors, intracellular signaling pathways, or nuclear oncoproteins (247,248). The second group of oncogenes immortalize cells by rescuing them from senescence and apoptosis (249).

A few inherited cancer syndromes are due to germline mutations in oncogenes (Table 2.9). However, the mutations in most oncogenes are somatic and are thus associated with sporadic malignancies. The type of mutation, as well as the involved oncogene, is nonetheless characteristic for many tumor types (Table 2.10).

TABLE 2.9
INHERITED CANCER SYNDROMES[a]

Syndrome	Primary Tumor in Hereditary Syndrome	Associated Tumors and Disease Traits in Hereditary Syndrome	Tumors Associated with Somatic Mutations	Gene	Mode of Inheritance	Function of Gene Product
Tumor suppressor genes—gatekeepers						
Familial retinoblastoma	Retinoblastoma	Osteosarcoma	Retinoblastoma; osteosarcoma; carcinoma of breast, lung, colon	RB1	AD	Cell cycle and transcriptional regulation
Li-Fraumeni syndrome	Multiple sarcomas and carcinomas		Mutated in about 50% of all sporadic malignancies	TP53	AD	Transcription factor; regulates cell cycle and apoptosis
Familial adenomatous polyposis[b]	Colorectal adenocarcinoma	Colorectal adenomas, jaw osteomas, desmoid tumors; Gardner syndrome; Turcot syndrome	Carcinomas of stomach, colon, pancreas, thyroid; melanoma	APC1	AD	Regulation of β-catenin; binding to microtubules
Juvenile polyposis coli[b,c]	Colorectal adenocarcinoma; upper gastrointestinal carcinomas	Multiple hamartomatous polyps of stomach, small intestine, colon		SMAD4 BMPR1A PTEN1	AD AD AD	Transcription factor Cell surface receptor Dual-specificity phosphatase
Neurofibromatosis type1[b]	Neurofibromas	Malignant peripheral nerve sheath tumors, neuroblastoma	Schwannomas	NF1	AD	GTPase
Neurofibromatosis type2[b]	Aucoustic schwannomas, meningiomas	Gliomas, ependymomas	Schwannomas and meningiomas	NF2	AD	Membrane link to cytoskeleton
Wilms tumor	Wilms tumor	WAGR syndrome (Wilms tumor, aniridia, genitourinary abnormalities, mental retardation); Denys-Drash syndrome	Wilms tumor	WT1	AD	Transcription factor
Nevoid basal cell carcinoma syndrome[b]	Basal cell carcinoma	Jaw cysts, medulloblastoma		PTCH	AD	Transmembrane receptor
Von Hippel-Lindau syndrome[b]	Renal carcinoma, clear cell type	Pheochromocytomas, hemangioblastomas	Renal carcinoma, clear cell type	VHL	AD	Regulation of transcriptional elongation by RNA polII
Familial melanoma	Melanoma	Pancreatic cancer, dysplastic nevi	Pancreatic and esophageal carcinomas	CDKN2A CDK4	AD AD	Cell cycle regulation at the G1/S checkpoint Unknown
Multiple endocrine neoplasia type 1	Endocrine tumors of the pancreas	Parathyroid adenomas, pituitary adenomas	Parathyroid adenomas; endocrine tumors of the pancreas; bronchial carcinoid	MEN1	AD	Unknown
Hereditary multiple exostoses	Exostoses	Chondrosarcomas		EXT1 EXT2 EXT3	AD AD AD	Unknown

(continued)

TABLE 2.9
continued

Disease	Cancer	Associated findings	Gene	Inheritance	Function
Cowden syndrome[b]	Breast carcinoma, follicular carcinomas of the thyroid	Hamartomatous intestinal polyps; mucocutaneous lesions; fibroadenomas	PTEN1	AD	Dual-specificity phosphatases
Hereditary prostate cancer	Adenocarcinoma of the prostate		HPC1	AD	Unknown
			HPCX	XR	Unknown
Hereditary diffuse gastric cancer	Diffuse gastric cancer	Carcinomas of stomach and breast	E-CAD/CDH1	AD	Transcriptional factor in TGF-β pathway
Rhabdoid predisposition syndrome	Renal or extrarenal malignant rhabdoid tumors, various CNS tumors		hSNF5/INI1	AD	Chromatin remodeling; transcriptional modulation
Tumor suppressor genes—caretakers					
Hereditary nonpolyposis colorectal cancer (HNPCC)[d]	Colorectal adenocarcinomas	Adenocarcinomas of the endometrium, ovary, stomach	hMSH2 hMLH1 hPMS1 hPMS2 hMSH6	AD AD AD AD AD	DNA mismatch repair
Ataxia telangiectasia[e]	Acute lymphocytic leukemia, T-cell prolymphocytic leukemia	Cerebellar ataxia; immunodeficiency; breast carcinoma in heterozygotes	ATM	AR	DNA double-strand break repair
		T-cell prolymphocytic leukemia			
Bloom syndrome[f]	Leukemias and lymphomas	Small status; immunodeficiency	BLM	AR	DNA helicase
Xeroderma pigmentosum[g]	UV-induced skin cancer	Pigmentation abnormalities, neurologic abnormalities	XPA through XPG	AR	DNA nucleotide excision repair
Fanconi anemia	Acute myelogenous leukemia	Pancytopenia, skeletal abnormalities	FANCA-FANCC, FANCD1, FANCD2/BRCA2, FANCE-FANCL	AR	DNA crosslink repair
Tumor suppressor genes—gatekeepers and caretakers					
Familial breast cancer 1	Breast carcinoma	Ovarian carcinoma	BRCA1	AD	DNA double-strand break repair
Familial breast cancer 2	Breast carcinoma	Breast carcinoma in both males and females; pancreatic adenocarcinoma	BRCA2	AD	DNA double-strand break repair
Oncogenes					
Multiple endocrine neoplasia type 2	Medullary carcinoma of the thyroid	Type 2A: pheochromocytomas; parathyroid adenomas Type 2B: pheochromocytomas; mucosal hamartomas	c-ret	AD	Tyrosine kinase
Hereditary papillary renal cancer	Papillary renal cell carcinoma		c-met	AD	Transmembrane receptor

Syndrome	Representative tumors	Associated disease traits	Other tumors/polyps	Gene	Inheritance	Function
Hereditary gastrointestinal stromal tumor syndrome	Gastrointestinal stromal tumors	Cutaneous hyperpigmentation? Systemic mast cell disease?	Gastrointestinal stromal tumors	*KIT*	AD	Transmembrane tyrosine kinase
Peutz-Jeghers syndrome[b]	Wide variety of gastrointestinal carcinomas; extraintestinal cancers	Mucocutaneous melanin pigmentation; gastrointestinal polyposis		*LKB1*	AD	Serine/threonine kinase
Tuberous sclerosis[b]	Giant cell astrocytomas	Autism, mental retardation; multiple hamartomas of brain, kidneys, lungs, heart, and skin		*TSC1* *TSC2*	AD AD	Unknown Unknown
Genes with other functions						
Multiple colorectal adenomas	Colorectal adenocarcinoma		Duodenal polyps	*MYH*	AR	Base excision repair gene
Hereditary paraganglioma and pheochromocytoma	Paragangliomas and pheochromocytomas	Leigh syndrome		*SDHD* *SDHC* *SDHB*	AD AD AD	Components of the mitochondrial respiratory chain
Carney complex	Thyroid carcinoma; extracardiac myxomas; testis tumors	Cardiac myxomas	Pituitary adenomas, thyroid adenomas; benign breast adenomas	*PRKAR1α*	AD	Roll in cAMP pathway

[a]This listing is not exhaustive in that only representative tumors and disease traits are given for each cancer syndrome. In addition, for some syndromes (such as Cowden syndrome, Peutz-Jeghers syndrome, hereditary diffuse gastric cancer, and Carney complex, the most appropriate functional classification of the responsible gene remains uncertain (149, 250–253).
[b]One of the phakomatoses.
[c]The diagnosis of familial juvenile polyposis is only made when pathognomonic features of Peutz-Jeghers syndrome and Cowden syndrome are not present (251,252).
[d]Muir-Torre syndrome (Table 2.7) could also be included.
[e]Ataxia telangiectasia–like disorder and Nijmegan breakage syndrome (Table 2.7) could also be included.
[f]The related Werner and Rothmund-Thomson syndromes (Table 2.7) could also be included.
[g]The related diseases X-P variant, Cockayne syndrome, and trichothiodystophy (Table 2.7) could also be included.
AD, autosomal dominant; AR, autosomal recessive; CNS, central nervous system; XR, X-linked recessive.

TABLE 2.10

EXAMPLES OF ONCOGENES ASSOCIATED WITH HUMAN MALIGNANCIES

Oncogene	Associated Neoplasms	Genetic Abnormality
Nuclear protein family		
C-myc	Leukemias and lymphomas; stomach, breast, lung, and colon carcinomas	Translocation; gene amplification
N-myc	Neuroblastoma; rhabdomyosarcoma; lung carcinomas	Gene amplification
L-myc	Lung carcinomas	Gene amplification
c-myb	Colon and breast carcinomas; leukemias	Gene amplification
Guanine nucleotide exchange factors		
rgr	T-cell lymphomas	Rearrangement
Cytoplasmic serine/threonine kinases		
b-raf	Melanoma; thyroid, squamous cell, and colonic carcinomas	Point mutation
Tyrosine kinases (growth factor receptors)		
c-erbB (EGRF)	CNS tumors; renal cell, squamous cell, breast, and esophageal carcinomas	Amplification
NEU (HER2)	Neuroblastoma	Point mutation
	Breast carcinoma	Amplification
Tyrosine kinases (membrane associated)		
src	Colonic carcinomas	Point mutation
c-abl	CML; subset of ALL	Translocation
Membrane-associated GTPases		
H-ras	Colon, lung, pancreas, and bladder carcinomas	Point mutation
K-ras	Exocrine pancreas and bile-duct carcinomas	Point mutation
N-ras	Carcinomas; melanoma	Point mutation
Growth Factors		
int-2	Breast carcinoma	Proviral insertion
int-1	Breast carcinoma	Proviral insertion

CNS, central nervous system; CML, chronic myelogenous leukemia; ALL, acute lymphoblastic leukemia.

REFERENCES

1. Gupta RC, Lutz WK. Background DNA damage from endogenous and unavoidable exogenous carcinogens: a basis for spontaneous cancer incidence? *Mutat Res* 1999;424:1–8.
2. Kawanishi S, Hiraku Y, Murata M, et al. The role of metals in site-specific DNA damage with reference to carcinogenesis. *Free Radic Biol Med* 2002;32:822–832.
3. Dizdaroglu M, Jaruga P, Birincioglu M, et al. Free radical-induced damage to DNA: mechanisms and measurement. *Free Radic Biol Med* 2002;32:1102–1115.
4. Beesk F, Dizdaroglu M, Schulte-Frohlinde D, et al. Radiation-induced DNA strand breaks in deoxygenated aqueous solutions: the formation of altered sugars as end groups. *Int J Radiat Biol Relat Stud Phys Chem Med* 1979;36:565–576.
5. Kasprzak, KS. Oxidative DNA and protein damage in metal-induced toxicity and carcinogenesis. *Free Radic Biol Med* 2002;10:958–967.
6. Box HC, Dawidzik JB, Budzinski EE. Free radical-induced double lesions in DNA. *Free Radic Biol Med* 2001;31:856–868.
7. Dizdaroglu M, Gajewski E, Reddy P, et al. Structure of a hydroxyl radical induced DNA-protein cross-link involving thymine and tyrosine in nucleohistone. *Biochemistry* 1989;28:3625–3628.
8. Margolis S, Coxon B, Gajewski E, et al. Structure of a hydroxyl radical induced cross-link of thymine and tyrosine. *Biochemistry* 1988;27:6353–6359.
9. Chung FL, Nath RG, Nagao Minako et al. Endogenous formation and significance of 1,N²-propanodeoxyguanosine adducts. *Mutat Res* 1999; 424:71–81.
10. Anastassopoulou J, Theophanides T. Magnesium–DNA interactions and the possible relation of magnesium to carcinogenesis: irradiation and free radicals. *Crit Rev Oncol Hematol* 2002;42:79–91.
11. Halliwell B. Oxygen radicals and human disease. *Ann Intern Med* 1987;107;526–545.
12. Hartwig A. Role of DNA repair inhibition in lead- and cadmium-induced genotoxicity: a review. *Environ Health Perspect* 1994;102:45–50.

13. Hartwig A. Carcinogenicity of metal compounds: possible role of DNA repair inhibition. *Toxicol Lett* 1998;102–103:235–239.
14. Snyder RD, Lachmann PJ. Thiol involvement in the inhibition of DNA repair by metals in mammalian cells. *Mol Toxicol* 1989;2:117–128.
15. Jin YH, Clark AB, Slebos RJC, et al. Cadmium is a mutagen that acts by inhibiting mismatch repair. *Nat Genet* 2003;34:326–329.
16. McMurray CT, Tainer JA. Cancer, cadmium and genome integrity. *Nat Genet* 2003;34:239–241.
17. Guengerich FP. Common and uncommon cytochrome P450 reactions related to metabolism and chemical toxicity. *Chem Res Toxicol* 2001;14:611–650.
18. Pfeifer GP, Denissenko MF, Olivier M, et al. Tobacco smoke carcinogens, DNA damage and p53 mutations in smoking-associated cancers. *Oncogene* 2002;21:7435–7451.
19. Poirer MC. Chemical-induced DNA damage and human cancer risk. *Nat Rev Cancer* 2004;4:630–637.
20. Pryor WA. Cigarette smoke radicals and the role of free radicals in chemical carcinogenicity. *Environ Health Perspect* 1997;105(suppl 4):875–882.
21. Arora A, Willhite CA, Liebler D. Interactions of β-carotene and cigarette smoke in human bronchial epithelial cells. *Carcinogenesis* 2001;22:1173–1178.
22. Tang D, Phillips DH, Stampfer M, et al. Association between carcinogen-DNA adducts in white blood cells and lung cancer risk in the physicians health study. *Cancer Res* 2001;61:6708–6712.
23. Sanderson BJ, Shield AJ. Mutagenic damage to mammalian cells by therapeutic alkylating agents. *Mutat Res* 1996;355:41–57.
24. Kartalou M, Essigmann JM. Recognition of cisplatin adducts by cellular proteins. *Mutat Res* 2001;478:1–21.
25. de Gruijl FR. Photocarcinogenesis: UVA vs. UVB radiation. *Skin Pharmacol Appl Skin Physiol* 2002;15:316–320.
26. Henner WD, Rodriguez LO, Hecht SM. γ Ray induced deoxyribonucleic acid strand breaks: 3′ glycolate termini. *J Biol Chem* 1983;258:711–713.

27. Dizdaroglu M, von Sonntag C, Schulte-Frohlinde D. Letter: Strand breaks and sugar release by gamma-irradiation of DNA in aqueous solution. *J Am Chem Soc* 1975;97:2277–2278.
28. Ward JF. Radiation mutagenesis: the initial DNA lesions responsible. *Radiat Res* 1995;142:362–368.
29. Little JB. Radiation carcinogenesis. *Carcinogenesis* 2000;21:397–404.
30. Rydberg B. Radiation-induced DNA damage and chromatin structure. *Acta Oncol* 2001;40:682–685.
31. Ward JF. Symposium on radical processes in radiobiology and carcinogenesis. *Radiat Res* 1981;86:185–195.
32. Millard JT. DNA modifying agents as tools for studying chromatin structure. *Biochimie* 1996;78:803–816.
33. Mendell JT, Dietz HC. When the message goes awry: disease-producing mutations that influence mRNA content and performance. *Cell* 2001;107:411–414.
34. Antonorakis SE, Krawczak M, Cooper DN. The nature and mechanisms of human gene mutation. In: Scriver CR, et al., eds. *Metabolic and Molecular Bases of Inherited Disease*, 8th ed. New York: McGraw-Hill; 2001;343–377.
35. Kunkel TA, Bebenek K. DNA replication fidelity. *Annu Rev Biochem* 2000;69:497–529.
36. Kunkel TA, Alexander PS. The base substitution fidelity of eukaryotic DNA polymerases. *J Biol Chem* 1986;261:160–166.
37. Burrows NP, Nicholls AC, Richards AJ, et al. A point mutation in an intronic branch site results in aberrant splicing of COL5A1 and in Ehlers-Danlos syndrome type II in two British families. *Am J Hum Genet* 1998;63:390–398.
38. Liu HX, Cartegni L, Zhang MQ, et al. A mechanism for exon skipping caused by non-sense or missense mutations in *BRCA1* and other genes. *Nat Genet* 2001;27:55–58.
39. Maquat LE. The power of point mutations. *Nat Genet* 2001;27:5–6.
40. Longley MJ, Nguyen D, Kunkel TA, et al. The fidelity of human DNA polymerase gamma with and without exonucleolytic proofreading and the p55 accessory subunit. *J Biol Chem* 2001;276:38555–38562.
41. Krawczak M, Reiss J, Cooper DN. The mutational spectrum of single base-pair substitutions in mRNA splice junctions of human genes: causes and consequences. *Hum Genet* 1992;90:41–54.
42. Guil S, Darzynkiewicz E, Bach-Elias M. Study of the 2719 mutant of the c-H-ras oncogene in a bi-intronic alternative splicing system. *Oncogene* 2002;21:5649–5653.
43. Mitchell GA, Labuda D, Fontaine G, et al. Splice-mediated insertion of an Alu sequence inactivates ornithine δ-aminotransferase: a role for Alu elements in human mutation. *Proc Natl Acad Sci USA* 1991;88:815–819.
44. Cartegni L, Chew SL, Krainer AR. Listening to silence and understanding nonsense: exonic mutations that affect splicing. *Nat Rev Genet* 2002;3:285–298.
45. Nishimura H, Yerkes E, Hohenfellner, et al. Role of the angiotensin type 2 receptor gene in congenital anomalies of the kidney and urinary tract, CAKUT, of mice and men. *Mol Cell* 1999;3:1–10.
46. Brand K, Dugi KA, Brunzell JD, et al. A novel A→G mutation in intron I of the hepatic lipase gene leads to alternative splicing resulting in enzyme deficiency. *J Lipid Res* 1996;37:1213–1223.
47. Hsu BY, Iacobazzi V, Wang Z, et al. Aberrant mRNA splicing associated with coding region mutations in children with carnitine-acylcarnitine translocase deficiency. *Mol Genet Metab* 2001;74:248–255.
48. Kuivenhoven JA, Weibusch H, Pritchard PH, et al. An intronic mutation in a lariat branchpoint sequence is a direct cause of an inherited human disorder (fish-eye disease). *J Clin Invest* 1996;98:358–364.
49. Zhu X, Chung I, O'Gorman, et al. Coexpression of normal and mutated CD40 ligand with deletion of a putative RNA lariat branchpoint sequence in X-linked hyper-IgM syndrome. *Clin Immunol* 2001;99:334–339.
50. Janssen RJ, Wevers RA, Haussler M, et al. A branch site mutation leading to aberrant splicing of the human tyrosine hydroxylase gene in a child with a severe extrapyramidal movement disorder. *Ann Hum Genet* 2000;64:375–382.
51. Fujimaru M, Tanaka A, Choeh K, et al. Two mutations remote from an exon/intron junction in the beta-hexosaminidase beta-subunit gene affect 3′-splice site selection and cause Sandhoff disease. *Hum Genet* 1998;103:462–469.
52. Wilkinson MF, Shyu AB. Multifunctional regulatory proteins that control gene expression in both the nucleus and the cytoplasm. *Bioessays* 2001;23:775–787.
53. Antonarakis SE, Krawczak M, Cooper DN. The nature and mechanisms of human gene mutation. In: Vogelstein B, Kuzler KW, eds. *The Genetic Basis of Human Cancer*. New York: McGraw-Hill; 2002;7–41.
54. Wong C, Dowling CE, Kaiki RJ, et al. Characterization of β-thalassaemia mutations using direct genomic sequencing of amplified single copy DNA. *Nature* 1987,330:384–386.
55. Culbertson MR. RNA surveillance: unforeseen consequences for gene expression, inherited genetic disorders and cancer. *Trends Genet* 1999;15:74–80.
56. Wang, J, Gudikote JP, Olivas OR, et al. Boundary-independent polar nonsense-mediated decay. *EMBO Rep* 2002;3:274–279.
57. Wilkinson MF, Shyu AB. RNA surveillance by nuclear scanning? *Nat Cell Biol* 2002;4:E144–E147.
58. Hentze MW, Kulozik AE. A perfect message: RNA surveillance and nonsense-mediated decay. *Cell* 1999;96:307–310.
59. Treistman R, Orkin SH, Maniatis T. Specific transcription and RNA splicing defects in five cloned β-thalassaemia genes. *Nature* 1983;302:591–596.
60. Martin DI, Tsai SF, Orkin SH. Increased γ-globin expression in a nondeletion HPFH mediated by an erythroid-specific DNA-binding factor. *Nature* 1989;338:435–438.
61. Flavell RA, Kooter JM, DeBoer E, et al. Analysis of the δβ globin gene loci in normal and Hb Lepore DNA: direct determination of gene linkage and intergene distance. *Cell* 1978;15:25–41.
62. Tanigawa G, Jarcho JA, Kass S, et al. A molecular basis for familial hypertrophic cardiomyopathy: an α/β cardiac myosin heavy chain hybrid gene. *Cell* 1990;62:991–998.
63. Nathans J, Piantanida TP, Eddy RL, et al. Molecular genetics of inherited variation in human color vision. *Science* 1986;232:203–210.
64. Smit AF. The origin of interspersed repeats in the human genome. *Curr Opin Gen Dev* 1996;6:743–748.
65. Lander ES, Linton LM, Birren B, et al. Initial sequencing and analysis of the human genome. *Nature* 2001;409:860–921.
66. Kolomietz E, Meyn S, Pandita A, et al. The role of *Alu* repeat clusters as mediators of recurrent chromosomal aberrations in tumors. *Genes Chromosomes Cancer* 2002; 35:97–112.
67. Petrij-Bosch A, Peelen T, van Vliet M, et al. *BRCA1* genomic deletions are major founder mutatins in Dutch breast cancer patients. *Nat Genet* 1997;17:341–345.
68. Van de Water N, Williams R, Ockelford P, et al. A 20.7 kb deletion within the factor VIII gene associated with LINE-1 element insertion. *Thromb Haemost* 1998;79:938–942.
69. Li X, Scaringe WA, Hill KA, et al. Frequency of recent retrotransposition events in the human factor IX gene. *Hum Mutat* 2001;17:511–519.
70. Shapiro LJ, Yen P, Pomerantz D, et al. Molecular studies of deletions at the human steroid sulfatase locus. *Proc Natl Acad Sci USA* 1989;86:8477–8881.
71. Yen PH, Li XM, Tsai SP, et al. Frequent deletions of the human X chromosome distal short arm result from recombination between low copy repetitive elements. *Cell* 1990;61:603–610.
72. Pizzuti A, Pieretti M, Fenwick RG, et al. A transposon-like element in the deletion-prone region of the dystrophin gene. *Genomics* 1992;13:594–600.
73. Shaihk TH, Kurahashi H, Emanuel BS. Evolutionarily conserved low copy repeats (LCRs) in 22q11 mediate deletions, duplications, translocations, and genomic instability: an update and literature review. *Genet Med* 2001;3:6–13.
74. Emanuel BS, Shaikh TH. Segmental duplications: an "expanding" role in genomic instability and disease. *Nat Rev Genet* 2001;2:791–800.
75. Zucman-Rossi J, Legoix P, Victor JM, et al. Chromosome translocation based on illegitimate recombination of human tumors. *Proc Natl Acad Sci USA* 1998;95:11786–11791.
76. Roix J, McQueen PG, Munson PJ, et al. Spatial proximity of translocation-prone gene loci in human lymphomas. *Nat Genet* 2003;34:287–291.
77. Parada L, McQueen P, Munson P, et al. Conservation of relative chromosome positioning in normal and cancer cells. *Curr Biol* 2002;12:1692–1697.
78. Pederson T. Gene territories and cancer. *Nat Genet* 2003;34:242–243.
79. Collier S, Tassabehji M, Strachan T. A *de novo* pathological point mutation at the 21-hydroxylase locus: implications for gene conversion in the human genome. *Nat Genet* 1993;3:260–265.
80. Sinnott P, Collier S, Costigan C, et al. Genesis by meiotic unequal crossover of a *de novo* deletion that contributes to steroid 21-hydroxylase deficiency. *Proc Natl Acad Sci USA* 1990;87:2107–2111.
81. Levinson G, Gutman GA. Slipped-strand mispairing: a major mechanism for DNA sequence evolution. *Mol Biol Evol* 1987;4:203–221.
82. Kunkel TA. The mutational specificity of DNA polymerase-β during in vitro DNA synthesis. *J Biol Chem* 1985;260:5787.
83. Huang Q, Xu F, Shen H. Mutation patterns at dinucleotide microsatellite loci in humans. *Am J Hum Genet* 2002;70:625–634.
84. Schlotterer C. Evolutionary dynamics of microsatellite DNA. *Chromosoma* 2000; 109:365–371.
85. Shoffner JM, Lott MT, Voljavec AS, et al. Spontaneous Kearns-Sayre/chronic external ophthalmoplegia plus syndrome associated with a mitochondrial DNA deletion: a slip-replication model and metabolic therapy. *Proc Natl Acad Sci USA* 1989;86: 7952–7956.
86. Ripley LS. Model for the participation of quasi-palindromic DNA sequences in frameshift mutation. *Proc Natl Acad Sci USA* 1982;79:4128–4132.
87. Ostertag EM, Kazazian Jr, HH. Biology of mammalian L1 retrotransposons. *Annu Rev Genet* 2001;35:501–538.
88. Miki Y, Katagiri T, Kusumi F, et al. Mutation analysis in the *BRCA2* gene in primary breast cancers. *Nat Genet* 1996;13:245–247.
89. Kazazian HH, Wong C, Youssoufian H, et al. Haemophilia A resulting from *de novo* insertion of L1 sequences represents a novel mechanism for mutation in man. *Nature* 1988;332:164–166.
90. Sukarova E, Dimovski AJ, Tchacarova P, et al. An *alu* insert as the cause of a severe form of hemophilia A. *Acta Haematol* 2001;106:126–129.
91. Suminaga R, Takeshima Y, Yasuda K, et al. Non-homologous recombination between *Alu* and LINE-1 repeats caused a 430-kb deletion in the dystrophin gene: a novel source of genomic instability. *J Hum Genet* 2000;45:331–336.
92. Wallace MR, Anderson B, Saulina AM, et al. A *de novo Alu* insertion results in neurofibromatosis type 1. *Nature* 1991;353:864–866.
93. Meischl C, de Boer M, Åhlin A, et al. A new exon created by intronic insertion of a rearranged LINE-1 element as the cause of chronic granulomatous disease. *Eur J Hum Genet* 2000;8:697–703.
94. Lutskiy MI, Jones LN, Rosen RS, et al. An *Alu*-mediated deletion at Xp11.23 leading to Wiskott-Aldrich syndrome. *Hum Genet* 2002;110:515–519.
95. Halling KC, Lazzaro CR, Honchel R, et al. Hereditary desmoid disease in a family with a germline *Alu* I repeat mutation of the APC gene. *Hum Hered* 1999;49:97–102.
96. Hagerman RJ, Hagerman PJ. The fragile X permutation: into the phenotypic fold. *Curr Opin Genet Dev* 2002;12:278–283.
97. Lalioti MD, Scott HS, Buresi C, et al. Dodecamer repeat expansion in cystatin B gene in progressive myoclonus epilepsy. *Nature* 1997;386:847–851.
98. Matsuura T, Yamagata T, Burgess DL, et al. Large expansion of the ATTCT pentanucleotide repeat in spinocerebellar ataxia type 10. *Nat Genet* 2000;26:191–194.
99. Cummings CJ, Zoghbi HY. Fourteen and counting: unraveling trinucleotide repeat diseases. *Hum Mol Genet* 2000;9:909–916.
100. Brais B, Bouchard JP, Xie YG, et al. Short GCG expansions in the PABP2 gene cause oculopharyngeal muscular dystrophy. *Nat Genet* 1998;18:164–167.
101. Muragaki Y, Mundlos S, Upton J, et al. Altered growth and branching patterns in synpolydactyly caused by mutations in HOXD13. *Science* 1996;272:548–551.
102. Oostra BA, Willemsen R. Diagnostic tests for fragile X syndrome. *Expert Rev Mol Diagn* 2001;1:226-232.
103. Willemsen R, Bontekoe CJ, Severijnen LA, et al. Timing of the absence of FMR1 expression in full mutation chorionic villi. *Hum Genet* 2002;110:601–605.
104. Stoppa-Lyonnet D, Duponchel C, Meo T, et al. Recombinational biases in the rearranged C1-inhibitor genes of hereditary angioedema patients. *Am J Hum Genet* 1991;49:1055–1062.
105. Tiller GE, Rimoin DL, Murray LW, et al. Tandem duplication within a type II collagen gene (COL2A1) exon in an individual with spondyloepiphyseal dysplasia. *Proc Natl Acad Sci USA* 1990;87:3889–3893.

106. Stoppa-Lyonnet D, Carter PE, Meo T, et al. Clusters of intragenic *Alu* repeats predispose the human C1 inhibitor locus to deleterious rearrangements. *Proc Natl Acad Sci USA* 1990;87:1551–1555.
107. Hu X, Ray PN, Worton RG. Mechanisms of tandem duplication in the Duchenne muscular dystrophy gene include both homologous and nonhomologous intrachromosomal recombination. *EMBO J* 1999;10:2471–2477.
108. Kornreich R, Bishop RF, Desnick RJ. Alpha-galactosidase A gene rearrangements causing Fabry disease: identification of short direct repeats at breakpoints in an *Alu*-rich gene. *J Biol Chem* 1990;265:9319–9326.
109. Bullock P, Champoux JJ, Botchan M. Association of crossover points with topoisomerase I cleavage sites: a model for non-homologous recombination. *Science* 1985;230:954–958.
110. Karathanasis SK, Ferris E, Haddad IA. DNA inversion within the apolipoproteins AI/CIII/AIV-encoding gene cluster of certain patients with premature atherosclerosis. *Proc Natl Acad Sci USA* 1987;84:7198–7202.
111. de Chadarevian JP, Dunn S, Malatack JJ, et al. Chromosome rearrangement with no apparent gene mutation in familial adenomatous polyposis and hepatocellular neoplasia. *Pediatr Dev Pathol* 2002;5:69–75.
112. Wagner A, van der Klift H, Wijnen FP. A 10-Mb paracentric inversion of chromosome arm 2p inactivates MSH2 and is responsible for hereditary nonpolyposis colorectal cancer in a North-American kindred. *Genes Chromosomes Cancer* 2002;35:49–57.
113. Kaneko Y, Kobayashi H, Handa M, et al. EWS-ERG fusion transcript produced by chromosomal insertion in a Ewing sarcoma. *Genes Chromosomes Cancer* 1997;18:228–231.
114. Lakich D, Kazazian Jr. HH, Antonarakis SE, et al. Inversions disrupting the factor VIII gene are a common cause of severe haemophilia A. *Nat Genet* 1993;5:236–241.
115. Bowen DJ. Haemophila A and haemophilia B: molecular insights. *Mol Pathol* 2002;55:1–18.
116. Bassing CH, Alt FW. Molecular biology: case of mistaken identity. *Nature* 2004;428: 29–31.
117. Raghavan SC, Swanson PC, Wu X, et al. A non-B-DNA structure at the Bcl-2 major breakpoint region is cleaved by the RAG complex. *Nature* 2004;428:88–93.
118. Richter C, Park JW, Ames BN. Normal oxidative damage to mitochondrial and nuclear DNA is extensive. *Proc Natl Acad Sci USA* 1988;85:6465–6467.
119. Wei YH, Lee HC. Oxidative stress, mitochondrial DNA mutation, and impairment of antioxidant enzymes in aging. *Exp Biol Med* 2002;227:671–682.
120. Marin-Garcia J, Goldenthal MJ, Sarnat HB. Kearns-Sayre syndrome with a novel mitochondrial DNA deletion. *J Child Neurol* 2000;15:555–558.
121. Musumeci O, Andreu AL, Ahanski S, et al. Intragenic inversion of mtDNA: a new type of pathogenic mutation in a patient with mitochondrial myopathy. *Am J Hum Genet* 2000;66:1900–1904.
122. Seneca S, Verhelst H, Meire F, et al. A new mitochondrial point mutation in the transfer RNA(Leu) gene in a patient with a clinical phenotype resembling Kearns-Sayre syndrome. *Arch Neurol* 2001;58:1113–1118.
123. Rachek LI, Grishko VI, Musiyenko SI, et al. Conditional targeting of the DNA repair enzyme hOGG1 into mitochondria. *J Biol Chem* 2002;277:44932–44937.
124. Zeviani M, Moraes CT, DiMauro S, et al. Deletions of mitochondrial DNA in Kearns-Sayre syndrome. *Neurology* 1988;38:1339–1346.
125. Awadalla P, Eyre-Walker A, Smith JM. Linkage disequilibrium and recombination in hominid mitochondrial DNA. *Science* 1999;286:2524–2525.
126. Kivisid T, Villems R, Jorde LB, et al. Questioning evidence for recombination in human mitochondrial DNA: technical comments. *Science* 2000;288:1931a.
127. Eyre-Walker A, Awadalla P. Does human mtDNA recombine? *J Mol Evol* 2001;53: 430–435.
128. Poulton J, Holt IJ. Mitochondrial DNA: does more lead to less? *Nat Genet* 1994;8:313–315.
129. Hoeijmakers JH. Genome maintenance mechanisms for preventing cancer. *Nature* 2001;411:366–374.
130. Tuteka M, Tuteka R. Unraveling DNA repair in human: molecular mechanisms and consequences of repair defect. *Crit Rev Biochem Mol Biol* 2001;36:261–90.
131. Bohr, VA. DNA damage and its processing: relation to human disease. *J Inherit Metab Dis* 2002;25:215–222.
132. Friedberg EC. DNA damage and repair. *Nature* 2003;421:436–440.
133. Ronen A, Glickman BW. Human DNA repair genes. *Environ Mol Mutagen* 2001;37:241–283.
134. Gerson SL. MGMT: its role in cancer aetiology and cancer therapeutics. *Nat Rev Cancer* 2004;4:296–307.
135. Begley TJ, Samson LD. Molecular biology: a fix for RNA. *Nature* 2003;421:795–796.
136. Aas PA, Otterlei M, Falnes PO, et al. Human and bacterial oxidative demethylases repair alkylation damage in both RNA and DNA. *Nature* 2003;421:859–863.
137. Sancar A. Structure and function of DNA photolyase. *Biochemistry* 1994;33:2–9.
138. van der Horst GT, Muijtjens M, Kobayashi K, et al. Mammalian Cry1 and Cry2 are essential for maintenance of circadian rhythms. *Nature* 1999;398:627–630.
139. Memisoglu A, Samson L. Base excision repair in yeast and mammals. *Mutat Res* 2000;451:39–51.
140. Cadet J, Bourdat AG, D'Ham C, et al. Oxidative base damage to DNA: specificity of base excision repair enzymes. *Mutat Res* 2000;462:121–128.
141. Frosina G, Fortini P, Rossi O, et al. Two pathways for base excision repair in mammalian cells. *J Biol Chem* 1996;271:9573–9578.
142. Al-Tassan N, Chmiel NH, Maynard J, et al. Inherited variants of MYH associated with somatic G:C→T:A mutations in colorectal tumors. *Nat Genet* 2002;30:227–232.
143. Jones S, Emmerson P, Maynard J, et al. Biallelic germline mutations in MYH predispose to multiple colorectal adenoma and somatic G:C→T:A mutations. *Hum Mol Genet* 2002;11:2961–2967.
144. Sieber OM, Lipton L, Crabtree M, et al. Multiple colorectal adenomas, classic adenomatous polyposis, and germ-line mutations in MYH. *N Engl J Med* 2003;348:791–799.
145. de Boer J, Joeijmakers HJ. Nucleotide excision repair and human syndromes. *Carcinogenesis* 2000;21:453–460
146. Shcherbakova PV, Bebenek K, Kunkel TA. Functions of eukaryotic DNA polymerases. Science's SAGE KE; http://sageke.sciencemag.org/cgi/content/full/sageke;2003/8/re3.
147. Levitt NC, Hickson ID. Caretaker tumour suppressor genes that defend genome integrity. *Trends Mol Med* 2002;8:179–186.
148. Cromie GA, Connelly JC, Leach. Recombination at double-strand breaks and DNA ends: conserved mechanisms from phage to humans. *Mol Cell* 2001;8:1163–1174.
149. Marsh DJ, Zori RT. Germline PTEN mutation in a family with Cowden syndrome and Bannayan-Riley-Ruvalcaba syndrome. *Am J Med Genet* 1998;80:399–402.
150. Hanks S, Coleman K, Reid S, et al. Constitutional aneuploidy and cancer predisposition caused by biallelic mutations in BUB1B. *Nat Genet* 2004;36:1159–1161.
151. Brooks PJ. DNA repair in neural cells: basic science and clinical implications. *Mutat Res* 2002;509:93–108.
152. Bootsma D, Kraemer KH, Cleaver JE, et al. Nucleotide excision repair syndromes: xeroderma pigmentosum, Cockayne syndrome, and trichothiodystrophy. In: Vogelstein B, Kinzler KW, eds. *The Genetic Basis of Human Cancer*, 2nd ed. New York: McGraw-Hill; 2002:211–237.
153. Coin F, Bergmann E, Tremeau-Bravard A, et al. Mutations in XPB and XPD helicases found in xeroderma pigmentosum patients impair the transcription function of TFIIH. *EMBO J.* 1999;18:1357–1366.
154. Vermeulen W, van Vuuren AJ, Chipoulet M, et al. Three unusual repair deficiencies associated with transcription factor BTF2(TFIIH): evidence for the existence of a transcription syndrome. *Cold Spring Harb Symp Quant Biol* 1994;59:317–329.
155. Bergmann E, Egly JM. Trichothiodystrophy, a transcription syndrome. *Trends Genet* 2001;17:279–286.
156. Ljungman M, Lane DP. Transcription: guarding the genome by sensing DNA damage. *Nat Rev Cancer* 2004;4:727–737.
157. van den Boom V, Jaspers NG, Vermeulen W. When machines get stuck: obstructed RNA polymerase II—displacement, degradation or suicide. *Bioessays* 2002; 24: 780–784.
158. Svejstrup JQ. Mechanisms of transcription-coupled DNA repair. *Nat Rev Mol Cell Biol* 2002;3:21–29.
159. Hanawalt PC. Subpathways of nucleotide excision repair and their regulation. *Oncogene* 2002,21:8949–8956.
160. Müller A, Fishel R. Mismatch repair and the hereditary non-polyposis colorectal cancer syndrome (HNPCC). *Cancer Invest* 2002;20:102–109.
161. Jiricny J, Nystrom-Lahti M. Mismatch repair defects in cancer. *Curr Opin Genet Dev* 2000;10:157–161.
162. Peltomaki P. DNA mismatch repair and cancer. *Mutat Res* 2001;488:77–85.
163. de la Chapelle A. Microsatellite instability. *N Engl J Med* 2003;349:209–210.
164. Fujiwara T, Stolker JM, Watanabe T, et al. Accumulated clonal genetic alterations in familial and sporadic colorectal carcinomas with widespread instability in microsatellite sequences. *Am J Pathol* 1998;153:1063–1078.
165. Guo G, Wang W, Bradley A. Mismatch repair genes identified using genetic screens in Blm-deficient embryonic stem cells. *Nature* 2004;429:891–895.
166. Boland CR. Hereditary nonpolyposis colorectral cancer (HNPCC). In: Vogelstein B, Kinzler KW, eds. *The Genetic Basis of Human Cancer*, 2nd ed. New York: McGraw-Hill; 2002:307–321.
167. Thomas DC, Roberts JD, Sabatino RD, et al. Fidelity of mammalian DNA replication and replicative DNA polymerases. *Biochemistry* 1991;30:11751–11759.
168. Goodman MF. Error-prone repair DNA polymerases in prokaryotes and eukaryotes. *Annu Rev Biochem* 2002;71:17–50.
169. Hubscher U, Maga G, Spadar S. Eukaryotic DNA polymerases. *Annu Rev Biochem* 2002;71:133–163.
170. Pages V, Fuchs RP. How DNA lesions are turned into mutations within cells. *Oncogene* 2002;21:8957–8966.
171. Lehmann AR. Replication of damaged DNA in mammalian cells: new solutions to an old problem. *Mutat Res* 2002;509:23–34.
172. Matsuda T, Bebenek K, Masutani C, et al. Error rate and specificity of human and murine DNA polymerase η. *J Mol Biol* 2001;312:335–346.
173. Zhang Y, Yuan F, Xin H, et al. Human DNA polymerase κ synthesizes DNA with extraordinarily low fidelity. *Nucleic Acids Res* 2000;28:4147–4156.
174. Nair DT, Johnson RE, Prakash S, et al. Replication by human DNA polymerase-iota occurs by Hoogsteen base-pairing. *Nature* 2004;430:377–380.
175. McCulloch SD, Kokoska RJ, Masutani C, et al. Preferential cis-syn thymine dimer bypass by DNA polymerase eta occurs with biased fidelity. *Nature* 2004;428:97–100.
176. Masutani C, Kusumoto R, Yamada A, et al. The XPV (xeroderma pigmentosum variant) gene encodes human DNA polymerase η. *Nature* 1999;399:700–704.
177. Johnson RE, Kondratick CM, Prakash S, et al. hRAD30 mutations in the variant form of xeroderma pigmentosum. *Science* 1999;285:263–265.
178. Thompson LH, Schild D. Homologous recombinational repair of DNA ensures mammalian chromosome stability. *Mutat Res* 2001;477:131–153.
179. Lowndes NF, Murguia JR. Sensing and responding to DNA damage. *Curr Opin Genet Dev* 2000;10:17–25.
180. Redon C, Pilch D, Rogakou E, et al. Histone H2A variants H2AX and H2AZ. *Curr Opin Genet Dev* 2002;12:162–169.
181. Zhou BB, Elledge SJ. The DNA damage response: putting checkpoints in perspective. *Nature* 2000;408:433–439.
182. Khanna RR, Jackson SP. DNA double-strand breaks: signaling, repair and the cancer connection. *Nature Genet* 2001;27:247–254.
183. Durocher D, Jackson SP. DNA-PK, ATM and ATR as sensors of DNA damage: variations on a theme? *Curr Opin Cell Biol* 2001;13:225–231.
184. Moggs JG, Grandi P, Quivy JP, et al. A CAF-1-PCNA-mediated chromatin assembly pathway triggered by sensing DNA damage. *Mol Cell Biol* 2000;20:1206–1218.
185. Zou L, Elledge SJ. Sensing DNA damage through ATRIP recognition of RPA-ssDNA complexes. *Science* 2003;300:1542–1548.
186. Iwabuchi K, Basu BP, Kysela B, et al. Potential role for 53BP1 in DNA end-joining repair through direct interaction with DNA. *J Biol Chem* 2003;278:36487–36495.
187. Huyen Y, Zgheib O, Ditullio RA Jr, et al. Methylated lysine 79 of histone H3 targets 53BP1 to DNA double-strand breaks. *Nature* 2004;432:406–411.
188. Karran P. DNA double strand break repair in mammalian cells. *Curr Opin Genet Dev* 2000;10:144–150.
189. Davies AA, Masson JY, McIlwraith MJ, et al. Role of *BRCA2* in control of the RAD51 recombination and DNA repair protein. *Mol Cell* 2001;7:273–282.
190. Venkitaraman AR. Cancer susceptibility and the functions of *BRCA1* and *BRCA2*. *Cell* 2002;108:171–182.

191. D'Andrea AD, Grompe M. The Fanconi anaemia/BRCA pathway. *Nat Rev Cancer* 2003;3:23–34.

192. McHugh PJ, Spanswick VJ, Hartley JA. Repair of DNA interstrand crosslinks: molecular mechanisms and clinical relevance. *Lancet Oncol* 2001;2:483–490.

193. Wang X, Peterson CA, Zheng H, et al. Involvement of nucleotide excision repair in a recombination-independent and error-prone pathway of DNA interstrand cross-link repair. *Mol Cell Biol* 2001;21:713–720.

194. Bessho T, Mu D, Sancar A. Initiation of DNA interstrand cross-link repair in humans: the nucleotide excision repair system makes dual incisions 5′ to the cross-linked base and removes a 22- to 28-nucleotide-long damage-free strand. *Mol Cell Biol* 1997;17:6822–6830.

195. De Silva IU, McHugh PJ, Clingen PH, et al. Defining the roles of nucleotide excision repair and recombination in the repair of DNA interstrand cross-links in mammalian cells. *Mol Cell Biol* 2000;20:7980–7990.

196. Akkani YM, Bateman RL, Reifsteck CA, et al. DNA replication is required to elicit cellular responses to psoralen-induced DNA interstrand cross-links. *Mol Cell Biol* 2000;20:8283–8289.

197. Thompson LH, Schild D. Recombinational DNA repair and human disease. *Mutat Res* 2002;509:49–78.

198. Gatti RA. Ataxia-telangiectasia. In: Vogelstein B, Kinzler KW, eds. *The Genetic Basis of Human Cancer*, 2nd ed. New York: McGraw-Hill; 2002:239–266.

199. Savitsky K, Bar-Shira A, Gilad S, et al. A single ataxia telangiectasia gene with a product similar to PI-3 kinase. *Science* 1995;268:1749–1753.

200. Rotman G, Shiloh Y. ATM: from gene to function. *Hum Mol Genet* 1998;7:1555–1563.

201. Kastan MB, Lim D, Kim S, et al. ATM—a key determinant of multiple cellular responses to irradiation. *Acta Oncol* 2001;40:686–688.

202. Lee JH, Paull TT. Direct activation of the ATM protein kinase by the Mre11/Rad50/Nbs1 complex. *Science* 2004;304:93–96.

203. Vorechovsky I, Luo L, Dyer MJ, et al. Clustering of missense mutatins in the ataxia-telangiectasia gene in a sporadic T-cell leukaemia. *Nat Genet* 1997;17:96–99.

204. Yuille MA, Coignet LJ, Abraham SM, et al. ATM is usually rearranged in T-cell prolymphocytic leukaemia. *Oncogene* 1998;16:789–796.

205. Carney JP, Maser RS, Olivares, et al. The hMre11/hRad50 protein complex and Nijmegen breakage syndrome: linkage of double-strand break repair to the cellular DNA damage response. *Cell* 1998;93:477–486.

206. Varon R, Vissinga C, Platzer M, et al. Nibrin, a novel DNA double-strand break repair protein, is mutated in Nijmegen breakage syndrome. *Cell* 1998;93:467–476.

207. Grompe M, D'Andrea A. Fanconi anemia and DNA repair. *Hum Mol Genet* 2001;10:2253–2259.

208. Meetei AR, Levitus M, Xue Y, et al. X-linked inheritance of Fanconi anemia complementation group B. *Nat Genet* 2004;36:1219–1224.

209. Rahman N, Ashworth A. A new gene on the X involved in Fanconi anemia. *Nat Genet* 2004;36:1142–1143.

210. Daniels MJ, Wang Y, Lee M, et al. Abnormal cytokinesis in cells deficient in the breast cancer susceptibility protein BRCA2. *Science* 2004;306:876–879.

211. Turner N, Tutt A, Ashworth A. Hallmarks of 'BRCAness' in sporadic cancers. *Nat Rev Cancer* 2004;4:814–819.

212. Narod SA, Foulkes WD. BRCA1 and BRCA2: 1994 and beyond. *Nat Rev Cancer* 2004;4:665–676.

213. Venkitaraman AR. Tracing the network connecting BRCA and Fanconi anaemia proteins. *Nat Rev Cancer* 2004;4:266–276.

214. Enomoto T. Functions of RecQ family helicases: possible involvement of Bloom's and Werner's syndrome gene products in guarding genome integrity during DNA replication. *J Biochem (Tokyo)* 2001;129:501–507.

215. Mohagheg P, Hickson ID. Premature aging in RecQ helicase-deficient human syndromes. *Int J Biochem Cell Biol* 2002;34:1496–1501.

216. Schellenberg GD, Miki T, Yu C, et al. Werner syndrome. In: Vogelstein B, Kinzler KW, eds. *The Genetic Basis of Human Cancer*, 2nd ed, New York: McGraw-Hill; 2002:323–335.

217. German J, Ellis NA. Bloom syndrome. In: Vogelstein B, Kinzler KW, eds. *The Genetic Basis of Human Cancer*, 2nd ed, New York: McGraw-Hill; 2002:267–288.

218. Wang LL, Gannavarapu A, Kozinetz CA, et al. Association between osteosarcoma and deleterious mutations in the RECQL4 gene in Rothmund-Thomson syndrome. *J Natl Cancer Inst* 2003;95:669–674.

219. Hickson ID. RecQ helicases: caretakers of the genome. *Nat Rev Cancer* 2003;3:169–178.

220. Wu L, Hickson ID. The Bloom's syndrome helicase suppresses crossing over during homologous recombination. *Nature* 2003;426:870–874.

221. Shen JC, Loeb LA. The Werner syndrome gene: the molecular basis of RecQ helicase-deficiency diseases. *Trends Genet* 2000;16:213–220.

222. Brosh RM Jr, Bohr VA. Roles of the Werner syndrome protein in pathways required for maintenance of genome stability. *Exp Gerontol* 2002;37:491–506.

223. Crabbe L, Verdun RE, Haggblom CI, et al. Defective telomere lagging strand synthesis in cells lacking WRN helicase activity. *Science* 2004;306:1951–1953.

224. Fishel ML, Seo YR, Smith ML, et al. Imbalancing the DNA base excision repair pathway in the mitochondria; targeting and overexpressing N-methylpurine DNA glycosylase in mitochondria leads to enhanced cell killing. *Cancer Res* 2003;63:608–615.

225. Agostino A, Valletta L, Chinnery PF, et al. Mutations of ANT1, Twinkle, and POLG1 in sporadic progressive external ophthalmoplegia (PEO). *Neurology* 2003;60:1354–1356.

226. Del Bo R, Bordoni A, Sciacco M, et al. Remarkable infidelity of polymerase gammaA associated with mutations in POLG1 exonuclease domain. *Neurology* 2003;61:903–908.

227. Trifunovic A, Wredenberg A, Falkenberg M, et al. Premature ageing in mice expressing defective mitochondrial DNA polymerase. *Nature* 2004;429:417–423.

228. Szczesny B, Hazra TK, Papaconstantinou J, et al. Age-dependent deficiency in import of mitochondrial DNA glycosylases required for repair of oxidatively damaged bases. *Proc Natl Acad Sci USA* 2003;100:10670–10675.

229. Mason PA, Matheson EC, Hall AG, et al. Mismatch repair activity in mammalian mitochondria. *Nucleic Acids Res* 2003;31:1052–1058.

230. Crouteau DL, Bohr VA. Repair of oxidative damage to nuclear and mitochondrial DNA in mammalian cells. *J Biol Chem* 1997;272:25409–25412.

231. Snyderwine EG, Bohr VA. Gene- and strand-specific damage and repair in Chinese hamster ovary cells treated with 4-nitroquinoline 1-oxide. *Cancer Res* 1992;52:4183–4189.

232. LeDoux SP, Wilson GL, Beecham EJ, et al. Repair of mitochondrial DNA after various types of DNA damage in Chinese hamster ovary cells. *Carcinogenesis* 1992;13:1967–1973.

233. Fearon ER. Tumor-suppressor genes. In: Vogelstein B, Kinzler KW, ed. *The Genetic Basis of Human Cancer*, 2nd ed. New York: McGraw-Hill; 2002:197–206.

234. Reinartz JJ. Cancer genes. In: Coleman WB, Tsongalis GJ, eds. *The Molecular Basis of Human Cancer*. Totowa, NJ: Humana Press Inc., 2001:45–64.

235. Kinzler KW, Vogelstein B. Familial cancer syndromes: the role of caretakers and gatekeepers. In: Vogelstein B, Kinzler KW, ed. *The Genetic Basis of Human Cancer*, 2nd ed. New York: McGraw-Hill; 2002:209–210.

236. Attardi LD, DePinho RA. Conquering the complexity of p53. *Nat Genet* 2004;36:7–8.

237. Knudson AG. Two genetic hits (more or less) to cancer. *Nat Rev Cancer* 2001;1:157–162.

238. Knudson AG. Mutation and cancer: statistical study of retinoblastoma. *Proc Natl Acad Sci USA* 1971;68:820–823.

239. Knudson AG, Hethcote HW, Brown BW. Mutation and childhood cancer: a probabilistic model for the incidence of retinoblastoma. *Proc Natl Acad Sci USA* 1975;72:5116–5120.

240. Park M. Oncogenes. In: Vogelstein B, Kinzler KW, ed. *The Genetic Basis of Human Cancer*, 2nd ed. New York: McGraw-Hill; 2002:177–196.

241. Weinberg RA. Oncogenes, antioncogenes, and the molecular bases of multistep carcinogenesis. *Cancer Res* 1989;49:3713–3721.

242. Hunter T. Oncoprotein networks. *Cell* 1997;88:333–346.

243. Parada LF, Land H, Weinberg RA, et al. Cooperation between gene encoding p53 tumour antigen and ras in cellular transformation. *Nature* 1984;312:649–651.

244. Yancopoulos GD, Nisen PD, Tesfaye A, et al. N-myc can cooperate with ras to transform normal cells in culture. *Proc Natl Acad Sci USA* 1985;82:5455–5459.

245. Kinzler KW, Vogelstein B. Lessons from hereditary colorectal cancer. *Cell* 1996;87:159–170.

246. Sellers WR, Kaelin WG Jr. Role of the retinoblastoma protein in the pathogenesis of human cancer. *J Clin Oncol* 1997;15:3301–3312.

247. Hartwell LH, Weinert TA. Checkpoints: controls that ensure the order of cell cycle events. *Science* 1989;246:629–634.

248. Pardee AB. G1 events and regulation of cell proliferation. *Science* 1989;246:603–608.

249. Kerr JF, Winterford CM, Harmon BV. Apoptosis: its significance in cancer and cancer therapy. *Cancer* 1994;73:2013–2026.

250. Erickson RP. Somatic gene mutation and human disease other than cancer. *Mutat Res* 2003;543:125–136.

251. Hanna NN, Mentzer RM. Molecular genetics and management strategies in hereditary cancer syndromes. *J Ky Med Assoc* 2003;101:100–107.

252. Yoo LI, Chung DC, Yuan J. LKB1: a master tumour suppressor of the small intestine and beyond. *Nat Rev Cancer* 2002;2:529–535.

253. Fearon ER. Human cancer syndromes: clues to the origin and nature of cancer. *Science* 1997;278:1043–1050.

Cytogenetics

3

The publication of Flemming's illustrations of human chromosomes in 1882 (1) is generally considered to mark the beginning of the field of human cytogenetics. Although the chromosome theory of inheritance was proposed in the early 1900s (2,3), the first demonstration of a chromosomal abnormality associated with a specific phenotype did not occur until 1959, when it was shown that the fibroblasts of patients with Down syndrome harbor an extra chromosome (4). Despite the description of several other chromosomal syndromes in the 1960s (reviewed in 5), cytogenetic analysis was severely limited by the lack of techniques that could identify specific chromosomes or chromosomal regions. The observation that plant chromosomes stained with fluorescent quinacrine compounds harbored a series of bright and dull regions, and that each chromosome pair had a different banding pattern, therefore had a profound impact on the field (6). The staining technique was quickly adapted for use with human chromosomes, and in 1971 a unique banding pattern for each human chromosome pair was reported (7,8). The development of banding techniques marks the emergence of clinical human cytogenetics, because banding methods not only permit identification of each chromosome but also make it possible to detect specific alterations associated with hereditary syndromes and neoplasms.

TRADITIONAL CYTOGENETIC ANALYSIS

Cytogenetic analysis is used in three general clinical settings. The first setting is the evaluation of congenital disorders, in which analysis is used to diagnose syndromes associated with abnormalities of chromosomal number or structure, to establish the chromosomal sex in cases of sexual ambiguity, and to screen for karyotypic abnormalities in patients with multiple birth defects (9–11).

The second clinical setting in which cytogenetics is widely used is prenatal diagnosis. Analysis to determine the karyotype of a fetus can be performed beginning at the 10th to 12th week of gestation by chorionic villus sampling, or beginning at about the 16th week of gestation by amniocentesis. There are many indications for prenatal cytogenetic testing, including advanced maternal age,

presence of a chromosomal abnormality in either parent, identification of a fetal abnormality by ultrasonography, and presence of a chromosomal abnormality in one or more of the parents' previous children.

Third, cytogenetic studies are used in the evaluation of neoplastic disorders. For example, a number of specific cytogenetic abnormalities have been recognized that are closely, and sometimes uniquely, associated with morphologically and clinically distinct subsets of lymphoma and leukemia (Chapter 13) and soft tissue neoplasms (Chapter 11).

Advantages

The power of conventional cytogenetics lies in its ability to provide simultaneous analysis of the entire genome without any foreknowledge of the chromosomal regions involved in the disease process. In most cases, the type or location of the identified chromosomal abnormalities can be used to direct additional testing and can even provide clues to the underlying gene-specific mechanisms.

Limitations

The overall clinical utility of traditional cytogenetic analysis is restricted by two general features of the method. From a technical standpoint, analysis can only be performed on viable tissue specimens that contain proliferating cells, as discussed in more detail later. From a sensitivity standpoint, analysis has a resolution of only about 3 to 4 mb at an 850-band level, and only about 7 to 8 mb at a 400-band level. Consequently, traditional cytogenetic analysis is suited only for detection of numerical abnormalities and gross structural rearrangements; the method does not have the sensitivity to detect mutations such as small deletions and insertions, small inversions, single base pair substitutions, and so on.

BASIC LABORATORY PROCEDURES

Chromosomes that can be individually distinguished by light microscopy can be obtained only during cell division; thus the fundamental requirement for traditional cytogenetic

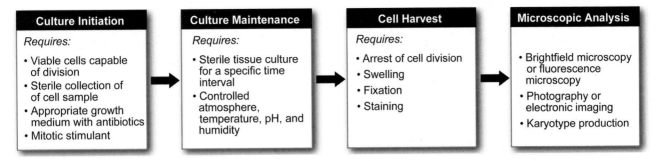

Figure 3.1 Overall scheme for the production of metaphase chromosomes for traditional cyto-genetic analysis.

TABLE 3.1		
SPECIMEN REQUIREMENTS		
Tissue Type	**Sample**	**Handling**
Peripheral blood	Collect in preservative-free sodium heparin	Transport refrigerated or at room temperature
Bone marrow aspirate	Collect in preservative-free sodium heparin; the first several milliliters of the aspirate usually contains the greatest proportion of cells and so is the optimal sample for cytogenetic analysis	Transport at room temperature
Amniotic fluid	Can be collected from about 16 weeks' gestation until term; the first several milliliters of the fluid should not be submitted, because it is most likely to be contaminated with maternal cells	Transport at room temperature; minimize transport time
Solid tissue	Fetal tissue: Collect and transport in sterile culture medium; tissue samples usually include skin biopsy, cord biopsy, amniotic biopsy, placental biopsy Solid neoplasms: Collect and transport in sterile culture medium containing broad-spectrum antibiotics; carefully select maximally viable tumor for analysis	Transport on ice to minimize autolysis and microbrial overgrowth
Chorionic villi	Collect at 10–12 weeks' gestation using a heparinized catheter	Transfer the sample to sterile transport medium; transport to laboratory as quickly as possible

analysis is a tissue specimen that contains actively proliferating cells. The overall scheme for the production of metaphase chromosomes for cytogenetic analysis is shown in Figure 3.1.

Culture Initiation

Cytogenetic analysis can be performed on many different cell types, although, as shown in Table 3.1, different specimen types have different sample and handing requirements. Because inappropriate handling, as well as delay between specimen collection and culture initiation, can markedly decrease the likelihood that the sample will grow in vitro, communication and coordination with the cytogenetics laboratory are essential.

Because in vitro culture relies on a sterile microenvironment, specimens should be collected under sterile conditions. In practice, sterility is most difficult to achieve when sampling solid tissues. In this setting, clean instruments and a clean cutting surface, together with transport of the specimen in medium supplemented with broad-spectrum antibiotics, can be used to minimize contamination (12).

Many tissues (e.g., bone marrow, chorionic villi, solid tissue neoplasms) consist of cell types that proliferate spontaneously in culture. Other tissues (e.g., lymph nodes) are composed of cells that have a low intrinsic proliferative rate but that can be induced to divide by the addition of mitogens. Phytohemagglutinin (PHA) stimulates proliferation of T-lymphocytes. Lipopolysaccharide (LPS), protein A, 12-O-tetradecanoly-phorbol-13-acetate (TPA), Epstein-Barr virus, and pokeweed mitogen induce proliferation of B-lymphocytes and are also required for successful culture of some leukemias and lymphomas of B-cell origin.

Culture Maintenance

The period of in vitro culture required depends on the cell type. Bone marrow cultures contain spontaneously proliferating cells, and they can be harvested after only a 24 to 48 hour culture interval, if not directly after specimen collection. Peripheral blood cultures usually require a 72-hour culture interval. The growth rate of amniotic fluid, chorionic villi, and solid tissue specimens is not easily predicted and may require culture periods of up to 2 weeks or longer.

Cell Harvest

Colcemide is used to block proliferating cells in metaphase by preventing separation of sister chromatids. (Colcemide is an analog of colchicine that binds to tubulin, obstructing the formation of mitotic spindle fibers and destroying

spindle fibers that have already formed). After exposure to colcemide, a hypotonic solution is used to swell the cells so that, after fixation, the chromosomes are adequately spread for microscopic analysis.

Synchronization of Cell Division

Cells in culture do not proceed through the cell cycle in synchrony. Because an extended colcemide treatment cannot be used to capture more cells in mitosis (exposure to the drug for more than about 30 minutes results in chromosome contraction that decreases the resolution of subsequent banding), chemical synchronization of cell division is often required to obtain an acceptable mitotic index. A common chemical approach involves addition of excess thymidine, which stalls cells at the S-phase of the cell cycle by decreasing the amount of dCTP available for DNA synthesis. When the excess thymidine is removed (or the effect of excess thymidine is eliminated by the addition of deoxycytidine), normal DNA replication resumes, and the collective release of the cells from S-phase produces a transiently high mitotic index. Alternatively, 5-fluorodeoxyuridine (FUdR, which inhibits the enzyme

TABLE 3.2

MAJOR CHROMOSOME STAINING AND BANDING TECHNIQUES

Method	Staining Pattern	Comments
Techniques that produce specific alternating bands along each chromosome		
Giemsa banding (G-banding)	Dark bands are AT-rich; light bands are CG-rich; widely used in the United States and Canada	G-banding performed with trypsin and Giemsa (GTG banding) is a common technical variation
Quinacrine banding (Q-banding)	Bright regions are AT rich	Utilizes fluorochromes for staining; because the stain is not permanent and requires specialized fluorescent microscopy hardware, technique is not widely used
Reverse banding (R-banding)	AT-rich regions stain lightly (have dull fluorescence), CG-rich regions stain darkly (have bright fluorescence); widely used in France	Fluorescent and nonfluorescent methods exist
4,6-Diamidino-2-phenylindole staining (DAPI staining)	DAPI binds AT-rich regions; produces a pattern similar to Q-banding	DAPI is a fluorescent dye; DAPI staining is widely used as a counterstain in FISH analysis
Techniques that stain selective chromosome regions		
Constitutive heterochromatin banding (C-banding)	Stains heterochromatin (α-satellite DNA) around the centromeres as well as some inherited polymorphisms	C-banding by barium hydroxide using Giemsa (CBG) is a variation used to detect dicentric and pseudodicentric chromosomes
Telomere banding (T-banding)	Technical variation of R-banding used to stain telomeres	Fluorescent and nonfluorescent methods exist
Silver staining for nucleolar organizer regions (NOR staining)	Stains the NORs (which contain the rRNA genes) on the satellite stalks of acrocentric chromosomes	Useful for identification of marker chromosomes, rearrangements, and polymorphisms of the acrocentric chromosomes
Fluorescent in situ hybridization (FISH)	Staining pattern is dependent on the probe	Useful with repetitive sequence probes, unique sequence probes, and whole chromosome probes

Compiled from references 13 and 14.

thymidylate synthetase) can be used to stall cells at the G_1/S boundary; in this method, addition of thymidine releases the block.

Banding

A number of different techniques can be used to stain metaphase chromosomes. The methods can be divided into two general categories: methods that produce specific alternating white and dark regions (bands) along the length of each chromosome and methods that stain only a defined region of specific chromosomes (Table 3.2).

The quality of staining depends on a number of technical factors, including sufficient separation of the chromosomes in the metaphase spread to allow clear visualization. Although there are no internationally accepted standards for banding resolution, ideograms (Fig. 3.2) are used as reference points. Some countries, including the United States, Canada, United Kingdom, France, Japan, and Australia, have established standards that specify the minimum requirements for the number and quality of cells that must be processed for chromosome analysis depending on sample type (reviewed in 15,16), but many cases require more detailed analysis.

Microscopic Analysis

The approach used to evaluate the metaphase chromosome spreads, whether brightfield microscopy or fluorescence

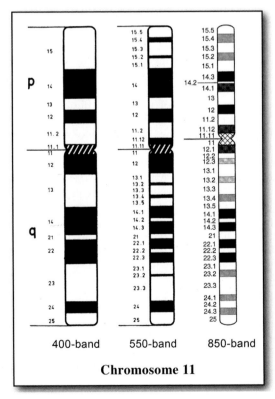

400-band   550-band   850-band

Chromosome 11

Figure 3.2 Ideograms for chromosome 11. The G-banding pattern from ISCN 1995 at three different band resolutions is shown. (Reprinted from Mitelman F (ed.) *ISCN 1995: An International System for Human Cytogenetic Nomenclature* (1995) Basel: S. Karger AG with permission.)

microscopy, is dictated by the method used to stain the chromosomes. Conventional photography has traditionally been used to produce high-resolution prints of the stained chromosomes, but electronic imaging systems are rapidly replacing conventional photographic processes, especially for fluorescence-based analysis.

The final step in cytogenetic analysis in most countries is the production of a karyotype. As shown in Figure 3.3, a karyotype consists of the chromosomal complement of the cell displayed in a standard sequence on the basis of size, centromere location, and banding pattern.

Assay Failure

The most common causes of failure to obtain a cytogenetic result are shown in Table 3.3. The table emphasizes the fact that many sources of failure can be avoided by careful selection of viable tissue, with prompt specimen transport to the cytogenetics laboratory in the appropriate medium. Nonetheless, it is important to stress that several causes of assay failure are inherent to in vitro culture and cannot be eliminated by even the most meticulous laboratory technique.

Cytogenetic analysis of solid tumors highlights a number of these intrinsic technical limitations. First, benign solid tumors contain few mitotic cells, so cultures are susceptible to overgrowth by non-neoplastic cells. Even high-grade malignant solid tumors often grow poorly in vitro, especially if grown without the appropriate culture medium and growth factor supplementation. Second, the number of neoplastic cells in a solid tumor sample can be difficult to determine based on gross examination, and the material submitted to the cytogenetics laboratory may consist primarily of stromal cells, inflammatory cells, and blood. Third, the viability of the neoplastic cells is often uncertain; even areas of the specimen that are not grossly necrotic may contain predominantly nonviable tumor cells. Fourth, in vitro culture select for subclones within the neoplastic population that have a growth advantage in the particular culture conditions, so it is often unclear whether an abnormal karyotype is representative of the entire neoplasm. Fifth, culture of solid tumors is particularly prone to microbial contamination when the tissue sample is collected in the frozen section area or gross room. Contamination is often unavoidable for specimens arising from anatomic sites normally colonized by bacteria, such as the oral cavity, gastrointestinal tract, or skin.

Since many different technical factors affect cytogenetic analysis, it is difficult to predict the overall failure rate of analysis for specific tissue types, neoplasms, and diseases. Consequently, it is often difficult to provide objective statements regarding the utility of cytogenetic analysis in routine diagnostic surgical pathology. In studies that specifically address this issue for hematolymphoid neoplasms, cytogentic analysis has a success rate for detecting characteristic chromosomal aberrations that varies from 33% to 100%, depending on the specific diagnosis, and about 70% overall (17). For prenatal diagnosis, success rates of over 99% have been reported (18).

However, for solid tumors, the clinical utility of cytogenetic analysis is less well characterized. Reports describing the cytogenetic abnormalities of many solid tumors suffer

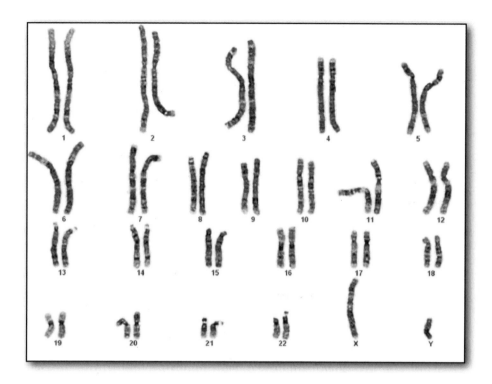

Figure 3.3 Example of a high-resolution G-banded karyotype (from peripheral blood lymphocytes) showing a normal 46,XY male chromosome complement. (Courtesy Dr. Diane Arthur, Head, Clinical Cytogenetics Section, U.S. National Institutes of Health.)

TABLE 3.3

COMMON REASONS FOR FAILURE OF TRADITIONAL CYTOGENETIC ANALYSIS

Culture failure

The sample contained no viable cells (e.g., because of a necrotic tumor sample or improper specimen handling)

Inappropriate sample (e.g., peripheral blood without blasts is submitted instead of bone marrow)

Overgrowth by non-neoplastic cells

Overgrowth by a nonrepresentative clone of tumor cells

Microbial overgrowth

Equipment or reagent failure (uncommon)

Postculture failure

Technical errors involving cell harvest, slide preparation, or staining

Misdiagnosis (e.g., the presence of an abnormality is missed or an abnormality is incorrectly interpreted)

from a reporting bias in that cases with recurring structural or numerical aberrations are described without accompanying data on assay failures. Published reports rarely indicate the percentage of cases that did not yield interpretable results or the reasons for the failed analyses. Objective measures of traditional cytogenetic analysis as a testing methodology in routine clinical practice (including sensitivity, specificity, predictive value of a positive or negative result, etc.; Chapter 8) are therefore usually unknown.

METAPHASE FLUORESCENCE IN SITU HYBRIDIZATION

Virtually all metaphase chromosome in situ hybridization (ISH) analysis is performed using probes that are directly or indirectly labeled with fluorescent labels, as initially described almost two decades ago (19). Guidelines and standards for the use of metaphase fluorescence in situ hybridization (FISH) in clinical laboratory testing have been developed by the American College of Medical Genetics (16), and standardized nomenclature for reporting the results has been developed, as discussed in more detail below. In principle, metaphase FISH is very straightforward and is essentially a modified Southern blot (Chapter 6) in which the target DNA consists of chromosomes rather than membrane-bound DNA. Technically, the method has four steps: the probe and metaphase target are denatured by a high temperature incubation, the probe (in great excess in order to drive the reaction kinetics) is hybridized to the chromosomal target; posthybridization washes are used to remove unbound probe; and, finally, the bound probe is detected by fluorescence microscopy. A fluorochrome-based counterstain is virtually always used to help detect the chromosomes during microscopic examination. Propidium iodide (PI), which binds DNA without any sequence preference, can be used to visualize the chromosomes, but cannot be used to identify specific chromosomes or chromosomal regions. In contrast, the use of DAPI (Table 3.2) as a counterstain makes it possible to localize the position of the bound probe to specific chromosomal bands.

Probes

A wide variety of fluorophores can be incorporated into metaphase FISH probes either directly or indirectly (Chapter 6; also see Table 6.4). The choice of labels is largely governed by practical issues, such as the excitation and emission filters on the microscope that will be used to view the chromosome spreads. For multiplex FISH, the set of fluorophores must not have significantly overlapping emission spectra.

A few probe kits have been approved by the United States Food and Drug Administration (FDA) for in vitro diagnostic testing. However, many of the probes for metaphase FISH are classified as analyte-specific reagents (ASRs) and so are exempt from FDA approval, although standards and guidelines for clinical use of ASRs have been established by the American College of Medical Genetics (16). Probe validation includes confirmation that the probe localizes to the correct chromosomal band in normal metaphase spreads, an evaluation of the probe's sensitivity and specificity, and continuous or at least biannual quality control testing to monitor the probe's performance characteristics (20–22). Recommendations have also been developed for interpretation of a metaphase FISH results that include both the number of cells that should be scored and the number of images saved for documentation (16).

Most FISH probes fall into one of three general categories, namely repetitive sequence probes, unique sequence probes, and whole chromosome probes (23).

Repetitive Sequence Probes

The most widely used repetitive sequence probes bind to α-satellite sequences of centromeres, and because α-satellite sequences are present in hundreds of thousands of copies, repetitive sequence probes produce strong signals. Chromosome-specific, centromere-specific probes have been developed for most human chromosomes (24) based on differences in the α-satellite sequences between the different chromosomes, and these probes are particularly useful for demonstrating aneuploidy in metaphase (as well as interphase) cells. Other repetitive sequence probes that are not as widely used include probes that recognize β-satellite sequences (located on the short arms of acrocentric chromosomes) and probes that recognize the telomeric repeat sequence TTAGGG.

Unique Sequence Probes

This class of probes is used to detect sequences that are present only once in the genome or at most at only one copy per chromosome. Unique sequence probes are usually derived from genomic clones, but also can be produced from cDNA or by PCR. A number of different cloning vectors have historically been used to produce genomic unique sequence probes, including plasmids (probes 1 to 10 kb long), bacteriophage λ (up to 25 kb long), bacterial artificial chromosomes (BACs, up to about 300 kb long), and yeast artificial chromosomes (YACs, from 100 kb to 2 mb long). The availability of mapped

BAC libraries, originally developed as part of the Human Genome Project, has greatly simplified the production of probes for any locus under study (25,26).

Unique sequence probes (Fig. 3.4) are used primarily to detect changes in the copy number of a specific locus (most commonly, to detect the presence of amplification), to confirm the presence of rearrangements involving a specific locus, or to detect so-called cryptic rearrangements that cannot be identified by examination of chromosomes stained by routine banding methods. The advantages and disadvantages of metaphase FISH analysis using unique sequence probes directly parallel those of interphase FISH (Chapter 4).

Whole Chromosome Probes

Whole chromosome probes (WCPs), also known as chromosome painting probes or chromosome libraries, consist of thousands of overlapping probes that recognize unique and moderately repetitive sequences along the entire length of individual chromosomes. Generation of WCPs requires isolation of the DNA from individual chromosomes, which has traditionally been accomplished by flow cytometric sorting of stained chromosomes, microdissection of specific chromosomes with subsequent PCR amplification, or construction of somatic cell hybrids that contain only a single human chromosome or chromosomal region (27). Not surprisingly, the cumbersome procedures required to generate WCPs has limited the use of this category of probes. However, because WCPs for each human chromosome are now commercially available, WCP FISH is likely to be more widely employed (28).

WCPs are used to identify rearrangements that are not evident by evaluation of metaphase chromosomes stained by routine banding methods, to confirm the interpretation of aberrations identified by routine banding methods, or to establish the chromosomal origin of rearrangements that are difficult to evaluate by other approaches (29).

Multiplex Metaphase FISH

Multiplex FISH (M-FISH, also known as multicolor FISH) and spectral karyotyping (SKY) are related techniques in which metaphase chromosome spreads are hybridized with a combination of probes labeled with different fluorophores. Since N different fluorophores can produce (2^N-1) different color combinations, five different fluorophores yield enough different color combinations to uniquely identify all 24 different human chromosomes. Although five different fluorophores is in theory sufficient to uniquely identify all human chromosomes, in practice a higher number of fluorophores is often required to provide sufficient resolution (30). Methods have recently been described that make it possible to label probes with multiple different fluorophores by the technique known as combined binary ratio labeling (COBRA), methods that markedly increase the theoretical number of different targets that can be recognized in a single M-FISH assay (31).

For both M-FISH and SKY, a cocktail consisting of labeled probes for each of the 24 chromosomes is

A.

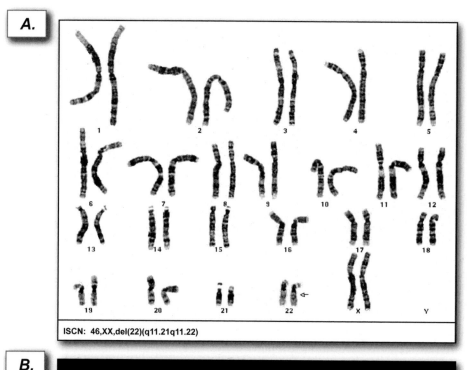

ISCN: 46,XX,del(22)(q11.21q11.22)

B.

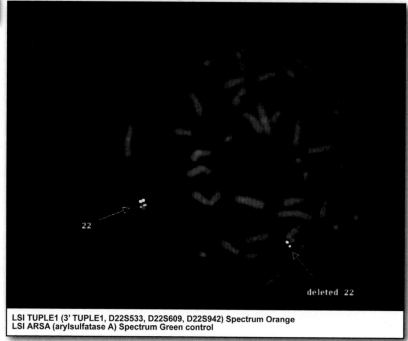

LSI TUPLE1 (3' TUPLE1, D22S533, D22S609, D22S942) Spectrum Orange
LSI ARSA (arylsulfatase A) Spectrum Green control

Figure 3.4 Example of metaphase FISH using a unique sequence probe. **A,** High-resolution G-banded karyotype (from peripheral blood lymphocytes) showing a microdeletion of the proximal long arm of one chromosome 22 *(arrow).* **B,** Metaphase FISH with the LSI TUPLE1 SpectrumOrange/LSI ARSA SpectrumGreen probe mixture (Vysis, Inc.) confirms deletion of the DiGeorge/velocardiofacial syndrome region (TUPLE1) of one chromosome 22. (Courtesy Dr. Diane Arthur, Head, Clinical Cytogenetics Section, U.S. National Institutes of Health.) (See color insert.)

hybridized to metaphase chromosome spreads and the fluorescent emissions are measured by computerized imaging systems (Fig. 3.5). For M-FISH, a composite image is obtained by multiple exposures using individual single bandpass filters (32), and specialized software is used to analyze the composite image to determine the combination of fluorophores present along the length of each chromosome. The software assigns a pseudocolor to each chromosome based on the pattern of fluorescence, which makes it possible to assemble a karyotype. For SKY, a specialized multibandpass filter permits simultaneous excitation of all the different fluorophores, which together with the use of specialized optics, makes it possible to measure the entire fluorescent emission spectrum in a single exposure (33). A mathematical algorithm based on Fourier transformation is used to convert the emitted light into spectral information, which is used to determine the combination of fluorophores present along the length of each chromosome. As with M-FISH, the software assigns a pseudocolor to each chromosome based on the pattern of

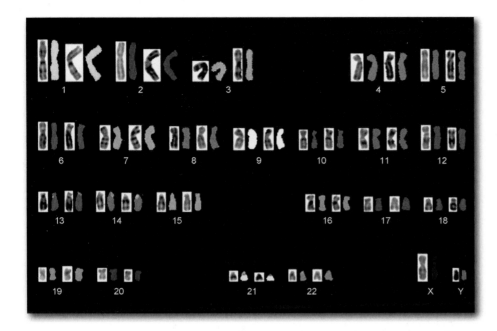

Figure 3.5 Spectral karyotype (SKY, Applied Spectral Imaging, Inc., Vista, CA) of peripheral blood lymphocytes from a normal 46,XY male. For each chromosome pair, black and white DAPI-banded chromosomes are shown on the *left* and SKY painted chromosomes are shown on the *right*. (Courtesy Dr. Diane Arthur, Head, Clinical Cytogenetics Section, U.S. National Institutes of Health.) (See color insert.)

fluorescence, which again makes it possible to produce a karyotype (34).

Advantages and Disadvantages

M-FISH and SKY are both useful for detection of aneuploidy and chromosome rearrangements. In many cases, M-FISH or SKY make it possible to establish the chromosomal origin of rearrangements that cannot be defined based on routine cytogenetic analysis (Fig. 3.6). A web-based database has been developed to facilitate the identification of recurrent tumor and stage-specific chromosomal aberrations detected by multiplex FISH (35); it contains links to other websites that can be used to integrate the cytogenetic map of human chromosomes with physical and sequence maps.

However, both M-FISH and SKY are still best considered screening approaches because the lower limit of the size of individual DNA chromosomal fragments that can be visualized by either technique is in the range of 1 to 2 mb (36). In addition, neither M-FISH nor SKY provides any information on the specific regions of the individual chromosomes that are involved in the translocation. Although M-FISH and SKY will reveal intrachromosomal deletions and duplications large enough to result in a change in size of the affected chromosome, small intrachromosomal changes (including duplications and inversions) will not be detected.

Modifications of Multiplex FISH

One recent modification of M-FISH and SKY employs mixtures of partial chromosome paints, each of which hybridizes to only a band or sub-band of an individual chromosome. When applied to metaphase chromosomes, this approach can be used to produce a pseudocolor banded karyotype at a resolution of about 550 bands (37). The use of partial chromosome paints makes it possible to use multiplex FISH

methodology to identify the break point of rearrangements and detect intrachromosomal rearrangements.

COMPARATIVE GENOMIC HYBRIDIZATION

Comparative genomic hybridization (CGH) is a variation of metaphase FISH that can be used to survey the entire genome for chromosomal deletions and amplifications (38,39).

For a typical CGH test, genomic DNA from a tumor sample is labeled with a green fluorophore by nick translation and genomic DNA from a paired normal tissue sample is labeled with a red fluorophore by nick translation. The green and red probes are mixed and used in a single hybridization to metaphase chromosomes prepared from normal cells (usually peripheral blood lymphocytes), and the ratio of the green to red fluorescent signals is measured along the length of each chromosome (38,40). Areas where the ratio deviates significantly from the expected one-to-one relationship indicate a change in DNA copy number in the tumor (Fig. 3.7). Areas where the green to red ratio is significantly greater than 1 are areas of chromosomal gain (usually amplifications) and regions where the green to red ratio is significantly lower than 1 are areas of chromosomal loss (deletions). Although metaphase CGH often has higher sensitivity than conventional cytogenetic analysis, in practice the smallest chromosomal alterations that can be reproducibly detected are about 3 mb long (41,42). As discussed in more detail in Chapters 6 and 9, array CGH offers higher resolution than metaphase CGH (43,44).

The fact that metaphase CGH (as well as array CGH) can be performed using DNA extracted from fixed as well as fresh tumor samples is a significant advantage of the technique. Consequently, CGH makes it possible to perform genomewide scans for a subset of structural alterations on even those cases for which conventional cytogenetic analysis is not possible or is unsuccessful. CGH essentially opens the

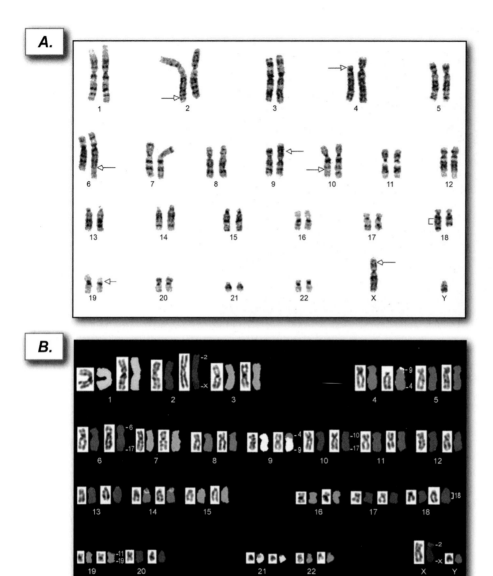

Figure 3.6 Example of SKY to establish the origin of rearrangements that cannot be defined based on routine cytogenetic analysis. G-banded karyotype from bone marrow of a patient with relapsed diffuse large B-cell non-Hodgkin's lymphoma showing a pseudodiploid male karyotype with complex structural rearrangements involving chromosomes X, 2, 4, 6, 9, 10, 18, and 19 (arrows). **B**, Spectral karyotyping is necessary to completely define the complex rearrangements noted with G-banding. **C**, Final karyotype. (Courtesy Dr. Diane Arthur, Head, Clinical Cytogenetics Section, U.S. National Institutes of Health.) (See color insert.)

ISCN: 46,Y,t(X;2)(p21;q33),t(4;9)(p14;p24),der(6)t(6;17)(q24;q11.2),der(10)t(10;17)(q24;q21), dup(18)(q21q23),der(19)t(11;19)(q25;p13.1)

entire formalin-fixed tissue archive to at least limited cytogenetic analysis.

HUMAN CHROMOSOME NOMENCLATURE

The initial guidelines for describing human chromosomes and chromosome abnormalities were published in 1960 (45). Technical advancements, together with a more complete understanding of human chromosomal structure, have necessitated periodic revision of the nomenclature guidelines. The document in current use is the International System for Human Cytogenetic Nomenclature from 1995, abbreviated ISCN 1995 (46,47); it includes ideograms for all of the chromosomes that serve as useful reference points

because of their universal acceptance and availability. An updated version of the ISCN nomenclature is scheduled for publication at the end of 2005.

Chromosome Region and Band Designations

The centromere divides each chromosome into a short or p arm and a long or q arm. Each chromosome arm ends in a terminus, designated pter and qter for the short and long arms, respectively. A list of the more frequent symbols and abbreviations used to describe human karyotypes is shown in Table 3.4.

Chromosome arms are divided into regions based on landmarks, defined as consistent and distinct morphologic

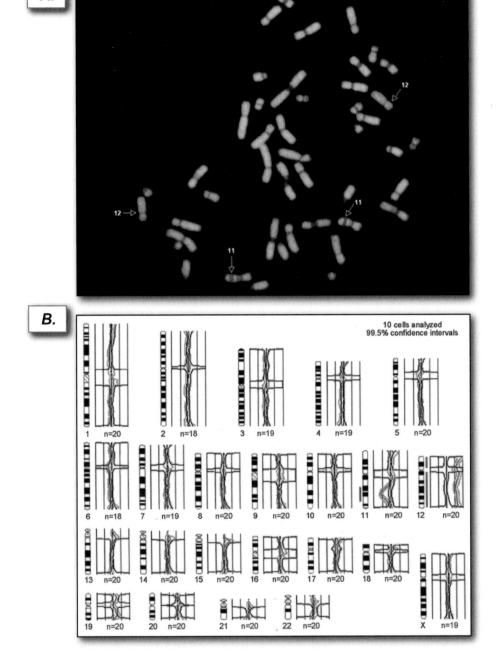

Figure 3.7 Example of comparative genomic hybridization (CGH). **A**, Metaphase spread hybridized for comparative genomic hybridization (GCH, Applied Imagining Corporation, San Jose, CA) showing interstitial deletion of part of the long arm of chromosome 11 and gain of chromosome 12 in a patient with chronic lymphocytic leukemia. **B**, CGH software analysis confirms 11q deletion and trisomy 12. (Courtesy Dr. Diane Arthur, Head, Clinical Cytogenetics Section, U.S. National Institutes of Health.) (See color insert.)

areas that aid in the identification of that chromosome. The regions adjacent to the centromere of the short arm and long arm are designated as p1 and q1, respectively, the next distal as p2 and q2, and so on (Fig. 3.2). Chromosome regions are divided into bands, and the bands are divided into sub-bands, both of which are numbered sequentially (for descriptive purposes, the portions of the chromosome that lie between the middle of the centromere and p1 and between the middle of the centromere and q1 are designated p10 and q10, respectively). Thus, the terminal band on the long arm of chromosome 11 is written as 11q25, indicating chromosome 11, long arm, region 2, band 5,

and is referred to as "eleven q two-five" and not as "eleven q twenty-five."

Description of Karyotypes

ISCN nomenclature also provides rules for karyotype designations. The first item of the designation is the total number of chromosomes (including the sex chromosomes) followed by the sex chromosomes; the normal female karyotype is therefore 46,XX and the normal male karyotype 46,XY. Chromosomal abnormalities follow the sex chromosome designations using established symbols

TABLE 3.4

SELECTED SYMBOLS AND ABBREVIATIONS USED IN KARYOTYPE DESIGNATIONS[a]

Abbreviation or Symbol	Description
add	Additional material of unknown origin
square brackets []	Number of cells in each clone
cen	Centromere
single colon (:)	Break
double colon (::)	Break and reunion
comma (,)	Separates chromosome number, sex chromosomes, and abnormalities
del	Deletion
der	Derivative chromosome
dmin	Double minute(s)
dup	Duplication
i	Isochromosome
idem	Identical abnormalities as in prior clone
inv	Inversion
ins	Insertion
mar	Marker chromosome
minus sign (−)	Loss
multiplication sign (×)	Multiple copies; also designates copy number with ish
plus sign (+)	Gain
question mark (?)	Uncertainty of chromosome identification or abnormality
r	Ring chromosome
rcp	Reciprocal
slash (/)	Separates cell lines or clones
semicolon (;)	Separates chromosomes and break points in rearrangements involving more than one chromosome
t	Translocation

[a] See references 46 and 47 for a complete list of symbols and abbreviations.

and abbreviations. The sex chromosomes are described first, followed by abnormalities in the autosomal chromosomes in numerical order. For each chromosome described, numerical changes are listed before structural aberrations. Table 3.5 provides a few examples of the karyotypic designation of numerical and structural abnormalities detected by traditional cytogenetic analysis.

The rules for designating the karyotype of constitutional abnormalities are also used for designating the abnormalities associated with neoplasms, although the biology of tumors requires additional definitions and guidelines. A clone is defined as two cells that share the same pattern of aberrations (unless the abnormality involves a chromosomal loss, in which case three cells are required); different clones are separated by slashes, with the number of cells observed in each clone given in square brackets. Several specific terms are used to designate the relationship between the clones in a tumor sample. The mainline (ML) is by definition the most common clone; because the mainline designation is based on the number of cells only, it does not necessarily bear any relationship to the underlying pattern of tumor progression from a biologic perspective. The clone that appears to be the most basic in terms of biologic tumor progression is referred to as the stemline (SL); clones that apparently evolved from the stemline are defined as sidelines (SDL). When clonal evolution is clearly present, the stemline is listed first, with sidelines listed in order of increasing complexity (when possible) or decreasing clone size; when no clear clonal progression is present, the mainline is listed first, followed by the additional clones listed in order of decreasing size (Table 3.5).

Prophase or Metaphase Chromosome ISH

ISCN 1995 also includes rules for designating cytogenetic findings derived from various ISH techniques. A summary of the more common symbols and abbreviations is shown in Table 3.6. The results of conventional cytogenetic analysis (if performed) are listed first, followed by the results of ISH analysis (even though ISH is virtually always performed by fluorescence microscopy, the abbreviation *ish* is used, not FISH). Abnormal ish results are presented in the following order: the abbreviation for the specific abnormality is listed first, followed by the chromosome number, the location of the break points, and the probe designation, all of which are separated by parentheses (Table 3.7). Ideally, loci are designated according to Genome Data Base (GDB) nomenclature (48), which consists of the letter D (for DNA), the chromosome number, the letter

TABLE 3.5

EXAMPLES OF KARYOTYPE DESIGNATIONS OF NUMERICAL AND STRUCTURAL ABNORMALITIES

Karyotype	Description
Constitutional sex chromosome aneuploidies[a]	
45,X	Turner syndrome
47,XXY	Klinefelter syndrome
48,XXYY	Variant of Klinefelter syndrome
Acquired sex chromosome aneuploidies	
47,XX,+X	Normal female with gain of one X chromosome in her tumor cells
45,XX,-X	Normal female with loss of one X chromosome in her tumor cells
46,XC,+X	Turner syndrome patient with gain of one X chromosome in her tumor cells
Autosomal chromosome aneuploidies	
47,XY,+21	Male with trisomy 21 (Down syndrome)
48,XY,+21C,+21	Male with trisomy 21, with gain of an additional chromosome 21 in his tumor cells
Abnormalities in neoplasms	
47,XY,+8,t(11;22)(q24;q12)	Male whose tumor cells have two cytogenetic abnormalities: an additional chromosome 8 and a translocation involving the long arms of chromosomes 11 and 22, at band q24 of chromosome 11 and band q12 of chromosome 22
47,XX,+mar[4]/50,idem,+6,+12,+19[8]/51,idem,+16[3]	Female whose tumor cells have three different clones. The first clone (which is the stemline) has a marker chromosome. The second clone contains the sex chromosomes and marker chromosome present in the first, plus an additional copy of chromosomes 6, 12, and 19; because it is the largest clone (with 8 cells), it is the mainline (although in terms of biologic progression it is a sideline). The third clone has abnormalities identical to those of the second, plus an additional copy of chromosome 16. In terms of biologic progression, it is a sideline.

[a] + and − signs are not needed to designate constitutional sex chromosome aneuploidies.

TABLE 3.6

EXAMPLES OF SYMBOLS AND ABBREVIATIONS USED FOR IN SITU HYBRIDIZATION NOMENCLATURE[a]

Abbreviation or Symbol	Description
plus sign (+)	Present on a specific chromosome
minus sign (−)	Absent on a specific chromosome
++	Duplication on a specific chromosome
period (.)	Separates cytogenetic results from ish results
con	Connected or adjacent signals
ish	When used by itself, refers to hybridization to chromosomes
nuc ish	Nuclear or interphase in situ hybridization
pcp	Partial chromosome paint
sep	Separated signals (which are usually adjacent in normal cells)
wcp	Whole chromosome paint

[a]See references 46 and 47 for a complete list of symbols and abbreviations.

S (segment), and the GDB probe number; when GDB designations are unavailable, probe names can be used. If more than one probe for the same chromosome is used, they are listed in order from pter to qter. If probes from different chromosomes are used, they are separated by a semicolon.

Interphase ISH

ISCN 1995 also introduced nomenclature to designate the results of chromosomal abnormalities detected by ISH performed on interphase nuclei. The results of conventional cytogenetic analysis (if performed) are listed

TABLE 3.7

EXAMPLES OF ISH CHROMOSOMES DESIGNATIONS IN NEOPLASMS

Designation	Description
Metaphase FISH	
47,XY,+mar.ish der(3)(wcp3+)	In this tumor, traditional cytogenetic analysis shows a marker chromosome; metaphase FISH using a whole chromosome paint for chromosome 3 shows that the marker is derived from chromosome 3.
Interphase FISH	
nuc ish 11p13(WT1x2),22q12(EWSx2) (WT1 con EWSx1)	Interphase FISH of a tumor cell using a probe for WT1 at 11q13 shows 2 signals, as does a probe for EWS at 22q12. However, one WT1 and one EWS signal are juxtaposed (or connected), suggesting they lie on the same chromosome, consistent with a t(11;22)(p13;q12) translocation.
nuc ish 22q12(EWSx4)(EWS sep EWSx1)	Interphase FISH of a tumor cell using a breakapart probe set for the EWS locus at 22q12. Four EWS signals are present, but on one copy of chromosome 22 the two probes are separated (most likely as a result of a rearrangement of the EWS locus).
nuc ish 22q12(EWSx4)(EWS con EWSx2)[169/200]	Interphase FISH using the same breakapart probe set as in the above example. However, in this tumor, the two probes remain juxtaposed on both copies of chromosome 22 (which provides no evidence of a rearrangement of the EWS locus). The indicated results are present in 169 of 200 nuclei evaluated.

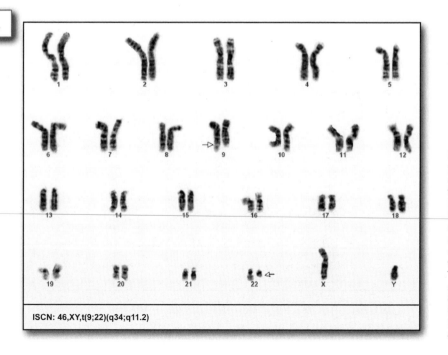

A.

ISCN: 46,XY,t(9;22)(q34;q11.2)

Figure 3.8 Example of interphase FISH using the probe fusion approach. **A**, G-banded karyotype from bone marrow showing a single Philadelphia chromosome (Ph) arising from the common t(9;22) translocation *(arrows)* in a patient with chronic myelogenous leukemia in chronic phase. **B**, Interphase FISH with the LSI BCR/ABL ES Dual Color Translocation Probe (Vysis, Inc.) showing the Ph BCR/ABL fusion. (Courtesy Dr. Diane Arthur, Head, Clinical Cytogenetics Section, U.S. National Institutes of Health.) (See color insert.)

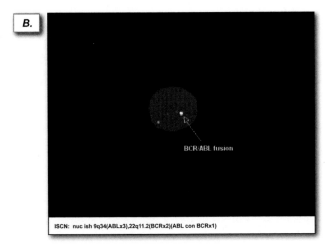

B.

BCR/ABL fusion

ISCN: nuc ish 9q34(ABLx3),22q11.2(BCRx2)(ABL con BCRx1)

Figure 3.8 (*continued*)

first, followed by a period, followed by the interphase ISH results presented in the following order: the abbreviation *nuc ish* is listed first, followed by a space, followed by the chromosome band to which the probe maps, followed by the locus designation, a multiplication sign, and the number of signals present (Table 3.7). Again, loci are designated according to GDB nomenclature, with substitution by probe names as required. If two or more probes for the same or different loci are used, they are separated by commas.

By interphase testing using the probe fusion approach (Chapter 4), simultaneous analysis of probes on different chromosomes is expected to produce separate signals in normal cells but juxtaposed signals in cells harboring the target rearrangement (Fig. 3.8). The abbreviation *con* (for connected) is used to indicate juxtaposed signals, a finding that suggests the target loci are present on the same chromosome.

By interphase testing via the probe splitting approach, probes that are juxtaposed in normal cells become separated in cells that harbor the target chromosomal rearrangement. The abbreviation *sep* is used to indicate separated signals, a finding that suggests a rearrangement of the target region.

REFERENCES

1. Flemming W. *Zellsubstanz, Kern and Zellteilung.* Vogel, Leipzig, 1882.
2. Sutton WS. The chromosomes in heredity. *Biol Bull Wood's Hole* 1903;4:231.
3. Boveri T. Über mehrpolige mitosen als mittle zur analyse des zellkerns. *Berh Phys-Med Ges* (*Wurzburg, N.F.*) 1902;35:67–90.
4. Lejune J, Gautier M, Turpin R. Etude des chromosomes somatiques de neuf enfants mongoliens. *CR Acad Sci* 1959;248:1721–1722.
5. Gersen SL. History of clinical cytogenetics. In: Gersen SL, Keagle MB, eds. *The Principles of Clinical Cytogenetics*, 2nd ed. Totowa, NJ: Humana Press; 2005:3–8.
6. Caspersson T, Farber S, Foley GE, et al. Chemical differentiation along metaphase chromosomes. *Exp Cell Res* 1968; 49:219–222.
7. Caspersson T, Zech L, Johansson C. Differential binding of alkylating fluorochromes. *Exp Cell Res* 1970;60:315–319.
8. Caspersson T, Lomakka G, Zech L. The 24 fluorescence patterns of the human metaphase chromosomes: distinguishing characters and variability. *Hereditas* 1971;67:89–102.
9. Vogel F, Motulsky AG. *Human Genetics: Problems and Approaches.* New York: Springer-Verlag; 1979.
10. Therman E. *Human Chromosomes: Structure, Behavior, Effects.* New York: Springer-Verlag; 1980.
11. deGrouchy J, Turleau C. *Clinical Atlas of Human Chromosomes.* New York: John Wiley & Sons; 1977.
12. Fletcher JA. Cytogenetics of solid tumors. In: Gersen SL, Keagle MB, eds. *The Principles of Clinical Cytogenetics*, 2nd ed. Totowa, NJ: Humana Press; 2005.
13. Keagle MB, Gersen SL. Basic laboratory procedures. In: Gersen SL, Keagle MB, eds. *The Principles of Clinical Cytogenetics*, 2nd ed. Totowa, NJ: Humana Press; 2005:63–79.
14. Benn PA, Tantravahi. Chromosome staining and banding techniques. Rooney DE, Czepulkowski B, eds. *Human Cytogenetics: Constitutional Analysis—A Practical Approach.* Oxford: Oxford Press; 2001:99–128.
15. Watson M, Gersen SL. Quality control and quality assurance. In: Gersen SL and Keagle MB, eds. *The Principles of Clinical Cytogenetics*, 2nd ed. Totowa, NJ: Humana Press; 2005:93–112.
16. http://www.acmg.net/Pages/ACMG_Activities/stds-2002/e.htm.
17. Cook JR, Shekhter-Levin S, Swerdlow SH. Utility of routine classical cytogenetic studies in the evaluation of suspected lymphomas: results of 279 consecutive lymph node/extranodal tissue biopsies. *Am J Clin Pathol* 2004;121:826–885.
18. Gunduz C, Cogulu O, Cankaya T, et al. Trends in cytogenetic prenatal diagnosis in a reference hospital in Izmir/Turkey: a comparative study for four years. *Genet Couns* 2004;15:53–59.
19. Pinkel D, Gray J, Trask B, et al. Cytogenetic analysis by in situ hybridization with fluorescently labeled nucleic acid probes. *Cold Spring Harbor Symp Quant Biol* 1986;51:151–157.
20. Cuthbert G, Thompson K, Breese G, et al. Sensitivity of FISH in detection of MLL translocations. *Genes Chromosomes Cancer* 2000;29:180–185.
21. McGrattan P, Humphreys MW. The prognostic value of FISH as an adjunct to conventional cytogenetics for the detection of cryptic gene rearrangements on chromosome 16: a retrospective investigation of 13 patients from Northern Ireland diagnosed with M4Eo acute myeloid leukaemia. *Ulster Med J* 2003;72:16–21.
22. Dewald GW, Stallard R, Bader PI, et al. Toward quality assurance for metaphase FISH: a multicenter experience. *Am J Med Genet* 1996;65:190–196.
23. Varella-Garcia M. Molecular cytogenetics in solid tumors: laboratorial tool for diagnosis, prognosis, and therapy. *Oncologist* 2003;8:45–58.
24. http://www.vysis.com/CEPProbes_19.asp.
25. http://genome.ucsc.edu/cgi-bin/hgGateway.
26. http://bacpac.chori.org/.
27. Jauch A, Daumer C, Lichter P, et al. Chromosomal in situ suppression hybridization of human gonosomes and autosomes and its use in clinical cytogenetics. *Hum Genet* 1990;85:145–150.
28. http://www.openbiosystems.com/human_whole_chromosome_specific_probes.php and http://www.cytocell.com/article.asp?title=whole%20chromosome%20painting%20probes and http://www.cambio.co.uk/13.php?l1_category_id=1&l2_category_id=2.
29. Bayani JM, Squire JA. Applications of SKY in cancer cytogenetics. *Cancer Invest* 2002;20:373–386.
30. Azofeifa J, Fauth C, Kraus J, et al. An optimized probe set for the detection of small interchromosomal aberrations by use of 24-color FISH. *Am J Hum Genet* 2000;66:1684–1688.
31. Tanke HJ, Wiegant J, van Gijlswijk RP, et al. New strategy for multi-colour fluorescence in situ hybridisation: COBRA: COmbined Binary RAtio labelling. *Eur J Hum Genet* 1999;7:2–11.
32. Speicher M, Ballard SG, Ward D.C. Karyotyping human chromosomes by combinatorial multi-fluor FISH. *Nat Genet* 1996;12:368–375.
33. Schröck E, du Manoir S, Veldman T, et al. Multicolor spectral karyotyping of human chromosomes. *Science* 1996;494–497.
34. Garini Y, Macville M, du Manoir S, et al. Spectral karyotyping. *Bioimaging* 1996; 4:65–72.
35. http://www.ncbi.nlm.nih.gov/sky/.
36. Speicher MR, Ward DC. The coloring of cytogenetics. *Nat Med* 1996;2:1046–1048.
37. Chudoba L, Plesch A, Sorch T, et al. High resolution multicolor-banding: a new technique for refined FISH analysis of human chromosomes. *Cytogenet Cell Genet* 1999;84:156–160.
38. Kallioniemi A, Kallioniemi O, Sudar D, et al. Comparative genomic hybridization for molecular cytogenetic analysis of solid tumors. *Science* 1992;258:818–821.
39. Forozan F, Karhu R, Kononen J, et al. Genome screening by comparative genomic hybridization. *Trends Genet* 1997;13:405–409.
40. du Manoir S, Schrock E, Bentz M, et al. Quantitative analysis of comparative genomic hybridization. *Cytometry* 1995;19:27–41.
41. Knuutila S, Bjorkqvist AM, Autio K, et al. DNA copy number amplifications in human neoplasms: review of comparative genomic hybridization studies. *Am J Pathol* 1998;152:1107–1123.
42. Knuutila S, Aalto Y, Autio K, et al. DNA copy number losses in human neoplasms. *Am J Pathol* 1999;155:683–694.
43. Pettus JA, Crowley BC, Maxwell T, et al. Multiple abnormalities detected by dye reversal genomic microarrays in prostate cancer: a much greater sensitivity than conventional cytogenetics. *Cancer Genet Cytogenet* 2004;154:110–118.
44. Smeets DF. Historical prospective of human cytogenetics: from microscope to microarray. *Clin Biochem* 2004;37:439–446.
45. Denver Conference: A proposed standard system of nomenclature of human mitotic chromosomes. *Lancet*, 1960;1063–1065.
46. Mitelman F. *An International System For Human Cytogenetic Nomenclature. ISCN.* Basel: Karger; 1995.
47. http://www.iscn1995.org/index.php.
48. http://gdbwww.gdb.org/.

Fluorescence In Situ Hybridization

4

Arie Perry

Although in situ hybridization (ISH) has been around for over three decades, its application to molecular diagnostics has only become commonplace relatively recently. In comparison to other molecular testing techniques, it is unique in its basis in morphology, utilizing direct microscopic visualization of probe-specific, intranuclear signals with either chromogenic (CISH) or fluorescence (FISH) detection (1). The latter is used most frequently because of its superior sensitivity and spatial resolution, as well as greater ease in applying multicolor probe combinations. Given that nonmitotic nuclei are analyzed and metaphase chromosomes are not required for interpretation, this technique has also been referred to as interphase cytogenetics. In many clinical cytogenetics laboratories, it is predominantly used for prenatal detection of germline alterations, such as aneusomies and microdeletion syndromes (Table 4.1). However, the detection of somatic cancer-associated alterations with

known diagnostic, prognostic, or therapeutic implications is also performed, particularly for leukemias, where cellular cytologic specimens are relatively easily obtained from the peripheral blood or bone marrow. In anatomic pathology laboratories, the oncology-associated applications for solid tumors are typically of greatest interest (Table 4.1). FISH essentially provides insight into intranuclear target DNA localization and copy number. Therefore, with the exception of XY sex-chromosome determinations in men, two signals per nucleus are normally expected and four common alterations are readily detectable by FISH: aneusomy (gain or loss of a chromosome), gene deletion, amplification, and translocation (Figs. 4.1, 4.2, 4.3 and 4.4). Additionally, sex-chromosome determinations can be useful in patients with sex-mismatched organ transplants to determine whether cellular populations are derived from the recipient or donor (Fig. 4.5). This is most commonly done in post–bone marrow transplant biopsies to monitor engraftment success or failure (2,3). In other words, the fraction of XX versus XY recipient and donor cells provides a reflection of hematopoietic activity generated by the donor marrow. Alternatively, if the transplant was done for a patient with leukemia, it may also provide insight into tumor relapse.

TABLE 4.1
EXAMPLES OF DIAGNOSTIC TESTS BY FISH

Prenatal testing
  Trisomies 13, 18, 21
  XY aneusomies
Microdeletion syndromes
  Cri-du-chat (5p)
  Prader-Willi/Angelman syndromes (15q)
  Di George syndrome (22q)
Transplant pathology
  XY FISH on sex-mismatched organ transplant
  Disease relapse using known genetic alterations in primary
Oncology (diagnostic, prognostic, and predictive markers)
  Chromosomal aneusomies
  Gene/locus deletions
  Gene amplifications
  Translocations

ADVANTAGES AND LIMITATIONS OF FISH

Specimens, Retained Morphology, and Combined FISH/Immunohistochemistry

FISH is applicable to a variety of specimen types, including fresh or frozen tissue, cytologic preparations, and formalin-fixed, paraffin-embedded (FFPE) tissue (Table 4.2). The latter provides a particularly rich source of archival material and may be performed using either thin (4 to 6 μ)

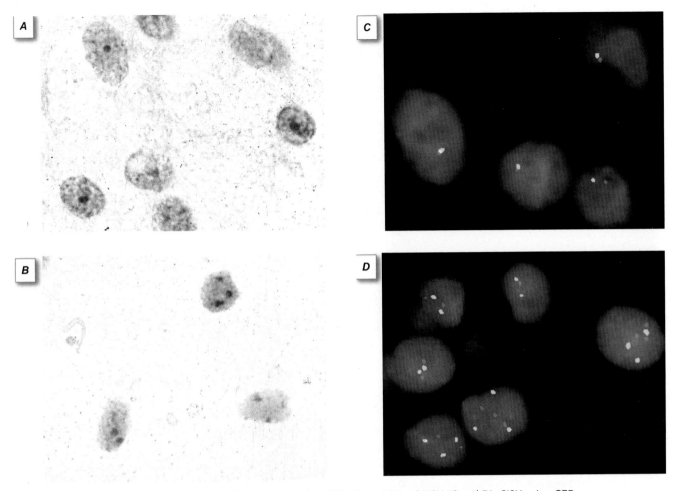

Figure 4.1 Examples of aneusomies using CISH (**A** and **B**) and FISH (**C** and **D**). CISH using CEP probes in a glioblastoma with monosomy 10 (**A**; only 1 brown signal per nucleus) and trisomy 7 (**B**; up to 3 brown intranuclear signals). Monosomy 10 (or 10q deletion) is similarly seen with FISH using locus-specific probes against *PTEN* on 10q23 (green) and *DMBT1* on 10q25-q26 (red) (**C**; 1 green and 1 red signal per nucleus). Trisomy 17 is seen in a subset of breast cancer cells with 3 CEP 17 (green) and 3 *HER-2/neu* (red) signals (**D**). (See color insert.)

sections, such as those cut for immunohistochemistry, or intact nuclei disaggregated from thick paraffin sections (e.g., 50 μ). Although adjustments must be made for nuclear truncation (discussed below), thin sections preserve architecture, are simpler to prepare, and waste less tissue from the block.

In clinical diagnostic testing and in translational research, morphologic preservation is one of the principal advantages, particularly attractive for studies on heterogeneous tissue samples, without the need for microdissection (Fig. 4.6). For example, a morphologically mixed tumor previously studied by FISH is the gliosarcoma (4,5). The finding of identical genetic alterations in both components refuted the notion of a biclonal collision tumor and supported the hypothesis that both elements arose from a single neoplastic clone, with the sarcomatous component likely resulting from mesenchymal metaplasia of the glioblastoma. An extension of this morphologic advantage comes from the possibility of combining FISH with immunohistochemistry, wherein separate assessments can be rendered in immunopositive and negative cellular

populations. For example, this approach, coined FICTION by one group (fluorescence immunophenotyping and interphase cytogenetics as a tool for investigation of neoplasms), was exploited to demonstrate numerical chromosomal alterations in the comparatively rare CD30-positive Reed-Sternberg cells of Hodgkin's lymphoma (6,7). Because these neoplastic cells typically constitute only a minor fraction of the lymphoid population, clonal alterations were not previously demonstrable by averaging techniques, such as flow cytometry and polymerase chain reaction (PCR). Also utilizing this dual FISH-immunohistochemistry approach, *NF1* deletions were found to be restricted to the S-100 protein–positive Schwann cell element in another heterogeneous neoplasm, the plexiform neurofibroma (8). Lastly, this technique has also been used to simultaneously visualize *HER-2/neu* gene amplification and protein overexpression in breast carcinomas (9), for which the acronym CODFISH (concomitant oncoprotein detection with FISH) has been proposed.

Another distinct advantage for diagnostic pathology laboratories is the similarity of FISH to immunohistochemistry.

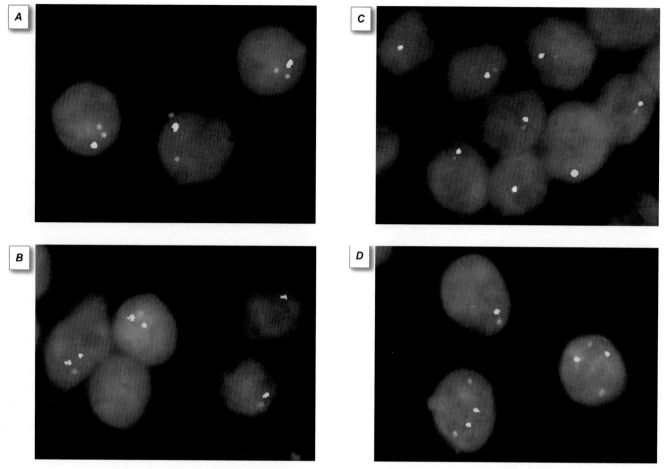

Figure 4.2 Examples of deletions detected by FISH, including an oligodendroglioma with 1p (**A**, 1 green 1p32 and 2 red 1q42 signals per nucleus) and 19q deletions (**B**, 1 red 19q13 and 2 green 19p13 signals), and an atypical teratoid/ rhabdoid tumor (**C**, 1 green *BCR* and 1 red *NF2* signal). A glioma with normal complements of chromosome 1 (2 green and 2 red signals in most nuclei) is shown for comparison (**D**). (See color insert.)

The two techniques are highly analogous, except that FISH uses DNA probes rather than antibodies. In contrast to the qualitative (e.g., positive versus negative) or semi-quantitative (e.g., 0 to 3+) interpretation schemes for immunohistochemistry, FISH provides quantitative data (i.e., copy numbers of target DNA per cell) and is therefore more objective overall. Nevertheless, FISH on paraffin tissue has at least as many artifacts as immunohistochemistry and experience with fluorescence microscopy is needed to avoid false positive and false negative results.

FISH versus Other Cytogenetic and Molecular Techniques

When compared with metaphase cytogenetics (i.e., karyotyping), FISH has several clear advantages, one of which is the lack of a requirement for mitotically active cells and culturing. For example, only actively proliferating cells are assessable on karyotype, and thus significant growth selection biases may occur in vitro, including overgrowth of non-neoplastic elements, such as stromal fibroblasts (particularly when analyzing benign or low-grade neoplasms).

On the other hand, FISH is not a genomic screening tool; it provides a targeted approach for alterations that have been initially identified by more global molecular techniques, such as classic cytogenetics, loss of heterozygosity (LOH) screening, comparative genomic hybridization (CGH), array CGH (aCGH), single nucleotide polymorphism (SNP) array, and gene expression profiling.

In terms of resolution, FISH is more sensitive than karyotyping and CGH but less sensitive than PCR-based assays for detecting small alterations. For example, the former is limited to alterations of several megabases in size, whereas the latter can be designed to detect even single base pair mutations. Because FISH probes are typically at least 20 kb and most average 100 to 200 kb in size, alterations need to be fairly large for reliable detection (i.e., molecular cytogenetic level). In other words, FISH cannot detect small intragenic mutations, deletions, or insertions. PCR of blood or fresh tissue specimens is also more sensitive than FISH for detecting abnormal fusion transcripts resulting from chromosomal translocations, picking up as few as one per million cells. This is particularly useful when attempting to detect "minimal residual disease" or early recurrence,

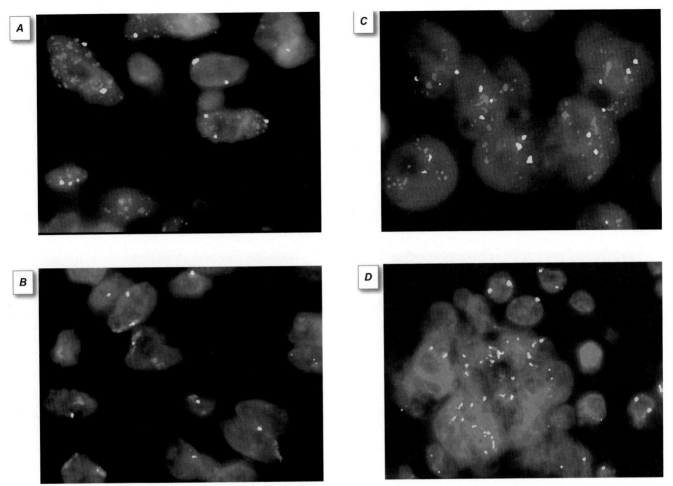

Figure 4.3 Examples of gene amplification, including glioblastomas with EGFR amplification (**A**, "double minute" pattern with small individual red signals; **B**, "homogenously staining region" pattern with large, coalescent red signals; CEP7 in green) and *HER-2/neu* amplification with numerous red gene signals and considerably fewer green CEP17 signals (**C**, *HER-2/neu* to CEP17 signal ratio >2.0). A dramatic example of polysomy 7 is shown for comparison with a multinucleated giant cell containing numerous copies of both the p16 gene on 9p21 in red and the CEP9 reference in green (**D**). In contrast to true gene amplification, the p16 to CEP9 signal ratio was close to 1.0 and several smaller, near diploid cells are seen nearby with 2 green and 2 red signals. (See color insert.)

though the biologic relevance of such small tumoral fractions is not always clear. In contrast, FISH is more sensitive than PCR at identifying gene deletions or amplifications from samples of mixed cellularity, such as neoplasms with clonal heterogeneity or contaminating non-neoplastic elements (10). It is estimated that sample purity must reach at least 70% tumor for quantitative PCR, and this is sometimes difficult to achieve in highly infiltrative neoplasms or tumors with abundant stroma or inflammation. FISH, on the other hand, can typically detect gains, translocations, or amplifications in as few as 5% and deletions in 15% to 30% of the cells within a sample. Lastly, whereas reverse-transcriptase PCR (RT-PCR) is quite reliable for identifying fusion transcripts in fresh frozen specimens, FISH may be less subject to false positive and false negative results in FFPE tissue.

In comparison to LOH studies by microsatellite analysis, FISH provides similar or complementary results, but is not identical and each method has advantages and disadvantages. A very common misconception is to equate the

two, stating that "FISH demonstrates LOH" for a particular region of interest. However, because FISH measures absolute copy number rather than allele status, this is inaccurate. Additionally, whereas LOH often reflects a simple deletion, the mechanism of loss can be more complicated. For example, James et al. (11) found that mitotic recombination of chromosome 17p leads to loss of the wild-type TP53 allele and duplication of the mutated allele in astrocytomas. In other words, although one "allele" (maternal or paternal) is lost (i.e., LOH), there are still two copies of the gene, yielding two signals per cell by FISH analysis and a false negative result for *TP53* loss. Therefore, FISH is not a suitable assay for detecting this type of loss in astrocytomas (12). Another advantage of the LOH studies is the ease of evaluating large numbers of markers spanning the entire length of a chromosome or chromosomal arm. As emphasized previously, however, morphologic correlation is not possible unless regions of interest are microdissected first. Additionally, LOH requires matching germline DNA

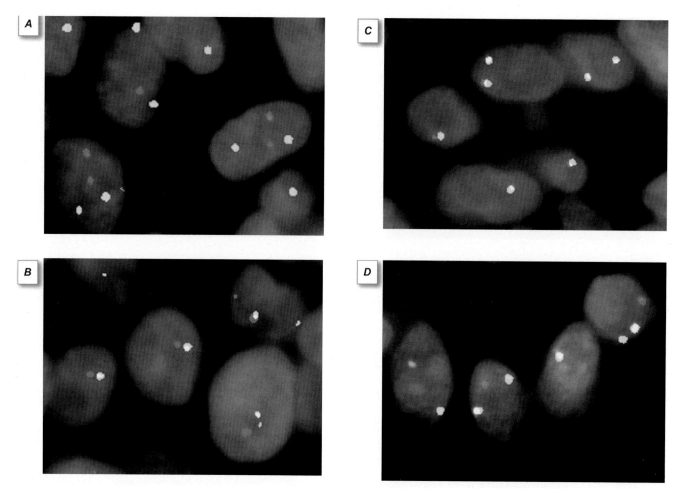

Figure 4.4 Examples of common FISH assays for translocation, including FISH-F negative (**A**, green and red signals split) and FISH-F positive cases (**B**, 1 yellow fusion signal and 1 pair of split red and green signals in most nuclei) tested with probes against *EWS* on 22q12 (red) and *FLI1* on 11q24 (green). The FISH-BA strategy for *SYT* is similarly illustrated with negative (**C**, only fused signals) and positive (**D**, 1 fusion signal and 1 pair of split red and green signals) cases. (See color insert.)

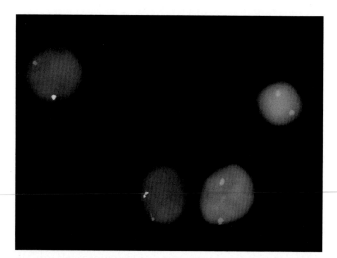

Figure 4.5 Chimeric bone marrow in patient with sex-mismatched transplant showing a mixture of donor and recipient, male (*left*) and female (*right*) cells (CEPX in red, CEPY in green). (See color insert.)

from the patient's leukocytes or microdissected normal tissue and this is often not readily available.

Tissue Microarray-FISH

A recent application of FISH uses high-throughput analysis via tissue microarray (TMA). This technology takes advantage of multispecimen paraffin blocks constructed from hundreds of 0.6 to 2.0-mm neoplastic, non-neoplastic, and control tissue cores of interest. TMA-FISH markedly increases efficiency by reducing data acquisition time, as well as probe, reagent, and storage space requirements. A recently popularized approach is to initially screen a small number of tumors with gene expression profiling and then verify the resulting candidate genes in a large number of tumors, using TMA-immunohistochemistry and TMA-FISH (13,14). TMA studies have shown excellent morphologic, antigenic, and genomic preservation with high levels of concordance compared to the traditional whole slide approach (14–18). As one might expect, however, tumor heterogene-

TABLE 4.2
EXAMPLES OF SPECIMEN TYPES APPLICABLE TO FISH

Fresh/frozen tissue
Cytology specimens
    Body fluids (urine)
    Intraoperative smears
    Cell culture preparations
Fresh-frozen, parafin-embedded tissue
    Thin sections (4–6 μ)
    Disaggregated nuclei
    Archived unstained sections
    Previously stained sections (e.g., negative immunohistochemistry controls)

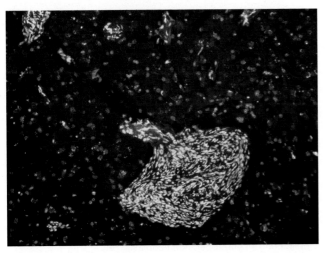

Figure 4.6 Low-magnification (100X) FISH image of a heterogeneous brain tissue sample involved by meningioangiomatosis. Because the morphology is retained, it is relatively simple to distinguish the perivascular spindled cells of interest *(lower center)* from the surrounding neocortex without the need for microdissection. (See color insert.)

ity can still be problematic, although adequate sampling can be optimized by incorporating multiple cores from each specimen. For gene amplifications, TMA-FISH is particularly appealing, because interpretations are rapid, typically requiring only seconds per tissue core. For aneusomies and deletions, manual signal counts still remain tedious and time consuming. However, early versions of automated spot counting software are now available from several vendors and promise to increase the efficiency of this technique further. Additionally, TMA-FISH is an excellent method for new probe validation, proficiency testing, interlaboratory comparisons, and quality assurance/quality control (19–22).

Disadvantages and Pitfalls of FISH

As discussed above, recent technical advances have greatly enhanced the clinical applicability of FISH, though a number of limitations remain. One of the main disadvantages of FISH is signal fading. Storing hybridized slides in a freezer and avoiding prolonged exposure to light can preserve hybridization signals for up to 2 to 3 years or longer. However, a permanent record is not currently possible unless chromogenic detection is used. Clinical labs typically circumvent this pitfall by capturing one or more digital images as a permanent record of each case. CISH is an alternative approach, although, unfortunately, multicolor CISH is not as simple as multicolor FISH and currently available chromogens lack the spectral versatility, sensitivity and spatial resolution attainable with fluorochromes. Some commercial CISH applications bypass this problem by providing the test (e.g., *Her-2/neu*) and reference (e.g., centromere 17) probes separately, so that in place of one dual-color FISH assay, two single-color CISH experiments are performed on serial sections and counts are obtained from the same basic regions of the two slides. The recently developed photostable quantum dots offer another potential alternative for permanent signals in future FISH applications (23).

Other limitations include a variety of artifacts, particularly common in paraffin sections. It is for this reason that although the FISH assay itself is mastered quickly, interpretation often requires significantly more experience. Most troublesome are nuclear truncation artifacts, aneuploid tumor populations, autofluorescence, and partial hybridization failures. Truncation artifact refers to the underestimation of copy numbers resulting from incomplete DNA complements within transected nuclei. Therefore it is important to assess controls cut at the same thickness. Definitions for hemizygous deletion are often based on the mean percentages of control nuclei with fewer than 2 signals plus 3 standard deviations. A requirement of greater than 20% nuclei with twice the number of tests to references probe signals is fairly typical (e.g., cells with 1 test and 2 reference signals, 2 test and 4 reference signals, etc.). However, other approaches have also been used and currently there are no widely sanctioned consensus criteria published. Homozygous deletions are defined by the complete lack of test probe signals in tumor cells. Partial hybridization failure is ruled out by the presence of reference probe signals in the tumor cells, as well as test probe signals in adjacent non-neoplastic elements, such as vascular endothelial cells.

Aneuploidy and polyploidy can result in confusing signal counts and is a particularly common finding in malignant and even some benign neoplasms. The inclusion of reference probes is helpful in such situations. Although the simplest approach is to interpret absolute losses (<2 copies) and gains (>2 copies), one may also opt to delineate "relative" losses and gains based on a reference ploidy, obtained either by flow cytometry or the assessment of multiple chromosomes by FISH. For example, the finding of 3 copies

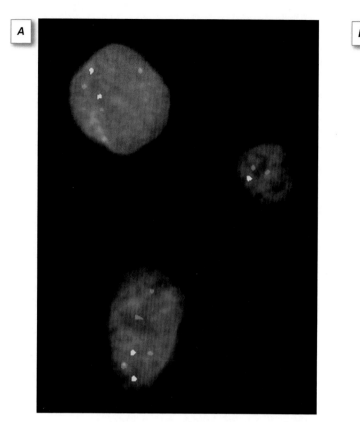 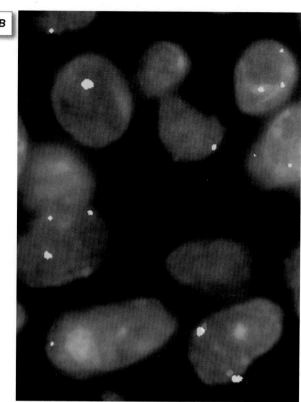

Figure 4.7 Relative 1p deletion within near-tetraploid cells of an oligodendroglioma with enlarged nuclei containing four copies of the red 1q32 reference probe signals and two copies of the green 1p32 test probe signals (**A**). A near-diploid tumor cell with 1 green and 2 red signals is also seen on the right. A homozygous deletion of the p16 gene on 9p21 is shown, wherein the majority of cells have retained green CEP9 signals, but no red p16 signals (**B**). A normal pattern of 2 paired red and green signals is seen in the lower right, likely representing an entrapped non-neoplastic cell. (See color insert.)

would be considered a relative gain in a diploid tumor, normal in a triploid tumor, and a relative loss in a tetraploid tumor. Similarly, one may combine a centromere or other reference probe (e.g., marker on opposite chromosomal arm) with a test probe of interest and determine their ratios. For example, cells with 4 chromosome 9 centromeres and 2 copies of the p16 region on 9p21 would be interpreted as having polysomy 9 and a hemizygous p16 deletion (Fig. 4.7A). A similar tumor with no p16 signals would be interpreted as polysomy 9 with homozygous p16 deletion (Fig. 4.7B). Similarly, cells with 6 copies of *HER-2/neu* might be interpreted as low-level amplification if there were only 2 chromosome 17 centromeres, but would represent polysomy 17 without gene amplification if there were 6 centromeres per cell (i.e., test to reference probe ratio of 1).

Lastly, autofluorescence is a particularly common problem in FFPE tissue sections. Autofluorescent tissue fragments are usually larger and more irregular than true signals, and thus they can be disregarded; however, some fragments have just the right size to mimic true signals. In this case, the use of multiple filters is helpful, because autofluorescence will often appear on both green and red filters, whereas true signals fluoresce only under one or the other. The problem of partial hybridization failure can be minimized by counting only in regions where the majority of cells have discernable signals. This issue is most problematic when combining a

highly robust probe (e.g., centromere) with a comparatively weak probe (e.g., small locus–specific [LSI] probe). Signals from both probes should be seen in normal cells (e.g., endothelial cells) within the region for the counts to be considered reliable.

FISH ASSAY: ADDITIONAL TECHNICAL CONSIDERATIONS

Many different FISH protocols are available and vary depending on individual preferences and specimen type. Overall, simple protocols are better, requiring less hands-on time, fewer opportunities for errors, and fewer troubleshooting requirements. Additionally, automated instruments are now available to minimize hands-on time, although they are fairly expensive. In general, the basic steps of the protocols are similar to those of immunohistochemistry and include deparaffinization, pretreatment/ target retrieval, probe and target DNA denaturation, hybridization (a few hours to overnight), posthybridization washes, detection, and microscopic interpretation/imaging. This is usually a 2-day assay, which requires roughly 3 to 4 hours the first day and 30 minutes the second day. Alternatively, same-day assays are possible if the probes are particularly robust (e.g., centromere probes).

Similar to immunohistochemistry, microwave or heat-induced target retrieval often works better than chemical forms of pretreatment, considerably enhancing hybridization efficiency (10,24,25). If this step is included, protein digestion times may be reduced or the step may be eliminated altogether. Nonetheless, optimal pretreatment and digestion varies from specimen to specimen and depends on a number of variables, including method of fixation/processing. Some hybridization buffers are also significantly more efficient and may lower probe concentration requirements considerably (e.g., DenHyb, Insitus*). This can be particularly beneficial with expensive commercial probes, because they may last 5 to 20 times as long as they would when using the manufacturer's recommended dilutions. Additional time-saving strategies include products such as "SkipDewax" (Insitus†), which deparaffinizes and pretreats all in one step. Lastly, a variety of amplification steps are available for enhancing weak signals. However, such steps are rarely necessary with good probes. The simpler protocol and generally cleaner background associated with directly labeled fluorochrome probes (e.g., fluorescein isothiocyanate [FITC], rhodamine) is a distinct advantage over indirectly labeled probes (e.g., digoxigenin, biotin) that require additional steps (e.g., fluorochrome-labeled secondary antibody) with or without further amplification. Nevertheless, dramatic levels of FISH signal amplification have been reported with tyramide signal amplification (TSA) or catalyzed reporter deposition (CARD) (26–29). This technique results in peroxidase-mediated deposition of haptenized tyramine molecules, not only in the precise site of hybridization, but also in the nearby vicinity, resulting in up to 1000-fold or greater amplification levels. Although one possible application is marked reductions of probe concentration requirements, the potentially more exciting possibility is the use of smaller probes, perhaps down to the level of 1 kb or less (30). Therefore TSA could potentially increase the sensitivity for small alterations, such as those detectable by PCR, while maintaining the morphologic advantages of FISH.

FISH PROBES AND PROBE DEVELOPMENT

Several basic probe types are used for FISH. Centromere enumerating probes (CEPs) were among the first to be developed and remain ideal for detecting whole chromosome gains and losses, such as monosomy, trisomy, and other polysomies. Targeting highly repetitive 171-bp sequences of α-satellite DNA, they are associated with excellent hybridization efficiencies, typically producing large, bright signals. Unfortunately, sequence similarities in some pericentromeric regions result in cross-hybridization artifacts with the potential for overestimating signal counts. For example, the cross-hybridization between centromeres 13 and 21 or between centromeres 14 and 22 is so extensive that these CEPs have been previously marketed with four expected signals rather than two. A better solution is to use LSI or painting probes to enumerate these individual

chromosomes. Cross-hybridization problems are occasionally encountered with other centromere probes as well, although the nonspecific signals are usually dimmer than the true signals and the use of either more stringent washes or lower probe concentrations often resolves this problem. Also, an interesting phenomenon observed in non-neoplastic brain specimens is that certain chromosomes are packaged into interphase nuclei with paired centromeres in close proximity, a concept known as somatic pairing (31,32). This phenomenon is most impressive with CEP17, but may be encountered to a lesser extent with other centromeres as well, including CEP1 and CEP8. Because of this close proximity, FISH yields an unexpected fraction of cells harboring a single large signal, rather than two smaller ones, potentially leading to overinterpretation of monosomy. For unknown reasons, somatic pairing is usually not seen in neoplasms of the brain. Nonetheless, determinations of chromosomal loss with these CEPs can be problematic if non-neoplastic brain specimens are used as controls to establish cutoffs. Despite these technical limitations, CEPs remain extremely useful for detecting aneusomies and are still among the best FISH probes available. The presence of similarly repetitive DNA sequences in subtelomeric regions has recently led to the development of commercially available probes for each chromosomal arm as well.

Another type of FISH probe is the whole chromosome paint (WCP), consisting of a cocktail of DNA fragments that targets all the nonrepetitive DNA sequences in an entire chromosome. Because it covers such a large region, it produces a more diffuse-appearing signal in interphase nuclei. Instead, it may be used on metaphase spreads for resolving complex structural alterations. However, some of the smaller, acrocentric chromosomes yield sufficiently discrete signals for enumeration, even in interphase nuclei. Also, the WCPs are primarily utilized in advanced molecular cytogenetics applications that are beyond the scope of this chapter, such as spectral karyotyping (SKY) and multiplex FISH (M-FISH), where each of the 24 human chromosomes or each of the 48 chromosomal arms is "painted" with a unique color, created by mixing a few basic fluorescent dyes in various combinations and ratios (i.e., combinatorial labeling). When applied to either a person's or a tumor's metaphase preparation and photographed, sophisticated software algorithms can accurately identify each specific chromosome or chromosomal fragment. This is particularly useful for identifying complex structural alterations, such as translocations involving multiple chromosomes, "marker chromosomes" that are unidentifiable on routine karyotype banding, and so on. In contrast, CGH applies an entire genome as the "probe." Genomic tumor DNA is labeled in one color (e.g., green dye), and normal genomic DNA is labeled in another color (e.g., red dye). Equal quantities of each are competitively hybridized to normal human metaphases to screen for regions of relative loss and gain in the tumor. In areas without loss or gain, there are relatively equal quantities of both genomic DNA signals and the chromosomal region will appear yellow. In contrast, regions of DNA gain or loss in the tumor will appear closer to green or red, because the signal from one of the genomic probes will predominate. As with SKY and M-FISH, software has been developed to quantitate the ratios of green to red throughout all

---

*DenHyb, Insitus, www.insitus.com.
†SkipDewax, Insitus, www.insitus.com.

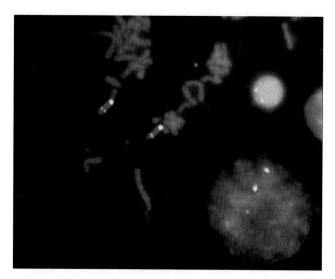

Figure 4.8 Interphase FISH study to verify the appropriate cytogenetic localization for a homemade DNA probe against the 4.1G gene on 6q23 (4.1G in red, CEP6 in green). (See color insert.)

chromosomal regions. This approach is very useful for cytogenetic screening of rare tumors in which nothing is known about the genetics. However, the resolution is fairly limited and therefore only large alterations are typically identified. Thus arrays (CGH) containing thousands of individual DNA probes throughout the genome have also been constructed to provide a modified approach with greatly enhanced resolution (33). Techniques such as FISH, CGH, M-FISH, and SKY are sometimes referred to collectively as "molecular cytogenetics" (34,35).

Today, the most versatile FISH probes are the LSI or gene-specific probes. These probes target distinct chromosomal regions of interest and use single copy rather than repetitive DNA sequences. Therefore, to yield signals of sufficient size in interphase FFPE nuclei, the probe typically needs to be at least 20 kb in size. The largest LSI probes are >1 mb, although most fall into the 100 to 300-kb range. Until recently, only a limited assortment of LSI probes has been commercially available, though the assortment has expanded greatly over the last few years. Nonetheless, cloning vectors remain excellent sources for developing homemade FISH probes, including cosmids, bacterial artificial chromosomes (BACs), P1 artificial chromosomes (PACs), and yeast artificial chromosomes (YACs). Whereas in the past, this required a rather lengthy and tedious process of screening vector libraries with PCR primers, the recent human genome project has completely sequenced entire BAC libraries, enabling rapid Internet screening, using DNA sequences of interest, gene names, or physical maps of individual chromosomes*. Similarly, mapped BAC clones spread throughout the human genome at 1-mb intervals have also become readily available†. Therefore it is now relatively simple to obtain a BAC clone localizing to virtually any region of interest, label the DNA with commercially available kits, and use it as a FISH probe. However, it is important to verify that the correct clone was obtained, either by screening for the DNA sequence of

interest by PCR or by performing metaphase FISH to determine that the probe localizes to the appropriate cytogenetic band (Fig. 4.8).

APPLICATION OF FISH TO CLINICAL AND TRANSLATIONAL RESEARCH

Over the past decade, FISH has been applied to many translational studies. Typical hypotheses tested include: (a) whether a cytogenetic alteration (deletion, gain, amplification, translocation) is highly sensitive and specific for a single tumor type (i.e., diagnostic biomarker); (b) within a single diagnostic category (e.g., ductal breast carcinoma), whether a specific cytogenetic alteration can predict which tumors will be either aggressive or indolent (i.e., prognostic biomarker); and (c) within a single diagnostic category, whether a cytogenetic alteration will predict which tumors will respond to either general, nontargeted forms of chemotherapy or molecularly targeted therapy (i.e., predictive biomarker). The most common applications today include *HER-2/neu* amplification testing in breast cancer, 1p/19q deletion testing in gliomas (a form of brain cancer), testing for signature translocations associated with specific hematologic, soft tissue, or pediatric malignancies. Each of these examples is covered in greater detail in their respective organ-specific chapters. However, clinically relevant examples for each alteration type detectable by FISH are summarized in Table 4.3, with several examples discussed below (36–78).

Aneusomies and Deletions

Aneusomies represent gains and losses of whole chromosomes, whereas deletions are losses of distinct chromosomal regions, varying in size from the targeted loss of a specific gene or portion of a gene to an entire chromosomal arm. Aneusomies and deletions are amongst the most common alterations detected in neoplasms by FISH (Table 4.3). Sometimes it is difficult to distinguish specific tumor-associated polysomies and monosomies from the nonspecific gains and losses associated with either an overall state of genomic instability that commonly occurs during the malignant progression of many solid tumors or with polyploidy. The latter often results from endoreduplication, wherein DNA is successfully replicated during a cell cycle, but the nucleus fails to divide. With one such event, the tumor cell converts from 2n to 4n (i.e., tetraploid), whereas several such cycles results in huge mononucleated or multinucleated giant cells with astonishing gains in chromosomal number (Fig. 4.3D). The use of reference probes helps to distinguish such chromosomal gains or high-level polysomies from true gene amplification (Fig. 4.3).

One of the most commonly used FISH applications for deletions is that of 1p and 19q testing in diffuse gliomas. The presence of 1p and 19q codeletion (typically one entire arm from each) has diagnostic, prognostic, and predictive value in that this genetic signature (Fig. 4.2A and B) is associated predominantly with pure oligodendrogliomas with enhanced therapeutic responsiveness and overall survival time (36,37). Also commonly encountered in such tumors is a population of near-tetraploid tumor

---

*For example, http://genome.ucsc.edu.
†For example, http://mp.invitrogen.com.

TABLE 4.3
CANCER-ASSOCIATED ALTERATIONS COMMONLY DETECTED BY FISH

Type	Tumor Type (References)	Alterations/Probes	Association
Aneusomies/deletions	Oligodendroglioma[36,37]	1p- with 19q-	Diagnostic, prognostic, predictive
	Urothelial carcinoma[38–40]	+3, 7, or 17; 9p-	Diagnostic
	Lung carcinoma[41]	+7p, 8q, 5p, or 6	Diagnostic
	CLL[41-44]	13q-, 11q-, 17q-	Diagnostic, prognostic
	GBM[45,46]	+7, -10	Diagnostic
	Prostatic carcinoma[47]	8p-, 8q+	Prognostic
	Medulloblastoma[48,49]	17p-, 17q+; (il7q)	Diagnostic
	Leukemias/MDS[50–52]	+8, +12; -5, -7	Diagnostic, prognostic
	MRT, AT/RT[53,54]	INI1/hSNF5 (22q-)	Diagnostic
	Meningioma[55]	NF2 (22q-)	Diagnostic
	Multiple myeloma[56,57]	RB1 (13q-), TP53 (17p-)	Prognostic
	MPNST[58]	NF1 (17q-)	Diagnostic
Amplifications	Breast carcinoma[59–62]	HER-2/neu	Prognostic, predictive
	Neuroblastoma[63,64]	N-myc	Diagnostic, prognostic
	GBM[45,46]	EGFR	Diagnostic
	Medulloblastoma[48,49]	MYCN, c-myc	Diagnostic, prognostic
Translocations	EWS/PNET[65,66]	EWS-FL11, EWS-BA	Diagnostic
	Synovial sarcoma[67]	SYT-SSX, SYT-BA	Diagnostic
	Alveolar RMS[68,69]	PAX3-FKHR, FKHR-BA	Diagnostic
	DSRCT	EWS-WT1, EWS-BA	Diagnostic
	M/RC liposarcoma	CHOP-BA	Diagnostic
	Clear cell sarcoma[70]	EWS-ATF1, EWS-BA	Diagnostic
	IMT[71–73]	ALK-TPM3, ALK-TPM4, ALK-CARS, ALK-BA	Diagnostic, prognostic
	Burkitt lymphoma[74]	MYC-IGH, MYC-BA	Diagnostic
	MALT lymphoma[74]	API2-MALT1, IGH-MALT1, MALT1-BA	Diagnostic
	Follicular lymphoma[74]	IGH-BCL2	Diagnostic
	ALCL[73,74]	ALK-BA	Diagnostic
	Mantle cell lymphoma[74]	IGH-CCND1	Diagnostic
	Multiple myeloma[56,57]	IGH-CCND1, IGH-FGFR3, IGH-BA	Prognostic
	CML[75]	BCR-ABL	Diagnostic, MRD
	AML[76,78]	AML1-ETO, CBFB-BA, PML-RARA, RARA-BA, MLL-BA, BCR-ABL	Diagnostic, prognostic, predictive
	ALL[77,78]	TEL-AML1, BCR-ABL, MLL-BA	Diagnostic, prognostic, predictive

CLL, chronic lymphocytic leukemia; GBM, glioblastoma; MDS, myelodysplastic syndrome; MRT, malignant rhabdoid tumor; AT/RT, atypical teratoid/rhabdoid tumor; MPNST, malignant peripheral nerve sheath tumor; EWS, Ewing sarcoma; PNET, primitive neuroectodermal tumor; RMS, rhabdomyosarcoma; DSRCT, desmoplastic small, round cell tumor; M/RC, myxoid/round cell; IMT, inflammatory myofibroblastic tumor; ALCL, anaplastic large cell lymphoma; CML, chronic myelogenous leukemia; AML, acute myelogenous leukemia; ALL, acute lymphoblastic leukemia; BA, break apart probe set; MRD, minimal residual disease assessment.

cells with four copies of the reference probes (1q and 19p) and two copies of the test probes (1p and 19q) (Fig. 4.7A). Common cutoffs for 1p or 19q loss include the presence of more than 20% cells with twice the number of reference versus test probe signals or an overall test to reference probe signal ratio of less than 0.8. There is no current consensus for the optimal way to enumerate signals for chromosomal losses and gains, though in clinical cases, a common approach is to use two individuals who count signals in 100 cells each. In the majority of cases, the counts are concordant and they are simply added for a total enumeration of 200 cells. If there is a discrepancy or the counts are borderline for an alteration, then either the same individuals count additional cells or a third enumerator is used. Despite the clinical utility of 1p and 19q testing, the precise gene targets on these chromosomes remain unclear. In other tumor types, a specific tumor suppressor is known to be targeted by various chromosomal deletions (Table 4.3). Notable examples include the INI1/hSNF5 gene on 22q11.2 in malignant rhabdoid tumors and atypical teratoid/rhabdoid tumors (53,54) (Fig. 4.2C), the NF2 gene on 22q12 in meningiomas (55), the RB1 gene on 13q14 and the TP53 gene on 17p13.1 in multiple myeloma (56,57), and the NF1 gene on 17q11.2 in malignant peripheral nerve sheath tumors (58).

In terms of tumor-specific chromosomal gains and losses, a number of new multicolor probe cocktails have recently become commercially available for clinical and translational studies,* each with different recommendations

_____

*Vysis, www.vysis.com.

for minimum numbers of nuclei counted and cutoffs for alterations. For example, the UroVysion and LAVysion probe sets have been shown to increase diagnostic sensitivities in body fluid cytology specimens for urothelial carcinoma (38–40) and lung carcinoma (41), respectively. Similarly, the CLL (Fig. 4.9) and ProVysion FISH assays have been shown to identify prognostically relevant subsets of chronic lymphocytic leukemia (42–44) and prostatic adenocarcinoma (47) patients, respectively. Lastly, the detection of specific aneusomies and deletions by FISH has been clinically useful in identifying diagnostically challenging cases of glioblastoma, particularly the small cell variant (45,46), medulloblastoma, especially the anaplastic/ large cell variant (48,49), and prognostically relevant subsets of leukemia/myelodysplastic syndrome (50–52).

Gene Amplifications

High-level gene amplifications are typically seen in one of two patterns. If the amplified gene is present on small extrachromosomal segments known as double minutes, FISH will show numerous individual signals (Fig. 4.3A and C). On the other hand, if gene amplifications consist of contiguously arranged gene copies within a single chromosomal region, then, by karyotyping, this amplified region is identified as a homogenously stained region (HSR) on chromosomal banding, whereas by FISH, the signals are so close together that they coalesce into abnormally large linear or globular signals (Fig. 4.3B). In the latter case, rough estimates are made regarding how many signals are contained within the coalescent signals based on their overall size. Lastly, CEP probes are often used as references to chromosome number, to distinguish polysomies (i.e., gains of the entire chromosome; Fig. 4.3D) from true gene amplification.

Of all the current clinical applications of FISH analysis in tumor pathology, the assessment of *HER-2/neu* amplification status in breast cancer is typically one of the highest volume tests and has attracted great attention and controversy (59–62). Although there is now agreement that *HER-2/neu* assessment provides clinically useful information, the optimal diagnostic approach is still widely debated (Chapter 20). *HER-2/neu* gene amplification has been identified in 20% to 35% of breast carcinomas (Fig. 4.3C) and provides both prognostic and predictive information, with the following associations for positive tumors: (a) reduced patient survival, especially in lymph node–positive, but also in node-negative, cases; (b) increased responsiveness to adriamycin-based therapeutic regimens; (c) increased responsiveness to trastuzumab (Herceptin), which specifically targets the overexpressed surface protein; and (d) decreased responsiveness to radiation therapy, cyclophosphamide, methotrexate, 5-fluorouracil, hormonal therapy, and taxol. Additionally, testing is justified by the fact that there is a significant risk of cardiotoxicity with combined adriamycin and trastuzumab therapy, and this should therefore be avoided in patients with a low probability of response. In pediatric pathology, testing of neuroblastomas for *MYCN* amplification has similarly become standard of care (Fig. 12.4), with positive cases typically showing an aggressive biology (63,64). A similar

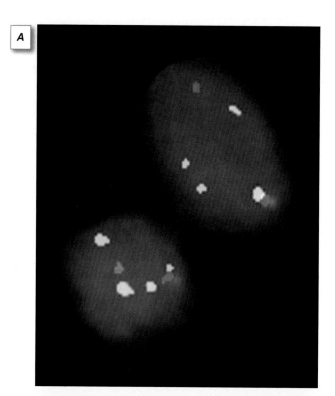

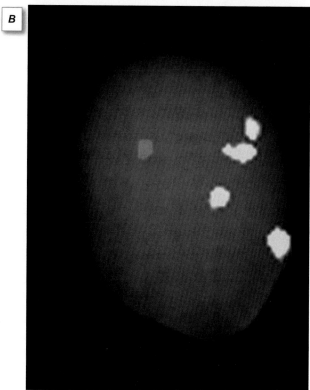

Figure 4.9 Three-color aneusomy/ deletion FISH cocktail for CLL in negative (**A**; 2 green CEP12, 2 red 13q14.3, and 2 aqua 13q34 signals) and positive (**B**; three green, 1 red, 1 aqua) examples. (See color insert.)

pattern is encountered in a subset of the central nervous system counterpart medulloblastoma; *MYCN* and *c-myc* amplifications are particularly common in the highly aggressive anaplastic/large cell variant (48,49). Lastly,

TABLE 4.4

EXPERIMENTAL DESIGN FOR TRANSLATIONAL FISH STUDIES

Identify a cytogenetic biomarker
    Chromosomal gain/loss
    Gene/locus deletion
    Gene amplification
    Translocation
Obtain test and reference DNA probes
    Commercial
    Homemade (e.g., BAC clones)
Assess potential clinical relevance
    Diagnostic aid
    Prognostic aid
    Predicts response or lack of response to patient therapy
Determine appropriate specimen cohort to test and clinical endpoints needed
    Archival paraffin-embedded tissue versus fresh/frozen versus cytology
    Retrospective versus prospective
    Morphologically overlapping tumor entities to assess specificity
    Times to disease progression, metastasis, or patient death
    Patient age or other demographically relevant prognosticators
    Extent of resection/surgical margin status
    Types of adjuvant therapy administered
    Biostatistics needed to answer study questions?
    Statistical power analysis: number of specimens needed for statistical significance

EGFR amplification (Fig. 4.2A and B), often in combination with monosomy 10 or chromosome 10q deletion (Fig. 4.1A and C) helps to distinguish the clinically aggressive and relatively therapeutically refractory small cell variant of glioblastoma from the more biologically favorable and chemotherapeutically responsive look-alike, anaplastic oligodendroglioma (45,46).

Translocations

The list of currently known tumor-associated chromosomal translocations is already impressive and continues to grow as new translocations are described. They are particularly useful as ancillary diagnostic aids in primitive-appearing hematopoietic and soft tissue malignancies, with most of the examples previously studied by FISH listed in Table 4.3. Some are already routinely used for clinical diagnosis (Chapters 11 and 13), and the applications are likely to expand in the future. Chromosomal translocations are unique among the FISH assays in that the interpretation relies more on the spatial relationships of the signals rather than their quantitation. For optimal probe design, detailed knowledge of the break points is often needed, though most of the common translocations now have reliable probes available commercially. One common strategy is fusion FISH (FISH-F), by which a probe localizing just centromeric to one chromosomal break point is combined with a second probe localizing just telomeric to the reciprocal break point (e.g., *BCR* on 22q and *ABL* on 9q). This yields separated, or "split," signals (e.g., 2 green, 2 red signals; Fig. 4.4A) in translocation-negative cells, but produces a "fusion" yellow or red-green signal when they are brought together by the translocation (e.g., 1 fusion, 1 green, 1 red signal; Fig. 4.4B). Nevertheless, one must avoid overinterpreting small cellular populations where green and red signals are overlapping purely by chance. The opposite or "break apart" strategy (FISH-BA) uses two probes localizing just proximal and distal to only one of the two breakpoints of interest. The two probes are normally in close proximity to one another; therefore this results in purely fusion signals in negative cases (e.g., 2 fusion signals; Fig. 4.4C), but at least one pair of split signals if there is a translocation (e.g., 1 fusion, 1 green, 1 red signal; Fig. 4.4D). The advantages of FISH-BA are that split signals should not occur purely by chance and it will still be positive in the variant translocations that may involve multiple partner genes (e.g., *EWS* can fuse with many other genes, as discussed in Chapter 11). Also, the commercial break apart probes are often more than 500 kb in size and therefore yield large, easy-to-interpret signals. The disadvantage to FISH-BA is that it provides no information regarding the identity of the fusion partner. Based on signal proximities in normal controls, we have typically used conservative cutoffs for positive test results of 30% cells with fused signals for FISH-F and 15% cells with split signals for FISH-BA (66). Another strategy to increase the sensitivity of FISH-F is to include one particularly large FISH probe that spans both sides of a break-point region. In the presence of a translocation, that DNA probe gets split, leading to an extra signal (FISH-ES) that is smaller than the remaining nonsplit, nonfused signal (e.g., 1 fusion, 1 green, 1 normal red, and 1 ES red signal). Because it is less likely that individual cells will contain both a fusion signal and an extra signal, smaller populations of tumor cells can be confidently identified in heterogeneous specimens (e.g., minimal residual disease in chronic myelogenous leukemia). Lastly, an even more reliable method to increase the sensitivity is to use two large probes that span both break-point regions, leading to two fusion or "double fusion" signals (D-FISH) (e.g., 2 fusion signals, marking the two derivative chromosomes). As one can imagine, if a positive tumor additionally has superimposed changes, such as polyploidy or the deletion of one of the derivative chromosomes (i.e., unbalanced translocation), the FISH pattern may be considerably more complex and difficult to interpret with certainty.

Designing a FISH Study

The basic format for designing a translational FISH study is outlined in Table 4.4. The first critical step is the identification of distinct molecular cytogenetic alterations known to be associated with a particular tumor type or a genetic syndrome. These data typically come from initial genomic screening studies. Next, the issue of DNA probe availability must be addressed. If commercially available, then acquisition is simple, but, if not, homemade probes can be fashioned as previously described. For deletions, regional chromosomal gains, or gene amplifications, the CEP from the same chromosome is often used as the reference probe, such that the copy number for the locus of interest can be compared with the copy number of the chromosome from which it originates. Alternatively, a marker on the opposite chromosomal arm may serve as a copy number reference. Depending on the frequencies of various translocations, break point inconsistencies, and variant translocations, FISH-F, FISH-BA, FISH-ES, D-FISH, or multiple strategies may be chosen, in addition to the consideration of alternative methods of detection, such as RT-PCR (Chapter 5).

Once the appropriate DNA probes are obtained, a clinically relevant question or hypothesis should be tested. If diagnostic accuracy is being evaluated, other tumor types with overlapping morphologic features should also be assessed to determine sensitivities and specificities. If prognostic value is the issue, testing can be done on only a single tumor type, but there must be sufficient clinical follow-up to accurately determine statistical associations to patient outcomes, such as time to tumor recurrence, presence or absence of metastases, and patient death. Lastly, if therapeutic responsiveness to a specific form of therapy is being tested, it is critical that patients are treated in a uniform manner in addition to knowing times to recurrence, radiographic parameters of response versus progression, or survival times. The latter type of study is often the most rewarding, but is also the most difficult to design, often requiring large multi-institutional clinical trials with multidisciplinary expertise and biostatistical support. Other confounding variables that often affect prognosis should also be considered (e.g., patient age, relevant demographics, extent of surgery, forms of adjuvant therapy, etc.). Depending on the clinical question addressed, it is often helpful to consult a biostatistician in order to determine the sample numbers that will be required to provide sufficient statistical power.

ACKNOWLEDGEMENTS

The author is grateful to Ruma Banerjee, Diane Robirds, and Julie Branson for their assistance with many of the FISH studies illustrated in this chapter.

REFERENCES

1. Fuller CE, Perry A. Fluorescence in situ hybridization (FISH) in diagnostic and investigative neuropathology. *Brain Pathol* 2002;12:67–86.
2. Najfeld V, Burnett W, Vlachos A, et al. Interphase FISH analysis of sex-mismatched BMT utilizing dual color XY probes. *Bone Marrow Transplant* 1997;19:829–834.
3. Tamura S, Saheki K, Takatsuka H, et al. Early detection of relapse and evaluation of treatment for mixed chimerism using fluorescence in situ hybridization following allogeneic hematopoietic cell transplant for hematological malignancies. *Ann Hematol* 2000;79:622–626.
4. Paulus W, Bayas A, Ott G, et al. Interphase cytogenetics of glioblastoma and gliosarcoma. *Acta Neuropathol* 1994;88:420–425.
5. Boerman RH, Anderl K, Herath J, et al. The glial and mesenchymal elements of gliosarcomas share similar genetic alteration. *J Neuropathol Exp Neurol* 1996; 55:973–981.
6. Weber-Matthiesen K, Deerberg J, Poetsch M, et al. Numerical chromosome aberrations are present within the CD30+ Hodgkin and Reed-Sternberg cells in 100% of analyzed cases of Hodgkin's disease. *Blood* 1995;86:1464–1468.
7. Nolte M, Werner M, Vonwasielewski R, et al. Detection of numerical karyotype changes in the giant cells of Hodgkins lymphomas by a combination of FISH and immunohistochemistry applied to paraffin sections. *Histochem Cell Biol* 1996;105:401–404.
8. Perry A, Roth KA, Banerjee R, et al. NF1 deletions in S-100 protein-positive and negative cells of sporadic and neurofibromatosis 1 (NF1)-associated plexiform neurofibromas and MPNSTs. *Am J Pathol* 2001;159:57–61.
9. Tubbs RR, Pettay J, Roche P, et al. Concomitant oncoprotein detection with fluorescence in situ hybridization (CODFISH): a fluorescence-based assay enabling simultaneous visualization of gene amplification and encoded protein expression. *J Mol Diag* 2000;2:78–83.
10. Perry A, Nobori T, Ru N, et al. Detection of p16 gene deletions in gliomas: fluorescence in situ hybridization (FISH) versus quantitative PCR. *J Neuropathol Exp Neurol* 1997;56:999–1008.
11. James CD, Carlbom E, Nordenskjold M, et al. Mitotic recombination of chromosome 17 in astrocytomas. *Proc Nat Acad Sci USA* 1989;86:2858–2862.
12. Perry A, Anderl KA, Borell TJ, et al. Detection of p16, RB, CDK4, and p53 gene deletion/amplification by fluorescence in situ hybridization (FISH) in 96 gliomas. *Am J Clin Pathol* 1999;112:801–809.
13. Sallinen S-L, Sallinen PK, Haapasalo HK, et al. Identification of differentially expressed genes in human gliomas by DNA microarray and tissue chip techniques. *Cancer Res* 2000;60:6617–6622.
14. Moch H, Kallioniemi O-P, Sauter G. Tissue microarrays: what will they bring to molecular and anatomic pathology? *Adv Anat Pathol* 2001; 8:14–20.
15. Kononen J, Bubendorf L, Kallioniemi A, et al. Tissue microarrays for high-throughput molecular profiling of tumor specimens. *Nature Med* 1998; 4:844–847.
16. Schraml P, Kononen J, Bubendorf L, et al. Tissue microarrays for gene amplification surveys in many different tumor types. *Clin Cancer Res* 1999; 5:1966–1975.
17. Camp RL, Charette LA, Rimm DL. Validation of tissue microarray technology in breast carcinoma. *Lab Invest* 2000;80:1943–1949.
18. Hoos A, Urist MJ, Stojadinovic A, et al. Validation of tissue microarrays for immunohistochemical profiling of cancer specimens using the example of human fibroblastic tumors. *Am J Pathol* 2001;158:1245–1251.
19. Fuller CE, Wang H, Zhang W, et al. High-throughput molecular profiling of high-grade astrocytomas: the utility of fluorescence *in situ* hybridization on tissue microarrays (TMA-FISH). *J Neuropathol Exp Neurol* 2002;61:1078–1084.
20. Zhang D, Salto-Tellez M, Do E, et al. Evaluation of *HER-2/neu* oncogene status in breast tumors on tissue microarrays. *Hum Pathol* 2003;34:362–368.
21. Brat DJ, Seiferheld W, Perry A, et al. Analysis of 1p, 19q, 9p, and 10q as prognostic markers for high-grade astrocytomas using FISH on tissue microarrays from RTOG trials. *Neuro-Oncology* 2004;6: 96–103.
22. Diaz LK, Gupta R, Kidwai N, et al. The use of TMA for interlaboratory validation of FISH testing for detection of HER2 gene amplification in breast cancer. *J Histochem Cytochem* 2004;52:501–507.
23. Ness JM, Akhtar RS, Latham CB, et al. Combined tyramide signal amplification and quantum dots for sensitive and photostable immunofluorescence detection. *J Histochem Cytochem* 2003;51:981–987.
24. Henke R-P, Ayhan N. Enhancement of hybridization efficiency in interphase cytogenetics on paraffin-embedded tissue sections by microwave treatment. *Analyt Cell Pathol* 1994;6:319–325.
25. Shi S-R, Cote RJ, Taylor CR. Antigen retrieval techniques: current perspectives. *J Histochem Cytochem* 2001;49:931–937.
26. van Gijlswijk RPM, Zijlmans HJ, Weigant J, et al. Fluorochrome-labeled tyramides: use in immunocytochemistry and fluorescence in situ hybridization. *J Histochem Cytochem* 1997;45:375–382.
27. Macechko PT, Krueger L, Hirsch B, et al. Comparison of immunologic amplification vs enzymatic deposition of fluorochrome-conjugated tyramide as detection systems for FISH. *J Histochem Cytochem* 1997;45:359–363.
28. Schmidt BF, Chao J, Zhu Z, et al. Signal amplification in the detection of single-copy DNA and RNA by enzyme-catalyzed deposition (CARD) of the novel fluorescent reporter substrate Cy3.29-tyramide. *J Histochem Cytochem* 1997;45:365–373.
29. Speel EJM, Hopman AHN, Komminoth P. Amplification methods to increase the sensitivity of in situ hybridization: play CARD(S). *J Histochem Cytochem* 1999; 47:281–288.
30. Schriml LM, Padilla-Nash HM, Coleman A, et al. Tyramide signal amplification (TSA)-FISH applied to mapping PCR-labeled probes less than 1 Kb in size. *Biotechniques* 1999;27:608–613.
31. Arnoldus EPJ, Peters ACB, Bots GTAM, et al. Somatic pairing of chromosome 1 centromeres in interphase nuclei of human cerebellum. *Hum Genet* 1989;83:231–234.
32. Arnoldus EPJ, Noordermeer IA, Peters ACB, et al. Interphase cytogenetics reveals somatic pairing of chromosome 17 centromeres in normal human brain tissue, but no trisomy 7 or sex-chromosome loss. *Cytogenet Cell Genet* 1991;56:214–216.
33. Wadlow R, Ramaswamy S. DNA microarrays in clinical cancer research. *Curr Mol Med* 2005;5:111–120.

34. Liehr T, Claussen U. Current developments in human molecular cytogenetic techniques. *Curr Mol Med* 2002;2:283–297.
35. Salman M, Jhanwar SC, Ostrer H. Will the new cytogenetics replace the old cytogenetics? *Clin Genet* 2004;66:265–275.
36. Perry A. New developments in the molecular diagnosis of gliomas. *Can J Neurol Sci* (in press).
37. Reifenberger G, Louis DN. Oligodendroglioma: toward molecular definitions in diagnostic neuro-oncology. *J Neuropathol Exp Neurol* 2003; 62:111–126.
38. Halling KC, Walter K, Sokolova IA, et al. A comparison of cytology and fluorescence in situ hybridization for the detection of urothelial carcinoma. *J Urol* 2000; 164:1768–1775.
39. Sarosdy MF, Schellhammer P, Bokinsky G, et al. Clinical evaluation of a multi-target fluorescent in situ hybridization assay for detection of bladder cancer. *J Urol* 2002;168:1950–1954.
40. Skacel M, Fahmy M, Brainard JA, et al. Multitarget fluorescence in situ hybridization assay detects transitional cell carcinoma in the majority of patients with bladder cancer and atypical or negative urine cytology. *J Urol* 2003; 169:2101–2105.
41. Bubendorf L, Muller P, Joos L, et al. Multitarget FISH analysis in the diagnosis of lung cancer. *Am J Clin Pathol* 2005;123:516–523.
42. Stilgenbauer S, Bullinger L, Lichter P, et al. Genetics of chronic lymphocytic leukemia: genomic aberrations and V_H gene mutation status in pathogenesis and clinical course. *Leukemia* 2002;16:993–1007.
43. Shanafelt TD, Call TG. Current approach to diagnosis and management of chronic lymphocytic leukemia. *Mayo Clin Proc* 2004;79:388–398.
44. Glassman AB, Hayes KJ. The value of fluorescence in situ hybridization in the diagnosis and prognosis of chronic lymphocytic leukemia. *Cancer Gen Cytogenet* 2005; 158:88–91.
45. Burger PC, Pearl DK, Aldape K, et al. Small cell architecture: a histological equivalent of EGFR amplification in glioblastoma multiforme? *J Neuropathol Exp Neurol* 2001;60:1099–1104.
46. Perry A, Aldape KD, George DH, et al. Small cell astrocytoma: an aggressive variant that is clinicopathologically and genetically distinct from anaplastic oligodendroglioma. *Cancer* 2004;101:2318–2326.
47. Tsuchiya N, Slezak JM, Lieber M, et al. Clinical significance of alterations of chromosome 8 detected by fluorescence in situ hybridization analysis in pathologic organ-confined prostate cancer. *Genes Chrom Cancer* 2002;34:363–371.
48. Leonard J, Cai DX, Rivet D, et al. Large cell/anaplastic medulloblastomas and medullomyoblastomas: clinicopathologic and genetic features. *J Neurosurg* 2001; 95:82–88.
49. Helton KJ, Fouladi M, Boop FA, et al. Medullomyoblastoma: a radiographic and clinicopathologic analysis of 6 cases and review of the literature. *Cancer* 2004; 101:1445–1454.
50. Yan J, Marceau D, Drouin R. Tetrasomy 8 is associated with a major cellular proliferative advantage and a poor prognosis: two cases of myeloid hematologic disorders and review of the literature. *Cancer Genet Cytogenet* 2001; 125:14–21.
51. Dickinson JD, Smith LM, Sanger WG, et al. Unique gene expression and clinical characteristics are associated with the 11q23 deletion in chronic lymphocytic leukaemia. *Br J Haematol* 2005;128:460–471.
52. Primo D, Tabernero MD, Perez JJ, et al. Genetic heterogeneity of BCR/ABL+ adult B-cell precursor acute lymphoblastic leukemia: impact on the clinical, biological and immunophenotypical disease characteristics. *Leukemia* 2005;19:713–720.
53. Fuller CE, Pfeifer J, Humphrey P, et al. Chromosome 22q dosage in composite extrarenal rhabdoid tumors: clonal evolution or a phenotypic mimic? *Hum Pathol* 2001;32:1102–1108.
54. Raisanen J, Biegel JA, Hatanpaa KJ, et al. Chromosome 22q deletions in adult atypical teratoid / rhabdoid tumors. *Brain Pathol* 2005;15:23–28.
55. Rajaram V, Brat DJ, Perry A. Anaplastic meningioma vs. meningeal hemangiopericytoma: immunohistochemical and genetic markers. *Hum Pathol* 2004;35:1413–1418.
56. Chang H, Li D, Zhuang L, et al. Detection of chromosome 13q deletions and IgH translocations in patients with multiple myeloma by FISH: comparison with karyotype analysis. *Leuk Lymph* 2004;45:965–969.
57. Pantou D, Rizou H, Tsarouha H, et al. Cytogenetic manifestations of multiple myeloma heterogeneity. *Genes Chrom Cancer* 2005;42:44–57.
58. Perry A, Kunz SN, Fuller CE, et al. Differential NF1, p16, and EGFR patterns by interphase cytogenetics (FISH) in malignant peripheral nerve sheath tumor (MPNST) and morphologically similar spindle cell neoplasms. *J Neuropathol Exp Neurol* 2002; 61:702–709.
59. Cell Markers and Cytogenetics Committees, College of American Pathologists. Clinical laboratory assays for HER-2/*neu* amplification and overexpression: quality assurance, standardization, and proficiency testing. *Arch Pathol Lab Med* 2002;126:803–808.
60. Zarbo RJ, Hammond EH. Conference summary, strategic science symposium. *HER-2/neu* testing of breast cancer patients in clinical practice. *Arch Pathol Lab Med* 2003; 127:549–553.
61. Taucher S, Rudas M, Mader RM, et al. Do we need HER-2/*neu* testing for all patients with primary breast carcinoma? *Cancer* 2003;98:2547–2553.
62. Lal P, Salazar PA, Hudis CA, et al. HER-2 testing in breast cancer using immunohistochemical analysis and fluorescence in situ hybridization: a single-institution experience of 2,279 cases and comparison of dual-color and single-color scoring. *Am J Clin Pathol* 2004;121:631–636.
63. Mathew P, Valentine MB, Bowman LC, et al. Detection of *MYCN* gene amplification in neuroblastoma by fluorescence in situ hybridization: a pediatric oncology group study. *Neoplasia* 2001;3:105–109.
64. Sartelet H, Grossi L, Pasquier D, et al. Detection of *N-myc* amplification by FISH in immature areas of fixed neuroblastomas: more efficient than Southern blot/PCR. *J Pathol* 2002;198:83–91.
65. Qian X, Jin L, Shearer BM, et al. Molecular diagnosis of Ewing's sarcoma/primitive neuroectodermal tumor in formalin-fixed paraffin-embedded tissues by RT-PCR and fluorescence in situ hybridization. *Diagn Mol Pathol* 2005;14:23–28.
66. Bridge RS, Rajaram V, Dehner LP, Pfeifer JD, Perry A. Molecular diagnosis of Ewing sarcoma/primitive neuroectodermal tumor in routinely processed tissue: a comparison of two FISH strategies and RT-PCR in 67 malignant round cell tumors. *Mod Pathol* (in press).
67. Yang P, Hirose T, Hasegawa T, et al. Dual-colour fluorescence in situ hybridization analysis of synovial sarcoma. *J Pathol* 1998;184:7–13.
68. Biegel JA, Nycum LM, Valentine V, et al. Detection of the t(2;13)(q35;q14) and PAX3-FKHR fusion in alveolar rhabdomyosarcoma by fluorescence in situ hybridization. *Genes Chrom Cancer* 1995; 12:186–192.
69. McManus AP, O'Reilly MA, Jones KP, et al. Interphase fluorescence in situ hybridization detection of t(2;13)(q35;q14) in alveolar rhabdomyosarcoma: a diagnostic tool in minimally invasive biopsies. *J Pathol* 1996;178:410–414.
70. Covinsky M, Gong S, Rajaram V, et al. EWS-ATF1 fusion transcripts in gastrointestinal tumors previously diagnosed as malignant melanoma. *Hum Pathol* 2005;36:74–81.
71. Lawrence B, Perez-Atayde A, Hibbard MK, et al. TPM3-ALK and TPM4-ALK oncogenes in inflammatory myfibroblastic tumors. *Am J Pathol* 2000;157:377–384.
72. Bridge JA, Kanamori M, Ma Z, et al. Fusion of the ALK gene to the clathrin heavy chain gene, CLTC, in inflammatory myofibroblastic tumor. *Am J Pathol* 2001;159:411–415.
73. Cools J, Wlodarska I, Somers R, et al. Identification of novel fusion partners of ALK, the anaplastic lymphoma kinase, in anaplastic large-cell lymphoma and inflammatory myofibroblastic tumor. *Genes Chrom Cancer* 2002;24:354–362.
74. Cook JR. Paraffin section interphase fluorescence in situ hybridization in the diagnosis and classification of non-Hodgkin lymphomas. *Diagn Mol Pathol* 2004;13:197–206.
75. Tefferi A, Dewald GW, Litzow ML, et al. Chronic myeloid leukemia: current application of cytogenetics and molecular testing for diagnosis and treatment. *Mayo Clin Proc* 2005;80:390–402.
76. Kelly L, Clark J, Gilliland DG. Comprehensive genotypic analysis of leukemia: clinical and therapeutic implications. *Curr Opin Oncol* 2002;14:10–18.
77. Greaves M. Childhood leukaemia. *Br Med J* 2002;324:283–287.
78. Pui CH, Relling MV, Downing JR. Acute lymphoblastic leukemia. *N Engl J Med* 2004;350:1535–1548.

Polymerase Chain Reaction

5

The polymerase chain reaction (PCR) is essentially a cell-free method of deoxyribonucleic acid (DNA) cloning. Since the original description of the technique (1,2), PCR has revolutionized molecular biology and genetics research. Because PCR is quick, reliable, and sensitive, it has also become a central technology of clinical molecular genetic testing. Variations of the basic PCR technique have made a broad range of specimen types and genetic aberrations amenable to testing by the method.

BASIS OF THE METHOD

Selective amplification of the target sequence by PCR is achieved through the use of oligonucleotide primers that hybridize to the 5' and 3' ends of the DNA target sequence (Fig. 5.1). In addition to the two primers and input (template) DNA, the reaction mixture also includes the four deoxynucleotide triphosphates (dATP, dCTP, dGTP, dTTP) and a heat-stable (thermostable) DNA polymerase, all mixed together in reaction buffer. The first step of the PCR itself involves heating the mixture to a high temperature (usually 95°C) to denature the target DNA; in the second step, the reaction is cooled to allow the primers to anneal to their complementary sequence in the target DNA; in the third step, the reaction is heated to a temperature at which the heat-stable DNA polymerase has optimal activity (usually in the range of 70° to 75°C). As a result of this three-step denaturation, annealing, and polymerization cycle, the two primers will initiate synthesis of new DNA molecules from opposite strands of the input DNA heteroduplex. With each repetition of the three-step cycle, each newly synthesized DNA strand can also act as a template for further DNA synthesis. Although new strands of variable length polymerized from primers that hybridize to the input DNA molecules accumulate linearly, DNA duplexes in which both strands have the fixed length of the target sequence (so-called amplicons) accumulate exponentially.

PCR makes it possible to selectively amplify a specific DNA target sequence within a background of heterogeneous DNA sequences such as total genomic DNA or cDNA derived from unfractionated cellular ribonucleic acid (RNA). However, each of the components in a PCR, including the input DNA, the oligonucleotide primers, the thermostable polymerase, the buffer, and the cycle parameters, has an effect on the sensitivity, specificity, and fidelity of the reaction.

Template DNA

As a result of the inherent sensitivity of PCR, template DNA must be neither abundant nor highly purified. In fact, in those settings in which the concentration of template DNA is intrinsically very high, unpurified DNA (from even live cells) can be added directly to the PCR. The high temperatures during the denaturation phase of each PCR cycle quickly inactivate cellular enzymes from even unpurified DNA preparations that could potentially interfere with the reaction.

Effect of Fixation

DNA extracted from fresh tissue or cell suspensions is the optimal template for PCR. The preferred method of preservation of fresh tissue before isolation of DNA (or RNA) is ultra–low-temperature frozen storage at −70°C, which permits indefinite preservation of tissue with virtually no effect on the quality of the extracted nucleic acids. Low-temperature frozen storage at around −20°C can adequately preserve DNA and RNA for several months (3). Successful PCR has been performed on DNA extracted from cell suspensions after nonfrozen storage at 4°C for weeks up to several years, although prolonged storage under these conditions is likely associated with a loss of PCR sensitivity. Room temperature storage of tissue at 23° to 25°C for a period of hours to days may have no significant

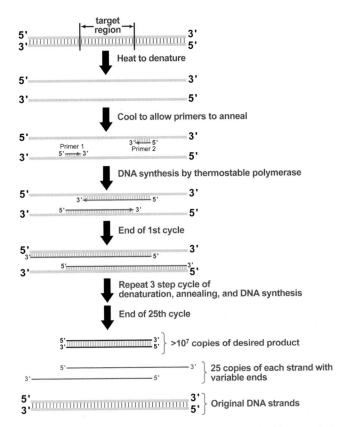

Figure 5.1 Schematic diagram of PCR. The double-stranded DNA template is denatured by heating and then cooled to permit annealing of the oligonucleotide primers to sequences that flank the region to be amplified. When hybridized, the oligonucleotides prime the synthesis of new DNA strands by the heat-stable polymerase. Each newly synthesized DNA strand then acts as a template for synthesis of the complementary strand in the subsequent three-step cycles of denaturation, annealing, and DNA synthesis. The target region undergoes exponential amplification according to the equation $X_n = X_o(1 + E_x)^n$ where X_n is the number of copies of the target at cycle n, X_o is the initial number of copies of the target, and E_x is the efficiency of target amplification (which not only varies by amplicon sequence and length, but also changes during the progress of the reaction).

effect on the quality of nuclear DNA for use in PCR, especially for some tissues such as peripheral blood lymphocytes that naturally occur as single cell suspensions (3), but mitochondrial DNA is apparently quite sensitive to degradation in thawed tissues (4).

Although there is no doubt that fresh tissue is the best source of DNA for testing by PCR-based methods, nucleic acids extracted from fixed tissue can also be used in PCR (5,6), although the type of fixative and length of fixation both have a profound effect on their recovery. Non-crosslinking fixatives such as ethanol provide the most consistent preservation of amplifiable DNA, with more variability from tissues fixed with formalin, Zamboni's and Clark's fixatives, paraformaldehyde, and formalin-alcohol-acetic acid; tissues processed in Carnoy's, Zenker's, Bouin's and B-5 fixatives are poor substrates for PCR testing because little amplifiable DNA can be recovered from them (6–14).

The affects of formalin fixation on subsequent PCR-based testing have been studied in great detail, not surprising given that most surgical specimens are fixed in formalin (15–19). These studies have demonstrated that the quality of DNA isolated from formalin-fixed tissue depends on the protocol used to extract the DNA and on the length of fixation, with a deterioration of PCR signal with increasing fixation time (7,8,16). Formaldehyde reacts with DNA and proteins to form labile hydroxymethyl intermediates that give rise to a mixture of end products. The end products include DNA–DNA and DNA–protein molecules covalently linked by methylene bridges, as well as cyclic base derivatives (Fig. 5.2). Purification of DNA from formalin-fixed tissue therefore usually includes heating to reverse the hydroxymethyl additions and treatment with a proteinase to hydrolyze the covalently linked proteins, steps designed to make the DNA a more accessible template. However, the DNA–DNA crosslinks that form in the presence of formalin are not significantly removed by current DNA extraction techniques. The steric inhibition of DNA polymerases caused by these crosslinks provides a likely explanation for the decreased

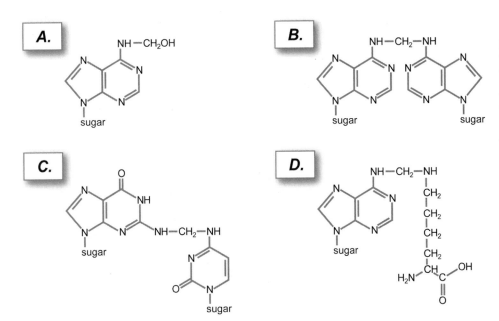

Figure 5.2 Crosslinks produced from formaldehyde-treated nucleic acids. Formaldehyde reacts with NH_2 groups of purine and pyrimidine bases to form labile intermediates, such as N^6-hydroxymethyladenosine (**A**). With time, the hydroxymethyl derivatives react to form crosslinked purine and pyrimidine bases, examples of which are adenosine–adenosine crosslinks (**B**) and guanosine–cytidine crosslinks (**C**). The hydroxymethyl base derivatives can also react with amino acids to form crosslinks, an example of which is an adenosine–lysine crosslink (**D**). Because the sugar can be either ribose or deoxyribose, the full range of reaction products includes DNA–DNA, DNA–RNA, and RNA–RNA crosslinks, as well as DNA–protein and RNA–protein crosslinks.

sensitivity that is a characteristic of PCR performed on formalin-fixed tissue and provides a rationale for the decrease in amplifiable DNA that occurs with increasing length of fixation (8,14). In general, tissue fixed in neutral buffered formalin for less than 8 hours contains DNA from which PCR products greater than 600 base pairs (bp) in length can be reliably amplified, but fixation extended for greater than 8 to 12 hours decreases the length of the PCR product that can consistently be amplified (16,17). Paraffin embedding itself apparently has no effect on DNA stability.

Because most fixatives have such a pronounced effect on the recovery of DNA (and RNA, as discussed later) for PCR-based studies, fresh tissue should be collected proactively in those cases in which the diagnosis will not be compromised if the entire specimen is not fixed. A portion of the lesion, as well as adjacent normal control tissue, should be rapidly frozen and stored at $-70\,^{\circ}$C to ensure that the optimal tissue substrate is available for testing should the need arise.

Amplicon Length

The target PCR sequence is 0.1 to 5 kb long, usually in the lower end of this range. Amplification of products in kilobase size range is absolutely dependent on the availability of fresh tissue because of the effects of fixation noted above. Recent methods for long-range PCR have extended the upper size limit for reliable PCR amplification to at least 35 kb (20,21). Long-range PCR methods have great clinical utility because they permit identification of deletions or insertions in large chromosomal regions (e.g., in Duchenne muscular dystrophy) in a single PCR reaction.

Oligonucleotide Primers

PCR depends on the specificity of the hybridization of the oligonucleotide primers to the intended target DNA sequences. By convention, the forward primer anneals to the DNA minus strand and directs synthesis in a 5' to 3' direction; consequently, the reverse primer is located downstream (or 3') from the forward primer and is complementary to the sequence on the DNA plus strand. Oligonucleotide primer sequences are always indicated in the 5' to 3' direction.

Melting temperature, T_m, a measure of the stability of the duplex formed between the primer and its complementary target DNA sequence, is an important consideration in primer design. T_m corresponds to the midpoint in the observed transition from a double-stranded to a single-stranded form, and a higher T_m permits an increased annealing temperature that helps ensure that only strongly matched primer:target duplexes are formed. The equations for calculating T_m presented in Table 5.1 demonstrate that T_m of a primer is dependent on both the length of the oligonucleotide and on its content of G and C bases.

Primers are usually designed to avoid matching known repetitive DNA sequences, including stretches of a single nucleotide. The two (or more) primers used in a PCR are not homologous to each other, especially at their 3' ends, because regions of complementarity between the primers themselves can lead to spurious amplification artifacts known as primer dimers. Because the 3' end of a primer is

TABLE 5.1

EQUATIONS FOR CALCULATING T_M FOR OLIGONUCLEOTIDE PRIMERS USED IN PCR

Length of Primer[a]	T_m in °C
Less than 20 nucleotides long	2(effective length[b])
20 to 35 nucleotides long	22 + 1.46(effective length)

[a]Assumes no mismatches.
[b]The effective length of the single-stranded oligonucleotide probe is defined as 2(number of G + C) + (number of A + T).

the most critical for initiating polymerization, accidental complementarity between the 3' end and the template DNA at sites other than the target sequence can also produce spurious amplification products even if the rest of the primer:template duplex shows substantial mismatching.

For complex DNA sources (such as total genomic DNA from a human cell), primers about 20 to 25 nucleotides long are usually sufficient to ensure specific amplification of the target sequence. For primers of this length, the likelihood of accidental matches elsewhere in the template by random chance is exceedingly low. However, primers are often longer to guarantee they have a T_m high enough to permit use of an annealing temperature that ensures only matched primer:target duplexes are formed.

Thermostable Polymerases

The first experiments describing PCR (1,2) used a modified version of *Escherichia coli* DNA polymerase I. Because the polymerase was not heat stable, it was necessary to add a fresh aliquot of the enzyme after the denaturation step of each cycle. In addition, the low annealing and extension temperatures required to preserve enzyme activity resulted in nonspecific hybridization of the primers to the template DNA and the production of abundant nonspecific reaction products. The development of thermostable polymerases that not only could survive extended incubation at temperatures as high as 95°C but also had optimal enzymatic activity at elevated temperatures (usually in the range of 70 to 75°C) was therefore a major advancement in PCR technology (22). The use of thermostable polymerases eliminated much of the nonspecific hybridization that occurred at lower annealing and extension temperatures and also made it possible to automate PCR.

All thermostable polymerases used for PCR, even those with a 3'→5' exonuclease proofreading function, have an intrinsic error rate that is highly dependent on buffer composition, dNTP concentration, and pH of the PCR, as well as the sequence of the template itself (23–32). The types of errors introduced by thermostable polymerases during PCR include single bp substitutions (transitions as well as transversions), frame shift mutations, and even spontaneous rearrangements. Frame shift mutations, thought to be due to slipped strand mispairing, include both deletions and insertions and are especially problematic at sites of mononucleotide and dinucleotide repeats (33–35). Table 5.2 shows the error rates of several thermostable polymerases and highlights the effect that a 3'→5'

TABLE 5.2

ERROR RATES OF VARIOUS THERMOSTABLE DNA POLYMERASES USED IN PCR

Polymerase	$3' \rightarrow 5'$ Exonuclease Activity	Base Substitution Error Rate[a]	Total Error Rate[b]
Taq	No	2.4×10^{-5}	—[c]
Pfu	Yes	6.0×10^{-7}	—
Pab	Yes	7.0×10^{-7}	—
Tfu	Yes	8.0×10^{-6}	—
Vent	Yes	3.2×10^{-5}	1.3×10^{-3}
Vent$_{Exo-}$[d]	No	4.4×10^{-4}	1.2×10^{-2}
Replinase	No	2.1×10^{-4}	5.9×10^{-3}

[a]Expressed as base substitutions per nucleotide per cycle, measured using each enzyme's optimal buffer, dNTP concentration, reaction pH, etc., using biologic assay for p53 mutations for Taq, Pfu, Pab and Tfu (25) and an in vitro gap-filling DNA synthesis reaction for Vent, VentExo− and Replinase (26).
[b]Expressed as errors per nucleotide per cycle, measured using a forward mutational assay that detects frame shifts, deletions, duplications, complex errors, and a broader range of base substitution errors (26).
[c]Not determined.
[d]A recombinant form of Vent lacking $3' \rightarrow 5'$ exonuclease activity.

exonuclease proofreading function has on enzyme fidelity. The data in Table 5.2 also emphasize the fact that base substitutions account for only a small percentage of the total errors introduced by thermostable polymerases.

The significance of the polymerase error rates can be put into context using the formulas in Table 5.3. For a polymerase with an error rate that is constant at one error per 10,000 nucleotides per cycle, the average frequency of a change in the PCR product is 1 change per 1,000 nucleotides after 20 cycles, but increases to one change per 400 nucleotides after 50 cycles. However, it is important to

TABLE 5.3

EQUATIONS FOR EVALUATING THE EFFECT OF POLYMERASE ERROR RATES ON SEQUENCE ALTERATIONS IN PCR PRODUCT DNA

Let b = number of bases per single strand in the amplicon.
Let n = number of PCR cycles.
Let p = polymerase error rate per base per cycle.
Assuming that all sequence alterations can be detected, and that each cycle produces a perfect doubling,

The average mutation frequency of f is:

$$f = np/2 \qquad \text{(Equation 1)}$$

The probability p' that a strand of DNA contains at least one error is:

$$p' = 1 - (1 - p)^b \qquad \text{(Equation 2)}$$

If π denotes the proportion of copies without a replication error, the mean proportion of copies without an error is:

$$\bar{X}_\pi = (1 - p'/2)^n \qquad \text{(Equation 3)}$$

The probability q that a specific base on a randomly chosen strand from the amplified population is an error is:

$$q = 1 - (1 - p/2)^n \qquad \text{(Equation 4)}$$

From references 23, 30, 32, 36.

realize that because of the exponential nature of PCR, the rare occurrence of an error in the early rounds of a PCR will produce an error frequency that is even higher (30,31,36–38). From a different perspective (Table 5.4), for a polymerase with an error rate of one error per 10,000 nucleotides per cycle, and a 1,000 base amplicon, the average proportion of product DNA molecules that will contain at least one error after just 20 cycles is 62%, while the proportion of the product DNA molecules that will contain at least one error after 50 cycles is 91%. Nonetheless, despite the very high percentage of product molecules that contain an error, the percentage of molecules that harbor an error at any given specific base is much lower, only 0.1% after 20 cycles and only 0.25% after 50 cycles.

PCR reactions therefore generate a population of DNA molecules that have extremely similar but not identical sequences. However, even though individual molecules in the PCR product contain errors, the approach used to evaluate the PCR product has a significant effect on the rate at which the sequence changes are detected. For example, in the above illustration, even if 62% of the product DNA molecules contain an error, direct analysis of the total PCR product is likely to give the correct sequence of the original template because the changes in the individual product strands occur on average randomly and so only 0.1% of the strands will have an error at a specific base. When all the PCR product strands are sequenced together, the incorrect base of a small number of strands will be overwhelmed by the contribution of the vast majority of strands that have the correct sequence at that position. However, if the PCR product DNA is cloned before analysis, the situation is entirely different. The cloning process selects for a single DNA molecule from the PCR product population, and so 62% of the sequenced PCR product strands will yield an incorrect sequence. Consequently, if PCR product DNA is cloned before analysis, multiple individual clones must be evaluated to determine the consensus sequence, especially if a putative mutation is detected.

TABLE 5.4					
DISTRIBUTION OF REPLICATION ERRORS IN PCR PRODUCT DNA[a]					
	Number of Cycles				
	10	**20**	**30**	**40**	**50**
Percentage of product DNA molecules that contain at least one error when the polymerase error rate is[b]:					
10^{-3} errors per base per cycle[c]	98%	>99%	100%	100%	100%
10^{-4} errors per base per cycle	39%	62%	77%	86%	91%
10^{-5} errors per base per cycle	5%	9%	14%	18%	22%
Percentage of product DNA molecules that contain an error at a specific base when the polymerase error rate is[d]:					
10^{-3} errors per base per cycle[c]	0.5%	1.0%	1.5%	2.0%	2.5%
10^{-4} errors per base per cycle	0.05%	0.1%	0.15%	0.20%	0.25%
10^{-5} errors per base per cycle	0.005%	0.01%	0.015%	0.02%	0.025%

[a]Assuming all errors are detected and a 1,000 base amplicon.
[b]From Equation 3 in Table 5.3.
[c]Compare with error rates in Table 5.2.
[d]From Equation 4 in Table 5.3.

Cycle Parameters

The temperature of the annealing phase of each cycle is the most critical for specific PCR amplification. The annealing temperature is typically about 5°C below the calculated T_m of the oligonucleotide primers, although annealing temperatures closer to T_m can be used to increase the stringency of the primer:target hybridization and minimize the formation of spurious PCR products. To reduce the effect of nonspecific binding of primer sequences before the first round of PCR, the polymerase is often not added to the reaction mixture until after the denaturation step of the first cycle, a method known as "hot-start PCR."

The extension, or DNA synthesis phase, of each cycle is typically performed at 70 to 75°C and is primarily determined by the optimum reaction temperature of the thermostable polymerase. The denaturation phase of each cycle is typically performed at about 95°C for human genomic DNA, a temperature high enough to effectively melt all DNA duplexes without significantly diminishing the enzymatic activity of the polymerase.

A typical PCR reaction involves from 25 to 35 cycles. A greater number of cycles usually does not significantly increase the amount of product, as discussed more fully in the quantitative PCR section below. Instead, greater sensitivity can be achieved by optimizing DNA template preparation or performing a second, nested PCR, as is also discussed more fully later.

Advantages of PCR

Simple, Quick, and Inexpensive

In many cases, PCR provides a method for detecting specific DNA sequences that is quicker and simpler than Southern or northern blot hybridization. A single PCR cycle of melting, annealing, and extension takes under 5 minutes, and consequently an entire PCR amplification of 25 to 35 cycles can be performed in only a few hours. Because of the high level of amplification achieved by PCR, the product DNA can be visualized by ethidium bromide staining after simple gel electrophoresis, eliminating the hazards and expense associated with the use of radioactivity.

High Sensitivity and Specificity

When optimized, PCR can detect one abnormal cell in a background of 10^5 normal cells (39) and can even be used to analyze single copy genes from individual cells (40–43). PCR can also be used to detect a broad range of genetic abnormalities ranging from gross structural alterations such as translocations and deletions to point mutations within a specific gene. With appropriate primer design and reaction conditions, the high level of sensitivity is achieved with no loss of specificity.

However, the high technical sensitivity and specificity of PCR must not be confused with diagnostic sensitivity and specificity. As discussed in detail in Chapter 8, the technical features of PCR testing often do not accurately reflect the diagnostic utility of the method when applied in routine clinical practice.

Ease of PCR Product Labeling

Direct labeling of PCR product DNA is easily accomplished, providing even greater test flexibility and sensitivity. For primer-mediated 5' endlabeling, the labeled chemical group (usually a fluorophore) is attached to the 5' end of either or both oligonucleotide primers. Alternatively, the PCR product can be directly labeled by including one or more modified nucleotide precursors into the PCR reaction mix; use of radiolabeled dNTPs (usually with ^{32}P or ^{35}S) enhances the sensitivity of PCR even further, and facilitates subsequent evaluation of PCR product for mutations by techniques such as single strand conformational polymorphism (SSCP) analysis and denaturing gradient gel electrophoresis (DGGE).

Phenotype–Genotype Correlations

As traditionally performed on a tissue fragment or tissue section, PCR provides only an indirect correlation of morphology and genetic abnormalities. A number of techniques permit better-defined phenotype–genotype correlations. Microdissection, in which the region of interest is simply carved out of the formalin-fixed, paraffin-embedded tissue block, scraped from tissue sections or cytology slides, or collected more precisely with a micromanipulator apparatus, affords some enrichment for morphologic–genetic correlations (44–48). More precise phenotypic–genotypic analysis is achieved by collecting individual cells by laser capture microdissection (42,43,49,50), by flow cytometry (51), or even immunomagnetic methods (52). Although these methods make it possible to analyze single cells, in situ PCR performed on histologic tissue sections themselves is perhaps the ultimate method for providing phenotypic–genotypic correlations (53–55). Although technically demanding (54,56,57), in situ PCR has a sensitivity that makes it possible to detect low-level gene expression in individual cells at a copy number below that which can be detected by conventional in situ hybridization (55,58,59).

Limitations of PCR

Polymerase Chain Reaction Analyzes Only the Target Region

PCR analysis of a segment of DNA is limited to the region amplified by the specific primer set employed. Unlike conventional cytogenetics and Southern or northern blot hybridization, PCR will fail to identify structural changes that do not alter the sequence of target region itself.

PCR Will Amplify Only Intact Target Regions

Some mutations (including very large insertions or inversions that include one of the primer binding sites) alter the structure of the target region in such a way that it cannot be amplified. Mutations that damage a primer binding site (including insertions, deletions, and even point mutations) will also preclude amplification of the target region by PCR and can easily lead to errors in test interpretation. For example, consider a patient heterozygous for a deletion that includes the binding site for one of the primers; PCR testing of the locus would show a DNA product from the wild-type allele but not from the mutated allele, an outcome that would be interpreted as indicating that the patient is homozygous wild-type, a false negative test result.

Amplification Bias

PCR bias refers to the fact that some DNA templates are preferentially amplified versus other templates within the same reaction. PCR bias can be caused by differences in template length (in general, shorter amplicons are preferentially amplified), random variations in template number (especially with very low target abundance, producing an artifact known as allele dropout), and random variations in PCR efficiency with each cycle (47,60–62).

Amplification bias can even result from differences in the target sequence itself that are as small as a single base change (61,63–64). The magnitude of PCR bias, which can cause 10- to 30-fold differences in amplification efficiency in some settings, is easily large enough to influence quantitative PCR test results and loss of heterozygosity analysis, and can be a particularly troublesome problem in multiplex PCR (65,66).

Spurious PCR Products

PCR occasionally produces nonspecific amplification artifacts, also known as spurious PCR products. Spurious DNA products occur at a low level even in reactions using well-designed primers and stringent amplification conditions and often consist of fragments of irrelevant genes.

Technical Issues

Technical factors in actual clinical practice decrease the sensitivity of PCR to levels below those in optimized research settings. Nonspecific inhibitors of PCR include detergents, phenol, heparin, dyes such as bromphenol blue, and other uncharacterized components commonly present in cerebrospinal fluid, urine, and sputum. However, the most important technical limitation is degradation of target nucleic acids, especially when extracted from fixed tissue, as discussed above.

Although the extreme sensitivity of PCR underlies its clinical utility, it also greatly increases the risk of erroneous test results from cross-contamination of samples, especially contamination resulting from PCR product carryover (67–69). The risk of contamination is an important technical issue, the significance of which cannot be overstated in terms of practical application of PCR testing in the clinical laboratory. Problems resulting from contamination can be largely avoided by strict attention to laboratory technique, physical separation of the various stages of testing, use of aerosol barrier pipette tips, regular ultraviolet radiation of laboratory workspaces and instruments to degrade any transient uncontained DNA, and rigorous use of appropriate positive and negative controls (67,68,70–73).

The use of the enzyme uracil DNA glycosylase (UNG), which degrades uracil-containing DNA, offers a particularly elegant anti-contamination technique (74). By this method, the nucleotide dUTP is substituted for dTTP in all PCR amplifications performed in the laboratory, and so all amplicons contain the pyrimidine base uracil in place of thymine. When clinical samples are tested, an initial incubation with UNG destroys any carryover contaminants that are DNA products from prior PCR amplifications while target sequences from the clinical specimens remain unaltered.

NESTED PCR

Nested PCR is the name of the technique in which two consecutive PCR reactions are performed on the same DNA sample, an initial amplification of a longer target sequence followed by a second amplification of a shorter sequence contained within the first amplicon (Fig. 5.3). The second PCR may involve two internal primers (fully

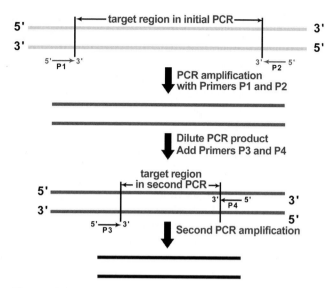

Figure 5.3 Nested PCR. The PCR product from an initial PCR amplification using external primers P1 and P2 is diluted and used as the target DNA in a second PCR. The internal (or nested) primers P3 and P4 in the second PCR are complementary to sequences located internal to those bound by P1 and P2.

nested) or one internal primer and one of the original primers (semi-nested). Either variant provides a markedly increased sensitivity and specificity compared with a single PCR and makes the technique ideal for those situations in which the target sequence is present at an extremely low copy number. Common settings for nested PCR include when the mutation is present in only a small subset of the cell population under study, when the nucleic acids have been degraded as a result of tissue fixation, or, for reverse transcriptase–PCR (RT-PCR) as discussed in the following section, when the target mRNA is expressed at extremely low levels.

However, the increased sensitivity of nested PCR carries an increased risk of contamination as a result of the additional manipulations that are required to perform the consecutive PCR reactions. Reliable, reproducible nested PCR results therefore require strict attention to laboratory technique, rigorous use of controls, and confirmation of product identity (68,70–73). Unexpected nested PCR results ideally should be confirmed by an independent technique such as Southern blot, FISH, or cytogenetic analysis (72,75).

REVERSE TRANSCRIPTASE PCR

RT-PCR makes it possible to amplify RNA, usually mRNA. For RT-PCR, RNA extracted from the tissue sample is purified and then converted into cDNA using reverse transcriptase, an enzyme that transcribes RNA into single-stranded complementary DNA. The cDNA then serves as the template in a conventional PCR. The primers for the cDNA synthesis reaction are either short random primers (often a mixture of random hexamers that includes virtually all possible six base sequences) that make it possible to synthesize cDNA from the entire RNA population without sequence specificity or an oligo-dT primer (which binds to the poly-A tail of mRNA molecules) that makes it possible

to synthesize cDNA from the entire mRNA population without sequence specificity or precise knowledge of the mRNA sequence (76).

There is no doubt that fresh tissue (or fresh frozen tissue) is the preferred source of RNA for RT-PCR. There is apparently no major decrease in the quality of mRNA isolated from samples stored in appropriate buffers for up to 1 week at room temperature, although longer periods of storage at room temperature do result in the deterioration of mRNA from many tissue types (77,78). However, RNA recovered from fixed tissue is degraded; the extent of degradation depends on the prefixation interval, the type of fixative, the length of fixation, and the method used to isolate the RNA (6,13,15,18,79–86). In reactions identical to those discussed above for DNA, formalin fixation results in the addition of labile hydroxymethyl groups to the bases of RNA, leading to methylene bridge crosslinks (15,18,79). Despite the fact that the majority of the methylol groups can be removed by heating, and that the majority of RNA protein crosslinks can be removed by proteinase digestion, RT-PCR performed on RNA isolated from formalin-fixed, paraffin-embedded (FFPE) tissue has a significantly lower sensitivity than when performed on RNA isolated from fresh tissue (6,8–10,15,18,70,87,88). Reproducible amplification of RNA from fixed tissue by RT-PCR is extremely dependent on the length of the amplicon, which in practice effectively excludes amplicons that are greater than 200 bp long (81,89,90).

Advantages of RT-PCR

RT-PCR analysis of RNA offers advantages over analysis of DNA. RT-PCR is a robust technique and can be performed on RNA isolated from fresh or fixed tissue, fresh or archival cytology specimens, and even cDNA synthesized directly from cell lysates without prior RNA purification (90). RT-PCR permits direct amplification of multiexon sequences by eliminating the intervening introns and thus greatly simplifies mutation scanning methods that would require multiple reactions to evaluate the exons individually from DNA. Similarly, RT-PCR makes it much simpler to demonstrate the presence of translocations that create fusion genes by making it possible to directly detect the fusion transcripts encoded by the translocations; because the precise break point often ranges over dozens of kilobases, detection of the translocations by standard PCR based on DNA would be unwieldy. RT-PCR can also be used to detect changes in mRNA structure that result from alternative splicing, to demonstrate aberrant splicing resulting from mutations, and to evaluate the level of gene expression through the quantitative methods discussed below. Using the methods described above for conventional PCR, RT-PCR can also be used to provide phenotypic–genotypic correlations from defined cell populations collected from cytology smears (92,93) or tissue sections (87,94,95).

Limitations of RT-PCR

RNA is a more technically demanding substrate than DNA. Tissue samples must be processed carefully to avoid mRNA degradation, especially because many mutations result in unstable mRNA (Chapter 1). Because a nested PCR approach is often necessary when the target RNA is present at very low levels, and because short amplicons are required when the RNA is degraded or recovered from fixed tissue, RT-PCR carries a much increased risk of contamination and amplification of nonspecific sequences (70,72,96). The recently described method for linear amplification of RNA before RT-PCR may provide an approach for detecting very low levels of mRNA that carries less of a risk of contamination or nonspecific amplification (97).

Strict attention to laboratory technique is required to reduce the risk of contamination, which can be monitored by the rigorous use of negative controls. Appropriate negative controls include "no RNA" controls (which lack input RNA and so address reagent contamination) and "no RT" controls from sham cDNA synthesis reactions (which are performed without reverse transcriptase enzyme and so address possible contamination of the RNA sample itself by DNA) (70–72,82,96). The increased risks of contamination underscore the need to confirm unexpected results by an independent technique (70,72).

Spurious PCR products occur even in reactions using well-designed primers and stringent amplification conditions,

and often consist of fragments of irrelevant genes (Fig. 5.4). A recent study demonstrated that in routine clinical use, RT-PCR based testing of soft tissue tumors for fusion transcripts generated spurious PCR products of the same size as the anticipated PCR product in approximately 6% of cases (70). Because the spurious PCR products were the same size as the expected products, the spurious products were only detected by DNA sequence analysis. Product confirmation steps are therefore an integral part of RT-PCR–based testing to avoid false positive test results (70,98).

QUANTITATIVE PCR

An ideal PCR would generate a perfect 2-fold increase in the number of copies of the amplicon in each cycle of the reaction. In reality, inhibitors of the reaction, accumulation of pyrophosphate molecules, decreasing polymerase activity, and reagent consumption all contribute to a plateau phase in the later stages of the reaction at which the amplicon is no longer increasing at an exponential rate (99). Quantitation is further complicated by the nonlinear signal

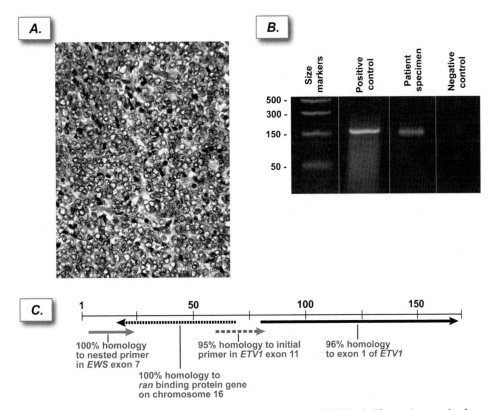

Figure 5.4 Example of a spurious PCR product occurring in RT-PCR. **A**, Photomicrograph of an undifferentiated round cell sarcoma arising in the cheek of a 5-year-old boy; the tumor had non-diagnostic morphologic and immunohistochemical features. **B**, Nested RT-PCR performed for fusion transcripts between *EWS* and *Ets* family members (70) characteristic of Ewing sarcoma/peripheral neuroectodermal tumor (Chapter 11) showed the presence of a band from the tumor tissue of a size consistent with an *EWS-ETV1* fusion transcript (*lane 1:* molecular weight standards; *lane 2:* positive control tumor expressing *EWS* exon 7 to *ETV1* exon 11 fusion transcript; *lane 3:* putative *EWS-ETV1* fusion transcript in check sarcoma; *lane 4:* negative control consisting of no input DNA). **C**, DNA sequence analysis of the PCR product from the tumor shows a haphazard amalgamation of sequences but no evidence of an *EWS-ETV1* fusion; the direction of the arrowheads indicates whether the homologous coding sequence is on the sense (→) or antisense (←) strand. Note that interpretation of the PT-PCR product as an *EWS-ETV1* fusion based on its size alone would have led to an erroneous (false positive) test result.

TABLE 5.5			
REPORTER AND QUENCHER GROUPS COMMONLY USED IN Q-PCR			

*Taq*Man system			
Reporters:	FAM,[a] HEX/JOE/VIC, TET	Quenchers:	TAMRA, DABCYL[b]
Molecular beacons			
Reporters:	BODIPY, Coumarin, EDANS, Eosine, Fluorescein, Lucifer Yellow, Tetramethylrhodamine, Texas Red	Quencher:	DABCYL
Scorpions			
Reporters:	Cy3, Cy5, FAM, Fluorescein, HEX/JOE/VIC, Rhodamine, TAMRA, TET, Texas Red	Quenchers:	Methyl red, DABCYL
Probe/Probe or Primer/Probe format:			
Reporters:	Cy5, LC Red640, LC Red705	Donor:	Fluorescein
Deoxyguanosine—quenching format:			
Reporters:	None required	Donors:	Fluorescein, BODIPY-FL

[a]The chemical structures of FAM, TAMRA, DABCYL, and EDANS are shown in Figure 5.6.
[b]A so-called dark quencher.

to target relationships of many detection systems, including autoradiography. Consequently, reliable quantitation of PCR involves more than simple measurement of the amount of product DNA present at the end of the reaction.

The quantitative competitive PCR method involves coamplification of an internal control (the competitor) with the unknown sample in the same tube; a standard curve produced by serial dilutions of the control sample is used to determine the starting concentration of the target sequence in the test sample (99–102). By the semi-quantitative method, the amount of accumulated amplicon is directly measured; because the measurement is performed early in the PCR, after an empirically determined optimum number of cycles, it can be used to calculate the starting concentration of the target sequence in the test sample with reasonable accuracy (103–105). However, these methods require post-PCR manipulations to detect the DNA product, steps that not only involve radioisotopes or hazardous chemicals such as ethidium bromide, but that also carry the potential risk for laboratory contamination of future reactions (106).

Real-time PCR, usually simply referred to as quantitative-PCR (Q-PCR), is a less cumbersome and much faster method for quantification. As the name implies, the method uses real-time measurements of DNA accumulation as the PCR progresses to provide a more precise estimate of the initial concentration of the target sequence. The initial description of Q-PCR used ethidium bromide intercalation to quantitate the increase in product DNA as the PCR progressed (107), but fluorescence-based methods are now used, most of which rely on the phenomenon of quenching. In fluorescence resonance energy transfer (FRET) quenching, the energy from the reporter fluorophore that would normally be released as light is instead transferred to the quencher (106,108); although the quencher group is often a fluorophore itself, it releases the

transferred energy at a longer wavelength and so does not interfere with measurement of light of the wavelength emitted by the reporter fluorophore. In proximal (or collisional) quenching, energy from the reporter fluorophore that would normally be released as light is transferred to a quencher that dissipates the energy as heat rather than as visible light (109). Proximal quenchers are therefore often referred to as "dark quenchers"; because they have a broad absorption spectrum, the same group can be used as the quencher for a number of different reporter fluorophores for multiplex analysis (110), as shown in Table 5.5.

Q-PCR Chemistries

Q-PCR using a *Taq*Man probe (also known as 5' exonuclease or hydrolysis real-time PCR) requires three oligonucleotide primers, the two primers used to amplify the target DNA as in conventional PCR, as well as a third primer that is the *Taq*Man probe itself (106,108,111). The *Taq*Man probe binds to an internal sequence in the target DNA sequence (Fig. 5.5), carries a blocking group at its 3' terminal nucleotide so that it cannot prime new DNA synthesis, and, most importantly, is dual-labeled with a reporter dye and a quencher dye (Fig. 5.6) to take advantage of FRET. As long as the probe is intact, FRET occurs and the fluorescence of the reporter dye is quenched. However, as *Taq* polymerase synthesizes a new DNA strand, its 5'→3' exonuclease activity degrades the internal *Taq*Man probe, the reporter and quencher dyes become unlinked, FRET ceases, and there is an increase in reporter fluorescence (note that since different thermostable polymerases have different levels of 5'→3' exonuclease activity, not all are equally suitable for real-time PCR using *Taq*Man probes). The labeled probe also functions as an internal specificity control; therefore the amplification plot not only confirms the presence of DNA product but also confirms its identity.

Like *Taq*Man probes, molecular beacons are single-stranded DNA probes that have a reporter dye linked to one end of the molecule and a quencher to the other. However, molecular beacons are designed to form a stem-and-loop structure stabilized by intramolecular bp hydrogen bonds that bring the reporter and quencher in such close proximity that fluorescence is quenched by proximal quenching (Figs. 5.5 and 5.6). When the molecular beacon hybridizes with a complementary sequence in the amplicon, the probe assumes a linear confirmation that separates the quencher and reporter by a distance that is sufficient to permit fluorescence (106,108). Molecular beacons can be

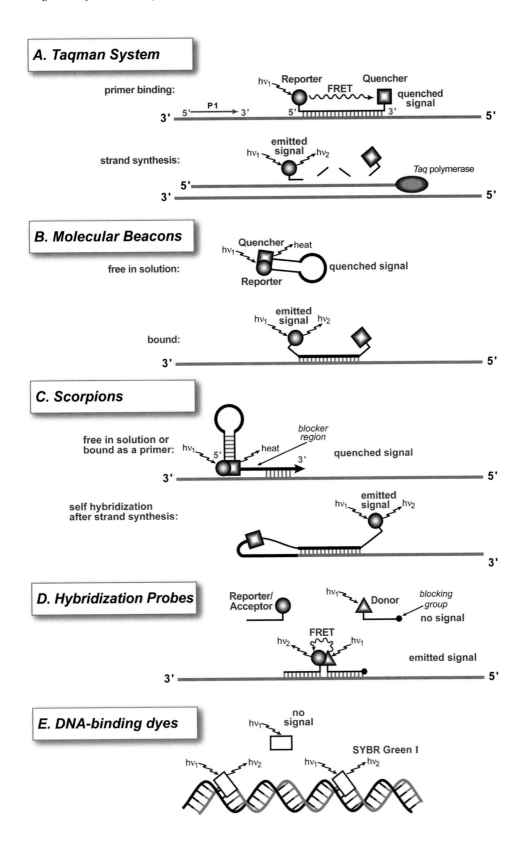

designed that distinguish targets differing by only a single nucleotide (109,112,113), which, together with the fact that a number of different fluorophores can be used simultaneously (110), makes this type of probe ideally suited for multiplex real-time PCR.

Scorpions, also known as self-probing amplicons, are conventional PCR primers with an additional 5' sequence that is designed to form a hair-pin loop with the region of the oligonucleotide that primes DNA polymerization of the amplicon (114–116). As with molecular beacons, the hair-pin loop brings the reporter and quencher together in a structure that is stabilized by intrastrand bp hydrogen bonds, inhibiting fluorescence by proximal quenching (Fig. 5.5). After primer extension, the scorpion self-anneals to a target region in the nascent DNA strand, the probe assumes a linear conformation, the reporter fluorophore and quencher are separated, and fluorescence is increased.

Q-PCR by the hybridization probe method employs four oligonucleotides: the two conventional PCR primers and two internal probes (117). In the probe/probe format (Fig. 5.5), one of the two probes is labeled with a donor dye and the other with a reporter/acceptor dye. Hybridization of the probes to the target sequence in a head-to-tail confirmation brings the dyes in close proximity, which permits energy transfer from the donor group to the reporter/acceptor group, resulting in fluorescence. The primer/probe format is a simple modification of the probe/probe format in which one of the external primers for the PCR amplification is labeled so that only one internal probe is needed to hybridize to the amplicon to generate increased reporter/acceptor group fluorescence. Still another format, the deoxyguanosine-quenching format, requires only a single probe labeled at either the 5' or 3' end with fluorescein or a fluorescein derivative (117–119); the probe is designed to hybridize with an area of the target sequence in which at least one deoxyguanosine is present on the target strand adjacent to the labeled end of the probe, which by itself produces reliable fluorescence quenching when the probe is hybridized to the target.

The dye SYBR Green I fluoresces when it intercalates into dsDNA and so can be used for quantitative PCR with any pair of primers for any target (120–122). However, the flexibility of SYBR Green is offset by its diminished specificity. Unlike the chemistries discussed previously, which have very high specificity because they involve a probe that binds to an internal sequence of the target amplicon, SYBR Green binds to any dsDNA, so nonspecific PCR products as well as the target amplicon will contribute to measured fluorescence. In practice, this nonspecificity is handled by an automated melting curve analysis of the PCR product that determines the fraction of fluorescence that originates from the target versus nonspecific amplification products. Once the melting curve is established, the PCR machine can be programmed to acquire fluorescence data only in the temperature range for which the target amplicon is annealed but not the nonspecific PCR products.

Calculation of DNA Levels by Q-PCR

Changes in fluorescence that result from target amplification are measured by a detector and used by a computer to construct an amplification plot of fluorescence versus the cycle number (Fig. 5.7). During the early cycles of PCR amplification, the specific fluorescence does not exceed the

Figure 5.5 Schematic diagram of some of the common methods used to produce fluorescent emissions in Q-PCR. **A,** In the *Taq*Man system, a labeled probe is designed to hybridize to the target sequence between the binding sites for the PCR primers. The proximity of the Reporter and Quencher groups in the probe permits FRET, so fluorescent emissions from the Reporter group do not occur from probes free in solution or bound to the target sequence. During the extension phase of each PCR cycle, the 5'→3' endonuclease activity of *Taq* polymerase cleaves the probe into many fragments; after cleavage, the Reporter and Quencher are no longer linked, FRET does not occur, and the Reporter fluoresces. **B,** When free in solution, molecular beacon probes have a stem-and-loop hair-pin structure stabilized by intramolecular bp hydrogen bonds that bring the Reporter and Quencher in such close proximity that proximal quenching prevents a fluorescent signal. The molecular beacon is linearized when it binds to the amplicon target, the Reporter and Quencher are separated, and Reporter fluorescence increases. Note that Q-PCR using a molecular beacon requires measurement of fluorescence during the annealing phase of the PCR cycle. **C,** Scorpions have a stem-and-loop hair-pin structure stabilized by intramolecular bp hydrogen bonds between self-complementary sequences, as well as a 3' region that functions as a conventional PCR primer. When the scorpion is free in solution or bound as a primer, the Reporter and Quencher are in such close proximity that proximal quenching prevents a fluorescent signal. After extension from the primer, the newly synthesized amplicon target region is connected to the same DNA strand as the probe, and can self-anneal during the next annealing phase of the PCR cycle. Self-annealing linearizes the scorpion, separates the Reporter and Quencher, and results in increased Reporter fluorescence. The presence of the blocker element (typically hexethylene glycol) prevents copying of the more 5' elements of the scorpion in subsequent PCR cycles. **D,** One of the three formats for Q-PCR using hybridization probes. When the two probes hybridize to adjacent sequences in the amplicon, the Donor and Reporter/Acceptor groups are brought in close proximity, allowing the Donor to transfer energy to the Reporter/Acceptor by FRET, which the Reporter/Acceptor then emits as fluorescence. A blocking group prevents extension of the 3' end of the 5'-labeled probe by the thermostable polymerase, and so the hybridization probes cannot function as primers themselves. Note that when the Donor is a fluorophore itself, Q-PCR could also be performed by simply measuring the decreased Donor emissions. **E,** DNA-binding dyes such as SYBR Green I show strong fluorescence when bound to double-stranded DNA, but have undetectable fluorescence in solution. Although use of DNA-binding dyes is the easiest and cheapest method for Q-PCR, the dyes do not discriminate between the target amplicon and non-specific PCR products.

A.

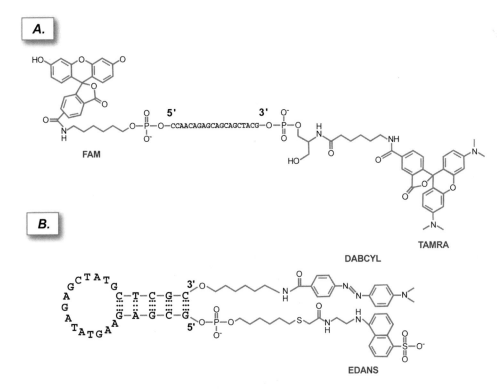

B.

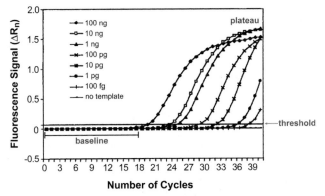

Figure 5.6 Examples of Q-PCR probes. **A**, A *Taq*Man probe dual-labeled with 5' FAM and 3' TAMRA. *Taq*Man probes have no significant secondary structure when free in solution. **B**, A molecular beacon dual-labeled with 5' EDANS and 3' DABCYL. As shown, when not hybridized to the complementary sequence in the amplicon, the molecular beacon forms a stem-and-loop structure stabilized by intramolecular bp hydrogen bonds.

Figure 5.7 An amplification plot illustrating the nomenclature used in Q-PCR. The baseline is defined as that portion of the amplification during which the amplicon is accumulating but has a fluorescence that is below the limit of detection. The threshold is usually related to the variability of the baseline and is often set at 10 times the standard deviation of the average fluorescence of the baseline. During the course of the Q-PCR, a computer program calculates $\Delta R_n = R_n^+ - R_n^-$, where R_n^+ is the fluorescence of the sample and R_n^- is the fluorescence of the baseline. The ΔRn values are then plotted versus the PCR cycle number as illustrated in this schematic plot. Fluorescence signals above the threshold are considered real signals and are used to determine the cycle threshold (C_t) for the sample, which by definition is therefore the fractional cycle at which the fluorescence signal is greater than the threshold. C_t values can therefore be used to calculate the relative abundance of the input template for different samples. Note that C_t is a better measure of the input abundance of the template than the quantity of the PCR product at the plateau phase of the amplification. (Reprinted from Leone F, Perissinotto E, Viale A, et al. Tumor cell contamination. Detection of breast cancer cell contamination in leukapheresis product by real-time quantitative polymerase chain reaction. *Bone Marrow Transplantation* 2001;27:517–523; with permission.)

background, and therefore a number of PCR cycles is required to generate a fluorescence signal strong enough to exceed the baseline. The number of PCR cycles at which the signal generated from the sample crosses the threshold (which can be calculated based on the variability of the baseline or manually determined) is defined as the cycle threshold C_t, and C_t values therefore decrease as the quantity of input target DNA increases. C_t is used to quantify the concentration of the input target DNA sequence by one of two methods, either standard curve quantitation or relative quantitation.

The standard curve method is used when absolute quantitation is essential, for example, when measuring viral load. A DNA sample of known concentration is serially diluted, and a plot of the resulting C_t values against input copy number produces a curve that can be used to determine the target concentration in the test sample based on its C_t.

By the relative quantitation method, comparison of the C_t of the test gene and the C_t of a control housekeeping gene in the same sample is used to calculate the difference in abundance between the two genes (Table 5.6). Ideally, the control housekeeping gene should be expressed at a constant level in all tissues under evaluation and have an efficiency of amplification that is the same as for the target gene. The genes most commonly used as housekeeping controls include β-actin, glyceraldehyde-3-phosphate dehydrogenase (GADPH), and rRNA (106). Comparison of separate assays can be made even more precise through the use of calibrator genes that control for underlying variations in housekeeping gene expression (101,106,123,124).

TABLE 5.6

EQUATIONS FOR RELATIVE QUANTITATION OF INPUT DNA USING Q-PCR

Simplest relative quantitation method (useful for comparing two genes within the same sample): The factor Y by which the quantity of a test gene has changed relative to the housekeeping gene is,

$$Y = 2^{-\Delta C_t}$$

Where $\Delta C_t = C_t$ (test gene) $- C_t$ (housekeeping gene)

Comparative C_t method (useful for comparing two genes under different experimental conditions[a]): The factor X by which the quantity of a test gene has changed normalized to the housekeeping gene and relative to the reference sample is,

$$X = 2^{-\Delta \Delta C_t}$$

Where $\Delta \Delta C_t = \Delta C_t$ (experimental sample) $- \Delta C_t$ (reference sample); ΔC_t (experimental sample) $= C_t$ (test gene) $- C_t$ (housekeeping gene) of the experimental tissue; and ΔC_t (reference sample) $= C_t$ (test gene) $- C_t$ (housekeeping gene) of the reference or control tissue.

Limitations of Q-PCR

Q-PCR can be applied to fresh as well as FFPE tissue, and phenotype–genotype correlations are possible through analysis of specific cell populations collected via microdissection, laser capture microdissection, and so on. However, just like conventional PCR, the reliability of Q-PCR is critically dependent on the fixative, purity of the input nucleic acid preparation, primer and probe design (greatly facilitated by a number of Internet websites [108]), choice of thermostable polymerase, cycle parameters, and buffer conditions (83,84,125). Consequently, real-time PCR assays must be optimized to ensure their reliability in routine use.

Even in optimized Q-PCR assays, testing can be complicated by amplification bias, which as noted above, is the preferential amplification of one target sequence over another. In the context of Q-PCR, amplification bias has two major sources, PCR drift and PCR selection (61,126,127). PCR drift is thought to be due to random fluctuations in amplification efficiency in the early cycles of the reaction when the templates are present at very low concentration. PCR selection encompasses the mechanisms that systematically favor amplification of one particular target, including target length and target sequence itself. In general, the shortest amplicon is more efficiently amplified than longer amplicons, but the bias introduced by PCR selection often exceeds theoretical predictions for nearly identical DNA sequences that differ by only a few bp in length or sequence (65,128).

One parameter of quantitative RT-PCR that is often overlooked is the reverse transcription step itself. Although a high level of RNA purity is of fundamental importance for generating reproducible data (108,124,130), a lack of attention to detail in the reverse transcription reaction can introduce additional variables into quantitative RT-PCR that prevent accurate measurement of the level of gene expression, regardless of the purity of the RNA preparation, the use of optimally designed primers and probes, and so on (76,108).

Use of Q-PCR in Nonquantitative Settings

Because the labeled probe used in real-time Q-PCR has specificity for the target amplicon, the amplification plot not only confirms the presence of the DNA product but also confirms its identity. Similarly, assuming that a melting curve analysis is performed, the use of a binding dye such as SYBR Green I can provide confirmation of both the presence and identity of the DNA product. Because it eliminates the need for gel electrophoresis to demonstrate successful amplification, and even further simplifies the assay by eliminating the need to confirm the identity of the product, Q-PCR is often used as a one-step alternative to conventional PCR or RT-PCR, even when quantitation is not required.

MULTIPLEX PCR

Multiplex PCR is the simultaneous amplification of multiple target sequences in a single PCR through the use multiple primer pairs. Considerable savings of both time and expense are achieved by the technique, and multiplex PCR is also ideal for conserving templates that are in short supply (126,127). The method has been successfully applied to many PCR techniques including allele-specific PCR, nested PCR, and Q-PCR, and in many different DNA testing scenarios including mutation and polymorphism analysis (131,132), solid tumor diagnosis (133,134), infectious disease testing (135–137), and identity determination (Chapter 23).

It is usually necessary to adjust the concentrations of the various PCR components (such as Mg^{++} concentration, dNTP concentrations, and buffer composition) to achieve reproducible amplification of each target sequence in combination (126,127). Multiplex PCR is inherently competitive; thus more efficiently amplified target sequences will negatively influence the yield from less efficiently amplified target sequences, and consequently reaction conditions that work well in individual PCR amplifications (sometimes referred to as monoplex or uniplex PCR) may still require empiric optimization in multiplex to achieve the same sensitivity and specificity. Primer redesign may even be required because it is not uncommon that primer pairs that work well in uniplex generate spurious amplification products when combined in multiplex. Although there is no theoretical limit to the number of reactions that can be combined into a single multiplex PCR, in practice, constraints on establishing conditions that retain the necessary sensitivity and specificity for each amplicon generally limit the number of different target sequences that can be amplified in a single reaction.

Even in optimized reactions, multiplex PCR is often complicated by amplification bias as a result of PCR drift and PCR selection. Careful primer design helps ensure that the different amplicons produced in a multiplex PCR are of similar enough length to avoid PCR bias but of sufficiently different length to be easily resolved by gel electrophoresis. Nonetheless, mutations that change the size of the amplicons can potentially produce a complicated mixture of products that requires more extensive analysis for definitive identification.

METHYLATION-SPECIFIC PCR

As discussed in more detail in Chapter 1, human DNA is methylated predominately at the cytosine in the CpG dinucleotide (the nomenclature used to indicate a 5'-CG-3' DNA sequence). CpG dinucleotides are not randomly distributed throughout the genome, but are clustered in CpG stretches called CpG islands. Methylation of CpG sites has been associated with transcriptional inactivation of imprinted genes, is important for X chromosome inactivation, and is an important mechanism for developmentally regulated and tissue-specific gene regulation (138). An altered pattern of methylation is also characteristic of

many human diseases; methylation of normally unmethylated CpG islands is a frequent event in the neoplastic transformation of cells (139–143), has been associated with transcriptional inactivation of tumor suppressor genes and DNA repair genes in human malignancies (144–146), and may predispose neoplastic cells to genomic instability (141). Changes in the CpG methylation pattern in some malignancies have been associated with differences in response to specific chemotherapeutic agents (147–150) and overall survival (147,151–153).

Traditional methods for DNA methylation analysis rely on digestion of genomic DNA with methylation-sensitive restriction enzymes that do not cleave their target sequence when it contains one or more methylated CpG sites (44). Although this approach provides an assessment of the overall methylation status of CpG islands, it evaluates only the small percentage of CpG sites that lie within sequences recognized by methylation-sensitive restriction endonucleases. Similarly, immunohistochemical analysis of the genome using antibodies against 5-methycytosine can provide an overall assessment of methylation patterns but lacks the sensitivity to evaluate individual genetic loci (154–156).

More sensitive and specific DNA methylation analysis is possible using the recently developed methylation-specific PCR technique that exploits the sequence differences that result when methylated and unmethylated CpG are treated with sodium bisulfite (157). Sodium bisulfite treatment converts unmethylated cytosine to uracil while 5'-methylcytosine remains unaltered, and, consequently, as shown in Fig. 5.8, the two strands of genomic DNA are no longer complementary after bisulfite treatment. With appropriate primer design, the presence or absence of a DNA product after PCR is performed on the bisulfite-treated template can be used to infer the methylation status of the original untreated DNA. Alternatively, upstream and downstream

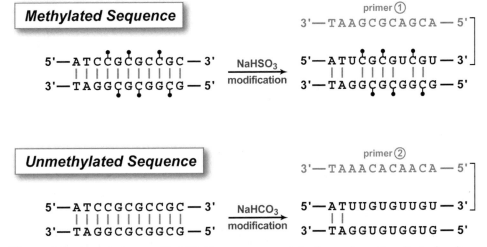

Figure 5.8   Methylation-specific PCR. The upper part of the figure shows the effect of sodium bisulfite treatment when the template is methylated (methylcytosines are indicated by the black knobs). Sodium bisulfite converts unmethylated cytosines to uracil, while methylcytosines remain unchanged. The lower part of the figure shows the effect of sodium bisulfite treatment of the same template when it is not methylated. Note that in both cases, bisulfite conversion changes the template sequence and destroys the self-complementarity of the double-stranded DNA. Also note that primers complementary to the treated methylated sequence (primer 1) or the treated unmethylated sequence (primer 2) of the same DNA strand have different sequences, a fact that is exploited in PCR amplifications designed to infer the methylation status of the target region.

primers can be used to amplify the target region regardless of any changes introduced by bisulfite treatment, and the DNA product can be directly sequenced, or evaluated by SSCP, denaturing gel electrophoresis, or other techniques to identify the sequence changes indicative of CpG methylation (158–162). Sodium bisulfite modification of template DNA is technically straightforward, and, when optimized, methylation-specific PCR has a very high sensitivity, reportedly capable of detecting an altered pattern of methylation involving only 0.1% of the target DNA (163), although amplification bias can complicate analysis under such limiting conditions (66).

Methylation-specific PCR has several advantages over the traditional methods of DNA methylation analysis (163). First, the technique makes it possible to evaluate the methylation status of individual CpG sites, whether or not they are within a sequence recognized by a methylation-sensitive restriction endonuclease. Second, methylation-specific PCR requires only small quantities of template DNA, which makes the method ideally suited to the analysis of small samples such as tissue biopsies. Third, the technique can be applied to DNA extracted from FFPE tissue or fresh tissue. Fourth, even archival cytology specimens can be evaluated by the method (164). Methylation-specific oligonucleotide arrays have been developed that even offer the potential for high-throughput genomewide analysis (165). For these reasons, methylation-specific PCR has found several applications in the clinical molecular genetics laboratory, including diagnostic tests for various imprinting disorders such as Prader-Willi and Angelman syndromes (166); prognostic

tests of a variety of malignancies, including non–small cell lung cancer (151), diffuse large B-cell lymphoma (152), and gastric carcinoma (153); and tests for the identification of tumor subgroups likely to respond to standard chemotherapy (147,150).

TELOMERASE REPEAT AMPLIFICATION PROTOCOL

The hexanucleotide TTAGGG repeat sequence of human telomeres is essential for the maintenance of chromosome stability and integrity (Chapter 1). Because abnormalities of telomere length have been associated with a number of developmental abnormalities and malignancies, accurate quantitative measurement of telomerase activity is of potential clinical importance as an adjunct in early diagnosis, for prognostic testing, or as a means to identify drugs that inhibit telomerase function (167,168). The PCR telomeric repeat amplification protocol (TRAP) assay (169) provides a simple, sensitive, and reproducible method to evaluate telomerase activity in even small tissue samples.

Technically, the TRAP assay is straightforward (Fig. 5.9). In the first step, a protein extract is prepared from the cell pellet or tissue specimen. An aliquot of the extract is added to a reaction mixture that includes a synthetic nontelomeric oligonucleotide that contains the telomeric repeat sequence recognized by telomerase; the synthetic oligonucleotide serves as an artificial telomere, and any telomerase enzyme present in the protein extract will add telomeric

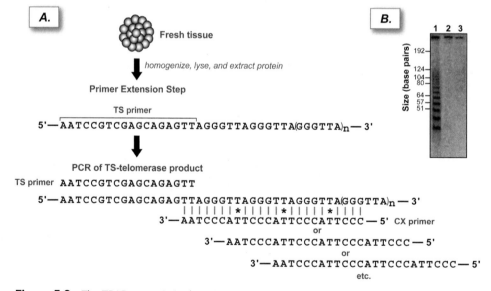

Figure 5.9 The TRAP assay. **A,** In the primer extension step, a protein extract of a fresh tissue is prepared and mixed with the TS primer, an oligonucleotide of nontelomeric sequence known to be extended by telomerase. Next, the TS-telomerase product is amplified in a PCR using the TS oligonucleotide itself as one primer, and the CX oligonucleotide as the downstream primer. The sequence of the CX primer results in amplification of only those TS-telomerase products containing 3 or more TTAGGG repeats, and because the CS primer binds at different positions along the TS-telomerase product, the PCR generates a ladder of TRAP assay products that vary in size by six nucleotides. The mismatches between the CX primer and the telomeric TTAGGG repeats (indicated by the asterisks) are designed to reduce artifacts from primer complementarity. **B,** Antoradiograph from a TRAP assay performed on an extract from an immortal renal cell line (lane 1). Pretreatment of the cell line extract with RNase destroys the internal RNA template of telomerase and abolishes the enzymatic activity of telomerase, producing a negative test result (lane 2). Control normal fibroblasts contain no measurable telomerase activity (lane 3). (Panel B is excerpted with permission from Kim NW, Platyszek MA, Prowse KR, et al. Specific association of human telomerase activity with immortal cells and cancer. Science 1994;266:2001–2015. Copyright 1994 AAAS.)

repeats to the 3′ end of the oligonucleotide. In the second step, an oligonucleotide complementary to the TTAGGG telomeric repeat sequence is added to the reaction mixture, and the subsequent PCR thus amplifies any synthetic non-telomeric oligonucleotides that have been extended in the first step of the assay. After simple gel electrophoresis, the PCR product DNA can be detected by autoradiography, direct staining with ethidium bromide or silver nitrate, or fluorescence, depending on assay design (170). Commercially available TRAP assay kits have made the technique widely accessible, and Q-PCR modifications have made the TRAP assay quantitative (170–173).

However, the technique does have limitations. The protein extract used for testing can be prepared only from fresh cells or tissue samples, a requirement that restricts the clinical utility of the method when evaluating tumor specimens. False negative and false positive reactions are commonly encountered in the standard TRAP assay (170, 174–176), and heterogeneity within a tumor can lead to significant variability in the test result (177–181). And, as with all PCR-based methods, there is always a risk of contamination and primer-dimer artifacts.

Although early studies suggested that altered telomerase activity is a characteristic finding in a variety of neoplasms (169,182), a growing body of evidence suggests that telomerase activity demonstrated by the TRAP assay is neither a consistent feature of malignancy nor specific for a malignant phenotype (183–190). Attempts to correlate a malignant phenotype with telomerase activity measured by other techniques have likewise produced mixed results. RT-PCR–based measurement of the level of expression of mRNA encoding the hTERT catalytic subunit of telomerase has been shown to provide increased sensitivity for distinguishing malignant versus reactive diseases in some (but not all) studies (173,191–196), results that may reflect the fact that assay variability is significantly influenced by tumor heterogeneity (196). Similarly, immunohistochemical analysis of hTERT provides a method for precise localization of the protein within tissues, but has not proved to be diagnostically useful because the catalytic subunit of hTERT is apparently expressed in both benign and malignant tissues (197–199), even though it may not be functionally active (200).

The recently described single telomere length analysis method (STELA) provides an approach to accurately measure the telomere length of a single chromosome arm (201), offering the opportunity for more precise correlation of telomere abnormalities and disease (202).

RAPID AMPLIFICATION OF cDNA ENDS

Rapid amplification of cDNA ends (RACE) is basically an RT-PCR used to obtain a full-length mRNA sequence when only a portion of the sequence of the transcript is known (203). The method takes two general forms, termed 3′ RACE when the unknown sequence is 3′ to the known region and 5′ RACE when the unknown sequence is 5′ to the known region. Although several modified approaches have been described (204–206), the basic RACE techniques are diagrammed in Figure 5.10.

The first step in RACE is cDNA synthesis. 3′ RACE is essentially a modification of RT-PCR in which the cDNA

synthesis step is primed by a modified poly(dT) primer that binds to the poly(A) tail of mRNA; subsequent PCR using a primer complementary to a region of known sequence in the transcript and the modified poly(dT) primer generates a DNA product that can be sequenced to characterize the 3′ end of the transcript. For 5′ RACE, the enzyme terminal deoxynucleotidyl transferase is used to add a poly-deoxynucleotide tail to the 3′ end of the cDNA molecules via a reaction performed in the presence of only one nucleotide, usually either dATP or dCTP. This tailing reaction makes it possible to amplify the uncharacterized 5′ region of the transcript in a PCR using a primer complementary to a region of known sequence in the message and a poly(dG) or poly(dT) primer.

RACE is not usually performed during clinical testing of patient specimens but instead is primarily used in research settings. It is mentioned here because, in the context of surgical pathology, RACE is one of the primary methods used in the initial discovery and characterization of fusion transcripts that result from chromosomal translocations shown by traditional cytogenetic analysis to be characteristic of specific neoplasms. RACE is easily performed, and thus it can be used as a screening method to identify fusion transcripts when large-scale mapping studies such as FISH have identified a set of candidate genes involved in the chromosomal translocation (207–211), eliminating the need for more precise localization of the break point by costly and time-consuming analysis of genomic DNA.

CLONALITY ASSAYS

According to the clonal model of carcinogenesis, all tumors arise from a single cell (212,213). The founder cell acquires an initial mutation that provides its progeny with a selective growth advantage, and from within this expanded population another single cell acquires a second mutation that provides an additional growth advantage, and so on, until a fully developed malignant tumor emerges. Demonstration that the cells in a lesion share a common genetic alteration therefore can be used to support classification as a neoplasm rather than as a polyclonal reactive process, but clonal neoplasms are not necessarily malignant (214).

Loss of Heterozygosity Assays

PCR-based approaches to loss of heterozygosity (LOH) can be used to identify a clonal pattern of gene inactivation at a target locus (X-linked assays) or detect clonal loss of one allele at a target locus (microsatellite-based assays).

X-linked Loss of Heterozygosity Assays

X-linked clonality assays have their basis in Lyon's hypothesis (215,216), which states that one of the two X chromosomes in every normal human female cell is inactivated on a random basis during early embryogenesis and that the pattern of inactivation is stable and perpetuated through subsequent cell cycles. Although skewing toward one chromosome has been documented in some individuals (217,218), for the vast majority of females the average lyonization ratio is close to 1:1 in large cell populations. Consequently, each X

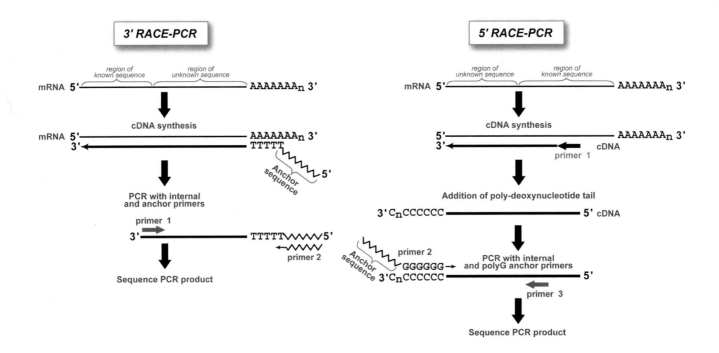

Figure 5.10 Schematic diagram of the basic methodology used for rapid amplification of cDNA ends (RACE). 3′ RACE: cDNA synthesis is performed using a poly(dT) primer with a 5′ extension sequence called the anchor sequence that is usually at least 15 to 20 nucleotides long. PCR amplification can then be performed using a primer complementary to the region of known sequence (primer 1) and a primer complementary to the anchor sequence (primer 2), which makes the PCR more specific. 5′ RACE: cDNA synthesis is performed using a primer complementary to the 3′ region of known sequence (primer 1), and a homopolymeric tail is added using the enzyme terminal deoxynucleotidyl transferase. PCR is then performed using a primer complementary to the homopolymeric tail (primer 2, which usually also has a 5′ anchor sequence) and an internal primer complementary to the region of known sequence (primer 3).

chromosome is inactivated in an approximately equal number of cells in normal tissues, and all cells in a neoplasm share the same X chromosome inactivation pattern as the founder cell. X-linked clonality assays are obviously only informative for female patients.

X chromosome inactivation has traditionally been evaluated by analysis of the phenotypic expression of X-linked isoenzymes such as glucose-6-phosphate dehydrogenase (219). However, the most frequently used PCR approach to X-clonality assays is based on differences in the DNA methylation pattern between the active and inactive X chromosomes. As discussed in Chapter 1, X chromosome inactivation is maintained via increased DNA methylation. Although different patterns of X inactivation in principle could be distinguished by gene expression analysis (mRNA would only be transcribed from genes on the active X chromosome), in practice it is much easier to distinguish the active and inactive X chromosomes at the DNA level using methylation-sensitive restriction endonucleases. The most commonly employed enzymes are HpaII and HhaI because both have recognition sequences that include the CpG dinucleotide but only cleave DNA when the CpG site is unmethylated (218,220).

The genes encoding hypoxanthine phosphoribosyl transferase (HPRT) and phosphoglycerate kinase (PGK) were the first targets for detection of differential methylation by restriction fragment length polymorphism analysis. However, because both HPRT and PGK are associated with a relatively low frequency of polymorphisms, they have limited usefulness in loss of heterozygosity assays (218,221). Consequently, the human androgen receptor gene (HUMARA) is the locus used for most methylation-sensitive restriction endonuclease assays because approximately 90% of women are heterozygous at the locus due to a trinucleotide repeat polymorphism (222,223). Because the trinucleotide repeat is close to HpaII and HhaI sites known to be methylated on the inactive X chromosome, restriction digestion of genomic DNA followed by PCR amplification of the region of the gene that includes the restriction sites can be used to determine the pattern of X chromosome inactivation in lesional and matched control tissues (44), as shown in Figure 5.11. And, because the PCR target sequence is less than 300 bp long, the assay can be reliably performed on both FFPE tissues and fresh tissue (224–226).

Following electrophoresis, a shift in the relative abundance of the DNA product from the different alleles (termed allelic imbalance) provides evidence for clonality. Shifts in abundance usually can be reliably interpreted visually, but approaches that use a radiolabled dNTP in the PCR amplification permit quantitative comparison of the intensity of the bands from the different alleles, as do recently described methods for quantitative analysis using fluorophores. In most studies, a minimum of a 1.5- to 2-fold shift in the intensity of one allele relative to the other, compared to the findings in normal tissue, has been required for a lesion

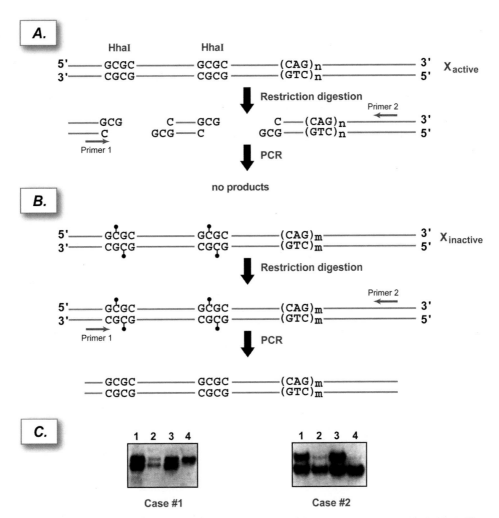

Figure 5.11   X-linked LOH analysis using the human androgen receptor gene (HUMARA). The region of exon 1 of the HUMARA gene contains several methylation-specific endonuclease sites within 100 bp of the polymorphic CAG repeat; for simplicity, only two *Hha1* sites are shown. **A**, The *Hha1* sites on the active X chromosome are cleaved because they are not methylated, and so no products are generated in the subsequent PCR using primers that flank the restriction sites and the CAG repeat. **B**, The *Hha1* sites on the inactive X chromosome are methylated (indicated by the black knobs) and are not cleaved, so a PCR product is generated in the subsequent PCR amplification. **C**, Examples of results from X-linked HUMARA of endometrial carcinomas. Both gels show autoradiographs of the PCR products of undigested *(lanes 1 and 3)* and *Hha1* digested DNA *(lanes 2 and 4)*, from normal myometrium *(lanes 1 and 2)* and carcinoma *(lanes 3 and 4)* after electrophoretic separation. For both cases, lanes 1 and 3 show allelic polymorphism in both the myometrium and tumor. For case 1, the tumor is interpreted as monoclonal because the tumor alleles (lane 4) are skewed versus the matched polyclonal normal myometrium (lane 2). For case 2, the clonality of the tumor is unknown because the normal myometrium and carcinoma have similar allelic ratios *(lanes 2 and 4)*. (Panel C is reprinted from Mutter GL, Chaponot ML, Fletcher JA. A polymerase chain reaction assay for nonrandom X chromosome inactivation identifies monoclonal endometrial cancers and precancers. *American Journal of Pathology* 1995;145;501–508; with permission.)

the to be interpreted as clonal. However, more stringent fold-change thresholds can affect interpretation of the assay result (as discussed more fully later).

Microsatellite-Based Loss of Heterozygosity Assays

As discussed in Chapter 1, microsatellites are hypervariable regions of DNA composed of repetitive short sequences that belong to the family of highly polymorphic and repetitive noncoding DNA sequences. Although the origin and function of microsatellites are not clear, they are particularly well suited for use in PCR-based clonality assays because of

their ubiquity in the genome, easy amplification by PCR-based techniques, mendelian codominant inheritance, and extreme polymorphism (227–230).

LOH at target loci usually represents hemizygosity from loss of one allele, generally as the result of a deletion. Although any microsatellite can function as a target, those linked to tumor suppressor genes involved in malignant transformation often provide the most information. Searchable databases that are accessible via the Internet* make it very easy to identify microsatellite markers linked to regions of interest.

_____

*For example, http://www.gdb.org/ or http://gai.nci.nih.gov/CHLC/.

Several facts have important implications for use of microsatellite LOH assays as a basis for assessment of clonality. First, although an individual tumor type may have a characteristic pattern of LOH at specific loci, the prevalence of LOH at each locus is variable and virtually always less than 100% (231–234). Second, a background level of LOH can be demonstrated in 4% to 20% of even normal tissues (235–238), implying the presence of a similar background frequency of LOH in tumor tissue. Third, microsatellite instability that results from defects in the DNA mismatch repair system (see below) can cause differences in the length of a microsatellite locus in different subpopulations of tumor cells; this instability can produce a pattern of heterogeneity that masks LOH when a tumor is actually hemizygous for the chromosomal region, or, conversely, can produce a pattern of overlapping alleles that mimicks LOH when a tumor remains heterozygous. Consequently, evaluation of LOH at a single locus usually does not provide enough evidence to classify a proliferation as monoclonal with a high degree of certainty (214,239–241).

In practice, test DNA derived from either fresh or FFPE tissue can be used in PCR-based assays for evaluation of LOH. Comparison of the abundance of the DNA product from the different alleles after PCR amplification is used to determine the presence of LOH, a comparison that can be made quantitative by either isotopic or nonisotopic methods. The use of fluorescence-based detection systems makes multiplex analysis possible (234,242–244). As with the HUMARA assay discussed above, a minimum of a 1.5- to 2-fold shift in the intensity of one allele relative to the other, compared to the findings in normal tissue, has generally been required for a lesion to be interpreted as clonal, but more stringent fold-change thresholds can effect interpretation of the assay result (234), as discussed below.

One technical problem with microsatellite-based LOH analysis is that the thermostable polymerases required for PCR are themselves responsible for variability in the pattern of products that can sometimes make typing less than definitive (242,245,246), variability that is usually manifested as a cluster of products of different lengths and abundance (Fig. 5.12). Slippage of the thermostable polymerases at short repeat sequences is responsible for some of the variability (33,248,249). The template-independent,

sequence-dependent terminal deoxynucleotidyl transferase activity of some thermostable polymerases, which adds one additional base to the PCR product (an activity that is especially prominent in the most widely used enzyme *Taq*), can produce additional variability in the population of products (247).

Pitfalls in LOH Clonality Assays

There are several technical aspects of LOH clonality assays that can lead to erroneous results. Lack of attention to these sources of error may explain the so-called zebra pattern of loss and retention of heterozygosity across a chromosomal region that has been reported for some tumor types, and is probably also a cause of conflicting results between different studies.

First, the quality of specimen-derived DNA has a marked influence on the reliability of clonality assays. DNA extracted from FFPE tissue often contains a low number of amplifiable DNA molecules, especially for amplicons longer than about 300 bp. Random deviations at high template dilutions can cause allelic dropout and lead to results that do not reflect tissue allelic ratios. Strict attention to the quantity of amplifiable DNA content, especially from archival samples, has been shown to improve the efficiency and reliability of LOH assays (243,244,250). Analytic and statistical methods have been developed to increase the reliability of assays performed with very low levels of input DNA (251).

Second, as discussed previously in the section on quantitative PCR, the amount of PCR product accurately reflects the abundance of input DNA only during the exponential phase of amplification. Overamplification can produce a plateau effect in which the quantity of PCR product formed is not proportional to the amount of input template DNA, and consequently the endpoint-based measurements of product DNA that are frequently used in LOH clonality assays can cause erroneous results. Quantitative PCR methods can be used to help ensure that allelic ratios are compared during the exponential phase of amplification.

Third, for most microsatellite markers, the longer allele is less efficiently amplified than the shorter allele. The amplification bias may exceed theoretical predictions and be significant even for DNA sequences that differ by only a few bp (64,128,251–253).

Fourth, although X-chromosome inactivation during development is random and usually produces a mosaic pattern, the size of regions that share inactivation of the same X-chromosome can still be a limiting factor in clonality assays. The size of a contiguous tissue region that shares inactivation of the same X-chromosome, sometimes referred to as the patch size, places a lower limit on the size of a tumor for which an X-linked clonality assay can provide a meaningful result. Analysis of a neoplasm smaller than the anticipated patch size will yield a clonal pattern of X-inactivation even if the lesion is polyclonal. Patch size is quite variable, but can be relatively large. Monoclonal X-chromosome inactivation regions can be up to 4 mm in diameter in large arteries (254,255), and about 2 mm in diameter in the colon (256). Even entire terminal ductal-lobular units in the breast can show monoclonal X-chromosome inactivation patterns (256,257).

Fifth, non-neoplastic cells in a tumor sample (including lymphocytes, macrophages, endothelial cells, and even

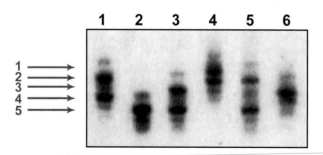

Figure 5.12 PCR-based typing of the D11S35 microsatellite locus, a (CA/GT)n dinucleotide repeat polymorphism. Arrows on the left mark the main band seen at different alleles which differ by one repeat unit. The genotypes (in parentheses) for the individuals in lanes 1 to 6 are as follows: 1(2,4); 2(5,5); 3(3,5); 4(1,2); 5(2,5); 6(3,3). Note that, because they are homozygous at D11S35, the locus would be uninformative in LOH assays performed on individuals 2 and 6. (Reprinted from Litt M, Hauge X, Sharma V. Shadow bands seen when typing polymorphic dinucleotide repeats: some causes and cures. *BioTechniques* 1993;15:280–284; with permission.)

residual normal parenchymal cells) can mask LOH within the neoplastic population of cells (241). Non-neoplastic cells can also contribute to LOH in some settings (258), not surprising given the discussion of patch size above. A wide variety of techniques has been used to try to overcome the problem of stromal contamination, including microdissection and flow cytometric purification of the tumor cells (259). However, it is important to recognize that heterogeneity within the tumor itself can also complicate analysis, creating a different pattern of LOH in different regions of the neoplasm (258,260).

Sixth, although shifts in the abundance of one allele relative to the other usually can be reliably interpreted, the minimum 1.5- to 2-fold shift that has been widely used as the threshold for a lesion to be classified as clonal is arbitrary (241). In general, test interpretations based on higher fold-change shifts are less likely to be affected by technical artifacts (214,218), and so higher-fold thresholds increase test specificity. On the other hand, test interpretations based on more stringent fold-change thresholds limit assay sensitivity. Although criteria have been proposed for quantitative evaluation of the ratio of PCR products, especially for marginal cases (245), there is no uniform standard for objective classification of a lesion as clonal.

Clonality Assays Based on Gene Rearrangements

The main PCR-based assays in this category are used to assess lymphoid infiltrates based on evaluation of immunoglobulin gene or T-cell receptor gene rearrangements (261,262). PCR primer design is an important component of these assays, because generation of immunoglobulin and T-cell receptors involves deletions, template-independent nucleotide additions, and single bp changes. To avoid false negative results, primers are designed to bind to less variable sequence regions, and multiple sets of primers are used to ensure that a broad range of rearrangements can be detected (261,262).

However, demonstration of a monoclonal or oligoclonal population of cells within an infiltrate is not always indicative of malignancy. As discussed in more detail in Chapter 13, oligoclonal and even monoclonal gene rearrangements can be detected in reactive lymphoid proliferations, as well as various disorders, including multiple sclerosis, idiopathic thrombocytopenic purpura, immunodeficiency-related lymphocytic infiltrates, and various dermatologic disorders (241,263–266). Conversely, a true monoclonal population may go undetected because of technical limitations of the analysis; most assays based on evaluation of immunoglobulin or T-cell receptor rearrangements can detect only clonal populations that constitute at least 1% of the total cell population (261,267,268). Fragmentation of the test DNA, a feature of nucleic acids extracted from formalin-fixed tissue, can further decrease test sensitivity.

Clonality Assays Based on Specific Gene Mutations

This class of assays focuses on detection of specific mutations in individual genes, including point mutations (usually in tumor suppressor genes or oncogenes) and larger scale structural changes (e.g., deletions, or insertions of viral genomes). Although this type of assay can be applied to a broad range of tumor types, the prevalence of mutations at test loci is often quite low, and so evaluation of a single locus usually does not provide enough evidence to classify a proliferation as monoclonal. Consequently, assessment of multiple loci is required to provide statistical confidence that a neoplasm is of monoclonal origin.

Analysis of specific gene mutations can be a useful approach for demonstrating the presence of two different clonal populations when attempting to show that two neoplasms represent synchronous or metachronous tumors rather than a single neoplasm with metastasis. Although PCR bias can complicate testing (62), this type of analysis has been successfully used to evaluate the clonal origin of tumors (269–271) and study the relationship between precursor lesions and subsequent tumors (272,273). Nonetheless, the approach is hindered by the low rates of mutations and larger scale structural changes at the test loci, and by the extensive analysis required to establish the mutation rates of the various test loci in different tumor types.

MICROSATELLITE INSTABILITY ASSAYS

As discussed in Chapter 2, defects in the DNA mismatch repair system result in a characteristic pattern of mutations known as microsatellite instability (MSI). Direct analysis of the genes responsible for mismatch repair is an inefficient approach for detecting mutations in the repair system because of the number of genes involved, because of the fact that the genes have no specific mutation "hot spots" (274–277), and because the genes may be inactive as a result of epigenetic silencing rather than mutation (278–282). PCR-based analysis is a more effective way to identify defects in the DNA mismatch repair system because PCR can easily detect the short increases or decreases in the length of microsatellite sequences that are the characteristic feature of microsatellite instability.

There is no uniform laboratory definition of MSI despite the fact that the phenomenon is a characteristic feature of many sporadic tumors as well as epithelial malignancies that arise in patients who have germline mutations in the DNA mismatch repair pathway. Similarly, the laboratory testing regimen itself is not standardized in terms of the number and identity of microsatellite loci that must be analyzed for a particular tumor type, or in terms of the number of loci that need to show alterations in length to be considered indicative of a particular tumor phenotype. A workshop that addressed these issues in the context of colorectal cancer is one of the few attempts to provide some standardization for MSI analysis (283); MSI was defined as a change of any length resulting from insertion or deletion of repeating units in a microsatellite within a tumor compared with normal tissue, distinct from LOH or allelic imbalance. Criteria proposed to define particular phenotypes required instability at two or more of a panel of five specific markers for a tumor to possess MSI high frequency, and a lack of instability at all loci for a tumor to be classified as microsatellite stable. Tumors with an intermediate test result were defined as MSI low frequency. Although these definitions of MSI and tumor phenotypes were proposed specifically in the context of MSI in colorectal cancer, they have been applied to many tumor types.

In actual practice, test DNA derived from either fresh or FFPE tissue can be used in the assay. Comparison of the size of the PCR products from microsatellite loci in the neoplasm versus normal tissue is used to detect changes in the length of the microsatellite sequences indicative of MSI, a comparison that can be made quantitative by either isotopic or nonisotopic methods (242,246). In most cases the profile of PCR-amplified sequences permits straightforward classification as indicative of MSI or not; however, there are no uniform criteria for interpretation of marginal test results, although standards have been proposed (245,283). The lack of uniform criteria for interpreting marginal cases is an important issue because, as discussed above for microsatellite-based LOH assays, variability introduced at microsatellite short repeat sequences by slippage of thermostable polymerases can produce a complicated result. This variability is, in fact, a technical artifact that mirrors the slippage by replication polymerases that is the fundamental cause of MSI (248,249).

Sources of Error in MSI Analysis

There are several technical sources of error in MSI analysis, some of which are identical to the potential pitfalls in LOH testing. First, the quality of specimen-derived DNA affects the reproducibility of MSI test results, although it is possible to obtain reliable MSI results using single cells from fresh tissue or very few cells from paraffin-archived specimens if PCR conditions are optimized for a limiting amount of DNA template (243,250). Second, the presence of contaminating non-neoplastic tissue can limit test reliability because demonstration of MSI in even the most sensitive testing regimens requires that lesional cells compose at least 10% of the total population (242,250,284). Biased amplification of one of the alleles of a microsatellite marker is a third source of artifacts that can complicate interpretation of the PCR product profile (128,244), as is tumor heterogeneity, which can lead to a different pattern of MSI in different regions of a neoplasm (260). And fourth, as noted above, slippage of the termostable polymerases used in the PCR amplification step often introduces variability in the pattern of products, which can complicate test interpretation (33,248,249).

MSI test results are also strongly affected by the choice of the microsatellite markers used in the analysis for several reasons. The susceptibility of a given microsatellite to instability is highly dependent both on the number of repeats and the length of the repeat units; MSI analysis of different microsatellite loci can lead to different results (285,286). The use of markers from regions known to display high levels of allelic loss can complicate test interpretation. Apart from any intrinsic differences in stability, microsatellites with alleles that vary in length by only a few nucleotides can produce a pattern that is indistinguishable from that of LOH, masking true MSI (245,283). Finally, presumably because of the terminal deoxynucleotidyl transferase activity of thermostable polymerases, MSI analysis of mononucleotide repeats may produce length variations that do not correlate with mutations in mismatch repair genes (287).

REFERENCES

1. Saiki RK, Scharf S, Faloona F, et al. Enzymatic amplification of beta-globin genomic sequences and restriction site analysis for diagnosis of sickle cell anemia. *Science* 1985;230:1350–1354.
2. Mullis KB, Faloona FA. Specific synthesis of DNA in vitro via a polymerase-catalyzed chain reaction. *Methods Enzymol* 1987;155:335–350.
3. Visvikis S, Schlenck A, Maurice M. DNA extraction and stability for epidemiological studies. *Clin Chem Lab Med* 1998;36:551–555.
4. Berger A, Bruschek M, Grethen C, et al. Poor storage and handling of tissue mimics mitochondrial DNA depletion. *Diagn Mol Pathol* 2001;10:55–59.
5. Gall K, Pavelic J, Jadro-Santel D, et al. DNA amplification by polymerase chain reaction from brain tissues embedded in paraffin. *Int J Exp Pathol* 1993;74:333–337.
6. Jackson DP, Lewis FA, Taylor GR, et al. Tissue extraction of DNA and RNA and analysis by the polymerase chain reaction. *J Clin Pathol* 1990;43:499–504.
7. Dubeau L, Chandler LA, Gralow JR, et al. Southern blot analysis of DNA extracted from formalin-fixed pathology specimens. *Cancer Res* 1986;46:2964–2964.
8. Greer CE, Peterson SL, Kiviat NB, et al. PCR amplification from paraffin-embedded tissues: Effects of fixative and fixation time. *Am J Clin Pathol* 1991;95:117–124.
9. Ben-Ezra J, Johnson DA, Rossi J, et al. Effect of fixation on the amplification of nucleic acids from paraffin-embedded material by the polymerase chain reaction. *J Histochem Cytochem* 1991;39:351–354.
10. Crisan D, Mattson JC. Hepatosplenic gamma/delta T-cell lymphoma in immunocompromised patients: report of two cases and review of literature. *Am J Clin Pathol* 2001;116:41–50.
11. Impraim CC, Saiki RK, Erlich HA, et al. Analysis of DNA extracted from formalin-fixed, paraffin-embedded tissues by enzymatic amplification and hybridization with sequence-specific oligonucleotides. *Biochem Biophys Res Commun* 1987;142:710–716.
12. Tubbs RR, AHsi ED, Hicks D, et al. Molecular pathology testing of tissues fixed in prefer solution (Letter). *Am J Surg Pathol* 2004;28:417–419.
13. Gillespie JW, Best CJ, Bichsel VE, et al. Evaluation of non-formalin tissue fixation for molecular profiling studies. *Am J Pathol* 2002;160:449–457.
14. Greer CE, Lund JK, Manos MM. PCR amplification from paraffin-embedded tissues: recommendations on fixatives for long-term storage and prospective studies. *PCR Methods Appl* 1991;1:46–50.
15. Feldman MY. Reactions of nucleic acids and nucleoproteins with formaldehyde. *Prog Nucleic Acid Res Mol Biol* 1973;13:1–49.
16. Karlsen F, Kalantari M, Chitemerere M, et al. Modifications of human and viral deoxyribonucleic acid by formaldehyde fixation. *Lab Invest* 1994;71:604–611.
17. Auerbach C, Moutschen-Dahmen M, Moutschen J. Genetic and cytogenetical effects of formaldehyde and related compounds. *Mutat Res* 1977;39:317–361.
18. Masuda N, Ohnishi T, Kawamoto S, et al. Analysis of chemical modification of RNA from formalin-fixed samples and optimization of molecular biology applications for such samples. *Nucleic Acids Res* 1999;27:4436–4443.
19. Inadome Y, Noguchi M. Selection of higher molecular weight genomic DNA for molecular diagnosis from formalin-fixed material. *Diagn Mol Pathol* 2003;12:231–236.
20. Barnes WM. PCR amplification of up to 35-kb DNA with high fidelity and high yield from lambda bacteriophage templates. *Proc Natl Acad Sci USA* 1994; 91: 2216–2220.
21. Cheng S, Fockler C, Barnes WM, et al. Effective amplification of long targets from cloned inserts and human genomic DNA. *Proc Natl Acad Sci USA* 1994;91:5695–5699.
22. Saiki RK, Gelfand DH, Stoffel S, et al. Primer-directed enzymatic amplification of DNA with a thermostable DNA polymerase. *Science* 1988;239:487–491.
23. Flaman JM, Frebourg T, Moreau V, et al. A rapid PCR fidelity assay. *Nucleic Acids Res* 1994;22:3259–3260.
24. Jacobs G, Tscholl E, Sek A, et al. Enrichment polymerase chain reaction for the detection of Ki-ras mutations: relevance of Taq polymerase error rate, initial DNA copy number, and reaction conditions on the emergence of false-positive mutant bands. *J Cancer Res Clin Oncol* 1999;125:395–401.
25. Dietrich J, Schmitt P, Zieger M, et al. PCR performance of the highly thermostable proof-reading B-type DNA polymerase from *Pyrococcus abyssi*. *FEMS Microbiol Lett* 2002;217:89–94.
26. Mattila P, Korpela J, Tenkanen T, et al. Fidelity of DNA synthesis by the *Thermococcus litoralis* DNA polymerase: an extremely heat stable enzyme with proofreading activity. *Nucleic Acids Res* 1991;19:4967–4973.
27. Bracho MA, Moya A, Barrio E. Contribution of Taq polymerase-induced errors to the estimation of RNA virus diversity. *J Gen Virol* 1998;79:2921–2928.
28. Cline J, Braman JC, Hogrefe HH. PCR fidelity of Pfu DNA polymerase and other thermostable DNA polymerases. *Nucleic Acids Res* 1996;24:3546–3551.
29. André P, Kim A, Khrapko K, et al. Fidelity and mutational spectrum of Pfu DNA polymerase on a human mitochondrial DNA sequence. *Genome Res* 1997;78:843–852.
30. Eckert KA, Kunkel TA. DNA polymerase fidelity and the polymerase chain reaction. *PCR Methods Appl* 1991;1:17–24.
31. Eckert KA, Kunkel TA. The fidelity of DNA polymerases used in the polymerase chain reactions. In: McPherson MJ, ed. *PCR: A Practical Approach*, vol 1. Oxford: IRL Press at Oxford, University Press Oxford; 1992:225–244.
32. Krawczak M, Reiss J, Schmidtke J, et al. Polymerase chain reaction: replication errors and reliability of gene diagnosis. *Nucleic Acids Res* 1989;17:2197–2201.
33. Hauge XY, Litt M. A study of the origin of 'shadow bands' seen when typing dinucleotide repeat polymorphisms by the PCR. *Hum Mol Genet* 1993;2:411–415.
34. Viguera E, Canceill D, Ehrlich SD. In vitro replication slippage by DNA polymerases from thermophilic organisms. *J Mol Biol* 2001;312:323–333.
35. Clarke LA, Rebelo CS, Goncalves J, et al. PCR amplification introduces errors into mononucleotide and dinucleotide repeat sequences. *Mol Pathol* 2001;54:351–353.
36. Reiss J, Krawczak M, Schloesser M, et al. The effect of replication errors on the mismatch analysis of PCR-amplified DNA. *Nucleic Acids Res* 1990;18:973–978.
37. Luria SE, Delbruck M. Mutations of bacteria from virus sensitivity to virus resistance. *Genetics* 1943;28:491–511.
38. Wagner A, Blackstone N, Cartwright P, et al. Surveys of gene families using polymerase chain reaction: PCR selection and PCR drift. *Syst Biol* 1994;43:250–261.

39. Kohler S, Galili N, Sklar JL, et al. Expression of bcr-abl fusion transcripts following bone marrow transplantation for Philadelphia chromosome-positive leukemia. *Leukemia* 1990;4:541–547.
40. Li H, Gyllensten UB, Cui X, et al. Amplification and analysis of DNA sequences in single human sperm and diploid cells. *Nature* 1988;335:414–417.
41. Chong SS, Gore-Langton RE, Hughes MR. Single-cell DNA analysis for applicaton to preimplantation genetic diagnosis. In: Dracopoli NC, Haines JL, Korf BR, et al., eds. *Current Protocols in Human Genetics*. New York: John Wiley and Sons; 1996: 9.10.1–9.10.26.
42. Hahn S, Zhong XY, Holzgreve W. Single cell PCR in laser capture microscopy. *Methods Enzymol* 2002;356:295–301.
43. Persson A, Backvall H, Ponten F, et al. Single cell gene mutation analysis using laser-assisted microdissection of tissue sections. *Methods Enzymol* 2002;356:334–343.
44. Mutter GL, Chaponot ML, Fletcher JA. A polymerase chain reaction assay for non-random X chromosome inactivation identifies monoclonal endometrial cancers and precancers. *Am J Pathol* 1995;146:501–508.
45. Maitra A, Wistuba II, Virmani AK, et al. Enrichment of epithelial cells for molecular studies. *Nat Med* 1999;5:459–463.
46. Serth J, Kuczyk MA, Paeslack U, et al. Quantitation of DNA extracted after micropreparation of cells from frozen and formalin-fixed tissue sections. *Am J Pathol* 2000;156:1189–1196.
47. Heinmoller E, Liu Q, Sun Y, et al. Toward efficient analysis of mutations in single cells from ethanol-fixed, paraffin-embedded, and immunohistochemically stained tissues. *Lab Invest* 2002;82:443–453.
48. Mattu R, Sorbara L, Filie AC, et al. Utilization of polymerase chain reaction on archival cytologic material: a comparison with fresh material with special emphasis on cerebrospinal fluids. *Mod Pathol* 2004;17:1295–1301.
49. Simone NL, Bonner RF, Gillespie JW, et al. Laser-capture microdissection: opening the microscopic frontier to molecular analysis. *Trends Genet* 1998;14:272–276.
50. Fend F, Quintanilla-Martinez L, Kumar S, et al. Composite low grade B-cell lymphomas with two immunophenotypically distinct cell populations are true biclonal lymphomas: a molecular analysis using laser capture microdissection. *Am J Pathol* 1999;154:1857–1866.
51. Thompson L, Chang B, Barsky SH. Monoclonal origins of malignant mixed tumors (carcinosarcomas): evidence for a divergent histogenesis. *Am J Surg Pathol* 1996; 20:277–285.
52. Yaremko ML, Kelemen PR, Kutza C, et al. Immunomagnetic separation can enrich fixed solid tumors for epithelial cells. *Am J Pathol* 1996;148:95–104.
53. Retzel E, Staskus KA, Embretson JE, et al. The in situ PCR: amplification and detection of DNA in a cellular context. In: Innis MA, Gelfand DH, eds. *PCR Strategies*. Academic Press: San Diego; 1995;199–212.
54. Cowlen MS. Nucleic acid hybridization and amplification in situ: principles and applications in molecular pathology. In: Coleman WB, Tsongalis GJ, eds. *Molecular Diagnostics: For the Clinical Laboratorian*. Totawa, NJ: Humana Press; 1997;163–191.
55. Haase AT, Retzel EF, Staskus KA. Amplification and detection of lentiviral DNA inside cells. *Proc Natl Acad Sci USA* 1990;87:4971–4975.
56. Nuovo GJ, MacConnell P, Gallery F. Analysis of nonspecific DNA synthesis during in situ PCR and solution-phase PCR. *PCR Methods Appl* 1994;4:89–96.
57. Zehbe I, Sallstrom JF, Hacker GW, et al. Indirect and direct in-situ PCR for the detection of human papillomavirus: an evaluation of two methods and a double staining technique. *Cell Vision* 1994;1:163–167.
58. Zehbe IE, Hacker GW, Sallstrom J, et al. Detection of single HPV copies in SiHa cells by in situ polymerase chain reaction (in situ PCR) combined with immunoperoxidase and immunogold-silver staining (IGSS) techniques. *Anticancer Res* 1992;12:2165–2168.
59. Patterson BK, Till M, Otto P, et al. Detection of HIV-1 DNA and messenger RNA in individual cells by PCR-driven in situ hybridization and flow cytometry. *Science* 1993;260:976–979.
60. Walsh PS, Erlich HA, Higuchi R. Preferential PCR amplification of alleles: mechanisms and solutions. *PCR Methods Appl* 1992;1:241–250.
61. Ogino S, Wilson RB. Quantification of PCR bias caused by a single nucleotide polymorphism in SMN gene dosage analysis. *J Mol Diagn* 2002;4:185–190.
62. Barnard R, Futo V, Pecheniuk N, et al. PCR bias toward the wild-type k-ras and p53 sequences: implications for PCR detection of mutations and cancer diagnosis. *Biotechniques* 1998;25:684–691.
63. Liu Q, Thorland EC, Sommer SS. Inhibition of PCR amplification by a point mutation downstream of a primer. *Biotechniques* 1997;22:292–294, 296, 298.
64. Mutter GL, Boynton KA. PCR bias in amplification of androgen receptor alleles, a trinucleotide repeat marker used in clonality studies. *Nucleic Acids Res* 1995;23:1411–1418.
65. Polz MF, Cavanaugh CM. Bias in template-to-product ratios in multitemplate PCR. *Appl Environ Microbiol* 1998;64:3724–3730.
66. Warnecke PM, Stirzaker C, Melki JR, et al. Detection and measurement of PCR bias in quantitative methylation analysis of bisulphite-treated DNA. *Nucleic Acids Res* 1997;25:4422–4426.
67. Niederhauser C, Hofelein C, Wegmuller B, et al. Reliability of PCR decontamination systems. *PCR Methods Appl* 1994;4:117–123.
68. Kwok S, Higuchi R. Avoiding false positives with PCR. *Nature* 1989;339:237–238.
69. Rys PN, Persing DH. Preventing false positives: quantitative evaluation of three protocols for inactivation of polymerase chain reaction amplification products. *J Clin Microbiol* 1993;31:2356–2360.
70. Hill DA, O'Sullivan MJ, Zhu X, et al. Practical application of molecular genetic testing as an aid to the surgical pathologic diagnosis of sarcomas: a prospective study. *Am J Surg Pathol* 2002;26:965–977.
71. Burkardt H. Standardization and quality control of PCR analyses. *Clin Chem Lab Med* 2000;38:87–91.
72. Ladanyi M, Bridge J. Contribution of molecular genetic data to the classification of sarcomas. *Hum Pathol* 2000 May;31:532–538.
73. Sarkar G, Sommer SS. Shedding light on PCR contamination. *Nature* 1990;343:27.
74. Longo MC, Berninger MD, Hartley JL. Use of uracil DNA glycosylase to control carry-over contamination in polymerase chain reactions. *Gene* 1990;93:125–128.
75. O'Sullivan MJ, Humphrey PA, Dehner LP, et al. (X;18) reverse transcriptase-polymerase chain reaction demonstrating a variant transcript. *J Mol Diagn* 2002;4:178–180.
76. Freeman WM, Walker SJ, Vrana KE. Quantitative RT-PCR: pitfalls and potential. *Biotechniques* 1999;26:112–122, 124–125.
77. Grotzer MA, Patti R, Geoerger B, et al. Biological stability of RNA isolated from RNAlater-treated brain tumor and neuroblastoma xenografts. *Med Pediatr Oncol* 2000;34:438–442.
78. Eikmans M, Baelde HJ, de Heer E, et al. Processing renal biopsies for diagnostic mRNA quantification: improvement of RNA extraction and storage conditions. *J Am Soc Nephrol* 2000;11:868–873.
79. Chaw YF, Crane LE, Lange P, et al. Isolation and identification of cross-links from formaldehyde-treated nucleic acids. *Biochemistry* 1980;19:5525–5531.
80. Macabeo-Ong M, Ginzinger DG, Dekker N, et al. Effect of duration of fixation on quantitative reverse transcription polymerase chain reaction analyses. *Mod Pathol* 2002;15:979–987.
81. Godfrey TE, Kim S, Chavira M, et al. Quantitative mRNA expression analysis from formalin-fixed, paraffin-embedded tissues using 5′ nuclease quantitative reverse transcription-polymerase chain reaction. *J Mol Diagn* 2000;2:84–91.
82. Lewis F, Maughan NJ, Smith V, et al. Unlocking the archive: gene expression in paraffin-embedded tissue. *J Pathol* 2001;195:66–71.
83. Gjerdrum LM, Abrahamsen HN, Villegas B, et al. The influence of immunohistochemistry on mRNA recovery from microdissected frozen and formalin-fixed, paraffin-embedded sections. *Diagn Mol Pathol* 2004;13:224–233.
84. Benchekroun M, DeGraw J, Gao J, et al. Impact of fixative on recovery of mRNA from paraffin-embedded tissue. *Diagn Mol Pathol* 2004;13:116–125.
85. Gloghini A, Canal B, Klein U, et al. RT-PCR analysis of RNA extracted from Bouin-fixed and paraffin-embedded lymphoid tissues. *J Mol Diagn* 2004;6:290–296.
86. Foss RD, Guha-Thakurta N, Conran RM, et al. Effects of fixative and fixation time on the extraction and polymerase chain reaction amplification of RNA from paraffin-embedded tissue: comparison of two housekeeping gene mRNA controls. *Diagn Mol Pathol* 1994;3:148–155.
87. Jin L, Majerus J, Oliveira A, et al. Detection of fusion gene transcripts in fresh-frozen and formalin-fixed paraffin-embedded tissue sections of soft-tissue sarcomas after laser capture microdissection and rt-PCR. *Diagn Mol Pathol* 2003;12:224–230.
88. Argani P, Zakowski MF, Klimstra DS, et al. Detection of the SYT-SSX chimeric RNA of synovial sarcoma in paraffin-embedded tissue and its application in problematic cases. *Mod Pathol* 1998;11:65–71.
89. Krafft AE, Duncan BW, Bijwaard KE, et al. Optimization of the isolation and amplification of RNA from formalin-fixed, paraffin-embedded tissue: the armed forces institute of pathology experience and literature review. *Mol Diagn* 1997;2:217–230.
90. Gilliland G, Perrin S, Blanchard K, et al. Analysis of cytokine mRNA and DNA: detection and quantitation by competitive polymerase chain reaction. *Proc Natl Acad Sci USA* 1990;87:2725–2729.
91. Klebe RJ, Grant GM, Grant AM, et al. RT-PCR without RNA isolation. *Biotechniques* 1996;21:1094–1100.
92. Schlott T, Nagel H, Ruschenburg I, et al. Reverse transcriptase polymerase chain reaction for detecting Ewing's sarcoma in archival fine needle aspiration biopsies. *Acta Cytol* 1997;41:795–801.
93. Inagaki H, Murase T, Otsuka T, et al. Detection of SYT-SSX fusion transcript in synovial sarcoma using archival cytologic specimens. *Am J Clin Pathol* 1999;111:528–533.
94. Fend F, Emmert-Buck MR, Chuaqui R, et al. Immuno-LCM: laser capture microdissection of immunostained frozen sections for mRNA analysis. *Am J Pathol* 1999; 154:61–66.
95. Kohda Y, Murakami H, Moe OW. Analysis of segmental renal gene expression by laser capture microdissection. *Kidney Int* 2000;57:321–331.
96. Ivell R. A question of faith: or the philosophy of RNA controls. *J Endocrinol* 1998;159:197–200.
97. Schumacher JA, Jenson SD, Elenitoba-Johnson KS, et al. Utility of linearly amplified RNA for RT-PCR detection of chromosomal translocations: validation using the t(2;5)(p23;q35) NPM-ALK chromosomal translocation. *J Mol Diagn* 2004;6:16–21.
98. van Huijsduijnen RH. PCR-assisted cDNA cloning: a guided tour of the minefield. *Biotechniques* 1998;24:390–392.
99. Jung R, Soondrum K, Neumaier M. Quantitative PCR. *Clin Chem Lab Med* 2000;38:833–836.
100. Raeymaekers L. Quantitative PCR: theoretical considerations with practical implications. *Anal Biochem* 1993;214:582–585.
101. Barth S, Kleinhappl B, Gutschi A, et al. In vitro cytokine mRNA expression in normal human peripheral blood mononuclear cells. *Inflamm Res* 2000;49:266–274.
102. Lehman U, Kreipe H. Real-time PCR analysis of DNA and RNA extracted from formalin-fixed and paraffin-embedded biopsies. *Methods* 2001;25:409–418.
103. Montgomery RA, Dallman MJ. Semi-quantitative polymerase chain reaction analysis of cytokine and cytokine receptor gene expression during thymic ontogeny. *Cytokine* 1997;9:717–726.
104. Kuschnaroff LM, Valckx D, Goebels J, et al. Effect of treatments with cyclosporin A and anti-interferon-gamma antibodies on the mechanisms of immune tolerance in staphylococcal enterotoxin B primed mice. *Scand J Immunol* 1997;46:459–468.
105. Fox CJ, Danska JS. IL-4 expression at the onset of islet inflammation predicts nondestructive insulitis in nonobese diabetic mice. *J Immunol* 1997;158:2414–2424.
106. Giulietti A, Overbergh L, Valckx D, et al. An overview of real-time quantitative PCR: applications to quantify cytokine gene expression. *Methods* 2001;25:386–401.
107. Higuchi R, Fockler C, Dollinger G, et al. Kinetic PCR analysis: real-time monitoring of DNA amplification reactions. *Biotechnology* 1993;11:1026–1030.
108. Ginzinger DG. Gene quantification using real-time quantitative PCR: an emerging technology hits the mainstream. *Exp Hematol* 2002;30:503–512.
109. Mhlanga MM, Malmberg L. Using molecular beacons to detect single-nucleotide polymorphisms with real-time PCR. *Methods* 2001;25:463–471.
110. Tyagi S, Bratu DP, Kramer FR. Multicolor molecular beacons for allele discrimination. *Nat Biotechnol* 1998;16:49–53.
111. Holland PM, Abramson RD, Watson R, et al. Detection of specific polymerase chain reaction product by utilizing the 5′→3′ exonuclease activity of *Thermus aquaticus* DNA polymerase. *Proc Natl Acad Sci USA* 1991;88:7276–7280.
112. Smit ML, Giesendorf BA, Vet JA, et al. Semiautomated DNA mutation analysis using a robotic workstation and molecular beacons. *Clin Chem* 2001;47:739–744.

113. Durand R, Eslahpazire J, Jafari S, et al. Use of molecular beacons to detect an antifolate resistance-associated mutation in *Plasmodium falciparum*. *Antimicrob Agents Chemother* 2000;44:3461–3464.
114. Whitcombe D, Theaker J, Guy SP. Detection of PCR products using self-probing amplicons and fluorescence. *Nat Biotechnol* 1999;17:804–807.
115. Hart KW, Williams OM, Thelwell N, et al. Novel method for detection, typing, and quantification of human papillomaviruses in clinical samples. *J Clin Microbiol* 2001;39:3204–3212.
116. Thelwell N, Millington S, Solinas A, et al. Mode of action and application of Scorpion primers to mutation detection. *Nucleic Acids Res* 2000;28:3752–3761.
117. Wittwer CT, Herrmann MG, Cundry CN, et al. Real-time multiplex PCR assays. *Methods* 2001;25:430–442.
118. SantaLucia J Jr. A unified view of polymer, dumbbell, and oligonucleotide DNA nearest-neighbor thermodynamics. *Proc Natl Acad Sci USA* 1998;95:1460–1465.
119. Torimura M, Kurata S, Yamada K, et al. Fluorescence-quenching phenomenon by photoinduced electron transfer between a fluorescent dye and a nucleotide base. *Anal Sci* 2001;17:155–160.
120. Schneeberger C, Speiser P, Kury F, et al. Quantitative detection of reverse transcriptase-PCR products by means of a novel and sensitive DNA stain. *PCR Methods Appl* 1995;4:234–238.
121. Becker A, Reith A, Napiwotzki J, et al. A quantitative method of determining initial amounts of DNA by polymerase chain reaction cycle titration using digital imaging and a novel DNA stain. *Anal Biochem* 1996;237:204–207.
122. Ponchel F, Toomes C, Bransfield K, et al. Real-time PCR based on SYBR-Green I fluorescence: an alternative to the TaqMan assay for a relative quantification of gene rearrangements, gene amplifications and micro gene deletions. *BMC Biotechnol* 2003;3:18.
123. Elenitoba-Johnson K, Bohling SD, Jenson SD, et al. Fluorescence PCR quantification of cyclin D1 expression. *J Mol Diagn* 2002;4:90–96.
124. Specht K, Richter T, Muller U, et al. Quantitative gene expression analysis in microdissected archival formalin-fixed and paraffin-embedded tumor tissue. *Am J Pathol* 2001;158:419–429.
125. Paska C, Bogi K, Szilak L, et al. Effect of formalin, acetone, and RNAlater fixatives on tissue preservation and different size amplicons by real-time PCR from paraffin-embedded tissue. *Diagn Mol Pathol* 2004;13:234–240.
126. Markoulatos P, Siafakas N, Moncany M. Multiplex polymerase chain reaction: a practical approach. *J Clin Lab Anal* 2002;16:47–51.
127. Edwards MC, Gibbs RA. Multiplex PCR: advantages, development, and applications. *PCR Methods Appl* 1994;3:S65–S75.
128. Liu J, Zabarovska VI, Braga E, et al. Loss of heterozygosity in tumor cells requires re-evaluation: the data are biased by the size-dependent differential sensitivity of allele detection. *FEBS Lett* 1999;462:121–128.
129. Godfrey TE, Kim SH, Chavira M, et al. Quantitative mRNA expression analysis from formalin-fixed, paraffin-embedded tissues using 5′ nuclease quantitative reverse transcription-polymerase chain reaction. *J Mol Diagn* 2000;2:84–91.
130. Lehmann U, Bock O, Glockner S. Quantitative molecular analysis of laser-microdissected paraffin-embedded human tissues. *Pathobiology* 2000;68:202–208.
131. Chamberlain JS, Gibbs RA, Ranier JE, et al. Deletion screening of the Duchenne muscular dystrophy locus via multiplex DNA amplification. *Nucleic Acids Res* 1988; 16:11141–11156.
132. Shuber AP, Skoletsky J, Stern R, et al. Efficient 12-mutation testing in the CFTR gene: a general model for complex mutation analysis. *Hum Mol Genet* 1993;2:153–158.
133. Peter M, Gilbert E, Delattre O. A multiplex real-time PCR assay for the detection of gene fusions observed in solid tumors. *Lab Invest* 2001;81:905–912.
134. Downing JR,Khandekar A, Shurtleff SA, et al. Multiplex RT-PCR assay for the differential diagnosis of alveolar rhabdomyosarcoma and Ewing's sarcoma. *Am J Pathol* 1995;146:626–634.
135. Zimmermann KD, Schogl B, Plaimauer B, et al. Quantitative multiple competitive PCR of HIV-1 DNA in a single reaction tube. *Biotechniques* 1996;21:480–484.
136. Markoulatos P, Georgopoulou A, Kotsovassilis C, et al. Detection and typing of HSV-1, HSV-2, and VZV by a multiplex polymerase chain reaction. *J Clin Lab* Anal;14:214–219.
137. Markoulatos P, Samara V, Siafakas N, et al. Development of a quadriplex polymerase chain reaction for human cytomegalovirus detection. *J Clin Lab Anal* 1999;13:99–105.
138. Paulsen M, Ferguson-Smith AC. DNA methylation in genomic imprinting, development, and disease. *J Pathol* 2001;195:97–110.
139. Antequera F, Boyes J, Bird A. High levels of de novo methylation and altered chromatin structure at CpG islands in cell lines. *Cell* 1990;62:503–514.
140. Graff JR, Herman JG, Nyohanen S, et al. Mapping patterns of CpG island methylation in normal and neoplastic cells implicates both upstream and downstream regions in de novo methylation. *J Biol Chem* 1997;272:22322–22329.
141. Hanahan D, Weinberg RA. The hallmarks of cancer. *Cell* 2000;100:57–70.
142. Baylin SB, Herman JG, Draff JR, et al. Alterations in DNA methylation: a fundamental aspect of neoplasia. *Adv Cancer Res* 1998;72:141–196.
143. Ehrlich M. DNA methylation in cancer: too much, but also too little. *Oncogene* 2002;21:5400–5413.
144. Merlo A, Herman JG, Mao L, et al. 5′ CpG island methylation is associated with transcriptional silencing of the tumour suppressor p16/CDKN2/MTS1 in human cancers. *Nat Med* 1995;1:686–692.
145. Herman JG, Latif F, Weng Y, et al. Silencing of the VHL tumor-suppressor gene by DNA methylation in renal carcinoma. *Proc Natl Acad Sci USA* 1994;91:9700–9704.
146. Esteller M. CpG island hypermethylation and tumor suppressor genes: a booming present, a brighter future. *Oncogene* 2002;21:5427–5440.
147. Esteller M, Garcia-Foncillas J, Andion E, et al. Inactivation of the DNA-repair gene MGMT and the clinical response of gliomas to alkylating agents. *N Engl J Med* 2000;343:1350–1354.
148. Widschwendter M, Jones PA. The potential prognostic, predictive, and therapeutic values of DNA methylation in cancer. *Clin Cancer Res* 2002;8:17–21.
149. Lapidus RG, Ferguson AT, Ottaviano YL, et al. Methylation of estrogen and progesterone receptor gene 5′ CpG islands correlates with lack of estrogen and progesterone receptor gene expression in breast tumors. *Clin Cancer Res* 1996;2:805–810.
150. Strathdee G, MacKean MJ, Illand M, et al. A role for methylation of the hMLH1 promoter in loss of hMLH1 expression and drug resistance in ovarian cancer. *Oncogene* 1999;18:2335–2341.
151. Tang X, Khuri FR, Lee JJ, et al. Hypermethylation of the death-associated protein (DAP) kinase promoter and aggressiveness in stage I non-small-cell lung cancer. *J Natl Cancer Inst* 2000;92:1511–1516.
152. Esteller M, Gaidano G, Goodman SN, et al. Hypermethylation of the DNA repair gene O(6)-methylguanine DNA methyltransferase and survival of patients with diffuse large B-cell lymphoma. *J Natl Cancer Inst* 2002;94:26–32.
153. Park TJ, Han S, Cho Y, et al. Methylation of O(6)-methylguanine-DNA methyltransferase gene is associated significantly with K-ras mutation, lymph node invasion, tumor staging, and disease free survival in patients with gastric carcinoma. *Cancer* 2001;92:2760–2768.
154. Bensaada M, Kiefer H, Tachdjian G, et al. Altered patterns of DNA methylation on chromosomes from leukemia cell lines: identification of 5-methylcytosines by indirect immunodetection. *Cancer Genet Cytogenet* 1998;103:101–109.
155. Montpellier C, Bourgeois C, Kokalj-Vokac N, et al. Detection of methylcytosine-rich heterochromatin on banded chromosomes: application to cells with various status of DNA methylation. *Cancer Genet Cytogenet* 1994;78:87–93.
156. Barbin A, Montpellier C, Kokallj-Vokac N, et al. New sites of methylcytosine-rich DNA detected on metaphase chromosomes. *Hum Genet* 1994;94:684–892.
157. Herman JG, Graff JR, Myohanen S, et al. Methylation-specific PCR: a novel PCR assay for methylation status of CpG islands. *Proc Natl Acad Sci USA* 1996;93:9821–9826.
158. Trinh BN, Long TI, Laird PW. DNA methylation analysis by MethyLight technology. *Methods* 2001;25:456–462.
159. Clark SJ, Harrison J, Paul CL, et al. High sensitivity mapping of methylated cytosines. *Nucleic Acids Res* 1994;22:2990–2997.
160. Frommer M, McDonald LE, Millar DS, et al. A genomic sequencing protocol that yields a positive display of 5-methylcytosine residues in individual DNA strands. *Proc Natl Acad Sci USA* 1992;89:1827–1831.
161. Maekawa M, Sugano K, Kashiwabara H, et al. DNA methylation analysis using bisulfite treatment and PCR-single-strand conformation polymorphism in colorectal cancer showing microsatellite instability. *Biochem Biophys Res Commun* 1999;262:671–676.
162. Uhlmann K, Marczinek K, Hampe J, et al. Changes in methylation patterns identified by two-dimensional DNA fingerprinting. *Electrophoresis* 1999;20:1748–1755.
163. Herman JG, Baylin SB. Methylation-specific PCR. *Curr Protocols Hum Genet* 1998;10.6.1–10.6.10.
164. Pu RT, Laitala LE, Alli PM, et al. Methylation profiling of benign and malignant breast lesions and its application to cytopathology. *Mod Pathol* 2003;16:1095–1101.
165. Gitan RS, Shi H, Chen CM, et al. Methylation-specific oligonucleotide microarray: a new potential for high-throughput methylation analysis. *Genome Res* 2002;12:158–164.
166. Zeschnigk M, Lich C, Buiting K, et al. A single-tube PCR test for the diagnosis of Angelman and Prader-Willi syndrome based on allelic methylation differences at the SNRPN locus. *Eur J Hum Genet* 1997;5:94–98.
167. Cong YS, Wright WE, Shay JW. Human telomerase and its regulation. *Microbiol Mol Biol Rev* 2002;66:407–425.
168. Hiyama E, Hiyama K. Clinical utility of telomerase in cancer. *Oncogene* 2002; 21:643–649.
169. Kim NW, Platyszek MA, Prowse KR, et al. Specific association of human telomerase activity with immortal cells and cancer. *Science* 1994;266:2011–2015.
170. Burger AM. Standard TRAP assay. *Methods Mol Biol* 2002;191:109–124.
171. Uehara H, Nardone G, Nazarenko I, et al. Detection of telomerase activity utilizing energy transfer primers: comparison with gel- and ELISA-based detection. *Biotechniques* 1999;26:552–558.
172. Hou M, Xu D, Bjorkholm M, et al. Real-time quantitative telomeric repeat amplification protocol assay for the detection of telomerase activity. *Clin Chem* 2001;47:519–524.
173. Buchler P, Conejo-Garcia JR, Lehmann G, et al. Real-time quantitative PCR of telomerase mRNA is useful for the differentiation of benign and malignant pancreatic disorders. *Pancreas* 2001;22:331–340.
174. Matthews P, Jones CJ. Clinical implications of telomerase detection. *Histopathology* 2001;38:485–498.
175. Yan P, Bosman FT, Benhattar J. Tissue quality is an important determinant of telomerase activity as measured by TRAP assay. *Biotechniques* 1998;25:660–662.
176. Braunschweig R, Guilleret I, Delacretaz F, et al. Pitfalls in TRAP assay in routine detection of malignancy in effusions. *Diagn Cytopathol* 2001;25:225–230.
177. Kleinschmidt-Demasters BK, Evans LC, Bobak JB, et al. Quantitative telomerase expression in glioblastomas shows regional variation and down-regulation with therapy but no correlation with patient outcome. *Hum Pathol* 2000;31:905–913.
178. DeMasters BK, Markham N, Lillehei KO, et al. Differential telomerase expression in human primary intracranial tumors. *Am J Clin Pathol* 1997;107:548–554.
179. Kleinschmidt-DeMasters BK, Hashizumi TL, Sze CI, et al. Telomerase expression shows differences across multiple regions of oligodendroglioma versus high grade astrocytomas but shows correlation with Mib-1 labelling. *J Clin Pathol* 1998;51: 284–293.
180. Wullich B, Rohde V, Oehlenschlager B, et al. Focal intratumoral heterogeneity for telomerase activity in human prostate cancer. *J Urol* 1999;161:1997–2001.
181. Carey LA, Hedican CA, Henderson GS, et al. Careful histological confirmation and microdissection reveal telomerase activity in otherwise telomerase-negative breast cancers. *Clin Cancer Res* 1998;4:435–440.
182. Hiyama E, Yokoyama T, Tatsumoto N, et al. Telomerase activity in gastric cancer. *Cancer Res* 1995;55:3258–3262.
183. Broccoli D, Young JW, de Lange T. Telomerase activity in normal and malignant hematopoietic cells. *Proc Natl Acad Sci USA* 1995;92:9082–9086.
184. Bryan TM, Englezou A, Gupta J, et al. Telomere elongation in immortal human cells without detectable telomerase activity. *EMBO J* 1995;14:4240–4248.
185. Counter CM, Hirte HW, Bacchetti S, et al. Telomerase activity in human ovarian carcinoma. *Proc Natl Acad Sci USA* 1994;91:2900–2904.
186. Counter CM, Gupta J, Harley CB, et al. Telomerase activity in normal leukocytes and in hematologic malignancies. *Blood* 1995;85:2315–2320.
187. Hsiao R, Sharma HW, Ramakrishnan S, et al. Telomerase activity in normal human endothelial cells. *Anticancer Res* 1997;17:827–832.

188. Brien TP, Kallakury BV, Lowry CV, et al. Telomerase activity in benign endometrium and endometrial carcinoma. *Cancer Res* 1997;57:2760–2764.

189. Hwang CF, Su CY, Kou SC, et al. Diagnostic usefulness of telomerase activity in nasopharyngeal carcinoma. *Jpn J Cancer Res* 2000;91:760–766.

190. Ince TA, Crum CP. Telomerase: promise and challenge. *Hum Pathol* 2004;35:393–395.

191. Yan P, Coindre JM, Benhattar J, et al. Telomerase activity and human telomerase reverse transcriptase mRNA expression in soft tissue tumors: correlation with grade, histology, and proliferative activity. *Cancer Res* 1999;59:3166–3170.

192. Jakupciak JP, Wang W, Barker PE, et al. Analytical validation of telomerase activity for cancer early detection: TRAP/PCR-CE and hTERT mRNA quantification assay for high-throughput screening of tumor cells. *J Mol Diagn* 2004;6:157–165.

193. Schneider-Stock R, Jaeger V, Rys J, et al. High telomerase activity and high HTRT mRNA expression differentiate pure myxoid and myxoid/round-cell liposarcomas. *Int J Cancer* 2000;89:63–68.

194. Takakura M, Kyo S, Kanaya T, et al. Expression of human telomerase subunits and correlation with telomerase activity in cervical cancer. *Cancer Res* 1998;58:1558–1561.

195. Wu A, Ichihashi M, Ueda M. Correlation of the expression of human telomerase subunits with telomerase activity in normal skin and skin tumors. *Cancer* 1999;86:2038–2044.

196. Yan P, Benhattar J, Coindre JM, et al. Telomerase activity and hTERT mRNA expression can be heterogeneous and does not correlate with telomere length in soft tissue sarcomas. *Int J Cancer* 2002;98:851–85.

197. Kawakami Y, Kitamoto M, Nakanishi T, et al. Immuno-histochemical detection of human telomerase reverse transcriptase in human liver tissues. *Oncogene* 2000;19:3888–3893.

198. Hiyama E, Hiyama K, Yokoyama T, et al. Immunohistochemical detection of telomerase (hTERT) protein in human cancer tissues and a subset of cells in normal tissues. *Neoplasia* 2001;3:17–26.

199. Wei R, Younes M. Immunohistochemical detection of telomerase reverse transcriptase in colorectal adenocarcinoma and benign colonic mucosa. *Hum Pathol* 2002;33:693–696.

200. Shroyer KR. Immunohistochemical markers of cell immortality. *Hum Pathol* 2002;33:683–685.

201. Baird D, et al. Extensive allelic variation and ultrashort telomeres in senescent human cells. *Nat Genet* 2003;33:203–207.

202. Sedivy JM, Shippen DE, Shakirov EV. Surprise ending. *Nat Genet* 2003;33:114–116.

203. Frohman MA, Dush MK, Martin GR. Rapid production of full-length cDNAs from rare transcripts: amplification using a single gene-specific oligonucleotide primer. *Proc Natl Acad Sci USA* 1988;85:8998–9002.

204. Ohara O, Dorit RL, Gilbert W. Direct genomic sequencing of bacterial DNA: the pyruvate kinase I gene of *Escherichia coli*. *Proc Natl Acad Sci USA* 1989;86:6883–6887.

205. Loh EY, Elliott JF, Cwirla S, et al. Polymerase chain reaction with single-sided specificity: analysis of T cell receptor delta chain. *Science* 1989;243:217–220.

206. Chenchik A, Moqadam F, Siebert P. Marathon cDNA amplification: a new method for cloning full-length cDNAs. *CLONTECHniques* 1995;10:5–8.

207. Zucman J, Delattre O, Desmaze C, et al. EWS and ATF-1 gene fusion induced by t(12;22) translocation in malignant melanoma of soft parts. *Nat Genet* 1993;4:341–345.

208. Hibbard MK, Kozakewich HP, Dal Cin P, et al. PLAG1 fusion oncogenes in lipoblastoma. *Cancer Res* 2000;60:4869–4872.

209. Lawrence B, Perez-Atayde A, Hibbard M, et al. TPM3-ALK and TPM4-ALK oncogenes in inflammatory myofibroblastic tumors. *Am J Pathol* 2000;157:377–384.

210. Kroll TG, Sarraf P, Pecciarini L, et al. PAX8-PPARgamma1 fusion oncogene in human thyroid carcinoma. *Science* 2000;289:1357–1360.

211. Reading NS, Jenson SD, Smith JK, et al. 5′-(RACE) identification of rare ALK fusion partner in anaplastic large cell lymphoma. *J Mol Diagn* 2003;5:136–140.

212. Nowell PC. The clonal evolution of tumor cell populations. *Science* 1976;194:23–28.

213. Fialkow PJ. Clonal origin of human tumors. *Biochim Biophys Acta* 1976;458:283–321.

214. Diaz-Cano SJ. Designing a molecular analysis of clonality in tumours. *J Pathol* 2000;191:343–344.

215. Lyon MF. Some milestones in the history of X-chromosome inactivation. *Annu Rev Genet* 1992;26:16–28.

216. Lyon MF. Sex chromatin and gene action in the mammalian X-chromosome. *Am J Hum Genet* 1962;14:135–148.

217. Fialkow PJ. Primordial cell pool size and lineage relationships of five human cell types. *Ann Hum Genet* 1973;37:39–48.

218. Gale RE, Wheadon H, Linch DC. X-chromosome inactivation patterns using HPRT and PGK polymorphisms in haematologically normal and post-chemotherapy females. *Br J Haematol* 1991;79:193–197.

219. Fialkow PJ. Use of genetic markers to study cellular origin and development of tumors in human females. *Adv Cancer Res* 1972;15:191–226.

220. McClelland M, Nelson M, Raschke E. Effect of site-specific methylation on restriction endonucleases and DNA modification methyltransferases. *Nucleic Acids Res* 1993;21:3139–3154.

221. Willman CL, Busque L, Griffith BB, et al. Langerhans'-cell histiocytosis (histiocytosis X): a clonal proliferative disease. *N Engl J Med* 1994;331:154–160.

222. Allen RC, Zoghbi HY, Moseley AB, et al. Methylation of HpaII and HhaI sites near the polymorphic CAG repeat in the human androgen-receptor gene correlates with X chromosome inactivation. *Am J Hum Genet* 1992;51:1229–1239.

223. Tilley WD, Marcelli M, Wilson JD, et al. Characterization and expression of a cDNA encoding the human androgen receptor. *Proc Natl Acad Sci USA* 1989;86:327–331.

224. Gaffey MJ, Iezzoni JC, Weiss LM. Clonal analysis of focal nodular hyperplasia of the liver. *Am J Pathol* 1996;148:1089–1096.

225. Walsh DS, Tsou HC, Harrington A, et al. Clonality of basal cell carcinoma: molecular analysis of an interesting case. *J Invest Dermatol* 1996;106:579–582.

226. Li M, Cardon-Cardo C, Gerald WL, et al. Desmoid fibromatosis is a clonal process. *Hum Pathol* 1996;27:939–943.

227. Boland CR. Setting microsatellites free. *Nat Med* 1996;2:972–974.

228. Brentnall TA. Microsatellite instability. Shifting concepts in tumorigenesis. *Am J Pathol* 1995;147:561–563.

229. Koreth J, O'Leary JJ, O'D McGee J. Microsatellites and PCR genomic analysis. *J Pathol* 1996;178:239–248.

230. Weber JL, May PE. Abundant class of human DNA polymorphisms which can be typed using the polymerase chain reaction. *Am J Hum Genet* 1989;44:388–396.

231. Califano J, van der Riet P, Westra W, et al. Genetic progression model for head and neck cancer: implications for field cancerization. *Cancer Res* 1996;56:2488–2492.

232. Jones PA, Droller MJ. Pathways of development and progression in bladder cancer: new correlations between clinical observations and molecular mechanisms. *Semin Urol* 1993;11:177–192.

233. Vogelstein B, Fearon ER, Hamilton SR. Genetic alterations during colorectal-tumor development. *N Engl J Med* 1988;319:525–532.

234. Liloglou T, Maloney P, Xinarianos G, et al. Sensitivity and limitations of high throughput fluorescent microsatellite analysis for the detection of allelic imbalance: application in lung tumors. *Int J Oncol* 2000;16:5–14.

235. Chen LC, Kurisu W, Ljung BM, et al. Heterogeneity for allelic loss in human breast cancer. *J Natl Cancer Inst* 1992;84:506–510.

236. Deng G, Lu Y, Zlotnikov G, et al. Loss of heterozygosity in normal tissue adjacent to breast carcinomas. *Science* 1996;274:2057–2059.

237. Sager R. Tumor suppressor genes: the puzzle and the promise. *Science* 1989;246:1406–1412.

238. Wolman SR, Heppner GH. Genetic heterogeneity in breast cancer. *J Natl Cancer Inst* 1992;84:469–470.

239. Diaz-Cano SJ. Clonality studies in the analysis of adrenal medullary proliferations: application principles and limitations. *Endocr Pathol* 1998;9:301–316.

240. Diaz-Cano SJ, Wolfe HJ. Clonality in Kaposi's sarcoma. *N Engl J Med* 1997;337:571–572.

241. Diaz-Cano SJ, Blanes A, Wolfe HJ. PCR techniques for clonality assays. *Diagn Mol Pathol* 2001;10:24–33.

242. Oda S, Oki E, Maehara Y, et al. Precise assessment of microsatellite instability using high resolution fluorescent microsatellite analysis. *Nucleic Acids Res* 1997;25:3415–3420.

243. Cui X, Feiner H, Li H. Multiplex loss of heterozygosity analysis by using single or very few cells. *J Mol Diagn* 2002;4:172–177.

244. Farrand K, Jovanovic L, Delahunt B, et al. Loss of heterozygosity studies revisited: prior quantification of the amplifiable DNA content of archival samples improves efficiency and reliability. *J Mol Diagn* 2002;4:150–158.

245. Maehara Y, Oda S, Sugimachi K. The instability within: problems in current analyses of microsatellite instability. *Mutat Res* 2001;461:249–263.

246. Berg KD, Glaser CL, Thompson RE, et al. Detection of microsatellite instability by fluorescence multiplex polymerase chain reaction. *J Mol Diagn* 2000;2:20–28.

247. Litt M, Hauge X, Sharma V. Shadow bands seen when typing polymorphic dinucleotide repeats: some causes and cures. *Biotechniques* 1993;15:280–284.

248. Bovo D, Rugge M, Shiao YH. Origin of spurious multiple bands in the amplification of microsatellite sequences. *Mol Pathol* 1999;52:50–51.

249. Walsh PS, Fildes NJ, Reynolds R. Sequence analysis and characterization of stutter products at the tetranucleotide repeat locus vWA. *Nucleic Acids Res* 1996;24:2807–2812.

250. Sieben NL, Ter Haar NT, Cornelisse CJ, et al. PCR artifacts in LOH and MSI analysis of microdissected tumor cells. *Hum Pathol* 2000;31:1414–1419.

251. Slebos R, Umbach DM, Sommer CA, et al. Analytical and statistical methods to evaluate microsatellite allelic imbalance in small amounts of DNA. *Lab Invest* 2004;84:649–657.

252. Findlay I, Matthews P, Quirke P. Multiple genetic diagnoses from single cells using multiplex PCR: reliability and allele dropout. *Prenat Diagn* 1998;18:1413–1421.

253. Ray PF, Handyside AH. Increasing the denaturation temperature during the first cycles of amplification reduces allele dropout from single cells for preimplantation genetic diagnosis. *Mol Hum Reprod* 1996;2:213–218.

254. Chung IM, Schwartz SM, Murry CE. Clonal architecture of normal and atherosclerotic aorta: implications for atherogenesis and vascular development. *Am J Pathol* 1998;152:913–923.

255. Murry CE, Gipaya CT, Bartosek T, et al. Monoclonality of smooth muscle cells in human atherosclerosis. *Am J Pathol* 1997;151:697–705.

256. Novelli M, Cossu A, Oukrif D, et al. X-inactivation patch size in human female tissue confounds the assessment of tumor clonality. *Proc Natl Acad Sci USA* 2003;100:3311–3314.

257. Tsai Y, Lu Y, Nichols PW, et al. Contiguous patches of normal human mammary epithelium derived from a single stem cell: implications for breast carcinogenesis. *Cancer Res* 1996;56:402–404.

258. Dietmaier W, Gansbauer S, Beyser K, et al. Microsatellite instability in tumor and non-neoplastic colorectal cells from hereditary non-polyposis colorectal cancer and sporadic high microsatellite-instable tumor patients. *Pathobiology* 2000;68:227–231.

259. Diaz-Cano S, et al. Are PCR artifacts in microdissected samples preventable? [Letter]. *Hum Pathol* 2001;32:1415–1416.

260. Wild P, Knuechel R, Dietmaier W, et al. Laser microdissection and microsatellite analyses of breast cancer reveal a high degree of tumor heterogeneity. *Pathobiology* 2000;68:180–190.

261. Bagg A, Braziel RM, Arber DA. Immunoglobulin heavy chain gene analysis in lymphomas: a multi-center study demonstrating the heterogeneity of performance of polymerase chain reaction assays. *J Mol Diagn* 2002;4:81–89.

262. Arber DA. Molecular diagnostic approach to non-Hodgkin's lymphoma. *J Mol Diagn* 2000;2:178–190.

263. Brady SP, Magro CM, Diaz-Cano SJ, et al. Analysis of clonality of atypical cutaneous lymphoid infiltrates associated with drug therapy by PCR/DGGE. *Hum Pathol* 1999;30:130–136.

264. Cossman J, Zenhbauer B, Garrett CT, et al. Gene rearrangements in the diagnosis of lymphoma/leukemia: guidelines for use based on a multi-institutional study. *Am J Clin Pathol* 1991;95:347–354.

265. Diaz-Cano S. PCR-based alternative for diagnosis of immunoglobulin heavy chain gene rearrangement: principles, practice, and polemics. *Diagn Mol Pathol* 1996;5:3–9.

266. Kroft SH. Monoclones, monotypes, and neoplasia pitfalls in lymphoma diagnosis. *Am J Clin Pathol* 2004;121:457–459.

267. Ritter JH, Wick MR, Adesokan PN, et al. Assessment of clonality in cutaneous lymphoid infiltrates by polymerase chain reaction analysis of immunoglobulin heavy chain gene rearrangement. *Am J Clin Pathol* 1997;108:60–68.

268. O'Sullivan MJ, Ritter JH, Humphrey PA, et al. Lymphoid lesions of the gastrointestinal tract: a histologic, immunophenotypic, and genotypic analysis of 49 cases. *Am J Clin Pathol* 1998;110:471–477.

269. Fujita M, Enomoto T, Wada H, et al. Application of clonal analysis: differential diagnosis for synchronous primary ovarian and endometrial cancers and metastatic cancer. *Am J Clin Pathol* 1996;105:350–359.
270. Jacobs IJ, Kohler MF, Wiseman RW, et al. Clonal origin of epithelial ovarian carcinoma: analysis by loss of heterozygosity, p53 mutation, and X-chromosome inactivation. *J Natl Cancer Inst* 1992;84:1793–1798.
271. Kounelis S, Jones MW, Papadaki H, et al. Carcinosarcomas (malignant mixed mullerian tumors) of the female genital tract: comparative molecular analysis of epithelial and mesenchymal components. *Hum Pathol* 1998;29:82–87.
272. Jiang X, Morland SJ, Hitchcock A, et al. Allelotyping of endometriosis with adjacent ovarian carcinoma reveals evidence of a common lineage. *Cancer Res* 1998;58:1707–1712.
273. Garrett AP, Lee KR, Colitti CR, et al. k-ras mutation may be an early event in mucinous ovarian tumorigenesis. *Int J Gynecol Pathol* 2001;20:244–251.
274. Beck N, Tomlinson I, Homfray T. Use of SSCP analysis to identify germline mutations in HNPCC families fulfilling the Amsterdam criteria. *Hum Genet* 1997;99:219–224.
275. Liu B, Parsons R, Papadopoulos N, et al. Analysis of mismatch repair genes in hereditary non-polyposis colorectal cancer patients. *Nat Med* 1996;2:169–174.
276. Nystrom-Lahti M, Wu Y, Moisio AL, et al. DNA mismatch repair gene mutations in 55 kindreds with verified or putative hereditary non-polyposis colorectal cancer. *Hum Mol Genet* 1996;5:763–769.
277. Weber TK, Conlon W, Petrelli NJ, et al. Genomic DNA-based hMSH2 and hMLH1 mutation screening in 32 eastern United States hereditary nonpolyposis colorectal cancer pedigrees. *Cancer Res* 1997;57:3798–3803.
278. Ahuja N, Mohan A, Li Q, et al. Association between CpG island methylation and microsatellite instability in colorectal cancer. *Cancer Res* 1997;57:3370–3374.
279. Cunningham JM, Christensen ER, Tester DJ, et al. Hypermethylation of the hMLH1 promoter in colon cancer with microsatellite instability. *Cancer Res* 1998;58:3455–3460.
280. Kane MF, Loda M, Gaida GM, et al. Methylation of the hMLH1 promoter correlates with lack of expression of hMLH1 in sporadic colon tumors and mismatch repair-defective human tumor cell lines. *Cancer Res* 1997;57:808–811.
281. Herman JG, Umar A, Polyak K, et al. Incidence and functional consequences of hMLH1 promoter hypermethylation in colorectal carcinoma. *Proc Natl Acad Sci USA* 1998;95:6870–6875.
282. Veigl ML, Kasturi L, Olechnowicz J, et al. Biallelic inactivation of hMLH1 by epigenetic gene silencing, a novel mechanism causing human MSI cancers. *Proc Natl Acad Sci USA* 1998;95:8698–8702.
283. Boland CR, Thibodeau SN, Hamilton SR, et al. A National Cancer Institute workshop on microsatellite instability for cancer detection and familial predisposition: development of international criteria for the determination of microsatellite instability in colorectal cancer. *Cancer Res* 1998;58:5248–5257.
284. Bohm M, Wieland I. Analysis of tumor-specific alterations in native specimens by PCR: how to procure the tumor cells. *Int J Oncol* 1997;15:63–67.
285. Tran HT, Keen JD, Kricker M, et al. Hypermutability of homonucleotide runs in mismatch repair and DNA polymerase proofreading yeast mutants. *Mol Cell Biol* 1997;17:2859–2865.
286. Green CN, Jinks-Robertson S. Frameshift intermediates in homopolymer runs are removed efficiently by yeast mismatch repair proteins. *Mol Cell Biol* 1997;17:2844–2850.
287. Percesepe A, Kristo P, Aaltonen LA, et al. Mismatch repair genes and mononucleotide tracts as mutation targets in colorectal tumors with different degrees of microsatellite instability. *Oncogene* 1998;17:157–163.

Nucleic Acid Electrophoresis and Hybridization

Gel electrophoresis is most commonly used to separate double-stranded DNA based on size, although some electrophoretic techniques make it possible to separate single-stranded or double-stranded DNA based on secondary structure. Nucleic acids labeled with fluorophores can be directly detected following electrophoresis or, if unlabeled, can be visualized by chemical stains. Nucleic acids can also be indirectly detected by hybridization with labeled probes. Hybridization with labeled probes also underlies methods used to detect specific nucleic acid sequences in settings that do not require prior electrophoresis, specifically tissue and chromosome in situ hybridization.

GEL ELECTROPHORESIS

The rate of migration of a molecule through a porous support medium or gel matrix by a sieving mechanism is dependent on several factors (Table 6.1). The forces acting to drive the molecule through the gel are the charge of the molecule and the electric field strength. The frictional force that acts to retard the molecule's movement is defined by Stokes' Law and is a function of the viscosity of the gel matrix, the radius of the molecule, and the velocity of the molecule's movement.

When applied to the electrophoresis of nucleic acids, the equations in Table 6.1 have several consequences. First, because the charge of the phosphate backbone is the dominant feature that determines the overall charge of a DNA or RNA molecule, nucleic acid electrophoresis is typically performed at a slightly alkaline pH to ensure ionization of all the phosphate residues. Second, because the shape and size of a nucleic acid affect its general radius, temperature

TABLE 6.1
EQUATIONS GOVERNING ELECTROPHORESIS

Electrophoretic driving force: $F = \dfrac{VQ}{L} = X \cdot Q$

where, F = force driving the ion forward
V = voltage drop
Q = charge on the analyte molecule
L = length of the gel
X = voltage drop per unit distance (electric field strength)

Stoke's law: $F' = 6\pi r \eta v$

where, F' = the counterforce retarding the ion
r = radius of the analyte
η = viscosity of the matrix
v = velocity of analyte movement

During electrophoresis at constant speed, $F = F'$, or

$X \cdot Q = 6\pi r \eta v$

When electrophoretic mobility μ is defined as the velocity of analyte movement through the gel matrix per unit electric field strength,

$$\mu = \frac{v}{X} = \frac{Q}{6\pi r \eta}$$

and buffer conditions that alter the formation of intramolecular and intermolecular hydrogen bonds will change the molecule's electrophoretic mobility. Third, since the viscosity of a gel matrix used for electrophoresis is dependent on the matrix's effective pore size, nucleic acids with a radius substantially smaller than the effective pore size of the gel will not be significantly retarded by the matrix.

Agarose and polyacrylamide are the two types of gel matrix used for nucleic acid electrophoresis. Agarose is a polysaccharide polymer consisting of multiple agarbiose molecules linked together into linear chains that have an average molecular weight of approximately 120 kDa (Fig. 6.1A). The ease of handling and preparation of agarose gels, and their utility in separating nucleic acids of a wide size range (from about 200 bp to 20 kb, depending on the concentration of agarbiose) are reasons for their widespread use.

Polyacrylamide gels are produced by adding a free radical initiator, usually tetraethylenediamine (TEMED) and ammonium persulfate (APS), to a solution of acrylamide monomer and crosslinker, usually *bis*-acrylamide (Fig. 6.1B). The starting concentration of the acrylamide monomer, together with the ratio of the crosslinker to the monomer, determines the effective pore size of the resulting gel. Because the pore sizes in polyacrylamide gels are much smaller than those in agarose gels, polyacrylamide gels are used to size fractionate smaller nucleic acids. Polyacrylamide gels are easy to prepare and use, but because acrylamide is a potent neurotoxin that is readily absorbed through the skin, adequate protective clothing is required.

Slab Gel Electrophoresis

Slab gel electrophoresis is performed under assay conditions designed to separate nucleic acids based on size alone or on variations in secondary structure caused by sequence changes.

Separation Based on Size

Electrophoretic separation of double-stranded nucleic acids based on their size alone (e.g., for verification of polymerase chain reaction (PCR) product size, separation of DNA before Southern hybridization analysis) is performed under non-denaturing conditions to ensure that the molecules remain double-stranded. On the other hand, electrophoretic separation of single-stranded nucleic acids based solely on their size (e.g., separation of RNA before northern hybridization analysis, separation of DNA during sequence analysis) must

be performed under denaturing conditions. Denaturing conditions prevent interstrand reannealing and intrastrand base pairing that create secondary structures with altered electrophoretic mobility.

Very large DNA fragments, typically from 20 kb to several megabases in length, can be size fractioned by the specialized technique of pulsed-field gel electrophoresis (1–3). The method is based on the fact that very long DNA molecules seem to orient themselves along an electric field and migrate end-first. Consequently, their movement through a gel matrix is not retarded by the sieving mechanism responsible for electrophoretic separation of smaller molecules. Instead, very long DNA molecules migrate end-first through the matrix pores and, once oriented with a pore, migrate at a rate independent of size. In pulsed-field electrophoresis, the electric field changes strength and direction over time, forcing the DNA molecules to periodically reorient in new directions. Since the rate of orientation to the changing electric field is related to size, excellent separation of the very large DNA molecules can be achieved.

Separation Based on Secondary Structure

Some electrophoretic techniques (e.g., single-stand conformational polymorphism [SSCP] analysis) exploit the fact that single-stranded DNA folds into complex three-dimensional structures stabilized by intrastrand base pairing. Because the three-dimensional structure of the molecule is dictated by its base sequence, wild-type and mutant molecules of the same length that differ in sequence by even a single nucleotide usually adopt different three-dimensional confirmations and exhibit different electrophoretic mobility. Once normal and mutant alleles at a locus have been characterized and correlated with disease, these techniques can be useful for detecting the presence of small sequence changes, including single base-pair (bp) changes, small deletions, small insertions, and polymorphisms.

Other methods (e.g., heteroduplex analysis, denaturing gradient gel electrophoresis) take advantage of the fact that sequence differences in double-stranded DNA also cause structural perturbations that result in an altered mobility when electrophoresed under appropriate temperature and buffer conditions. Electrophoretic techniques used to

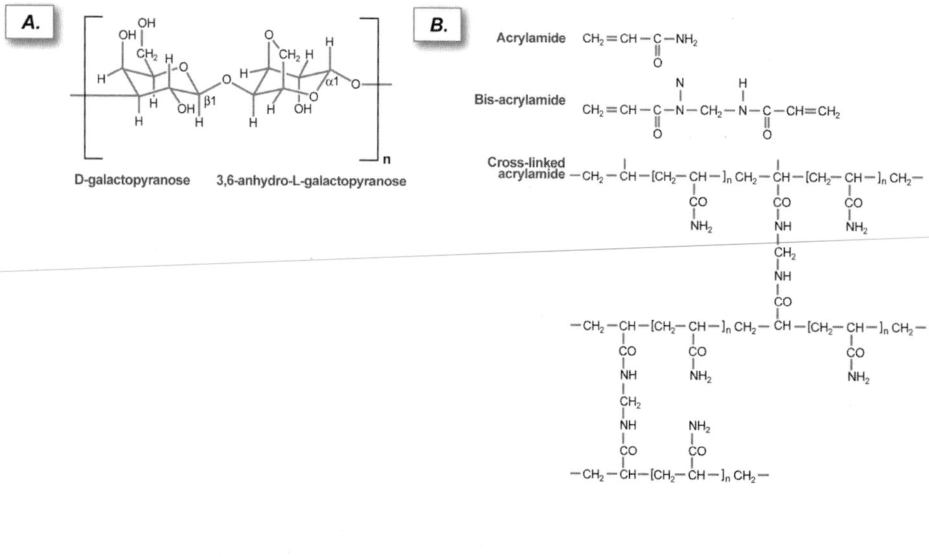

Figure 6.1 **A,** Agarose (agarbiose) is a linear polymer consisting of alternating residues of D-galactopyranose and 3,6-anhydro-L-galactopyranose. **B,** In the presence of free radicals, usually generated by the reaction of ammonium persulfate with tetraethylenediamine, monomers of acrylamide are polymerized into long chains crosslinked by *bis*-acrylamide. The porosity of the gel is determined by the length of the acrylamide chains and the degree of crosslinking.

separate molecules based on secondary structure are discussed more fully in Chapter 7.

Capillary Electrophoresis

Although slab gel electrophoresis has been in use for over 100 years (4), the feasibility of electrophoretic separations in thin glass tubes (or capillaries) was not demonstrated until 1967 (5). Most commercial instruments on the market employ a narrow internal diameter (typically less than 100 μm) fused-silica tube and high voltage (in the range of 30 kV), with on-column detection using fluorophores.

Capillary electrophoresis has several advantages compared with traditional slab gel electrophoresis (6–9). Capillary electrophoresis has a higher resolving power (a result of the physics of flow through the narrow tube with associated minimal diffusion, both of which are augmented by the short assay time) and is faster (a typical assay takes only about 30 to 60 minutes). In addition, capillary electrophoresis yields quantitative data (based on the detection of emitted light or ultraviolet [UV] absorbance), can be automated, and requires a much smaller sample for analysis (10–13).

Separation of nucleic acid fragments by capillary electrophoresis occurs by the same sieving mechanism as in conventional slab gel electrophoresis (9,14). The ease of filling the tubes makes a broad range of liquid gels amenable to use, including hydroxymethyl cellulose, methyl cellulose, polyvinyl alcohol, and liquid polyacrylamide (12). Methods have been developed in which a thermal gradient, chemical denaturing gradient, or porosity gradient can be formed within the capillary, modifications that have made capillary gel electrophoresis a suitable method in a wide range of settings, especially DNA mutation detection (7,8,10,11,15–17).

Denaturing High Performance Liquid Chromatography

Separation of DNA fragments by denaturing high performance (or high pressure) liquid chromatography (DHPLC) (18,19) is dependent on the differential retention of double-stranded DNA under conditions of partial thermal denaturation. Positively charged triethylammonium ions adsorbed to the stationary phase column matrix pair with the negatively charged phosphate groups of the DNA backbone; because the number of ion pairs formed increases with increasing DNA fragment size, an increasingly higher concentration of organic solvent is required to elute longer DNA fragments. Within this trend, heteroduplex DNA tends to elute earlier than the corresponding homoduplex DNA because a "bubble" of unpaired bases in heteroduplex DNA diminishes binding to the stationary phase of the column. Alkylated 2-μM nonporous poly(styrene-divinylbenzene) beads were the initial matrix used for DHPLC, although a number of novel matrices have been produced (20). Several characteristics of DHPLC make it a useful clinical technique, including high sensitivity, rapid analysis times (analysis usually takes only 5 or 6 minutes, including column regeneration and reequilibration), online detection of the DNA fragments (usually by UV absorbance, which can be quantitated), and relatively low cost.

In practice, DHPLC consists of two stages. First, DNA fragments generated by PCR from patient DNA and wild-type DNA are mixed, heated, and allowed to reanneal to form heteroduplexes and homoduplexes. Second, the mixture is fractionated by DHPLC. The sequence composition flanking the region near a mismatch greatly influences the optimum temperature to detect the heteroduplex, which can be determined either computationally (21), when the primary sequence of the candidate mutations has already been established, or empirically for those samples that may harbor novel mutations (19).

DHPLC detects all combinations of nucleotide mismatches, independent of their location within the DNA fragment, and can also detect small insertions and deletions. However, DHPLC does not define the nature of the mutation, which must be determined by formal DNA sequence analysis. The sensitivity for detection of single bp mismatches in DNA fragments that range from 100 to 1500 bp long is over 90% (21–25), although the sensitivity for the detection of other types of mutations has not been as well studied.

DETECTION OF NUCLEIC ACIDS AFTER ELECTROPHORESIS

The most convenient method for visualizing DNA after standard electrophoresis is ethidium bromide staining (26). Ethidium bromide intercalates between the stacked bases of double-stranded DNA, and the intercalated dye has a much increased fluorescence compared with dye in free solution (specifically, UV light of wavelength 254 nm is absorbed by DNA and reemitted by the dye as red-orange light of wavelength 590 nm). Ethidium bromide is not sequence specific but instead binds to double-stranded DNA stoichiometrically, and so the intensity of fluorescence provides a rough quantitation of the amount of DNA. The dye also binds to single-stranded DNA and RNA, although the affinity of the dye is weaker for single-stranded nucleic acids. Staining a gel with the dye takes only 15 to 20 minutes, but because ethidium bromide is moderately toxic and a powerful mutagen, protective clothing must be worn when working with the dye and used solutions must be decontaminated before disposal.

The nonisotopic silver staining assay (27,28), which also is not sequence specific, is another technically straightforward and reproducible method for visualization of nuclei acids after standard electrophoresis. For silver staining, the gel is first oxidized in a nitric acid solution and then incubated in a silver nitrate solution, a process that takes about 20 minutes. Silver nitrate must be disposed of according to hazardous waste regulations.

Isotopically labeled nucleic acids, usually produced by incorporating radiolabeled nucleotides during their synthesis (see below), can be directly detected by autoradiography. Autoradiographs can be quantitated by a scanning densitometer, which measures the relative density of the bands in the x-ray film. Alternatively, labeled nucleic acids can be detected by a phosphorimager, which directly quantitates the rate of radioactive emissions from each band in the gel. Because of the risks and disposal costs involved with the use of radioisotopes, nonisotopic methods for detecting nucleic acids are used more often. Nonisotopic techniques are quantitative and have a sensitivity that approaches that of isotopic methods. Nonisotopically labeled nucleic acids are produced by incorporating chemically modified nucleotides during their synthesis, and widely used labels for quantitative detection include fluorophores and chemical groups that can be linked to enzymatic reactions (see later discussion).

PRINCIPLES OF NUCLEIC ACID HYBRIDIZATION

The fundamental principle underlying nucleic acid hybridization assays is that complementary single-stranded nucleic acid strands will, under appropriate temperature and buffer conditions, anneal based on the Watson-Crick base-pairing rules. The sequence specificity of the complementary basepairing underlies the utility of nucleic acid hybridization assays, and makes it possible for a labeled probe to identify target sequences even in complex, heterogeneous mixtures of nucleic acids.

Factors Influencing Nucleic Acid Hybridization

The energy required to separate, or denature, two perfectly complementary DNA strands depends on base composition, strand length, and chemical environment. Because G:C bp have three hydrogen bonds and A:T bp only two, duplexes with a higher percentage of GC composition are more difficult to separate. Even among duplexes with the same percentage of GC composition, a longer double-stranded molecule will contain a greater number of hydrogen bonds overall and will therefore require more energy to separate.

The chemical environment of the buffer used in hybridization assays influences the stability of duplexes. Monovalent cations (e.g., Mg^+ ions) stabilize nucleic acid duplexes, whereas chemical denaturants (such as formamide

and urea) destabilize duplexes by disrupting the hydrogen bonds between bp.

A useful measure of the stability of the nucleic acid duplex is its melting temperature (T_m), the temperature that corresponds to the midpoint in the observed transition from a double-stranded to a single-stranded form. The T_m of perfect DNA, RNA, or oligonucleotide probe hybrids can be calculated using numerous formulas (Table 6.2).

Hybridization Stringency

Heteroduplexes formed between the probe and target sequences are most thermodynamically stable when the region of duplex formation contains perfect base matches. Mismatches between the two strands of the heteroduplex reduce the T_m; for most DNA probes, each 1% of mismatching reduces T_m by approximately 1° to 1.5°C, although a significant degree of mismatching can be tolerated if the overall region of base complementarity is long.

In practice the conditions of hybridization are often manipulated to influence the stringency of hybridization. Stability of mismatched heteroduplexes is enhanced when hybridization is performed under low stringency conditions, specifically reduced temperature, decreased urea or formamide concentration, and increased salt concentration (Table 6.2). Low stringency hybridization permits stable heteroduplex formation between sequences that may have significant differences, for example, between members of a multigene family, repetitive DNA families, pseudogenes, and so on. In contrast, high stringency conditions—specifically increased temperature, increased urea or formamide concentration, and low salt concentration—destabilize mismatched heteroduplexes. Under high stringency conditions, when using a small oligonucleotide probe, even a single mismatch will render a heteroduplex unstable, and, consequently, high stringency hybridizations are performed in assays designed to detect only a single specific sequence.

TABLE 6.2

EQUATIONS GOVERNING T_M FOR PERFECT HYBRIDS[a]

Hybrid	T_M in °C
For hybrids at least 100 nucleotides long[b]	
DNA-DNA	$81.5 + 16.6(\log_{10}[Na^+]) + 0.41(\% \ G + C) - 0.63(\% \ \text{formamide}) - (600/L)$
DNA-RNA	$79.8 + 18.5(\log_{10}[Na^+]) + 0.58(\% \ G + C) + 11.8(\% \ G + C)^2 - 0.50(\% \ \text{formamide}) - (820/L)$
RNA-RNA	$79.8 + 18.5(\log_{10}[Na^+]) + 0.58(\% \ G + C) + 11.8(\% \ G + C)^2 - 0.35(\% \ \text{formamide}) - (820/L)$
For hybrids 20–35 nucleotides long	$1.46(\text{effective length}^c) + 22$
For hybrids <20 nucleotides long	$2(\text{effective length}^c)$

[a]For more details see references 29–32.
[b]For concentrations of Na^+ or any other monovalent cation in the range of 0.01 M to 0.4 M; for DNA with a G + C content in the range of 30% to 75%; and where L is the length of the hybrid in base pairs.
[c]The effective length of a single-stranded oligonucleotide probe is defined as 2(number of G + C) + (number of A + T).

NUCLEIC ACID PROBES

Single-stranded oligonucleotide DNA probes in the range of 15 to 50 bp long are chemically synthesized. The sequence of an oligonucleotide probe is generally 100% identical to the target DNA sequence. However, degenerate oligonucleotide probes, a mixture of probes that share a consensus sequence but differ at a small number of specific positions, are sometimes used to increase sensitivity, identify all numbers of a gene family, or detect related sequences that have not yet been characterized. PCR provides a method to generate DNA probes in the range of 100 to several thousand bp long. Probes prepared from cloned genome DNA are typically much larger, in the range of 100 bp to over 100 kb long.

RNA probes have traditionally been synthesized using wild-type DNA or cDNA as the template (33). In practice, this requires cloning of the DNA template into a vector that provides the promoter sequences necessary for RNA transcription. However, a much simplified method of probe generation has recently been developed that eliminates the cloning step: the DNA template is amplified using primers that include T7 and SP6 bacterial promoter sequences, primer design features that make it possible to produce large quantities of both sense and antisense RNA via in vitro transcription of the PCR product DNA (34,35).

Figure 6.2 provides a summary of the characteristics of different types of probes.

Probe Labeling

DNA and RNA probes are either labeled during in vitro synthesis or end-labeled after synthesis.

Labeling During Synthesis

Labeling during in vitro synthesis requires that at least one of the four nucleotides carries a labeled group. Several different approaches have been developed.

Nick translation employs an endonuclease (usually pancreatic DNase I) to generate single-strand breaks (called nicks) in double-stranded DNA, which then serve as the starting point for DNA synthesis by *Escherichia coli* DNA polymerase I. Polymerization proceeds from the 3' terminus created by the nick as existing nucleotides are removed by the 5'→3' exonuclease activity of the enzyme. The elimination of nucleotides from the 5' side, with addition of nucleotides to the 3' side, results in movement of the nick along the DNA. Although there is no net DNA synthesis, the reaction incorporates labeled nucleotides in the newly synthesized region of DNA.

For randomly primed DNA labeling, denatured DNA is slowly cooled in the presence of a mixture of virtually all possible hexadeoxynucleotides (or 8-mers, or 9-mers, etc.). Individual hexadeoxynucleotides will bind to their complementary sequence within the DNA strands and function as primers for synthesis of new complementary DNA

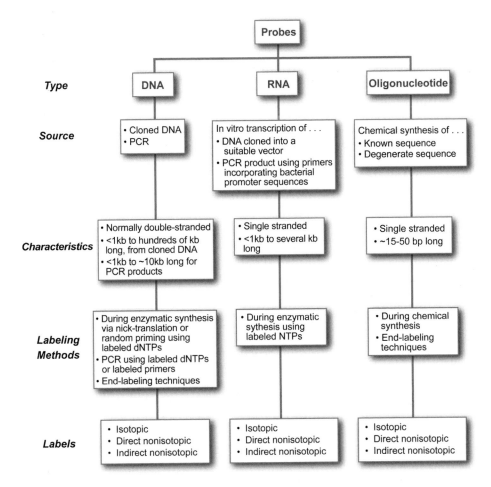

Figure 6.2 Characteristics of the different types of hybridization probes.

strands by *E. coli* DNA polymerase I. Because all sequence combinations are represented in the hexadeoxynucleotide mixture, primers bind throughout the entire length of the template DNA, and labeling is therefore uniform and of high specific activity (36).

Standard PCR provides a very easy method to label DNA. The PCR can be modified to include at least one labeled dNTP, which becomes incorporated into the product DNA throughout its entire length, producing a very highly labeled probe. Alternatively, labeled primers can be used in the PCR, an approach that produces a less highly labeled probe. Riboprobes, whether produced from cloned or PCR-generated templates, are labeled by including at least one labeled NTP in the transcription reaction.

End-labeling of DNA

The enzyme polynucleotide kinase catalyzes an exchange reaction between the γ-phosphate position of ATP and the 5′-terminal phosphate of DNA. This method is most often used to label chemically synthesized single-stranded oligonucleotides, although the same procedure can be used to label double-stranded DNA. Because polynucleotide kinase only transfers one labeled phosphate group, the specific activity of the probe is much lower than that achieved by labeling during in vitro synthesis.

In Situ Enzymatic Labeling

Some of the enzymatic methods used to label nucleic acid probes for hybridization studies can also be applied in situ to tissue sections. One of the best examples of this technique in surgical pathology is the measurement of apoptosis, important because apoptotic rates correlate with prognosis in a number of diseases and malignancies (37–41).

Although necrosis is a passive process associated with cell death resulting from noxious injuries such as trauma, apoptosis is a regulated active process initiated by a diverse range of cellular insults, as well as normal developmental events (37,42,43). Regardless of the cause, apoptosis occurs by a stereotypical program of cellular events that leads to characteristic morphologic changes including cell shrinkage with increased cytoplasmic density, nuclear pyknosis, chromatin condensation, and blebbing of the cytoplasmic membrane. However, one of the most striking features of apoptosis is the activation of endogenous endonucleases that cleave genomic DNA between nucleosomes producing DNA fragments that are multiples of approximately 185 bp in length (44,45). These fragments give rise to a characteristic DNA ladder by simple gel electrophoresis. Even though the DNA ladder is specific for apoptotic cells, the electrophoretic result is difficult to quantitate and does not permit identification of the population of cells undergoing apoptosis.

In situ methods for labeling apoptotic cells are used to demonstrate the DNA fragments produced by endonucleolytic cleavage directly within tissue sections. The in situ methods make use of enzymes that label the 3′-OH ends that result from endonucleolytic cleavage; the terminal deoxynucleotidyl transferase–mediated UTP nick end-labeling (TUNEL) reaction employs, obviously, terminal deoxynucleotidyl transferase (TdT); the in situ end labeling (ISEL) reaction uses the Klenow fragment of DNA poly-

merase (46–48). A variety of radioactive or nonisotopically labeled dideoxy nucleotides can be used to visualize the reaction products, and commercial kits are available that greatly simplify the use of either enzyme. And because either enzyme can be used for in situ labeling of individual apoptotic cells in tissue sections, enzymatic approaches make phenotypic–genotypic correlations possible, although tissue fixation can create technical artifacts (43,47,49).

However, the specificity of in situ methods has always been uncertain. The enzymes label 3′-OH ends regardless of their origin and consequently mark apoptotic cells as well as a subset of necrotic cells, cells with DNA damage, replicating cells, and cells undergoing some types of DNA repair (43,48,50–52). There are also significant differences in the sensitivity between the TUNEL and ISEL methods (46) because the TdT enzyme can label 3′ recessed, 5′ recessed, and blunt ends of DNA, whereas the Klenow fragment can only label 3′ recessed ends. Paired labeling using immunohistochemistry in addition to TUNEL/ISEL permits a more stringent correlation of the genetic result with phenotypic changes by direct microscopy (38,40,47,53,54) or flow cytometry (55,56), but it is difficult to compare individual studies because of the lack of a uniform standard for quantitation (46).

It remains unclear as to whether in situ methods offer any advantage over more traditional approaches to assess apoptosis. Direct light microscopic identification of apoptotic cells based on the presence of characteristic morphologic changes is sensitive and specific and, though tedious, may actually be a quicker and more reproducible approach for quantitation of apoptosis than the use of in situ enzymatic methods (57). Immunohistochemical methods used to evaluate apoptotic pathways (43,46,47,58–61) often show limited specificity because apoptosis involves the activation of preexisting proteins whose constitutive level of expression often shows little correlation with the apoptotic pathway of cell death (46,47).

Functional Groups Used to Label Probes

The denaturation and renaturation properties of probes labeled with either radioactive or nonradioactive subgroups are essentially identical to those of unsubstituted probes, a fundamental property that underlies their utility in molecular genetic testing.

Isotopic Labels and Their Detection

As indicated in Table 6.3, ^{32}P-labeled and ^{33}P-labeled nucleotides used to label DNA during strand synthesis have the radioisotope at the α-phosphate position, because the β- and γ-phosphate groups are cleaved to provide the energy for incorporation of the nucleotide into the growing nucleic acid strand. For the same reason, the isotope in ^{35}S-labeled nucleotides replaces a nonbridge oxygen atom of the α-phosphate group. However, ^{32}P-labeled ATP used in end-labeling reactions has the isotope at the γ-phosphate position because end-labeling is an exchange reaction between the 5′-terminal phosphate of the oligonucleotide and the γ-phosphate of ATP. Nucleotides can be substituted with the ^{3}H isotope at several different positions.

The intensity of the signal produced by a radiolabeled probe depends on the type of radioisotope and the time of

TABLE 6.3

RADIOISOTOPES COMMONLY USED TO LABEL RNA AND DNA PROBES

Radioisotope	Half-life	Emission	Energy	Position of Label in NTPs or dNTPs
^{3}H	12.4 years	β	0.019 MeV	Multiple positions
^{32}P	14.3 days	β	1.710 MeV	α-Phosphate position for strand synthesis reactions; γ-phosphate position for end-labeling reactions
^{33}P	25.4 days	β	0.249 MeV	α-Phosphate position for strand synthesis reactions
^{35}S	87.4 days	β	0.167 MeV	Replaces an oxygen of the α-phosphate

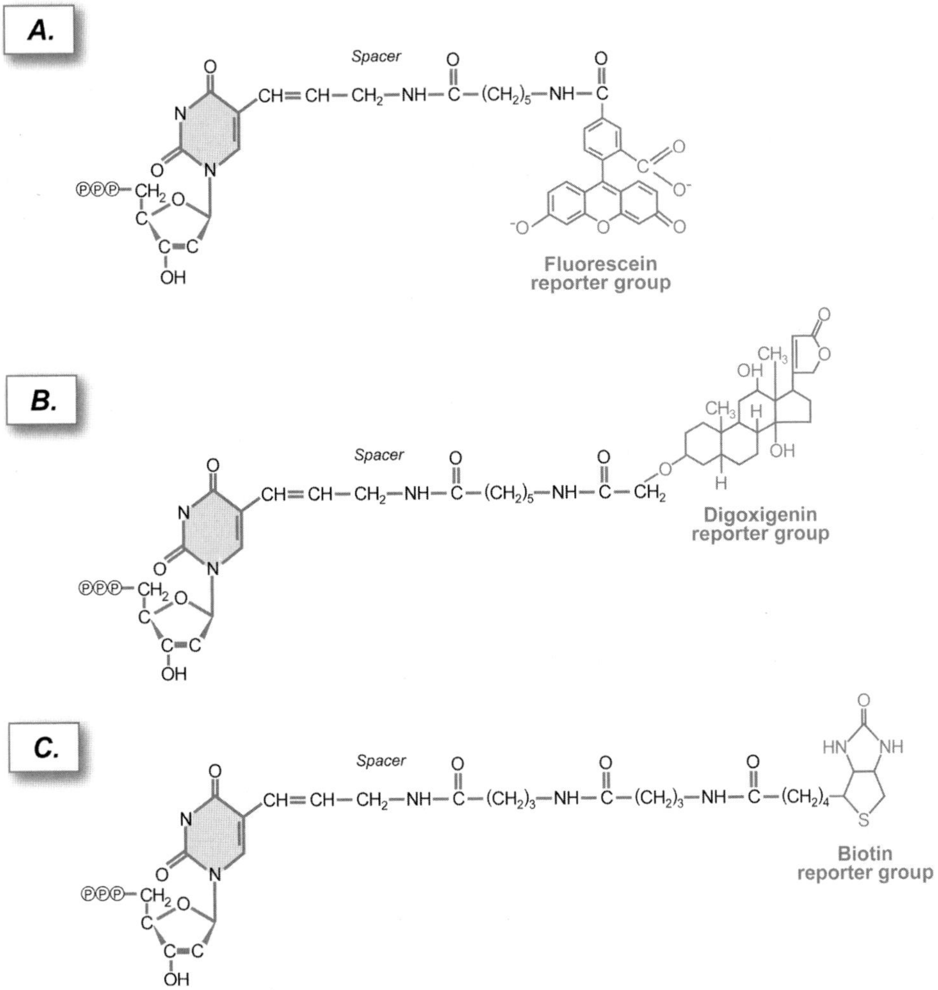

Fluorescein
reporter group

Digoxigenin
reporter group

Biotin
reporter group

Figure 6.3 Examples of the structure of nucleotides modified with direct or indirect labels. **A,** Fluorescein-dUTP. The fluorophore fluorescein, a direct label, is linked to the carbon atom at position 5 of uracil. The spacer ensures that when the labeled nucleotide is incorporated into a nucleic acid probe it does not interfere with the structure or hybridization properties of the probe. **B,** Digoxigenin-dUTP. **C,** Biotin-dUTP. Both digoxigenin and biotin are indirect labels; for these labels, the spacer group also ensures that the label is readily accessible for recognition by antibodies or streptavidin, respectively.

exposure (which is usually at least 1 day and may be longer). The high-energy β particle emitted by ^{32}P affords a high degree of sensitivity, but the increase in scatter that accompanies autoradiographic detection of the particle inhibits resolution. Consequently, radioisotopes that emit less energetic β particles are used in many applications, including ^{35}S-labeled and ^{33}P-labeled nucleotides for manual DNA sequence analysis and in situ hybridization. ^{35}S and ^{33}P also have longer half-lives than ^{32}P, which provides greater flexibility in routine use.

Nonisotopic Labels and Their Detection

Nonisotopic labels can be grouped into two classes based on whether they are directly or indirectly detected. Nonisotopic labels can be linked to the 5' or 3' carbon atom at the ends of oligonucleotides or to various carbon atoms in the purine or pyrimidine bases. For example, chemical groups are often linked to the carbon atom at position 5 of uridine (Fig. 6.3) to produce labeled precursors that can be incorporated into probes by standard PCR. Similarly,

TABLE 6.4
COMMON FLUOROPHORES

Fluorophore	Excitation Maximum[a] (Absorbance Maximum)	Emission Maximum[a]	Color
AMCA	399	446	Blue
DABCYL[b]	453	None	—
CY3	550	570	Yellow-orange
CY5	649	670	Far red
CY7	743	767	Near infrared
FAM (6-carboxy fluorescein)	494	525	Green
HEX/JOE/VIC[c]	535/527/528	556/548/546	Green
Malachite Green[b]	630	None	—
Methyl Red[b]	410	None	—
Rhodamine	555	580	Red
SYBR Green	497	520	Green
TAMRA[d]	565	580	Orange-red
TET	521	536	Green
Texas Red	590	615	Red

[a]Wavelength in nm.
[b]A dark quencher, which absorbs light over a relatively broad spectrum but releases the energy as heat rather than as light in the visible spectrum (Chapter 5).
[c]Widely used derivatives of fluorescein.
[d]Widely used as a quencher in quantitative PCR applications (Chapter 5).

chemical groups incorporated into NTPs can be used to produce labeled RNA probes.

Only one family of directly detected nonisotopic labels, fluorophores, is in widespread use. Because different fluorophores demonstrate maximum excitation and emission at different wavelengths of light (Table 6.4), multiple probes, each labeled with a different fluorophore, can be used in the same assay.

Two indirect nonisotopic labeling systems are in wide use. For both, nucleotides that are chemically coupled to a reporter molecule are incorporated into the probe. Biotin (a naturally occurring vitamin) is the reporter in the biotin-streptavidin system; although biotin cannot be directly detected, it is bound with extremely high affinity by streptavidin (a bacterial protein), which itself can be easily conjugated to a variety of so-called marker groups. In the other widely employed indirect nonisotopic labeling system, digoxigenin (a steroid obtained from *Digitalis* plants) is the reporter molecule; an antibody conjugated with a marker group is then used to recognize digoxigenin. The most common marker groups in use include fluorophores and enzymes (e.g., alkaline phosphatase and peroxidase), which are detected via colorimetric or chemiluminescence assays (62,63).

HYBRIDIZATION ASSAYS

Southern blot hybridization and northern blot hybridization are similar in principal. Negatively charged, purified nucleic acids (DNA for Southern blots, RNA for northern

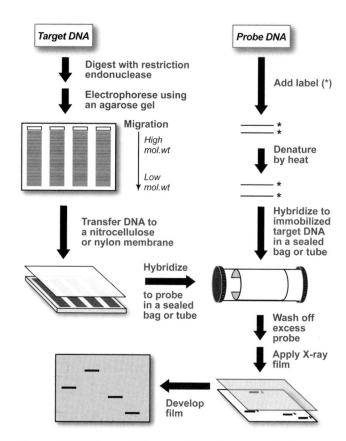

Figure 6.4 Schematic diagram of Southern blot hybridization. DNA fragments that are first size-fractionated by gel electrophoresis are transferred to a membrane and then hybridized to a labeled probe. The bound probe indicates the presence of the target sequence complementary to the probe. In this example, the probe is radiolabeled and detected by autoradiography, but nonisotopic labels and probe detection methods have also been developed. (Modified with permission from Dr. Tom Strachan and Dr. Andrew Read, *Human Molecular Genetics*, 3rd edition, Taylor and Francis Group, New York, © 2003.)

blots) are size-fractionated separated by gel electrophoresis, transferred to and then immobilized on a nitrocellulose or nylon membrane, and then hybridized to a specific nucleic acid probe; the bound probe is then visualized by one of several methods. In situ hybridization methods are technical variations of this same process in which specific labeled probes are used to detect DNA or RNA sequences directly in chromosomal preparations or tissue sections.

Southern Blot Hybridization

Developed by Southern in 1975, this technique remains the method of choice for reliable quantitative detection of specific DNA sequences. The DNA sample is first cut, by digestion with one or more restriction endonucleases, into fragments that can be efficiently size-fractioned by gel electrophoresis. Following electrophoresis, the DNA fragments are denatured, immobilized on a membrane, and then detected by hybridization with a labeled probe (Fig. 6.4).

The denatured single-stranded DNA is physically transferred to the membrane through a variety of methods. Capillary transfer, by which the nucleic acid fragments are eluted from the gel and deposited on the membrane by buffer drawn through the gel by capillary action, is the most common method and takes a minimum of 10 to 12 hours. Electrophoretic transfer (64) is an alternative that takes only 2 to 3 hours, and vacuum blotting (65,66), in which the nucleic acids are eluted from the gel by buffer drawn through the gel by negative pressure, can be accomplished in 3 to 4 hours.

Following transfer, the individual DNA fragments are immobilized on the membrane at a location that corresponds to their position after size separation by electrophoresis. For nitrocellulose, historically the first type of membrane used for Southern blotting, the DNA is affixed by simply baking the damp membrane at high temperature (80°C for 2 hours) in a vacuum oven; because nucleic acids attach to nitrocellulose membranes by hydrophobic rather than covalent interactions, they slowly leach out of the nitrocellulose matrix during hybridization and washing, especially at high temperatures. For nylon membranes, low-level UV irradiation (at a wavelength of 254 nm) is used to create crosslinks between the nucleotides and the positively charged amine groups on the membrane surface (67,68). Because nucleic acids bind covalently to nylon membranes, and because nylon membranes are much more durable than nitrocellulose, the same membrane can be used and reused in sequential hybridizations with different probes.

Hybridization of the immobilized single-stranded target DNA sequence on the membrane with a labeled DNA probe is performed in a sealed plastic bag or tube that contains the membrane, probe, and hybridization buffer. Following hybridization, unbound and non-specifically bound probe is removed by sequential washes of the appropriate stringency. Bound probe indicates the presence of the target DNA sequence.

Southern blot hybridization is a reliable and versatile method for sequence-specific DNA analysis, although it requires a large sample (most standard Southern blot hybridization protocols require about 10 to 50 mcg of DNA per gel lane; for comparison, the usual yield from peripheral blood lymphocytes in 20 ml of human blood is approximately 250 mcg of DNA; 100 mg of fresh tissue contains about 100 mcg of DNA). Southern blots provide information about gene integrity, including the presence of deletions, insertions, and rearrangements, and because the method is quantitative, it can provide information on gene copy number. Traditionally, Southern blot hybridization was the method employed to detect pathogenic point mutations (through restriction fragment length polymorphism analysis), perform linkage analysis, monitor variable number of tandem repeat (VNTR) polymorphisms, etc. However, PCR-based methods have replaced the routine use of Southern blot hybridizations in these settings because PCR-based methods are faster and less cumbersome, require less tissue, and have a similar sensitivity and reliability.

Northern Blot Hybridization

Northern blotting is a variant of Southern blotting in which the target nucleic acid is RNA instead of DNA. The method simultaneously provides information on both transcript abundance (a measure of the gene's level of expression) and transcript structure (reflecting utilization of alternative transcription initiation or termination sites, alternative splicing patterns, and mutations). Because the method is quantitative, northern blots also provide the relative proportion of the different transcripts.

Northern blot analysis can be technically demanding. It is necessary to minimize the activity of cellular RNases released during cell lysis and to avoid contamination by RNases that are ubiquitously present in the laboratory environment. Because mRNA accounts for only about 2.5% of total cellular RNA, enrichment for mRNA before electrophoresis is often required. And, because RNA molecules are single-stranded, they must be denatured by heating to abolish any secondary structure that would alter their electrophoretic mobility. Electrophoresis itself must also be performed under denaturing conditions, usually employing a buffer containing formaldehyde, although glyoxal and dimethyl sulfoxide or methylmercuric hydroxide (which is very toxic) have also been used (69,70).

As with Southern blots, the RNA is transferred to a nitrocellulose or nylon membrane after electrophoresis and then hybridized with a labeled probe. For analyses evaluating differences in mRNA expression, normalization of the target gene signal relative to the quantity of mRNA present in that particular lane of the gel can be accomplished by probing the blot for the mRNA of the target gene under investigation, stripping the blot of the labeled probe, and then rehybridizing with a new probe for a housekeeping gene.

Northern blot analysis is widely used in basic science laboratories to determine the range of cell types in which a gene is expressed, measure the level of expression, and detect the presence of alternative transcripts (which may indicate the presence of different functional isoforms of the encoded protein). One caveat to the interpretation of northern blots, as discussed in Chapter 1, is that there are a number of post-transcriptional mechanisms that regulate mRNA translation, and consequently the level of detected mRNA may not be highly correlated with the level of expression of the encoded protein.

Tissue In Situ Hybridization (ISH)

In situ hybridization (ISH) makes it possible to detect mRNA or DNA in histologic sections of tissue that have been fixed and processed by standard techniques (71–73), providing the opportunity to directly correlate the morphology of individual cells with the presence of the target sequence. ISH is widely used to detect abnormalities in chromosomal structure; detect DNA associated with infectious agents such as Epstein-Barr virus and human papilloma virus (74–78); measure mRNA levels for gene expression analysis (79,80); and detect transgene mRNA from expression vectors under development in gene therapy regimens (81–83).

ISH for Measurement of mRNA

For hybridization to mRNA, single-stranded complementary RNA (cRNA) riboprobes, also known as antisense riboprobes, are widely used. Probes for ISH were originally labeled with radioisotopes, but they have largely been replaced by nonradioactive probes that are as just as sensitive, have a lower background, provide greater resolution, and eliminate the health hazards and disposal problems associated with radioactive probes (84,85).

Although the hybridization is performed on the tissue section itself, the stability of the hydrogen bonds between the probe and the target mRNA remains dependent on temperature, buffer composition, length, and GC content of the hybrid, as in any other hybridization technique. Important controls in ISH assays include pretreatment of the tissue sections with RNase or DNase for demonstration of the specificity of target sequence binding, parallel Southern or northern blot hybridization assays to demonstrate that the probe is specific for the target sequence, and the use of sense probes (which are homologous to the mRNA under study and should therefore show no hybridization) for detection of nonspecific binding.

In many clinical settings, the simple demonstration of mRNA is of diagnostic or prognostic significance, irrespective of an exact correlation with protein levels. However, use of ISH for precise evaluation of gene expression is subject to the same limitations noted above for northern blots; specifically, because there are a number of post-transcriptional mechanisms that regulate mRNA translation, the level of detected mRNA may not be an accurate measure of the level of expression of the encoded protein. Discrepancies between ISH measures of mRNA abundance and immunohistochemically detectable protein levels have in fact been noted (86).

The correlation between cell morphology and the presence of the target sequence (and the target's subcellular localization) that is provided by ISH makes the technique extremely powerful. However, ISH is technically demanding, and optimization of the probe for each specific mRNA can be time consuming, as can detection of labeled probes by autoradiography, immunohistochemistry, or fluorescence microscopy (although commercially available kits have simplified many assays). In addition, even when optimized, ISH can detect only about 10 copies of mRNA or foreign DNA (87,88) per cell, a level of sensitivity below that of PCR-based methods. These practical issues have limited the use of ISH in clinical molecular pathology laboratories.

ISH Analysis of Chromosomes

Conventional chromosome in situ hybridization is performed on air-dried microscope preparations of metaphase chromosomes produced from peripheral blood lymphocytes or from cultured cells of solid tumors by standard techniques, as discussed in Chapter 3.

A useful modification of chromosome ISH is its application to interphase cells, in which context it is referred to as fluorescence in situ hybridization (FISH). FISH analysis of interphase cells is a straightforward and remarkably versatile technique that has revolutionized the direct detection of genetic abnormalities by chromosome in situ hybridization. FISH eliminates the need for in vitro cell culture, which not only reduces the turn around time of chromosome ISH but also makes possible analysis of a much broader range of cell types.

A wide variety of abnormalities can be evaluated by FISH, including insertions, deletions, amplifications, and complex rearrangements that are difficult to assess by the chromosome banding techniques of traditional karyotypic analysis. Of most importance, because FISH can be performed on sections of formalin-fixed, paraffin-embedded tissue, FISH makes it possible to correlate cellular morphology with the underlying chromosomal abnormalities. FISH has become an indispensable component of the laboratory evaluation of a number of human malignancies and is discussed in detail in Chapter 4.

Three general classes of nucleic acid probes for chromosome ISH have been employed. Repetitive sequence probes (which hybridize to chromosome-specific repetitive DNA sequences located near the centromere) are particularly useful for detecting aneuploidy. Unique sequence probes are complementary to single-copy loci and are used to detect amplifications, deletions, or translocations; multiple unique sequence probes, each labeled with a different fluorophore, are often used in the same assay to permit more detailed analysis of genetic abnormalities. Whole chromosome probes or library probes hybridize to sequences throughout the entire length of a specific chromosome and are used for so-called spectral karyotyping (89). Chromosome probes are particularly useful for accurate identification of the components of complex rearrangements and marker chromosomes (89–91). However, chromosome probes are largely restricted to use in the analysis of metaphase chromosomes because many regions of interphase chromosomes exist as euchromatin and thus produce a very diffuse pattern of labeling which is difficult to interpret.

Chromosome ISH is more sensitive than traditional cytogenetics for evaluation of karyotypic alterations (92), and the use of multiple specific probes, each labeled with a different fluorophore, permits simultaneous evaluation of multiple loci (93,94). Chromosome ISH can detect karyotypic alterations below the level of resolution of conventional cytogenetic analysis and can be used to analyze complex rearrangements and other structural alterations that are difficult to assess by conventional banding techniques (92,95–99). Nevertheless, it is important to emphasize that chromosome ISH detects abnormalities of only the target chromosomal regions; structural alterations in sequences that are not complementary to the probe(s), which may nonetheless be clinical significant, will not be detected.

Despite the ease and flexibility of chromosome ISH methods, in some settings they are less sensitive than PCR, for example, in the detection of minimal residual disease in patients with leukemia (100,101). There are also limitations on the minimum size of the probe that can be successfully hybridized and therefore on the minimum size of the chromosomal abnormalities that can be detected. Although published techniques indicate that it is possible to detect unique gene sequences (102,103) or low copy number gene sequences as small as 500 bp long (104,105), the efficiency of small probes is quite low (106). Regardless, whether performed on metaphase chromosomes or interphase nuclei, ISH cannot detect small deletions, small insertions, or mutations at the single bp level.

Because only a limited number of probes are commercially available, a sophisticated molecular biology laboratory has traditionally been required to perform the cloning, screening, and mapping steps required to generate probes needed to test patient specimens for most of the chromosomal alterations characteristic of specific neoplasms or diseases. Not surprisingly, this constraint restricted the clinical utility of chromosome ISH. However, the availability of bacterial artificial chromosome (BAC) clones, produced as part of the human genome project, now makes it possible to quickly and easily produce a probe for any locus that is of clinical interest. Each BAC clone contains an insert from the human genome that is typically in the range of 150 to 250 kb long, a size that is ideally suited for use as a probe in chromosome ISH. Searchable computer databases (107,108) can be used to identify a BAC clone whose insert corresponds to the region of clinical interest. It is then a simple process, using basic techniques available in most clinical molecular genetics laboratories, to generate a labeled probe from the DNA extracted from bacterium harboring the BAC.

COMPARATIVE GENOMIC HYBRIDIZATION

Comparative genomic hybridization (CGH) is a powerful genetic technique that can be used to survey the entire genome for chromosomal deletions and amplifications (109,110). For a typical CGH test, genomic DNA from the tumor sample is labeled with a green fluorophore by nick translation, and genomic DNA from a paired normal tissue sample is labeled with a red fluorophore by nick translation. The green and red probes are mixed and then used in a single hybridization.

Standard CGH is merely a variation of chromosomal FISH. The mixture of green and red probes is hybridized to metaphase chromosome spreads prepared from normal peripheral blood lymphocytes, and the ratio of the green to red fluorescence signal is measured along the length of each chromosome (109,111). Regions where the ratio deviates significantly from the expected one-to-one relationship are areas where there has been a change in DNA copy number in the tumor versus the paired normal tissue; regions where the green to red ratio is significantly greater than 1 are areas of chromosomal gain (amplifications), and regions where the green to red ratio is significantly lower than 1 are areas of chromosomal loss (deletions). In practice, the smallest chromosomal alterations that can be detected by standard CGH are about 3 megabases.

For array CGH, DNA from BACs is ordered on a support, and the mixture of green and red probes is hybridized to the microarray. Because each BAC in the array has been mapped to a specific region of the genome, the ratio of the green to red fluorescence signal for each individual BAC provides information on the gain or loss of the corresponding chromosomal region. Array CGH therefore potentially offers much higher resolution than standard CGH and is in theory limited only by the number of BACs in the array; current arrays that contain 3,000 BACs give approximately 1-mb resolution (112).

Although CGH often has a higher sensitivity than conventional cytogenetic analysis (113,114), of even greater significance is the fact that CGH can be performed using DNA extracted from fixed as well as fresh tumor samples. Consequently, the technique makes it possible to perform a genomewide scan for structural alterations even on those cases for which conventional cytogenetic analysis is not feasible or is unsuccessful. CGH essentially opens the entire formalin-fixed tissue archive to at least limited cytogenetic analysis.

REFERENCES

1. Burmeister M, Ulanovsky L. *Pulsed-Field Gel Electrophoresis.* Totowa, NJ: Humana;1992.
2. Schwartz DC, Cantor CR. Separation of yeast chromosome-sized DNAs by pulsed field gradient gel electrophoresis. *Cell* 1984;37:67–75.
3. Schwartz DC, Saffran W, Welsh J, et al. New techniques for purifying large DNAs and studying their properties and packaging. *Cold Spring Harb Symp Quant Biol* 1983;47:189–195.
4. Camilleri P. In: *Camilleri P, ed. Capillary Electrophoresis, Theory and Practice.* Boca Raton, FL: CRC Press; 1997:1–22.
5. Hjerten S. Free zone electrophoresis. *Chromatogr Rev* 1967;9:122–219.
6. Righetti PG, Gelfi C, D'Acunto MR. Recent progress in DNA analysis by capillary electrophoresis. *Electrophoresis* 2002;23:1361–1374.
7. Mitchelson KR. The application of capillary electrophoresis for DNA polymorphism analysis. *Methods Mol Biol* 2001;162:3–26.
8. Kourkine IV, Hestekin CN, Barron AE. Technical challenges in applying capillary electrophoresis-single strand conformation polymorphism for routine genetic analysis. *Electrophoresis* 2002;23:1375–1385.
9. von Heeren F, Thormann W. Capillary electrophoresis in clinical and forensic analysis. *Electrophoresis* 1997;18:2415–2426.
10. Greiner TC, Rubocki RJ. Effectiveness of capillary electrophoresis using fluorescent-labeled primers in detecting T-cell receptor gamma gene rearrangements. *J Mol Diagn* 2002;4:137–143.
11. Issaq HJ. A decade of capillary electrophoresis. *Electrophoresis* 2000;21:1921–1939.
12. Schmalzing D, Koutny L, Salas-Solano O, et al. Recent developments in DNA sequencing by capillary and microdevice electrophoresis. *Electrophoresis* 1999;20:3066–3077.
13. Dorschner MO, Barden D, Stephens K. Diagnosis of five spinocerebellar ataxia disorders by multiplex amplification and capillary electrophoresis. *J Mol Diagn* 2002;4:108–113.
14. Issaq HJ, Chan KC, Muschik GM. The effect of column length, applied voltage, gel type, and concentration on the capillary electrophoresis separation of DNA fragments and polymerase chain reaction products. *Electrophoresis* 1997;18:1153–1158.
15. Kourkine IV, Hestekin CN, Magnusdottier SO, et al. Optimized sample preparation for tandem capillary electrophoresis single-stranded conformational polymorphism/heteroduplex analysis. *Biotechniques* 2002;33:318–320, 322, 324–325.
16. Righetti, Gelfi C. Capillary electrophoresis of DNA for molecular diagnostics: an update. *J Capillary Electrophor* 1999;6:119–124.
17. Atha DH, Kasprzak W, O'Connell CD, et al. Prediction of DNA single-strand conformation polymorphism: analysis by capillary electrophoresis and computerized DNA modeling. *Nucleic Acids Res* 2001;29:4643–4653.
18. Oefner PJ, Underhill PA. Comparative DNA sequence by denaturing high performance liquid chromatography (DHPLC). *Am J Hum Genet* 1995;57:A266.
19. Oefner PJ, Underhill PA. DNA mutation detection using denaturing high-performance liquid chromatography (DHPLC). *Curr Protocols Hum Genet* 1998;7.10.1–7.10.12.
20. Xiao W, Oefner PJ. Denaturing high-performance liquid chromatography: a review. *Hum Mutat* 2001;17:439–474.
21. http://insertion.stanford.edu/melt.html.
22. Roberts PS, Jozwiak S, Kwiatkowski DJ, et al. Denaturing high-performance liquid chromatography (DHPLC) is a highly sensitive, semi-automated method for identifying mutations in the TSC1 gene. *J Biochem Biophys Methods* 2001;47:33–37.
23. Taliani MR, Roberts SC, Dukek BA, et al. Sensitivity and specificity of denaturing high-pressure liquid chromatography for unknown protein C gene mutations. *Genet Test* 2001;5:39–44.
24. Liu W, Smith DI, Rechtzigel KJ, et al. Denaturing high performance liquid chromatography (DHPLC) used in the detection of germline and somatic mutations. *Nucleic Acids Res* 1998;26:1396–1400.
25. Oldenburg J, Ivaskevicius V, Rost S, et al. Evaluation of DHPLC in the analysis of hemophilia A. *J Biochem Biophys Methods* 2001;47:39–51.
26. Sharp PA, Sugden B, Sambrook J. Detection of two restriction endonuclease activities in *Haemophilus parainfluenzae* using analytical agarose-ethidium bromide electrophoresis. *Biochemistry* 1973;12:3055–3063.
27. Budowle B, Chakraborty R, Giusti A, et al. Analysis of the VNTR locus D1S80 by the PCR followed by high-resolution PAGE. *Am J Hum Genet* 1991;48:137–144.
28. Bender B, Wiestler OD, von Deimling A. A device for processing large acrylamide gels. *Biotechniques* 1994;16:204–206.
29. Bodkin DK, Knudson DL. Assessment of sequence relatedness of double-stranded RNA genes by RNA-RNA blot hybridization. *J Virol Methods* 1985;10:45–52.
30. Bolton ET, McCarthy BJ. A general method for the isolation of RNA complementary to DNA. *Proc Natl Acad Sci USA* 1962;48:1390–1397.
31. Bonner TI, Brenner DJ, Neufeld BR, et al. Reduction in the rate of DNA reassociation by sequence divergence. *J Mol Biol* 1973;81:123–135.
32. Casey J, Davidson N. Rates of formation and thermal stabilities of RNA:DNA and DNA:DNA duplexes at high concentrations of formamide. *Nucleic Acids Res* 1977;4:1539–1552.
33. Melton DA, Krieg PA, Rebagliati MR, et al. Efficient in vitro synthesis of biologically active RNA and RNA hybridization probes from plasmids containing a bacteriophage SP6 promoter. *Nucleic Acids Res* 1984;12:7035–7056.
34. Goldrick MM, Kimball GR, Martin LA, et al. NIRCA: a rapid robust method for screening for unknown point mutations. *Biotechniques* 1996;21:106–112.
35. Goldrick M, Prescott J. Detection of mutations in human cancer using nonisotopic RNase cleavage assay. *Methods Mol Med* 2002;68:141–155.

36. Feinberg AP, Vogelstien B. A technique for radiolabeling DNA restriction endonuclease fragments to high specific activity. *Anal Biochem* 1983;132:6–13.

37. Kerr JF, Winterford CM, Harmon BV. Apoptosis: its significance in cancer and cancer therapy. *Cancer* 1994;73:2013–2026.

38. Kawauchi S, Goto Y, Ihara K, et al. Survival analysis with p27 expression and apoptosis appears to estimate the prognosis of patients with synovial sarcoma more accurately. *Cancer* 2002;94:2712–2718.

39. Zorc M, Vraspir-Porenta O, Zorc-Pleskovic R, et al. Apoptosis of myocytes and proliferation markers as prognostic factors in end-stage dilated cardiomyopathy. *Cardiovasc Pathol* 2003;12:36–39.

40. Grabenbauer GG, Suckorada O, Niedobitek G, et al. Imbalance between proliferation and apoptosis may be responsible for treatment failure after postoperative radiotherapy in squamous cell carcinoma of the oropharynx. *Oral Oncol* 2003;39:459–469.

41. Houston A, Waldron-Lynch FD, Bennett MW, et al. Fas ligand expressed in colon cancer is not associated with increased apoptosis of tumor cells in vivo. *Int J Cancer* 2003;107:209–214.

42. Cohen JJ. Apoptosis. *Immunol Today* 1993;14:126–30.

43. Loro LL, Vintermyr OK, Johannessen AC. Cell death regulation in oral squamous cell carcinoma: methodological considerations and clinical significance. *J Oral Pathol Med* 2003;32:125–138.

44. Arends MJ, Morris RG, Wyllie AH. Apoptosis: the role of the endonuclease. *Am J Pathol* 1990;136:593–608.

45. Wyllie AH. Glucocorticoid-induced thymocyte apoptosis is associated with endogenous endonuclease activation. *Nature* 1980;284:555–556.

46. Hall PA. Assessing apoptosis: a critical survey. *Endocr Relat Cancer* 1999;6:3–8.

47. Valavanis C, Naber S, Schwartz LM. In situ detection of dying cells in normal and pathological tissues. *Methods Cell Biol* 2001;66:393–415.

48. Baima B, Sticherling M. How specific is the TUNEL reaction? An account of a histochemical study on human skin. *Am J Dermatopathol* 2002;24:130–134.

49. Jerome KR, Vallan C, Jaggi R. The TUNEL assay in the diagnosis of graft-versus-host disease: caveats for interpretation. *Pathology* 2000;32:186–190.

50. Yasuda M, Umemura S, Osamura RY, et al. Apoptotic cells in the human endometrium and placental villi: pitfalls in applying the TUNEL method. *Arch Histol Cytol* 1995;58:185–190.

51. Grasl-Kraupp B, Ruttkay-Nedecky B, Koudelka H, et al. In situ detection of fragmented DNA (TUNEL assay) fails to discriminate among apoptosis, necrosis, and autolytic cell death: a cautionary note. *Hepatology* 1995;21:1465–1468.

52. Kanoh T, Fujiwara T, Fukuda K, et al. Significance of myocytes with positive DNA in situ nick end-labeling (TUNEL) in hearts with dilated cardiomyopathy: not apoptosis but DNA repair. *Circulation* 1999;99:2757–2764.

53. Kurrer MO, Pakala SV, Hanson HL, et al. Beta cell apoptosis in T cell-mediated autoimmune diabetes. *Proc Natl Acad Sci USA* 1997;94:213–218.

54. Nagler RM, Kerner H, Ben-Eliezer S, et al. Prognostic role of apoptotic, Bcl-2, c-erbB-2 and p53 tumor markers in salivary gland malignancies. *Oncology* 2003;64:389–398.

55. Koopman G, Reutelingsperger CP, Kuijten GA, et al. Annexin V for flow cytometric detection of phosphatidylserine expression on B cells undergoing apoptosis. *Blood* 1994;84:1415–1420.

56. Sgonc R, Gruber J. Apoptosis detection: an overview. *Exp Gerontol* 1998;33:525–533.

57. Vagunda V, Kalabis J, Vagundova M. Correlation between apoptotic figure counting and the TUNEL technique. *Anal Quant Cytol Histol* 2000;22:307–310.

58. Martin SJ, Reutelingsperger CP, McGahon AJ, et al. Early redistribution of plasma membrane phosphatidylserine is a general feature of apoptosis regardless of the initiating stimulus: inhibition by overexpression of Bcl-2 and Abl. *J Exp Med* 1995;182:1545–1556.

59. Cummings M. Apoptosis of epithelial cells in vivo involves tissue transglutaminase upregulation. *J Pathol* 1996;179:288–293.

60. Fesus L, Thomazy V, Autuori F, et al. Apoptotic hepatocytes become insoluble in detergents and chaotropic agents as a result of transglutaminase action. *FEBS Lett* 1989;245:150–154.

61. Wang S, Pudney J, Song J. Mechanisms involved in the evolution of progestin resistance in human endometrial hyperplasia: precursor of endometrial cancer. *Gynecol Oncol* 2003;88:108–117.

62. Nicolas JC. Applications of low-light imaging to life sciences. *J Biolumin Chemilumin* 1994;9:139–144.

63. Musiani M, Pasini P, Zerbini M, et al. Chemiluminescence: a sensitive detection system in in situ hybridization. *Histol Histopathol* 1998;13:243–248.

64. Smith MR, Devine CS, Cohn SM, et al. Quantitative electrophoretic transfer of DNA from polyacrylamide or agarose gels to nitrocellulose. *Anal Biochem* 1984;137:120–124.

65. Kroczek R, Siebert E. Optimization of northern analysis by vacuum-blotting, RNA-transfer visualization, and ultraviolet fixation. *Anal Biochem* 1990;184:90–95.

66. Stacey J, Isaac PG. Restriction enzyme digestion, gel electrophoresis, and vacuum blotting of DNA to nylon membranes. *Methods Mol Biol* 1994;28:25–36.

67. Van Oss CJ, Good RJ, Chaudhury MK. Mechanism of DNA (Southern) and protein (western) blotting on cellulose nitrate and other membranes. *J Chromatogr* 1987;391:53–65.

68. Khandjian EW. UV crosslinking of RNA to nylon membrane enhances hybridization signals. *Mol Biol Rep* 1986;11:107–115.

69. Lehrach H, Diamond D, Wozney JM, et al. RNA molecular weight determinations by gel electrophoresis under denaturing conditions, a critical reexamination. *Biochemistry* 1977;16:4743–4751.

70. McMaster GK, Carmichael GG. Analysis of single- and double-stranded nucleic acids on polyacrylamide and agarose gels by using glyoxal and acridine orange. *Proc Natl Acad Sci USA* 1977;74:4835–4838.

71. Wilkinson D. *In Situ Hybridization: A Practical Approach.* Oxford UK: IRL Press; 1998.

72. Szakacs JG, Livingston SK. mRNA in-situ hybridization using biotinylated oligonucleotide probes: implications for the diagnostic laboratory. *Ann Clin Lab Sci* 1994;24:324–338.

73. Lloyd RV, Jin L, Bonnerup MK. In situ hybridization in diagnostic pathology. *Mayo Clin Proc* 1994;69:597–598.

74. Negro F, Pacchioni D, Mondardini A, et al. In situ hybridization in viral hepatitis. *Liver* 1992;12:217–226.

75. Morey AL, Fleming KA. The use of in situ hybridization in studies of viral disease. In: Coulton GR, de Belleroche J, eds. *In Situ Hybridization: Medical Applications.* Boston: Kluwer, 1992:66–96.

76. Ambinder RF, Mann RB. Epstein-Barr-encoded RNA in situ hybridization: diagnostic applications. *Hum Pathol* 1994;25:602–605.

77. Gowans EJ, Arthur J, Blight K, et al. Application of in situ hybridization for the detection of virus nucleic acids. *Methods Mol Biol* 1994;33:395–408.

78. Dictor M, Siven M, Tennvall J, et al. Determination of nonendemic nasopharyngeal carcinoma by in situ hybridization for Epstein-Barr virus EBER1 RNA: sensitivity and specificity in cervical node metastases. *Laryngoscope* 1995;105:407–412.

79. Uner AH, Hutchison RE, Davey FR. Applications of in situ hybridization in the study of hematologic malignancies. *Hematol Oncol Clin North Am* 1994;8:771–784.

80. DeLellis RA. In situ hybridization techniques for the analysis of gene expression: applications in tumor pathology. *Hum Pathol* 1994;25:580–585.

81. Andersen JK, Frim DM, Isacson O, et al. Herpesvirus-mediated gene delivery into the rat brain: specificity and efficiency of the neuron-specific enolase promoter. *Cell Mol Neurobiol* 1993;13:503–515.

82. Hyde SC, Gill Dr, Higgins CF, et al. Correction of the ion transport defect in cystic fibrosis transgenic mice by gene therapy. *Nature* 1993;362:250–255.

83. Gazit G, Kane SE, Nichols P, et al. Use of the stress-inducible grp78/BiP promoter in targeting high level gene expression in fibrosarcoma in vivo. *Cancer Res* 1995;55:1660–1663.

84. Komminoth P. Digoxigenin as an alternative probe labeling for in situ hybridization. *Diagn Mol Pathol* 1992;1:142–150.

85. Matsuno A, Teramoto A, Takekoshi S, et al. Expression of plurihormonal mRNAs in somatotrophic adenomas detected using a nonisotopic in situ hybridization method: comparison with lactotrophic adenomas. *Hum Pathol* 1995;26:272–279.

86. Lloyd RV, Long J. In situ hybridization analysis of chromogranin A and B mRNAs in neuroendocrine tumors with digoxigenin-labeled oligonucleotide probe cocktails. *Diagn Mol Pathol* 1995;4:143–151.

87. Nuovo GJ. *PCR In Situ Hybridization: Protocols and Applications.* 2nd ed. New York: Raven; 1994.

88. Zehbe I, Sallstrom JF, Hacker GW, et al. Indirect and direct in situ PCR for the detection of human papillomavirus: an evaluation of two methods and a double staining technique. *Cell Vision* 1994;1:163–167.

89. Hilgenfeld E, Montagna C, Padilla-Nash H, et al. Spectral karyotyping in cancer cytogenetics. *Methods Mol Med* 2002;68:29–44.

90. Kearney L, Tosi S, Jaju RJ. Detection of chromosome abnormalities in leukemia using fluorescence in situ hybridization. *Methods Mol Med* 2002;68:7–27.

91. Tchinda J, Neumann TE, Volpert S, et al. Characterization of chromosomal rearrangements in hematological diseases using spectral karyotyping. *Diagn Mol Pathol* 2004;13:190–195.

92. Sandberg AA. Cancer cytogenetics for clinicians. *CA Cancer J Clin* 1994;44:136–159.

93. Ried T, Baldini A, Rand TC, et al. Simultaneous visualization of seven different DNA probes by in situ hybridization using combinatorial fluorescence and digital imaging microscopy. *Proc Natl Acad Sci USA* 1992;89:1388–1392.

94. Morrison LE. Chromosome analysis by multicolor fluorescence in situ hybridization using direct-labeled fluorescent probes. *Clin Chem* 1993;39:733–734.

95. Wang YL, Bagg A, Pear W, et al. Chronic myelogenous leukemia: laboratory diagnosis and monitoring. *Genes Chromosomes Cancer* 2001;32:97–111.

96. Geurts van Kessel A, de Bruijn D, Hermsen L, et al. Masked t(X;18)(p11;q11) in a biphasic synovial sarcoma revealed by FISH and RT-PCR. *Genes Chromosomes Cancer* 1998;23:198–201.

97. Birch NC, Antonescu CR, Nelson M, et al. Inconspicuous insertion 22;12 in myxoid/round cell liposarcoma accompanied by the secondary structural abnormality der(16)t(1;16). *J Mol Diagn* 2003;5:191–194.

98. Batanian JR, Bridge JA, Wickert R, et al. EWS/FLI-1 fusion signal inserted into chromosome 11 in one patient with morphologic features of Ewing sarcoma, but lacking t(11;22). *Cancer Genet Cytogenet* 2002;133:72–75.

99. Hattinger CM, Rumpler S, Kovar H, et al. Fine-mapping of cytogenetically undetectable EWS/ERG fusions on DNA fibers of Ewing tumors. *Cytogenet Cell Genet* 2001;93:29–35.

100. Campana D, Pui CH. Detection of minimal residual disease in acute leukemia: methodologic advances and clinical significance. *Blood* 1995;85:1416–1434.

101. Lion T. Clinical implications of qualitative and quantitative polymerase chain reaction analysis in the monitoring of patients with chronic myelogenous leukemia. *Bone Marrow Transplant* 1994;14:505–509.

102. Gerhard DS, Kawasaki ED, Carter-Bancroft F, et al. Localization of a unique gene by direct hybridization in situ. *Proc Natl Acad Sci USA* 1981;78:3755–3759.

103. Harper ME, Ullrich A, Sanders GF. Localization of the human insulin gene to the distal end of the short arm of chromosome 11. *Proc Natl Acad Sci USA* 1981;78:4458–4460.

104. Mathew S, Murty VV, Hunziker W, et al. Subregional mapping of 13 single-copy genes on the long arm of chromosome 12 by fluorescence in situ hybridization. *Genomics* 1992;14:775–779.

105. Bhatt B, Burns J, Flannery D, et al. Direct visualization of single copy genes on banded metaphase chromosomes by nonisotopic in situ hybridization. *Nucleic Acids Res* 1988;16:3951–3961.

106. Lichter P, Boyle AL, Cremer T, et al. Analysis of genes and chromosomes by nonisotopic in situ hybridization. *Genet Anal Tech Appl* 1991;8:24–35.

107. http://www.genome.ucsc.edu/.

108. http://www.ncbi.nlm.nih.gov/Entrez.

109. Kallioniemi A, Kallioniemi O, Sudar D, et al. Comparative genomic hybridization for molecular cytogenetic analysis of solid tumors. *Science* 1992;258:818–821.

110. Forozan F, Karhu R, Kononen J, et al. Genome screening by comparative genomic hybridization. *Trends Genet* 1997;13:405–409.

111. du Manoir S, Schrock E, Bentz M, et al. Quantitative analysis of comparative genomic hybridization. *Cytometry* 1995;19:27–41.

112. Ishkanian AS, Malloff CA, Watson SK, et al. A tiling resolution DNA microarray with complete coverage of the human genome. *Nat Genet* 2004;36:299–303.

113. Knuutila S, Bjorkqvist AM, Autio K, et al. DNA copy number amplifications in human neoplasms: review of comparative genomic hybridization studies. *Am J Pathol* 1998;152:1107–1123.

114. Knuutila S, Aalto Y, Autio K, et al. DNA copy number losses in human neoplasms. *Am J Pathol* 1999;155:683–694.

DNA Sequence Analysis

7

The chemical degradation and enzymatic techniques for direct DNA sequence analysis were developed at about the same time. The chemical degradation method developed by Maxam and Gilbert (1,2) makes use of five separate chemical modification reactions, each specific for a particular base or type of base, to partially cleave end-labeled fragments of DNA. The enzymatic technique developed by Sanger et al. (3,4) utilizes an oligonucleotide primer that is extended by DNA polymerase in the presence of one or more labeled nucleotides. The enzymatic technique is the method currently used for virtually all routine DNA sequence analysis because it is simpler, quicker, less expensive, and requires far less template DNA than the chemical degradation approach. Other techniques for direct sequence analysis have recently been introduced, including array-based hybridization approaches and mass spectrometry, but they remain largely experimental.

Although the exact base sequence of a locus can only be obtained through direct DNA sequence analysis, once the normal and mutant alleles have been characterized, indirect methods often can be used to provide sequence information. These indirect techniques for DNA sequence analysis include restriction fragment length polymorphism (RFLP) analysis, allele-specific polymerase chain reaction (PCR), single-strand conformational polymorphism analysis, heteroduplex analysis (HA), denaturing gradient gel electrophoresis (DGGE), chemical cleavage analysis, ligase chain reaction, and the protein truncation test, all of which are used either alone or in combination.

DNA SEQUENCING BY THE DIDEOXY-MEDIATED CHAIN TERMINATION

Priming of enzymatic DNA synthesis by the chain termination method of DNA sequencing is achieved by the use of synthetic oligonucleotide primers complementary to a known sequence of the template strand to be analyzed, and the method is greatly simplified by the use of chain-terminating dideoxynucleoside triphosphates. $2',3'$ Dideoxynucleotides (ddNTPs) differ from conventional ddNTPs by their lack of a hydroxyl residue at the $3'$ of dioxyribose (Fig. 7.1). Although ddNTPs can be incorporated by DNA polymerases into elongating DNA chains through their $5'$ triphosphate groups, the absence of the

$3'$-hydroxyl group prevents formation of a phosphodiester bond with the succeeding dNTP; consequently, after a ddNTP is incorporated into an elongating DNA chain, further extension of the DNA chain is impossible. If a very low concentration of one ddNTP is included with a much higher concentration of the four conventional dNTPs in a DNA sequencing reaction, competition for incorporation into the growing DNA chain between the ddNTP and its normal dNTP analog results in competition between extension of the chain and infrequent but specific chain termination at positions where the ddNTP is incorporated into the growing DNA strand (Fig. 7.2A). The reaction product is therefore a population of DNA strands of assorted lengths that have a common $5'$ end (defined by the sequencing primer), but a different $3'$ end depending on the specific site of incorporation of the ddNTP. Four separate parallel enzymatic reactions, each using a different ddNTP, followed by electrophoretic size-fractionation of the products, make it possible to determine the sequence of the template strand.

As initially described, enzymatic extension of the primer is performed only once per sequencing reaction. However, the utility of the method is greatly increased by the modification known as cycle sequencing (or linear amplification sequencing). Cycle sequencing is similar to conventional PCR in that it employs a thermostable DNA polymerase and a temperature cycling format for DNA denaturation, annealing, and enzymatic DNA synthesis. However, unlike standard PCR, only one primer (the

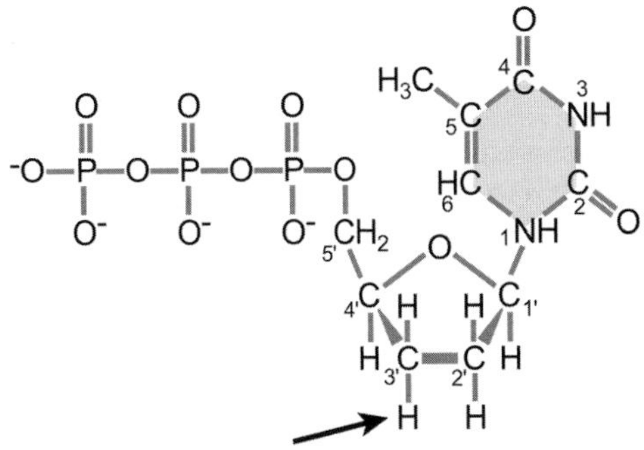

Figure 7.1 $2',3'$-Dideoxythymidine $5'$-triphosphate (ddTTP), an example of a dideoxynucleotide. Note that the hydroxyl group attached to carbon $3'$ in conventional nucleotides (Figure 1.1) is replaced by a hydrogen (arrow).

sequencing primer) is added to the reaction mixture. The use of thermostable polymerases and cycle sequencing protocols typically generates higher quality sequence than single extension protocols because the elevated reaction temperatures eliminate sequencing problems caused by DNA secondary structure, tracts rich in G and C, and homopolymeric tracts. Of equal importance, because of the linear accumulation of the population of labeled DNA fragments, cycle sequencing reactions require a much lower amount of template DNA to generate enough product for subsequent automated DNA sequence analysis, making the technique particularly well suited for sequence analysis of DNA from tissue specimens. Multiple targets can be sequenced simultaneously via a multiplex PCR format using primers designed to ensure that the labeled products from the different targets are of different sizes (5).

Dideoxy sequencing methods traditionally employed ^{35}S- or ^{33}P-labeled primers or nucleotides for visualization of the size-fractionated bands by autoradiography. However, automated procedures for DNA sequencing utilize nucleotides or primers that are labeled by fluorophores. In the dye terminator method, a different fluorophore is attached to each of the four different ddNTPs, allowing all four enzymatic sequencing reactions to be performed in a single tube. In the dye primer method, four primers, each labeled with a different fluorescent dye, are used in four parallel sequencing reactions, each with a different ddNTP. For both techniques, the use of four different fluorophores in the four base-specific reactions makes it possible to electrophorese all the reactions in a single gel lane (Fig. 7.2B). For automated sequencing, a laser at the bottom of the gel excites the fluorescent dyes in the ladderlike pattern of fragments as they pass and detectors measure the emission intensities at the wavelengths that correspond to the maximum fluorescence for each of the four different dyes. The emission intensities are electronically recorded, and computer analysis is used to convert the pattern of measured emission intensities to an electropherogram and inferred base sequence.

SOURCES OF ERROR IN DIRECT DNA SEQUENCE ANALYSIS

Errors Introduced During Production of the DNA Template

Errors introduced into the DNA template to be sequenced are almost exclusively the result of template production by PCR-based protocols.

One class of errors is due to the intrinsic error rate of the thermostable DNA polymerases (Chapter 5). Even polymerases with a proofreading function have an intrinsic error rate that is highly dependent on the precise reaction conditions, including the buffer composition, salt concentration, dNTP concentration, reaction pH, and even the template sequence itself (6–13). Consequently, PCR product DNA consists of a population of DNA molecules that contains many different sequence changes, a fact that explains why different approaches used to sequence PCR products will have a significant effect on the rate at which sequence changes are detected. As an illustration, for a poly-

merase with an error rate of one error per 10,000 bases, and a 20-cycle PCR amplification of a 1,000-base long amplicon, 62% of the product DNA strands will harbor at least one error, but only about 0.1% of the products strands will harbor a change at any given specific base (refer to Table 5.4). Direct analysis of the total PCR product is therefore likely to give the correct sequence of the original template because the changes in the individual PCR product strands occur essentially randomly, and, as a result, for each individual base position, the contribution of an incorrect base in only a subset of product DNA strands will be overwhelmed by the huge majority of strands that have the correct base. However, if the PCR product DNA is cloned before analysis, the situation is entirely different. The cloning process selects for a single DNA molecule from the PCR product population, and consequently on average 62% of the clones will harbor a sequence change. Clearly, if PCR product DNA is cloned before analysis, multiple individual clones must be evaluated to determine the consensus sequence, especially when a putative mutation is detected.

Another class of errors in DNA templates produced by PCR arises when there is biased amplification of the two different alleles at a heterozygous locus, a well-documented PCR outcome even for alleles that have sequences that vary by as little as a single base (Chapter 5). The PCR product may be so skewed toward one allele that the presence of the second may go unrecognized by direct sequence analysis of the total PCR product. When biased amplification is a problem, the PCR primers and reaction conditions must be redesigned.

Errors Introduced during Conversion of Measured Emission Intensities into the Inferred Base Sequence

The computer analysis used to convert the pattern of measured emission intensities to an inferred base sequence typically involves four distinct steps: lane tracking (identification of the boundaries of each lane within the gel), lane profiling (summation of each of the four fluorescence signals across the lane to produce a profile or trace of the signal intensities as a function of time during the gel run), trace processing (mathematical processing of the profile to smooth signal estimates, reduce noise, and correct for dye effects on fragment mobility and long-range electrophoratic trends), and base-calling (translation of the processed trace into a sequence of bases). An idealized processed trace (consisting of noise-free, evenly spaced, nonoverlapping Gaussian-shaped peaks of equal height, each corresponding to the labeled fragments that terminate at a particular base in the sequenced strand) would optimize conversion of the measured emission intensities to an inferred base sequence by the base-calling software. However, real processed traces deviate from the ideal because of imperfections in the sequencing reactions, gel electrophoresis, and trace processing steps (14–16). Base-calling programs therefore employ algorithms to produce a sequence that is as accurate as possible in the face of imperfect data, and an integral part of many existing algorithms is an estimate of the quality or confidence of each assigned base (14,17,18).

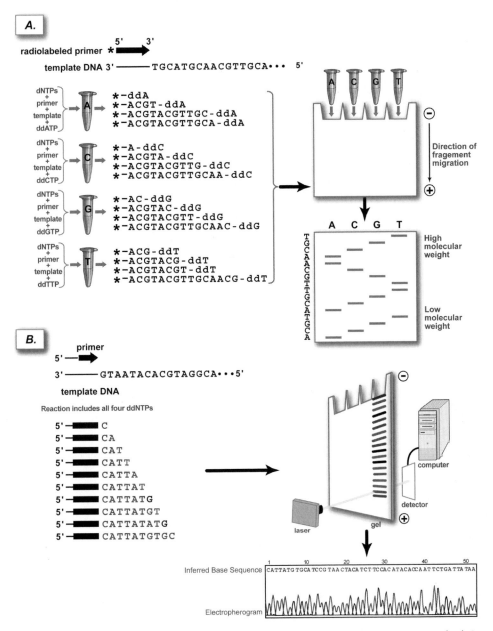

Figure 7.2 Schematic diagram of enzymatic DNA sequencing by the chain termination method. **A**, Traditional method. Four parallel base-specific reactions are performed, each with the same primer and all four dNTPs; each reaction is radiolabeled either by use of a labeled primer (illustrated here by asterisks) or much more commonly by use of labeled dNTPs. Each reaction also includes a low concentration of one ddNTP. Competition for incorporation into the growing DNA strand between the ddNTP and its conventional dNTP analog results in infrequent but specific chain termination at the position where the ddNTP is incorporated, generating a population of DNA strands of assorted lengths that all have the same 5′ end defined by the sequencing primer. The four separate enzymatic reactions are size-fractioned in parallel lanes in a denaturing polyacrylimide gel. The pattern of bands produced by autoradiography of the gel (read from smallest to largest) yields the sequence of the complementary strand. **B**, Automated method. In the dye terminator method (illustrated), all four base-specific reactions are performed simultaneously in a single tube in which each ddNTP is labeled with a different fluorescent dye. The reaction products are size-fractionated in a single lane, and a laser beam focused at a constant position of the gel causes the dyes to fluoresce as they migrate past. The fluorescence emissions are recorded, and computer analysis converts the electropherogram into an inferred base sequence. The illustrated sequence is from human papilloma virus type 6. (See color insert.)

Regardless of the algorithm, all currently available base-calling programs have an error rate in the range of less than 0.3% to over 4%. The error rates vary by base position in the sequencing run and include both base substitution errors and insertion and deletion errors (18–20). Sequencing chemistry can influence the frequency of base-calling errors, but overall the source of the template DNA, specific sequencing polymerase, automated sequencing apparatus, and gel length have only a relatively minor influence on the error rate of base-calling software (19). Careful visual inspection of the

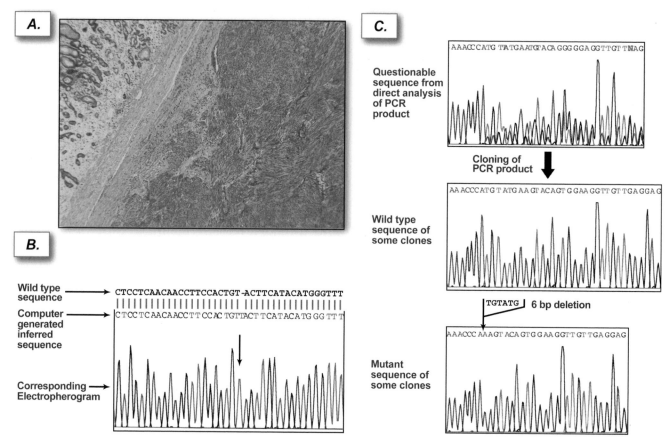

Figure 7.3 Errors in automated sequence analysis. **A**, Photomicrograph of a gastric gastrointestinal stromal tumor (GIST), a tumor type that often harbors mutations in exon 11 of the *c-kit* gene (Chapter 15). **B**, Exon 11 was amplified by PCR and subjected to automated sequence analysis. A homology search of the computer-generated inferred base sequence search identified a putative single base pair insertion. Inspection of the actual electropherogram demonstrates that the putative mutation is a base-calling error *(arrow, bottom)*. **C**, Automated sequence analysis of the total DNA product from PCR amplification of exon 11 from another GIST. Visual inspection of the electropherogram *(top)* shows a complicated pattern of overlapping peaks that calls into question the validity of the inferred base sequence. Sequence analysis of the cloned PCR products shows that some of the DNA molecules have a wild-type sequence *(middle)*, whereas others have a mutant sequence containing a 6-bp deletion involving codons 562 to 564 *(bottom)*. This result indicates that the tumor is actually heterozygous for an exon 11 deletion. (See color insert.)

electropherogram and corresponding inferred base sequence identifies many base-calling errors and minimizes the possibility that a base-calling error is misinterpreted as a mutation (Fig. 7.3), but one of the most critical components of sequence analysis is determination of the sequence from both DNA strands. Although sequencing of both strands will confirm the presence of mutations and call attention to many base-calling errors, it will not discriminate between a true mutation versus a change resulting from an error that arose during production of the template.

When PCR amplification of a heterozygous locus produces a roughly equivalent amount of DNA from both alleles, direct sequence analysis of the total PCR product will produce a pattern of overlapping peaks in the electropherogram. In many cases, especially if the sequences vary at a small number of bases, visual inspection of the electropherogram will suggest the presence of two alleles, the presence of which may not be apparent based on the sequence produced by the base-calling software. However, if the difference between the alleles is due to an insertion or deletion, the electropherogram is quite complicated and the sequence produced by base-calling software is unreliable (Fig. 7.3C).

Although base-calling software designed to decipher areas of overlapping sequence has been developed* (21), sequence analysis of the cloned PCR product is the only way to definitively determine the sequence of both alleles.

INDIRECT METHODS OF DNA SEQUENCE ANALYSIS

Once normal and mutant alleles at a specific locus have been characterized and correlated with disease, indirect methods can often provide enough DNA sequence information to be of clinical utility. These indirect techniques include allelic discrimination by size, RFLP analysis, allele-specific PCR, single-strand conformational

---

*Factura, Applied Biosystem (*http://home.appliedbiosystems.com/*), Foster City, CA; Sequencher, GeneCodes Corporation (*http://www.genecodes. com/*), Ann Arbor, MI; Lasergene, DNAStar, Inc., (*http://dnastar.com/*), Madison, WI; PolyBayes, Washington University School of Medicine Genome Sequencing Center (*http://genome.wustl.edu/groups/inform ratics/software/polybayes/*).

polymorphism analysis, heteroduplex analysis, denaturing gradient gel electrophoresis, cleavage of mismatched nucleotides, ligase chain reaction, the protein truncation test, and numerous variants, used either alone or in combination. Because these indirect methods are based on PCR, they can be applied to a broad range of clinical specimens. The advantages and disadvantages of the different methods are summarized in Table 7.1.

Allelic Discrimination by Size

Variant and normal alleles that vary by small insertions or deletions can be distinguished based on the size of the PCR product after gel electrophoresis, perhaps the most straightforward method for indirect DNA sequence analysis. The method is especially useful for analysis of regions that contain short tandem repeat (STR) polymorphisms, even though PCR amplification of STRs often produces a mixture of products because of slipped strand mispairing that can be a source of error in test interpretation (22–24).

Allelic Discrimination Based on Susceptibility to a Restriction Enzyme

Using the RFLP analysis technique, mutations that either create or destroy a restriction endonuclease site can be easily distinguished by a two-step process that involves DNA digestion with the restriction endonuclease followed by gel electrophoresis to size-fractionate the digested DNA (25). The size of the DNA fragments after gel electrophoresis indicates the presence or absence of a mutation at the restriction site. Although RFLP analysis can be performed using genomic DNA followed by Southern blot hybridization to detect the restriction fragments, currently virtually all RFLP analysis is performed on PCR product DNA followed by direct visualization of the restriction products after electrophoresis. As shown in Figure 7.4, in those cases in which a mutation does not directly create or destroy a restriction site polymorphism, RFLP analysis can still be performed if one of the PCR primers is designed to introduce a restriction site in either the mutant or wild-type

TABLE 7.1
METHODS FOR DNA SEQUENCE ANALYSIS

Method	Advantages	Disadvantages
Direct methods		
Dideoxy enzymatic sequencing	Detects and fully characterizes all changes; inexpensive and quick; can be automated	Computer-generated inferred base sequence can contain errors

Oligonucleotide arrays
  Hybridization-based arrays
  Mini-sequencing–based arrays
	Both types of arrays provide quick, high-throughput analysis	Both types or arrays require expensive equipment; individual arrays are also expensive and are available for only a limited number of genes; arrays do not characterize all changes

Mass spectrometry	Quick; high throughput	Novel technology still under development; requires expensive instrumentation
Indirect methods		
Allelic discrimination based on size	Quick; simple; high throughput	Only detects insertions or deletions, does not reveal position of change
Allelic discrimination based on restriction fragment length polymorphism analysis	Quick; simple; high throughput	Only detects targeted change
Allele-specific polymerase chain reaction	Quick; simple, useful for screening	Only detects targeted change
Single-strand conformational polymorphism analysis	Simple; useful for screening	Limited sensitivity; limited to sequences <200 bp long; does not reveal position or type of change
Heteroduplex analysis	Simple; inexpensive	Limited sensitivity; limited to sequences <200 bp long; does not reveal position or type of change
Denaturing gradient gel electrophoresis	High sensitivity; useful for screening	Requires optimization for each individual DNA region; does not reveal position or type of change
Ligase chain reaction	Quick; simple; useful for screening	Only detects targeted changes
Protein truncation test	High sensitivity for truncating mutations; indicates general position of change; useful for screening	Only detects terminating mutations; technically difficult
Cleavage of mismatched nucleotides Chemical	High sensitivity; indicates general position of change; useful for screening	Toxic chemicals; technically difficult
Enzymatic (ribonuclease-based)	Greatly simplified by nonisotopic methodology	Cumbersome methodology; does not reveal position or type of change

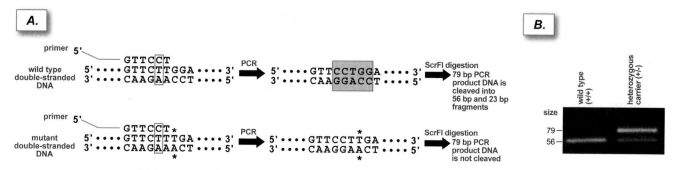

Figure 7.4 Mutation detection by PCR-mediated site-directed alterations of the nonsense mutation G542X in the *CFTR* gene in cystic fibrosis. **A**, PCR is used to introduce a *Scr*FI site (*shaded box*) into the wild-type sequence via the mismatch between the primer and the wild-type sequence (*unshaded box*). Use of the same primer in a PCR with the mutant G542X sequence (the G→T transversion is highlighted by asterisks) still introduces a sequence change via the mismatch (*unshaded box*), but does not produce a *Scr*FI site. **B**, Example of analysis of a wild-type control and a heterozygous carrier of the G542X mutation. Amplification of the 79-bp region that flanks the restriction site is followed by *Scr*FI digestion, electrophoresis, and ethidium bromide staining of the DNA product. The presence of the mutation is visualized by the presence of the 79-bp band that is not cleaved by *Scr*FI because of loss of the restriction site. The 23-bp fragment migrates quickly through the gel and is not visible in this cropped image. (Panel B is adapted from Gasparini P, Bonizzato A, Dognini M, et al. Restriction site generating polymerase chain reaction (RG-PCR) for the probeless detection of hidden genetic variation: application to the study of some common cystic fibrosis mutations. *Molecular and Cellular Probes* 1992;6:1–7; with permission from Elsevier.)

allele (26–29). An important technical detail of this approach is use in the PCR step of a thermostable polymerase without 3'-exonuclease proofreading activity; otherwise, the enzyme will simply correct the mismatches between the primers and the template.

Allele-specific PCR

Allele-specific PCR (also known as the amplification refractory mutation system [ARMS]) employs oligonucleotide primers designed to discriminate between target DNA sequences that differ by a single base (30). Allele-specific PCR takes advantage of the fact that extension of each primer during the DNA synthesis step in each cycle of PCR is critically dependent on correct base-pairing at the 3' end of the primer (Fig. 7.5). The primers for allele-specific PCR are therefore designed so that the site of the base change corresponds to the extreme 3' terminus of one of the primers, and the presence or absence of the PCR product can then be correlated with the sequence at that particular base (30–32); the assay also requires a polymerase without 3'-exonuclease activity, or the terminal mismatch will simply be corrected. Simultaneous analysis of multiple loci via a multiplex PCR format is possible if the amplicons from the different loci are of different sizes (33,34).

The PCR-clamping technique is a variant of allele-specific PCR that employs peptide nucleic acids (PNAs). PNAs are different from conventional oligonucleotides in that they have a peptide backbone instead of a ribose-phosphate backbone. They recognize and hybridize to their complementary DNA sequences by hydrogen bonding as do conventional oligonucleotides, but have a higher thermal stability and specificity than conventional oligonucleotides. However, PNAs cannot serve as primers for DNA synthesis by the thermostable polymerases used in PCR (35,36). Consequently, a PNA/DNA hybrid complex can block formation of a PCR product when the PNA is targeted against a primer sequence (or even an internal sequence in

the amplicon). This blockage makes it possible to selectively suppress amplification of specific target sequences during PCR that differ by as little as one base (35).

Single-Strand Conformational Polymorphism Analysis

Single strand conformational polymorphism (SSCP) analysis is one of the most simple and widely used techniques for mutation scanning (37–39). The technique is based on the fact that under nondenaturing conditions single-stranded DNA molecules fold into complex three-dimensional structures that are stabilized primarily by base-pairing hydrogen bonds and that alter the DNA's mobility during nondenaturing gel electrophoresis. Because the three-dimensional structure of the molecule is dictated by the DNA sequence, wild-type and mutant molecules of the same length that differ in sequence, by even a single nucleotide, will likely adopt different three-dimensional conformations and therefore exhibit different electrophoretic mobility (Fig. 7.6).

In practice, the DNA fragments evaluated by SSCP are generated by PCR. The double-stranded PCR product is heat denatured, and then fractionated via nondenaturing polyacrylamide gel electrophoresis or capillary electrophoresis (40,41) in which the concentration of DNA loaded to the gel is kept very low to prevent complementary DNA strands from reannealing. Visualization of the band after electrophoretic separation was traditionally achieved via silver staining or radiolabeling of the PCR product (37,38,42), but fluorescence-based methods of detection (43,44) are now more widely used.

The sensitivity of SSCP analysis for detecting mutations in PCR product DNA is controversial. Because there is no theoretical model for predicting the secondary and tertiary structure of single-stranded DNA, attempts to empirically evaluate the sensitivity of SSCP analysis have used different models systems without standardization of variables that

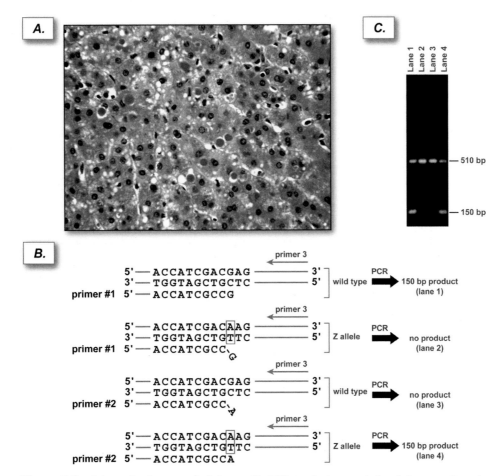

Figure 7.5 Schematic diagram of allele-specific PCR applied to analysis of the α_1-antitrypsin gene. **A,** Photomicrograph of the liver from a 2-year-old child with the ZZ genotype and resulting α_1-antitrypsin deficiency. Note that many hepatocytes contain the round cytoplasmic globular inclusions that are a characteristic finding in patients homozygous for the Z allele. **B,** Primers 1 and 2 differ at the 3' nucleotide and so are specific for the wild-type and variant alleles, respectively, while the third common primer is not allele specific (the site of the G → A transition in the variant allele is boxed; the mismatch three bases from the 3' end of primers 1 and 2 has been empirically shown to increase the specificity of the PCR amplifications). Because Taq polymerase cannot extend a primer with a 3'-terminal base mismatch, PCR amplification does not occur with mismatched primers. **C,** Example of PCR amplification of the α_1-antitrypsin gene using the illustrated primers. The PCR product DNA was electrophoresed and visualized by ethidium bromide staining. For a wild-type individual, successful PCR occurs with primers 1 + 3 (lane 1) but not primers 2 + 3 (lane 3); for an individual homozygous for the Z allele, successful PCR occurs with primers 2 + 3 (lane 4) but not primers 1 + 3 (lane 2). The 510-bp band present in all lanes is an internal positive control PCR product. (Panel C is adapted from Newton CR, Graham A, Heptinstall LE, et al. Analysis of any point mutation in DNA: the amplification refractory mutation system (ARMS). *Nucleic Acids Research* 1989;17:2503–2516; by permission of Oxford University Press.)

likely influence the technique's sensitivity (including pH, ionic strength of the buffer, temperature, length and G + C content of DNA fragment examined, type of sequence variation, and location of the sequence variation relative to the ends of the DNA fragment). The lack of standardization makes comparison of different studies difficult, but some trends have emerged. First, the sensitivity of SSCP analysis is more affected by the position of a mutation and its flanking sequence than the type of mutation itself (45,46). Second, the size of the analyzed DNA fragment appears to dramatically affect the test; sensitivity approaches 100% for detection of base substitutions in DNA fragments in the 100 to 150-bp range, but drops when fragment size increases to 500 bp or longer (46–49). Third, because it is so difficult to predict whether a specific

sequence change will be detected under a given set of electrophoresis conditions, increased sensitivity can be achieved by varying the assay conditions (48–52). Fourth, in practice, the sensitivity of SSCP analysis is most often limited by technical factors, such as loading excessive amounts of DNA per well (which leads to reannealing of complementary DNA strands to form double-stranded DNA), electrophoresis at an excessively high voltage (which leads to gel overheating with resulting denaturation of the weak intramolecular hydrogen bonds), and the presence of spurious PCR products which complicate the interpretation of the electrophoretic pattern (52–55).

Although SSCP analysis can be particularly useful for demonstrating the presence of small sequence changes, including single bp changes, small deletions, small

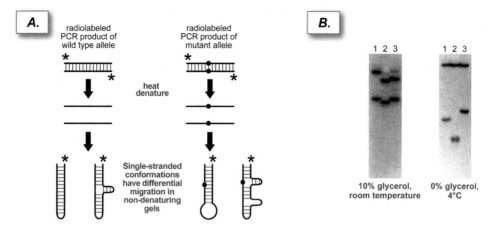

Figure 7.6   Single-strand conformational analysis. **A**, Schematic diagram of the principle of SSCP. The labeled PCR product DNAs are heat denatured, and, during electrophoresis in a nondenaturing gel, the single strands assume a three-dimensional conformation that is dependent on their primary sequence. Different sequences that cause different three dimensional conformations have different electrophoretic mobilities. In this diagram, the *asterisks* represent a radiolabeled nucleotide, the *closed circle* on the mutant allele is a point mutation, and the *crosshatches* represent intrastrand base-pairing hydrogen bonds that help stabilize the three-dimensional conformations. **B**, SSCP analysis of *K-ras* in a lung carcinoma cell line *(lane 1)*, a colon carcinoma cell line *(lane 2)*, and a wild-type normal control *(lane 3)*. The cell lines each harbor a different mutation, as indicated by their altered mobility from the control and from each other. Note that changes in the electrophoresis conditions (denaturant and temperature in this example) cause changes in the single-strand conformation of the PCR products that are reflected by different mobilities. (Panel C is adapted from Orita M, Iwahana H, Kanazawa H, et al. Detection of polymorphisms of human DNA by gel electrophoresis as single-strand conformation polymorphisms. *Proceedings of the National Academy of Sciences of the United States of America* 1989;86:2766–2770; with permission from Elsevier.)

insertions, and polymorphisms, the method does not reveal the type or position of the sequence change. Complementary methods (such as direct DNA sequence analysis) are required to define the sequence that is responsible for the altered electrophoretic mobility.

Because SSCP analysis is performed on PCR product DNA, mutations that affect the PCR itself will have an indirect effect on the SSCP analysis and can be a source of errors in test interpretation. Mutations in the target DNA that preclude its amplification in the initial PCR reaction can lead to a false negative result, a problem most often resulting from base substitutions, insertions, or deletions that significantly alter the binding site of one of the primers used in the PCR. In addition, as discussed above for direct sequence analysis, errors introduced by thermostable polymerases during PCR are scattered throughout the product DNA, and these errors will behave as DNA sequence mutations in the subsequent analysis that can result in a background smear that complicates test interpretation.

Heteroduplex Analysis

HA is a method of identifying DNA sequence variation that is based on gel electrophoresis of double-stranded DNA. Control (wild-type) and patient DNA samples are mixed together, the mixture is heated to denature the double-stranded DNA, and the mixture is then slowly cooled to reanneal the single-stranded molecules, a procedure that leads to the formation of four types of DNA duplexes, namely a homoduplex of control DNA, a homoduplex of

patient DNA, and two heteroduplex species formed when a strand of control DNA reanneals with a strand of patient DNA. Sequence differences in the DNA strands that form the heteroduplexes cause structural perturbations (a "bubble" when the sequence difference between the two DNA fragments consists of one or more point mutations, or a "bulge" when the sequence difference between the two fragments is a small insertion or deletion [56]) that result in an altered mobility when electrophoresed in a nondenaturing gel. Alternatively, the structural perturbations can be detected by melting in the presence of a dye that binds stoichiometrically to regions of only double-stranded DNA (57).

Although not extensive, studies evaluating the sensitivity of HA have demonstrated that, for short fragments of DNA less than about 200 bp long, the technique can identify most insertions, deletions, and single base substitutions (58–60). Several reports suggest that HA has a slightly higher rate of mutation detection than SSCP, although optimum sensitivity may actually be achieved using a combination of both SSCP and HA (42,54,58,61).

Note that for patients expected to be heterozygous at the locus of interest, heteroduplexes can be produced by simply heating the PCR product from the patient, obviating the need for added wild-type DNA. However, for patients with homozygous mutations, as well as male patients with X-linked mutations, it is always necessary to add wild-type DNA to generate heteroduplexes. Finally, because HA analysis is performed on PCR product DNA, mutations that affect the PCR amplification, as well as intrinsic features of PCR itself, can have an effect on the test result and can be a source of errors in test interpretation (see previous discussion of SSCP).

Denaturing Gradient Gel Electrophoresis

Introduced 25 years ago (62), DGGE is another scanning method used to identify sequence variations in DNA. The method is based on the fact that the denaturation of double-stranded DNA, whether by heat or by chemical reagents such as urea and formamide, does not occur in a single step. Instead, melting occurs in a series of steps, each of which represents melting of a discrete segment (termed a melting domain) of the double-stranded DNA. DNA molecules usually contain several melting domains, typically from 25 to 300 contiguous bp long with a melting temperature (T_m) between 60° and 85°C, and because the behavior of each melting domain is a function of its base sequence, changes in the base sequence usually alter the melting profile (62–64). For maximum sensitivity, DGGE usually employs DNA heteroduplexes formed between wild-type DNA and patient DNA.

The standard gel used in DGGE contains a uniform concentration of polyacrylamide throughout, but a gradient of a denaturing agent, usually a combination of urea and formamide. Because a high concentration of denaturant alone is usually not sufficient to produce DNA melting, the gel is immersed in an electrophoretic buffer kept at an elevated temperature that is just below the T_m of the lowest melting domain. As the DNA fragment migrates through the gel, it initially moves with a velocity determined solely by its length. When the fragment reaches the point in the gel at which the level of denaturant corresponds to the T_m of the lowest melting domain, the domain is destabilized and the altered confirmation of the partially melted intermediate results in a lower velocity of migration; small changes in the T_m of the domain resulting from sequence alterations cause destabilization of the domain at a slightly different concentration of the denaturants, corresponding to a different position in the gel, providing the basis for the physical separation by electrophoresis (Fig. 7.7). As the DNA fragment migrates to the region of increased denaturant concentration corresponding to the T_m of the next higher melting domain, the fragment will be further partially melted and migrate even more slowly, providing additional physical separation. When the domain with the highest T_m melts, the two strands of the DNA fragment completely disassociate and the resolving power of the gel is lost. To eliminate this constraint, a GC-rich sequence (called a GC-clamp) is added to one end of the DNA fragment, introducing an artificial highest melting domain that makes it possible to analyze of all the original domains (65–67).

Commercially available computer programs provide a simple and accurate method to determine the melting profile of a DNA molecule (68). Once the T_m of a melting domain is known, the corresponding denaturant concentration can be approximated using the simple formula $X = (T_m - T_b)/0.3$, where X is the percentage of denaturant at which the domain melts, T_m is the melting temperature of the domain, and T_b is the bath temperature (69). Typically, a 30% to 40% difference in the concentration of the denaturant centered about X gives satisfactory resolution.

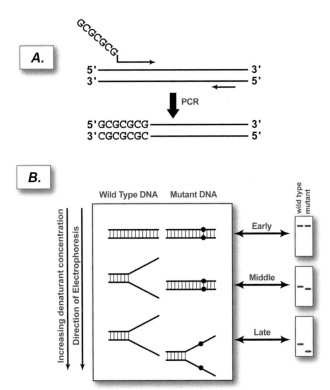

Figure 7.7 Denaturing gradient gel electrophoresis. **A**, PCR is used to generate an amplicon that contains the DNA region of interest. Note the use of a GC-clamp (which in actual practice is 30 to 60 bp long) on one PCR primer. **B**, Schematic representation of three stages during electrophoresis. Early in the run, neither the wild-type amplicon nor mutant amplicon (indicated by the *closed circles*) has melted and so both bands have migrated the same distance. In the middle of the run, the wild-type amplicon has melted while the mutant has not, and so the mutant migrates slightly faster. Late in the run the mutant amplicon melts, and the cumulative difference in melting behavior is reflected by a different mobility between wild-type and mutant. Note how the GC-clamp introduces an artificial highest-melting domain that prevents complete disassociation of the two strands, thereby maintaining the resolving power of the gel.

DGGE is a highly flexible technique, especially suited to screening samples for the presence of mutations. When optimized for evaluation of a specific DNA fragment, DGGE is reported to have a sensitivity for mutation detection that approaches 100% (63,67,69–72), and has been shown to be capable of detecting a clonal population that constitutes only 0.1% to 1% of a DNA mixture (73). Nonetheless, an altered electrophoretic mobility does not provide any direct information on the nature of the sequence change. Reference DNA run in parallel can identify mutations that have been previously characterized, but the nature of a sequence change that produces a novel electrophoretic mobility must be determined by some other technique, such as direct sequence analysis. And, as with SSCP and HA analysis, because DGGE is performed on PCR product DNA, mutations that affect the PCR amplification can have an indirect effect on the test result and be a source of errors in test interpretation (see previous discussion of SSCP).

Several variations of DGGE have been described, an indication of the flexibility and clinical utility of the technique. All are based on the principle of identifying DNA sequence differences based on melting behavior (63). Double-gradient DGGE analysis uses a gel that contains two colinear gradients, one of the denaturant and one of polyacrylamide concentration, a modification that results in considerable improvement in band focusing during electrophoretic separation (74,75). In broad-range DGGE, the denaturing gradient typically ranges from 0 to 80% to accommodate DNA fragments with a broad spectrum of melting temperatures (76), and, as its name implies, temperature gradient gel electrophoresis makes use of a temperature gradient rather than a denaturing gradient (77). Genomic DGGE and bisulfite-DGGE are modifications used to detect mutations and altered methylation patterns in GC-rich regions of DNA (78,79).

Chemical Cleavage of Mismatched Nucleotides

Mutation screening by the chemical cleavage assay takes advantage of the fact that pyrimidines in DNA that are incorrectly paired by the Watson and Crick rules for hydrogen bonding are much more reactive with specific modifying chemical reagents (80). In double-stranded DNA, T mismatched with G or C is hypersusceptible to chemical modification by osmium tetroxide and C mismatched with A or T is hypersusceptible to modification by hydroxylamine. DNA strands containing T or C nucleotides modified by either reaction can be cleaved by piperidine.

In practice, the chemical cleavage of mismatched nucleotides (CCM) assay involves mixing patient DNA (usually amplified by PCR) with a 5- to-10 fold excess of wild-type DNA (also amplified by PCR) that has been radiolabeled on one strand. After melting and reannealing, the DNA is divided into two aliquots. One aliquot is treated with osmium tetroxide and the other with hydroxylamine, followed by piperidine treatment of both. After separation by electrophoresis, the presence of mutations is indicated by appearance of extra smaller bands. By performing the assay twice, once with each strand of the wild-type DNA labeled, the sensitivity of CCM for detection of mutations is very high, in the range of 95% to 100% (80–83).

Although the CCM assay is very sensitive, it does not define the exact nature of the mutation, although the size of the novel bands provides some indication of the position of the mutation. The technique was primarily developed to screen for point mutations, but deletions and insertions can also be detected. Despite the sensitivity of the CCM technique, the number of steps involved in the assay and the toxicity of the reagents has limited its use.

Ribonuclease Cleavage Assay

This technique takes advantage of the fact that ribonucleases can specifically cleave RNA at the site of sequence mismatches in RNA-DNA or RNA-RNA duplexes. The assay was initially developed using the enzyme ribonuclease A (RNase A), which efficiently cleaves single-stranded RNA resulting from mismatches involving pyrimidines (C and U), as well as larger areas of single-stranded RNA (84,85). However, RNase A does not efficiently recognize single-stranded RNA resulting from mismatches involving purines, a technical limitation that was overcome through the use of RNase I, which more efficiently recognizes mismatches involving any of the four bases, and through the use of mixtures of RNases with complementary cleavage specificity (86).

The RNA probe (known as the riboprobe) is synthesized using wild-type DNA as the template and is traditionally radiolabeled by ^{32}P. In actual practice, the wild-type DNA or cDNA must therefore first be cloned into a vector that provides the promoter sequences necessary for transcription. Patient DNA produced by PCR is denatured and then hybridized to the riboprobe to produce RNA-DNA hybrids; the hybrids are digested with RNase, denatured, and then separated by gel electrophoresis. The presence of cleavage fragments smaller than the full-length riboprobe indicates the presence of a mutation, although DNA sequence analysis is required to formally define the type of mutation. Parallel analysis of the patient DNA with both sense and antisense riboprobes increases the likelihood that sites of mismatch caused by mutations will be digested by RNase and increases the sensitivity of the technique.

Even though the technique has a high sensitivity for detecting single base substitutions and most small insertions and deletions (87), the number of steps involved in the assay, as well as the hazards and expense involved with the use of radioisotopes, has limited the utility of the assay. However, a much simplified nonisotopic RNase cleavage assay (NIRCA) has recently been developed that eliminates the need for radioisotopes and, just as important, provides a method to produce the riboprobe that does not require cloned DNA (88). For NIRCA, both the wild-type DNA and the patient DNA are amplified by PCR using primers that include T7 and SP6 bacterial promoter sequences, a primer design feature that makes it possible to produce large quantities of both strands of target and wild-type RNA via in vitro transcription of the PCR product DNA. The patient and wild-type RNA are hybridized to form RNA-RNA heteroduplexes that are treated with RNase and separated by gel electrophoresis as in the conventional RNase cleavage assay, but because large quantities of RNA are generated by the in vitro transcription protocol, the cleavage products can be visualized by ethidium bromide staining. Because the primer design ensures that RNA is produced from both DNA strands during in vitro transcription, reciprocal mismatches are automatically created in the RNA-RNA duplexes, eliminating the need for parallel analysis using separate sense and antisense riboprobes and optimizing the likelihood that mismatches will be cleaved by RNase.

Ligase Chain Reaction

Ligase chain reaction (LCR) is based on the observation that DNA ligases catalyze the formation of a phosphodiester bond between two adjacent oligonucleotides when there is perfect complementary basepairing between the target and the two hybridized probes, whereas a nucleotide mismatch within two bases of the probe joining site will inhibit the reaction (89,90). Because two probes must lie directly adjacent to one another to be joined, the technique can be used to identify insertions, deletions, and point mutations (Fig. 7.8).

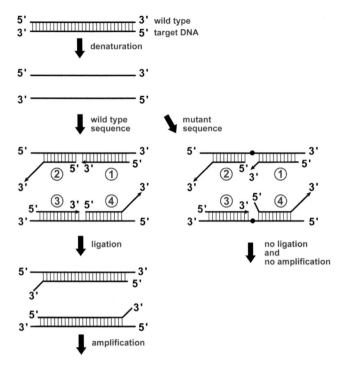

Figure 7.8 Schematic diagram of the basic ligase chain reaction. The target DNA is denatured, and two sets of primers (in this example, designed to recognize the wild-type sequence) anneal at immediately adjacent regions of the target template, one pair for each DNA strand. When there is complete complementarity with the target sequence (*left*), the gap between the primers is sealed by the thermostable DNA ligase, additional copies of the target sequence are thereby produced, and subsequent cycles of the reaction produce exponential amplification of the target sequence. When a mutation is present (*right*; the *closed circle* signifies a point mutation) ligation does not occur, and no products are formed.

In practice, LCR employs two sets of probes that anneal at immediately adjacent regions of the target template, one pair for each of the two DNA strands of the target sequence. The probes are mixed with the test sample and a thermostable DNA ligase, followed by 20 to 30 cycles of the LCR itself. Analogous to PCR, each cycle of the LCR consists of a denaturation or melting phase (usually at 95°C), an annealing phase (at a temperature dependent on the melting temperature of the probes), and a ligation phase (usually at 65°C). If the target sequence has complete complementarity with the probes, it will undergo exponential amplification because the ligated probes can function as target templates in subsequent cycles of the reaction (90,91). By incorporating biotinylated probes into the LCR, it is possible to detect the reaction products by fluorescence or enzyme-based techniques. However, for maximum sensitivity, the 5'-oligonucleotide probes can be end-labeled with ^{32}P and the reaction product visualized by autoradiography after gel electrophoresis (92).

Several different approaches can enhance the sensitivity and specificity of the basic LCR technique (90,91,93–95). Multiplex LCR has been described in which different probe sets labeled with different fluorophores make it possible to perform simultaneous analysis of different mutations in the same assay (96,97), and the technique has even been adapted for use in genomewide screens (98,99).

Protein Truncation Test

The protein truncation test (PrTT) is used to detect frame shift mutations, splice site mutations, and nonsense mutations that truncate a protein product (100). In the first step of the assay, the coding sequence of interest from either genomic DNA or cDNA is amplified by PCR. The forward primer used in the PCR is composed of a T7 bacterial promoter sequence, a translation initiation site, and an initiation codon in continuity with the target-specific sequence. Although only the target-specific region of the oligonucleotide anneals to the DNA template to prime DNA polymerization, the 5'sequence elements are incorporated into the amplicon, and the PCR product can therefore serve as the template in the second step of the assay, an in vitro transcription and translation assay (conveniently available as a commercial kit). Radiolabeled amino acids (usually ^{35}S-methionine or ^{3}H-leucine) are most often used to label the nascent proteins during the in vitro transcription and translation step, but biotinylated amino acids provide an alternative for nonradioactive detection. The labeled proteins are then separated by SDS-polyacrylamide gel electrophoresis, and mutations that produce a shortened or truncated protein are identified by altered electrophoretic mobility. Although the assay does not provide precise information on the type or location of the mutation, the estimated size of the truncated protein can be used to direct analysis to the corresponding portion of the gene.

PrTT performed on cDNA greatly simplifies the analysis of large genes with numerous exons, and because it is possible to evaluate larger PCR products by PrTT than by other techniques such as SSCP or heteroduplex analysis, fewer reactions are required for analysis of an entire gene. Nonetheless, in most cases the gene of interest is too large to be analyzed by PrTT in one PCR, even from cDNA, and consequently the coding region is usually split into partially overlapping segments of 1 to 2 kb in length that together span the coding region. Interpretation of the protein products after SDS-PAGE analysis can be difficult because several bands of varying intensity are usually present, a result of alternative splicing, internal methionines that act as additional start sites, or incomplete transcription or translation. Variants of the technique that incorporate immunoprecipitation of the protein products before electrophoresis often produce a cleaner electrophoretic pattern that is easier to interpret (101).

PrTT is a useful clinical test for diseases such as Duchenne muscular dystrophy, familial adenomatous polyposis, neurofibromatosis type 1, and *BRCA1*-related breast cancer, which have a high incidence of pathogenic truncating mutations (102–108). However, because PrTT does not detect missense mutations, it is not a useful genetic test for diseases such as cystic fibrosis in which only a minority of pathogenic mutations introduce premature termination codons.

SEQUENCE ANALYSIS BY DNA MICROARRAY TECHNOLOGY

High-density DNA micoarrays have found their greatest use in hybridization-based evaluation of gene expression (Chapter 9), but chip-based hybridization analysis is also a promising technology for sequence analysis. Hybridization-based and mini-sequencing–based approaches to microarray sequence analysis are the two methods that have been most widely employed, although a number of additional strategies for chip-based DNA sequence analysis have also been described (109,110). Hybridization-based and mini-sequencing–based methods both employ custom-designed arrays to evaluate specific sequences, and both have a variety of applications, including de novo sequencing, mutation and single nucleotide polymorphism (SNP) discovery, and genotyping (109,111,112). Both have been shown to have a high concordance with DNA sequence obtained by dideoxy-mediated chain termination methods (113,114)

Hybridization-based Approaches

There are two different methods of hybridization-based microarray sequence analysis. In the loss of hybridization signal approach, patient samples and wild-type reference samples are hybridized to the oligonucleotide array and sequence variations are scored by quantitation of relative losses in the hybridization signal between the two samples. Although this method can detect the presence of a mutation, the identity of the sequence change must be determined by subsequent formal DNA sequence analysis (112,115). The gain of hybridization signal approach permits a partial scan of a DNA region for all possible sequence variations through the use of oligonucleotide probes complementary to each of the four possible nucleotides present on a DNA strand at a particular location (Fig. 7.9A). Although the gain of signal approach has been successfully employed to detect both germline mutations and somatic mutations in neoplasms (109,114, 116–119), the number of probes required to screen for mutations other than single base substitutions is prohibitive. In practice, a combination of both loss and gain of signal approaches often achieves the highest sensitivity of mutation detection (112,120,121).

Mini-sequencing–based Assays

Mini-sequencing chips are arrayed with oligonucleotide primers that are tethered to the chip surface via a 5'-end linkage that leaves an exposed free 3'-OH group (Fig. 7.9B). Unlabeled test DNA is hybridized to the array, and a mixture of DNA polymerase and all four ddNTPs (each labeled with a different fluorophore) is added. The chip-bound oligonucleotide probe and the hybridized test DNA therefore serve as primer and template, respectively, in a DNA extension reaction. As in allele-specific PCR, addition of a nucleotide will occur only if the 3' end of the bound primer exactly matches the test DNA, and because only ddNTPs are used, only a single nucleotide will be added to each primer. The sequence of the target then can be determined by the pattern of fluorescence emissions (122).

Mini-sequencing–based assays are especially useful for evaluation of single base substitutions in either homozygous or heterozygous individuals, and have been developed for analysis of nuclear and mitochondrial genes (122–124). Direct comparison has shown that mini-sequencing–based analysis is at least an order of magnitude more sensitive than hybridization-based approaches for discriminating between homozygous and heterozygous genotypes (125).

MASS SPECTROMETRY FOR DNA SEQUENCE ANALYSIS

Nucleic acids have traditionally been difficult to evaluate by mass spectrometry because their susceptibility to adduct formation and fragmentation complicates highly accurate mass measurements. However, the development of matrix-associated laser desorption/ionization time of flight mass spectrometry (MALDI-TOF-MS) has made it possible to analyze nucleic acids up to about 450 bp long (126–131). Advanced matrixes have broadened the range of mass spectrometry applications to include oligonucleotide sequence analysis (132), PCR or ligase chain reaction product detection (133,134), PCR product sequence analysis (127,128,135), and rapid screening of genetic polymorphisms (130,136), applications that all have clear utility for clinical testing. Although the high specificity and rapid analysis times of mass spectrometry make the technique amenable to laboratory use, the sophisticated instrumentation required has limited its use to only a few research centers. Nonetheless, mass spectrometry may have a future role in mutation analysis, SNP discovery, and genotyping.

INTERNET RESOURCES FOR DNA SEQUENCE ANALYSIS

Numerous Internet resources are available that greatly simplify the process of DNA sequence interpretation and mutation identification (Table 7.2). The utility of these sites is enhanced by the fact that DNA sequence from automated analysis can be submitted electronically, eliminating the need for error-prone and time-consuming manual entry. The www.ncbi.nlm.nih.gov/BLAST website is particularly useful for identifying sequence changes (137), and an example of the output from the site is presented in Figure 7.10.

However, there are several caveats regarding the use of Internet resources for sequence analysis. First, the accuracy of many accessioned sequences in the databases is unknown, and some accessioned sequences contain outright errors. Because sequences produced as part of the human genome project were subjected to rigorous quality control standards, they are some of the most reliable. Second, the accessioning information that accompanies each sequence may not provide detailed information on

Wild type 5'•••TTTGCTCCGTTTTCA•••3'
Variant 5'•••TTTGCTCTGTTTTCA•••3'
*

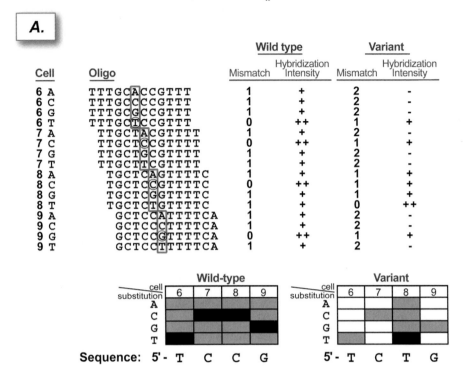

A.

Cell	Oligo	Wild type		Variant	
		Mismatch	Hybridization Intensity	Mismatch	Hybridization Intensity
6 A	TTTGCACCGTTT	1	+	2	-
6 C	TTTGCCCCGTTT	1	+	2	-
6 G	TTTGCGCCGTTT	1	+	2	-
6 T	TTTGCTCCGTTT	0	++	1	+
7 A	TTGCTACGTTTT	1	+	2	-
7 C	TTGCTCCGTTTT	0	++	1	+
7 G	TTGCTGCGTTTT	1	+	2	-
7 T	TTGCTTCGTTTT	1	+	2	-
8 A	TGCTCAGTTTTC	1	+	1	+
8 C	TGCTCCGTTTTC	0	++	1	+
8 G	TGCTCGGTTTTC	1	+	1	+
8 T	TGCTCTGTTTTC	1	+	0	++
9 A	GCTCCATTTTCA	1	+	2	-
9 C	GCTCCCTTTTCA	1	+	2	-
9 G	GCTCCGTTTTCA	0	++	1	+
9 T	GCTCCTTTTTCA	1	+	2	-

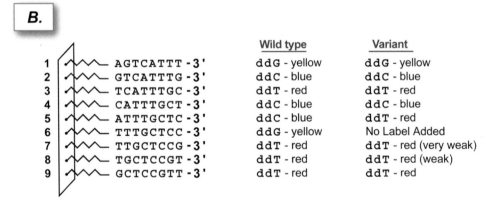

Wild-type

cell substitution	6	7	8	9
A				
C				
G				
T				

Sequence: 5'- T   C   C   G

Variant

cell substitution	6	7	8	9
A				
C				
G				
T				

5'- T   C   T   G

B.

		Wild type	Variant
1	AGTCATTT-3'	ddG - yellow	ddG - yellow
2	GTCATTTG-3'	ddC - blue	ddC - blue
3	TCATTTGC-3'	ddT - red	ddT - red
4	CATTTGCT-3'	ddC - blue	ddC - blue
5	ATTTGCTC-3'	ddC - blue	ddT - red
6	TTTGCTCC-3'	ddG - yellow	No Label Added
7	TTGCTCCG-3'	ddT - red	ddT - red (very weak)
8	TGCTCCGT-3'	ddT - red	ddT - red (weak)
9	GCTCCGTT-3'	ddT - red	ddT - red

Figure 7.9 Oligonucleotide array sequence analysis of the wild-type *BRCA-1* gene and a variant sequence (the C→T transition is indicated by an *asterisk*). **A,** Schematic diagram of the gain of signal approach. Oligonucleotides are arrayed in sets of four that are identical except at the single substitution position (the substitution position for each set is boxed; within the set, the match to the wild-type sequence is indicated by a circle). Oligos with one mismatch hybridize weakly, whereas oligos with two mismatches do not hybridize. The number of mismatches and strength of the hybridization signal are shown on the right for both wild-type and variant DNA. Note that when hybridized to the variant sequence, probes in adjacent sets that overlap the substitution site have either one or two mismatches (instead of zero or one) because they are designed to match the wild-type sequence. Consequently, for the variant DNA, the chip will show an area of diminished hybridization with one strongly hybridizing cell marking the single base pair substitution *(bottom)*. **B,** Schematic diagram of mini-sequencing approach. Oligonucleotides are tethered to the chip surface via a 5'-end linkage that leaves an exposed free 3'-OH group. A mixture of all four ddNTPs, each labeled with a different fluorophore, is added along with the target DNA. The bound oligos and hybridized target DNA act as primer and template, respectively, in a primer extension reaction in which each primer is extended by only a single ddNTP. Note that primer 5 identifies the altered base in the variant sequence. No extension will occur with primer 6 because of the mismatched 3' end. (Modified with permission from Dr. Tom Strachan and Dr. Andrew Read, *Human Molecular Genetics*, 3rd edition, Taylor and Francis Group, New York, © 2003).

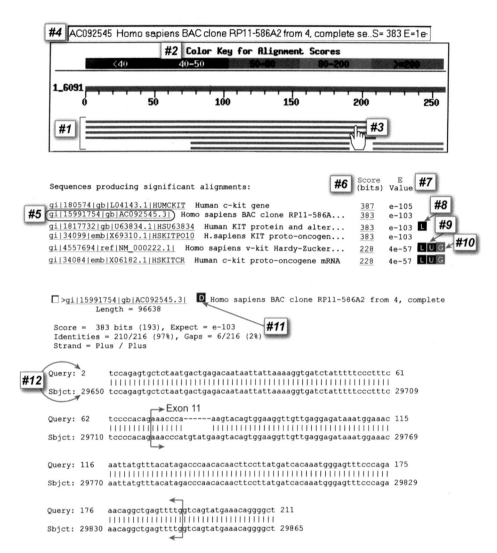

Figure 7.10 Partial output of a nucleotide similarity search using the NCBI Basic Local Alignment Search Tool (BLAST) at www.ncbi.nlm.nih.gov/BLAST for the query sequence of exon 11 of the *c-kit* gene illustrated in the lower panel of Figure 7.3C. The upper region of the output graphically summarizes the BLAST alignment results; each horizontal bar (#1) indicates the region of the query sequence that is homologous to individual sequences in the Entrez Nucleotides database; the bar's color indicates the degree of homology (#2). Mouse-over of a bar (#3) displays the name of the matching sequence in the textbox (#4). The middle region of the output provides a brief description of sequences with significant homology. The output includes the identifier for the database sequence linked to the GenBank entry (#5), the "bit score" measure of the homology in the alignment that is higher the better the alignment (#6), and an E value that provides a statistical measure of the significance of the alignment (#7). The output also provides links, where applicable, to curated sequence and descriptive information about genetic loci at NCBI LocusLink (#8), nonredundant gene-oriented clusters at UniGene (#9), and expression and hybridization array data at the Gene Expression Omnibus GEO (#10). The lower region of the output shows the actual alignments for the sequences with significant homology. For simplicity, the only alignment shown is the one that corresponds to the moused-over sequence at #3 and #4 and highlighted at #5. In addition to the identifier and brief description, the output includes a link to the full homologous subject sequence in the database (#11) and indicates the position of the nucleotides in the query and subject sequences that delineate the region of homology (#12). The horizontal dashes indicate the site of the 6-bp deletion. The boundaries of exon 11 have been added for clarity. (See color insert.)

the experimental or tissue source, which can complicate interpretation of the significance of putative differences. Third, identification of even genuine sequence differences is of little use in vacuo. Sequence differences may not be mutations; single base pair substitutions may merely represent polymorphisms; insertions or deletions in a cDNA may

simply reflect alternative mRNA processing that is a normal component of developmental or tissue-specific gene regulation; and so on. All these uncertainties emphasize that it is difficult to evaluate the importance of a putative mutation in a patient sample without detailed knowledge of the biology of the gene product and associated disease process.

TABLE 7.2

INTERNET RESOURCES FOR SEQUENCE ANALYSIS

www.ncbi.nlm.nih.gov/	National Center for Biotechnology Information homepage; links to PubMed, Entrez, BLAST, OMIM, and other sites
www.ncbi.nlm.nih.gov/Entrez	A versatile cross-database search engine
www.ncbi.nlm.nih.gov/entrez/query.fcgi	PubMed homepage; provides links to other NCBI sites
www.ncbi.nlm.nih.gov/BLAST/	BLAST nucleotide similarity search homepage
www.ncbi.nlm.nih.gov/entrez/query.fcgi?db	Experimental system for automatically partitioning GenBank sequences into a nonredundant set of gene-oriented clusters
www.ncbi.nlm.nih.gov/geo	The Gene Expression Omnibus, a gene expression and hybridization array data repository
www.ncbi.nlm.nih.gov/LocusLink/	Interface to curated sequence and descriptive information about genetic loci
www.girinst.org	Homepage of Genetic Information Research Institute, focused on repetitive sequence elements
www.ncbi.nlm.nih.gov/omim	Online Mendelian Inheritance in Man (OMIM), a catalog of human genes and genetic disorders
www.ncbi.nlm.nih.gov/genome/guide/	Views of chromosomes, maps, and loci with links to other NCBI resources
www.ncbi.nlm.nih.gov/SNP	A database of single nucleotide polymorphisms (SNPs) and other nucleotide variations
snp.cshl.org/	Provides a variety of methods to query for SNPs in the human genome
genome.ucsc.edu/	University of California Santa Cruz Genome Bioinformatics homepage; links to Human BLAT homology search and genome browser
genome.wustl.edu/	Washington University School of Medicine Genome Sequencing Center homepage; links to multiple human genome sites
www.ensembl.org	Ensemble genome browser at the Wellcome Trust Sanger Institute
www.gdb.org	A genome database useful for identifying microsatellite loci
gai.nci.nih.gov/CHLC/	Useful for identifying microsatellites linked to loci of interest

REFERENCES

1. Maxam AM, Gilbert W. A new method for sequencing DNA. *Proc Natl Acad Sci* 1977;74:560–565.
2. Maxam AM, Gilbert W. Sequencing end-labeled DNA with base-specific chemical cleavages. *Methods Enzymol* 1980;65:499–560.
3. Sanger F, Coulson AR. A rapid method for determining sequences in DNA by primed synthesis with DNA polymerase. *J Mol Biol* 1975;94:441–448.
4. Sanger F, Nicklen S, Coulsen AR. DNA sequencing with chain-terminating inhibitors. *Biotechnology* 1992;24:104–108.
5. Murphy KM, Eshleman JR. Simultaneous sequencing of multiple polymerase chain reaction products and combined polymerase chain reaction with cycle sequencing in single reactions. *Am J Pathol* 2002;161:27–33.
6. Flaman JM, Frebourg T, Moreau V, et al. A rapid PCR fidelity assay. *Nucleic Acids Res* 1994;22:3259–3260.
7. Jacobs G, Tscholl E, Sek A, et al. Enrichment polymerase chain reaction for the detection of Ki-ras mutations: relevance of *Taq* polymerase error rate, initial DNA copy number, and reaction conditions on the emergence of false-positive mutant bands. *J Cancer Res Clin Oncol* 1999;125:395–401.
8. Dietrich J, Schmitt P, Zieger M, et al. PCR performance of the highly thermostable proof-reading B-type DNA polymerase from *Pyrococcus abyssi*. *FEMS Microbiol Lett* 2002;217:89–94.
9. Mattila P, Korpela J, Tenkanen T, et al. Fidelity of DNA synthesis by the *Thermococcus litoralis* DNA polymerase: an extremely heat stable enzyme with proofreading activity. *Nucleic Acids Res* 1991;19:4967–4973.
10. Bracho MA, Moya A, Barrio E. Contribution of Taq polymerase-induced errors to the estimation of RNA virus diversity. *J Gen Virol* 1998;79:2921–2928.
11. Cline J, Braman JC, Hogrefe HH. PCR fidelity of pfu DNA polymerase and other thermostable DNA polymerases. *Nucleic Acids Res* 1996;24:3546–3551.
12. André P, Kim A, Khrapko K, et al. Fidelity and mutational spectrum of Pfu DNA polymerase on a human mitochondrial DNA sequence. *Genome Res* 1997;78:843–852.
13. Eckert KA, Kunkel TA. DNA polymerase fidelity and the polymerase chain reaction. *PCR Methods Appl* 1991;1:17–24.
14. Ewing B, Hillier L, Wendl MC, et al. Base-calling of automated sequencer traces using phred. I. Accuracy assessment. *Genome Res* 1998;8:175–185.
15. Parker LT, Zakeri H, Deng Q, et al. AmpliTaq DNA polymerase, FS dye-terminator sequencing: analysis of peak height patterns. *Biotechniques* 1996;21:694–699.
16. Rosenblum BB, Lee LG, Spurgeon SL, et al. New dye-labeled terminators for improved DNA sequencing patterns. *Nucleic Acids Res* 1997;25:4500–4504.
17. Ewing B, Green P. Base-calling of automated sequencer traces using phred. II. Error probabilities. *Genome Res* 1998;8:186–194.
18. Walther D, Bartha G, Morris M. Basecalling with LifeTrace. *Genome Res* 2001;11:875–888.
19. Richterich P. Estimation of errors in "raw" DNA sequences: a validation study. *Genome Res* 1998;8:251–259.
20. Durbin R, Dear S. Base qualities help sequencing software. *Genome Res* 1998;8:161–162.
21. Feoli-Fonseca JC, Oligny LL, Yotov WV. New method for automatic identification identification and typing of single and multiple superimposed human papillomavirus sequences. *Diagn Mol Pathol* 1999;8:216–221.

22. Hauge XY, Litt M. A study of the origin of 'shadow bands' seen when typing dinucleotide repeat polymorphisms by the PCR. *Hum Mol Genet* 1993;2:411–415.
23. Clarke LA, Rebelo CS, Goncalves J, et al. PCR amplification introduces errors into mononucleotide and dinucleotide repeat sequences. *Mol Pathol* 2001;54:351–353.
24. Viguera E, Canceill D, Ehrlich SD. In vitro replication slippage by DNA polymerases from thermophilic organisms. *J Mol Biol* 2001;312:323–333.
25. Kan YW, Dozy AM. Antenatal diagnosis of sickle-cell anaemia by D.N.A. analysis of amniotic-fluid cells. *Lancet* 1978;2:910–912.
26. Gasparini P, Bonizzato A, Dognini M, et al. Restriction site generating-polymerase chain reaction (RG-PCR) for the probeless detection of hidden genetic variation: application to the study of some common cystic fibrosis mutations. *Mol Cell Probes* 1992;6:1–7.
27. Haliassos A, Chomel JC, Tesson L, et al. Modification of enzymatically amplified DNA for the detection of point mutations. *Nucleic Acids Res* 1989;17:3606.
28. Friedman KJ, Highsmith WE, Silverman LM. Detecting multiple cystic fibrosis mutations by polymerase chain reaction-mediated site-directed mutagenesis. *Clin Chem* 1991;37:753–755.
29. Lindeman R, Hu SP, Volpato F, et al. Polymerase chain reaction (PCR) mutagenesis enabling rapid non-radioactive detection of common beta-thalassaemia mutations in Mediterraneans. *Br J Haematol* 1991;78:100–104.
30. Newton CR, Graham A, Heptinstall LE, et al. Analysis of any point mutation in DNA: the amplification refractory mutation system (ARMS). *Nucleic Acids Res* 1989;17:2503–2516.
31. Bugalho MJ, Domingues R, Sobrinho L. The minisequencing method: a simple strategy for genetic screening of MEN 2 families. *BMC Genet* 2002;3:8–12.
32. Hasegawa Y, Takeda S, Ichii S, et al. Detection of K-ras mutations in DNAs isolated from feces of patients with colorectal tumors by mutant-allele-specific amplification (MASA). *Oncogene* 1995;10:1441–1445.
33. Shapero MH, Leuther KK, Nguyen A, et al. SNP genotyping by multiplexed solid-phase amplification and fluorescent minisequencing. *Genome Res* 2001;11:1926–1934.
34. Krone N, Braun A, Weinert S, et al. Multiplex minisequencing of the 21-hydroxylase gene as a rapid strategy to confirm congenital adrenal hyperplasia. *Clin Chem* 2002;48:818–825.
35. Orum H, Nielsen PE, Egholm M, et al. Single base pair mutation analysis by PNA directed PCR clamping. *Nucleic Acids Res* 1993;21:5332–5336.
36. Buchardt O, Egholm M, Berg RH, et al. Peptide nucleic acids and their potential applications in biotechnology. *Trends Biotechnol* 1993;11:384–386.
37. Orita M, Suzuki Y, Sekiya T, et al. Rapid and sensitive detection of point mutations and DNA polymorphisms using the polymerase chain reaction. *Genomics* 1989;5:874–879.
38. Orita M, Iwahana H, Kanazawa H, et al. Detection of polymorphisms of human DNA by gel electrophoresis as single-strand conformation polymorphisms. *Proc Natl Acad Sci USA* 1989;86:2766–2770.
39. Jaeckel S, Epplen JT, Kauth M, et al. Polymerase chain reaction-single strand conformation polymorphism or how to detect reliably and efficiently each sequence variation in many samples and many genes. *Electrophoresis* 1998;19:3055–3061.
40. Andersen PS, Jespersgaard C, Vuust J, et al. High-throughput single strand conformation polymorphism mutation detection by automated capillary array electrophoresis: validation of the method. *Hum Mutat* 2003;21:116–122.
41. Ren J. High-throughput single-strand conformation polymorphism analysis by capillary electrophoresis. *J Chromatogr B Biomed Sci Appl* 2000;741:115–128.

42. Wallace AJ. SSCP/heteroduplex analysis. *Methods Mol Biol* 2002;187:151–63.
43. Moore L, Godfrey T, Eng C, et al. Validation of fluorescent SSCP analysis for sensitive detection of p53 mutations. *Biotechniques* 2000;28:986–992.
44. Ellis LA, Taylor CF, Taylor GR. A comparison of fluorescent SSCP and denaturing HPLC for high throughput mutation scanning. *Hum Mutat* 2000;15:556–564.
45. Ravnik-Glavac M, Glavac D, Dean M. Sensitivity of single-strand conformation polymorphism and heteroduplex method for mutation detection in the cystic fibrosis gene. *Hum Mol Genet* 1994;3:801–807.
46. Sheffield VC, Beck JS, Kwitek AE, et al. The sensitivity of single-strand conformation polymorphism analysis for the detection of single base substitutions. *Genomics* 1993;16:325–332.
47. Jordanova A, Kalaydjieva, Savov A, et al. SSCP analysis: a blind sensitivity trial. *Hum Mutat* 1997;10:65–70.
48. Hayashi K, Yandell DW. How sensitive is PCR-SSCP? *Hum Mutat* 1993;2:338–346.
49. Jaeckel S, Epplen JT, Kauth M, et al. Polymerase chain reaction-single strand conformation polymorphism or how to detect reliably and efficiently each sequence variation in many samples and many genes. *Electrophoresis* 1998;19:3055–3061.
50. Lin-Goerke J, Ye S, Highsmith WE, et al. Effects of gel matrix on the sensitivity of single strand conformational polymorphism (SSCP) analysis: a study of the effects of novel gel matrices, fragment size GC content, and base alteration. *Am J Human Genet* 1994;55(suppl):A188.
51. Leren TP, Solberg K, Rodningen OK, et al. Evaluation of running conditions for SSCP analysis: application of SSCP for detection of point mutations in the LDL receptor gene. *PCR Methods Appl* 1993;3:159–162.
52. Vorechovsky I. Mutation analysis of large genomic regions in tumor DNA using single-strand conformation polymorphism: lessons from the ATM gene. *Methods Mol Med* 2002;68:115–124.
53. Wikman FP, Katballe N, Christensen M, et al. Efficient mutation detection in mismatch repair genes using a combination of single-strand conformational polymorphism and heteroduplex analysis at a controlled temperature. *Genet Test* 2000;4:15–21.
54. Reiss J, Krawczak M, Schloesser M, et al. The effect of replication errors on the mismatch analysis of PCR-amplified DNA. *Nucleic Acids Res* 1990;18:973–978.
55. Eng C, Brody LC, Wagner TM, et al. Interpreting epidemiological research: blinded comparison of methods used to estimate the prevalence of inherited mutations in *BRCA1*. *J Med Genet* 2001;38:824–833.
56. Bhattacharyya A, Lilley DM. The contrasting structures of mismatched DNA sequences containing looped-out bases (bulges) and multiple mismatches (bubbles). *Nucleic Acids Res* 1989;17:6821–6840.
57. Gundry CN, Vandersteen JG, Reed GH, et al. Amplicon melting analysis with labeled primers: a closed-tube method for differentiating homozygotes and heterozygotes. *Clin Chem* 2003;49:396–406.
58. Rossetti S, Corra S, Biasi MO, et al. Comparison of heteroduplex and single-strand conformation analyses, followed by ethidium fluorescence visualization, for the detection of mutations in four human genes. *Mol Cell Probes* 1995;9:195–200.
59. Keen J, Lester D, Inglehearn C, et al. Rapid detection of single base mismatches as heteroduplexes on Hydrolink gels. *Trends Genet* 1991;7:5.
60. Korkko J, Kaitila I, Lonnqvist L, et al. Sensitivity of conformation sensitive gel electrophoresis in detecting mutations in Marfan syndrome and related conditions. *J Med Genet* 2002;39:34–41.
61. Glavac D, Dean M. Applications of heteroduplex analysis for mutation detection in disease genes. *Hum Mutat* 1995;6:281–287.
62. Fischer SG, Lerman LS. DNA fragments differing by single base-pair substitutions are separated in denaturing gradient gels: correspondence with melting theory. *Proc Natl Acad Sci USA* 1983;80:1579–1583.
63. Fodde R, Losekoot M. Mutation detection by denaturing gradient gel electrophoresis (DGGE). *Hum Mutat* 1994;3:83–94.
64. Abrams ES, Murdaugh SE, Lerman LS. Intramolecular DNA melting between stable helical segments: melting theory and metastable states. *Nucleic Acids Res* 1995;23:2775–2783.
65. Sheffield VC, Cox DR, Lerman LS, et al. Attachment of a 40-base-pair G + C-rich sequence (GC-clamp) to genomic DNA fragments by the polymerase chain reaction results in improved detection of single-base changes. *Proc Natl Acad Sci USA* 1989;86: 232–236.
66. Myers RM, Fischer SG, Maniatis T, et al. Modification of the melting properties of duplex DNA by attachment of a GC-rich DNA sequence as determined by denaturing gradient gel electrophoresis. *Nucleic Acids Res* 1985;13:3111–3129.
67. Myers RM, Fischer SG, Lerman LS, et al. Nearly all single base substitutions in DNA fragments joined to a GC-clamp can be detected by denaturing gradient gel electrophoresis. *Nucleic Acids Res* 1985;13:3131–3145.
68. Lerman LS, Silverstein K. Computational simulation of DNA melting and its application to denaturing gradient gel electrophoresis. *Methods Enzymol* 1987;155:482–501.
69. Guldberg P, Gronbaek K, Worm J, et al. Mutational analysis of oncogenes and tumor suppressor genes in human cancer using denaturing gradient gel electrophoresis. *Methods Mol Med* 2002;68:125–139.
70. Theophilus BD, Latham T, Grabowski GA, et al. Comparison of RNase A, a chemical cleavage and GC-clamped denaturing gradient gel electrophoresis for the detection of mutations in exon 9 of the human acid beta-glucosidase gene. *Nucleic Acids Res* 1989;17:7707–7722.
71. Dolinsky LC, de Moura-Neto RS, Falcao-Conceicao DN. DGGE analysis as a tool to identify point mutations, de novo mutations and carriers of the dystrophin gene. *Neuromuscul Disord* 2002;12:845–848.
72. Gejman PV, Cao Q, Guedj F, et al. The sensitivity of denaturing gradient gel electrophoresis: a blinded analysis. *Mutat Res* 1998;382:109–114.
73. Wood GS, Uluer AZ. Polymerase chain reaction/denaturing gradient gel electrophoresis (PCR/DGGE): sensitivity, band pattern analysis, and methodologic optimization. *Am J Dermatopathol* 1999;21:547–551.
74. Cremonesi L, Firpo S, Ferrari M, et al. Double-gradient DGGE for optimized detection of DNA point mutations. *Biotechniques* 1997;22:326–330.
75. Dhanda RK, Smith WM, Scott CB, et al. A simple system for automated two-dimensional electrophoresis: applications to genetic testing. *Genet Test* 1998;2:67–70.
76. Guldberg P, Guttler F. 'Broad-range' DGGE for single-step mutation scanning of entire genes: application to human phenylalanine hydroxylase gene. *Nucleic Acids Res* 1994;22:880–881.
77. Wartell RM, Hosseini S, Powell S, et al. Detecting single base substitutions, mismatches and bulges in DNA by temperature gradient gel electrophoresis and related methods. *J Chromatogr A* 1998;806:169–185.
78. Guldberg P, Gronbaek K, Aggerholm A, et al. Detection of mutations in GC-rich DNA by bisulphite denaturing gradient gel electrophoresis. *Nucleic Acids Res* 1998;26:1548–1549.
79. Uitterlinden AG, Slagboom PE, Knook DL, et al. Two-dimensional DNA fingerprinting of human individuals. *Proc Natl Acad Sci USA* 1989;86:2742–2746.
80. Cotton RG, Rodrigues NR, Campbell RD. Reactivity of cytosine and thymine in single-base-pair mismatches with hydroxylamine and osmium tetroxide and its application to the study of mutations. *Proc Natl Acad Sci USA* 1988;85:4397–4401.
81. Saleeba JA, Ramus SJ, Cotton RG. Complete mutation detection using unlabeled chemical cleavage. *Hum Mutat* 1992;1:63–69.
82. Grompe M. The rapid detection of unknown mutations in nucleic acids. *Nat Genet* 1993;5:111–117.
83. Orita M, Iwahana H, Hayashi K, et al. Detection of polymorphisms of human DNA by gel electrophoresis as single-strand conformation polymorphisms. *Proc Natl Acad Sci USA* 1989;86:2766–2770.
84. Myers RM, Larin Z, Maniatis T. Detection of single base substitutions by ribonuclease cleavage at mismatches in RNA:DNA duplexes. *Science* 1985;230:1242–1246.
85. Winter E, Yamamoto F, Almoguera C, et al. A method to detect and characterize point mutations in transcribed genes: amplification and overexpression of the mutant c-Ki-ras allele in human tumor cells. *Proc Natl Acad Sci USA* 1985;82:7575–7579.
86. Goldrick M. Detection of mutations by RNase cleavage (alternative protocol). In: Dracopoliu NC, Haines JL, Korf BR, eds. *Current Protocols in Human Genetics*. Suppl. 14. New York: John Wiley & Sons; 1996:7.2.5–7.2.17.
87. Goldrick M, Prescott J. Detection of mutations in human cancer using nonisotopic RNase cleavage assay. *Methods Mol Med* 2002;68:141–155.
88. Goldrick MM, Kimball GR, Martin LA, et al. NIRCA: a rapid robust method for screening for unknown point mutations. *Biotechniques* 1996;21:106–112.
89. Wu DY, Wallace RB. Specificity of the nick-closing activity of bacteriophage T4 DNA ligase. *Gene* 1989;76:245–254.
90. Barany F. Genetic disease detection and DNA amplification using cloned thermostable ligase. *Proc Natl Acad Sci USA* 1991;88:189–193.
91. Wu DY, Wallace RB. The ligation amplification reaction (LAR): amplification of specific DNA sequences using sequential rounds of template-dependent ligation. *Genomics* 1989;4:560–569.
92. Wiedmann M, Barany F, Batt CA. Detection of *Listeria monocytogenes* by PCR-coupled ligase chain reaction. In: Innis MA, Gelfand DH eds. *PCR Strategies*. San Diego: Academic Press; 1995:347–361.
93. Abravaya K, Carrino JJ, Muldoon S, et al. Detection of point mutations with a modified ligase chain reaction (Gap-LCR). *Nucleic Acids Res* 1995;23:675–682.
94. Wiedmann M, Wilson WJ, Czajka J, et al. Ligase chain reaction (LCR): overview and applications. *PCR Methods Appl* 1994;3:S51–S64.
95. Wiedmann M, Czajka J, Barany F, et al. Discrimination of *Listeria monocytogenes* from other *Listeria* species by ligase chain reaction. *Appl Environ Microbiol* 1992;58: 3443–3447.
96. Dong SM, Traverso G, Johnson C, et al. Detecting colorectal cancer in stool with the use of multiple genetic targets. *J Natl Cancer Inst* 2001;93:858–865.
97. Eggerding FA. A one-step coupled amplification and oligonucleotide ligation procedure for multiplex genetic typing. *PCR Methods Appl* 1995;4:337–345.
98. Liu D, Liu C, DeVries S, et al. LM-PCR permits highly representative whole genome amplification of DNA isolated from small number of cells and paraffin-embedded tumor tissue sections. *Diagn Mol Pathol* 2004;13:105–115.
99. van Dijk MC, Rombout PD, Boots-Sprenger SH, et al. Multiplex ligation-dependent probe amplification for the detection of chromosomal gains and losses in formalin-fixed tissue. *Diagn Mol Pathol* 2005;14:9–16.
100. Roest PA, Roberts RG, Sugino S, et al. Protein truncation test (PTT) for rapid detection of translation-terminating mutations. *Hum Mol Genet* 1993;2:1719–1721.
101. Rowan AJ, Bodmer WF. Introduction of a myc reporter tag to improve the quality of mutation detection using the protein truncation test. *Hum Mutat* 1997;9:172–176.
102. Bateman JF, Freddi S, Lamande SR, et al. Reliable and sensitive detection of premature termination mutations using a protein truncation test designed to overcome problems of nonsense-mediated mRNA instability. *Hum Mutat* 1999;13:311–317.
103. Gardner RJ, Bobrow M, Roberts RG. The identification of point mutations in Duchenne muscular dystrophy patients by using reverse-transcription PCR and the protein truncation test. *Am J Hum Genet* 1995;57:311–320.
104. Roest PA, Roberts RG, van der Tuijn AC, et al. Protein truncation test (PTT) to rapidly screen the DMD gene for translation terminating mutations. *Neuromuscul Disord* 1993;3:391–394.
105. Heim RA, Kam-Morgan LN, Binnie CG, et al. Distribution of 13 truncating mutations in the neurofibromatosis 1 gene. *Hum Mol Genet* 1995;4:975–981.
106. Hogervorst FB, Cornelis RS, Bout M, et al. Rapid detection of BRCA1 mutations by the protein truncation test. *Nat Genet* 1995;10:208–212.
107. van der Luijt R, Khan PM, Vasen H, et al. Rapid detection of translation-terminating mutations at the adenomatous polyposis coli (APC) gene by direct protein truncation test. *Genomics* 1994;20:1–4.
108. Side L. Mutational analysis of the neurofibromatosis type 1 gene in childhood myelodysplastic syndromes using a protein truncation assay. *Methods Mol Med* 2002;68:157–170.
109. McGall GH, Christians FC. High-density genechip oligonucleotide probe arrays. *Adv Biochem Eng Biotechnol* 2002;77:21–42.
110. Goto S, Takahashi A, Kamisango K, et al. Single-nucleotide polymorphism analysis by hybridization protection assay on solid support. *Anal Biochem* 2002;307:25–32.
111. Warrington JA, Shah NA, Chin X, et al. New developments in high-throughput resequencing and variation detection using high density microarrays. *Hum Mutat* 2002;19:402–409.
112. Hacia JG. Resequencing and mutational analysis using oligonucleotide microarrays. *Nat Genet* 1999;21:42–47.

113. Gunthard HF, Wong JK, Ignacio CC, et al. Comparative performance of high-density oligonucleotide sequencing and dideoxynucleotide sequencing of HIV type 1 pol from clinical samples. *AIDS Res Hum Retroviruses* 1998;14:869–876.

114. Ahrendt SA, Halachmi S, Chow JT, et al. Rapid p53 sequence analysis in primary lung cancer using an oligonucleotide probe array. *Proc Natl Acad Sci USA* 1999;96: 7382–7387.

115. Drmanac R, Drmanac S, Chui G, et al. Sequencing by hybridization (SBH): advantages, achievements, and opportunities. *Adv Biochem Eng Biotechnol* 2002;77:75–101.

116. Kozal MJ, Shah N, Shen N, et al. Extensive polymorphisms observed in HIV-1 clade B protease gene using high-density oligonucleotide arrays. *Nat Med* 1996;2: 753–759.

117. Wikman FP, Lu ML, Thykjaer T, et al. Evaluation of the performance of a p53 sequencing microarray chip using 140 previously sequenced bladder tumor samples. *Clin Chem* 2000;46:1555–1561.

118. Cronin MT, Fucini RV, Kim SM, et al. Cystic fibrosis mutation detection by hybridization to light-generated DNA probe arrays. *Hum Mutat* 1996;7:244–255.

119. Hacia JG, Sun B, Hunt N, et al. Strategies for mutational analysis of the large multiexon ATM gene using high-density oligonucleotide arrays. *Genome Res* 1998;8:1245–1258.

120. Hacia JG, Brody LC, Chee MS, et al. Detection of heterozygous mutations in *BRCA1* using high density oligonucleotide arrays and two-colour fluorescence analysis. *Nat Genet* 1996;14:441–447.

121. Chee M, Yang R, Hubbell E, et al. Accessing genetic information with high-density DNA arrays. *Science* 1996;274:610–614.

122. Syvanen AC. From gels to chips: "minisequencing" primer extension for analysis of point mutations and single nucleotide polymorphisms. *Hum Mutat* 1999;13:1–10.

123. Huber M, Losert D, Hiller R, et al. Detection of single base alterations in genomic DNA by solid phase polymerase chain reaction on oligonucleotide microarrays. *Anal Biochem* 2001;299:24–30.

124. Maitra A, Cohen Y, Gillespie SE, et al. The Human MitoChip: a high-throughput sequencing microarray for mitochondrial mutation detection. *Genome Res* 2004; 14:812–819.

125. Pastinen T, Kurg A, Metspalu, et al. Minisequencing: a specific tool for DNA analysis and diagnostics on oligonucleotide arrays. *Genome Res* 1997;7:606–614.

126. Jurinke C, van den Boom D, Cantor CR, et al. The use of MassARRAY technology for high throughput genotyping. *Adv Biochem Eng Biotechnol* 2002;77:57–74.

127. Little DP, Braun A, Darnhofer-Demar B, et al. Detection of RET proto-oncogene codon 634 mutations using mass spectrometry. *J Mol Med* 1997;75:745–750.

128. Higgins GS, Little DP, Koster H. Competitive oligonucleotide single-base extension combined with mass spectrometric detection for mutation screening. *Biotechniques* 1997;23:710–714.

129. Pieles U, Zurcher W, Schar M, et al. Matrix-assisted laser desorption ionization time-of-flight mass spectrometry: a powerful tool for the mass and sequence analysis of natural and modified oligonucleotides. *Nucleic Acids Res* 1993;21:3191–3196.

130. Braun A, Little DP, Koster H. Detecting CFTR gene mutations by using primer oligo base extension and mass spectrometry. *Clin Chem* 1997;43:1151–1158.

131. Leushner J, Chiu NH. Automated mass spectrometry: a revolutionary technology for clinical diagnostics. *Mol Diagn* 2000;5:341–348.

132. Faulstich K, Worner K, Brill H, et al. A sequencing method for RNA oligonucleotides based on mass spectrometry. *Anal Chem* 1997;69:4349–4353.

133. Jurinke C, Zollner B, Feucht H, et al. Application of nested PCR and mass spectrometry for DNA-based virus detection: HBV-DNA detected in the majority of isolated anti-HBc positive sera. *Genet Anal* 1998;14:97–102.

134. Jurinke C, van den Boom D, Jacob A, et al. Analysis of ligase chain reaction products via matrix-assisted laser desorption/ionization time-of-flight-mass spectrometry. *Anal Biochem* 1996;237:174–181.

135. Koster H, Tang K, Fu D, et al. A strategy for rapid and efficient DNA sequencing by mass spectrometry. *Nat Biotechnol* 1996;14:1123–1128.

136. Lechner D, Lathrop GM, Gut IG. Large-scale genotyping by mass spectrometry: experience, advances and obstacles. *Curr Opin Chem Biol* 2002;6:31–38.

137. Altschul SF, Madden TL, Schaffer AA, et al. Gapped BLAST and PSI-BLAST: a new generation of protein database search programs. *Nucleic Acids Res* 1997;25:3389–3402.

Sensitivity and Specificity Issues

The familiar probabilistic model used to define the likelihood that a particular patient is correctly classified based on a test result (Table 8.1) can be applied to molecular genetic tests just as with any other laboratory test. However, it is important to recognize that the quantitative performance of a laboratory test can be evaluated at four different levels (Table 8.2) and that test performance at one of the four levels does not necessarily predict performance at the other levels (1). The technical sensitivity and specificity of a test may be unrelated to its diagnostic sensitivity and specificity, both of which may not accurately reflect the utility of the test in clinical practice when applied, for

example, to groups of patients with different disease prevalence. Differences between these four levels of analysis are often overlooked, even though they account for many of the confusing or seemingly conflicting results regarding the utility of molecular genetic testing in surgical pathology.

FACTORS THAT AFFECT TESTING ON AN ANALYTICAL/TECHNICAL LEVEL

The features of the various molecular genetic methods that influence their sensitivity and specificity for purely technical

TABLE 8.1

NOMENCLATURE WHEN BAYES' THEOREM FOR ONE VARIATE IS APPLIED IN LABORATORY TESTING

	Number of Subjects with Positive Test Result	Number of Subjects with Negative Test Result
Number of subjects with disease	TP	FN
Number of subjects without disease	FP	TN

TP, true positive results *or* number of diseased patients correctly classified by the test; FP, false positive results *or* number of patients without the disease misclassified by the test; FN, false negative results *or* number of diseased patients misclassified by the test; TN, true negative results *or* number of patients without the disease correctly classified by the test.

Diagnostic sensitivity = $\dfrac{TP}{TP + FN}$

Diagnostic specificity = $\dfrac{TN}{FP + TN}$

Predictive value of a positive result = $\dfrac{TP}{TP + FP}$

Predictive value of a negative result = $\dfrac{TN}{TN + FN}$

Efficiency of the test *or* number fraction of patients correctly classified = $\dfrac{TP + TN}{TP + FP + FN + TN}$

Youden index = [(sensitivity + specificity) − 1].

TABLE 8.2

FOUR LEVELS AT WHICH A LABORATORY TEST CAN BE EVALUATED

Level	Measures
Analytic/technical	Technical sensitivity, technical specificity, precision, accuracy
Diagnostic	Diagnostic sensitivity, diagnostic specificity, Youden index
Operational	Predictive value of a positive result, predictive value of a negative result, efficiency
Medical decision-making	Cost–benefit analysis

reasons are discussed in detail in the chapters that deal with the methods individually. However, additional technical limitations on test performance are introduced when the methods are used to evaluate patient samples.

Cytogenetic Analysis

Cytogenetic testing is precise (i.e., there is a small distribution of results when the assay is performed repeatedly on the same specimen) and accurate (there is a close correlation between the reported test result and the actual gross cytogenetic abnormality present). The sensitivity of traditional cytogenetic analysis, which is especially limited when relatively small or complex structural arrangements are present (2–6), can be markedly improved by the use of methods such as spectral karyotyping (7).

One feature of cytogenetic analysis that has a significant impact on the method's sensitivity when applied to testing of patient samples is the requirement for fresh viable tissue that can be induced to proliferate during in vitro culture in order to generate a karyotype. Many studies include only the cases from which a karyotype was successfully produced and thus ignore this aspect of testing. Nevertheless, a candid appraisal of the method's sensitivity in actual clinical practice must take into account the fact that metaphase spreads can be generated from only a subset of even those cases for which fresh tissue is available (8).

The impact that the requirement for in vitro culture has on the sensitivity of analysis depends on tissue type. Culture of hematolymphoid cells for the production of a karyotype is straightforward; therefore cytogenetic testing has high sensitivity when used to evaluate most leukemias and lymphomas for the presence of characteristic translocations. However, cytogenetic testing has a much lower sensitivity for the evaluation of solid tissue tumors, explained in part by the fact that solid tissues are much harder to culture (8). Most studies do not provide information on the types or percentage of cases for which the tumor failed to grow; thus it is difficult to estimate the sensitivity of the method in routine clinical practice.

Southern and Northern Blot Hybridization

With appropriately designed assays, both methods can be used to detect gross structural abnormalities, as well as

smaller chromosomal alterations such as small deletions, small insertions, and even point mutations. Optimized assays used to evaluate lymphoid proliferations are capable of detecting a clonal population that represents only 1% to 5% of the analyzed population of cells, and in recent multicenter studies Southern blot analysis performed at least as well as polymerase chain reaction (PCR) for detection of immunoglobulin rearrangements and T cell receptor rearrangements in lymphoid neoplasms (9,10). However, optimum sensitivity requires up to about 0.5g of fresh tissue, an aspect of testing that is often overlooked. Many reported series include only cases for which sufficient fresh tissue was available and do not provide information on the types or percentage of cases for which tissue was not available; therefore it is difficult to estimate the magnitude of the impact the requirement for fresh tissue has on the use of the method in routine clinical practice

Fluorescence in Situ Hybridization

Although fluorescence in situ hybridization (FISH) can be applied to a broad range of specimen types because of its intrinsic flexibility, its sensitivity and specificity in routine practice can be influenced by the tissue substrate because tissue fixation has been shown to adversely affect hybridization (11). However, there is an even stronger relationship between test performance and assay design. For example, the specificity of testing interphase nuclei in sections of formalin-fixed, paraffin-embedded (FFPE) tissue using probes that become opposed by the target translocation (the probe-fusion or fusion-signal approach) is limited by random colocalization of the two signals that occurs in about 5% to 10% of nuclei (12–15); consequently, testing using probes that are split by the target translocation (the probe-split or split-signal approach) has a better performance (16,17). On the other hand, when testing metaphase chromosomes, colocalization of signals occurs much less frequently (18,19) and so there is less of a difference in specificity using probe-fusion versus probe-split probes.

PCR-based methods

When optimized, PCR is precise and accurate. And, from a purely technical point of view, PCR is extremely sensitive. When fresh tissue is the substrate for testing, PCR can detect one abnormal cell in a background of 10^5 to 10^6 normal cells (20–23), can be used to analyze single copy genes from individual cells (24), and has an analytic specificity that is virtually 100% in well-designed assays. However, several technical factors lower the performance of PCR when testing tissue specimens in routine clinical practice. The most important limitation is introduced when fixed tissue is used for testing (Chapter 5) because of the degradation of DNA and mRNA that occurs during fixation (25–28). It has repeatedly been shown that analysis of fixed tissue is unsuccessful in a higher percentage of cases than for fresh tissue (9,10,29).

From a technical perspective, tissue fixation also limits PCR-based test specificity. Because nucleic acids recovered from fixed tissue are degraded, amplification of shorter target sequences is necessary, often via a nested PCR approach, and both of these technical adjustments increase the risk of amplification of nonspecific sequences and contamination (25–27,29–31). Two recent studies of malignant round cell tumors emphasize the effect of tissue fixation on amplification of nonspecific sequences: no nonspecific PCR products were detected in over 100 cases when fresh tissue was the substrate for testing (32), but dominant nonspecific PCR products were present in about 6% of over 125 cases when FFPE tissue was the substrate for testing (29).

It is more difficult to objectively evaluate the effect that tissue fixation has on the risk of contamination. As discussed more fully below, when only a subset of tumors of a specific histologic type harbors a characteristic mutation, unless all cases are confirmed by an independent method, some presumed true positive results may actually represent false positive results. Similarly, unless confirmed by an independent method, it is often unclear whether an unexpected result is due to contamination or is merely a reflection of the biologic heterogeneity of disease. To date, no studies have specifically addressed these issues.

Additional technical specificity issues are due to the fact that PCR and reverse transcription PCR (RT-PCR) can amplify target DNA and RNA sequences from cellular debris as well as viable cells. In fact, one well-controlled model system has been used to demonstrate that, following injection, cell-free DNA can be detected in draining lymph nodes or systemic lymph nodes by PCR for up to 4 days (33). Consequently, in the absence of histologic confirmation of the presence of live tumor cells, the significance of PCR-based detection of tumor-derived nucleic acids in lymph nodes or even peripheral blood is unclear (see later discussion of illegitimate transcripts).

FACTORS THAT AFFECT TESTING ON A DIAGNOSTIC LEVEL

The intrinsic biologic variability of disease has the greatest impact on the diagnostic sensitivity and specificity of testing. Only a subset of cases of a specific disease often harbors the characteristic mutation, more than one genetic abnormality can be associated with a specific disease, more than one disease can share the same mutation, and so on; thus even a molecular genetic method with perfect analytic performance will have a lower sensitivity and specificity when used for diagnostic testing of patient samples.

More than one mutation can cause the same disease. Abnormalities in the *c-kit* gene associated with gastrointestinal stroma tumor (GIST) are a good example of how tumors caused by one of a number of different mutations in the same gene can affect the diagnostic sensitivity of testing. As discussed in more detail in Chapter 15, dozens of different gain-of-function mutations in four different exons of *c-kit* have been described in GIST, activating mutations that include missense mutations, small in-frame insertions, and small deletions. However, even when extensive analysis is performed to detect all the relevant *c-kit* mutations, testing still only has a sensitivity of 85% for causative mutations because a subset of GISTs harbor gain-of-function mutations in *PDGFRA*. Similarly, *EWS-FLI1* fusion transcripts that result from the t(11;22)(q24;q12) characteristic of Ewing sarcoma/peripheral neuroectodermal tumor (EWS/PNET) are present in only 85% to 90% of cases; *EWS-ERG*

transcripts that result from the t(21;22)(q22;q12) are present in another 5% of cases, and *EWS-E1AF*, *EWS-ETV1*, *EWS-FEV*, *EWS-ZSG*, or *TLS-ERG* are present in rare cases (Chapter 11). In both of these examples, unless extensive analysis of multiple loci is performed, diagnostic testing will not approach 100% sensitivity.

Heterogeneity in the pattern of mutations can even lead to differences in test sensitivity, depending on the phase of disease. For example, because about 5% of cases of chronic myeloid leukemia (CML) have translocation break points that are not detectable by the standard primers used for RT-PCR testing, FISH has a somewhat higher sensitivity for demonstrating the presence of the translocation t(9;22)(q34;q11) for initial diagnosis of CML (34,35). However, once the break point in an individual patient has been characterized, RT-PCR has a higher sensitivity for monitoring disease because PCR can detect 1 abnormal cell in 10^4 to 10^6 normal cells, whereas interphase FISH can detect only 1 abnormal cell in 200 to 500 normal cells (35).

A subset of cases lacks the mutation(s) characteristic of the disease. For many diseases, exhaustive testing, by even the most technically sensitive methods, fails to demonstrate the distinctive genetic aberration in a subset of cases. Some of these negative cases may be due to loss of the defining genetic aberration as a consequence of therapy or tumor progression (36); other negative cases are likely due to causative mutations that have yet to be described. Whatever the reason, this genetic heterogeneity influences the diagnostic performance of many tests regardless of their analytic performance.

The difference between the diagnostic and technical performance of testing due to genetic heterogeneity is often overlooked in studies evaluating the utility of molecular analysis in surgical pathology. The sensitivity of a method when used to test cases known to harbor the disease-associated mutation is often confused with, or assumed to be an accurate estimate of, the sensitivity of the method when used prospectively on unselected cases. Testing of cases known to harbor the mutation can provide an estimate of the analytic performance of the method, but often overestimates the diagnostic performance of the method when it is used prospectively in clinical practice (29).

The same mutation may be characteristic of more than one disease. The translocation t(9;22)(q34;q11) that produces the chimeric *BCR-ABL* fusion transcript and the Philadelphia (Ph) chromosome is a good example of a mutation that is not specific for a particular disease, even within the same tissue type. The translocation is present in about 95% of cases of CML, in 15% to 25% of adult and 3% to 5% of pediatric cases of acute lymphoblastic leukemia (ALL), and in rare cases of acute myeloblastic leukemia (AML). As discussed in Chapter 13, even precise characterization of the translocation break point is insufficient to provide absolute specificity for diagnosis, because in approximately one third of Ph+ ALL and virtually all Ph+ CML the chromosome 22 break point is located in the major break point cluster region (37).

The existence of the same oncogenic mutations in tumors of different tissue types is also well established (38). *ETV6-NTRK3* fusions have been documented in congenital fibrosarcoma/cellular mesoblastic nephroma (39), acute myeloid leukemia (40,41), and secretory carcinoma of the breast (42). Inflammatory myofibroblastic tumor and anaplastic large cell lymphoma share four (so far) of the exact same gene fusions, including *TPM3-ALK, TPM4-ALK, CLTC-ALK,* and *ATIC-ALK* (43–47). *TLS-ERG* fusions have been identified in EWS/PNET and acute myeloid leukemia (48).

Some rare neoplasms even simultaneously harbor genetic aberrations characteristic of two distinct tumor types. For example, several hematolymphoid malignancies, including angioimmunoblastic T cell lymphoma, mature B cell lymphoma, and mature T cell lymphoma, contain cells that have monoclonal rearrangements of both *IgH* and *TCRγ* loci (49,50). Rare sarcomas have also been shown to have a dual genotype. A biphenotypic small cell sarcoma has been described that harbored *EWS-FLI1* and *PAX3-FKHR* fusion transcripts characteristic of EWS/PNET and alveolar rhabdomyosarcoma, respectively (51), and rare cases of EWS/PNET have been shown to harbor both *EWS-FLI1* and *SYT-SSX* fusion transcripts characteristic of EWS/PNET and synovial sarcoma, respectively (52).

Finally, for those tumors that develop through a stepwise accumulation of mutations, it is possible for a neoplasm to harbor a specific genetic aberration characteristic of malignancy yet retain a benign phenotype because of the absence of other mutations required for full transformation (53). Conversely, it is possible that a malignancy contains a particular genetic aberration merely as an epiphenomenon reflecting chromosomal instability and clonal evolution within the neoplasm (54–58); in this situation, the presence of the mutation is unrelated to the genetic alterations initially responsible for malignant transformation and so would be unrelated to the tumor type.

From a practical standpoint, testing can be of diagnostic utility even when two diseases share the same mutation provided that the clinicopathologic features of the two illnesses are different. However, the lack of diagnostic specificity for many diseases and tumor types provides a cautionary note against attempts to interpret molecular genetic test results in the absence of the clinical history and without knowledge of the histopathologic features of the case.

A mutation characteristic of a disease may be present in healthy individuals. One of the best illustrations of biologic heterogeneity associated with a specific mutation is provided by the observation that the leukocytes of up to two thirds of healthy individuals harbor *BCR-ABL* fusion transcripts characteristically associated with CML (23,59), although healthy individuals who test positive do not have a higher risk for developing leukemia than the general population. Similarly, *Bcl2-IgH* fusion transcripts that result from t(14;18) characteristic of follicular lymphomas can be detected in the peripheral blood, benign lymph nodes, and tonsils of up to 88% of healthy adults (60–64). Admittedly, the assays used to identify fusion transcripts in healthy individuals are capable of detecting one abnormal cell in at least 10^5 normal cells (22,23,60,62), a level of analytic sensitivity that is one or two orders of magnitude greater than that of the protocols used in routine diagnostic assays. However, the presence of mutations in healthy individuals emphasizes that indexes of test performance from a purely analytic standpoint can be markedly different from the test sensitivity and specificity from a diagnostic point of view,

and that correct interpretation of a result (whether from an individual patient or a reported series of patients) requires awareness of the technical parameters of the method employed.

Microscopic disease detection (or minimal residual disease detection) is a related scenario in which the presence of submicroscopic disease may not correlate with prognosis or even disease progression. Examples of settings in which a positive PCR result does not predict outcome include demonstration of *BCR-ABL* transcripts in peripheral blood of CML patients in remission (37,65,66), *AML-ETO* transcripts in peripheral blood of patients with AML type M2 in continuous remission (67), *TLS-CHOP* or *EWS-CHOP* transcripts in peripheral blood of patients with myxoid liposarcoma (68), and *EWS-FLI1* and *EWS-ERG* transcripts in peripheral blood of patients with EWS/PNET (69,70). The assays used to detect residual disease are often far more sensitive than those used in routine testing (21,37), illustrating again that test performance from a purely analytic perspective may not reflect test performance from a diagnostic point of view.

Illegitimate transcripts may complicate detection of disease. A number of well-controlled studies have demonstrated that mRNA encoding markers of various epithelial malignancies, including carcinoembryonic antigen, cytokeratins 19 and 20, mucin-1 (MUC-1), and prostate specific antigen, can be detected in lymph nodes, blood, and even bone marrow samples of patients with no history of malignancy (20,22,71–77). The mRNAs are thought to arise from illegitimate transcription of wild-type genes or transcription of nonfunctional pseudogenes (73,78,79). Regardless of the mechanism, their presence has likely contributed to the conflicting results regarding the utility of RT-PCR testing for assessing the status of surgical margins or the presence of lymphovascular spread (33,80–85). Quantitative RT-PCR analysis of the level of mRNA expression tissue may not provide an easy technical solution to this lack of specificity because very low expression resulting from illegitimate transcription by nonmalignant cells may be difficult to distinguish from physiologic expression by very few tumor cells.

Benign anatomic variants or developmental anomalies also compromise the specificity of RT-PCR testing designed to detect metastatic disease based on the presence of particular mRNAs. For example, lymph nodes can contain benign nodal nevi, as well as benign inclusions of müllerian epithelium, breast tissue, thyroid follicles, and mesothelium. Similarly, the specificity of RT-PCR designed to evaluate the status of surgical margins after excision of a segment of bowel could be compromised by endometriosis involving the muscularis propria or serosa.

FACTORS THAT AFFECT TESTING ON AN OPERATIONAL LEVEL

Verification of Results

Verification of test results (Fig. 8.1) is not a consistent design feature of all studies so it is not surprising that different groups have reported different test specificities and

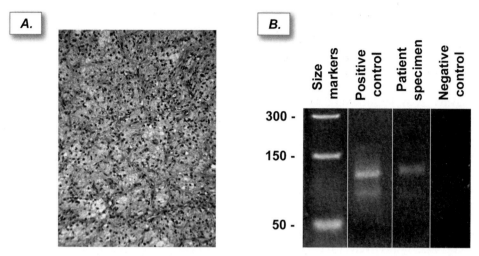

Figure 8.1 Example of how verification of test results can influence estimates of specificity and sensitivity. **A**, Biopsy of parapharyngeal tumor in a 13-year-old boy showed a cellular myxoid neoplasm for which the differential diagnosis included myxoid liposarcoma. **B**, RT-PCR based testing for the *TLS-CHOP* fusion transcript produced by the translocation t(12;16) characteristic of myxoid liposarcoma showed a band consistent with a type II *TLS-CHOP* fusion transcript (*lane 1:* molecular weight standards; *lane 2:* positive control tumor expressing a type II TLS-CHOP fusion transcript; *lane 3:* putative *TLS-CHOP* fusion in the parapharyngeal tumor; *lane 4:* no reverse transcriptase negative control). However, verification of the test result by DNA sequence analysis showed that the RT-PCR product actually consisted of primer concatamers and was therefore a spurious product that fortuitously had the same size as a type II transcript. Testing that relied on band size alone would have produced a false positive result.

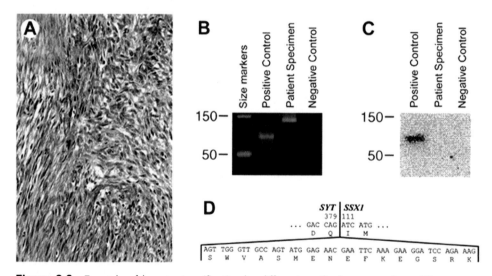

Figure 8.2 Example of how test verification by different methods can produce different outcomes. **A**, Biopsy of an antecubital soft tissue mass in a 43-year-old man showed broad, sweeping fascicles of spindle cells consistent with synovial sarcoma. **B**, RT-PCR based testing for *SYT-SSX* fusion transcripts produced by the translocation t(X;18) characteristic of synovial sarcoma showed an atypically sized product. **C**, The PCR product from the tumor did not hybridize to a [32P]-radiolabeled probe specific for the *SYT-SSX* fusion junction. **D**, DNA sequence analysis showed that the PCR product was an in-frame variant fusion transcript that harbored a 48-bp insert between the usual fusion boundaries of *SYT* and *SSX1*. Testing that relied on band size alone or verification by Southern blot hybridization would have produced a false negative result. (Panels B, C, and D reprinted from O'Sullivan MJ, Humphrey PA, Dehner, LP, et al. t(X;18) reverse transcriptase-polymerase chain reaction demonstrating a variant transcript. *Journal of Molecular Diagnostics* 2002;4:178–180; with permission.)

sensitivities. Furthermore, not all methods to verify test results are equivalent, as Figure 8.2 shows, and so different methods used to confirm test results can also produce different estimates of test performance.

The impact that product verification can have on estimates of test performance, especially when FFPE tissue is the substrate for analysis, is emphasized in a recent study of fusion transcripts in sarcomas (29). DNA sequence analysis of the RT-PCR products demonstrated that in 6% of cases the products were spurious amplification artifacts, and that had the analysis been limited to apparent size based on electrophoresis, these cases would have given false positive results. The same study demonstrated that the PCR product in 4.6% of cases was an atypically sized variant of a diagnostically relevant translocation-related transcript, and that had the analysis been limited to apparent size based on standard electrophoresis, these cases would have given false negative results.

It is important to note that when the probability that a case is subjected to additional analysis depends on the initial test result itself, clinical variables, or both, selection bias is introduced into estimates of test sensitivity and specificity. Selection bias (also called verification bias, post-test referral bias, and workup bias) significantly distorts evaluation of diagnostic test accuracy, causing systematic errors in estimates of diagnostic sensitivity and specificity (87–89).

Discrepant Analysis

Discrepant analysis (also known as discordant analysis or review bias) is an approach used to evaluate the performance of a new testing method. The method uses a combination of reference tests applied in two stages. In the first stage, the result of the new "candidate test" is compared to the result of a single "reference test." When the candidate and reference tests agree, no additional analysis is performed. When the two methods produce different results (a discrepant result), and only when the two methods produce different results, a second stage of testing is performed in which the specimen is retested with a "confirmatory test" or series of tests (90–95).

Discrepant analysis is intrinsically flawed because it generates significant overestimates of test performance (96–99), as illustrated in Table 8.3. Nonetheless, discrepant analysis is sometimes used to estimate the performance of molecular genetic tests in surgical pathology. In this setting, discrepant cases are those that are shown to have the mutation by the candidate molecular test although they are of a tumor type not expected to harbor the genetic alteration (presumed false positive results), or those cases that lack the mutation but are of a tumor type expected to harbor the change (presumed false negative results). The confirmatory tests include morphologic review, additional immunohistochemical stains, or additional genetic analysis. However, it is often impossible to determine the magnitude of the overestimate of test performance introduced by the discrepant analysis because the sensitivity and specificity of the confirmatory tests are usually unknown (96).

It is important to emphasize the difference between clinical review of cases with unexpected test results and discrepant analysis. In routine clinical practice, review of the morphology and immunohistochemical findings, with or without additional genetic testing, is essential for those cases in which there is an unanticipated molecular test result (29,30,52,100–102). However, in studies designed to evaluate the sensitivity and specificity of a test, additional review limited to only those cases with an unexpected result constitutes discrepant analysis. The distinction between review of cases with unexpected findings that is a routine part of surgical pathology versus review as part of a flawed experimental design is a frequent source of confusion (30,96,103–107).

TABLE 8.3
EXAMPLE OF BIAS INTRODUCED BY DISCREPANT ANALYSIS

		Test Results			
A.	**True Status of Specimen**	**Candidate Test**[a]	**Reference Test**[a]	**Confirmatory Test**[b]	**Classification of Specimen after Discrepant Analysis**
	+	+	+	ND[c]	+
	+	+	—	+	+
	+	—	+	+	+
	+	—	—	ND	—
	—	+	+	ND	+
	—	+	—	—	—
	—	—	+	—	—
	—	—	—	ND	—

B.	**Test**	**Sensitivity**	**Specificity**
	Candidate Test	50%	50%
	Reference Test	50%	50%
	Candidate Test with Discrepant Analysis	75%	75%

[a]Both the Candidate Test and Reference Test are simple fair coin flips.
[b]Perfect test with 100% sensitivity and 100% specificity.
[c]No discrepancy, so the Confirmatory Test is not done.

Sample Size

The sample size of many studies evaluating the role of molecular genetic testing is relatively small, often as a reflection of the rarity of the tumor type for which a characteristic genetic abnormality has been described. Many reports involve only a handful of cases, and series of more than 100 cases are relatively rare. Although sample size does not affect test performance, it does influence the statistical confidence of the measured sensitivity and specificity, and so studies that have relatively small sample sizes can generate estimates for test performance that are numerically quite different yet still statistically consistent. This fact is nicely illustrated by two reports of RT-PCR–based detection of *ETV6-NTRK3* fusion transcripts in cases of congenital fibrosarcoma using FFPE tissue. The two studies produced estimates of test sensitivity of 67% (108) and 25% (109). Because only 3 cases were evaluated in the former study, the exact 95% binomial confidence interval of the measured sensitivity is 9.4 to 99%, and because only 12 cases were evaluated in the latter study,

the 95% confidence interval of the measured sensitivity is 5.4 to 57%. Consequently, the difference in sensitivity between the two reports is not statistically significant ($p > 0.05$ by Fisher's exact test). Studies that do not include the confidence interval for the reported test performance can therefore engender unwarranted speculation over the cause of numerically different results that merely reflect small sample sizes. Table 8.4 illustrates the marked effect that relatively small samples sizes have on the confidence intervals of measured test performance and also emphasizes that at the extreme of 0% or 100% disease prevalence, no estimate of test sensitivity or specificity is possible, respectively.

Disease Prevalence

Even for tests with a high sensitivity and high specificity, disease prevalence has a marked effect on the predictive value of positive and negative test results, as shown in Table 8.5. The mathematical relationships between

---

TABLE 8.4

EFFECT OF SAMPLE SIZE ON THE CONFIDENCE INTERVAL OF MEASURED TEST PERFORMANCE INDEXES

Sample Size	Experimentally Determined Sensitivity or Specificity[a]					
	0%[b]	10%	20%	80%	90%	100%[b]
5	0–52%	NA[c]	1%–72%	28%–99%	NA	48%–100%
10	0–31%	0–45%	3%–56%	44%–97%	55%–100%	69%–100%
20	0–17%	1.2%–32%	6%–44%	56%–94%	68%–99%	83%–100%
50	0–7%	3.3%–22%	10%–34%	66%–90%	78%–97%	93%–100%
100	0–4%	4.9%–18%	13%–29%	71%–87%	82%–95%	96%–100%

[a]Data are presented as exact 95% binomial confidence intervals.
[b]When all cases are positive or negative, the value is a 97.5% confidence interval.
[c]Not applicable; binomial confidence intervals cannot be calculated for a fractional numerator.

TABLE 8.5

PREDICTIVE VALUE OF POSITIVE AND NEGATIVE TEST RESULTS AS A FUNCTION OF DISEASE PREVALENCE[a]

Prevalence of Disease (%)	Predictive Value of a Positive Result (%)[b]	Predictive Value of a Negative Result (%)[c]
1	16.1	99.9
5	50.0	99.7
10	67.9	99.4
20	82.6	98.7
50	95.0	95.0
80	98.7	82.6
90	99.4	67.9
95	99.7	50.0
99	99.9	16.1

[a]Assuming a test with 95% sensitivity and 95% specificity.

[b]Predictive value of a positive test result $= \dfrac{(\text{Prevalence}) \cdot (\text{Sensitivity})}{[(\text{Prevalence}) \cdot (\text{Sensitivity})] + [(1 - \text{Prevalence}) \cdot (1 - \text{Specificity})]}$

[c]Predictive value of a negative test result $= \dfrac{(1 - \text{Prevalence}) \cdot (\text{Specificity})}{[(\text{Prevalence}) \cdot (1 - \text{Sensitivity})] + [(1 - \text{Prevalence}) \cdot (\text{Specificity})]}$

predictive value, sensitivity, specificity, and disease prevalence explain how conflicting results regarding the utility of molecular genetic tests can arise because of simple differences in disease prevalence in the series of cases evaluated.

Preselection of Cases

Any preselection of cases that changes the distribution of disease (as opposed to disease prevalence) in the study population will affect measured sensitivity and specificity. Although the measured performance will be valid for the study population, it may not be an accurate estimate of the sensitivity and specificity of the test for a more general population from which the study cases are drawn. For example, in the setting of RT-PCR–based testing for fusion transcripts in soft tissue tumors, preselection of cases based on the presence of adequate fresh tissue, amplifiable nucleic acids, or a consensus diagnosis results in a statistically significant overestimate of the sensitivity of testing compared with unselected cases (29). The practical implication of this finding is that laboratories that use different criteria to preselect cases for testing will often generate different estimates of test performance even when the testing regimens themselves are identical.

IMPLICATIONS FOR CLINICAL TESTING

Taken together, the technical features of molecular genetic assays, biologic variability, assay design, distribution of disease in the study population, and so on, have a number of implications for testing applied to patients in routine clinical practice.

Type of Tissue Tested

There is no doubt that technical limitations inherent in analysis of FFPE tissue make fresh tissue the preferred substrate for testing. As noted above, analysis of FFPE tissue places significant constraints on methodology that lower test sensitivity and specificity. In practical terms, the limitations of FFPE tissue underscore the importance of proactively collecting fresh tissue in order to ensure that molecular genetic testing can achieve its full potential.

Nonetheless, the practice setting of individual pathology groups will dictate the type of tissue that is available for testing. Some laboratories will be provided with the opportunity to test primarily fresh tissue (103,110–112). Other pathology practices, especially those with a rich referral or consult service, may be forced to perform testing primarily on FFPE tissue (29,113). Consequently, even though molecular genetic testing is optimized when performed on fresh tissue, testing limited to only those cases for which frozen tissue is available would exclude a significant number of cases from analysis in many practice settings.

Discordant Cases

Consider two different patterns of referral of surgical pathology cases for molecular genetic testing. On one extreme, testing is performed only on those cases expected to harbor a mutation based on routine histopathologic evaluation, and so there is high disease prevalence in the population of analyzed cases (testing is only performed to confirm the diagnosis). On the other extreme, testing is only performed on those cases not expected to harbor a mutation, and so there is low disease prevalence in the population of analyzed cases (testing is only performed to

TABLE 8.6

EFFECT OF DISEASE PREVALENCE ON THE NUMBER OF FALSE POSITIVE AND FALSE NEGATIVE TEST RESULTS

	Testing to Confirm the Diagnosis (99% Disease Prevalence)*			Testing to Exclude a Diagnosis (1% Disease Prevalence)*	
A	Number of patients with a positive test result	Number of patients with a negative test result	**B**	Number of patients with a positive test result	Number of patients with a negative test result
Number of patients with disease	TP = 94	FN = 5	Number of patients with disease	TP = 1	FN = 0
Number of patients without disease	FP = 0	TN = 1	Number of patients without disease	FP = 5	TN = 94
	Predictive value of a positive test = 100%			Predictive value of a positive test = 17%	
	Predictive value of a negative test = 17%			Predictive value of a negative test = 100%	

*Both tables assume 100 cases tested, 95% test sensitivity, and 95% test specificity.
TP, True Positive; FN, False Negative; FP, False Positive; TN, True Negative.

exclude a diagnosis). As shown in Table 8.6, the difference in disease prevalence between the two sets of cases referred for testing will change the expected number of false positive and false negative test results, that is, the number of cases for which the molecular test result is discordant with the morphologic diagnosis. Although the pattern of molecular test utilization in actual practice will be somewhere in between for most laboratories, the two scenarios emphasize the fact that, for purely mathematical reasons, the mixture of tested cases has an unavoidable impact on the number and type of discrepant cases encountered.

In larger studies, there is a lack of concordance between the diagnosis suggested by the genetic findings and the morphologic diagnosis in about 4% to 6% of cases (29,92–94). The lively debate over the best approach to resolve the ambiguity presented by these cases, especially those that demonstrate presumed false positive results, reflects the fundamental impact of molecular genetics on the classification of disease as well as the power of morphology as the historical standard of pathologic diagnosis by which new methods of classification must be measured

(30,100,102–104,114). Rather than arbitrarily assuming that genetic testing or morphology is superior in all cases, many authors have suggested that the most reasonable way to handle discordant cases is to acknowledge the presence of the discrepancy and, in consultation with the patient's treating physicians, to reappraise all the clinical data, pathologic findings, and therapeutic implications (29,30, 52,56,100–102,109,111,115). This approach acknowledges that there is uncertainty as to the gold standard most appropriately used to define diagnostic categories (see later discussion), which itself highlights the difficulty in estimating test performance indexes when the correct classification of individual cases is uncertain.

In the end, discordant cases are the result of intrinsic limitations in histopathologic diagnosis and molecular methods (30). It is inappropriate to dismiss all unexpected test results as simple laboratory errors resulting from some systematic technical problem that remains undetected and uncorrected, because unanticipated results also occur as the result of factors that affect testing on a diagnostic or operational level, as discussed above. And, at least in the

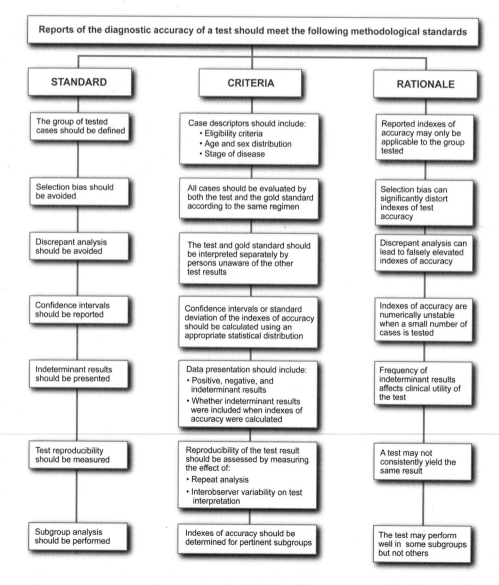

Figure 8.3 Proposed methodological standards for the evaluation of diagnostic tests. (Modified from reference 119).

setting of PCR-based analysis, it is important to remember that detection of a mutation says nothing about the number of cells that harbor the change (116).

Gold Standard

Traditionally, the test defined as the gold standard (or reference standard) has been thought to have the highest diagnostic accuracy and provide results that show the highest correlation with clinical outcome. However, it has recently been shown that, at least from an epidemiologic standpoint, there is a distinction between testing used for diagnosis versus testing used to predict prognosis or response to therapy, and that different study designs are required to assess the performance of tests in these two different settings (117,118). For the large majority of cases in which the

morphologic diagnosis is in agreement with the diagnosis suggested by molecular genetic testing, this distinction is a moot point. However, for those cases in which the diagnosis suggested by morphology and genetic testing are different, prospective clinical trials are needed to access whether prognosis and response to treatment are more accurately predicted by the molecular test than by the morphologic findings on which current staging and treatment protocols are based. Although it is often assumed that molecular testing can provide a more objective basis for diagnosis or therapy in those cases in which there is a disagreement with traditional morphology, it is important to recognize that, as of yet, there are no formal prospective randomized studies that have demonstrated that this conjecture is true.

Some molecular tests will certainly become gold standards for diagnostic or prognostic testing, but their role

---

TABLE 8.7

THE STARD CHECKLIST FOR THE REPORTING OF STUDIES OF DIAGNOSTIC ACCURACY[a]

Section	Standard
Title/Abstract/Keywords	Identify the article as a study of diagnostic accuracy.
Introduction	State the research questions or study aims, such as estimating diagnostic accuracy or comparing accuracy between tests.
Methods	
Participants	Define the study population, including the inclusion and exclusion criteria, setting, and locations where the data were collected.
	Participant recruitment: Was recruitment based on results from previous tests or the fact that the participants had received an index test or the reference standard?
	Participant sampling: Was the study population a consecutive series of participants defined by the selection criteria? If not, specify how participants were further selected.
	Data collection: Were data collected planned before the index test and reference standard were performed (prospective study) or after (retrospective study)?
Test methods	The reference standard and its rationale.
	Technical specifications of the materials and methods.
	Definition of the categories of the results, of the index tests, and the reference standard.
	The number, training, and expertise of the persons executing and reading the tests and the reference standard.
	Whether or not the readers of the index tests and reference standard were blinded (masked) to the results of the other test.
Statistical methods	Methods for calculating or comparing measures of diagnostic accuracy, and the statistical methods used to quantify uncertainty (e.g., 95% confidence intervals).
	Methods for calculating test reproducibility.
Results	
Participants	When the study was done, including beginning and ending dates of recruitment.
	Clinical and demographic characteristics of the study population (e.g., age, sex, spectrum of presenting symptoms, comorbidity, current treatments, recruitment centers).
	The number of participants satisfying the criteria for inclusion that did or did not undergo the index tests and/or the reference standard; describe why participants failed to receive either test.
Test results	Time interval from the index tests to the reference standard.
	Distribution of severity of disease in those with the target condition; other diagnoses in participants without the target condition.
	A cross tabulation of the results of the index tests (including indeterminate and missing results) by the results of the reference standard.
Estimates	Estimates of diagnostic accuracy and measures of statistical uncertainty (e.g., 95% confidence intervals).
	How indeterminate results, missing responses, and outliers of the index tests were handled.
	Estimates of variability of diagnostic accuracy between subgroups of participants, readers, or centers.
	Estimates of test reproducibility.
Discussion	Clinical applicability of the study findings.

(Reprinted from Bossuyt PM, Reisma JB, Bruns DE, et al. Towards complete and accurate reporting of studies of diagnostic accuracy: the STARD initiative. *Annals of Internal Medicine* 2003;138:40–44; with permission.)
[a]STARD, Standards for Reporting Diagnostic Accuracy.

will be decided method by method, disease by disease, based on the performance of the test when applied in routine clinical practice. Sweeping generalizations promoting molecular analysis as the new reference standard in diagnostic surgical pathology ignore the realities of testing outlined in this chapter.

Implications for Studies Designed to Evaluate the Performance of Molecular Genetic Testing

It is not surprising that it is often difficult to evaluate published studies reporting the performance of molecular genetic testing in surgical pathology because there are so many factors that affect the analytical/technical, diagnostic, and operational aspects of the analysis. This problem is not unique to molecular genetic testing in surgical pathology, but is instead shared by all studies of novel diagnostic tests, whether laboratory-based or clinic-based. Keys to the validity of studies evaluating the accuracy of diagnostic tests (Fig. 8.3) include independent blind comparison of the test results with the reference standard among consecutive patients suspected but not known to have the disease, inclusion of missing as well as indeterminate results, and replication of the study in other practice settings to evaluate how specificity and sensitivity of testing may change as the test is applied in other patient populations (117,120).

Methodologic standards have recently been proposed that are helpful guides for independently evaluating the design, conduct, analysis, and results of studies on the performance of novel diagnostic tests in all fields of medicine (121,122). One recent set of standards is presented in Table 8.7, standards that also serve as guidelines for study design. Unfortunately, many reports of molecular genetic testing in surgical pathology do not fare well when evaluated by these standards.

REFERENCES

1. Galen RS. Chapter 4. Statistics. In: Sonnenwirth AC, Jarett L, ed. *Gradwohl's Clinical Laboratory Methods and Diagnosis.* 8th ed. St. Louis: Mosby; 1980:41–68.
2. Geurts van Kessel A, de Bruijn D, Hermsen L, et al. Masked t(X;18)(p11;q11) in a biphasic synovial sarcoma revealed by FISH and RT-PCR. *Genes Chromosomes Cancer* 1998; 23:198–201.
3. Wagner A, van der Klift H, Franken P, et al. A 10-Mb paracentric inversion of chromosome arm 2p inactivates MSH2 and is responsible for hereditary nonpolyposis colorectal cancer in a North-American kindred. *Genes Chromosomes Cancer* 2002;35:49–57.
4. Kaneko Y, Kobayashi H, Handa M, et al. EWS-ERG fusion transcript produced by chromosomal insertion in a Ewing sarcoma. *Genes Chromosomes Cancer* 1997;18:228–231.
5. Batanian JR, Bridge JA, Wickert R, et al. EWS/FLI-1 fusion signal inserted into chromosome 11 in one patient with morphologic features of Ewing sarcoma, but lacking t(11;22). *Cancer Genet Cytogenet* 2002;133:72–75.
6. Merchant SH, Haines S, Hall B, et al. Fluorescence in situ hybridization identifies cryptic t(16;16)(p13;q22) masked by del(16)(q22) in a case of AML-M4 Eo. *J Mol Diagn* 2004;6:271–274.
7. Mrozek K, Iliszko M, Rys J, et al. Spectral karyotyping reveals 17;22 fusions in a cytogenetically atypical dermatofibrosarcoma protuberans with a large marker chromosome as a sole abnormality. *Genes Chromosomes Cancer* 2001;31:182–186.
8. Sandberg AA, Chen Z. Chromosome abnormalities in solid tumors: an overview. In: Mark HF, ed. *Medical Cytogenetics.* NewYork: Marcel Dekker, Inc.; 2000:413–435.
9. Bagg A, Braziel RM, Arber DA, et al. Immunoglobulin heavy chain gene analysis in lymphomas: a multi-center study demonstrating the heterogeneity of performance of polymerase chain reaction assays. *J Mol Diagn* 2002;4:81–89.
10. Arber DA, Braziel RM, Bagg A, et al. Evaluation of T cell receptor testing in lymphoid neoplasms: results of a multicenter study of 29 extracted DNA and paraffin-embedded samples. *J Mol Diagn* 2001;3:133–140.
11. Kumar S, Pack S, Kumar D, et al. Detection of EWS-FLI-1 fusion in Ewing's sarcoma/peripheral primitive neuroectodermal tumor by fluorescence in situ hybridization using formalin-fixed paraffin-embedded tissue. *Hum Pathol* 1999;30:324–330.
12. Biegel JA, Nycum LM, Valentine V, et al. Detection of the t(2;13)(q35;q14) and PAX3-FKHR fusion in alveolar rhabdomyosarcoma by fluorescence in situ hybridization. *Genes Chromosomes Cancer* 1995;12:186–192.
13. Covinsky M, Gong S, Rajaram V, et al. EWS-ATF1 fusion transcripts in gastrointestinal tumors previously diagnosed as malignant melanoma. *Hum Pathol* 2005;36:74–81.
14. Bentz M, Cabot G, Moos M, et al. Detection of chimeric BCR-ABL genes on bone marrow samples and blood smears in chronic myeloid and acute lymphoblastic leukemia by in situ hybridization. *Blood* 1994;83:1922–1928.
15. Seong DC, Song MY, Henske EP, et al. Analysis of interphase cells for the Philadelphia translocation using painting probe made by inter-Alu-polymerase chain reaction from a radiation hybrid. *Blood* 1994;83:2268–2273.
16. van der Burg M, Poulsen TS, Hunger SP, et al. Split-signal FISH for detection of chromosome aberrations in acute lymphoblastic leukemia. *Leukemia* 2004;18:895–908.
17. Qian X, Jin L, Shearer B, et al. Molecular diagnosis of Ewing's sarcoma/primitive neuroectodermal tumor in formalin-fixed paraffin-embedded tissues by RT-PCR and fluorescence in situ hybridization. *Diagn Mol Pathol* 2005;14:23–28.
18. Garcia-Isidoro M, Tabernero MD, Garcia JL, et al. Detection of the Mbcr/abl translocation in chronic myeloid leukemia by fluorescence in situ hybridization: comparison with conventional cytogenetics and implications for minimal residual disease detection. *Hum Pathol* 1997;28:154–159.
19. Zhao L, Kantarjian HM, Van Oort J, et al. Detection of residual proliferating leukemic cells by fluorescence in situ hybridization in CML patients in complete remission after interferon treatment. *Leukemia* 1993;7:168–71.
20. Stenman J, Lintula S, Hotakainen K, et al. Detection of squamous-cell carcinoma antigen-expressing tumour cells in blood by reverse transcriptase-polymerase chain reaction in cancer of the uterine cervix. *Int J Cancer* 1997;74:75–80.
21. Kelly KM, Womer RB, Barr FG. Minimal disease detection in patients with alveolar rhabdomyosarcoma using a reverse transcriptase-polymerase chain reaction method. *Cancer* 1996;78:1320–1327.
22. Zippelius A, Kufer P, Honold G, et al. Limitations of reverse-transcriptase polymerase chain reaction analyses for detection of micrometastatic epithelial cancer cells in bone marrow. *J Clin Oncol* 1997;15:2701–2708.
23. Bose S, Deininger M, Gora-Tybor J, et al. The presence of typical and atypical BCR-ABL fusion genes in leukocytes of normal individuals: biologic significance and implications for the assessment of minimal residual disease. *Blood* 1998;92:3362–3367.
24. Chong SS, Gore-Langton RE, Hughes MR. Single-cell DNA analysis for application to preimplantation genetic diagnosis. In: Dracopoli NC, Haines JL, Korft BR, et al., eds. *Current Protocols in Human Genetics.* New York: John Wiley & Sons; 1996:9.10.1–9.10.26.
25. Ben-Ezra J, Johnson DA, Rossi J, et al. Effect of fixation on the amplification of nucleic acids from paraffin-embedded material by the polymerase chain reaction. *J Histochem Cytochem* 1991;39:351–354.
26. Foss RD, Guha-Thakurta N, Conran RM, et al. Effects of fixative and fixation time on the extraction and polymerase chain reaction amplification of RNA from paraffin-embedded tissue: Comparison of two housekeeping gene mRNA controls. *Diagn Mol Pathol* 1994;3:148–155.
27. Greer CE, Peterson SL, Kiviat NB, et al. PCR amplification from paraffin-embedded tissues: effects of fixative and fixation time. *Am J Clin Pathol* 1991;95:117–124.
28. Benchekroun M, DeGraw J, Gao J, et al. Impact of fixative on recovery of mRNA from paraffin-embedded tissue. *Diagn Mol Pathol* 2004;13:116–125.
29. Hill DA, O'Sullivan MJ, Zhu X, et al. Practical application of molecular genetic testing as an aid to the surgical pathologic diagnosis of sarcomas: a prospective study. *Am J Surg Pathol* 2002;26:965–977.
30. Ladanyi M, Bridge J. Contribution of molecular genetic data to the classification of sarcomas. *Hum Pathol* 2000;31:532–538.
31. Ivell R. A question of faith: or the philosophy of RNA controls. *J Endocrinol* 1998; 159:197–200.
32. Delattre O, Zucman J, Melot T, et al. The Ewing family of tumors: a subgroup of small-round-cell tumors defined by specific chimeric transcripts. *N Engl J Med* 1994; 331:294–299.
33. Yamamoto N, Kato Y, Yanagisawa A, et al. Predictive value of genetic diagnosis for cancer micrometastasis: histologic and experimental appraisal. *Cancer* 1997;80:1393–1398.
34. Cox MC, Maffei L, Buffolino S, et al. A comparative analysis of FISH, RT-PCR, and cytogenetics for the diagnosis of bcr-abl-positive leukemias. *Am J Clin Pathol* 1998; 109:24–31.
35. Wang YL, Bagg A, Pear W, et al. Chronic myelogenous leukemia: laboratory diagnosis and monitoring. *Genes Chromosomes Cancer* 2001;32:97–111.
36. Knezevich SR, Hendson G, Mathers JA, et al. Absence of detectable EWS/FLI1 expression after therapy-induced neural differentiation in Ewing sarcoma. *Hum Pathol* 1998;29:289–294.
37. Bagg A. Chronic myeloid leukemia: a minimalistic view of post-therapeutic monitoring. *J Mol Diagn* 2002;4:1–10.
38. Ladanyi M. Aberrant ALK tyrosine kinase signaling: different cellular lineages, common oncogenic mechanisms. *Am J Pathol* 2000;157:341–345.
39. Knezevich SR, McFadden DE, Tao W, et al. A novel ETV6-NTRK3 gene fusion in congenital fibrosarcoma. *Nat Genet* 1998;18:184–187.
40. Eguchi M, Eguchi-Ishimae M, Tojo A, et al. Fusion of ETV6 to neurotrophin-3 receptor TRKC in acute myeloid leukemia with t(12;15)(p13;q25). *Blood* 1999;93:1355–1363.
41. Eguchi M, Eguchi-Ishimae M. Absence of t(12;15) associated ETV6-NTRK3 fusion transcripts in pediatric acute leukemias [Letter]. *Med Pediatr Oncol* 2001;37:417.
42. Tognon C, Knezevich SR, Huntsman D, et al. Expression of the ETV6-NTRK3 gene fusion as a primary event in human secretory breast carcinoma. *Cancer Cell* 2002;2:367–376.
43. Lawrence B, Perez-Atayde A, Hibbard MK, et al. TPM3-ALK and TPM4-ALK oncogenes in inflammatory myofibroblastic tumors. *Am J Pathol* 2000;157:377–384.
44. Bridge JA, Kanamori M, Ma Z. Fusion of the ALK gene to the clathrin heavy chain gene, CLTC, in inflammatory myofibroblastic tumor. *Am J Pathol* 2001;159:411–415.
45. Debiec-Rychter M, Marynen P, Hagemeijer A, et al. ALK-ATIC fusion in urinary bladder inflammatory myofibroblastic tumor. *Genes Chromosomes Cancer* 2003;38:187–190.
46. Reading MS, Jenson SD, Smith JK, et al. 5′-(RACE) identification of rare ALK fusion partner in anaplastic large cell lymphoma. *J Mol Diagn* 2003;5:136–140.
47. Liang X, Meech SJ, Odom LF, et al. Assessment of t(2;5)(p23;q35) translocation and variants in pediatric ALK+ anaplastic large cell lymphoma. *Am J Clin Pathol* 2004; 121:496–506.
48. Shing DC, McMullan DJ, Roberts P, et al. FUS/ERG gene fusions in Ewing's tumors. *Cancer Res* 2003;63:4568–4576.

49. Smith JL, Hodges E, Quin CT, et al. Frequent T and B cell oligoclones in histologically and immunophenotypically characterized angioimmunoblastic lymphadenopathy. *Am J Pathol* 2000;156:661–669.
50. Vergier B, Dubus P, Kutschmar A, et al. Combined analysis of T cell receptor gamma and immunoglobulin heavy chain gene rearrangements at the single-cell level in lymphomas with dual genotype. *J Pathol* 2002;198:171–180.
51. de Alava E, Lozano MD, Sola I, et al. Molecular features in a biphenotypic small cell sarcoma with neuroectodermal and muscle differentiation. *Hum Pathol* 1998;29:181–184.
52. Fritsch MK, Bridge JA, Schuster AE. Performance characteristics of a reverse transcriptase-polymerase chain reaction assay for the detection of tumor-specific fusion transcripts from archival tissue. *Pediatr Dev Pathol* 2003;6:43–53.
53. Michor F, Iwasa Y, Nowak MA. Dynamics of cancer progression. *Nat Rev Cancer* 2004;4:197–205.
54. Sandberg AA, Turc-Carel C, Gemmill RM. Chromosomes in solid tumors and beyond. *Cancer Res* 1988;48:1049–1059.
55. Lengauer C, Kinzler KW, Vogelstein B. Genetic instabilities in human cancers. *Nature* 1998;396:643–649.
56. Teixeira MR, Ribeiro FR, Cerveira N, et al. Karyotypic divergence and convergence in two synchronous lung metastases of a clear cell sarcoma of tendons and aponeuroses with t(12;22)(q13;q12) and type 1 EWS/ATF1. *Cancer Genet Cytogenet* 2003;145:121–125.
57. Thorner P. Intra-abdominal polyphenotypic tumor. *Pediatr Pathol Lab Med* 1996;16:161–169.
58. Nowell PC. Mechanisms of tumor progression. *Cancer Res* 1986;46:2203–2207.
59. Biernaux C, Loos M, Sels A, et al. Detection of major *bcr-abl* gene expression at a very low level in blood cells of some healthy individuals. *Blood* 1995;86:3118–3122.
60. Fuscoe JC, Setzer RW, Collard DD, et al. Quantification of t(14;18) in the lymphocytes of healthy adult humans as a possible biomarker for environmental exposures to carcinogens. *Carcinogenesis* 1996;17:1013–1020.
61. Aster JC, Kobayashi Y, Shiota M, et al. Detection of the t(14;18) at similar frequencies in hyperplastic lymphoid tissues from American and Japanese patients. *Am J Pathol* 1992;141:291–299.
62. Summers KE, Goff LK, Wilson AG, et al. Frequency of the Bcl-2/IgH rearrangement in normal individuals: implications for the monitoring of disease in patients with follicular lymphoma. *J Clin Oncol* 2001;19:420–424.
63. Ji W, Qu G, Ye P, et al. Frequent detection of bcl-2/JH translocations in human blood and organ samples by a quantitative polymerase chain reaction assay. *Cancer Res* 1995;55:2876–2882.
64. Limpens J, de Jong D, van Krieken JH, et al. Bcl-2/JH rearrangements in benign lymphoid tissues with follicular hyperplasia. *Oncogene* 1991;6:2271–2276.
65. Molldrem JJ, Lee PP, Wang C, et al. Evidence that specific T lymphocytes may participate in the elimination of chronic myelogenous leukemia. *Nat Med* 2000;6:1018–1023.
66. Bagg A. Commentary: minimal residual disease: how low do we go? *Mol Diagn* 2001; 6:155–160.
67. Nucifora G, Larson RA, Rowley JD. Persistence of the 8;21 translocation in patients with acute myeloid leukemia type M2 in long-term remission. *Blood* 1993;82:712–715.
68. Panagopoulos I, Aman P, Mertens F, et al. Genomic PCR detects tumor cells in peripheral blood from patients with myxoid liposarcoma. *Genes Chromosomes Cancer* 1996; 17:102–107.
69. de Alava E, Lozano MD, Patino A, et al. Ewing family tumors: potential prognostic value of reverse-transcriptase polymerase chain reaction detection of minimal residual disease in peripheral blood samples. *Diagn Mol Pathol* 1998;7:152–157.
70. Fagnou C, Michon J, Peter M, et al. Presence of tumor cells in bone marrow but not in blood is associated with adverse prognosis in patients with Ewing's tumor. Societe Francaise d'Oncologie Pediatrique. *J Clin Oncol* 1998;16:1707–1711.
71. Bostick PJ, Chatterjee S, Chi DD, et al. Limitations of specific reverse-transcriptase polymerase chain reaction markers in the detection of metastases in the lymph nodes and blood of breast cancer patients. *J Clin Oncol* 1998;16:2632–2640.
72. Traweek ST, Liu J, Battifora H. Keratin gene expression in non-epithelial tissues: detection with polymerase chain reaction. *Am J Pathol* 1993;142:1111–1118.
73. Burchill SA, Bradbury MF, Pittman K, et al. Detection of epithelial cancer cells in peripheral blood by reverse transcriptase-polymerase chain reaction. *Br J Cancer* 1995; 71:278–281.
74. Hoon D, Doi F, Giuliano AE, et al. The detection of breast carcinoma micrometastases in axillary lymph nodes by means of reverse transcriptase-polymerase chain reaction. *Cancer* 1995;76:533–535.
75. Novaes M, Bendit I, Garicochea B, et al. Reverse transcriptase-polymerase chain reaction analysis of cytokeratin 19 expression in the peripheral blood mononuclear cells of normal female blood donors. *Mol Pathol* 1997;50:209–211.
76. Krismann M, Todt B, Schroder J, et al. Low specificity of cytokeratin 19 reverse transcriptase-polymerase chain reaction analyses for detection of hematogenous lung cancer dissemination. *J Clin Oncol* 1995;13:2769–2775.
77. Yun K, Gunn J, Merrie AE, et al. Keratin 19 mRNA is detectable by RT-PCR in lymph nodes of patients without breast cancer. *Br J Cancer* 1997;76:1112–1113.
78. Bader BL, Magin TM, Hatzfeld M, et al. Amino acid sequence and gene organization of cytokeratin no. 19, an exceptional tail-less intermediate filament protein. *EMBO J* 1986;5:1865–1875.
79. Savtchenko ES, Schiff TA, Jiang CK, et al. Embryonic expression of the human 40-kD keratin: evidence from a processed pseudogene sequence. *Am J Hum Genet* 1988; 43:630–637.
80. de Graaf H, Maelandsmo GM, Ruud P, et al. Ectopic expression of target genes may represent an inherent limitation of RT-PCR assays used for micrometastasis detection: studies on the epithelial glycoprotein gene EGP-2. *Int J Cancer* 1997;72:191–196.
81. Bustin S, Dorudi S. Molecular assessment of tumour stage and disease recurrence using PCR-based assays. *Mol Med Today* 1998;4:389–396.
82. Liefers GJ, Cleton-Jansen AM, van de Velde CJ, et al. Micrometastases and survival in stage II colorectal cancer. *N Engl J Med* 1998;339:223–228.
83. Merrie AE, Yun K, McCall JL. Re: Detection of carcinoembryonic antigen messenger RNA in lymph nodes from patients with colorectal cancer [Letter]. *N Engl J Med* 1998;339:1642.
84. Ghossein RA. Re: Detection of carcinoembryonic antigen messenger RNA in lymph nodes from patients with colorectal cancer [Letter]. *N Engl J Med* 1998;339:1642.
85. Bostick PJ, Hoon DS, Cote RJ. Re: Detection of carcinoembryonic antigen messenger RNA in lymph nodes from patients with colorectal cancer [Letter]. *N Engl J Med* 1998;339:1642.
86. O'Sullivan MJ, Humphrey PA, Dehner LP, et al. t(X;18) reverse transcriptase-polymerase chain reaction demonstrating a variant transcript. *J Mol Diagn* 2002;4:178–180.
87. Diamond GA. Affirmative actions: can the discriminant accuracy of a test be determined in the face of selection bias? *Med Decis Making* 1991;11:48–56.
88. Begg CB, Greenes RA. Assessment of diagnostic tests when disease verification is subject to selection bias. *Biometrics* 1983;39:207–215.
89. Punglia RS, D'Amico AV, Catalona WJ, et al. Effect of verification bias on screening for prostate cancer by measurement of prostate-specific antigen. *N Engl J Med* 2003; 349:335–342.
90. Quinn TC, Welsh L, Lentz A, et al. Diagnosis by AMPLICOR PCR of *Chlamydia trachomatis* infection in urine samples from women and men attending sexually transmitted disease clinics. *J Clin Microbiol* 1996;34:1401–1406.
91. Smith KR, Ching S, Lee H, et al. Evaluation of ligase chain reaction for use with urine for identification of *Neisseria gonorrhoeae* in females attending a sexually transmitted disease clinic. *J Clin Microbiol* 1995;33:455–457.
92. Tamborini E, Agus V, Perrone F, et al. Lack of SYT-SSX fusion transcripts in malignant peripheral nerve sheath tumors on RT-PCR analysis of 34 archival cases. *Lab Invest* 2002;82:609–618.
93. Naito N, Kawai A, Ouchida M, et al. A reverse transcriptase-polymerase chain reaction assay in the diagnosis of soft tissue sarcomas. *Cancer* 2000;89:1992–1998.
94. Hiraga H, Nojima T, Abe S, et al. Diagnosis of synovial sarcoma with the reverse transcriptase-polymerase chain reaction: analyses of 84 soft tissue and bone tumors. *Diagn Mol Pathol* 1998;7:102–110.
95. Dagher R, Pham TA, Sorbara L, et al. Molecular confirmation of Ewing sarcoma. *J Pediatr Hematol Oncol* 2001;23:221–224.
96. Lipman HB, Astles JR. Quantifying the bias associated with use of discrepant analysis. *Clin Chem* 1998;44:108–115.
97. Hadgu A. The discrepancy in discrepant analysis. *Lancet* 1996;348:592–593.
98. Hadgu A. Discrepant analysis is an inappropriate and unscientific method. *J Clin Microbiol* 2000;38:4301–4302.
99. Miller WC. Bias in discrepant analysis: when two wrongs don't make a right. *J Clin Epidemiol* 1998;51:219–231.
100. Pfeifer JD, Hill DA, O'Sullivan MJ, et al. Diagnostic gold standard for soft tissue tumours: morphology or molecular genetics? *Histopathology* 2000;37:485–500.
101. Chang CC, Snidham VB. Molecular genetics of pediatric soft tissue tumors: clinical application. *J Mol Diagn* 2003;5:143–154.
102. Fletcher CD, Fletcher JA, Cin PD, et al. Diagnostic gold standard for soft tissue tumours: morphology or molecular genetics? [Letter]. *Histopathology* 2001;39:100–103.
103. Ladanyi M, Woodruff JM, Scheithauer BW, et al. Re: Malignant peripheral nerve sheath tumors with t(X;18): a pathologic and molecular genetic study [Letter]. *Mod Pathol* 2001;14:733–735.
104. O'Sullivan MJ, Wick MR, Kyriakos M, et al. Re: Malignant peripheral nerve sheath tumors with t(X;18): a pathologic and molecular genetic study [Letter]. *Mod Pathol* 2001;14:735–737.
105. O'Sullivan MJ, Pfeifer JD, Dehner LP. Re: Lack of SYT-SSX fusion transcripts in malignant peripheral nerve sheath tumors on RT-PCR analysis of 34 archival cases, by Tamborini E., et al. [Letter]. *Lab Invest* 2003;83:301–302.
106. Pilotti S, Tamborini E, Pierotti M. Re: Lack of SYT-SSX fusion transcripts in malignant peripheral nerve sheath tumors on RT-PCR analysis of 34 archival cases, by Tamborini E., et al. [Letter]. *Lab Invest* 2003;83:303.
107. Sandberg AA. "SHOW ME"—Eliza Doolittle in My Fair Lady. *Cancer Genet Cytogenet* 2001;128:93–96.
108. Bourgeois JM, Knezevich SR, Mathers JA, et al. Molecular detection of the *ETV6-NTRK3* gene fusion differentiates congenital fibrosarcoma from other childhood spindle cell tumors. *Am J Surg Pathol* 2000;24:937–946.
109. Agani P, Fritsch MK, Shuster AE, et al. Re: Reduced sensitivity of paraffin-based RT-PCR assays for *ETV6-NTRK3* fusion transcripts in morphologically defined infantile fibrosarcoma [Letter]. *Am J Surg Pathol* 2001;25:1461–1463.
110. Ladanyi M. Re: Translocation-based molecular diagnosis of sarcomas [Letter]. *Am J Surg Pathol* 2003;27:414–415.
111. Sorensen PH, Mathers J. Re: Reduced sensitivity of paraffin-based RT-PCR assays for *ETV6-NTRK3* fusion transcripts in morphologically defined infantile fibrosarcoma [Letter]. *Am J Surg Pathol* 2001;25:1464.
112. Barr FG, Chatten J, D'Cruz CM, et al. Molecular assays for chromosomal translocations in the diagnosis of pediatric soft tissue sarcomas. *JAMA* 1995;273:553–557.
113. Hill DA, Dehner LP, Humphrey PA, et al. Re: Translocation-based molecular diagnosis of sarcomas [Letter]. *Am J Surg Pathol* 2003;27:415–416.
114. Pfeifer JD, Dehner LP, Hill DA, et al. Re: Diagnostic gold standard for soft tissue tumours: morphology or molecular genetics? [Letter]. *Histopathology* 2001;39:101–103.
115. de Alava E. Transcripts, transcripts, everywhere. *Adv Anat Pathol* 2001;8:264–272.
116. Barr FG, Qualman SJ, Macris MH, et al. Genetic heterogeneity in the alveolar rhabdomyosarcoma subset without typical gene fusions. *Cancer Res* 2002;62:4704–4710.
117. Ransohoff DF. Challenges and opportunities in evaluating diagnostic tests. *J Clin Epidemiol* 2002;55:1178–1182.
118. Deyo RA, Jarvik JJ. New diagnostic tests: breakthrough approaches or expensive addons? *Ann Intern Med* 2003;139:950–951.
119. Reid MC, Lachs MS, Feinstein AR. Use of methodological standards in diagnostic test research: getting better but still not good. *JAMA* 1995;274:645–651.
120. Sackett DL, Haynes RB. The architecture of diagnostic research. *Br Med J* 2002; 324:539–541.
121. Bossuyt PM, Reitsma JB, Bruns DE, et al. Towards complete and accurate reporting of studies of diagnostic accuracy: the STARD initiative. *Ann Intern Med* 2003;138:40–44.
122. Bossuyt PM, Reitsma JB, Bruns DE, et al. The STARD statement for reporting studies of diagnostic accuracy: explanation and elaboration. *Ann Intern Med* 2003;138:W1–12.

Microarrays

Mark A. Watson

9

MICROARRAY TECHNOLOGY

In simplest terms, a microarray can be defined as ordered arrangement of a large number of objects in two- or three-dimensional space. Each object is referred to as a feature. Depending upon the type of microarray, a feature may range in size from an 800-μ-diameter tissue spot to a 5-μ-square area containing a single oligonucleotide sequence. Microarrays themselves are usually flat surfaces that range in size from 2 × 5 cm (e.g., a conventional glass microscope slide) to less than 1 cm square. Therefore, depending upon the microarray design, several hundred to over 1 million unique features may be represented on the array surface. For biomedical applications, microarrays may be conceptualized in two major categories (Fig. 9.1). In the first category, a large number of patient biospecimens are arranged in a grid and then assayed using a single biomarker probe, such as an antibody. Tissue microarrays are the most common application of this type (1,2). This class of specimen or reverse-phase microarray represents a powerful tool for performing clinical correlative studies that validate novel biomarkers on a large number of individual samples (3,4), but has limited application in a diagnostic laboratory and will not be discussed further. The second category of microarray uses an ordered arrangement of hundreds or thousands of biomarker probes upon which a single patient biospecimen is assayed. These forward-phase or probe microarrays will be the focus of this chapter. Although the most common form of probe microarray uses nucleic acid (usually DNA), it is important to note that antibody arrays are also a useful tool for simultaneously measuring the quantity of multiple proteins in a patient sample. Although they will not be discussed further in this chapter, several comprehensive reviews exist on the emerging technology of antibody arrays (5,6).

The power of nucleic acid microarray technology has been harnessed primarily for basic science studies that involve whole genome analyses to identify novel biomarkers or elucidate biologic signaling pathways. However, as this technology continues to mature, nucleic acid microarrays are now being used as a clinical diagnostic platform. This chapter will review basic principles of nucleic acid microarray fabrication, utilization, and data analysis. Results from clinical correlative studies to date will be highlighted, and the future of microarray technology in diagnostic clinical pathology will be discussed.

NUCLEIC ACID MICROARRAYS

Nucleic acid microarrays involve the ordered arrangement of DNA molecules (probes) on a solid surface. A sample of patient DNA or RNA (target) is then hybridized to the array to quantify the level of nucleic acid corresponding to each probe. The type and source of DNA probes on the microarray can vary, depending upon the intended application (Fig. 9.2). Bacterial artificial chromosome (BAC) arrays are composed of individual BAC clones that are deposited onto a solid surface (7,8). Each BAC clone generally represents a large stretch of genomic DNA from a specific chromosomal region, several megabases in length. As discussed below, BAC arrays have been particularly useful in assessing genomewide DNA copy number changes in tumor specimens and have enhanced the resolution of traditional cytogenetic studies using the array comparative genomic hybridization (aCGH) approach.

Some of the earliest microarray designs utilized cDNA probes (9,10). In this approach, messenger RNA from a defined tissue or cell source is converted into double-stranded cDNA. The cDNAs are transformed into a library of plasmids, where a single clone harbors a single cDNA, which in turn is derived from a single RNA. Plasmid DNA from each clone is then spotted onto the microarray surface. cDNA-based microarrays offer two major advantages over other array designs. First, genome sequence information is not required to fabricate the microarray. This is particularly

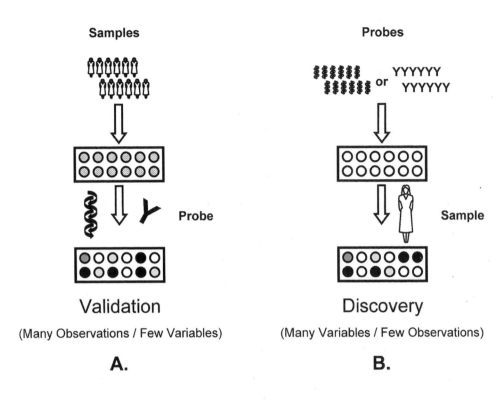

Samples

Probes

or

Probe

Sample

Validation

(Many Observations / Few Variables)

A.

Discovery

(Many Variables / Few Observations)

B.

Figure 9.1 Microarray applications. Sample, or reverse phase, microarrays **(A)** contain a large number of study samples, such as tissue cores, to which a single biomarker probe (nucleic acid or antibody) is applied. These arrays are excellent tools for biomarker validation. Probe, or forward-phase, microarrays **(B)** contain a large number of biomarker probes such as antibodies or nucleic acid sequences to which a single study sample is applied. They are generally used as biomarker discovery tools, but are also most applicable to the clinical laboratory.

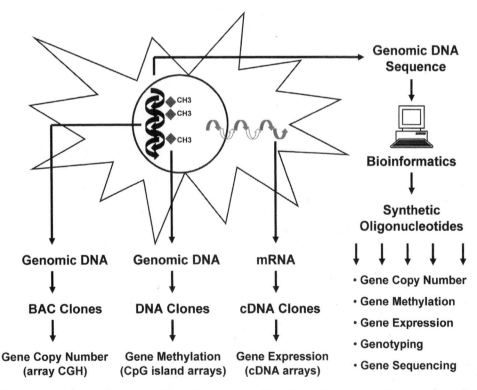

Genomic DNA Sequence

Bioinformatics

Synthetic Oligonucleotides

- Gene Copy Number
- Gene Methylation
- Gene Expression
- Genotyping
- Gene Sequencing

Genomic DNA

Genomic DNA

mRNA

BAC Clones

DNA Clones

cDNA Clones

Gene Copy Number (array CGH)

Gene Methylation (CpG island arrays)

Gene Expression (cDNA arrays)

Figure 9.2 Approaches to nucleic acid microarray fabrication. Molecular constituents of a cell (genomic DNA or mRNA) may be isolated and cloned (bacterial artificial chromosome [BAC] clones, DNA clones, cDNA clones). Libraries of clones are then spotted as probes onto the microarray surface to be used for genome copy number assessment (array comparative genomic hybridization [CGH]), DNA methylation analysis (CpG island arrays), or gene expression profiling (cDNA arrays). Alternatively, genome sequence information may be used with bioinformatics algorithms to design and synthesis oligonucleotides that may be spotted or synthesized directly on the array surface. Oligonucleotide probes may be used to perform a wide variety of microarray-based genomic assays. (See color insert.)

advantageous for studying experimental organisms where highly annotated genome sequence information is not available. Given the current quality and completeness of the human genome sequence, however, this is not a particular advantage for the design of diagnostic microarrays. A second advantage of cDNA microarrays is that they can be purposefully biased toward assaying for gene transcripts that are known to be expressed in a cell or tissue type of interest. For example, early efforts to develop a diagnostic lymphoma microarray ("lymphochip") used cDNAs obtained from a set of lymphocyte cell sources (11,12). This approach ensured that genes expressed by lymphoid cells and tissues, and hence potentially most diagnostic for lymphoid malignancies, would be adequately represented on the microarray. Again, however, an increasingly annotated human genome has now made this approach somewhat unnecessary, because genes with known functional attributes or disease-associations can be selected and represented as oligonucleotide sequence probes on the microarray (13,14). Because cDNA probes correspond to relatively long stretches of transcribed mRNA, often containing homologous sequences between gene family members, cross-hybridization and lack of specificity often can limit the accuracy of cDNA microarray results. The ability to assess subtle changes in transcriptional splicing patterns is also not possible using cDNA probes, because individual gene exons cannot be represented in the assay. Similarly, cDNA probes (often 400 to 2,000 nucleotides in length) do not have sufficient specificity to distinguish single nucleotide changes, such as might be sought in genotyping or sequencing assays (see later discussion). Finally, the effort and management infrastructure necessary to store, grow, purify, quality control, and track individual cDNA clones is considerable and not easily standardized. It is perhaps this last constraint that has and will continue to limit the use of cDNA microarrays as clinical diagnostic tools.

In recent years, design of nucleic acid microarrays has shifted toward the use of synthetic oligonucleotide probes. Two main factors have influenced this change. First, particularly for human diagnostic applications, a completely sequenced and annotated human genome has allowed investigators to specify probes for specific genes, gene transcripts, or gene transcript segments using absolute, defined nucleic acid sequences. This has been aided by sophisticated bioinformatics programs that can select optimized oligonucleotide sequences for any gene or transcript of interest while minimizing cross-reactivity with other sequences and standardizing hybridization properties such as melting temperature and G/C sequence content (15). The nucleic acid chemistry associated with oligonucleotide synthesis has also become increasingly more efficient and less expensive. The ability to generate large quantities of nucleic acid oligomers that are 60 to 70 nucleotides in length at the cost of only several dollars per oligonucleotide has resulted in standardized libraries of 20,000 to 40,000 probe sequences that can be commercially prepared and rapidly utilized for array construction (16,17). Oligonucleotides have provided a new level of standardization and flexibility to the design of sequence content on nucleic acid microarrays and for this reason are aptly suited for clinical diagnostic assays.

The use of oligonucleotide probes has also provided flexibility in the way in which nucleic acid microarrays are

constructed. There are two major approaches to microarray design. Spotted microarrays involve the "off-site" production of nucleic acid (e.g., BAC clones, cDNA clones, or oligonucleotides) followed by the deposition of the nucleic acid onto the microarray surface (10,18). In some applications, robotic units equipped with metallic quills or pins are used to collect nanoliter quantities of nucleic acid solution from a source plate and deposit it upon the surface of a specially treated glass microscope slide. Technical advances have enhanced the speed and uniformity with which material can be spotted to the microarray surface. Although many research core facilities continue to rely on spotted microarray technology because of the relatively low "per array" production cost (generally $25 to $200 per array), this approach is still plagued by sporadic mechanical failures and nonuniform probe deposition (Fig. 9.3).

Several proprietary alternatives have been developed to create spotted microarrays (19). For example, Agilent has utilized its ink-jet printer technology to spray oligonucleotides

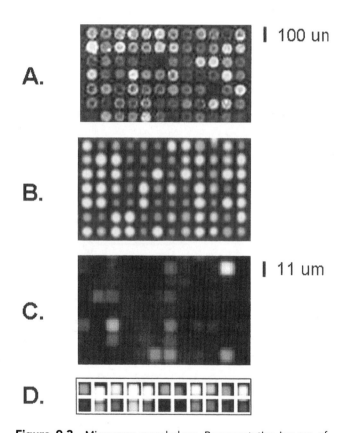

Figure 9.3 Microarray morphology. Representative images of scanned nucleic acid gene expression microarrays are shown. **(A)** Image from two-color spotted microarray. Independent red and green signals reflect the hybridization intensities of the two different target samples. Note the extensive nonuniformity ("doughnut holes") associated with the pin-based spotting process. **(B)** Image from two-color Agilent ink-jet array, demonstrating greater uniformity of hybridization intensity across each feature. **(C)** Image from Affymetrix single-color GeneChip microarray. Note the regular, grid-shaped hybridization feature pattern that reflects the mask-based in situ synthesis of oligonucleotides using photolithography. **(D)** In the GeneChip technology platform, 11 pairs of features that are randomly distributed across the array are electronically aggregated. The composite single of 11 probes and 11 negative control (mismatch) probes are used to generate a single intensity value for a transcript. (See color insert.)

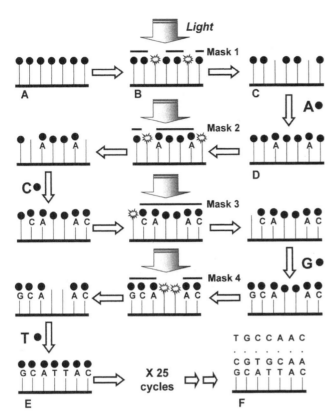

Figure 9.4 Schema for in situ oligonucleotide microarray synthesis. Photochemical sites on a solid phase **(A)** are selectively activated by shining light through a patterned mask or grid **(B)**. A photoreactive nucleotide is added to the surface **(C)**, which is covalently bound to each activated site **(D)**. This cycle is repeated four times with four independent masks for each possible nucleotide (A, C, G, T), until every site on the array is occupied **(E)**. The entire cycle of four can then be repeated with four new sets of masks to build a unique oligonucleotide sequence at every position on the array **(F)**. Depending upon the technology used, each address on the array may be as small as 11 μ^2. Using this scheme, 25 sets of masks could be used to build 1×10^{15} unique sequences while 9×10^6 of these sequences could be arranged within a single 1 cm^2 microarray.

array surface in the presence of each mask. Depending upon the mask pattern, a specific nucleotide is added to the growing chain of oligonucleotides at a specific position. In this combinatorial method, the use of 25 different masks sets (A, C, G, T) in 100 sequential nucleotide addition steps can result in 4^{25} (1×10^{15}) different sequences that are simultaneously created on the array surface. This is more than sufficient to represent every nucleotide in the human genome (3×10^9 nucleotides) as a unique probe sequence on the array surface. Because of the limited efficiency of each synthesis step and the inherent expense of each mask set, however, oligonucleotides fabricated on this platform are limited to 25 nucleotides in length. Because a single 25 nucleotide sequence has insufficient specificity for a single nucleic acid target, the GeneChip uses a collection of 22 probe sequences to interrogate a single genetic locus (Fig. 9.3). An alternative, "maskless" approach to in situ probe synthesis has also been developed (26). Using this technology, a sheet composed of micron-scale electronic mirrors can be programmed to direct light to specific areas of the microarray during sequential steps of photochemical oligonucleotide synthesis. The method is similar to GeneChip fabrication, but does not rely on the creation of fixed lithographic masks and therefore allows for flexible design on a single array basis.

Although methods for microarray fabrication will continue to evolve in a manner following Moore's Law (a tenet from the semi-conductor industry that states that technology will continually create increasing computing power in a smaller space for decreasing cost), one design consideration now seems well established—that defined oligonucleotide sequences provide the most flexible, standardized assay format for both sensitivity and reproducibility. With the eventual capability of routinely synthesizing and scanning nucleic acid microarrays with feature sizes as small as 1 μ^2, it will be possible to represent as many as 4×10^8 unique sequences on a conventional 2-cm^2 microarray surface. As discussed later in this chapter, this technical advance will allow for whole genome resequncing and genotyping of clinical samples using sequence tiling arrays.

SAMPLE REQUIREMENTS

Because of the inherent complexity of microarray-based assays, specimen quality and corresponding quality assurance are essential. The requisite quality of pathology specimens for microarray analysis depends, in part, on the target analyte. For example, DNA-based assays for copy number, sequencing, or methylation analysis may be more tolerant of sample degradation than RNA-based gene expression microarray assays.

Generally, diagnostic surgical pathology tissue specimens are subjected to crosslinking (e.g., formalin) fixative solutions and paraffin embedding. This process results in chemical crosslinking and degradation of nucleic acid (27,28). Using appropriate protocols (29–31), DNA extracted from formalin-fixed, paraffin embedded (FFPE) tissue can certainly be used for PCR assays, but also may be suitable for microarray-based DNA analysis if sufficient quantities of DNA are available (32,33). Despite improved protocols for the isolation of RNA from FFPE tissue (34,35), such RNA is still significantly degraded (Fig. 9.5).

onto a microarray surface (20), resulting in high-throughput microarray fabrication with more uniform features (Fig. 9.3). Other vendors have utilized electronically addressable microarrays, which allow customizable arrangement of probes (21). One of the newer and perhaps most innovative approaches to microarray design involves the use of microarray beads (22). In this approach, micron-sized beads, each containing a unique oligonucleotide gene sequence in tandem with a unique nucleotide address sequence, are allowed to randomly assemble onto a solid surface. By repeated interrogation of each bead address sequence, the identity of each bead at each position is deduced. The "decoded" array can then be used for its intended assay (23).

Another strategy for microarray design involves simultaneously synthesizing specific oligonucleotide probes in situ using combinatorial photochemistry. This method was pioneered by Affymetrix for the design of their GeneChip microarrays (24,25). In this method (Fig. 9.4), a series of micron-scale "masks" are used to direct light to specific locations on the microarray surface. Photoreactive nucleotides (A, C, G, T) are sequentially passed over the

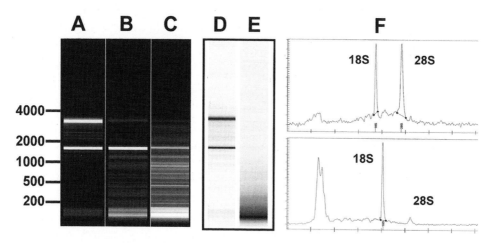

Figure 9.5 Assessment of RNA quality for microarray experiments. Pseudo-electrophoretogram images of RNA samples derived from differentially processed clinical tissue specimens. RNA was analyzed using the Agilent Technologies, "Lab-On-A-Chip" RNA microelectrophoresis system. High-quality RNA derived from freshly snap-frozen tissue (**A** and **D**) is indicated by sharp 28S and 18S ribosomal RNA bands in an intensity ratio of approximately 2:1 and the absence of low molecular weight nucleic acid. Slightly degraded RNA prepared from tissue fixed in 70% ethanol for 14 hours (**B**) demonstrates a relative decrease in 28S ribosomal RNA band intensity and the appearance of low molecular weight RNA fragments. Highly degraded RNA isolated from ethanol-fixed and paraffin-embedded tissue blocks (**C**) is characterized by a low molecular weight smear and the complete absence of detectable, full-length ribosomal RNA. Although RNA derived from ethanol-fixed, paraffin-embedded tissue is more degraded than that obtained from snap-frozen tissue, it still maintains a much higher median molecular weight than RNA isolated from archived, formalin-fixed, paraffin-embedded tissue blocks (**E**). **F**, in chromatographic plots of RNA samples in lanes **A (top)** and **C (bottom)**, the intensity of nucleic acid signal is plotted as a function of migration time, from fastest (smallest) to slowest (largest) nucleic acid fragments. Note the decrease in 28S ribosomal RNA intensity and increase in fragmented RNA that corresponds with the sample in lane **C**. Molecular weight markers (in base pairs) are indicated at left.

With rare exceptions (36), most investigators have found RNA derived from FFPE tissue to be unsuitable for traditional gene expression microarray-based assays.

For experimental studies, freshly procured, snap-frozen biospecimens remain the gold standard sample for microarray analysis, particularly for RNA-based gene expression assays. When properly processed, both DNA and RNA derived from such specimens are of the highest possible quality (Fig. 9.5). In a routine clinical environment, however, fresh-frozen specimens may not be so easy to procure. Many clinical centers may not have access to liquid nitrogen, dry ice, ultra-low freezers, or other resources needed for the processing and storage of frozen samples. For many organ sites, frozen tissue histology is vastly inferior to that of routinely fixed and embedded specimens and, therefore, when the diagnostic specimen is limiting or required in its entirety for accurate diagnosis (e.g., primary malignant melanoma) and the acquisition of frozen tissue specimens is not possible. It is also possible that a microarray-based analysis of a clinical specimen is requested retrospectively, long after all available specimen has been fixed and embedded.

In the context of research studies, a number of solutions have been proposed to circumvent the limited availability of fresh-frozen biospecimens for microarray analysis (37–39). One proposal involves abandoning the use of traditional crosslinking fixatives in exchange for more "molecularly friendly" precipitating fixatives such as ethanol or acetone derivatives (40–42). In general, these precipitating fixatives, coupled with low-temperature embedding techniques (43), result in more highly preserved DNA and RNA (Fig. 9.5). Although the histological detail achievable with such protocols is apparently comparable to that obtained from routine tissue processing (38), it is unlikely that decades of institutionalized standard operating procedures in clinical laboratories will be rapidly and universally replaced by these newer, less tested approaches. In cases in which fresh tissue is available, but there is no means for preservation by freezing, novel molecular fixatives have been created and are continually under development that allow for the preservation of nucleic acid in clinical specimens at ambient temperature (39,44,45). These reagents have performed well in research studies (46,47) and are rapidly making their way into the clinical laboratory. This advance should enable routine prospective analysis of clinical specimens collected at small clinical centers for RNA- or DNA-based microarray assays.

In addition to the actual specimen source required for microarray analysis, careful consideration must also be given to specimen collection and processing. Although DNA and DNA methylation patterns are relatively stable and probably less sensitive to environmental conditions, the same is not true for mRNA populations that may be the target of microarray-based gene expression profile assays. For example, global changes in gene expression may occur in tissue biospecimens as a result of tissue warm ischemia time (48–50). Therefore, artificial differences in gene expression patterns may be seen between specimens based on collection procedures rather than important clinical differences (Fig. 9.6). For peripheral blood and bone marrow

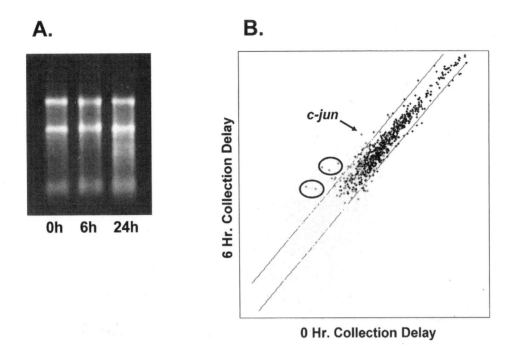

Figure 9.6 Specimen processing and microarray data results. In this experiment, three biopsies from nonmalignant splenic tissue were either snap-frozen immediately after surgical removal (0 hr) or stored in normal saline solution for 6 hours or 24 hours before freezing. RNA was isolated from each of the three specimens and analyzed by conventional agarose gel electrophoresis **(A)** and ethidium bromide staining. Based on ribosomal RNA band intensity, RNA derived from snap-frozen tissue or tissue maintained in saline at room temperature appear equally intact, whereas tissue maintained at room temperature for 24 hours shows evidence of slight RNA degradation. RNAs from 0-hour and 6-hour time points were then subjected to gene expression profiling using Affymetrix GeneChip microarrays. Expression values of ~1,500 transcripts are represented as a scatter plot **(B)**, where level of transcript expression in the snap-frozen sample is plotted on the x-axis and corresponding transcript levels in the 6-hour sample are plotted on the y-axis. Note that blue diagonal lines denote the limits of ± two-fold change between samples. Gray points represent transcripts that were undetected in either sample. Black points correspond to transcripts that were detected in both samples; red points denote transcripts whose expression was detected in one sample but not the other. Although the majority of gene transcript levels remained unchanged between the 0-hour and 6-hour samples, several transcripts (e.g., c-jun) demonstrate greater than two-fold differences in expression between tissue specimens that have been frozen after differing warm ischemia times. (See color insert.)

specimens, the method in which a specimen is collected and processed (e.g., frozen whole blood, molecularly preserved whole blood, Ficoll-enriched buffy coat, flow cytometry fractionated cell population) can also influence gene expression signatures (51,52). Finally, most tissue specimens are inherently heterogeneous collections of many cell types. Variable cellular composition between tissue specimens may lead to differences in genomic and transcriptional profiles based upon microarray assay data. For example, two prostate "tumor" samples, one of which contains 5% neoplastic cellularity and a second that contains 70% neoplastic cellularity, may demonstrate two different gene expression signatures, not based on biologic or clinical differences between the specimens, but simply based on the content of neoplastic epithelial cells present in the tissue. Similarly, measurement of a tumor-associated change in DNA copy number will vary considerably depending upon whether 5% or 70% of the tissue specimen contains tumor cells. For this reason, many investigators have sought to use techniques such as laser microdissection (53,54) to isolate more homogeneous cell populations for both gene expression and DNA copy number microarray analysis (55,56).

Overall, the specimen requirements discussed above are usually possible in the context of a relatively limited and controlled research investigation setting. In the environment of routine pathology practice, however, such control over specimen quality may not always be possible. Therefore, as microarray technology enters the medical laboratory, assays will need to be sufficiently robust to perform well on specimens that are processed in uncontrolled circumstances (57). As discussed later in this chapter, this is perhaps the key contingency for adopting microarray technology into clinical practice.

MICROARRAY ASSAYS

Figure 9.7 outlines the procedural steps involved in a typical gene expression–based microarray assay. Assays for DNA-based microarrays share many similarities. In some of the earliest and simplest protocols, RNA derived from a tissue or cell specimen is converted into cDNA in the presence of labeled deoxynucleotides. The labeled cDNA target is then hybridized to the microarray for a period of 12 to 24 hours under fixed temperature and buffer conditions.

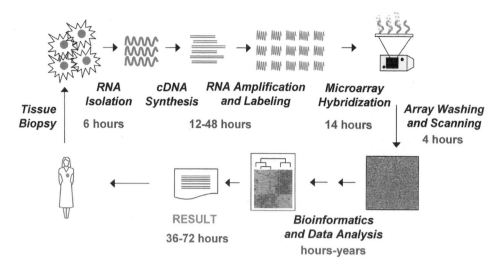

Figure 9.7   Outline of a gene expression microarray experiment. The experimental steps involved in performing a gene expression profiling experiment are outlined, along with estimates of time required for each step in the process, from patient biopsy to end results. If a prevalidated microarray-based assay is being used for clinical diagnostics, data analysis may require only several minutes to 1 hour to complete. Otherwise, as described in the text, data analysis of research studies for biomarker discovery may require months or years to complete and validate. (See color insert.)

Much like other hybridization assays (Chapter 6), the microarray is washed to remove non–specifically bound target and specifically bound target is detected by signal emission from the label. The intensity of the signal emission is proportional to mass of target bound to the specific microarray probe, which in turn is proportional to the level of corresponding mRNA transcript present in the original specimen.

Although RNA can be directly converted to labeled cDNA and hybridized to the microarray, this simple approach has a serious technical disadvantage. Because messenger RNA represents only 5% to 10% of the total cellular RNA content, large quantities of RNA are required for target synthesis, sometimes as much as 50 mcg of total RNA or 2 mcg of polyadenylated-enriched mRNA. This requirement generally precludes the analysis of clinical specimens containing small amounts of cellular material, such as diagnostic core or needle aspiration biopsies. For this reason, most protocols for microarray target synthesis now employ some method of molecular amplification.

Traditionally, the polymerase chain reaction (PCR) is used to quantitatively amplify specific gene targets in DNA or RNA (Chapter 5). However, when used to nonspecifically amplify an entire population of transcripts, PCR methods can create biased amplification products, resulting in under-representation or over-representation of specific transcripts and a distortion of the original mRNA population. More recently, modifications to PCR protocols have achieved unbiased amplification of mRNA transcript pools, allowing the generation of labeled targets from the mRNA population of a single cell (58,59). Another approach for mRNA amplification has involved the use of a proprietary isothermal polymerization procedure to create single-stranded DNA amplicons from RNA templates (60). This approach has the advantage of being simple,

rapid, and scalable and is therefore very attractive for use in diagnostic clinical laboratories.

To date, however, the most widely employed and extensively validated method for mRNA transcript amplification for microarray assays involves the use of T7 RNA polymerase, as originally described by VanGelder et al. (61,62). In this approach (Fig. 9.8), sample mRNA is converted into double-stranded cDNA using a poly-T oligomer to which is added a T7 RNA polymerase priming site. The cDNA created from each initial mRNA contains a T7 RNA polymerase promoter site, which, in the presence of T7 RNA polymerase, can be used to in vitro transcribe thousands of copies of synthetic RNA from each individual cDNA. This amplified, antisense, or complementary RNA (aRNA or cRNA) can then be used as a substrate for labeling or an additional round of linear amplification. Because a theoretical amplification of 1,000-fold can be achieved with each round of synthesis, 1 to 5 mcg of total cellular RNA (approximately 50 to 250 ng of mRNA) can generate sufficient target for hybridization using a single round of amplification, whereas two successive rounds of amplification can generate labeled target from as little as 1 to 5 ng of starting total cellular RNA (62–64).

For microarray assays that involve the use of genomic DNA targets, similar whole genome amplification (WGA) strategies have been developed (65–68). Most recently, isothermal amplification of genomic DNA using the Phi129 DNA polymerase has been used to generate targets for microarray-based copy number analysis (69). This method, as outlined in Figure 9.8, produces relatively uniform amplification of the entire genome from nanogram quantities of starting genomic DNA (70) and has sufficient sequence replication fidelity to allow accurate sequence analysis of amplified material (71). As discussed above, the need to dissect homogeneous cell subpopulations from

A.

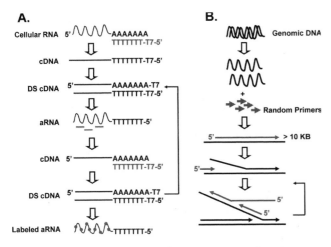

Figure 9.8 Nucleic acid amplification strategies for microarray analysis. In amplifying small quantities of mRNA for gene expression microarray analysis **(A)**, cellular RNA is converted into first-strand cDNA using an oligo-dT/T7 RNA polymerase promoter primer and double-stranded (DS) cDNA is then made using a standard Gubler-Hoffman synthesis protocol. The resulting cDNA template is used for in vitro transcription to generate cRNA. Amplified cRNA is converted back into first-strand cDNA using random primers and then into double-stranded DNA using the dT/T7 primer. The amplified cDNA can be used again for in vitro transcription to generate labeled cRNA target for microarray hybridization. Alternatively, another round of transcript amplification may be performed. For whole genome amplification (WGA) using strand-displacing Phi29 DNA polymerase **(B)**, genomic DNA is denatured and annealed to random primers. In the presence of Phi29 polymerase and dNTPs, primers are extended along the denatured, single-stranded DNA template for at least 10 kb. Subsequent primers can bind again to single-stranded DNA, displace the first synthesized strand, and generate additional single-stranded DNA copies. In the meantime, single-stranded DNA copies that are generated from template genomic DNA can themselves serve as templates for additional priming and polymerization in the opposite direction. This process continues in a linear and isothermal manner until reagents (primers, dNTPs, enzyme activity) are exhausted or the reaction is halted. Amplified, single-stranded genomic fragments can then be labeled for microarray hybridization using a wide variety of techniques. (See color insert.)

histologically complex tissues for array-based genomic analysis will undoubtedly require robust amplification strategies such as this for the preparation of clinical samples.

After amplification, the nucleic acid target must be labeled before hybridization to the microarray. Radioactive nucleotides were some of the first labels employed for detecting microarray hybridization events, drawing from their extensive use in blot hybridization procedures (Chapter 6). However, because of their relative inconvenience, safety concerns (particularly for a clinical laboratory), limited spatial resolution, and single emission signal, radionucleotides have been largely abandoned in favor of fluorescently labeled molecules. Target samples may be labeled directly or indirectly with fluorescent moieties (72–79). For example, nucleotide derivatives containing the fluorescent molecules Cy3 or Cy5 can be incorporated during target synthesis. Each fluorescent dye has its own unique absorption and emission spectrum, thus allowing more than one target sample to be hybridized to a microarray simultaneously. However, because each dye is an integral

part of the nucleotide molecule, incorporation rates for Cy3 and Cy5 into the synthesized target can vary, thus creating different specific activities of samples labeled with different dyes (80). Fluorescent dyes are also unstable, being sensitive to both photobleaching and chemical degradation. Therefore, once labeled targets are created, they have a limited half-life. An alternative strategy involves the incorporation of a single, nonfluorescent moiety into the synthesized target. Aminoallyl derivatives of nucleotides are available that demonstrate high incorporation rates (79). Biotinylated nucleotides can be used as well (72). Once target is synthesized, samples can be independently modified to accept Cy3, Cy5, or other fluorescent labels. Biotinylated targets can actually be conjugated to streptavidin fluorophores after hybridization to the microarray. These indirect labeling procedures prevent bias associated with incorporating different fluorescent molecules during target synthesis and allow unlabeled targets to be created and stored for long periods (months to years) before being labeled and hybridized to the microarray assay.

The final steps of a microarray assay—hybridization, washing, and detection—are very similar to those employed for other membrane hybridization assays (Chapter 6). Labeled target samples (either single-stranded DNA or RNA) are added to a hybridization solution optimized to enhance hybridization kinetics and minimize nonspecific binding to the array surface. The hybridization "cocktail" (usually 100 to 500 μL in volume) is briefly heated to denature nucleic acid and then applied to the microarray, where it is circulated over the microarray surface for 12 to 18 hours at a fixed temperature. After hybridization, the microarray is washed in solutions of defined ionic strength and temperature to remove nonspecifically bound target. Microarray washing can be accomplished manually, as in other membrane-based hybridization assays, or can be carried out in highly automated, programmatically controlled fluidics units, such as utilized in the Affymetrix GeneChip microarray platform. A particular constraint of microarray assays is that hybridization and washing conditions must be simultaneously optimized for thousands of different target/probe hybridization events. This is generally achievable using bioinformatic sequence design programs to create specific oligonucleotide sets with relatively uniform hybridization characteristics (15). The use of cloned cDNA and BAC probes with variable length and sequence content, however, is much more problematic and again illustrates the advantage of oligonucleotide-based microarray designs.

There are generally two assay formats for microarray hybridization: one channel and two channel assays (Fig. 9.3). In single-channel assays, a single target sample is hybridized to the microarray and hybridization intensity is detected via a single fluorophore. Signal intensities between multiple samples and (optionally) a reference sample are compared electronically using various interassay normalization procedures (see later discussion). In two-channel assays, two target samples, each labeled with a different fluorophore, are simultaneously hybridized to the microarray. The signal intensities of each sample (usually the experimental sample and a reference sample) are measured sequentially using different excitation frequencies, and the relative intensities from the two signals are expressed as a ratio. The major advantage of two-color assays is that two samples can be analyzed simultaneously on the same microarray. This not only decreases the cost of the assay, but is convenient for assays that measure relative expression directly between two samples (e.g., a pretreatment sample and a post-treatment sample from the same patient). However, when each experimental sample is paired with its own reference sample, this advantage of two-color arrays over single color arrays is no longer realized.

The entire microarray analysis procedure, from RNA isolation and quality review to target preparation and array hybridization, can realistically require 3 to 5 days to complete under the best possible circumstances (Fig. 9.7). Although advances in RNA isolation and target preparation chemistries may decrease assay turnaround time to some extent (60), for the purposes of clinical diagnostics, it should be emphasized that microarray assays are still considerably more complex and time consuming than other gene-targeted, PCR-based assay formats.

MICROARRAY DATA ANALYSIS AND VALIDATION

Perhaps the greatest challenge to investigators using microarray technology is not generating data, but rather analyzing it. Traditionally, microarrays have been used as discovery tools and hypothesis generation engines. In a diagnostic setting, microarray data analysis is likely to present somewhat different challenges. In this section, steps and considerations for microarray data analysis, both in an investigative and diagnostic environment, are reviewed. Although this chapter will focus on analysis of gene expression microarray data, similar tools and techniques have become increasingly available for analysis of data generated for array comparative genomic hybridization (CGH) (copy number assessment) and array genotyping data. Principal steps in microarray data analysis involve data collection and storage, image analysis and feature extraction, data conditioning, statistical analysis, and biologic interpretation.

Current microarray technology allows for laser scanning of several square centimeters of microarray surface at the resolution of several micron-sized image elements. The result is a primary image data file that can be hundreds of megabytes in size. Storage, transfer, and manipulation of microarray image data requires considerable computer infrastructure. Although a variety of software solutions and data repositories have been developed to hold and distribute experimental microarray data (81,82), regulatory issues related to storage and transfer of data in a clinical setting have yet to be addressed (83).

The first step in microarray analysis involves the conversion of raw, pixilated images into numerical values that relate to hybridization signal intensity at each feature (probe). Because the pixilated image is not uniform over the entire feature (Fig. 9.3), this step involves data averaging and smoothing algorithms. For two-color arrays, the fluorescence intensity must be sequentially captured and analyzed for each emission spectra at each feature (84). In most gene expression microarray platforms, a single probe (e.g., a cDNA or long oligonucleotide) represents a single

transcript. In other microarray platforms such as the Affymetrix GeneChip, however, multiple probes are used to assay for a single transcript. For this reason, the signal from multiple different probes must be integrated to create a single, averaged intensity value for the represented transcript (85). Because of the widespread use of the Affymetrix platform, several different algorithms have been developed to translate raw hybridization data into gene expression values (86–88). Using a standardized gene expression data set, the sensitivity and specificity of each of these algorithms to detected known changes in transcript copy number between samples has been calculated and discussed at length (89).

Once image data have been converted into numerical values for each probe or probe set represented on the array, the composite set of data is usually normalized to a reference point, to allow for comparison between sets of array data (Fig. 9.9). For example, interarray normalization algorithms compensate for global differences in the signal intensity of arrays. If gene X has a signal intensity of 500 on array 1, with a total average intensity of 1,000, and gene X has a signal intensity of 1,000 on array 2, with a total average intensity of 2,000, interarray normalization would correct signal intensities for gene X so that expression appeared equivalent between array 1 and array 2. Intergene normalization algorithms are useful for identifying common patterns of gene expression between study samples, even when absolute gene expression values are considerably different. One common transformation technique is

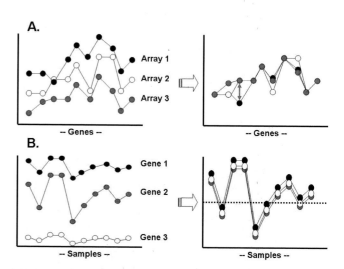

Figure 9.9 Microarray data normalization. **(A)** To compare patterns of gene expression (or gene copy number) across multiple microarrays, each associated with differing overall intensity as a result of technical variability, data may be normalized across arrays (samples). The effect of the interarray normalization process (*arrow*) is to make all data sets comparable so that true biologic changes in gene expression between samples (*green arrow*) can be appreciated. **(B)** To compare patterns of gene expression between different genes, where the absolute level of gene expression may be quite different, data for a given gene may be normalized across samples. The effect of the intergene normalization process (*arrow*) is to make all genes comparable by transforming their expression level relative to a mean (*dotted line*), so that similar patterns of gene expression can be identified across samples, irrespective of absolute hybridization signal. (See color insert.)

the z-score calculation. For each probe or probe set on the array, the average signal for that probe across all arrays in a set of samples is transformed to the value of zero, with a standard deviation of 1.0. After such a transformation, gene X with signal values of 100, 500, 2,000, and 1,000 on arrays 1 to 4 is made comparable to gene Y with signal values of 1,000, 5,000, 20,000, and 10,000 on arrays 1 to 4. Other types of data transformation techniques, such as log transformation of two-color signal ratios, may also be appropriate depending upon the nature of the primary microarray data set (90,91).

After normalization, data must be visualized and statistically analyzed to address the specific question that is being asked. There are now a number of relatively standard methods in which voluminous and multidimensional microarray data may visualized (Fig. 9.10). The choice of visualization tools depends partly on the question to be addressed (92,93). In hierarchical clustering, samples (targets) are organized based on their similarity in gene expression and genes (probes) based on their similarity in expression across samples. Several different measures of similarity can be used (e.g., Pearson correlation) and several different methods can be applied to perform the clustering (94). However, no

particular algorithm can be considered more correct. In fact, although hierarchical clustering is a useful tool to provide a manageable view of immense data sets, it does not necessarily impart any underlying truth to microarray data. Heat maps are a colorimetric representation of numerical data, usually presented in combination with hierarchical clustering. This visualization scheme provides a convenient method to identify patterns or blocks of similarity between gene expression values or samples. The use of k-means clustering or self-organizing maps is particularly useful for reducing the level of microarray data complexity. In these approaches, a large number of variables (i.e., microarray probe expression values) are placed into a finite number of "bins" based on their similarity of expression values across a much smaller number of observations (i.e., RNA target samples). The number of bins created (the k in k-means or the number of nodes in the self-organizing map) can be adjusted to create a much smaller set of similar, collective values that can then be used as the basis for further analysis (95,96). Principal components analysis and multidimensional scaling are two other similar methods used to perform data reduction. In principal components analysis, for example, samples may be plotted in "gene expression

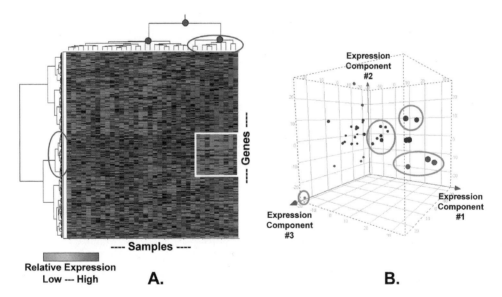

Figure 9.10   Microarray data visualization. When using hierarchical clustering and heat-map representation of gene expression microarray data **(A)**, samples (represented as 36 columns in this data set) are organized based on similarity of gene expression while genes (represented by approximately 9,000 rows) are simultaneously organized based on similarity of expression across all samples. In the heat-map image, *green lines* represent transcripts that are relatively less expressed in a sample while *red lines* represent transcripts that are relatively overexpressed in a sample. The tree (dendrogram) at top quantifies the relative similarity between samples. Each blue node is associated with a correlation coefficient that describes the relatedness of samples among the two subsequent branches of the dendrogram. Samples with higher similarity to each other based on gene expression are depicted as lower branches on the tree (*horizontal ellipse*). Similarly, the tree on the left quantifies the relative similarity between gene expression patterns. Genes that show similar patterns of expression across all samples are depicted as smaller branches on the tree (*vertical ellipse*). Note subgroups of genes that demonstrate identical patterns of expression in subgroups of samples (*white box*). In principle components analysis **(B)**, gene expression values may be condensed into two or three principle components that represent the majority of variation in gene expression across all samples. Each sample is plotted in two- or three-dimensional space (as shown here) based on the value of its principle expression components. Each point may be further color-coded based on other features of the sample (e.g., tumor grade, patient age, etc.). In this view, it is easy to demonstrate clusters of samples (*green ellipses*) that are very distinct in their gene expression profiles. (Visualizations generated using DecisionSite for Functional Genomics software, Spotfire, Inc., Somerville, MA). (See color insert.)

space," where the distance between samples in this space is related to their similarity based on gene expression. However, for a 47,000-element microarray, gene expression space is represented in 47,000 different dimensions. Therefore, the goal of principal component analysis is to reduce 47,000 dimensions into two to three principle components. Then, relatedness between samples can be plotted.

In experimental studies, one approach to the statistical analysis of microarray data involves unsupervised clustering or class discovery (97). In this approach, experimental specimens are classified based solely on their microarray data values and the results of this classification are reviewed to identify new, previously unappreciated clinical or pathologic classifications. Perhaps the most elegant illustration of this approach has been the reclassification of breast adenocarcinoma based on microarray-generated gene expression profiles (98,99). From a diagnostic perspective, this approach is of value only if the new classification scheme can be associated with a clinically relevant parameter or biologic phenotype (11,12). Otherwise, without some gold standard clinical parameter to compare against, it is difficult to determine whether such newly discovered classes are statistical artifacts or important new clinical features.

To date, most clinical microarray studies have been investigational or discovery-based, where patterns of gene expression are sought that demonstrate a correlation to a known parameter such as pathologic stage or clinical outcome. This type of supervised or class distinction (97) analysis is designed to identify novel predictive biomarkers. In principle, this type of analysis is no different than evaluating a single gene transcript at a time and calculating whether expression values for that gene are statistically significant between the defined sample classes using traditional statistics (i.e., ANOVA analysis). This approach, however, cannot be readily applied to microarray data. By definition, using a traditional significance threshold of $p = 0.05$ allows for a 5% false positive (false discovery) rate. Therefore, when analyzing 47,000 independent gene expression values obtained by a microarray assay, over 2,000 gene expression values will appear to be significant by chance alone. To contend with this problem of multiple testing, several methods have been applied to calculate a true significance threshold when analyzing thousands of variables in relatively few numbers of samples (100,101). Although these approaches minimize false positive results for a given sample set, they can in no way substitute for data validation using multiple, independent sets of samples across different technology platforms and laboratories.

A second problem involved in applying traditional statistical tests to microarray data is the consequence of data over-reduction. The true power of microarray data is that it allows for the examination of multiple, independent biomarker values rather than examination of one gene at a time. However, traditional statistical analysis considers only a single gene at a time. Therefore, whereas three single sets of gene expression values may not discriminate between classes on their own, their combined expression pattern may be a statistically significant discriminator (Fig. 9.11). One approach to this problem uses the concept of metagenes, or groups of genes whose composite expression pattern provides discriminatory power (102).

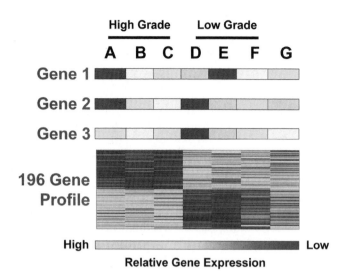

Figure 9.11 Synergism of gene expression signatures. In this study, seven oligodendroglioma tumors of low (**A** to **C**), high (**D** to **F**), and intermediate (**G**) histologic grade were analyzed on a gene expression microarray representing approximately 1,500 transcripts. When examined individually, the expression of three different genes appears to have little correlation with tumor grade. However, when the same three genes are examined in the context of 193 other genes, the composite gene expression signature clearly delimits a molecular difference between tumor grades. (See color insert.)

As discussed below, an obvious application of microarray assays is to provide a diagnostic result based upon a predetermined gene signature (103–105). In this approach, a specific subset of probes on the microarray is examined and a weighted discriminate index is calculated. Usually, this index is the summation of a set of expression values, where each expression value is weighted for its class prediction strength based on a training set. The resulting index provides a probability measure that a given specimen falls into a specific diagnostic category (Fig. 9.12). As more diagnostic gene signatures are identified and validated, algorithms such as weighted discrimination tests will become increasingly more useful. For purposes of clinical diagnostic assays, such algorithms will need to be heavily validated and standardized for each assay.

For clinical assays, the biology associated with microarray data results is probably less important than its diagnostic validity. However, for investigators conducting microarray assays in a research environment, a significant conundrum pertains to how patterns of gene expression can be related to biologically meaningful results. In other words, although the product of feature extraction, data normalization, and statistical analysis results in a list of biomarkers of interest, it is still a challenge to relate a biomarker list to a specific biologic pathway that might provide insight into the disease process. As annotation and our understanding of the human genome continue to advance, investigators have been able to classify a large number of human genes into ontologies based on function, cellular location, and structural determinants (106). Several software programs are now available that can map lists of biomarkers to these ontologies, which can result in

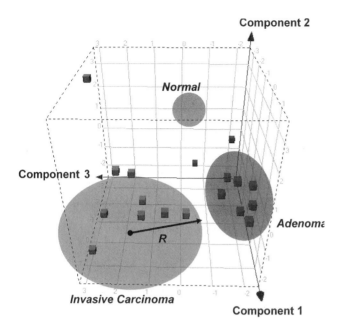

Figure 9.12 Utilization of gene expression profiles as a diagnostic index. In this graphical example, a validated set of biomarkers (i.e., gene expression, DNA copy number, methylation status, sequence mutation) have been used to develop an algorithm to map the results from any clinical sample into a three-dimensional biomarker space, based on the composite value of three principle components. The gene classifier may predict one or more classes of pathologic disease (*shaded areas*), but the power for prediction may vary among classes (compare the size of shaded areas). When a given sample is mapped to within one of the shaded areas, a diagnosis is made. The distance of the sample from the center of the prediction zone (*R*) indicates the certainty of the prediction. In some cases, samples that fall outside of any diagnostic zone will be labeled indeterminate by the algorithm, even if they have been classified by traditional histopathology or immunohistochemical review (*boxes outside of diagnostic zones*).

a clearer view of altered biologic processes associated with differential gene expression (107,108). For single cellular and simple multicellular organisms, this approach has led to sophisticated models for cell signaling and transcriptional regulatory networks (109,110) whereas for other mammalian species, this type of analysis is only in its infancy (111). A related approach involves utilizing the existing scientific literature to identify common themes between lists of biomarkers with no otherwise appreciated association. In this way, literature relevancy networks can sometimes be used to transform lists of biomarkers into more meaningful biologic events (112).

Ultimately, as with any other diagnostic test, the results of any microarray assay must be validated through independent testing. Although data validation is relatively straightforward for many new assays, it is particularly problematic for microarrays for three reasons. First, the cost of performing a microarray assay is still relatively expensive ($200 to $800 per sample), which creates financial constraints on the number of samples that can be analyzed. Second, given the stringent specimen requirements needed to perform most microarray assays, the simple availability

of suitable specimens is often limiting. Finally, as discussed above, the large number of variables associated with a microarray experiment requires that a relatively large number of observations (e.g., samples) be analyzed to create any degree of statistical confidence. To provide data validation for microarray results in the face of these limitations, investigators have devised a number of approaches. One of the most popular approaches is the sequential sampling or "leave-one-out" cross-validation analysis (113). In an analysis of N study samples, $N-1$ samples are used for the initial statistical analysis to identify groups of signature genes. The ability of these genes to correctly classify the Nth sample is then calculated and the gene list modified, discarding biomarkers that perform poorly and solidifying those with the best performance. This process is repeated, removing all N samples, one at a time, until a list of genes with the best class prediction score is created. The advantage of this method is that no additional data or experimentation are needed for validation. However, because the cross-validation is still applied to a single set of samples (i.e., the Test and Validation sets are one in the same), the ability to generalize conclusions to independent or larger sample sets may still be limited. If an initial microarray sample set is large enough, it is also possible to divide the experiment into independent sets of test data and validation data. In this scheme, patterns of significant gene expression are identified using the first set of samples and patterns are validated in a second set of arrays. Although this approach uses two truly independent data sets, it necessarily limits the number of independent samples available for the discovery phase and validation phase. The desire to split a limited number of samples into test and validation sets raises the question of appropriate sample size requirements for performing microarray analyses with sufficient statistical power (114,115). Although multiple methods have been proposed to calculate required sample sizes to validate gene expression signatures, ultimately the number of samples required will depend on the expected biologic effect. For example, relatively few study samples may be necessary to identify fundamental differences in gene expression between acute myelogenous leukemia (AML) and acute lymphocytic leukemia (ALL), because these tumor cell types are biologically very distinct (97). On the other hand, a considerably larger study set may be required to identify reliable differences in gene expression associated with clinical outcome within AML patients, if the intrinsic biologic basis for patient outcome is more subtle (116).

Microarray data results may be validated electronically as well. As an increasing number of microarray studies are published and corresponding data sets are made publicly available in microarray data repositories (81,82), it has become increasingly possible to validate patterns of gene expression identified in one experiment using other microarray experiments in the published literature. In fact, meta-analyses of microarray data are becoming more frequent, and while some studies demonstrate that significant patterns of gene expression can be validated in experiments conducted by independent investigators (99), other such analyses have demonstrated clear differences between studies (117,118). Based on a growing number of microarray meta-analyses, it is clear that any microarray-derived diagnostic signature, like any biomarker assay, requires independent validation in a large and randomly selected sample set. Continuing advances that improve microarray-associated technology and decrease its associated cost will likely make such independent validation routine in the near future.

APPLICATIONS OF MICROARRAY TECHNOLOGY

Microarrays have now been used in a wide variety of applications. This includes assessment of transcript abundance, gene copy number, DNA methylation status, genotyping, and sequencing. Measurement of transcript abundance (i.e., gene expression profiling) has been the most common use of microarray technology in investigative and diagnostic pathology, and this application has been mainly in the field of cancer.

Perhaps one of the most useful applications of gene expression microarray technology has been its use in the diagnosis of histologically ambiguous tumor specimens. Several studies have demonstrated that gene expression profiles can define the cell lineage of metastases of unknown origin (particularly adenocarcinoma) and that this diagnosis is 80% to 90% accurate, based on thorough retrospective analysis of clinical data (119–121). Gene expression data also can be used to discriminate histologic look-alikes with distinct cell origins, such as small round blue cell tumors (105). Each of these studies demonstrates the enhanced resolution of a microarray microscope over standard histopathology examination. Practically, however, most of these study results define a limited set of overlapping molecular markers that can just as easily be assayed using more traditional immunohistochemical methods in FFPE tissue specimens (121). Of greater interest are study results demonstrating that molecular profiling can subclassify histologically indistinguishable tumors into biologically relevant subtypes. The first study to define this principle was conducted in diffuse large B-cell lymphoma, where gene expression patterns clearly segregated tumors with aggressive and indolent molecular profiles that also had significance for patient survival (11,12). More recently, this has been elegantly demonstrated for breast adenocarcinoma. Gene expression profiles of invasive ductal carcinoma can clearly define basal cell and luminal cell tumor types (among others) that have unique biologic characteristics and therapeutic response profiles (98,99). An even more intriguing application of microarray-based molecular profiling involves complete tumor reclassification based not on anatomic site or histopathologic features, but by patterns or modules of gene expression (122). Given that the phenotypic behavior of tumor cells and their response to molecular therapies may be more dependent on molecular profiles than organ site of origin, this approach has the potential to completely reinvent the role of pathology and the practice of clinical oncology.

Many studies have also used gene expression profiles of primary tumor samples to develop predictive signatures of clinical behaviors such as local and distance metastases. Several studies have defined expression signatures that predict the subsequent development of nodal metastases,

both for specific tumor types (123–125) and more globally (126). The ability of primary tumor gene expression profiles to predict the presence of bone marrow micrometastases in breast cancer has also been examined (127). The concept that a primary tumor, before any evidence of metastatic behavior, is molecularly primed to metastasize has been controversial and those few metastasis signatures that have been identified have not been extensively validated in other, independently generated sample sets. Therefore, the validity of these signatures and their absolute clinical significance is still under investigation. In principle, the validation of such signatures would create a new diagnostic category of lymph node potential positive tumors, which could play an equal if not more important role for staging cancer patients for therapeutic decision making than the current use of histologically positive lymph nodes.

The ability of tumor gene expression signatures to predict patient survival has generated the greatest amount of attention in the literature. Several large clinical studies have identified expression signatures that predict absolute patient survival in breast cancer (128–130), lung cancer (131,132), leukemia (133), lymphoma (134) and many other tumor types. Results from these studies are usually individually validated using statistical methodology or in independent training and test patient populations. However, an increasingly worrisome finding is that clinically predictive gene expression signatures are not reproducible across multiple studies of the same tumor type (117,118,135,136). There have been several proposed explanations for this finding, which include the use of differing and nonstandardized microarray platforms, the examination of patient cohorts that are not matched for clinical and treatment parameters, and the relatively complex phenotype of survival, which can be dependent on many variables in addition to tumor molecular signatures. Although microarray analysis has led to the discovery of apparently robust markers that seem to predict clinical outcome in select group of patients (57), it is not clear whether this approach will be generally applicable for defining molecular signatures associated with clinical prognosis.

More recent studies have used microarray technology to define biomarkers that predict specific tumor response to therapy. In the context of neoadjuvant chemotherapy, investigators have performed gene expression microarray analysis of pretreatment tumor biopsy specimens and used this information to develop predictive signatures of treatment response (137,138). To date, most of these studies have been small and are performed retrospectively. However, molecular signatures hold great promise for stratifying patients to therapies that will be most effective for treating their tumors. This approach will prevent patients from receiving toxic chemotherapies from which they are unlikely to benefit and suggest alternative therapies that might not otherwise be considered based on standard clinical criteria. The ability to use tumor gene expression data to prospectively manage patient treatment will be an important step toward the concept of "personalized medicine" (139). With the advent of therapies such as imatinib (Gleevec) and gefitinib (Iressa), which target specific signaling pathways in tumor cells, the ability to predict the effectiveness of such therapies in patient tumors will be extremely important. For example, researchers have already begun to identify specific gene expression profiles that predict response to these drugs in myeloid leukemia and lung cancer, respectively (140,141).

Although the application of gene expression microarrays has been most predominant in the field of clinical oncology, this technology is rapidly finding its way into other fields of clinical medicine such as neurology (Alzheimer's, Parkinson's, epilepsy, schizophrenia), autoimmunity (systemic lupus, multiple sclerosis), organ transplantation, reproductive endocrinology, trauma and sepsis, and cardiovascular disease (142–150). Use of this technology in the clinical management of other disease pathology, however, may be somewhat limited. In many of these multiorgan disease processes, it may be difficult to identify the appropriate target cell population for study. In cancer research, the tumor itself is usually the target of molecular analysis. In more systemic diseases such as diabetes or cardiovascular disease, the target cell population is less well defined. Unlike cancer studies, in which large collections of surgically resected, fresh tumor tissue specimens may be readily available, acquisition of large numbers of specimens may be difficult for diseases such as Parkinson's, diabetic nephropathy, and idiopathic cardiac hypertrophy. Because of the cost of current microarray technology and limited access to adequate clinical specimens, most translational microarray studies focusing on noncancer disease processes have been limited to very small sample sizes. Together with the fact that studies have been performed using a wide variety of microarray platforms and technologies, it has been difficult to collect a sufficiently large enough number of study samples to make statistically valid conclusions regarding associations between gene expression patterns and disease phenotype. Known and unknown variability within disease processes and between patient participants makes establishing definitive patterns of gene expression associated with disease phenotype difficult as well. In the future, therefore, it will be important for microarray-based research studies to address specific diagnostic questions, to carefully consider what and how biospecimens are collected for analysis, and to use a sufficient number of clinical samples on a standardized microarray platform to ensure that statistically meaningful gene expression data can be generated that relate to specific clinical issues in treatment and diagnosis of human disease.

Another major application of microarray technology involves assessment of genome copy number. A fundamental attribute of cancer that is not frequently seen in other human disease processes is a high degree of genome instability. As discussed in Chapter 2, tumor cells experience a wide variety of chromosomal gains and losses. Although these events have been traditionally measured using cytogenetic techniques (Chapter 3), microarrays are becoming an increasingly powerful method to correlate gene copy number changes with clinical and pathologic features of tumors. BAC arrays can provide a view of genome copy number alterations at megabase resolution; however, newer, oligonucleotide-based arrays have increased this resolution to the kilobase level. This resolution will continue to increase to the 40 to 100-nucleotide

level with the development of high-density tiling arrays. Already, microarray-based gene copy number assessment has been used to define critical regions or even single genes whose gain or loss had previously been measured only on the scale of chromosome arm losses or gains (151). This has led to the rapid identification of new oncogenes and tumor suppressor genes that are subsequent targets of future biomarker and therapeutic studies (152,153). Microarray analysis of gene copy number has also identified genomic alterations that are characteristic of particular tumor types (154) and can be associated with clinical outcome (155). Perhaps the most intriguing use of microarray assessment of genome copy number variability will be independent of any associated tissue pathology. Sebat et al. (156) have demonstrated that the germline genomes of normal populations contain many copy number polymorphisms. This normal variability in locus copy number is likely to have enormous significance for disease predisposition and pharmacogenomics, making the use of copy number–based microarray analysis a likely tool for future patient management (157).

Although microarray-based gene copy number assessment is not currently as advanced as gene expression–based analyses, it holds even greater promise as a clinical tool for several reasons. First, the analyte of interest, genomic DNA, is more chemically stable than mRNA and can be extracted from tissue specimens that have not been optimally preserved, such as FFPE (158). Second, compared to mRNA populations, genomic DNA is more biologically stable, meaning that variability related to environmental conditions (e.g., in vivo stress response, in vitro tissue warm ischemia time) is less prominent and thus creates less biologic noise or variability. Finally, as discussed above, methods exist for whole genome amplification (69) that are currently more robust than methods for unbiased transcript amplification. This allows for simple and clinically applicable methods to use vanishingly small amounts of DNA that can be isolated from purified cell populations. All of these aspects suggest that microarray-based gene copy number assessment may soon rival gene expression profiling as a clinical tool for patient management.

A relatively recent appreciation for DNA methylation (epigenomics) and its role in human cancer and other diseases has heralded a third new application for microarray technology. As discussed in Chapters 1 and 2, methylation of CpG dinucleotides occurs frequently in tumor genomes and is associated with transcriptional silencing of key tumor suppressor genes. Although several PCR-based assays exist to interrogate the methylation of specific CpG residues as biomarkers for the detection of cancer (Chapter 5), microarray technology offers the potential to perform whole genome methylation profiling of diseased tissue. To date, microarray-based methylation analysis has been used to distinguish subtypes of leukemia (159) and identify patterns of methylation associated with treatment response (160). Microarray-based methylation profiling has many potential advantages over analysis of the transcriptome or the genome using similar methods. Like assessment of genome copy number status, assessment of methylation profiles are relatively stable and can be analyzed using genomic DNA. However, like transcriptional profiling, DNA methylation can be a functional readout of a cell's molecular pathologic state and complex patterns of somatic alterations in DNA methylation may be associated with disease processes other than cancer (161). Therefore, although the field of epigenomics is still in its infancy and corresponding microarray-based methylation assays are still rudimentary, it is likely that this approach will rapidly become an important tool for research and clinical diagnostics.

DNA sequence alterations, either single nucleotide polymorphisms (SNPs) present in germline DNA or somatic point mutations, which occur in tumor cells, are important diagnostic markers for disease predisposition, diagnosis, and treatment. As discussed in Chapters 5 and 7, numerous PCR and sequencing methods exist for detecting sequence alterations at defined genetic loci. Many of these assays can be multiplexed to genotype several hundred or several thousand loci simultaneously. However, microarray technology is now becoming an extremely powerful alternative approach to genotype individuals at as many as 500,000 loci across the genome. The ability to perform genomewide, high-resolution genotyping using these "SNP Chips" is beginning to have enormous implications for clinical genetics. For example, familial linkage studies designed to identify inherited disease genes associated with tumor syndromes have greatly benefited from this technology (162,163). Microarray-based genotyping has also been used in genetic association studies, to define loci associated with disease predisposition and clinical phenotype (164,165). Although most applications of genotyping microarrays have been used to discover a single disease locus of interest, it is easy to imagine how complex, multigenic diseases may eventually require genotyping at multiple loci to accurate classify a genetic phenotype.

A final, but perhaps most promising, application of microarrays involves their use in gene resequencing. Oligonucleotide microarrays can be constructed to interrogate individual bases of DNA sequence, thus providing a method for sequencing by hybridization of a clinical sample (Chapter 7). For example, microarrays have been designed to sequence the genomes of the severe acute respiratory syndrome (SARS) virus and human immunodeficiency virus (HIV) for the purposes of strain classification and predicting response to antiviral agents, respectively (166,167). In other applications, investigators have developed "MitoChip," a microarray designed to sequence the entire mitochondrial genome (168). Specific mitochondrial mutations occur frequently in human cancer cells and therefore have become intriguing candidates for tumor biomarkers. Likewise, a microarray designed to resequence the *p53* tumor suppressor gene has been used to predict clinical outcome and therapeutic response in patients based on the spectrum of somatic *p53* sequence alterations in their primary tumors (169,170). The sensitivity of this approach is greater than 90% and, with the exception of detecting nucleotide insertions and deletions, is comparable to that of traditional dideoxy sequencing (171). Although initial attempts to perform array-mediated sequencing of DNA isolated from FFPE specimens have been disappointing (172), it is likely that further refinements to DNA preparation (29–31) will enhance this technique. It is only recently that the sequence of the cancer genome has been explored to any degree of detail (173–175). However, there is already compelling evidence that specific gene sequence alterations in tumors will predict vulnerability and resistance to specific therapies such as the epidermal growth factor receptor inhibitor gefitinib (176,177). As more of these clinically relevant somatic sequence alterations are identified in viruses, tumor cells, and other pathologic specimens, the ability to perform rapid resequencing of multiple genetic loci on a single clinical specimen will be incredibly important. In this respect, compared to traditional sequencing methodologies, microarrays and the sequencing by hybridization approach should become routine clinical molecular diagnostic tools that will supplement traditional histopathologic and immunohistochemical analysis of pathology specimens.

STRENGTHS AND LIMITATIONS OF MICROARRAY-BASED ASSAYS IN THE CLINICAL LABORATORY

DNA microarrays have been used for numerous, exciting research discovery investigations; however, their routine use in a clinical laboratory requires considerable consideration, particularly with respect to their use for gene expression signature assays (178–180). On the one hand, microarray technology is well suited for performing highly multiplexed assays. The utility of this is obvious in discovery paradigms in which whole genome analyses are necessary to discover new biomarkers. However, in a clinical laboratory, this also means that several genetic targets can be evaluated using multiple probe sets to enhance assay reproducibility. A microarray used for discovery purposes may assay 10,000 genes using a single set of probes; a similar sized array could also assay 100 genes using 100 different probe measurements. The ability to create large number of redundant probe sets and control sequences should provide a level of precision not currently available from most research-based arrays. To date, many individual gene expression microarray studies have identified a limited number of transcripts that may be diagnostically useful (57,129,181), but in practice it is likely that a much larger number of gene targets will be required to define a diagnostic signature that is generalizable to larger populations of heterogeneous patient samples. This will be true not only for gene transcript analysis, but particularly for DNA resequencing by microarray. Thus, although the objectives of research-based and clinical-based microarray assays will differ, they both can effectively capitalize on the technology's ability to perform highly multiplexed assays. The microarray format is best suited to measure multiple analytes from a single sample; therefore it is ideal for the clinical laboratory that performs sporadic, prospective analysis on clinical specimens. Another potential advantage of microarray technology is that it can be highly automated and regulated, attributes that are critical for any clinical laboratory test. Newer sample (target) preparation methods utilize single-tube, "hands-off" chemistries that will facilitate their routine use in the clinical laboratory (60). Self-contained, microarray cassettes, such as those manufactured by Affymetrix and other vendors, also provide an acceptable format for regulated clinical tests.

Despite the potential advantages of using microarray technology in the clinical laboratory, there are a number of important caveats that should be considered. Some of these have been referenced throughout this chapter. First, microarrays are indisputably high-complexity assays, and, although streamlined protocols, automation, and standardized array manufacturing can mitigate some of the inherent technical complexity associated with microarrays as research tools, this technology may still remain in the hands of specialized clinical laboratories. As demonstrated in Figure 9.7, like most hybridization-based methods, the time required to perform microarray analysis even in its most automated format may still be 3 to 4 days. Assay turn-around time could be problematic for protocols in which microarray data must be used to guide therapy and the therapy must be initiated quickly. Because microarray assays are based on signal detection by hybridization, there is an inherent limit to sensitivity compared to amplification-based PCR detection assays. Microarrays are a powerful tool to assay thousands of genetic markers at once, but in being able to do this, each marker is not optimized for sensitivity. This may be particularly problematic for measuring low levels or subtle alterations of gene expression that are clinically relevant or for detecting genetic alterations that may be present in only a subset of cell populations. By focusing on fewer markers, optimizing hybridization conditions for each marker, and placing redundant probes for each marker on the same array, it may be possible to increase the sensitivity and precision of microarray assays, although this has only recently been a consideration in their design (182). A final technical limitation of microarray technology is the requirement for high sample quality. Although exact specimen requirements depend on the analyte measured (mRNA, genomic DNA, DNA methylation), as discussed throughout this chapter, the use of formalin-fixed tissue or other specimens that have been collected under routine hospital conditions may limit the use of microarray technology in a number of circumstances.

The biggest challenge for implementing microarray technology in the clinical laboratory, however, is not array technology itself but rather the clinical validity of the array biomarker content. To date, the majority of microarray platforms have been designed as whole genome, discovery tools. Studies have used a relatively small number of observations (patients) and a large number of variables (genes), which consistently leads to high false positive rates that are unacceptable for clinical assay validation. Most microarray data generated and reported in the literature (particularly gene expression data) have not been reproducible (135, 136). Therefore, although microarray technology itself holds great promise for use in a clinical laboratory, a great deal more clinical correlative data need to be validated to identify probe content that will be most universally applicable and diagnostically relevant.

THE FUTURE OF MICROARRAY TECHNOLOGY

Advances in microarray synthesis technology should soon allow comprehensive human transcriptome or genome analysis on a single array for minimal cost. Complex analyses such as quantification of alternative mRNA splicing events, simultaneous detection of SNPs at over 500,000 independent loci, and direct sequencing of over 500 kb of DNA sequence using a single array will be possible, limited only by data storage and analysis capabilities. Methods for fast and flexible creation of customized arrays continue to improve and will allow for the mass production of arrays to assay-specific sets of gene targets at the genomic, epigenomic, or transcriptional level for disease-specific assays.

Methods are now available for amplifying and labeling nanogram quantities of nucleic acids samples (both DNA and RNA) derived from microscopic biopsy specimens that are either fresh or archived in paraffin. These advances will be tremendously important for application of microarray technology in a clinical environment. The ability to use small numbers of cells obtained from minimally invasive procedures such as fine needle aspiration, swabs, and lavages will allow microarray-based assays to be used for diagnostics in a variety of different clinical scenarios. Utilization of routine pathology tissue specimens, fixed and embedded in paraffin, will allow full integration of this technology with routine histopathologic assessment.

Continuing annotation of the human genome will provide new information about relevant disease-related SNPs. Similarly, knowledge of gene exon structure and alternative mRNA splicing patterns will allow for independent quantification of multiple mRNA transcripts originating from a single genomic locus. The advances in microarray fabrication discussed above will be necessary to harness this explosion of genomic information and develop assays that can detect these more subtle genetic alterations and relate them to human pathology.

Finally, as diagnostic biomarkers become more well established, microarray platforms will need to evolve into clinical diagnostic tools that meet all regulatory requirements of standard clinical tests. This will require additional standardization and interlaboratory assay validation, which only recently has received appropriate attention (182). Already, several assays have been validated and are being adopted to an in vitro diagnostic platform for use in clinical laboratories (e.g., Roche Diagnostics AmpliChip CYP450 Test). As additional biomarker targets are validated, these assays should become increasingly more prevalent in clinical laboratories and microarray technology will become integrated within the standard practice of diagnostic pathology.

REFERENCES

1. Packeisen J, Korsching E, Herbst H, et al. Demystified . . . tissue microarray technology. *Mol Pathol* 2003;56:198–204.
2. Simon R, Mirlacher M, Sauter G. Tissue microarrays in cancer diagnosis. *Expert Rev Mol Diagn* 2003;3:421–430.
3. Sauter G, Simon R, Hillan K. Tissue microarrays in drug discovery. *Nat Rev Drug Discov* 2003;2:962–972.
4. Hao X, Sun B, Hu L, et al. Differential gene and protein expression in primary breast malignancies and their lymph node metastases as revealed by combined cDNA microarray and tissue microarray analysis. *Cancer* 2004;100:1110–1122.
5. Liotta LA, Espina V, Mehta AI, et al. Protein microarrays: meeting analytical challenges for clinical applications. *Cancer Cell* 2003;3:317–325.
6. Angenendt P. Progress in protein and antibody microarray technology. *Drug Discov Today* 2005;10:503–511.
7. Albertson DG, Pinkel D. Genomic microarrays in human genetic disease and cancer. *Hum Mol Genet* 2003;12 Spec No 2:R145–152.
8. Davies JJ, Wilson IM, Lam WL. Array CGH technologies and their applications to cancer genomes. *Chromosome Res* 2005;13:237–248.

9. Schulze A, Downward J. Navigating gene expression using microarrays: a technology review. *Nat Cell Biol* 2001;3:E190–E195.
10. Holloway AJ, van Laar RK, Tothill RW, et al. Options available—from start to finish—for obtaining data from DNA microarrays II. *Nat Genet* 2002;32 (suppl):481–489.
11. Alizadeh AA, Eisen MB, Davis RE, et al. Distinct types of diffuse large B-cell lymphoma identified by gene expression profiling. *Nature* 2000;403:503–511.
12. Wright G, Tan B, Rosenwald A, et al. A gene expression-based method to diagnose clinically distinct subgroups of diffuse large B cell lymphoma. *Proc Natl Acad Sci USA* 2003;100:9991–9996.
13. Takemasa I, Higuchi H, Yamamoto H, et al. Construction of preferential cDNA microarray specialized for human colorectal carcinoma: molecular sketch of colorectal cancer. *Biochem Biophys Res Commun* 2001;285:1244–1249.
14. Ohira M, Oba S, Nakamura Y, et al. Expression profiling using a tumor-specific cDNA microarray predicts the prognosis of intermediate risk neuroblastomas. *Cancer Cell* 2005;7:337–350.
15. Gordon PM, Sensen CW. Osprey: a comprehensive tool employing novel methods for the design of oligonucleotides for DNA sequencing and microarrays. *Nucleic Acids Res* 2004;32:e133.
16. Carter MG, Sharov AA, VanBuren V, et al. Transcript copy number estimation using a mouse whole-genome oligonucleotide microarray. *Genome Biol* 2005;6:R61.
17. Kronick MN. Creation of the whole human genome microarray. *Expert Rev Proteomics* 2004;1:19–28.
18. Wrobel G, Schlingemann J, Hummerich L, et al. Optimization of high-density cDNA-microarray protocols by 'design of experiments'. *Nucleic Acids Res* 2003;15:e67.
19. Venkatasubbarao S. Microarrays: status and prospects. *Trends Biotechnol* 2004;22:630–637.
20. Hughes TR, Mao M, Jones AR, et al. Expression profiling using microarrays fabricated by an ink-jet oligonucleotide synthesizer. *Nat Biotechnol* 2001;19:342–347.
21. Santacroce R, Ratti A, Caroli F, et al. Analysis of clinically relevant single-nucleotide polymorphisms by use of microelectronic array technology. *Clin Chem* 2002;48:2124–2130.
22. Kuhn K, Baker SC, Chudin E, et al. A novel, high-performance random array platform for quantitative gene expression profiling. *Genome Res* 2004;14:2347–2356.
23. Gunderson KL, Kruglyak S, Graige MS, et al. Decoding randomly ordered DNA arrays. *Genome Res* 2004;14:870–877.
24. Lipshutz RJ, Fodor SP, Gingeras TR, et al. High density synthetic oligonucleotide arrays. *Nat Genet* 1999;21:20–24.
25. Fodor SP, Read JL, Pirrung MC, et al. Light-directed, spatially addressable parallel chemical synthesis. *Science* 1991;251:767–773.
26. Nuwaysir EF, Huang W, Albert TJ, et al. Gene expression analysis using oligonucleotide arrays produced by maskless photolithography. *Genome Res* 2002;12:1749–1755.
27. Srinivasan M, Sedmak D, Jewell S. Effect of fixatives and tissue processing on the content and integrity of nucleic acids. *Am J Pathol* 2002;161:1961–1971.
28. Masuda N, Ohnishi T, Kawamoto S, et al. Analysis of chemical modification of RNA from formalin-fixed samples and optimization of molecular biology applications for such samples. *Nucleic Acids Res* 1999;27:4436–4443.
29. Fang SG, Wan QH, Fujihara N. Formalin removal from archival tissue by critical point drying. *Biotechniques* 2002;33:604, 606, 608–610.
30. Sato Y, Sugie R, Tsuchiya B, et al. Comparison of the DNA extraction methods for polymerase chain reaction amplification from formalin-fixed and paraffin-embedded tissues. *Diagn Mol Pathol* 2001;10:265–271.
31. Coombs NJ, Gough AC, Primrose JN. Optimisation of DNA and RNA extraction from archival formalin-fixed tissue. *Nucleic Acids Res* 1999;27:e12.
32. Devries S, Nyante S, Korkola J, et al. Array-based comparative genomic hybridization from formalin-fixed, paraffin-embedded breast tumors. *J Mol Diagn* 2005;7:65–71.
33. van Dekken H, Paris PL, Albertson DG, et al. Evaluation of genetic patterns in different tumor areas of intermediate-grade prostatic adenocarcinomas by high-resolution genomic array analysis. *Genes Chromosomes Cancer* 2004;39:249–256.
34. Specht K, Richter T, Muller U, et al. Quantitative gene expression analysis in microdissected archival formalin-fixed and paraffin-embedded tumor tissue. *Am J Pathol* 2001;158:419–429.
35. Korbler T, Grskovic M, Dominis M, et al. A simple method for RNA isolation from formalin-fixed and paraffin-embedded lymphatic tissues. *Exp Mol Pathol* 2003;74:336–340.
36. Bibikova M, Talantov D, Chudin E, et al. Quantitative gene expression profiling in formalin-fixed, paraffin-embedded tissues using universal bead arrays. *Am J Pathol* 2004;165:1799–1807.
37. Emmert-Buck MR, Strausberg RL, Krizman DB, et al. Molecular profiling of clinical tissues specimens: feasibility and applications. *J Mol Diagn* 2000;2:60–66.
38. Bostwick DG, al Annouf N, Choi C. Establishment of the formalin-free surgical pathology laboratory: utility of an alcohol-based fixative. *Arch Pathol Lab Med* 1994;118:298–302.
39. Florell SR, Coffin CM, Holden JA, et al. Preservation of RNA for functional genomic studies: a multidisciplinary tumor bank protocol. *Mod Pathol* 2001; 14:116–128.
40. Vincek V, Nassiri M, Nadji M, et al. A tissue fixative that protects macromolecules (DNA, RNA, and protein) and histomorphology in clinical samples. *Lab Invest* 2003; 83:1427–1435.
41. Shibutani M, Uneyama C. Methacarn: a fixation tool for multipurpose genetic analysis from paraffin-embedded tissues. *Methods Enzymol* 2002;356:114–125.
42. Wiedorn KH, Olert J, Stacy RA, et al. HOPE: a new fixing technique enables preservation and extraction of high molecular weight DNA and RNA of > 20 kb from paraffin-embedded tissues—hepes-glutamic acid buffer mediated organic solvent protection effect. *Pathol Res Pract* 2002;198:735–740.
43. Finkelstein SD, Dhir R, Rabinovitz M, et al. Cold-temperature plastic resin embedding of liver for DNA- and RNA-based genotyping. *J Mol Diagn* 1999;1:17–22.
44. Mutter GL, Zahrieh D, Liu C, et al. Comparison of frozen and RNALater solid tissue storage methods for use in RNA expression microarrays. *BMC Genomics* 2004;5:88.
45. Dunmire V, Wu C, Symmans WF, et al. Increased yield of total RNA from fine-needle aspirates for use in expression microarray analysis. *Biotechniques* 2002;33:890–892,894,896.
46. Jhavar SG, Fisher C, Jackson A, et al. Processing of radical prostatectomy specimens for correlation of data from histopathological, molecular biological, and radiological studies: a new whole organ technique. *J Clin Pathol* 2005;58:504–508.
47. Ellis M, Davis N, Coop A, et al. Development and validation of a method for using breast core needle biopsies for gene expression microarray analyses. *Clin Cancer Res* 2002;8:1155–1166.
48. Dash A, Maine IP, Varambally S, et al. Changes in differential gene expression because of warm ischemia time of radical prostatectomy specimens. *Am J Pathol* 2002; 161:1743–1748.
49. Ohashi Y, Creek KE, Pirisi L, et al. RNA degradation in human breast tissue after surgical removal: a time-course study. *Exp Mol Pathol* 2004;77:98–103.
50. Huang J, Qi R, Quackenbush J, et al. Effects of ischemia on gene expression. *J Surg Res* 2001;99:222–227.
51. Feezor RJ, Baker HV, Mindrinos M, et al. Whole blood and leukocyte RNA isolation for gene expression analyses. *Physiol Genomics* 2004;19:247–254.
52. Szaniszlo P, Wang N, Sinha M, et al. Getting the right cells to the array: gene expression microarray analysis of cell mixtures and sorted cells. *Cytometry A* 2004;59:191–202.
53. Hunt JL, Finkelstein SD. Microdissection techniques for molecular testing in surgical pathology. *Arch Pathol Lab Med* 2004;128:1372–1378.
54. Best CJ, Emmert-Buck MR. Molecular profiling of tissue samples using laser capture microdissection. *Expert Rev Mol Diagn* 2001;1:53–60.
55. Ernst T, Hergenhahn M, Kenzelmann M, et al. Decrease and gain of gene expression are equally discriminatory markers for prostate carcinoma: a gene expression analysis on total and microdissected prostate tissue. *Am J Pathol* 2002;160:2169–2180.
56. Lieberfarb ME, Lin M, Lechpammer M, et al. Genome-wide loss of heterozygosity analysis from laser capture microdissected prostate cancer using single nucleotide polymorphic allele (SNP) arrays and a novel bioinformatics platform dChipSNP. *Cancer Res* 2003;63:4781–4785.
57. Paik S, Shak S, Tang G, et al. A multigene assay to predict recurrence of tamoxifen-treated, node-negative breast cancer. *N Engl J Med* 2004;351:2817–2826.
58. Iscove NN, Barbara M, Gu M, et al. Representation is faithfully preserved in global cDNA amplified exponentially from sub-picogram quantities of mRNA. *Nat Biotechnol* 2002;20:940–943.
59. Chiang MK, Melton DA. Single-cell transcript analysis of pancreas development. *Dev Cell* 2003;4:383–393.
60. Dafforn A, Chen P, Deng G, et al. Linear mRNA amplification from as little as 5 ng total RNA for global gene expression analysis. *Biotechniques* 2004;37:854–857.
61. Van Gelder RN, von Zastrow ME, Yool A, et al. Amplified RNA synthesized from limited quantities of heterogeneous cDNA. *Proc Natl Acad Sci USA* 1990;87:1663–1667.
62. Glanzer JG, Eberwine JH. Expression profiling of small cellular samples in cancer: less is more. *Br J Cancer* 2004;90:1111–1114.
63. Luzzi V, Mahadevappa M, Raja R, et al. Accurate and reproducible gene expression profiles from laser capture microdissection, transcript amplification, and high density oligonucleotide microarray analysis. *J Mol Diagn* 2003;5:9–14.
64. Li L, Roden J, Shapiro BE, et al. Reproducibility, fidelity, and discriminant validity of mRNA amplification for microarray analysis from primary hematopoietic cells. *J Mol Diagn* 2005;7:48–56.
65. Stoecklein NH, Erbersdobler A, Schmidt-Kittler O, et al. SCOMP is superior to degenerated oligonucleotide primed-polymerase chain reaction for global amplification of minute amounts of DNA from microdissected archival tissue samples. *Am J Pathol* 2002;161:43–51.
66. Kittler R, Stoneking M, Kayser M. A whole genome amplification method to generate long fragments from low quantities of genomic DNA. *Anal Biochem* 2002;300:237–244.
67. Dietmaier W, Hartmann A, Wallinger S, et al. Multiple mutation analyses in single tumor cells with improved whole genome amplification. *Am J Pathol* 1999;154:83–95.
68. Cheung VG, Nelson SF. Whole genome amplification using a degenerate oligonucleotide primer allows hundreds of genotypes to be performed on less than one nanogram of genomic DNA. *Proc Natl Acad Sci USA* 1996;93:14676–14679.
69. Dean FB, Hosono S, Fang L, et al. Comprehensive human genome amplification using multiple displacement amplification. *Proc Natl Acad Sci USA* 2002;99:5261–5266.
70. Luthra R, Medeiros LJ. Isothermal multiple displacement amplification: a highly reliable approach for generating unlimited high molecular weight genomic DNA from clinical specimens. *J Mol Diagn* 2004;6:236–242.
71. Paez JG, Lin M, Beroukhim R, et al. Genome coverage and sequence fidelity of phi29 polymerase-based multiple strand displacement whole genome amplification. *Nucleic Acids Res* 2004;32:e71.
72. Cole K, Truong V, Barone D, et al. Direct labeling of RNA with multiple biotins allows sensitive expression profiling of acute leukemia class predictor genes. *Nucleic Acids Res* 2004;32:e86.
73. Gupta V, Cherkassky A, Chatis P, et al. Directly labeled mRNA produces highly precise and unbiased differential gene expression data. *Nucleic Acids Res* 2003;31:e13.
74. Hegde P, Qi R, Abernathy K, et al. A concise guide to cDNA microarray analysis. *Biotechniques* 2000;29:548–550, 552–554, 556.
75. Badiee A, Eiken HG, Steen VM, et al. Evaluation of five different cDNA labeling methods for microarrays using spike controls. *BMC Biotechnol* 2003;3:23.
76. Beier V, Bauer A, Baum M, et al. Fluorescent sample labeling for DNA microarray analyses. *Methods Mol Biol* 2004;283:127–135.
77. Richter A, Schwager C, Hentze S, et al. Comparison of fluorescent tag DNA labeling methods used for expression analysis by DNA microarrays. *Biotechniques* 2002; 33:620–628, 630.
78. Manduchi E, Scearce LM, Brestelli JE, et al. Comparison of different labeling methods for two-channel high-density microarray experiments. *Physiol Genomics* 2002; 10: 169–179.
79. Xiang CC, Kozhich OA, Chen M, et al. Amine-modified random primers to label probes for DNA microarrays. *Nat Biotechnol* 2002;20:738–742.
80. Dobbin KK, Kawasaki ES, Petersen DW, et al. Characterizing dye bias in microarray experiments. *Bioinformatics* 2005;21:2430–2437.
81. Barrett T, Suzek TO, Troup DB, et al. NCBI GEO: mining millions of expression profiles—database and tools. *Nucleic Acids Res* 2005;33:D562–D566.
82. Ball CA, Awad IA, Demeter J, et al. The Stanford Microarray Database accommodates additional microarray platforms and data formats. *Nucleic Acids Res* 2005; 33:D580–582.
83. Petricoin EF 3rd, Hackett JL, Lesko LJ, et al. Medical applications of microarray technologies: a regulatory science perspective. *Nat Genet* 2002;32 (suppl): 474–479.

84. Yang YH, Buckley MJ, Speed TP. Analysis of cDNA microarray images. *Brief Bioinform* 2001;2:341–349.

85. Irizarry RA, Bolstad BM, Collin F, et al. Summaries of Affymetrix GeneChip probe level data. *Nucleic Acids Res* 2003;31:e15.

86. Li C, Wong WH. Model-based analysis of oligonucleotide arrays: expression index computation and outlier detection. *Proc Natl Acad Sci USA* 2001;98:31–36.

87. Irizarry RA, Hobbs B, Collin F, et al. Exploration, normalization, and summaries of high density oligonucleotide array probe level data. *Biostatistics* 2003;4:249–264.

88. Gentleman RC, Carey VJ, Bates DM, et al. Bioconductor: open software development for computational biology and bioinformatics. *Genome Biol* 2004;5:R80.

89. Shedden K, Chen W, Kuick R, et al. Comparison of seven methods for producing Affymetrix expression scores based on false discovery rates in disease profiling data. *BMC Bioinformatics* 2005;6:26.

90. Churchill GA. Fundamentals of experimental design for cDNA microarrays. *Nat Genet* 2002;32(suppl):490–495.

91. Quackenbush J. Microarray data normalization and transformation. *Nat Genet* 2002; 32(suppl):496–501.

92. Gilbert DR, Schroeder M, van Helden J. Interactive visualization and exploration of relationships between biological objects. *Trends Biotechnol* 2000;18:487–494.

93. Hibbs MA, Dirksen NC, Li K, et al. Visualization methods for statistical analysis of microarray clusters. *BMC Bioinformatics* 2005;6:115.

94. Quackenbush J. Computational analysis of microarray data. *Nat Rev Genet* 2001; 2:418–427.

95. Dougherty ER, Barrera J, Brun M, et al. Inference from clustering with application to gene-expression microarrays. *J Comput Biol* 2002;9:105–126.

96. Garge NR, Page GP, Sprague AP, et al. Reproducible clusters from microarray research: whither? *BMC Bioinformatics* 2005;6(suppl 2):S10.

97. Golub TR, Slonim DK, Tamayo P, et al. Molecular classification of cancer: class discovery and class prediction by gene expression monitoring. *Science* 1999;286:531–537.

98. Sorlie T, Perou CM, Tibshirani R, et al. Gene expression patterns of breast carcinomas distinguish tumor subclasses with clinical implications. *Proc Natl Acad Sci USA* 2001; 98:10869–10874.

99. Sorlie T, Tibshirani R, Parker J, et al. Repeated observation of breast tumor subtypes in independent gene expression data sets. *Proc Natl Acad Sci USA* 2003;100:8418–8423.

100. Cui X, Churchill GA. Statistical tests for differential expression in cDNA microarray experiments. *Genome Biol* 2003;4:210.

101. Tusher VG, Tibshirani R, Chu G. Significance analysis of microarrays applied to the ionizing radiation response. *Proc Natl Acad Sci USA* 2001;98:5116–5121.

102. Pittman J, Huang E, Dressman H, et al. Integrated modeling of clinical and gene expression information for personalized prediction of disease outcomes. *Proc Natl Acad Sci USA* 2004;101:8431–8436.

103. Simon R. Using DNA microarrays for diagnostic and prognostic prediction. *Expert Rev Mol Diagn* 2003;3:587–595.

104. Dai H, van't Veer L, Lamb J, et al. A cell proliferation signature is a marker of extremely poor outcome in a subpopulation of breast cancer patients. *Cancer Res* 2005;65:4059–4066.

105. Khan J, Wei JS, Ringner M, et al. Classification and diagnostic prediction of cancers using gene expression profiling and artificial neural networks. *Nat Med* 2001;7:673–679.

106. Lee JS, Katari G, Sachidanandam R. GObar: a Gene Ontology based analysis and visualization tool for gene sets. *BMC Bioinformatics* 2005;6:189.

107. Doms A, Schroeder M. GoPubMed: exploring PubMed with the Gene Ontology. *Nucleic Acids Res* 2005;33:W783–W786.

108. Khatri P, Sellamuthu S, Malhotra P, et al. Recent additions and improvements to the Onto-Tools. *Nucleic Acids Res* 2005;33:W762–W765.

109. Lee TI, Rinaldi NJ, Robert F, et al. Transcriptional regulatory networks in *Saccharomyces cerevisiae*. *Science* 2002;298:799–804.

110. van Steensel B. Mapping of genetic and epigenetic regulatory networks using microarrays. *Nat Genet* 2005;37(suppl):S18–S24.

111. Stuart JM, Segal E, Koller D, et al. A gene-coexpression network for global discovery of conserved genetic modules. *Science* 2003;302:249–255.

112. Djebbari A, Karamycheva S, Howe E, et al. MeSHer: identifying biological concepts in microarray assays based on PubMed references and MeSH terms. *Bioinformatics* 2005; 21:3324–3326.

113. Braga-Neto U, Hashimoto R, Dougherty ER, et al. Is cross-validation better than resubstitution for ranking genes? *Bioinformatics* 2004;20:253–258.

114. Yang MC, Yang JJ, McIndoe RA, et al. Microarray experimental design: power and sample size considerations. *Physiol Genomics* 2003;16:24–28.

115. Betensky RA, Nutt CL, Batchelor TT, et al. Statistical considerations for immunohistochemistry panel development after gene expression profiling of human cancers. *J Mol Diagn* 2005;7:276–282.

116. Bullinger L, Dohner K, Bair E, et al. Use of gene-expression profiling to identify prognostic subclasses in adult acute myeloid leukemia. *N Engl J Med* 2004;350:1605–1616.

117. Michiels S, Koscielny S, Hill C. Prediction of cancer outcome with microarrays: a multiple random validation strategy. *Lancet* 2005;365:488–492.

118. Ntzani EE, Ioannidis JP. Predictive ability of DNA microarrays for cancer outcomes and correlates: an empirical assessment. *Lancet* 2003;362:1439–1444.

119. Tothill RW, Kowalczyk A, Rischin D, et al. An expression-based site of origin diagnostic method designed for clinical application to cancer of unknown origin. *Cancer Res* 2005;65:4031–4040.

120. Dennis JL, Vass JK, Wit EC, et al. Identification from public data of molecular markers of adenocarcinoma characteristic of the site of origin. *Cancer Res* 2002;62:5999–6005.

121. Shedden KA, Taylor JM, Giordano TJ, et al. Accurate molecular classification of human cancers based on gene expression using a simple classifier with a pathological treebased framework. *Am J Pathol* 2003;163:1985–1995.

122. Segal E, Friedman N, Koller D, Regev A. A module map showing conditional activity of expression modules in cancer. *Nat Genet* 2004;36:1090–1098.

123. Xi L, Lyons-Weiler J, Coello MC, et al. Prediction of lymph node metastasis by analysis of gene expression profiles in primary lung adenocarcinomas. *Clin Cancer Res* 2005; 11:4128–4135.

124. Roepman P, Wessels LF, Kettelarij N, et al. An expression profile for diagnosis of lymph node metastases from primary head and neck squamous cell carcinomas. *Nat Genet* 2005;37:182–186.

125. Lee YF, John M, Falconer A, et al. A gene expression signature associated with metastatic outcome in human leiomyosarcomas. *Cancer Res* 2004;64:7201–7204.

126. Ramaswamy S, Ross KN, Lander ES, et al. A molecular signature of metastasis in primary solid tumors. *Nat Genet* 2003;33:49–54.

127. Woelfle U, Cloos J, Sauter G, et al. Molecular signature associated with bone marrow micrometastasis in human breast cancer. *Cancer Res* 2003;63:5679–5684.

128. van de Vijver MJ, He YD, van't Veer LJ, et al. A gene-expression signature as a predictor of survival in breast cancer. *N Engl J Med* 2002;347:1999–2009.

129. Ma XJ, Wang Z, Ryan PD, et al. A two-gene expression ratio predicts clinical outcome in breast cancer patients treated with tamoxifen. *Cancer Cell* 2004;5:607–616.

130. Huang E, Cheng SH, Dressman H, et al. Gene expression predictors of breast cancer outcomes. *Lancet* 2003;361:1590–1596.

131. Beer DG, Kardia SL, Huang CC, et al. Gene-expression profiles predict survival of patients with lung adenocarcinoma. *Nat Med* 2002;8:816–824.

132. Bhattacharjee A, Richards WG, Staunton J, et al. Classification of human lung carcinomas by mRNA expression profiling reveals distinct adenocarcinoma subclasses. *Proc Natl Acad Sci USA* 2001;98:13790–13795.

133. Valk PJ, Verhaak RG, Beijen MA, et al. Prognostically useful gene-expression profiles in acute myeloid leukemia. *N Engl J Med* 2004;350:1617–1628.

134. Dave SS, Wright G, Tan B, et al. Prediction of survival in follicular lymphoma based on molecular features of tumor-infiltrating immune cells. *N Engl J Med* 2004; 351:2159–2169.

135. Reid JF, Lusa L, De Cecco L, et al. Limits of predictive models using microarray data for breast cancer clinical treatment outcome. *J Natl Cancer Inst* 2005;97:927–930.

136. Ein-Dor L, Kela I, Getz G, et al. Outcome signature genes in breast cancer: is there a unique set? *Bioinformatics* 2005;21:171–178.

137. Chang JC, Wooten EC, Tsimelzon A, et al. Gene expression profiling for the prediction of therapeutic response to docetaxel in patients with breast cancer. *Lancet* 2003;362:362–369.

138. Chang JC, Wooten EC, Tsimelzon A, et al. Patterns of resistance and incomplete response to docetaxel by gene expression profiling in breast cancer patients. *J Clin Oncol* 2005;23:1169–1177.

139. Langheier JM, Snyderman R. Prospective medicine: the role for genomics in personalized health planning. *Pharmacogenomics* 2004;5:1–8.

140. Ohno R, Nakamura Y. Prediction of response to imatinib by cDNA microarray analysis. *Semin Hematol* 2003;40:42–49.

141. Kakiuchi S, Daigo Y, Ishikawa N, et al. Prediction of sensitivity of advanced non-small cell lung cancers to gefitinib (Iressa, ZD1839). *Hum Mol Genet* 2004;13:3029–3043.

142. Blalock EM, Geddes JW, Chen KC, et al. Incipient Alzheimer's disease: microarray correlation analyses reveal major transcriptional and tumor suppressor responses. *Proc Natl Acad Sci USA* 2004;101:2173–2178.

143. Hauser MA, Li YJ, Xu H, et al. Expression profiling of substantia nigra in Parkinson disease, progressive supranuclear palsy, and frontotemporal dementia with parkinsonism. *Arch Neurol* 2005;62:917–921.

144. Sugai T, Kawamura M, Iritani S, et al. Prefrontal abnormality of schizophrenia revealed by DNA microarray: impact on glial and neurotrophic gene expression. *Ann N Y Acad Sci* 2004;1025:84–91.

145. Lock C, Hermans G, Pedotti R, et al. Gene-microarray analysis of multiple sclerosis lesions yields new targets validated in autoimmune encephalomyelitis. *Nat Med* 2002;8:500–508.

146. Sarwal M, Chua MS, Kambham N, et al. Molecular heterogeneity in acute renal allograft rejection identified by DNA microarray profiling. *N Engl J Med* 2003;349:125–138.

147. Kao LC, Tulac S, Lobo S, et al. Global gene profiling in human endometrium during the window of implantation. *Endocrinology* 2002;143:2119–2138.

148. Cobb JP, O'Keefe GE. Injury research in the genomic era. *Lancet* 2004;363:2076–2083.

149. Chen Y, Park S, Li Y, et al. Alterations of gene expression in failing myocardium following left ventricular assist device support. *Physiol Genomics* 2003;14:251–260.

150. Kittleson MM, Minhas KM, Irizarry RA, et al. Gene expression analysis of ischemic and nonischemic cardiomyopathy: shared and distinct genes in the development of heart failure. *Physiol Genomics* 2005;21:299–307.

151. Buckley PG, Jarbo C, Menzel U, et al. Comprehensive DNA copy number profiling of meningioma using a chromosome 1 tiling path microarray identifies novel candidate tumor suppressor loci. *Cancer Res* 2005;65:2653–2661.

152. Tagawa H, Karnan S, Suzuki R, et al. Genome-wide array-based CGH for mantle cell lymphoma: identification of homozygous deletions of the proapoptotic gene BIM. *Oncogene* 2005;24:1348–1358.

153. Cheng KW, Lahad JP, Kuo WL, et al. The RAB25 small GTPase determines aggressiveness of ovarian and breast cancers. *Nat Med* 2004;10:1251–1256.

154. Wilhelm M, Veltman JA, Olshen AB, et al. Array-based comparative genomic hybridization for the differential diagnosis of renal cell cancer. *Cancer Res* 2002; 62:957–960.

155. Mehta KR, Nakao K, Zuraek MB, et al. Fractional genomic alteration detected by arraybased comparative genomic hybridization independently predicts survival after hepatic resection for metastatic colorectal cancer. *Clin Cancer Res* 2005;11:1791–1797.

156. Sebat J, Lakshmi B, Troge J, et al. Large-scale copy number polymorphism in the human genome. *Science* 2004;305:525–528.

157. Buckley PG, Mantripragada KK, Piotrowski A, et al. Copy-number polymorphisms: mining the tip of an iceberg. *Trends Genet* 2005;21:315–317.

158. Paris PL, Albertson DG, Alers JC, et al. High-resolution analysis of paraffin-embedded and formalin-fixed prostate tumors using comparative genomic hybridization to genomic microarrays. *Am J Pathol* 2003;162:763–770.

159. Scholz C, Nimmrich I, Burger M, et al. Distinction of acute lymphoblastic leukemia from acute myeloid leukemia through microarray-based DNA methylation analysis. *Ann Hematol* 2005;84:236–244.

160. Martens JW, Nimmrich I, Koenig T, et al. Association of DNA methylation of phosphoserine aminotransferase with response to endocrine therapy in patients with recurrent breast cancer. *Cancer Res* 2005;65:4101–4117.

161. Richardson B. DNA methylation and autoimmune disease. *Clin Immunol* 2003; 109:72–79.

162. Carrasquillo MM, McCallion AS, Puffenberger EG, et al. Genome-wide association study and mouse model identify interaction between RET and EDNRB pathways in Hirschsprung disease. *Nat Genet* 2002;32:237–244.

163. Sellick GS, Longman C, Tolmie J, et al. Genomewide linkage searches for Mendelian disease loci can be efficiently conducted using high-density SNP genotyping arrays. *Nucleic Acids Res* 2004;32:e164.

164. Sellick GS, Webb EL, Allinson R, et al. A high-density SNP genomewide linkage scan for chronic lymphocytic leukemia-susceptibility loci. *Am J Hum Genet* 2005;77:420–429.

165. Hu N, Wang C, Hu Y, et al. Genome-wide association study in esophageal cancer using GeneChip mapping 10K array. *Cancer Res* 2005;65:2542–2546.

166. Wong CW, Albert TJ, Vega VB, et al. Tracking the evolution of the SARS coronavirus using high-throughput, high-density resequencing arrays. *Genome Res* 2004;14:398–405.

167. Gonzalez R, Masquelier B, Fleury H, et al. Detection of human immunodeficiency virus type 1 antiretroviral resistance mutations by high-density DNA probe arrays. *J Clin Microbiol* 2004;42:2907–2912.

168. Maitra A, Cohen Y, Gillespie SE, et al. The Human MitoChip: a high-throughput sequencing microarray for mitochondrial mutation detection. *Genome Res* 2004;14:812–819.

169. Ahrendt SA, Hu Y, Buta M, et al. p53 mutations and survival in stage I non-small-cell lung cancer: results of a prospective study. *J Natl Cancer Inst* 2003;95:961–970.

170. Takahashi Y, Ishii Y, Nagata T, et al. Clinical application of oligonucleotide probe array for full-length gene sequencing of TP53 in colon cancer. *Oncology* 2003;64:54–60.

171. Wen WH, Bernstein L, Lescallett J, et al. Comparison of TP53 mutations identified by oligonucleotide microarray and conventional DNA sequence analysis. *Cancer Res* 2000;60:2716–2722.

172. Cooper M, Li SQ, Bhardwaj T, et al. Evaluation of oligonucleotide arrays for sequencing of the *p53* gene in DNA from formalin-fixed, paraffin-embedded breast cancer specimens. *Clin Chem* 2004;50:500–508.

173. Parsons DW, Wang TL, Samuels Y, et al. Colorectal cancer: mutations in a signaling pathway. *Nature* 2005;436:792.

174. Wang Z, Shen D, Parsons DW, et al. Mutational analysis of the tyrosine phosphatome in colorectal cancers. *Science* 2004; 304:1164–1166.

175. Stephens P, Edkins S, Davies H, et al. A screen of the complete protein kinase gene family identifies diverse patterns of somatic mutations in human breast cancer. *Nat Genet* 2005;37:590–592.

176. Lynch TJ, Bell DW, Sordella R, et al. Activating mutations in the epidermal growth factor receptor underlying responsiveness of non-small-cell lung cancer to gefitinib. *N Engl J Med* 2004;350:2129–2139.

177. Kobayashi S, Boggon TJ, Dayaram T, et al. EGFR mutation and resistance of non-small-cell lung cancer to gefitinib. *N Engl J Med* 2005;352:786–792.

178. Dobbin KK, Beer DG, Meyerson M, et al. Interlaboratory comparability study of cancer gene expression analysis using oligonucleotide microarrays. *Clin Cancer Res* 2005; 11:565–572.

179. Dumur CI, Nasim S, Best AM, et al. Evaluation of quality-control criteria for microarray gene expression analysis. *Clin Chem* 2004;50:1994–2002.

180. Campbell G. Some statistical and regulatory issues in the evaluation of genetic and genomic tests. *J Biopharm Stat* 2004;14:539–552.

181. Bieche I, Tozlu S, Girault I, et al. Identification of a three-gene expression signature of poor-prognosis breast carcinoma. *Mol Cancer* 2004;3:37.

182. Shi L, Tong W, Goodsaid F, et al. QA/QC: challenges and pitfalls facing the microarray community and regulatory agencies. *Expert Rev Mol Diagn* 2004;4:761–777.

Clinical Testing

of Patient's Specimens

Barbara A. Zehnbauer

Genetics is becoming important to nearly every medical specialty as the molecular pathology underlying many clinical conditions is defined at the genomic level. Clinical application of insights derived from molecular genetic research studies has become increasingly important in the clinical care of patients. Clinical molecular diagnostic methods have been integrated into many laboratory disciplines, and there are many published guidelines and recommendations from both professional societies and regulatory agencies to assist laboratory directors in the development and operations of clinical molecular pathology testing (1–10, Table 10.1). Molecular diagnostic tools and approaches to disease pathology encompass numerous laboratory specialties, including medical genetics, microbiology, histocompatibility testing, forensics, oncology, and pharmacogenetics (Table 10.2). These analyses can provide information to aid in diagnosis of disease, identification of prognostic indications, stratification to effective treatment options, monitoring of minimal residual disease (treatment efficacy), disease predisposition, and detection of therapeutic targets in gene-specific therapy (Table 10.3).

What is a molecular pathology test? In one sense, molecular testing has been practiced for some time in surgical pathology in the context of immunohistochemistry, in which antibodies are used to detect and quantify protein expression. More recently, however, molecular pathology refers to the use of molecular detection of changes in nucleic acids, either DNA or RNA, and most frequently implies direct mutation testing. Genetic testing usually provides for detection of heritable DNA variations, whereas most surgical pathology tests focus on somatic or acquired DNA variations limited to specific cells of the disease process. This chapter will address the practical features of clinical molecular pathology analysis of solid tumors and hematolymphoid malignancies via the analytic techniques and instrumentation most commonly found in clinical chemistry or laboratory medicine divisions of pathology departments.

SPECIMEN REQUIREMENTS, HANDLING, AND PROCESSING

Clinical molecular testing in the setting of surgical pathology must observe the same criteria for efficient specimen identification, preparation, and routing as in any pathology laboratory venue (2–5). Preanalytic conditions can significantly influence the detection of nucleic acid variants, which may markedly affect the test outcome. Examples include accurate identification of patient; the type, condition, and delivery of specimens submitted for analysis; specific requests for appropriate testing (consent forms, detailed requisitions, pedigree); work flow patterns within the laboratory; and records of equipment maintenance and effective operations.

Three general aspects of isolated nucleic acid specifically influence the performance of molecular pathology assays. First, the isolated nucleic acids must be of sufficient purity, which usually requires absence of contamination with nucleases (particularly ribonuclease) and other proteins, and an absence of excess salts and metal ions in the isolation buffers. Second, there must be a sufficient quantity of the specific target cell, and therefore target genome, in the patient sample. For example, a clonal tumor admixed with normal polyclonal cells, or a heterogeneous tissue specimen with many different gene expression patterns are frequently encountered and require definition of detection threshold criteria. Third, the size of the nucleic acid molecules after isolation from the cells can dramatically affect the sensitivity of the detection of specific alterations. Degradation, either enzymatic, related to heat or pH, or resulting from mechanical shear forces can reduce the size of the nucleic acid fragments.

Tissue Types

Specimen requirements are first dictated by disease pathology, including the type of tissue, the amount of tissue, type of sample (fresh, frozen or formalin-fixed, paraffin-embedded [FFPE] tissue, cytology specimen, etc.), and the extent of the

TABLE 10.1

RESOURCES FOR CLINICAL MOLECULAR PATHOLOGY LABORATORY OPERATIONAL GUIDELINES

Entity	Site	Tool(s)
Clinical Laboratory Improvement Amendments '88	http://www.cms.hhs.gov/clia/ Centers for Medicare and Medicaid Services	Clinical laboratory accreditation requirements and compliance lists *Fed Register* 1992; 57:7137–7186.
College of American Pathologists (CAP)	http://www.cap.org	Laboratory accreditation (LAP) Molecular Pathology Laboratory Inspection Checklist Proficiency surveys • Molecular oncology (MO) • Medical genetics (MGL) • Monitoring engraftment (ME) • Molecular microbiology (HIV, HCV, ID) • Microsatellite instability (MSI) • Sarcoma translocation (SARC) • Nucleic acid testing (viral; NAT)
Clinical and Laboratory Standards Institute (CLSI; formerly National Committee for Clinical Laboratory Standards, NCCLS)	http://www.nccls.org	Molecular methods guidelines • Genetic diseases • IGH and TCR gene rearrangements • Nucleic acid amplification • Nucleic acid sequencing • Collection and handling of specimens • Proficiency testing
American College of Medical Genetics (ACMG)	http://www.acmg.net	Standards and guidelines for clinical genetics laboratories Policy statements for molecular Testing of genetic diseases
The New York State Department of Health	http://www.wadsworth.org/labservices.htm	Laboratory Quality Assurance Program
U.S. Food and Drug Administration (FDA)	http://www.fda.gov	Medical devices 21CFR809.30 In vitro diagnostic products for human use • Analyte-specific reagents
Secretary's Advisory Committee for Genetics, Health, and Society (SACGHS)	http://www4.od.nih.gov/oba/SACGHS/	Genetic test definitions and oversight
Association for Molecular Pathology (AMP)	http://www.amp.org	Molecular pathology professional organization (including genetics, hematopathology, infectious disease, solid tumors) CHAMP listserve for AMP members Test directories • Solid tumors • Hematopathology • Infectious disease
American Association for Clinical Chemistry (AACC)	http://www.aacc.org	Molecular Pathology Division (including pharmacogenetics)
Genetests	http://www.genetests.org	Test directory for heritable genetic disorders

disease pathology in the sample submitted for analysis. Most (but not all) molecular diagnostic techniques will be based on PCR amplification; therefore the amount of tissue required can be relatively small and many routine pathology specimens can be analyzed effectively. Appropriate handling of the tissue postexcision and pretesting should include specific transport conditions and nucleic acid preparation procedures in order to maximize detection limits of the molecular test (4). Prompt preservation of solid tissue samples by freezing or fixation will minimize degradation and loss of nucleic acid integrity. Hematologic specimens (peripheral blood, bone marrow) should be collected in the presence of an anticoagulant, preferably ethylenediamine tetraacetic acid (EDTA) or acid citrate dextrose (ACD), but not heparin, because heparin carryover after nucleic acid isolation can inhibit subsequent polymerase chain reaction (PCR) steps. Efforts to minimize cell lysis in fresh specimens will reduce release of nucleases that can degrade nucleic acids before isolation or testing. The amount of tissue required will depend on the proportion of cells present in the sample with the

TABLE 10.2

CLINICAL LABORATORY SPECIALTIES THAT USE MOLECULAR DIAGNOSTICS

Specialty	Example
Inherited disease (medical genetics)	Cystic fibrosis, fragile X syndrome
Histocompatibility	Bone marrow transplantation
Infectious disease (microbiology, virology)	HIV, HCV viral load
Hematology	Factor V Leiden
Hematopathology/oncology	Chronic myelogenous leukemia, follicular lymphoma
Solid tumors	Ewing sarcoma, synovial sarcoma
Forensics	Criminal investigation, autopsy confirmation
Identity testing	Paternity testing, monitoring engraftment
Blood bank	Rh typing
Pharmacology/pharmacogenetics	Cytochrome P450 genes, thiopurine methyltransferase

TABLE 10.3

CLINICAL UTILITY OF MOLECULAR DIAGNOSTIC TESTING

Role of Testing	Example	Gene Tested
Diagnosis	Ewing sarcoma	*EWS* translocations
Prognosis	Acute lymphocytic leukemia	*BCR-ABL*
Stratify to treatment	Acute promyelocytic leukemia	*PML-RARα*
Treatment efficacy (minimal residual disease)	Chronic myelogenous leukemia (CML)	*BCR-ABL*
Carrier detection	Cystic fibrosis	*CFTR*
Prenatal testing	Down syndrome	Trisomy 21
Presymptomatic testing	Huntington's disease	*huntingtin* gene
Disease predisposition/risk assessment	Multiple endocrine neoplasia, type 2	*RET*
Gene-targeted treatment	Tyrosine kinase inhibitors in CML	*BCR-ABL*

suspected genetic signature, that is, detection threshold. One percent of lymphoma cells in 10^9 cells of a lymph node section will be more readily detected than the same proportion of tumor cells in a section containing 1,000 total cells.

Specimen Quality and Collection Conditions

Fresh peripheral blood, bone marrow, solid tissue biopsies, or enriched cell populations (from flow cytometry or antibody selection) should be collected, prepared, and presented to the molecular pathology laboratory using aseptic techniques. Judgments about the specimen quality should be made at intake and recorded by the clinical molecular laboratory personnel (3,4). Any problems related to specimen collection (proper labeling and identification; type and condition of specimen tubes; presence and type of anticoagulants, transport solutions, or transport conditions), quantity (insufficient), or quality (cell lysis, clotting, frozen) must be documented for quality management purposes. These findings must also be communicated to the referring physician because they may be indications for test cancellation or new specimen collection. Every effort should be made to main-

tain the integrity of the cells and the nucleic acid in the sample. Cell lysis before receipt in the laboratory will lead to nucleic acid degradation (by nucleases released from the cells) and reduction of both the overall yield and average size of the molecules recovered from the specimen. Transporting the sample on ice (4°C) will reduce cell lysis and minimize nuclease activity to reduce nucleic acid degradation.

Specimen Processing

For most DNA isolation methods from peripheral blood, the red blood cells and white blood cells are separated by centrifugal fractionation (Ficoll or gel barrier tubes) or hypotonic lysis of the red cells, with recovery of the white cells. Removing the red cells reduces the large amount of globin gene messenger RNA (mRNA) and hemoglobin protein. The high viscosity of lysed cells through the release of large macromolecules (proteins and nucleic acids) physically retards the efficient cell lysis, protein digestion, and molecular separation that are necessary to ensure quality nucleic acid preparations. Hemoglobin can inhibit the activity of emzymes used in subsequent analysis, including restriction endonucleases and thermostable polymerases used for PCR amplification. Residual protein contamination may also produce errors in nucleic acid quantification and reduce nucleic acid mobility in gel electrophoresis. Clotted samples present protein complexes that hinder pure nucleic acid isolation even with exogenous protease digestion.

Solid tissue specimens that are frozen soon after excision yield good preservation of nucleic acid in both size and quantity because the nucleases are inactivated. Such specimens should be transported in the frozen state to the laboratory for nucleic acid isolation. There the cells can be lysed under defined conditions to further minimize nucleic acid degradation. Cells will lyse upon thawing (in the absence of dimethyl sulfoxide [DMSO]) and release nucleases, but if the cells are placed in buffer-containing proteases, ionic salts, or detergents, the nucleic acid yield and quality will be maximized. Frozen cell pellets may be handled in a similar manner.

Frozen whole blood or bone marrow presents distinct obstacles to the preparation of good-quality nucleic acid and should generally be avoided unless additives such as DMSO are present to prevent cell lysis upon thawing. The lysis of combined red and white blood cells releases large quantites of hemoglobin and globin mRNA, forming a very high macromolecule concentration with high viscosity in the lysis solution. The high viscosity hinders effective separation of proteins and hemoglobin from the nucleic acids.

FFPE tissue sections are suitable sources of nucleic acid for molecular pathology testing. The FFPE block is the most prevalent form of specimen provided in referrals for surgical pathology consultation and must be included in the repertoire of the molecular diagnostic laboratory. Advantages of the FFPE section as a source of nucleic acid is that the tissue fixation process suspends degradation of nucleic acids, the specimen is readily transported, and the specimen can be stored at room temperature ($\sim$25°C) for long periods. The limitations of FFPE are that, before fixation, nucleic acids may degrade significantly; very limited amounts of nucleic acid are recovered from a thin tissue section; and the paraffin must be removed before nucleic acid isolation. Paraffin is usually removed from the sections by xylene followed by phenol-chloroform extraction to remove the xylene. Then the cellular material is digested with a protease, following which nucleic acid is isolated. Molecular analyses that employ PCR methods to amplify DNA targets of 100 to 400 base pairs (bp) coupled with sensitive detection methods (fluorescence or radioisotope based) are suitable for testing FFPE samples.

Tissue Quantity

Minimum sample requirements are determined by the assay methodology and extent of target cell involvement in the submitted tissue. Genomic Southern hybridization requires at least 10^6 cells (6 to 10 mcg of genomic DNA) for each enzyme digest for detection of single copy genomic DNA targets. Hybridization signals to detect smaller molecular weight DNA fragments (<1kb) may be enhanced by using more DNA per each digestion ($\sim$20 mcg). PCR amplification has significantly reduced DNA requirements, and typically only 20 to 200 ng are needed per reaction for many applications. Multiplexed PCR may require a bit more DNA to equally represent all targets. The sensitivity of

PCR for detection of a few variant target molecules in a large background of unaltered DNA molecules (1 in 100,000) is one of the principal strengths of this methodology in molecular pathology. Detection of DNA isolated from just 1 to 10 cells alone is much more challenging and is not routinely performed in the clinical laboratory.

Analyte Isolation and Storage

DNA

In general, DNA is more stable than RNA and will survive brief storage under refrigeration conditions (4°C) in fresh specimens. Disruption of the hydrogen bonds between the strands of the DNA duplex, either by chemical or high temperature denaturation, before molecular testing may not be desirable, for example, if the assay methodology includes genomic DNA restriction enzyme digestion rather than PCR.

Absence of proteins that may nonspecifically bind to the DNA sequence and reduce access to enzyme recognition or cleavage sites is critical to producing complete digestion products. Hemoglobin contamination can inhibit *Taq* polymerase activity, thus reducing PCR amplification. DNA preparations should be relatively free of RNA contamination, because RNA as well as protein contamination can produce inaccurate DNA quantification.

The quantity of DNA contained in each human cell type is fairly consistent in the nondisease state. Many cancers exhibit disease-specific DNA aneuploidy or genomic instability caused by the underlying mutations. Thus the extent of DNA-specific variation is roughly equivalent to the proportion of cells in the specimen that are cancer cells.

DNA is sheared during routine handling and isolation thus the size of DNA isolated from most methods ranges from 20 to 50 kb. This is suitable for most molecular pathology applications, including genomic Southern hybridization and PCR, even long-range PCR.

RNA

RNA is less stable than DNA within intact cells, and ribonucleases are both ubiquitous and difficult to inactivate. Specimens collected for RNA isolation therefore require the addition of stabilization reagents at the time of collection or prompt isolation (within a couple of hours) to preserve RNA integrity and increase yield. Refrigeration alone is not sufficient to slow this process. The amount of specific mRNA per cell is more variable than DNA because of cell type differences in transcriptional activity. For example, mature red blood cells do not contain DNA but do contain abundant globin gene transcripts. Although mRNA does not generally interfere with most gene detection methods, RNA contributes to the overall nucleic acid concentration and may produce inaccurate DNA quantification values.

CLINICAL LABORATORY TESTING VERSUS INVESTIGATIONAL TESTING

Definition

"Under state and federal regulations, only licensed clinical laboratories (i.e., certified under the Clinical Laboratory

Improvement Amendments [CLIA]([2]) are legally permitted to perform testing on patients in which the results are released directly to patients or their physicians and used for medical management. This arrangement works well and is generally adhered to throughout clinical practice, even for esoteric testing areas such as molecular pathology and diagnostic molecular genetics" (3).

Among the extraordinary diversity of techniques and methodologies, what distinguishes research investigations from clinical applications of molecular pathology techniques? First and foremost, molecular testing performed on a clinical specimen that yields information that may be used to direct the care of that same patient defines clinical testing (2). If the information is more likely to guide diagnosis or treatment of future patients by insight into mechanisms of the disease, then this is research testing. Second, specific performance standards that are regulated and monitored are required in clinical laboratory testing. Third, findings are conveyed to the requesting medical professional in a concise document. This formal reporting highlights the clinical utility of the laboratory findings with an interpretive summary that is integrated with other laboratory results for the same patient or specimen. Fourth, continuing medical education ensures that pathology professionals are informed about state-of-the-art clinical laboratory service delivery and advances in molecular technology.

Clinical laboratory testing is required when the findings of the assay will be used to make decisions about the care of the patient whose specimen was directly analyzed (2). When the patient's immediate treatment course will be influenced by the test findings, assays must be performed under clinical laboratory standards. However, clinical laboratory operations may also support clinical research studies; however, investigational or research laboratory testing holds the promise of clinical utility, which may benefit future patients (with similar clinical conditions), but at the time of testing this is not yet proven nor validated. Both clinical and research testing require proper informed consent but differ in the potential to provide defined indications for medical decision making, that is, immediate clinical utility.

Clinical laboratory testing has defined utility to distinguish alternatives in algorithms of disease diagnosis, prognosis, or treatment options. Clinical and research laboratory operations are not determined by whether the laboratory charges fees for testing services, but by whether the information produced is used to make patient care decisions. When research observations demonstrate utility for disease diagnosis, prognosis, treatment stratification, or monitoring treatment efficacy, clinicians may decide to use these data to direct decisions about patient care following appropriate clinical laboratory test validation. Research laboratories should not provide results that become part of a patient's medical record because testing by research laboratory procedures rarely meet standards of practice required for reliable patient care testing.

Specific guidelines, regulations, and laboratory practices dictate the facility, personnel, and required performance standards of clinical laboratory tests (2,3,5,6). Although techniques and instrumentation are rapidly emerging, most mutation detection instruments and reagents resemble the original research laboratory methods. Nonetheless, evolving technology presents a considerable challenge to routine and standardized test performance in the clinical molecular diagnostic laboratory. Home-brew reagents, gene patents, and availability of suitable assay controls are just some of the obstacles to routine clinical implementation of genetic testing (1–3,5,6). As noted above, there are many resources in the literature of published guidelines and recommendations from both professional societies and regulatory agencies to assist laboratory directors in the development of procedures and operations in clinical molecular pathology testing (Table 10.1).

Analytical Validation

Clinical laboratories have the responsibility to validate assays through detailed documentation of the analytical performance characteristics and clinical correlation(s) (2,3,5). This is not only good laboratory practice; it is required by CLIA guidelines that describe the federal certification requirements for all laboratories that perform testing on patients' specimens to generate results that may be included in clinical care decisions. According to CLIA Regulation 493.1253(b)(1):

"Each laboratory that introduces an unmodified, FDA-cleared or approved test system must do the following before reporting patient test results:

i Demonstrate that it can obtain performance specifications comparable to those established by the manufacturer for the following performance characteristics: (A) accuracy, (B) precision, (C) reportable range of test results for the test system.
ii Verify that the manufacturer's reference intervals (normal values) are appropriate for the laboratory's patient population."

Extensive validation of new disease markers in the clinical laboratory is an integral element of good patient care, but how is testing validated? Essential features that distinguish clinical molecular testing from research studies of gene-disease association are rigorous quality control, quality assurance, and both analytical and clinical validation. Each laboratory must characterize *and provide detailed documentation of* the analytical performance characteristics of sensitivity, specificity, and reproducibility (Table 10.4). Central to this validation process is the evaluation of well-characterized control samples, both positive and negative controls, as well as comparison of the assay performance with a gold standard test that may already be published. The characteristics of assay validation should be defined before reporting patient test results. In the absence of available standards (as in rare genetic disorders), sharing of samples with another laboratory for evaluation with an established clinical assay is another validation approach (2,3,5).

The data collected in a typical validation procedure include the incidence of detection of true positive, false positive, true negative, and false negative results (Table 10.4). For each test, the laboratory must have ongoing review of test accuracy to assess how much error and what type of error might be present in the test results produced. Measures must be included that describe the laboratory's ability to detect and minimize these errors. The thresholds of test

TABLE 10.4
CHARACTERISTICS OF CLINICAL LABORATORY TEST VALIDATION

Term	Definition	Example
Accuracy	The ability to generate a correct measurement of the "true" value as detected by an accepted standard technique.	Proficiency testing.
Precision	The consistent production of the same test results on independent testing of the same sample.	Reproducibility of values produced in replicate samples or controls within an assay or between runs of an assay.
True positive	Positive test result in the presence of mutation/disease = A.	
False positive	Positive test result in the absence of mutation/disease = B.	
False negative	Negative test result in the presence of mutation/disease = C.	
True negative	Negative test result in the absence of mutation/disease = D.	
Analytical sensitivity	The probability that the method will detect the DNA sequence change of interest. [Variant detected/total samples with variant detected by gold standard method] = A/(A + C)	PCR-RFLP detects the same DNA variation as direct DNA sequencing.
Analytical specificity	The probability that the method will correctly detect the absence of a DNA sequence change. [Variant not detected / total samples with no variant detected by gold standard method] = D/(B + D)	Absence of detection of clonal gene rearrangements in normal cell lines.
Clinical sensitivity	The probability of a positive test result in the presence of disease (as confirmed by another standard diagnostic assay).	Greater than 90% of patients with CML have the *BCR-ABL* fusion transcript as detected by reverse transcription-PCR.
Clinical specificity	The probability of a negative test result in the absence of disease.	Absence of clonal IGH gene rearrangements in normal functional T lymphoid cell populations.
Positive predictive value (PPV)	Disease present / total with positive results = A/(A + B).	
Negative predictive value (NPV)	Disease absent / total with negative results = D/(C + D).	

performance must provide margins to ensure that errors will not affect the interpretation of the test result and thereby compromise patient care.

There are many different molecular methods available and a variety of analytical instruments for monitoring and detection (1,3, 7–10). Some are more adaptable to the quality measures and performance documentation required of clinical testing. Ideally, a molecular test would be performed in a closed-system, single-tube reaction vessel with complete data manipulation, archiving, and reporting capacities. In contrast, many molecular biology methods in the research laboratory are labor intensive and of high complexity, requiring many steps that are completed in several days or weeks.

Proficiency survey for laboratory test accuracy, peer inspection of all aspects of laboratory operations, and certification of personnel, procedures, and policies are required elements of reliable clinical laboratory functions (2,3,5,9). Specific and detailed descriptions of all aspects of laboratory performance are recorded and examined to ensure technical accuracy and clinical utility similar to a premarket review of commercial tests for precision, interference, and accurate ranges of analyte measurement.

Steps in the evaluation of a laboratory method include a thorough survey of the literature, definition of the purpose of the test, specification of the analyte to be tested, choice of a reference method (gold standard) that suits the application, definition of the test performance requirements, demonstration of the test characteristics, and determination of clinical or public health usefulness of the test results (3,5). Ongoing test validation includes quality control, proficiency testing, instrument calibration, historical data documentation, and competency testing of personnel (see later discussion).

Reagents

Each clinical molecular laboratory must verify and document that all reagents used, whether purchased or prepared in house, have the necessary biochemical reactivity (5). Several methods may be appropriate for this purpose, including "direct analysis with reference materials, parallel testing of old vs. new reagents, and checking against routine controls" (5). Where individually packaged reagents or kits are used, written criteria must be established to monitor reagent quality and stability. All reagents and solutions must be properly identified by labeling that includes content, concentration, storage conditions, date prepared, and an expiration date, either on the container or recorded in a separate log book. Molecular probes and PCR primers are considered reagents that also require detailed documentation (sequence type [genomic, cDNA, synthetic oligonucleotide], origin [human, microbial, viral], sequence position in the target gene, restriction enzyme map, and known polymorphisms) to facilitate interpretation and troubleshooting of test results (2,3,5). It is essential to guarantee comparable assay performance in different laboratories even when a commercial reagent kit is used. The performance characteristics under optimum conditions described by manufacturers may differ significantly with specimen type, specimen age, instrumentation, and operator expertise. Clinical laboratories regulated by CLIA 88 may use analyte specific reagents (ASRs) specified by the Food and Drug Administration (FDA) for in-house assay development (6). The clinical laboratory must include a disclaimer in the formal laboratory report stating that the performance characteristics of the ASRs were determined by that laboratory and have not been approved by the FDA.

Accuracy

Accuracy of the assay describes the ability to correctly identify a known molecular variation, usually defined by a separate method (1,9,11). This is frequently assessed using cell lines to represent both positive controls (with the molecular variation) and negative controls (absence of the molecular variation). Previously tested specimens that have been evaluated by other methods or by other laboratories may also be employed. The availability of these control materials is essential to the evaluation of the method and to the optimization of the assay conditions.

Precision

Precision refers to the reproducibility of the assay for a specific test result, usually by replicate analysis of the same sample (1, 5, 11). The agreement should be assessed within replicates of the assay (within-run), across replicates in separate assays (between-run), and by within-technologist and between-technologist assay performance. How many replicates are done commonly ranges from 10 to 50, but additional statistical considerations beyond the scope of this chapter are often required (11). All technologists in the laboratory should be trained and monitored to return good precision for each molecular laboratory test.

Quality Management: Maintenance and Calibration

Ensuring the fundamentally favorable performance of all laboratory systems increases the reliability and acceptance of laboratory data (12). This requires at least three levels of monitoring: analysis of control materials at the time of clinical specimen analysis; maintenance and evaluation of proper function of all laboratory facilities and equipment; and established calibration procedures to specify the relationship between the measured event (mutation) and the actual event, concentration, or activity (5). Each laboratory must define limits for acceptance or rejection of test results based on the calibration values. Usually this is ascertained by monitoring the results obtained from control samples (positive, negative, and contamination controls) that are included in each assay run. Unacceptable or unusual control results render clinical specimen findings questionable and unsatisfactory for reporting. The assay may be repeated, or a more detailed examination of all test parameters may be required to identify the source of the aberrant control values.

In addition, control materials are evaluated during test validation before clinical reporting. This demonstrates the reliability of the assay performance (precision) relative to the initial assay validation conditions (5). This is also critical in monitoring the calibration and function of the equipment and procedures.

Product Confirmation

PCR products are frequently detected by electrophoresis using an agarose or acrylamide gel matrix in a slab or capillary separation chamber. Comparison of the specific DNA fragment size to a molecular weight ladder is the first step to confirm that the correct target has been amplified (3,5). Additional confirmation of DNA fragment identity may be achieved by DNA sequencing, oligonucleotide hybridization, or melting curve profiles. These measures discriminate possible spurious or cross-reacting molecular profiles that may be produced from reduced specificity of the reaction or contamination of assay components.

Availability of Control Materials

Control materials are essential to assay development and accurate assay performance. The limited application of many tests is due to a lack of well-characterized and easily maintained control samples. Numerous commercial sources are available for many human cell lines, microbial and viral strains, isolated nucleic acids (DNA and RNA), and synthetic oligonucleotides (1,3,9). Manufacturers of diagnostic kits also may include these types of controls in addition to assay reagents. Interlaboratory exchanges of confirmed samples, or exchanges with authors who have published accounts of controls analyzed with the same or related molecular methods, may also be sources of suitable controls. Archived patient specimens previously analyzed by other methods also may be used as controls provided that the patient has given specific consent for this use, the institutional review board (IRB) has approved this use, or the sample material is completely anonymized and cannot be linked to personal identifiers (Health Insurance Portability and Accountability Act, HIPAA) (13) as approved by IRB safeguards. Each laboratory must document proficiency and quality performance with materials from these sources.

Variety of Technologies

The molecular techniques in use in many molecular diagnostic laboratories are very similar to the research laboratory applications of these same methods. The burden of the clinical molecular pathology laboratory is to apply these methods in well-defined and validated procedures that will ensure a high level of accuracy coupled with a low level of repeat analyses. There are many detailed guidelines for the application of common molecular methods to clinical testing, including Southern blot hybridization analysis, electrophoresis, nucleic acid amplification, direct DNA sequencing, DNA conformation analysis, and quantitative real-time PCR (1,3–, 7-10).

Clinical Validation

Clinical validation of molecular pathology assays requires that a clear disease phenotype can be ascertained and confirmed with another assay type, whether molecular or nonmolecular (biopsy findings, clinical examination, etc). Clinical sensitivity refers to the ability to detect the molecular signature in the presence of disease, clinical specificity refers to the absence of the molecular variation when disease is not present (1,5,11). Similar to analytical validation, clinical validation parameters balance the true positive and false negative findings (sensitivity) with the true negative and false positive (specificity) observations.

Clinical validation and analytical validation may not exhibit the same extent of sensitivity, as discussed in more detail in Chapter 8. This can arise because the genetic variation detected in the control samples is more limited than the biologic variation of the disease presentation. The analytical sensitivity may be high but the clinical sensitivity reduced in patients with disease pathology but no molecular variation. Multiple disease-causing genes may be the cause and require additional technical design. DNA polymorphisms that adversely affect the annealing of PCR primers and reduce PCR amplification efficiency may also reduce clinical sensitivity of the assay.

However, with the increased sensitivity of PCR amplification to detect rare cells or molecules, molecular pathology studies may detect DNA changes in the absence of overt disease. This may be a useful feature for presymptomatic diagnosis providing the opportunity for early intervention or treatment. Or this may create a dilemma when a positive result is detected in a patient who either has no pathogenic disease in evidence or has a distinctly different phenotype from patients in the affected test population. Interactions with other gene products (receptors, ligands, cofactors, modifiers) can attenuate the function of the abnormality detected in the single gene assay. Unanticipated biologic roles for the gene of interest or relatively mild and uncharacterized disease presentation may explain seemingly discordant positive genetic test findings in atypical phenotypic presentations. For some disorders, it may be very difficult to identify large numbers of patients with the disease to establish the clinical sensitivity of the test. In this case, the laboratory should evaluate as many cases as are available to validate the method and cite scientific publications that describe similar investigations of the same disorder (3,5).

Laboratory Accreditation

The requirements for accurate and reliable test performance are specified by the Federal Centers for Medicare and Medicaid Services (CMS) in the Clinical Laboratory Improvement Amendments '88 (CLIA), Public Law 100-578 (2). CMS regulates all laboratory testing (except research) performed on humans in the United States through the Clinical Laboratory Improvement Amendments (CLIA), and in total, CLIA covers approximately 175,000 laboratory entities. Recommendations of CLIA-acceptable laboratory practices (Table 10.1) are usually monitored by inspectors certified by the College of American Pathologists (CAP) through their Laboratory Accreditation Program (LAP) using the Molecular Pathology Checklist inspection guidelines (5). "Testing that involves DNA/RNA probe hybridization or amplification constitutes molecular testing. The Molecular Pathology Checklist covers most aspects of clinical molecular testing including oncology, hematology, infectious disease, inherited disease, HLA typing, forensics, and parentage applications." It does not include cytogenetics or anatomic pathology applications for fluorescence in situ hybridization (FISH) or in situ hybridization (ISH). Microbiology laboratory molecular methods that are not FDA approved or that modify an FDA-approved method will also be inspected with the Molecular Pathology Checklist. A list of FDA-approved molecular tests is published online by the Association for Molecular Pathology (www.amp.org).

All aspects of effective molecular pathology laboratory operations are measured, including test requisitions, specimen handling, reagent integrity, instrument maintenance and calibration, reports of laboratory data, personnel qualifications, and proficiency assessment. It is notable that no particular molecular technique or equipment is specifically recommended, but instead provisions for inspection of a wide variety of methodologies are accommodated (2,3,5). The contents described in the CAP Laboratory General Checklist also apply to molecular pathology laboratory practices covering such aspects as information that must be included in laboratory test requisitions, procedures, and reports (3, 5). The CAP further recognizes that "inspection of a molecular pathology laboratory requires special knowledge of the science [such that] the inspector should be an actively practicing molecular scientist familiar with the Checklist and possessing the technical and interpretive skills necessary to evaluate the quality of the laboratory's performance" (5).

The CAP Commission on Laboratory Accreditation (CLA) and CLIA guidelines describe requirements that must be fulfilled, but do not specify methods or techniques to achieve these conditions. Individual laboratories may devise different procedures and policies for collecting and organizing the data required for certification inspections. Concise and easily accessed documentation is essential to the inspection process. Linking the documentation to the specific checklist item helps to focus the inspection. Favorable CAP inspection findings are usually sufficient to satisfy CLIA accreditation requirements, but separate unannounced CLIA-led inspections may also take place. The New York State Department of Health also performs inspections of molecular pathology/genetics laboratories to fulfill requirements for New York State Laboratory accreditation. This applies not only to New York laboratories, but to testing of specimens from patients with New York medical insurance coverage, even if the testing is performed in another state (14).

Personnel Certification

For optimal patient care, only qualified personnel should perform molecular pathology testing (2). Professional qualification for molecular pathology laboratory directors are described by CLIA as "commensurate with the responsibilities of a high complexity laboratory director" to include pathologists, board-certified physicians in other specialties, or doctoral scientists in a biologic science with specialized training or experience in molecular pathology. In addition, starting in 2003, new doctoral degreed directors of molecular pathology ("high-complexity") laboratories were also required to obtain board certification. Professional board certification provides a measure of expertise in laboratory-based medical science or clinical practice by assessing comprehensive knowledge of molecular pathology and laboratory principles. Although many medical specialties are recognized for physician laboratory directors, only the American Board of Medical Genetics (ABMG), American Board of Clinical Chemistry (ABCC), American Board of Bioanalysis (ABB), and the National Credentialing Agency (NCA) will certify Ph.D.-trained scientists (Table 10.5) (15). Molecular pathology technologists may obtain certification from the American Society of

Clinical Pathology (ASCP) or the or the NCA. Training for these boards involves education regarding molecular test design and validation. These certificates also require continued educational assessment at specified intervals to maintain current knowledge.

TECHNICAL ISSUES OF TEST IMPLEMENTATION

Procedure Manual

An instructional manual that precisely describes the procedures currently in use is essential and must be available to laboratory personnel at the workbench (2,3,5). Complete procedure manuals not only ensure that all laboratory personnel can refer to the same well-defined steps for each test but also provide an excellent instructional tool for training new technologists. The elements that must be included in each assay procedure are as follows (1–3,5):

- Name of the procedure
- Indications for testing
- Clinical significance
- The principle of the test method
- Specimen requirements
- Required reagents and equipment
- Test calibration
- Procedural steps
- Quality control measures
- Calculations
- Reference values
- Interpretation of results
- Pertinent literature references that are the basis for the procedure methods.

TABLE 10.5

SPECIALTY CERTIFICATION IN MOLECULAR PATHOLOGY/ MOLECULAR DIAGNOSTICS*

Specialty	Board	Eligibility
Clinical Molecular Genetics	American Board of Medical Genetics (ABMG)	M.D. and Ph.D.; residency or fellowship required
Molecular Genetic Pathology	American Board of Pathology (ABP)	M.D.; fellowship required
Molecular Diagnostics	American Board of Clinical Chemistry (ABCC)	M.D. and Ph.D.; prior general board certification required
Bioanalyst Clinical Laboratory Director;	American Board of Bioanalysis (ABB)	M.D. and Ph.D., B.A. and B.S.
High-complexity Clinical Laboratory Director;		
Moderate-complexity Clinical Laboratory Director		
Certified Laboratory Specialist in Molecular Biology (CLSp(MB))	National Credentialing Agency for Laboratory Personnel (NCA)	B.A. and B.S., Clinical Laboratory Scientist (CLS)

*Non-physicians with doctoral degrees and certification by the American Board of Medical Microbiology or the American Board of Medical Laboratory Immunology may work as laboratory directors (per CLIA'88) but specific molecular pathology certification is not available.

Considerations of both preanalytic and postanalytic critical factors that affect test reliability are also necessary. Manufacturers' package inserts and instrument operations manuals may be included in the procedure manual but are not sufficient substitutes for a complete procedure as performed in the laboratory (5). Electronic procedure manuals are acceptable, provided there are appropriate document control measures in place to limit alterations of the procedures to only authorized personnel (laboratory director or designate), and provided there is documentation of annual review of each procedure.

Reporting of Results

Many molecular tests yield primary data that must be interpreted in context before the results can be clearly stated. For example, a base change is evidence of DNA mutation, but whether the change alters protein function or is pathogenic must be interpreted in the context of the gene sequence. The position of the base change within the gene (regulatory region, intron, exon) or within the codon influences the effect on the protein expressed. An amino acid substitution that results from the mutation may change the protein function to cause severe disease or may not be associated with disease. Reporting is separate from the analysis, but links the analytical detection and understanding of the limitations of the test methodology to the interpretation of the biologic significance of the molecular findings.

Reporting the results of clinical molecular pathology tests should be concise and use terminology that aids the physician in the care of the patient. It must provide sufficient background and context for the results to provide the physician with the knowledge to explain the findings to the patient. Ideally, the report should merge molecular findings with other diagnostic findings of the surgical pathology consult report. The degree of integration of these features may vary widely across laboratories because there are no standards of practice to describe this interaction and many laboratory information systems do not provide this interface. Clinical laboratories do have specific and essential elements that must be included in laboratory reports as defined by CLIA and CAP (2,3,5), but reports should nonetheless be consistent with the practices of both the molecular and the surgical pathology laboratories acting in a consultative role in the care of the patient.

Turn-around Time

Adapting molecular diagnostic research methods to yield results within a time frame that will facilitate effective clinical management (12) can be a significant technologic obstacle. Most molecular pathology procedures have many steps, which may not be automated and may require several days to complete. Many laboratory equipment manufacturers are developing instruments and reagent combinations that will significantly shorten some analysis steps, but sample preparation, appropriate clinical laboratory documentation, and reporting of assay results are not frequently automated.

The nature of molecular tests rarely permits STAT performance. In some instances of urgent clinical need, many laboratories can assign personnel to focus on a single specimen with direct processing in less than 1 day, if the impact and clinical utility of the molecular findings justifies the expense. With the increasing role of molecular pathology to define effective treatment stratification, particularly with gene-targeted drugs, the need for accurate genotyping before initiation of therapy will increase the requirement for rapid analyses. For example, before treating a leukemia patient with the tyrosine kinase inhibitor imatinib mesylate, the oncologist will need molecular verification that the patient's leukemia cells harbor the *BCR-ABL* fusion gene that is specifically targeted by this chemotherapy (Chapter 13).

Cost Analysis, Billing Considerations, and Reimbursement

Physicians' Current Procedural Terminology (CPT) codes, descriptions, and other data are defined by the American Medical Association (16). This system of terminology is the most widely accepted medical nomenclature used to report medical procedures and services under public and private health insurance programs. CPT is also used for administrative management purposes such as claims processing and developing guidelines for medical care review. The uniform language is likewise applicable to medical education and research by providing a useful basis for local, regional, and national utilization comparisons. CPT codes were adopted as part of the Centers for Medicare and Medicaid Services (CMS) Healthcare Common Procedure Coding System (HCPCS) (17). With this adoption, CMS mandated the use of HCPCS to report services for Part B of the Medicare Program. In October 1986, CMS also required state Medicaid agencies to use HCPCS in the Medicaid Management Information System. In July 1987, as part of the Omnibus Budget Reconciliation Act, CMS mandated the use of CPT for reporting outpatient hospital surgical procedures. Today, in addition to use in federal programs (Medicare and Medicaid), CPT is used extensively throughout the United States as the preferred system of coding and describing health care services.

Reimbursement for clinical laboratory services is related to and depends on accurate descriptions of laboratory procedures and methods. However, reimbursement rates will vary significantly among third-party payers, insurance companies, and Medicare/Medicaid. Clinical Laboratory Fee Schedules consider both technical and professional components of laboratory testing (1,16,17). Fees are assigned to CPT codes by CMS for Medicare/Medicaid reimbursement, but many institutions may derive different fee schedules from different insurance providers. Professional laboratory organizations frequently designate experts to represent the interests of their members in negotiations for fair and reasonable recovery of test costs. Molecular pathology tests are perceived as high-cost relative to many clinical laboratory tests because they are comparatively labor intensive rather than highly automated and because they require costly specialty reagents, royalty and license payments, and rapidly changing instrumentation designs.

Quality Assurance (QA) and Proficiency Testing (PT)

Quality assurance is defined by policies and procedures designed to monitor and evaluate clinical laboratory test performance to ensure production of highly accurate data. These criteria include descriptions of the proper values in each assay, as well as interpretation of positive and negative control analytes (3,5). Monitoring and documention of assay turn-around time, incidence, cause and resolution of assay failures, and detailed technical standards for each technique (3–5,7–10) are aspects of laboratory practice that contribute to quality assurance.

Proficiency testing is required as an indicator of laboratory test accuracy (1,2,5,11). This may be accomplished by participating in formal CAP programs relevant to the laboratory test capabilities (Table 10.1). If a laboratory is unable to enroll in a proficiency survey program, alternative assessment of laboratory test accuracy must be implemented. These may include split sample analysis with another established in-house reference method or split sample analysis with other laboratories (5). The opportunities to share knowledge, control materials, and experiences with other laboratory professionals enhances the laboratory practice of each pathologist who participates in these activities.

CHARACTERISTICS OF TESTS WITH CLINICAL UTILITY

Clinical Utility

One definition of clinical utility states: "The value of a test, including risks and benefits, for the purposes of confirmation of diagnosis in a symptomatic patient, presymptomatic analysis, treatment, family planning, and prenatal testing (when relevant)" (3). In most aspects, the same criteria that evaluate the clinical utility of other hospital laboratory tests can and should be applied when considering the role of the molecular pathology laboratory in patient care (Table 10.6).

- The relative merit of the molecular testing should focus on the ability of the test findings to improve patient care rather than the presence of the technical capacity to perform the test.
- General characteristics of the molecular tests must consider practical aspects of clinical prevalence, test run frequency, turn-around time, sensitivity and specificity.
- Routine laboratory methods by which molecular tests are validated must include positive and negative assay controls, confirmation of the identity of the product, specifications for instrument calibration and maintenance, definition of the details and limits of interpretation of test results, and provisions for proficiency testing of the method and the technologists.
- Models for reporting results should not only explain the molecular assay data but also integrate these findings with other pathology results to avoid seemingly contradictory reports from other laboratory tests with different levels of resolution or detection.
- Biosafety, legal, ethical, and privacy issues must consistently be observed, documented, and reviewed at regular intervals.

When is clinical molecular testing beneficial? Genetic testing can take the pathologist beyond the characterization of cell biology, protein expression, or chromosomal abnormalities to the resolution of single nucleotide changes in the DNA molecule. The most obvious benefit of application of genetic testing is sensitive identification of subclinical conditions. Molecular genetics tests can indicate disease risk in presymptomatic individuals, assess recurrence risk, or determine carrier status and risk for affected offspring. Molecular pathology tests may also contribute to more precise diagnosis, refine prognostic categories, stratify patients

TABLE 10.6
CHARACTERISTICS OF MOLECULAR TESTS WITH CLINICAL UTILITY

Criterion	Utility
The disorder must be a significant health problem.	Disease prevalence and adverse effect on affected individuals are measurable and serious.
Treatment alternatives are available to alter disease course.	The genotype does affect the patient's clinical outcome.
A reliable molecular test is available to distinguish true positive and false positive results.	Focus on molecular changes known to be associated with disease pathology.
Pre-test and Post-test counseling resources are available.	Interpretation of molecular findings with the data from the clinical presentation and other pathology tests.
The test is cost-effective and /or cost-beneficial.	More costly or invasive disease monitoring methods are unnecessary. Specific treatment options and/or prognostic outcomes are indicated by the molecular results.
Referring clinicians accept the test as worthwhile to aid their decision-making.	Diagnosis, treatment, and/or clinical outcome are enhanced by the addition of the molecular pathology results to other medical tests.

to optimal treatment choices, and monitor the efficacy of the treatment by detection of minimal residual disease.

For clinical utility, the molecular diagnostic test must be an improvement in the standard of patient care. It may provide new or redefined information with the potential for clinical stratification of disease subtypes, prognostic categories, survival statistics, and disease progression. Molecular pathology should complement the findings of established testing, such as cytogenetics, immunohistochemistry, cell surface marker analysis, and routine histopathologic analysis. This may require the interpretation by a qualified anatomic pathologist in concert with the molecular laboratory specialist. Molecular pathology testing that has utility in clinical decision making has several hallmarks common to other clinical laboratory analyses, including reproducibility, accuracy, clinically relevant turn-around time, and cost-effectiveness. Improved patient care is the primary goal and directs all aspects of test selection, design, and performance. With increasing knowledge of gene–disease associations deduced from the Human Genome Project and other basic science research studies, the challenge of the molecular pathology laboratory director is to focus his or her practice, expertise, and resources on the most significant clinical problems. The definition of what assays fulfill the "significant" criterion may be quite variable in different laboratory settings.

The disease should represent a significant health problem (or diagnostic dilemma). Diseases that are common and frequent in many populations (cancer, microbial infections, genetic predispositions) and that have well-defined molecular causes will be the subject of assay development in many laboratories. Molecular genetic associations for rare disorders usually will not develop into clinical diagnostic assays except at a few select laboratories representing specific clinical programs or areas of institutional focus and expertise. For example, cancer is a very common diagnosis in the pathology laboratory for which many molecular assays are available. Patients with leukemia or lymphoma are frequently diagnosed, assigned to prognostic groups, stratified to treatment options, and followed for minimal residual disease by molecular pathology testing. Sarcomas with similar morphologic features but distinct genetic abnormalities and different treatment alternatives may be more accurately diagnosed and treated based on the findings of molecular testing. Cancer recurrence or progression may be more sensitively detected at earlier stages and lower tumor burden using specific molecular signatures.

Familial cancer syndromes, however, usually represent only a small percentage of total cases of a specific tumor type. Although the genetic factors that contribute to inherited predisposition to cancer have been intensely studied to elucidate biologic mechanisms of tumorigenesis and identify targets for cancer treatment, testing for the associated mutations has not significantly affected the clinical care of patients in the general population with sporadic forms of the tumors. Only academic or commercial reference laboratories that focus their molecular testing on some of the less frequent familial presentations and that have active partnerships with clinical colleagues with specific interest or expertise in the disorder (e.g., a registry of patients, a clinical trial, a program project grant) will generate enough referrals to justify assay development.

The molecular pathology results affect clinical outcome. Molecular results may provide a basis for the selection of a specific treatment regimen. Detection of a molecular mutation detection may correlate with favorable prognostic outcome (response to treatment or disease-free survival) or may indicate treatment choices that have previously been most beneficial to patients with that molecular signature. Stratification of treatment based on molecular characteristics emerge only as a result of understanding the unique biologic features conferred by the genetic variant and relies on the results of previous clinical trials that have demonstrated treatment efficacy in patients with the same clinical features and molecular disease characteristics.

A reliable molecular test is available. Multiple assay platforms may be available for detection of a specific type of mutation, or a variety of techniques may be required for detection of different mutation types. The choice of assay methodology will be determined by the spectrum of mutations represented in the disease, the performance characteristics of the methods, the time and expense of the methods, and the availability of control materials. No single assay methodology will efficiently identify all possible types of mutation or be best suited to all laboratories.

For example, direct DNA sequencing may be regarded as the gold standard in the detection of nucleotide changes because it provides the highest level of resolution of genetic variation. But in the clinical laboratory setting, DNA sequencing is very labor intensive and expensive. For genes with many different mutations, sequencing may be a very direct method of evaluating many nucleotide positions with a single assay. But if the most common mutations are large deletions or rearrangements, DNA sequencing may be very difficult to apply because the regions required for PCR amplification may no longer be present. Complete gene sequencing may be more feasible and cost-effective with current high-throughput technologies, but predicting the function of the expressed protein or disease phenotype from the primary DNA sequence data can be imperfect or misleading. Conserved amino acid substitutions may exist as normal functional variations within the population, and, conversely, nonconserved substitutions may confer mild or severe phenotype dependent on which region of the protein is affected (active site, cofactor binding site, dimerization domain, external surface domain, etc.). Furthermore, the same base change may be associated with different phenotypes when other modifier gene functions attenuate the target gene expression or function. One example of this phenomenon is provided by the *RET* proto-oncogene, a tyrosine kinase receptor in which identical mutations are associated with familial medullary thyroid carcinoma in some families but cause multiple endocrine neoplasia type 2A (MEN2A; MTC plus pheochromocytoma and parathyroid hyperplasia) in other kindreds (Chapter 12). Genetic variations in other genes in these different families may attenuate the affect of the *RET* mutation to produce these distinct clinical presentations.

Many mutation detection assays are available as commercial kits, which include quality-controlled reagents and appropriate control samples. Some of these are designed to be coupled with specific instrumentation, whereas others may interface with a variety of detection techniques (fluorescence, bioluminescence, slab gel electrophoresis, capillary gel electrophoresis), formats (manual, automatic, or robotic), and analytic scales (single sample, 12 samples, 16 samples, 96 samples). Many new platforms are emerging and guidelines for reliable implementation in the clinical laboratory will be necessary.

Laboratory space and design must also be considered when selecting test methodologies. Physical separation of preanalytical, analytical, and postanalytical operations is important to prevent contamination and safety hazards. These features are described in greater detail elsewhere (3–5, 7–10).

For each application, the molecular pathologist should focus on DNA changes known to be consistent with disease expression. DNA variation without consistent pathogenic consequences may indicate reduced penetrance of the abnormal gene function associated with disease phenotype or may indicate that the gene product represents one possible downstream result generated by abnormal function of the true causative gene. Molecular testing to detect disease-associated nucleic acid changes currently refers to DNA-and mRNA-based analysis, but may soon include RNAi or microRNA applications.

The molecular diagnostic test must clearly distinguish true positive from false positive results. Specific interpretive guidelines must be described by each clinical testing laboratory (2,3,5). These guidelines are developed with consideration of the technical limitations of the test methodology, variable presentation of disease phenotypes, and a distinct understanding of possible contaminating substances that can interfere with test accuracy or precision. Test validation and characterization require thorough literature review, clinical correlation studies of the genetic variant, definition of test performance to ensure consistent and reliable accuracy, establishment of the clinical utility of the test findings in directing patient care, careful delineation of the parameters that must be observed to maintain test performance, and specification of the limitations of the test methodology (2,3,5).

Pretest and posttest counseling resources are available for contextual interpretation of the molecular test findings. For inherited disorders, a genetic counseling session to explain the implications and limitations of molecular genetics test is conducted both before a patient consents to the test and when the patient is informed of the test results (3). Molecular pathology results should also be conveyed to the patient in an informative and supportive context.

Clinical and investigational testing both require informed consent before testing but with very different implications. In research testing, informed consent explains the relative risk of specimen collection, the biologic hypothesis tested in the study, and the future promise for improved diagnosis or treatment for future patients. Clinical testing requires informed consent that includes explanation of the risks of specimen collection, but also includes a description of the direct implications of the test findings for treatment selection or prognostic outcome. Limitations of the testing procedures should also be conveyed, along with the implications of a positive or negative test finding. Through this approach, each patient should be able to understand how the test results will be used by their physician to formulate the immediate and future course of treatment.

Proper referral of cases for molecular testing requires resources to integrate the molecular findings with the results of other clinical and diagnostic tools. This may be accomplished thorough shared electronic laboratory information systems, case conferences attended by a variety of clinical specialists, and informative laboratory newsletters for physician clients. Molecular pathology assays are significant tools in disease diagnosis and will be more broadly accepted and requested when supported by collegial educational programs.

LEGAL ISSUES

Ethical Issues

The National Human Genome Research Institute (NHGRI; 18) created the Ethical, Legal and Social Implications (ELSI) Research Program in 1990 as an integral part of the Human Genome Project. Through the ELSI Research Program, NHGRI supported numerous ethics- and policy-related forums to explore and address such issues. One outcome of this program was the development of current U.S. legislation, the Genetic Nondiscrimination Act, which safeguards against misuse of genetic information.

Perceptions that genetic discrimination in health insurance and employment may occur continue to persist even though very few cases have actually been documented. Both federal and state laws for Genetic Information Nondiscrimination have been implemented in nearly every state of the United States, although the provisions for health care and employment vary across states (19). The Health Insurance Portability and Accountability Act (HIPAA) prohibits the use of genetic information in denying or limiting health insurance coverage for members of a group health plan (19). Nonetheless, the public continues to voice fears about the use and storage of molecular genetic information with trepidation regarding misuse of this data extending to potential discrimination in disability insurance, life insurance, access to education, adoption, and immigration policy (20), even though the majority of testing in many molecular pathology laboratories involves detection of acquired rather than inherited genetic variations and the risk for disease predisposition in other family members in this setting is minimal. Nonetheless, the very promise of the Human Genome Project to apply genetic information to the development of individualized medical treatment, the expansion of preventive measures, and the improvement of human health may not be realized if patients fear that the same test results may exclude them from affordable insurance coverage (19).

Patient Safety and Privacy

The provisions of HIPAA apply to molecular pathology laboratory findings as part of a patient's medical record. Therefore measures must be implemented to restrict access to and provide confidentiality for these laboratory test results. Some genetics professionals further assert the issue of "genetic exceptionalism" to maintain that genetic or DNA information is special and should be afforded distinct safeguards in addition to those usually associated with medical records (20), because genetic sequence is a unique identifier, is heritable, has relevance to other family members, can predict future disease risk, and has the potential to be used to stigmatize, discriminate, or psychologically affect individuals who may not express symptoms of disease. Opponents of this view claim that the uniqueness of genetic material is also present in other types of medical information, thus no unique safeguards are required. In purely practical terms, separating genetic information from other information in the medical record or chart is not feasible in routine clinical practice.

FDA Regulation

A laboratory that develops an in-house test using an analyte-specific reagent (ASR) must inform the medical professional who requests the test in a statement appended to the test report that "This test was developed and its performance characteristics determined by [Laboratory name]. It has not been cleared or approved by the U.S. Food and Drug Administration." Even though specimens may cross state boundaries, the in-house assays are not distributed beyond the testing laboratory. The FDA accepts the CLIA'88 oversight program standards for verification of method performance, but because CLIA'88 requirements are more stringent for in-house developed assays than for FDA-reviewed assays (1), separate FDA approval is not required. The Association for Molecular Pathology has a table of FDA-approved molecular diagnostics tests.*

Patents

Patent law was developed to create incentives for technologic innovation by granting the inventor exclusive rights for making, using, or selling the invention for 20 years from the date of the patent application (21,22). The patent, as an item of intellectual property, is a contract issued to the inventor by the U.S. Patent and Trademark Office (USPTO) of the Department of Commerce. There are similar patent offices throughout the world. The patent applicant must demonstrate that the invention is useful, nonobvious, and novel. By granting a patent, the government allows the inventor to restrict others from making, using, selling, or importing the invention. Permission is granted to others to practice the patent when the inventor issues a license, which may be exclusive or limited. U.S. patent laws were also designed to ensure that the public could benefit from a new invention in exchange for the monopoly granted to the inventor (23,24).

The USPTO has upheld broad claims to patents of genes not as products of nature but as manmade chemicals. Initial concerns about gene patents have gone beyond the moral issues of patentability of genes as products of nature, and have broadened into issues of impeding the practice of medicine and scientific research (23,24). Although the initial goal of the patent process is to encourage invention by public disclosure of knowledge, many diagnostic laboratories that provide molecular testing services may not be able

*Association for Molecular Pathology FDA approved table, at http://amp.org/FDATable/FDATableNov04.doc.

to afford the expensive licensing fees imposed by both commercial and academic patent holders. The net effect currently is to inhibit further research and interfere with patient care (24). There are four basic types of licensing (22), as follows:

Sole: Patent holder is the only designated testing facility
Exclusive: Patent holder designates one laboratory to perform all testing
Limited: Licenses are sold to any laboratory deemed qualified by the patent holder. Prices of these licenses may be prohibitive for some laboratories, prompting specimen send out to a licensed laboratory rather than performing the test in house, particularly if the test is a low volume request. Some have argued that this scenario may actually encourage referral centers of excellence and expertise for tests that are infrequently requested at many locations (23,24).
Royalties: Patent holder may require laboratory to pay a fee to run the test in house *or* they may purchase an entire testing kit that includes the royalty fee in the cost. The fee is directly related to the volume of testing performed by the diagnostic laboratory.

The real and perceived effects of patents and licenses on the provision of clinical genetic testing services have been assessed by surveys of laboratory directors through several professional organizations including American Society of Human Genetics (ASHG), American College of Medical Genetics (ACMG), and Association for Molecular Pathology (AMP) (Table 10.1) (23). Most of these studies indicate that a significant negative impact on the ability of clinical laboratories to develop and provide both genetic testing services and clinical research has already been experienced. The fact that fewer laboratories are able to perform the tests may reduce the availability of testing for patients, which could lead to reductions in test quality, test innovation, and clinical research. Although patents originally are intended to provide incentives for conducting the discovery phase of basic research, inhibition of clinical testing research may restrict the full and efficient translation of Human Genome Project insights into effective clinical practice.

Gene Patents

Patents have been issued for complete gene sequences or parts of genes, antisense and sense gene sequences, specific gene mutations, and polymorphisms within genes. Gene patents currently must include more than DNA sequence and must describe some idea of the potential function of the gene product as a potential pharmaceutical agent, as the underlying cause of a particular disease (useful as a diagnostic tool), or as providing a function that may be targeted in assays for treatment development. There is very limited testing available for some molecular variations, for example mutation detection for *BRCA1*, *BRCA2*, *MLH1*, *MSH2*, and the genes responsible for hemochromatosis or Canavan disease (23). Disease-gene patents present unique problems for clinical laboratories because they result in increased costs to cover payment of royalty or licensing fees (24). Some patents enforce a limited monopoly (exclusive license) to prevent other laboratories from performing the test (22), using legal notification ("cease and desist orders") to force nonlicensed laboratories to discontinue testing (23).

Methodology Patents

Patents have been issued for a broad variety of molecular medicine approaches, including recombinant DNA and proteins; transgenomic animals; PCR, RT-PCR, quantitative PCR, multiplex PCR, and related amplification technologies; cell lines, enzymes, probes, and primers; automated DNA sequencing with four different fluorophore-labeled nucleotides; gene delivery systems; and many other common molecular techniques. Laboratories comply with these patents by either paying licensing fees or royalty fees for each test performed or each kit purchased.

ACKNOWLEDGMENTS

BAZ is supported by CA62773 NIH/NCI; CA91842 NIH/NCI; GM62809 NIH/NIGMS; and GM63340 NIH/NIGMS.

REFERENCES

1. Association for Molecular Pathology Recommendations for in-house development and operation of molecular diagnostic tests. *Am J Clin Pathol* 1999;111:449–463.
2. Department of Health and Human Services, Centers for Medicare and Medicaid Services. Clinical laboratory improvement amendments of 1988; final rule. *Federal Register*. 1992:7170 [42CFR493.1265], 7176 [42CFR493.1445(e)(5)].
3. American College of Medical Genetics, Standards and Guidelines for Clinical Genetics Laboratories. *Clinical Molecular Genetics*; 2005. http://www.acmg.net/pages/acmg_activities/stds-2002/g.htm Accessed June 14, 2005.
4. Clinical Laboratory Standards Institute. *Collection, Transport, Preparation, and Storage of Specimens for Molecular Methods: Proposed Guideline*. CLSI document MM13-P, Vol 25, No. 9. Wayne, PA: Clinical Laboratory Standards Institute; 2005.
5. College of American Pathologists. Commission on Laboratory Accreditation. *Molecular Pathology Checklist*. http://www.cap.org/apps/docs/laboratory_accreditation/checklists/molecular_pathology_april2005.doc. Accessed June 14, 2005.
6. U.S. Food and Drug Administration. *Code of Federal Regulations (CFR)*, Title 21, Vol. 8 (21CFR809.30). *In Vitro Diagnostic Products for Human Use*. http://www.accessdata. fda.gov/scripts/cdrh/cfdocs/cfcfr/CFRSearch.cfm?FR=809.30. Accessed June 14, 2005.
7. National Committee for Clinical Laboratory Standards. *Molecular Diagnostic Methods for Genetic Diseases: Approved Guideline*. NCCLS document MM1-A, Vol. 20, No. 7. Wayne, PA: NCCLS; 2000.
8. National Committee for Clinical Laboratory Standards. *Nucleic Acid Amplification Assays for Molecular Hematopathology: Approved Guideline*. NCCLS document MM5-A, Vol. 23, No. 17. Wayne, Pa: NCCLS; 2003.
9. National Committee for Clinical Laboratory Standards. *Proficiency Testing for Molecular Methods*: Proposed Guideline. NCCLS document MM14-P, Vol 24, No. 27. Wayne, Pa: NCCLS; 2004.
10. National Committee for Clinical Laboratory Standards. *Nucleic Acid Sequencing Methods in Diagnostic Laboratory Medicine: Approved Guideline*. NCCLS document MM9-A, Vol, 24 No. 40. Wayne, Pa: NCCLS; 2004.
11. Koch DD, Peters T Jr. Evaluation of methods: with an introduction to statistical techniques. In: Burtis CA, Asherwood ER, eds. *Tietz Fundamentals of Clinical Chemistry*, 5th ed. Philadelphia: WB Saunders; 2001: 233–250.
12. Westgard, JO, Klee, GG. Quality management. In: Burtis CA, Asherwood ER, eds. *Tietz Fundamentals of Clinical Chemistry*, 5th ed. Philadelphia: WB Saunders; 2001: 285–298.
13. Health Insurance Portability and Accountability Act (HIPAA). *Medical Privacy: National Standards to Protect the Privacy of Personal Health Information*. http://www.hhs.gov/ocr/hipaa/finalreg.html. Accessed June 15, 2005.
14. *Clinical Laboratory Evaluation Program*. The Wadsworth Center, NY State Department of Health. http://www.wadsworth.org/labcert/clep/clep.html. Accessed June 15, 2005.
15. Killeen AA, Leung W-C, Payne D, et al. Certification in molecular pathology in the United States. *J Mol Diag* 2002;4:181–184.
16. American Medical Association. *CPT 2005: Current Procedural Terminology for Pathology and Laboratory Medicine*. Chicago, IL: American Medical Association. https://catalog.ama-assn.org/Catalog/product/. Accessed June 15, 2005.
17. Center for Medicare and Medicaid Services. *Healthcare Common Procedure Coding System*. https://www.amaassn.org/ama/pub/category/3662.html. Accessed June 14, 2005.
18. National Human Genome Research Institute. National Institutes of Health. Policy and Legislation Database by U.S. State. http://www.genome.gov/PolicyEthics/LegDatabase/pubMapSearch.cfm. Accessed June 14, 2005.
19. National Human Genome Research Institute. National Institutes of Health. *Summary of Genetic Information Non-Discrimination Act of 2003* (S. 1053). http://www.genome.gov/11508845. Accessed June 14, 2005.
20. Secretary's Advisory Committee on Genetics, Health, and Society. March 2004. http://www4.od.nih.gov/oba/sacghs/. Accessed June 14, 2005.
21. American College of Medical Genetics. *Patent Primer*. http://www.acmg.net/resources/patent.asp. Accessed June 14, 2005.
22. Caulfield T, Gold ER, Cho MK. Patenting human genetic material: refocusing the debate. *Nat Rev Genet* 2000;1:227–236.
23. Cho MK, Illangasekare S, Weaver MA, et al. Effects of patents and licenses on the provision of clinical genetic testing services. *J Mol Diag* 2003;5:3–8.
24. Merz JF. Disease gene patents: overcoming unethical constraints on clinical laboratory medicine. *Clin Chem* 1999;45:324–330.

Tumors of Soft Tissue and Bone

11

Nonrandom mutations have been described in a number of benign and malignant soft tissue tumors. These mutations have been used to reclassify many sarcomas into categories that more accurately reflect tumor biology, which has in turn led to a more complete description of the clinicopathologic profile of many soft tissue tumors. The molecular consequences of the mutations have not only provided insight into oncogenic mechanisms, but have also been used to develop new diagnostic tests and novel drug therapies.

Molecular genetic testing has emerged as an important component in the diagnosis of many soft tissue neoplasms for several reasons. First, because many translocations are characteristic of specific soft tissue tumor types, molecular analysis can help confirm or exclude a specific diagnosis. Second, molecular genetic testing can be a source of prognostic information that is not provided by microscopic examination; for example, variation in the structure of the characteristic fusion gene provides prognostic information independent from the clinical and histomorphologic features of the case. Third, specific mutations are correlated with a response to particular chemotherapy regimens; thus testing can be used to direct patient therapy. Fourth, submicroscopic disease that is detected by molecular analysis may, in some settings, correlate with prognosis or accurately predict early disease recurrence.

For many soft tissue tumor types, a fusion gene produced by a characteristic translocation underlies tumor development. Much of the molecular genetic analysis of soft tissue neoplasms therefore centers on detection of translocations, fusion genes, or fusion gene transcripts by conventional cytogenetic analysis, Southern blot hybridization, fluorescence in situ hybridization (FISH), or reverse transcription polymerase chain reaction (RT-PCR). However, for some soft tissue neoplasms, gene deletions or gene inactivation by point mutations are responsible for tumor development. Although routine cytogenetic analysis or FISH can demonstrate the gross structural abnormalities in these cases, identification of the point mutation requires DNA sequence

analysis. For still other tumor types, activating mutations are responsible for oncogenesis, and for these neoplasms, the mutations can be detected only by DNA sequence analysis.

MALIGNANT ROUND CELL TUMORS

Ewing Sarcoma/Peripheral Neuroectodermal Tumor

Ewing sarcoma/peripheral neuroectodermal tumor (EWS/PNET) is a prototypic malignant round cell tumor of childhood and adolescence (1–3) that classically arises in the soft tissue of bone in children and young adults. Once thought to be an uncommon tumor, EWS/PNET now accounts for approximately 20% of malignant soft tissue tumors in children (4) and has been described in patients of all ages (5,6). The clinical pathologic spectrum of EWS/PNET has been broadened even further by the demonstration that EWS/PNET also can involve a wide variety of sites besides soft tissue and bone, including the pancreas, biliary tract, esophagus, small intestine, uterus, ovary, central nervous system, and skin (5,7–19).

Molecular characterization of the genetic features of EWS/PNET has had a significant impact on tumor classification, and, in fact, the current diagnostic grouping of EWS, PNET, and Askin tumor is based on the recognition that all three share the same pattern of genetic abnormalities (20). However, despite description of the genetic basis of EWS/PNET, the identity of the progenitor cell from which the tumor arises remains unknown.

Genetics

The genetic abnormality that is the hallmark of EWS/PNET is a balanced translocation that forms a chimeric gene in which the *EWS* gene at 22q12 is fused with a member

TABLE 11.1

SUMMARY OF RECURRENT GENETIC ABERRATIONS IN MALIGNANT ROUND CELL TUMORS[a]

Tumor	Aberration	Gene(s) Involved	Estimated Prevalence
Ewing sarcoma/peripheral neuroectodermal tumor	t(11;22)(q24;q12)	EWS-FLI1	85%–95%
	t(21;22)(q22;q12)	EWS-ERG	5%–10%
	t(7;22)(p22;q12)	EWS-ETV1	Rare
	t(17;22)(q21;q12)	EWS-E1AF	Rare
	t(2;22)(q33;q12)	EWS-FEV	Rare
	Inversion of 22q	EWS-ZSG	Rare
	t(16;21)(p11;q22)	TLS-ERG	Rare
Desmoplastic small round cell tumor	t(11;22)(p13;q12)	EWS-WT1	>80%
	t(21;22)(q22;q12)	EWS-ERG	Rare
Embryonal rhabdomyosarcoma	Gains of 2, 7, 8, 12, 13; losses of 1, 6, 9, 14, and 17	IGF2, GOK, PTCH, p53 Unknown	—
Alveolar rhabdomyosarcoma	t(2;13)(q35;q14)	PAX3-FKHR	75%
	t(1;13)(p36;q14)	PAX7-FKHR	10%

[a]See text for references.

of the *ETS* family of transcription factors (Table 11.1). The most common translocation, present in over 90% of cases, is t(11;22)(q24;q12), which results in an *EWS-FLI1* fusion gene (21–24). About 5% of tumors result from a translocation that produces an *EWS-ERG* fusion gene (23,25). Fusion genes between *EWS* and other members of the *ETS* family, including *ETV1, E1AF, FEV,* and *ZSG,* each account for less than 1% of cases of EWS/PNET (26–29). Given the extensive similarity between *TLS* and *EWS* (30,31), it is not surprising that cases of EWS/PNET have recently been described that harbor a t(16;21)(p11;q22) translocation in which *TLS* (also known as *FUS*) is fused to *ERG* (32).

Because the exact position of the genomic break can vary, structural heterogeneity is a prominent feature of the fusion genes (Fig. 11.1). For example, at least 18 different in-frame *EWS-FLI1* chimeric transcripts can be produced from break points between the conventional exons of *EWS* and *FLI1* (most of which have been detected in vivo), and cryptic exons contribute even greater structural diversity (33). Because the exonic structure of *ERG* and *FLI1* is very similar, it is not surprising that several variants of *EWS-ERG* fusion transcripts have also been described (23,34,35). Detailed sequence analysis of *EWS* and *FLI1* genomic break points has shown that the fusion genes arise through illegitimate recombination, a finding that suggests the translocations responsible for EWS/PNET are essentially random, with subsequent selection for those that create a fusion gene encoding a functional protein product. Although translocations that result in *EWS-ETS* fusion genes are the characteristic genetic abnormality in EWS/PNET, secondary chromosomal aberrations including trisomy 8, trisomy 12, and gain of 1q are present in more than half of the cases and have been associated with an unfavorable outcome (36–38).

EWS-ETS fusion genes encode a chimeric protein in which the N-terminal region of EWS that contains a strong transcription transactivation domain is fused to a DNA-binding domain located in the C-terminal region of the

ETS family member (39). The novel protein can initiate and maintain EWS/PNET tumorigenesis (40–42), presumably through an altered pattern of gene expression resulting from juxtaposition of the two functional domains in a single protein (43,44). Because *EWS* transcription is driven by a strongly and broadly active promoter, the chimeric protein is highly expressed (45–47). Recent observations indicate that the EWS-FLI1 protein many also influence 5'-splice site selection, which suggests another mechanism by which the chimeric proteins characteristic of EWS/PNET may exert their oncogenic effect (48).

Technical Issues in Molecular Genetic Analysis of EWS/PNET

Because the genomic break points in *EWS* are clustered within a 7–kilobase (kb) region (49–51), Southern blots can be used to detect the presence of the characteristic translocations. However, because the amount of DNA required for analysis can be obtained only from a reasonably large amount of fresh tissue, the method is poorly suited for evaluation of clinical specimens. It is worth noting that a polymorphism consisting of a deletion of 2.5 kb within a stretch of *Alu* repeats in intron 6 of the *EWS* gene is occasionally observed by Southern blotting (52); although this deletion has thus far been observed only in individuals of African origin, it can complicate test interpretation.

RT-PCR has been shown to be an extremely useful method for demonstrating the fusion transcripts characteristic of EWS/PNET. Given the number of different *ETS* family genes that can partner with *EWS,* and the structural heterogeneity that results from the exact translocation break point, the maximum sensitivity of the assay depends on the comprehensiveness of testing. Exhaustive testing is simplified by the use of consensus primers for *FLI1* and *ERG,* and for *ETV1* and *E1AF,* made possible by the high degree of sequence homology between the gene pairs (5), but testing for the rare fusion partners *FEV* and *ZSG* is

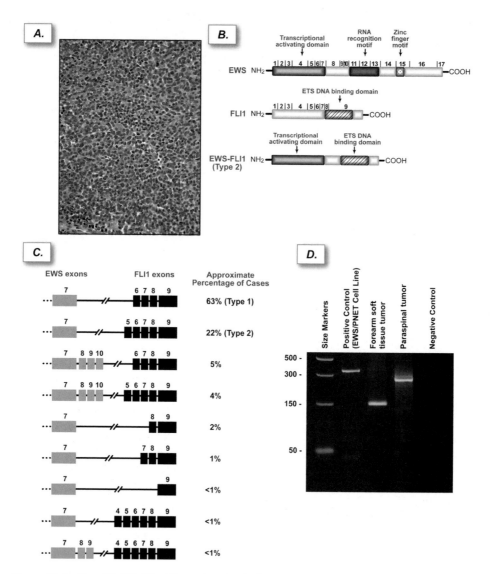

Figure 11.1 The t(11;22)(q24;q12) translocation is the most common of the rearrangements characteristic of Ewing's sarcoma/peripheral neuroectodermal tumor (EWS/PNET). **A**, Photomicrograph of an EWS/PNET arising in the forearm of a 20-year-old woman. **B**, Schematic diagram of the EWS-FLI1 chimeric protein, which includes the N-terminal transcriptional activation domain of EWS linked to the ETS DNA binding domain of FLI1 (the small numbers indicate the regions of the proteins encoded by each exon of the native genes). **C**, Because the translocation break point can be located within different introns of *EWS* and *FLI1*, the fusion gene and resulting transcripts (and chimeric proteins) show marked structural heterogeneity. **D**, Example of reverse-transcriptase polymerase chain reaction (RT-PCR) analysis of formalin-fixed, paraffin-embedded tissue for *EWS-FLI1* fusion transcripts. The structural heterogeneity of the fusion genes is reflected in the different sizes of the PCR products; the band size of 343 base pairs (bp) indicates that the positive control cell line harbors a fusion between exon 7 of *EWS* and exon 5 of *FLI1*, the band size of 150 bp from the forearm tumor indicates a fusion between exon 7 of *EWS* and exon 8 of *FLI1*, and the band size of 277 bp from the paraspinal tumor indicates a fusion between exon 7 of *EWS* and exon 6 of *FLI1*.

usually performed separately. The clinical utility of multiplex real-time PCR for the detection of fusion transcripts associated with EWS/PNET in the diagnostic workup of sarcomas has also been demonstrated (53).

EWS-FLI1 and related fusion transcripts can be detected by RT-PCR from both fresh and formalin-fixed, paraffin-embedded (FFPE) tissue. However, testing FFPE tissue places significant constraints on methodology, including amplification of shorter target sequences often via a nested approach (22,54), both of which increase the risk of con-

tamination and amplification of nonspecific sequences (55–58). In addition, analysis of FFPE tissue has lower sensitivity (59–62). Two large studies have shown that an *EWS-FLI* or related fusion transcript can be demonstrated in 90% to 95% of cases when fresh tissue is tested, but in only about 70% to 85% of cases when FFPE tissue is tested (59,60), a statistically significant difference in sensitivity. Every attempt should therefore be made to obtain fresh tissue to help ensure that testing can achieve its full potential (24,59).

The type I fusion gene (the most common type, EWS exon 7-FLI1 exon 6) and the type II fusion gene (the second most common, EWS exon 7-FLI1 exon 5) can both usually be recognized after simple gel electrophoresis of the RT-PCR product because of their characteristic size. However, because such a wide variety of fusion transcripts is possible as a result of the structural heterogeneity of the possible fusion genes, it is prudent to confirm the identity of the RT-PCR product directly by Southern blot, DNA sequence analysis, or indirectly by FISH. The importance of a product confirmation step in routine testing of clinical specimens is emphasized by a recent study in which DNA sequence analysis was performed on all RT-PCR products (59). This study, which focused on analysis of soft tissue tumors using established primers and reaction conditions, showed that about 6% of the RT-PCR products were amplification artifacts; had analysis of the RT-PCR products been limited to gel electrophoresis, these cases would have produced false positive results.

Cytogenetic analysis can be used to demonstrate the rearrangements characteristic of EWS/PNET, but it is difficult to accurately estimate the percentage of cases that can be shown to harbor one of the typical translocations, by routine cytogenetic analysis because most series are biased by selective reporting of positive cases. FISH has also proven useful for demonstrating the translocations characteristic of EWS/PNET, especially in those cases with complex cytogenetic abnormalities, masked translocations, or an atypical clinical presentation (63–72). However, many different loci can combine with EWS to produce a fusion gene characteristic of EWS/PNET; thus, comprehensive probe-fusion FISH is cumbersome because it requires a separate probe for each of the partner loci. Probe-split FISH, also known as break-apart FISH, using probes that bracket EWS, is much simpler to perform and yields results that are concordant with RT-PCR based analysis in 83% of cases (73).

Immunohistochemistry

Immunohistochemical detection of the chimeric EWS-FLI1 protein using an antibody directed against FLI1 shows positive nuclear staining in 70% to 100% of EWS/PNET, depending on the antibody preparation employed (74,75). Although rhabdomyosarcoma, neuroblastoma, Wilms' tumor, and high-grade pleomorphic sarcomas show no immunoreactivity, up to 100% of various vascular neoplasms, 88% of lymphoblastic lymphomas, 100% of desmoplastic small round cell tumors, and 30% of synovial sarcoma show at least weak immunoreactivity, as do 100% of Merkel's carcinomas and 60% of malignant melanomas (74–76). The use of immunohistochemistry to detect other chimeric proteins that are characteristic of EWS/PNET has not been described.

Diagnostic Issues in Molecular Genetic Analysis of EWS/PNET

Although there is no doubt that gene fusions between EWS and a member of the ETS family are characteristic of EWS/PNET, they have also been described in isolated cases of a variety of other tumor types, including biphenotypic sarcomas with myogenic and neural differentiation (also known as malignant ectomesenchymoma) and other polyphenotypic tumors (77–81), malignant rhabdoid tumor (70), mesenchymal chondrosarcoma (82), desmoplastic small round cell tumor (83), typical neuroblastoma (84), mixed embryonal and alveolar rhabdomyosarcoma (78), giant cell tumor of bone (85), and even synovial sarcoma (60). Such a long list of other tumor types highlights several important points. First, the detection of the gene fusions in tumor types other than EWS/PNET is, not surprisingly, dependent on the method employed. For example, after RT-PCR, Southern blot analysis can be used to demonstrate the presence of EWS-FLI1 fusion transcripts that are present at such extremely low levels that they are not evident based on routine gel electrophoresis (60). However, the significance of gene fusions that are detected only by extremely sensitive testing protocols is unclear. Second, the presence of EWS-FLI1 and related fusion genes in tumor types other than EWS/PNET may reflect the chromosomal instability that is characteristic of malignant tumors rather than a genetic alteration responsible for tumor development (86–88). Fusion genes that are an epiphenomenon of a tumor's clonal evolution may be present in only a very small subset of cells and still be detected by PCR-based methods. Third, given the acknowledged risks of contamination and amplification of nonspecific products by RT-PCR, especially when testing FFPE tissue by a nested approach, it is likely that demonstration of fusion transcripts in some tumor types is, in fact, the result of contamination, especially if the result has not been verified by an independent method or by other investigators (58). Fourth, detection of EWS-FLI1 and related fusion genes in occasional tumors other than EWS/PNET does not undermine the utility of molecular genetic analysis. The lack of 100% specificity simply emphasizes that diagnoses should be based on all the clinical and histopathologic features of a case, rather than the molecular genetic test result alone (58–60,89–91).

Prognostic Features of Transcript Type

The role of molecular genetic analysis of EWS/PNET extends beyond diagnosis. Several studies have shown that the heterogeneity of the fusion genes is clinically significant, specifically that patients whose tumors harbor the type I fusion have a significantly better survival compared with those of other fusion types (92,93). This clinical feature of EWS/PNET is consistent with the basic science observation that type I fusion genes encode a protein that has weaker transactivation activity and that is associated with a lower proliferative rate (42,94).

Detection of Minimal Disease

Submicroscopic bone marrow involvement detected by RT-PCR is associated with tumor stage (95,96), and the presence of an RT-PCR–positive bone marrow at the time of diagnosis is significantly associated with an adverse outcome in univariant analysis (97). In the subgroup of patients with localized disease based on routine histopathologic evaluation, RT-PCR detection of submicroscopic bone marrow involvement is also correlated with an adverse outcome, although the trend is not statistically significant, likely because of the small number of patients thus far evaluated (97).

However, the significance of submicroscopic disease in peripheral blood detected by RT-PCR is uncertain. One study that employed serial blood sampling indicated that the presence of fusion transcript–positive cells in the peripheral blood was associated with, and possibly predictive of, disease progression (98). In contrast, another larger study found no correlation between the detection of fusion transcript–positive cells and tumor size, primary site, metastasis, or survival (97). One factor that can complicate the analysis of peripheral blood samples for minimal disease is tumor cell mobilization as a result of a recent biopsy procedure (99).

RT-PCR has also been used to detect minimal residual disease in bone marrow stem cells harvested from patients with EWS/PNET. Although 11% to 54% of stem cell collections are RT-PCR positive in different studies (100–102), testing has a low reproducibility (102) likely as a result of random variations in whether sample aliquots contain even a single target cell given the highly diluted tumor cell population in the stem cell collections. In any event, the clinical significance of submicroscopic disease in bone marrow stem cell collections is unknown.

Desmoplastic Small Round Cell Tumor

Desmoplastic small round cell tumor (DSRCT) is a primitive sarcoma with a growth pattern that includes striking desmoplasia and an immunophenotype that shows multilineage differentiation (103,104). Although the initial description of DSRCT highlighted the fact that most patients with DSRCT are young men in their second or third decade who present with widespread peritoneal involvement, molecular characterization of DSRCT has broadened the clinical spectrum of disease. DSCRT has been recognized at a number of sites outside the peritoneum, including the pleura, hand, parotid gland, pancreas, ovary, testes, bone, and brain (58,104–106), and the tumor has been shown to occur in patients of all ages, even the elderly (107).

Genetics

Regardless of the tumor's anatomic location, the characteristic genetic abnormality in DSRCT is the t(11;22)(p13;q12) translocation that produces a fusion gene between the *EWS* gene on chromosome 22 and the *WT1* Wilms' tumor gene on chromosome 11 (108–110). Variation in the precise site of the translocation results in a limited number of recurring structural variants of the *EWS-WT1* fusion gene (Fig. 11.2). Unique nonrecurring structural variants have also been described (98).

The fusion gene encodes a chimeric protein in which the N-terminal transactivation domain of EWS is fused to the WT1 DNA-binding domain; however, the oncogenic mechanism of the chimeric protein is unknown, as is the identity of the target cell. It is interesting to note that the *WT1* gene is expressed in the developing urogenital tract by renal cells during their transition from a mesenchymal to an epithelial phenotype, and by fetal abdominal and pelvic mesothelium (111), a pattern of expression that may be related to both the polyphenotypic nature of DSRCT and its propensity to involve mesothelial surfaces (110,112).

Technical Issues in the Molecular Diagnosis of DSRCT

Most molecular genetic testing is performed by RT-PCR. Taken together, published reports show that when fresh tissue is the substrate for RT-PCR testing, *EWS-WT1* fusion transcripts can be detected in about 80% of cases (59). However, when FFPE tissue is used as the substrate for RT-PCR testing, fusion transcripts can be detected in an average of only about 60% of cases, a statistically significant decrease in sensitivity (59). Multiplex PCR designed to detect a variety of fusion transcripts characteristic of several different malignant round cell tumors has also been shown to have clinical utility for detecting *EWS-WT1* fusion transcript characteristic of DSRCT (53).

The *EWS* and *WT1* genomic breaks are easily detected by Southern blot analysis (108), but the relatively large amount of fresh tissue that is required limits the clinical utility of this approach. As yet, no studies have formally evaluated the utility of FISH-based testing for detecting the translocation characteristic of DSRCT, but it can be anticipated that interphase FISH will turn out to be quite useful for molecular genetic analysis of DSRCT in routine clinical practice.

Immunohistochemistry

DSRCT is an excellent example of how molecular characterization of a tumor's underlying genetic abnormality can guide development of an immunohistochemical assay. Because the chimeric EWS-WT1 protein does not contain the amino terminal region of the wild-type WT1 protein, and because the full-length native WT1 protein is not expressed in most cases of DSRCT (108), antibodies to the amino-terminal region of WT1 do not typically stain cases of DSRCT (104,113) while antibodies to the carboxy-terminal region of WT1 typically show strong immunoreactivity (114–117). The clinical utility of an immunohistochemical approach based on the underlying molecular biology of DSRCT has been emphasized in a study that showed immunostaining using an antibody against the carboxy terminal region of WT1 reliably differentiates DSRCT from EWS/PNET (118).

Diagnostic Issues in Molecular Genetic Analysis of DSRCT

The *EWS-WT1* fusion gene is regarded as specific for DSRCT because the fusion gene is not a characteristic feature of any other tumor type. However, a case of DSRCT has been reported that harbored an *EWS-ERG* fusion gene (83). Consequently, although the diagnostic specificity of molecular testing for *EWS-WT1* gene fusions may be virtually 100%, testing limited to *EWS-WT1* has a somewhat lower sensitivity.

Alveolar Rhabdomyosarcoma

Alveolar rhabdomyosarcoma (ARMS) is a primitive malignant round cell tumor that shows partial skeletal muscle differentiation. The tumor occurs in all age-groups, most

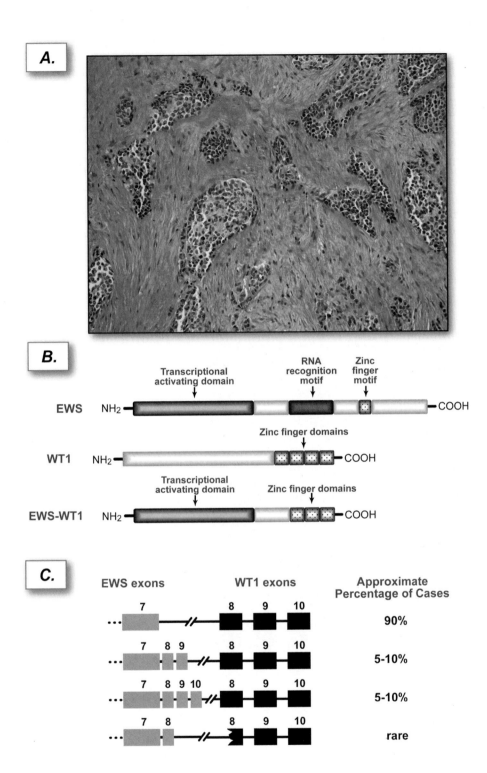

A.

B.

EWS   NH₂ ── Transcriptional activating domain ── RNA recognition motif ── Zinc finger motif ──COOH

WT1   NH₂ ── Zinc finger domains ──COOH

EWS-WT1   NH₂ ── Transcriptional activating domain ── Zinc finger domains ──COOH

C.

EWS exons	WT1 exons	Approximate Percentage of Cases
7	8 9 10	90%
7 8 9	8 9 10	5-10%
7 8 9 10	8 9 10	5-10%
7 8	8 9 10	rare

Figure 11.2 The EWS-WT1 chimeric protein produced by the t(11;22)(p13;q12) is the hallmark of desmoplastic small round cell tumor. **A,** Photomicrograph of an abdominal desmoplastic small round cell tumor (DSRCT) from a 29-year-old man showing the typical nests of cells within a highly desmoplastic stroma. **B,** Schematic diagram of the EWS-WT1 chimeric protein in which the N-terminal transcriptional activation domain of EWS is linked to the WT1 DNA binding domain. **C,** Differences in the site of the translocation break point cause limited heterogeneity in the structure of the *EWS-WT1* fusion gene and resulting transcripts (and chimeric proteins).

often in adolescents and young adults. ARMS commonly arises in the extremities, although the tumor also frequently involves the paraspinal and perineal regions and the paranasal sinuses. ARMS accounts for about 20% of rhabdomyosarcomas overall (119,120).

Genetics of ARMS

About 75% of cases of ARMS harbor the t(2;13)(q35;q14) translocation that results in a fusion gene in which the 5′ end of the *PAX3* gene on chromosome 2 is fused with the 3′ end of the *FKHR* gene on chromosome 13 (121,122). About 10% of cases harbor the t(1;13)(p36;q14) translocation in which the 5′ end of the *PAX7* gene on chromosome 1 is fused with the *FKHR* gene (123). The chromosomal break points that produce *PAX3-FKHR* fusion genes are always located in intron 7 of *PAX3* and intron 1 of *FKHR*, and the break points that produce *PAX7-FKHR* genes are always located in intron 7 of *PAX7* and intron 1 of *FKHR*, and consequently there is no structural heterogeneity in the encoded chimeric proteins (124–126). Southern blot hybridization has demonstrated that *PAX7-FKHR* fusion genes are often amplified on double minute chromosomes, although amplification of *PAX3-FKHR* fusion genes is less common (127); whether or not this finding is responsible for the difference in prognosis (discussed later) between tumors harboring the two types of fusion genes remains unknown. Although transcripts from the reciprocal *FKHR-PAX* fusion genes can be detected, the encoded proteins are not thought to be involved in the pathogenesis of *ARMS* (121). The 15% to 20% of ARMS that does not harbor *PAX3-FKHR* or *PAX7-FKHR* gene fusions is apparently a heterogeneous group; this subset of cases includes tumors with low expression of the standard *PAX3-FKHR* and *PAX7-FKHR* fusions, variant fusions of *PAX3* or *PAX7* with other genes, and cases without any detectable rearrangements in *PAX3*, *PAX7*, or *FKHR* (128).

The chimeric PAX-FKHR proteins consist of an N-terminal DNA binding domain (composed of paired-box and homeobox domains) encoded by the 5' region of the *PAX* gene and a C-terminal transactivation domain encoded by the 3' region of the *FKHR* gene (Fig. 11.3). The proteins apparently act as aberrant transcription factors that cause excessive activation of genes with PAX binding sites (129), a mechanism of oncogenesis that is consistent with the fact that *PAX3* and *PAX7* are highly homologous members of a family of genes that encode transcription factors important for normal embryonal development (130). A possible explanation for the involvement of these genes specifically in rhabdomyosarcoma is suggested by the finding that both *PAX3* and *PAX7* are expressed in developing myotomes. Although cell culture experiments have shown that the *PAX3-FKHR* fusion gene has oncogenic activity (131), the fact that *PAX3-FKHR* transgenic mice do not

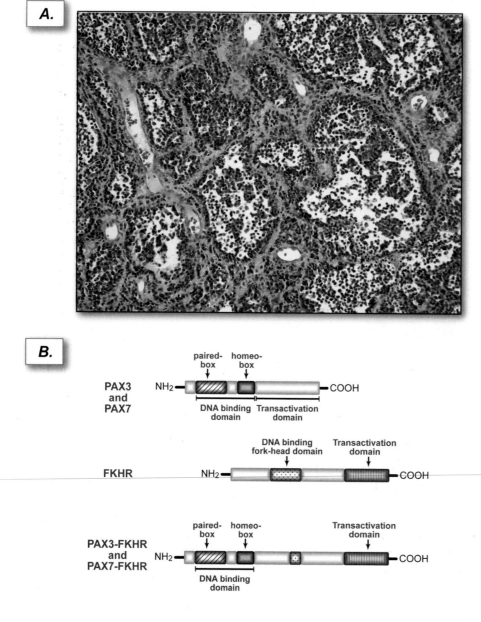

Figure 11.3 PAX-FKHR chimeric proteins are the hallmark of alveolar rhabdomyosarcoma. **A**, Photomicrograph of an ARMS from a 4-year-old boy that shows broad nests of small cells with minimal cytoplasm separated by fibrous septa; the cells in the center of the nests are typically discohesive, as is prominent in this example. **B**, Schematic diagram of the PAX-FKHR proteins formed by the t(2;13) and t(1;13) translocations in which the N-terminal paired-box and homeobox domains of the native PAX protein are linked to the C-terminal transactivation domain of native FKHR.

develop tumors implies that the role of *PAX3-FKHR* fusion gene in carcinogenesis is more complicated (132).

Comparative genomic hybridization analysis has demonstrated that several amplification events also are characteristic of ARMS, including amplification of chromosomal region 12q13–15 in about one third of cases and amplification of chromosomal region 2p24 in about one third of cases (86,133). It is noteworthy that region 2p24 harbors the *MYCN* oncogene, characteristically amplified in several other tumors, most notably neuroblastoma. However, the clinical significance of these other amplifications has yet to be established.

Technical Issues in Molecular Genetic Analysis of ARMS

Southern blot hybridization can be used to detect the translocations associated with ARMS (124,126,134). However, the utility of the method in routine clinical practice is limited by the large amount of fresh tumor that is required and by the fact that the translocation break points, though limited to specific introns, are nonetheless distributed over large genomic regions (intron 7 of *PAX3* is 20 kb long, intron 7 of *PAX7* is 30 kb long, and intron 1 of *FKHR* is 130 kb long). Southern blot analysis that surveys the entire break point region therefore requires digestion of genomic DNA with multiple restriction enzymes and hybridization with multiple probes.

Despite the variability in the translocation break points at a genomic level, the lack of structural heterogeneity of the encoded chimeric proteins makes RT-PCR based assays for *PAX-FKHR* fusion transcripts very straightforward. Primer pairs that are specific for *PAX3-FKHR* or *PAX7-FKHR* fusion transcripts have been described (135–138), but the use of consensus primers that bind to highly homologous 5' regions of *PAX3* and *PAX7* make it possible to amplify either fusion transcript in a single RT-PCR reaction (139). Multiplex analysis for the fusion transcripts characteristic of ARMS, as well as other malignant small round cell tumors, also has been described (53). Taken together, the published data indicate that RT-PCR–based testing of fresh tissue demonstrates *PAX-FKHR* fusion transcripts in slightly less than 75% of ARMS (59). RT-PCR has been adapted for use with FFPE tissue (138,140,141), although only about 55% of cases can be shown to harbor *PAX-FKHR* fusion transcripts when fixed tissue is used for analysis, a statistically significant decrease in test sensitivity (59). The modified RT-PCR strategy in which the reverse transcription step is performed using an oligonucleotide specific for the 3'-*FKHR* region, instead of random hexamers or oligo(dT) primers (141), makes a nested PCR strategy unnecessary and consequently diminishes the risk of contamination or amplification of nonspecific products. Nonetheless, it must be emphasized that the relatively low technical sensitivity of RT-PCR–based testing of ARMS is a direct consequence of the fact that about 15% to 20% of cases do not harbor either the t(2;13) or t(1;13), which limits the utility of RT-PCR (or any other molecular genetic method), regardless of technical modifications to the testing protocol.

FISH has also been used to detect the t(2;13) and t(1;13) translocations characteristic of ARMS. By the probe-fusion approach, which employs probes adjacent to the 5' regions of the *PAX* genes and a probe adjacent to the 3' region of *FKHR*, translocations that generate *PAX-FKHR* fusions are identified as apposed or overlapping hybridization signals (127,142,143). By the probe-split approach, which employs two probes that flank *FKHR*, translocations are identified as splitting of the two hybridization signals. Both assays can be performed on either metaphase chromosomes or interphase nuclei, and comparison of FISH-based assays with RT-PCR analysis has demonstrated excellent concordance between the two different testing methods (135).

Diagnostic Issues in Molecular Genetic Analysis of ARMS

Because *PAX-FKHR* rearrangements are not a hallmark of any other tumor type, including embryonal rhabdomyosarcoma (ERMS), the demonstration of a *PAX-FKHR* fusion is thought to be specific for ARMS (135,136,144,145). The rare cases of ERMS that do contain *PAX-FKHR* fusions are therefore interpreted as representing ARMS with mixed embryonal and alveolar histology in which only the embryonal pattern was present in the areas sampled for microscopic evaluation, ARMS with solid alveolar histology that were misclassified as ERMS, or true ERMS for which the rearrangement is an epiphenomenon (136).

As an interesting aside, a *PAX3-FKHR* fusion gene has also been detected in a biphenotypic small cell sarcoma with both neuroectodermal and muscle differentiation (146). The particularly fascinating aspect of this tumor was its simultaneous expression of both *EWS-FLI1* and *PAX3-FKHR* fusion transcripts, the clinical and biologic significance of which is unknown.

Prognostic Features of Transcript Type

There are several differences between the clinical behavior of ARMS that harbor *PAX3-FKHR* fusion genes and those that harbor *PAX7-FKRH* fusion genes. Tumors with *PAX7-FKHR* fusion genes occur in younger patients and are less invasive locally (147–149), and although there are no differences in the rate of metastases between the two groups, tumors with *PAX7-FKHR* show a lower propensity for bone marrow involvement. Even though survival between the two categories of ARMS is comparable when disease is localized at presentation, the estimated 4-year overall survival rate is 8% for tumors that harbor the *PAX3-FKHR* rearrangement versus 75% for tumors that harbor the *PAX7-FKHR*. These differences suggest that, whatever the role of molecular genetic testing in the diagnosis of ARMS, identification of the *PAX-FKHR* fusion type can provide important prognostic information.

Detection of Minimal Disease

Using a RT-PCR–based assay capable of detecting one tumor cell in 10^5 normal cells, molecular evidence of bone marrow involvement can be demonstrated in 15% of bone marrow samples that show no evidence of metastatic disease by routine histologic evaluation (150). The clinical significance of this finding is suggested by the fact that patients with submicroscopic bone marrow involvement detectable only by molecular methods tend to have a worse outcome, although a much larger number of cases must be evaluated to establish whether the trend is statistically significant. There is apparently no role for RT-PCR–based testing for tumor cells in peripheral blood samples from patients with ARMS (150).

Undifferentiated Soft Tissue Sarcoma

Undifferentiated soft tissue sarcomas (USTS), also often termed poorly differentiated malignant round cell neoplasms, undifferentiated sarcomas, or small round cell sarcomas of indeterminate type, are a group of tumors that show a diffuse hypercellular pattern consisting of sheets of medium-sized cells that have a minimal to moderate amount of cytoplasm and a variable nuclear morphology (151). Consistent with the lack of identifying morphologic features, the tumors do not have a diagnostic histochemical or immunohistochemical profile and have no diagnostic ultrastructural features (151,152).

Technical Issues in Molecular Genetic Analysis of USTS

When RT-PCR is used to screen USTS, a fusion transcript characteristic of a specific sarcoma type can be detected in about 40% of cases, regardless of whether fresh or FFPE tissue is used for testing (22,59,135,153). Not unexpectedly, RT-PCR has a higher sensitivity for detecting the presence of a rearrangement in USTS than routine cytogenetic analysis (59,135).

Diagnostic Issues in Molecular Genetic Analysis of USTS

The demonstration of a fusion gene characteristic of a specific sarcoma type in USTS can be used to guide patient management even if a more precise pathologic classification remains uncertain (59). However, it is important to recognize that prospective clinical trials have yet to demonstrate that USTS classified as a specific sarcoma type based solely on the results of molecular analysis have the same prognosis and response to therapy as cases of the specific sarcoma type diagnosed on the basis of their morphologic and immunohistochemical features.

From a more general perspective, the fact that only about 40% of USTS harbor a rearrangement typical of a specific sarcoma type indicates that molecular genetic testing for a small number of fusion genes falls short as a gold standard for classification of USTS. This result should probably have been anticipated. Given that the phenotype of a tumor is ultimately determined by its genotype, the fact that USTSs lack histomorphologic features diagnostic of the well-defined sarcoma types is likely an indication that USTSs do not harbor the same patterns of genetic alterations associated with the well-defined sarcoma types. Even though molecular genetic testing limited to a small number of fusion genes is insufficient, analysis of a larger number of cases, a broader range of mutations, and patterns of gene expression may ultimately provide enough information to permit more precise classification of USTS.

SPINDLE CELL TUMORS

Synovial Sarcoma

Synovial sarcoma (SS) accounts for about 10% of all soft tissue sarcomas. SS typically arises in periarticular regions in adolescents and young adults, but despite the name, no biologic or pathologic relationship between SS and synovium has been demonstrated. Histologically, SS is divided into two major subtypes. Biphasic SS contains spindle cells as well as epithelial cells (often arranged in glandular structures); immunohistochemical analysis shows that the epithelial component expresses epithelial membrane antigen and, less frequently, cytokeratins. Monophasic SS is composed entirely of spindle cells.

Although over 80% of SS arises in deep soft tissues of the extremity, molecular characterization of the genetic abnormalities characteristic of SS has markedly expanded the clinicopathologic spectrum of disease. SS has been shown to occur in patients of all ages (including newborns and the elderly) at a wide variety of anatomic sites, including the head and neck, kidney, prostate, skin, vulva, and penis tumors arising in intrathoracic, intraneural, and intraosseus sites have also been reported (154–160).

Genetics

The t(X;18)(p11;q11) translocation is the genetic hallmark of SS (Table 11.2). The translocation fuses the SYT gene from chromosome 18 to a member of the SSX gene family (161,162). The SSX gene family at Xp11 contains five highly homologous members, SSX1 through SSX5 (163,164). SSX1 and SSX2 are involved in most SS (161,165); biphasic tumors usually harbor an SYT-SSX1 fusion gene, while most tumors with an SYT-SSX2 transcript are monophasic (166,167). SYT-SSX4 fusions have been described in rare cases of SS (168–170), but tumors that harbor fusions with SSX3 or SSX5 have not been described (163,165). There is little heterogeneity in the structure of SYT-SSX fusion transcripts; the rare variant SYT-SSX fusion transcripts that have been reported reflect unique and nonrecurring break points (161,162,171–175).

SYT-SSX fusion genes encode a chimeric protein (Fig. 11.4) in which a transcription activation domain of SYT is juxtaposed to a repressor domain in the C-terminal region of the SSX proteins (176), replacing the Kruppel-associated box (KRAB) transcription repression domain in the N-terminal region of SSX (177,178). Because the native SYT and SSX proteins lack recognizable DNA-binding domains, the chimeric SYT-SSX protein is thought to be oncogenic as a result of aberrant transcriptional regulation mediated through protein–protein interactions, although the identity of dysregulated genes is presently unknown. Nonconservative sequence differences between SSX1 and SSX2 suggest that the different SYT-SSX fusion proteins may induce different patterns of altered gene regulation (179–181).

Finally, it should be noted that although the t(X;18) is the sole cytogenetic abnormality in about one third of cases of SS, more complex translocations and aneuploidy are often also present, most often loss of chromosome 3 with gains of chromosome 7, 8, and 12.

TABLE 11.2

SUMMARY OF RECURRENT GENETIC ABERRATIONS IN SPINDLE CELL TUMORS[a]

Tumor	Aberration	Gene(s) involved	Estimated Prevalence
Synovial sarcoma	t(X;18)(p11;q11)	*SYT-SSX1*	65%
	t(X;18)(p11;q11)	*SYT-SSX2*	35%
	t(X;18)(p11;q11)	*SYT-SSX4*	Rare
Congenital/infantile fibrosarcoma	t(12;15)(p13;q25)	*ETV6-NTRK3*	Up to 100%
Inflammatory myofibroblastic tumor	Rearrangements of 2p23 (Table 11.4)	*ALK*; (Table 11.4)	50%–60%
Malignant peripheral nerve sheath tumor	Complex changes	Not yet identified; *SYT-SSX* in rare cases	—
Dermatofibrosarcoma protuberans (DFSP)	t(17;22)(q22;q13) and derivative ring chromosomes	*COLIA1-PDGFB*	>95%
Giant cell fibroblastoma (juvenile form of DFSP)	t(17;22)(q22;q13) and derivative ring chromosomes	*COLIA1-PDGFB*	>95%
Angiomatoid fibrous histiocytoma	t(12;16)(q13;p11)	*TLS-ATF1*	Unknown
Low-grade fibromyxoid sarcoma	t(7;16)(q34;p11)	*TLS-CREB3L2*	Unknown
Extragastrointestinal (soft tissue) stromal tumors	Activating mutations	*c-kit* or *PDGFRA*	Up to 100%

[a]See text for references.

Technical Issues in Molecular Genetic Analysis of SS

RT-PCR–based demonstration of *SYT-SSX* chimeric transcripts is a highly sensitive and widely used method to detect the fusion genes characteristic of SS, even in cases that have a masked translocation by conventional cytogenetic analysis (182). Fusion transcripts can be detected in well over 90% of SS when fresh tissue is used for analysis and in over 90% of cases when FFPE tissue is used for analysis (59,60,183,184), one of the few settings in which analysis of fixed tissue is not associated with diminished test sensitivity (59). RT-PCR–based analysis can be performed using consensus primers that will detect *SYT-SSX1* and *SYT-SSX2* fusions, which can then be distinguished by direct sequence analysis (185), by restriction enzyme digestion of the PCR product (186), or by Southern blot hybridization with probes specific for the individual *SSX* genes (187). Alternatively, RT-PCR or real-time PCR can be performed using primers that are specific for the different *SSX* genes (162,188). Multiplex PCR designed to simultaneously detect the fusion transcripts characteristic of several different sarcomas has been shown to be a straightforward approach for evaluation of SS, especially poorly differentiated SS for which the differential diagnosis often includes malignant round cell tumors (53). Up to 10% of cases of SS harbor both *SYT-SSX1* and *SYT-SSX2* fusion genes that can be detected at the genomic level, as well as by RT-PCR (189), although the clinical significance of this heterogeneity is unknown. Finally, it should be noted that the rare variant *SYT-SSX* fusion genes produce atypically sized PCR products that can lead to errors in test interpretation (175); although DNA sequence analysis can unequivocally confirm the identity of these PCR products, and conventional cytogenetic analysis or FISH can be used to verify the presence of the t(X;18) translocation, Southern blot analysis of the PCR product can be misleading (Fig. 8.2).

FISH has also been widely used to demonstrate the presence of the t(X;18) translocation in SS, using either metaphase chromosomes or interphase nuclei (66,68,166, 190–193). With appropriately designed probes, FISH can even be used to distinguish which *SSX* gene is involved in the translocation (194), which is important given that different *SYT-SSX* fusions may be associated with differences in clinical outcome (see later discusssion).

The use of Southern blot hybridization to detect *SYT-SSX* rearrangements is rarely used in clinical molecular genetic testing for several technical reasons. First, as is true for Southern blotting in general, analysis requires a large amount of fresh tissue. Second, use of *SSX* probes is hampered by cross hybridization resulting from the high homology between the various *SSX* genes and pseudo-genes. Third, it is cumbersome to survey the *SYT* intron involved in the translocation because it is greater than 13 kb long (186).

Immunohistochemistry

SYT is broadly expressed, and *SSX* is expressed in a wide variety of tumor types (195). Consequently, immuno-histochemical analysis of SYT and SSX in an attempt to

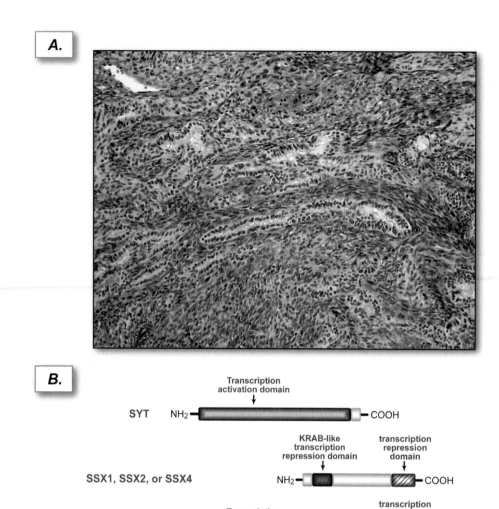

A.

B.

SYT — NH2 [Transcription activation domain] COOH

SSX1, SSX2, or SSX4 — NH2 [KRAB-like transcription repression domain | transcription repression domain] COOH

SYT-SSX — NH2 [Transcription activation domain | transcription repression domain] COOH

Figure 11.4 *SYT-SSX* fusion genes are produced by the translocation t(X;18)(p11.2;q11) characteristic of synovial sarcoma. **A**, Photomicrograph of a biphasic SS arising in the abdominal wall of a 27-year-old woman. **B**, Schematic diagram of SYT-SSX chimeric proteins in which the transactivation domain of SYT is linked to a C-terminal transcription repression domain common to SSX1, SSX2, and SSX4.

demonstrate the presence of chimeric SYT-SSX fusion proteins is of little utility in the diagnosis of SS.

Diagnostic Issues in Molecular Genetic Analysis of SS

The rarity of tumors other than SS that harbor *SYT-SSX* rearrangements makes molecular genetic analysis for *SYT-SSX* fusion genes very useful, especially in problematic cases (184–196). Nonetheless, rare tumors other than SS have been shown to harbor *SYT-SSX* fusions. *SYT-SSX* fusion transcripts have been detected by RT-PCR in malignant peripheral nerve sheath tumors (154,197,198), the significance of which remains controversial (see the discussion of MPNST below). *SYT-SSX* fusion transcripts also have been detected in rare cases of EWS/PNET via an approach in which Southern blot was used to detect RT-PCR products present at very low levels (189), although the diagnostic significance of such weak bands is admittedly unknown (189). Because tumors other than SS that harbor *SYT-SSX* rearrangements are apparently uncommon, the unexpected finding of an *SYT-SSX* fusion in a tumor type other than SS should lead to a review of all the

clinical and pathologic aspects of the case to ensure that the tumor is not just a misdiagnosed SS.

Prognostic Significance of Transcript Type

In most clinical series the *SYT-SSX2* fusion is associated with a better clinical outcome than the *SYT-SSX1* fusion, although the prognostic implications of *SYT-SSX4* fusions, atypical *SYT-SSX* fusions, and heterogeneous patterns of fusion transcripts are unknown (165,171,189,199–202). In one study, the *SYT-SSX2* transcript type was the only independent statistically significant factor for overall survival in patients with localized disease at presentation (202). Even though patient therapy is not (yet) stratified on the basis of fusion transcript type, differences in clinical outcome indicate that prognostic information can be obtained from determination of the fusion gene type, even when testing is not required for diagnosis. On the other hand, cytogenetic complexity based on karyotypic findings has not been shown to predict clinical outcome (199), and genomic imbalances detected by comparative genomic hybridization also do not correlate with overall survival (203).

Detection of Minimal Disease

Circulating tumor cells can be detected by nested RT-PCR in patients who have SS, but the clinical significance of the finding is uncertain because of the small number of patients thus far evaluated (204,205). Other studies have assessed the potential role of RT-PCR testing for fusion transcripts in the evaluation of surgical resection margins, and have found that molecular genetic evidence of positive margins can be detected in a subset of cases that have uninvolved margins by routine histologic examination, but again the clinical significance of the submicroscopic disease is unclear because of the limited number of cases thus far evaluated (205,206).

Malignant Peripheral Nerve Sheath Tumor

Malignant peripheral nerve sheath tumor (MPNST) is a spindle cell sarcoma that is traditionally associated with peripheral nerves, especially in patients with neurofibromatosis.

Genetics

Conventional cytogenetic analysis has shown that cases of MPNST typically have a complex karyotype without any recurring translocations. However, SYT-SSX fusion transcripts have been detected in a subset of MPNST by RT-PCR (154,197,198), in some cases by both RT-PCR and FISH in paired analysis (197,198). SYT-SSX fusion transcripts have also been identified in tumors accepted as bona fide examples of MPNST at the initiation of molecular analysis, although the cases were later reclassified to retain the presumed specificity of the SYT-SSX rearrangement for SS (207–209). Still other studies have failed to detect SYT-SSX fusions in MPNST altogether (210,211).

Diagnostic Issues in Molecular Genetic Analysis of MPNST

There is still no consensus on the significance of SYT-SSX fusion genes detected by RT-PCR in MPNST (212–216), and the debate highlights several features of molecular genetic analysis that can cause uncertainty in the interpretation of test results. First, the technical sensitivity of a test may affect its diagnostic utility. For example, some tumors harbor SYT-SSX transcripts at such low abundance that, after electrophoresis of the RT-PCR product, the fusions are not evident by routine ethidium bromide staining, even though they can be detected by Southern blot hybridization (60). Whether transcripts present at such low levels that they can be detected only by an additional hybridization step carry the same diagnostic significance as transcripts that can be detected by less sensitive methods remains unclear (60,154). Second, there is often confusion between review of cases with unexpected findings that is a routine part of diagnostic surgical pathology and review of cases that constitutes discrepant analysis. In studies designed to evaluate the sensitivity and specificity of testing (e.g., of RT-PCR analysis of MPNST for SYT-SSX fusions), review limited to those cases with an unexpected result (207–209) is a form of discrepant analysis that can lead to significant overestimates of test performance (Chapter 8). Third, an individual

neoplasm may harbor a specific genetic aberration merely as a reflection of the chromosomal instability and clonal evolution that is a hallmark of malignancy (86–88), in which case the mutation is unrelated to the genetic alterations responsible for tumor development, but is instead a nonspecific epiphenomenon. Chromosomal instability may explain not only the presence of the t(X;18) in MPNST, but also the presence of the t(2;5)(p23;q35) characteristic of anaplastic large cell lymphoma in MNPST (217). Fourth, for problematic cases, it is not always clear what test should function as the reference standard. Given the extensive clinical, morphologic, and immunohistochemical overlap between SS and MPNST (218–220), it is unclear whether an MPNST shown to harbor an SYT-SSX fusion is merely an indication that the t(X;18) translocation is not 100% specific for SS (which assumes traditional histopathologic evaluation is the reference standard) or is instead an example of a misdiagnosed SS (which assumes molecular testing is the reference standard). The presence of the SYT-SSX fusion in cases for which the diagnosis of MPNST versus SS is unclear may be an indication that the two tumor types are actually related (154,221), a conjecture supported by gene expression analysis (222).

Although the interpretation of SYT-SSX fusion transcripts demonstrated by RT-PCR in MPNST remains controversial, what is clear from the cumulative data is that such cases are uncommon. Consequently, when faced with the unexpected finding of an SYT-SSX fusion in an MPNST, it is prudent to review all the clinical and pathologic aspects of the case to ensure that the tumor is not just a misdiagnosed SS.

Congenital/Infantile Fibrosarcoma

Congenital/infantile fibrosarcoma (CIF), also known as juvenile fibrosarcoma, most commonly involves the superficial or deep soft tissues of the distal extremities, although tumors of the trunk, as well as the head and neck, do occur. As the name suggests, most cases are congenital, and the tumor is virtually never encountered after 2 years of age (223,224).

Genetics

The translocation t(12;15)(p13;q25) that produces an ETV6-NTRK3 fusion gene is the most common cytogenetic abnormality in CIF (225). Although trisomies of chromosomes 8, 11, 17, and 20 are nearly as common as the t(12;15), the translocation is thought to be the initial transforming event, and the polysomies are thought to represent acquired aberrations responsible for tumor progression to a more mitotically active phenotype (225,226).

The ETV6-NTRK3 fusion gene encodes a protein in which the N-terminal helix-loop-helix dimerization domain of the highly expressed ETV6 transcription factor (also known as TEL) is fused to the tyrosine kinase domain of NTRK3 (also known as TRKC) (Fig. 11.5). The chimeric protein is thought to undergo ligand-independent, helix-loop-helix–mediated dimerization with subsequent activation of the tyrosine kinase activity of NTRK3 (225), producing a constitutively active protein tyrosine kinase that has potent transforming activity through a number of different cell activation pathways (227,228).

A.

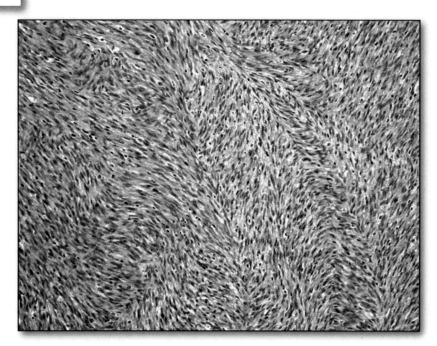

B.

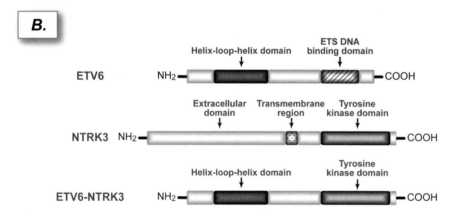

Figure 11.5 The ETV6-NTRK3 chimeric protein that results from the t(12;15)(p13;q25) is the hallmark of congenital/infantile fibrosarcoma (CIF). **A**, Photomicrograph of a CIF from the abdominal wall of a 3-year-old girl. The tumor is composed of elongate, minimally pleomorphic cells arranged in a herring-bone pattern. **B**, Schematic diagram of the ETV6-NTRK3 protein in which the N-terminal helix-loop-helix dimerization domain of native ETV6 is fused with the C-terminal tyrosine kinase domain of native NTRK3.

The t(12;15) translocation break point occurs in intron 5 of *ETV6* and intron 12 of *NTRK3* (225). Although variation in the translocation break point has not been described, alternative splicing produces variation in the structure of *ETV6-NTRK3* fusion transcripts (229). The clinical significance of alternatively spliced transcripts encoding an ETV6-NTRK3 protein isoform that contains a 14 amino acid insertion is uncertain, but wild-type NTRK3 proteins that include the 14 amino acid insertion have decreased tyrosine kinase activity (230). Similarly, the functional significance of fusion transcripts in which the 3' terminal 462 bases of *NTRK3* are missing from the fusion transcripts remains unknown (229).

Technical Issues in Molecular Genetic Analysis of CIF

In the original reports that described the t(12;15)(p13;q25) translocation as a recurrent finding in CIF, cytogenetic analysis was used to detect the rearrangement (225,231,232). However, because the regions that are exchanged between chromosomes 12 and 15 are so similar in size and banding characteristics, the translocation can be easily overlooked when evaluated by conventional banding methods (225,231,233). In fact, review of karyotypes from cases of CIF with the expressed purpose of identifying the t(12;15)(p13;q25) has shown that in most cases the translocation was overlooked at the time of the initial cytogenetic analysis (231). Because the translocation is so difficult to identify by conventional cytogenetic analysis, FISH-based testing is especially useful for demonstrating the rearrangement. In a study designed specifically to address the sensitivity of FISH-based analysis, testing using probe-splitting methodology detected the t(12;15) translocation in 80% of cases of CIF (233).

Although northern blot hybridization was used to demonstrate *ETV6-NTRK3* fusion transcripts in the early reports describing the t(12;15) translocation (225,234), the method has been replaced by RT-PCR in routine laboratory testing. When performed on cases of CIF in which fresh tissue is available for testing, RT-PCR demonstrates an *ETV6-NTRK3* fusion transcript in 83% to 100% of cases (225,229,231,232). However, the sensitivity of RT-PCR analysis of FFPE tissue is less certain; because RT-PCR analysis of FFPE tissue has only been evaluated in series that tested small numbers of cases, it is not surprising that the estimates of test sensitivity are widely different, ranging from 25% to over 90% (232,235–238). However, when the studies are taken together, RT-PCR–based testing of FFPE tissue for *ETV6-NTRK3* fusion transcripts apparently has a statistically significant lower sensitivity than RT-PCR testing of fresh tissue (59).

Immunohistochemistry

Molecular testing for *ETV6-NTRK3* fusion transcripts has been compared with immunohistochemical staining using antisera specific for the carboxy-terminal domain of the NTRK3 protein in a number of reports (229,232,238). All of these studies have shown that although CIFs consistently express NTRK3 protein that can be detected by immunohistochemical methods, NTRK3 is also expressed in a wide variety of other spindle cell tumors. RT-PCR for *ETV6-NTRK3* fusion transcripts therefore provides a more specific assay that is of greater utility for the diagnosis of CIF (229,232,238).

Diagnostic Issues in Molecular Genetic Analysis of CIF

The *ETV6-NTRK3* fusion gene is present in congenital mesoblastic nephroma of both the cellular and mixed types (231,234,235), a finding that essentially establishes these two neoplasms as renal forms of CIF. Neither the t(12;15)(p13;q25) translocation nor the *ETV6-NTRK3* fusion gene has been detected in a wide variety of other pediatric and adult spindle cell lesions (229,232,238) or in a variety of other renal tumors in the differential diagnosis of congenital mesoblastic nephroma (235).

However, the t(12;15) translocation and *ETV6-NTRK3* fusion gene have been described in tumors of other cellular lineages (Table 11.3), including rare cases of acute myeloid leukemia (239,240,242) and the distinct variant of invasive ductal carcinoma known as secretory carcinoma (241,243). The *ETV6-NTRK3* fusion in acute leukemia and secretory breast carcinoma is identical at both the cytologic and molecular levels to that in CIF, a result that emphasizes that aberrant tyrosine kinase signaling by a chimeric ETV6-NTRK3 protein is a common oncogenetic mechanism across a number of different cell types (228,241).

Inflammatory Myofibroblastic Tumor

Inflammatory myofibroblastic tumor (IMT) is composed of myofibroblastic spindled cells accompanied by an inflammatory infiltrate of plasma cells, lymphocytes, and eosinophils. The tumor occurs primarily in the soft tissue and viscera of children and young adults, although cases also occur throughout adulthood (1–3).

Genetics

Cytogenetic abnormalities that involve the *ALK* receptor tyrosine kinase gene at chromosome band 2p23 are a characteristic feature of IMT in children and young adults (244). The *ALK* gene has been shown to be fused to a variety of other genes in IMT (Table 11.4), paralleling the genetics of anaplastic large cell lymphoma (ALCL) in which translocations involving *ALK* were first described (hence the name *ALK* for anaplastic lymphoma kinase) (251). In fact, IMT and ALCL share four (thus far) identical gene fusions, including *TPM3-ALK*, *TPM4-ALK*, *CLTC-ALK*, and *ATIC-ALK* (246,247,250,252). It is noteworthy that the characteristic rearrangements are present only in myofibroblasts, a finding that indicates that the myofibroblasts are the neoplastic component of IMT.

Whereas translocations that form *ALK* fusion genes are common in IMT arising in children and young adults, the rearrangements are much less frequent in IMT that arise in adults more than 40 years old (253–255). Overall, therefore, 40% to 50% of IMTs do not harbor a fusion gene involving the *ALK* locus (253,255); the molecular abnormality in these cases remains unknown, although a chromosomal rearrangement involving the *HMGA2* locus on chromosome 12 has been described in a single case (256).

All of the *ALK* fusion genes encode proteins in which the N-terminal dimerization or oligomerization domain of a strongly or ubiquitously expressed protein is fused to the C-terminal tyrosine kinase domain of ALK, producing cytoplasmic instead of membrane proteins. All the apparently unrelated ALK partners share the ability to cause oligomerization of the encoded chimeric protein with consequent activation of the ALK tyrosine kinase activity, mimicking the kinase activation normally mediated by ligand binding to the native ALK protein (228).

TABLE 11.3
TUMOR TYPES THAT CAN HARBOR *ETV6-NTRK3* FUSION GENES

Neoplasm	Estimated Prevalence	References
Congenital/infantile fibrosarcoma	83%–100%	225, 229, 231, 232
Mesoblastic nephroma (cellular and mixed types)	>90%	231, 234
Acute myeloid leukemia	Rare	239, 240
Secretory carcinoma of the breast	>90%	241

TABLE 11.4

ALK FUSIONS IN INFLAMMATORY MYOFIBROBLASTIC TUMOR

Fusion	Rearrangement	Fusion Partner	Presence in a Subset of Anaplastic Large Cell Lymphomas	References
RANBP2-ALK	t(2;2)(p23;q13)	Ran-binding protein 2	No	245
TPM3-ALK	t(1;2)(q25;p23)	Tropomyosin 3	Yes	246
TPM4-ALK	t(2;19)(p23;p13.1)	Tropomyosin 4	Yes	246
CLTC-ALK	t(2;17)(p23;q23)	Clathrin	Yes	247
CARS-ALK	t(2;11)(p23;p15)	Cysteinyl-tRNA synthetase	No	248, 249
ATIC-ALK	inv(2)(p23;q35) and other complicated structural changes	Amino terminus of 5-aminoimidazole-4-carboxamide ribonucleotide formyltransferase	Yes	250

Technical Issues in Molecular Genetic Analysis of IMT

Conventional cytogenetic analysis is a reliable method for detecting translocations involving the *ALK* locus in IMT. In fact, all of the rearrangements involving the 2q23 locus that are characteristic of IMT were first detected by cytogenetic analysis (245–250).

Given the genetic heterogeneity of IMT, FISH analysis using probes that border the *ALK* locus in a probe-splitting approach is a very practical way to screen for *ALK* rearrangements that indicate the presence of a fusion gene. Some case reports have shown that break-apart FISH is a sensitive method for detecting *ALK* rearrangements in both metaphase chromosomes and interphase nuclei (244–250, 255). When applied more broadly, break-apart FISH can be used to detect *ALK* rearrangements in about 47% of cases of IMT (253). Note that because probe-splitting FISH will detect *ALK* rearrangements regardless of the fusion partner, novel rearrangements that have yet to be described (which are almost certain to exist given the oncogenic mechanism of *ALK* fusion genes) will also be detected by the method. When necessary, probe-fusion FISH can be used to confirm the probe-splitting result or to identify the specific *ALK* fusion partner (245,246,250), as can RT-PCR.

Although RT-PCR can be used to detect fusion transcripts that arise from *ALK* rearrangements (245–250), optimal test sensitivity requires a panel of PCR primers to detect all of the different *ALK* fusion genes that have been described in IMT. And, even with a comprehensive panel of primers, novel ALK rearrangements will still not be detected.

Immunohistochemistry

All of the chimeric proteins characteristic of IMT contain the C-terminal protein kinase domain of native ALK; thus, immunohistochemistry using either monoclonal antibodies or a polyclonal antiserum for the C-terminal region of ALK provides another method to demonstrate the presence of *ALK* rearrangements. Three distinct patterns of cytoplasmic immunohistochemical staining have been observed that appear to correlate with specific ALK fusion protein types (245,255). However, the proportion of cases that show cytoplasmic immunopositivity varies widely between different studies, ranging from 0 to 62% (244,245,253–257), which may be a reflection of nonstandardized assay conditions or differences in the age distribution of the patients whose tumors were tested. Nonetheless, the immunohistochemical assay is highly specific; one study demonstrated a 90% correlation between immunohistochemical expression of ALK and the presence of an *ALK* rearrangement based on probe-splitting FISH (253).

The lack of cytoplasmic immunopositivity for the C-terminal protein kinase domain of ALK in nodular fasciitis, desmoid fibromatosis, gastrointestinal stromal tumors, infantile myofibromatosis, CIF, SS, leiomyoma, and myofibrosarcoma indicates that immunohistochemistry for ALK is useful in the differential diagnosis of IMT (217,255). However, ALK immunopositivity is not specific for IMT; a significant percentage of cases of MPNST, rhabdomyosarcoma, leiomyosarcoma, malignant fibrous histiocytoma, and alveolar rhabdomyosarcoma have all been demonstrated to show ALK immunoreactivity (217).

Diagnostic Issues in Molecular Genetic Analysis of IMT

The demonstration that *ALK* fusion genes are a characteristic feature of IMT provides evidence that at least a subset of IMT are neoplastic. Proof of an *ALK* fusion gene fusion is of diagnostic utility, as discussed above, but only about 50% to 60% of IMT harbor abnormalities at the 2p23 locus overall, and *ALK* rearrangements are still less frequent in IMT that arise in adults over the age of 40 years. Consequently, the predictive value of a positive result for an *ALK* rearrangement is quite high, but the predictive value of a negative result is quite low, and the results of molecular testing (and immunohistochemistry) must be interpreted in the context of the clinicopathologic and morphologic features of each individual case.

The possible diagnostic uncertainty introduced by the fact that ALCL and IMT can share the same specific fusion gene and have the same pattern of ALK immunoreactivity is highlighted by a recent report of a sarcomatoid variant of ALCL that expressed both cytoplasmic ALK and α-smooth muscle actin (258). Given the broad morphologic spectrum of ALCL, which includes a fibroblastic as well as a sarcomatoid variant with spindle-shaped lymphoma cells (259,260), the lack of specificity of ALK rearrangements is diagnostically relevant.

Prognostic Features of ALK Rearrangements

For IMT, there does not appear to be any statistical association between patient sex, tumor site, tumor histology, tumor recurrence, or malignant transformation and the presence of an *ALK* rearrangement (253).

A.

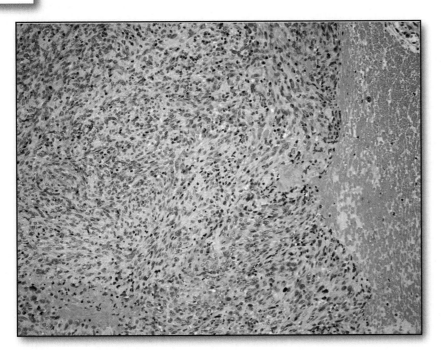

B.

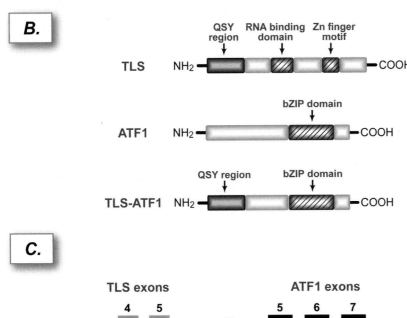

C.

Figure 11.6 The *TLS-ATF1* fusion gene is a recurring feature of angiomatoid fibrous histiocytoma (AFH). **A,** Photomicrograph of a posterior scalp AFH composed of a compact proliferation of oval to spindle cells; note the associated cystic spaces that are lined by lesional cells and filled with red blood cells, a typical feature of the tumor (*right hand region of micrograph*). **B,** Schematic diagram of the TLS-ATF1 chimeric protein in which the glutamine-serine-tyrosine region (QSY region) of TLS is linked to the bZIP DNA binding and dimerization domain of ATF1. **C,** Only one fusion transcript type has (thus far) been described in AFH.

Angiomatoid Fibrous Histiocytoma

Angiomatoid fibrous histiocytoma (AFH) is a slowly grow-ing hemorrhagic, multicystic tumor that usually arises in the lower dermis or subcutis of the limbs, trunk, or head and neck in children and young adults, although rare cases are encountered in older adults. Morphologically, the tumor is composed of solid to lobulated sheets of plump to spindled cells adjacent to areas of hemorrhage (1–3).

Genetics

Two case reports have documented the presence of *TLS-ATF1* fusion genes in AFH (261,262). In the *TLS-ATF1* fusion tran-scripts of both of the described cases (Fig. 11.6), *TLS* is inter-rupted at exactly the same site (between the first and second position of codon 175) as in type 2 *TLS-CHOP* fusion tran-scripts of myxoid liposarcoma (see Fig. 11.9), and *ATF1* is interrupted at exactly the same site (between the first and second position of codon 110) as in types 2 and 3 *EWS-ATF1* fusion transcripts of clear cell sarcoma (see Fig. 11.11). Consequently, the *TLS-ATF1* fusion encodes a chimeric pro-tein in which the strong transcriptional activation domain in the N-terminal region of the native TLS protein (30,31) is fused to the bZIP DNA binding and dimerization domain of the C-terminal region of ATF1 (263–266).

AFH is one of the five tumor types that result from translocations involving the *TLS* gene at 16p11 (Fig. 11.7). In all five tumor types, the general structure of the result-ing TLS fusion protein is the same; the C-terminal RNA binding domain of the native TLS protein is replaced by the DNA binding domain of a transcription factor.

Technical Issues in Molecular Genetic Analysis of AFH

In both of the reported cases of AFH, RT-PCR was used to demonstrate the presence of the *TLS-ATF1* fusion gene (261,262). FISH-based analysis of metaphase chromosomes was performed on only one of cases and was successful in confirming the presence of the *TLS-ATF1* fusion gene (261). Only one of the cases was evaluated by conventional

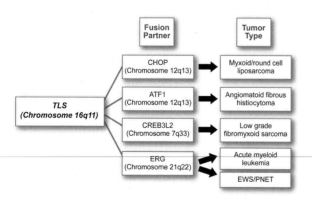

Figure 11.7 Translocations involving the *TLS* gene are character-istic of a number of different tumor types. Note that despite the homology between *EWS* and *TLS*, *TLS-ATF1* and *TLS-ERG* gene fusions are associated with different tumor types than *EWS-ATF1* and *EWS-ERG* fusions (Figure 11.10).

cytogenetics (261), and so it is unknown whether the com-plex rearrangements involving four different chromosomes that were present in the case are a typical feature of AFH.

Given that the *TLS-ATF1* fusion gene has been described in only two case reports, the percentage of cases of AFH that harbor the rearrangement is unknown, as is the sensitivity of the various molecular genetic techniques for identifying the fusion. Similarly, it is unknown whether the presence of the gene fusion correlates with particular histologic features of the tumor or has any prognostic significance.

Low-Grade Fibromyxiod Sarcoma

Low-grade fibromyxoid sarcoma (LGFMS) is a rare variant of fibrosarcoma. The tumor usually has a distinctive bland architectural pattern characterized by alternating heavily collagenized fibrous regions and more cellular myxoid areas. Cytologically, the tumor is composed of bland spindle cells with a very low mitotic rate. LGFMS usually presents as a painless deep soft tissue mass in young to middle-aged adults; in a minority of cases, the tumor has been present for many years (267,268). LGFMS has the potential to locally recur and even metastasize.

The presence of the same translocation in both LGFMS and hyalinizing spindle cell tumor with giant rosettes (269) has provided proof that the two tumor types are vari-ants of the same entity, as has been assumed based on the similar clinicopathologic and histologic features of the two tumors (270,271).

Genetics

The t(7;16)(q34;p11) translocation is a hallmark of LGFMS (269,272) and produces a fusion gene in which the 5' region of *TLS* at 16p11 is linked to the 3' region of *CREB3L2* (also known as *BBF2H7*) at 7q34 (272,273). As noted above, the 5' region of *TLS* encodes a strong transcriptional activation domain. The 3' region of *CREB3L2* encodes a basic DNA binding and leucine zipper dimerization (bZIP) domain (272). The strongly and broadly activated upstream promoter of *TLS* is thought to lead to high-level expression of a chimeric protein that causes dysregulated gene expression, an oncogenic mechanism for the TLS-CREB3L2 protein in LGFMS that mirrors the oncogenic mechanism of chimeric TLS proteins in the three other tumor types that harbor *TLS* fusion genes (Fig. 11.7).

Although *TLS-CREB3L2* fusions are present in the vast majority of cases of LGFMS, one case has recently been described that harbored a *TLS-CREB3L1* fusion, which pre-sumably results from a t(11;16)(p11;p11) translocation (274). Because *CREB3L1* shows strong homology to *CREB3L2*, the rearrangement is thought to promote tumorigenesis through a pathway analogous to that of TLS-CREB3L2 (274).

The break points that give rise to the t(7;16) transloca-tion usually occur within a relatively small region of the *TLS* and *CREB3L2* genes and remarkably are most often located within exons rather than introns (273,274). Variability in the precise site of the translocation break point results in heterogeneity in the structure of *TLS-CREB3L2* fusion transcripts (Fig. 11.8), and rare tumors

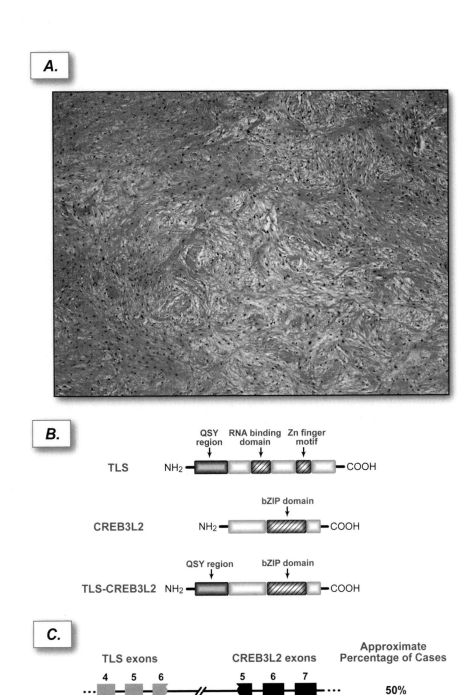

A.

B.

C.

Figure 11.8 The *TLS-CREB3L2* fusion gene is characteristic of low-grade fibromyxoid sarcoma. **A**, Photomicrograph of an LGFMS from the axillary region of a 13-year-old boy, consisting of bland cells with a swirling growth pattern within a myxoid stroma. **B**, Schematic diagram of the TLS-CREB3L2 chimeric protein in which the glutamine-serine-tyrosine (QSY region) of TLS is linked to the basic DNA binding and leucine zipper dimerization motif (bZIP) of CREB3L2. **C**, Structural heterogeneity in the *TLS-CREB3L2* fusion genes and fusion transcripts is due to differences in the precise site of the translocation break point.

also show alternative splicing of *TLS-CREB3L2* transcripts (273). However, no specific fusion type appears to be preferentially expressed in LGFMS versus hyalinizing spindle cell tumor with giant rosettes, and no individual fusion types appear to have clinical significance with respect to the development of metastatic disease or patient outcome (273,274).

Technical Issues in Molecular genetic Analysis of LGFMS

The t(7;16)(q34;p11) translocation characteristic of LGFMS can be easily identified by conventional cytogenetic analysis (269,272,275). Although the sensitivity of cytogenetic analysis in routine clinical practice has not been formally evaluated, retrospective review of cases of LGFMS known to harbor *TLS-CREB3L2* fusion transcripts has demonstrated that 75% have an abnormal karyotype that includes either a rearrangement of 7q or a ring chromosome (273). FISH analysis has also been used to detect chromosomal rearrangements in LGFMS. Using a probe-fusion approach on metaphase chromosome spreads, the t(7;16) translocation can be detected in virtually 100% of cases known to harbor *TLS-CREB3L2* fusion transcripts (273).

RT-PCR has been used to detect *TLS-CREB3L2* or *TLS-CREB3L1* fusion transcripts in virtually 100% of cases of LGFMS and hyalinizing spindle cell tumor with giant rosettes (272–274). However, because these studies evaluated only cases preselected on the basis of amplifiable RNA, the sensitivity of RT-PCR in routine practice will undoubtedly be somewhat lower. Given the heterogeneity in the location of the translocation break points that give rise to *TLS-CREB3L2* fusions, the size of the RT-PCR product can be quite variable, and so the studies reported to date have all used DNA sequence analysis to confirm the identity of the amplification product.

Diagnostic Issues in Molecular Genetic Analysis of LGFMS

Based on standardized expert review, no other low-grade (or even high-grade) soft tissue sarcomas have been shown to harbor *TLS-CREB3L2* or *TLS-CREB3L1* fusion transcripts (273,274). Consequently, molecular analysis is considered to be a reliable method for distinguishing LGFMS from a variety of other soft tissue neoplasms, including fibroma, hemangiopericytoma, malignant fibrous histiocytoma, perineurioma, and myxofibrosarcoma (273).

Extragastrointestinal (Soft Tissue) Stromal Tumors

Gastrointestinal stromal tumors (GIST) are tumors of mesenchymal origin and are the most common nonepithelial tumor of the gastrointestinal tract. The stomach is the most common site for GIST, followed by the small intestine, rectum, and colon. Primary GISTs have also been recognized outside the gastrointestinal tract at sites including the omentum and mesentery (276–279), and these tumors are often referred to as extragastrointestinal (soft tissue) stromal tumors (EGIST). Although GIST is thought to be derived from the interstitial cells of Cajal, the cell of origin of EGIST remains uncertain, although it has recently been proposed that EGIST arise from KIT-positive mesenchymal cells in the omentum that may be the counterpart of interstitial cells of Cajal (280).

Genetics

As discussed in more detail in Chapter 15, GIST are characterized by gain-of-function mutations in the *c-kit* gene that encodes the KIT receptor tyrosine kinase (281), or gain-of-function mutations in the related *PDGFRA* gene that encodes the platelet-derived growth factor receptor α tyrosine kinase (282,283). In GIST, the activating mutations in *c-kit* occur in exons 9, 11, 13, and 17, which encode the

extracellular, juxtamembrane, tyrosine kinase I (TKI), and TKII domains, respectively, of the KIT protein (Chapter 17), and the activating mutations in *PDGFRA* occur in exons 12, 14, and 18 that encode the juxtamembrane, TKI, and TKII domains, respectively, of the PDGFRA protein (283–289). The pattern of mutations in EGIST parallels that of conventional GIST in that the majority of tumors harbor mutations in exons 9 or 11 of *c-kit*, while the minority harbor mutations in exons 12 or 18 of *PDGFRA* (278–280,286,290,291)

Technical Issues in Molecular Genetic Analysis of EGIST

Because the activating mutations in *c-kit* and *PDGFRA* in EGIST (and likewise in GIST) are small insertions, deletions, and single base substitutions, they can be detected only by DNA sequence analysis. In most studies, individual exons of the genes are amplified by PCR from genomic DNA, and direct DNA sequence analysis is then performed on those samples shown to harbor mutations by SSCP or denaturing high-pressure liquid chromatography (278–280,290). The fact that DNA extracted from FFPE tissue has been used for analysis in most studies emphasizes the applicability of the approach in routine practice. In the studies performed to date, a mutation in one of the two genes has been identified in 49% to 100% of EGIST.

Diagnostic and Prognostic Issues in Molecular Genetic Analysis of EGIST

The phenotypic and immunohistochemical features of EGIST, together with the clinical setting of the tumor, are usually sufficient for diagnosis without the need for molecular analysis (276,277). The presence of *c-kit* or *PDGFRA* mutations is not a highly sensitive or specific predictor of malignant behavior in GIST (292), and thus it is likely that molecular analysis of EGIST also will not provide any independent prognostic information.

However, molecular evaluation of EGIST may be important from a therapeutic standpoint. The drug imatinib mesylate (Gleevec) is a potent inhibitor of the KIT and PDGFRA receptor tyrosine kinases (293), but the degree of inhibition depends on which functional domain of the receptor is mutated. For GIST, imatinib mesylate has the greatest therapeutic effect on tumors with juxtamembrane mutations in KIT; the drug has less efficacy on tumors that harbor extracellular or TKII domain mutations in KIT and on tumors without KIT mutations (294–296). These differences in efficacy of imatinib mesylate therapy of GIST suggest that molecular evaluation of EGIST may be necessary to identify patients who are most likely to benefit from drug therapy.

TUMORS OF ADIPOSE TISSUE

Lipoma

Lipoma is the most common mesenchymal neoplasm in adults and occurs most frequently in obese individuals. Conventional lipomas occur over a wide age range, usually in individuals between the 40 and 60 years of age. About 5% of patients have multiple lipomas (1–3).

Genetics

Conventional cytogenetic analysis of a large number of lipomas has demonstrated karyotypic abnormalities in 55% to 75% of cases (297–299). The cytogenetic abnormalities are quite heterogeneous, but cluster into three defined subgroups (Table 11.5): rearrangements of 12q14–15, rearrangements of 6p21–22, and deletions of 13q12–14 and 13q22. Although the frequency of abnormal karyotypes is higher in lipomas from older patients, there are no other consistent correlations between the clinical features of lipomas and their cytogenetic aberrations.

In lipomas with aberrations involving 12q14–15, the gene encoding the high mobility group protein HMGA2 (previously known as HMGIC) is consistently rearranged (297,321). High mobility group proteins are small, acidic, nonhistone chromatin-associated proteins that form a number of families. HMGA2 contains three DNA binding domains and an acidic C-terminal domain, and it has an important role during growth and development (322). The DNA binding domains specifically bind to the minor groove of adenine and thymine-rich (AT-rich) DNA sequences and are therefore referred to as AT hooks (300). Although HMG proteins do not exhibit transcriptional activity themselves, through protein–DNA and protein–protein interactions they facilitate formation of transcriptional complexes.

The most frequent rearrangement involving 12q14–15 is the translocation t(3;12)(q29;q15) which is present in approximately 20% of tumors with 12q14–15 abnormalities. However, a number of other HMGA2 translocation partners in lipomas have been characterized (Table 11.6), and virtually all other chromosomes (including X and Y) can be involved in rearrangements with region 12q14–15 (297,301). The diversity of translocation partners, together with the fact that the coding sequence of some of the partner genes is out of frame (Table 11.6), suggests that the partners in HMGA2 rearrangements have no specific role in tumor development beyond merely separating the DNA-binding domains from the acidic C-terminal region of the HMGA2 protein (328), or beyond simple deregulation of the level of expression of HMGA2 itself (297,322,329). The demonstration that some lipomas result from rearrangements with break points that lie 3' or 5' to the coding region of HMGA2 (301) offers additional support for a model in which deregulation of HMGA2 expression is alone sufficient to promote tumor development.

The HMGA1 gene (also known as HMGIY) is located at 6p21, and encodes a high mobility group protein that belongs to the same HMG family as HMGA2. Translocations involving 6p21 are present in about 7% of lipomas, and

---

TABLE 11.5

SUMMARY OF RECURRENT GENETIC ABERRATIONS IN LIPOMATOUS NEOPLASMS

Tumor	Aberration	Gene(s) Involved	Estimated Prevalence	References
Lipoma	Rearrangements of 12q14-15 (Table 11.6)	HMGA2 (Table 11.6)	<40%	300, 301
	Rearrangements of 6p21–22	HMGA1	<10%	302
	Interstitial deletions of 13q12-14 and 13q22	Not yet identified	<10%	297
Hibernoma	Rearrangements of 11q13	MEN1; PPP1A	—	303
Chondroid lipoma	t(11;16)(q13;p12-13)	Not yet identified	—	304, 305
Lipoblastoma	Intrachromosomal 8q rearrangements	HAS2-PLAG1	Combined, 8q11-13 rearrangements are present in up to 90%	307, 308
	t(7;8)(q22;q12)	COLIA2-PLAG1		
	t(3;8)(q13.1;q12)	Unknown		
	Other rearrangements of 8q11-13; polysomy 8	Unknown		308, 309
Spindle cell/ pleomorphic lipoma	Deletions of 16q13-qter; interstitial deletions of 13q	Not yet identified	—	297
Atypical lipomatous tumor (ALT/WDLPS)	Supernumerary ring chromosomes; giant marker chromosomes	Amplification of region 12q14-15, including MDM2, CDK4, HMGA2, SAS	Up to 100%	310–312
Dedifferentiated liposarcoma	Sames as for ALT/WDLPS	Same as for ALT/WDLPS	Up to 100%	313–316
Myxoid/round cell liposarcoma	t(12;16)(q13;p11)	TLS-CHOP	95%	317, 318
	t(12;22)(q13;q12)	EWS-CHOP	5%	319
Pleomorphic liposarcoma	Complex changes	Not yet identified	—	320

TABLE 11.6

RECURRENT RECOMBINATION PARTNERS IN LIPOMAS WITH 12q14–15 REARRANGEMENTS

Fusion	Rearrangement	Fusion Partner	References
HMGA2-LPP	t(3;12)(q27;q15)	Contains LIM domains	323, 324
HMGA2-?	t(12;15)(q15;q24)	Unknown	300
HMGA2-RDC1	t(2;12)(q35-37;q15)	G-protein coupled receptor	325
HMGA2-LHFP	t(12;13)(q15;q12)	Unknown; the rearrangement creates an out of frame sequence that encodes 69 amino acids	326
HMGA2-?	inv(12)(p11.2;q15)	Unknown; only 7 amino acids added	327

because HMGA1 is structurally and functionally very similar to HMGA2, rearrangements involving 6p21 are also thought to cause lipomas by simple deregulation of gene expression rather than through formation of fusion genes that encode chimeric proteins with novel biologic activity (297,302,322). The observation that many of the break points in the 6p21–22 region lie outside the coding region of HMGA1 is consistent with this model (321).

Technical Issues in Molecular Genetic Analysis of Lipomas

Routine cytogenetic evaluation of lipomas demonstrates a karyotypic abnormality in 55% to 75% of cases. About 20% to 40% of lipomas have rearrangements at 12q14–15, less than 10% have rearrangements at 6p21–22, and less than 10% have rearrangements at 13q12–14 or 13q22 (297). Given the marked heterogeneity in the cytogenetic aberrations associated with lipomas, the genomewide screen provided by conventional cytogenetic analysis makes the method ideally suited for evaluating the tumor.

FISH was an essential component of the experimental approach used to identify many of the 12q14–15 rearrangements characteristic of lipomas (300,301,323–325,327), which indicates the usefulness of the method in the evaluation of lipomas. In the studies to date, FISH has been primarily performed on metaphase chromosomes, so the utility of interphase FISH for the demonstration of 12q14–15 rearrangements remains to be formally evaluated. Given the wide range of translocations that can involve the 12q14–15 region in lipomas, probe-splitting FISH will likely turn out to be a much more sensitive approach in routine use than probe-fusion FISH. FISH-based testing of metaphase chromosomes has been also used to demonstrate rearrangements of the HMGA1 locus (302) and to characterize 13q12–22 deletions in lipomas (314).

PCR-based methods, including 3'-RACE and RT-PCR, have been used to evaluate the break points and fusion genes characteristics of lipomas (300,301,323–327). RT-PCR has been used to confirm the presence of HMGA2-LPP fusion transcripts in a subset of cases known to harbor translocations involving chromosome region 12q13-q15, and to demonstrate HMGA2-LPP fusion transcripts in

occasional cases that have a normal karyotype (324). However, given the heterogeneity of the cytogenetic aberrations associated with lipoma, and the large number of recombination partners that have been described for even the HMGA2 and HMGA1 loci, PCR is obviously not ideally suited for comprehensive evaluation of lipomas.

Immunohistochemistry

Whereas both HMGA2 and HMGA1 are expressed during development, HMGA2 is not expressed in normal adult tissues and HMGA1 is expressed at only very low levels (322,330–332). Consequently, the aberrant expression of HMGA2 or HMGA1 detected immunohistochemically in from 44% to 64% of lipomas correlates with chromosomal alterations at 12q14–15 or 6p21–22 (333,334). Because immunoreactivity for HMGA2 and HMGA1 is observed in about 20% of lipomas without evidence of rearrangements involving 12q14–15 or 6p21–22 (331,333), immunohistochemistry may actually be a more sensitive method than cytogenetics or FISH for demonstrating deregulated expression of the genes in lipoma. However, because about 85% of cases of atypical lipomatous tumor/well-differentiated liposarcoma (ALT/WDLPS) also express HMGA2 (333,334), the clinical utility of immunohistochemical evaluation of HMGA2 and HMGA1 alone is limited. Immunohistochemical evaluation of MDM2 and CDK4 may provide a more reliable way for differentiating lipomas from ALT/WDLS as discussed in the section devoted to ALT/WDLPS below.

Diagnostic Issues in Molecular Genetic Analysis of Lipomas

As is shown in Table 11.7, one of the remarkable features of rearrangements involving the 12q14–15 and 6p21–22 regions is that translocations involving the same loci are characteristic of a wide variety of benign mesenchymal tumors in many anatomic locations (301,322), and can even be detected in rare malignant mesenchymal tumors (306,335). Some of these other benign mesenchymal neoplasms harbor the exact same fusion genes that are present in lipomas (e.g., HMGA2-LPP fusions have been

TABLE 11.7

TUMOR TYPES WITH REARRANGED HIGH MOBILITY GROUP (*HMG*) LOCI

Tumor types with rearranged *HMGA2*[a]

Common
    Lipoma
    Pulmonary chondroid hamartoma
    Uterine leiomyoma
    Renal leiomyoma
    Pleomorphic adenoma of salivary glands
    Benign endometrial polyp
    Aggressive angiomyxoma
    Breast hamartoma
    Breast fibroadenoma
    Skeletal chondroma
    Extraskeletal chondroma
    Chondrosarcoma
Rare[b]
    Uterine leiomyosarcoma
    Inflammatory myofibroblastic tumor

Tumor types with rearranged *HMGA*[c]

Common
    Lipoma
    Pulmonary chondroid hamartoma
    Uterine leiomyoma
    Benign endometrial polyp

[a]*HMGA2* was previously known as *HMGIC*.
[b]For these tumor types, rearrangements of *HMGA2* are not a recurring finding but instead are primarily the subject of case reports (306).
[c]*HMGA1* was previously known as *HMGIY*.

demonstrated in lipomas, as well as a chondroma and a pulmonary chondroid hamartoma) (335,336), whereas others harbor *HMGA2* fusion genes that have not (at least, not yet) been documented in lipomas (387,338). However, from a diagnostic point of view, the fact that the *HMGA2* and *HMGA1* loci are also involved in the development of a number of benign and malignant mesenchymal neoplasms other than lipoma is of limited relevance, because most of the neoplasms listed in Table 11.7 do not usually enter into the differential diagnosis of lipoma. Finally, it is interesting to note that in biphasic tumors with *HMGA2* or *HMGA1* fusion genes, such as endometrial polyps and pulmonary hamartomas, the rearrangement is present in the stroma but not the epithelial component of the lesion.

Lipoblastoma

Lipoblastoma is a benign tumor of adipose tissue that has two patterns: a localized, well-circumscribed pattern (lipoblastoma) and a diffuse infiltrative pattern (lipoblastomatosis). Lipoblastoma is usually diagnosed in children under the age of 5 years, occurs most often in the soft tissues of the extremities, and is more common in males. Histologically, the tumor is composed of an admixture of cell types, including mature and immature adipocytes, a variable number of lipoblasts, and stellate mesenchymal cells.

Genetics

The genetic hallmark of lipoblastoma is the rearrangement of chromosomal region 8q12 that generates a *PLAG1* fusion gene (307). So far, two different fusion genes have been described. The majority of lipoblastomas harbor an intrachromosomal 8q rearrangement that produces an *HAS2-PLAG1* fusion gene in which the partner is the hyaluronic synthase 2 gene at 8q24; the minority of cases harbor a translocation that produces a *COLIA2-PLAG1* fusion gene in which the partner is the collagen Iα2 gene at 7q22 (307–309). The chromosomal break point in both fusion genes is located in intron 1 of *PLAG1*, and so the rearrangements are essentially promoter-swapping events in which the upstream 5' regulatory elements of *PLAG1* are replaced by the promoter regions of the fusion partner. Because *PLAG1* encodes a zinc finger transcription factor that is normally developmentally regulated, increased expression of *PLAG1* as a result of the promoter-swapping is thought to be responsible for the development of lipoblastoma, even when the structure of protein is unaltered by the associated translocation (307,308).

The *PLAG1* alterations are present in many of the different mesenchymal cell types in lipoblastoma, including lipoblasts, mature adipocytes, primitive mesenchymal cells, and fibroblast-like cells, which suggests that lipoblastomas originate from a primitive mesenchymal precursor cell with variable differentiation to a mature adipocyte endpoint (309). This hypothesis is consistent with the finding that *PLAG1* alterations are present in classic as well as myxoid and lipoma-like lipoblastoma (309).

Chromosome 8 polysomy is also a characteristic feature of lipoblastoma. Polysomy 8 is present in almost 20% of lipoblastomas without rearrangements of 8q12, and even in a subset of tumors with 8q12 rearrangements (309). *PLAG1* dosage alterations that result from polysomy 8 are thought to possibly represent an alternative mechanism for lipoblastoma tumorigenesis (309).

Technical Issues in Molecular Genetic Analysis of Lipoblastoma

Rearrangements of 8q11–13 are present in 50% to over 80% of lipoblastomas by routine cytogenetic analysis (297,308,309). However, this estimate of the prevalence of 8q rearrangements is based on analysis of a relatively small number of preselected cases; therefore, it may not accurately predict the frequency of rearrangements in cases prospectively evaluated in routine clinical practice.

FISH, using either metaphase chromosomes or interphase nuclei, can be used to detect rearrangements of *PLAG1* or the 8q12 region, or chromosome 8 polysomy, in 87% of lipoblastomas, including some cases that are normal by routine cytogentic analysis (309,339).

Consistent with the hypothesis that 8q12 rearrangements cause increased expression of *PLAG1*, northern blot analysis has demonstrated an increased abundance of *PLAG1* transcripts in lipoblastomas (307,308), but the requirement for fresh tissue and the cumbersome methodology limit the usefulness of this approach in routine practice. Immunohistochemistry with a polyclonal anti-PLAG1 antibody has shown increased nuclear staining in two lipoblastomas (308), but because PLAG1 expression has been demonstrated in other tumors (340), the utility of PLAG immunohistochemistry in the diagnosis of lipoblastomas needs to be evaluated in larger case series. Similarly, although 5′ RACE and RT-PCR were used in the initial characterization of the *HAS2-PLAG1* and *COLIA2-PLAG1* fusion genes, the role of RT-PCR in routine pathologic evaluation of lipoblastomas has not been evaluated.

Diagnostic Issues in Molecular Genetic Analysis of Lipoblastoma

Rearrangements of 8q12 and polysomy 8 are uncommon in other tumors of adipose tissue (320), including the neoplasms most likely to enter into the differential diagnosis of lipoblastoma (e.g., lipoma, atypical lipomatous tumor/well-differentiated liposarcoma, and myxoid/round cell liposarcoma). The utility of cytogenetic analysis and FISH-based demonstration of rearrangements of the *PLAG1* gene in the distinction of lipoblastoma with an atypical presentation from atypical lipomatous tumor/well-differentiated liposarcoma has recently been emphasized (339).

Even though 8q12 rearrangements have not been described in mesenchymal neoplasms other than lipoblastoma, approximately 40% of salivary gland pleomorphic adenomas harbor *PLAG1* fusion genes, although the *PLAG1* fusion partners in pleomorphic adenomas are different from those in lipoblastoma (340–342). Although the presence of *PLAG1* fusion genes in both lipoblastomas and salivary gland pleomorphic adenomas is interesting from the perspective of tumor biology, it obviously has little impact on the diagnostic utility of molecular genetic analysis of fatty tumors.

Atypical Lipomatous Tumor/ Well-Differentiated Liposarcoma

Atypical lipomatous tumor/well-differentiated liposarcoma (ALT/WDLPS) is a malignant soft tissue neoplasm that most commonly arises in adults in the fifth to seventh decade of life. Histologically, the tumor is composed of cells that show adipocyte differentiation with variation in cell size and at least focal nuclear atypia; scattered hyperchromatic, often multinucleated stromal cells are also often present. ALT/WDLPS has no metastatic potential unless it undergoes dedifferentiation, and so the prognosis of ALT/WDLPS is largely determined by the tumor site. Lesions arising at surgically amenable locations such as the limbs and trunk that can be excised with wide uninvolved margins rarely reoccur and virtually never metastasize. However, because it is often impossible to achieve wide surgical excision of lesions that arise in the retroperitoneum, mediastinum, or spermatic cord, tumors of these sites frequently recur, and uncontrolled recurrences can cause death even in the absence of dedifferentiation or metastasis (3).

Genetics

The defining cytogenetic feature of ALT/WDLPS is the presence of supernumerary ring or giant marker chromosomes (320,343) or, much less commonly, supernumerary marker chromosomes (344), all of which have the common feature of containing amplifications of the 12q14-15 region. The 12q14-15 region contains several putative and established oncogenes, including *MDM2*, *CDK4*, *SAS*, and *HMGA2* (310,321). Several other chromosomal regions, the most frequent of which are 12q21–22 and 1q21–25, are often co-amplified with the 12q14–15 region (311,345). The *CHOP* gene at 12q13 involved in the t(12;16) and t(12;22) translocations characteristic of myxoid/round cell liposarcoma is centromeric to the 12q14–15 region and thus is not one of the genes amplified in ALT/WDLPS.

The exact mechanism of tumorigenesis of ALT/WDLPS remains to be described, and no one particular gene of the *MDM2*, *CDK4*, *SAS*, and *HMGA2* group seems to play a more important role than the others. However, it is hypothesized that they promote tumor development via a direct or indirect control of cell proliferation. Both *MDM2* and *CDK4* encode proteins that are directly involved in regulation of the cell cycle (MDM2 by binding and inhibiting p53 activity, CDK4 by regulating phosphorylation of the retinoblastoma tumor suppressor encoded by the *RB1* gene), and, as noted previously, HMGA2 has an indirect role over cell proliferation (mediated by modification of DNA structure that facilitates formation of transcriptional complexes).

Technical Issues in Molecular Genetic Analysis of ALT/WDLPS

The vast majority of of ALT/WDLPS contain supernumerary ring or giant marker chromosomes (311,321). Conventional cytogenetic techniques such as G- and R-banding do not reveal the chromosomal origin of the supernumerary chromosomes, but FISH can be used to confirm their identity when necessary (344,346). Supernumerary ring chromosomes are not absolutely specific for ALT/WDLPS and have also been described in some sporadic lipomas (310,311), although the ring chromosomes in lipomas apparently do not harbor 12q14–15 rearrangements.

Quantitative PCR and RT-PCR analysis has shown the level of MDM2 and CDK4 gene amplification or gene expression can be used to reliably distinguish lipoma from ALT/WDLPS (347,348). In the larger of these two series, the specificity of MDM2 and CDK4 gene amplification for ALT/WDLPS was 98% and 82%, respectively, and the specificity of the absence of MDM2 and CDK4 amplification for lipoma was 97% and 94%, respectively (347). Given the large number of tumors evaluated, these estimates of test performance are likely very reliable. The results were obtained using FFPE tissue as the substrate for testing; therefore, the quantitative PCR approach seems especially well suited for routine use in the evaluation of ALT/WDLPS. Comparative genomic hybridization has also been used to evaluate the genetic abnormalities in ALT/WDLPS (349), but the method is poorly suited for everyday use in diagnostic surgical pathology because it is so time consuming and technically complex.

Immunohistochemistry

Consistent with quantitative RT-PCR results showing increased transcription of the genes in the 12q14–15 region (347,348), immunohistochemistry demonstrates overexpression of the corresponding proteins in ALT/WDLPS. MDM2 and CDK4 are overexpressed in 50% and 100% of ALT/WDLPS, respectively, but only 0% and 11% of lipomas, respectively (330,334), and so immunohistochemistry has been proposed as a reliable way to distinguish the two tumor types (312,350). However, the MDM2 gene is also frequently amplified or overexpressed in several other sarcomas, including malignant fibrous histiocytoma, osteosarcoma, and even rare leiomyosarcomas (348,351–355).

Diagnostic Issues in Molecular Genetic Analysis of ALT/WDLPS

Amplification of MDM2 has been described in three ordinary lipomas that harbored ring chromosomes (356), as well as in four deep-seated lipomas (355). These rare cases indicate that amplification of the 12q14–15 region can occur in ordinary lipomas, especially deep-seated lipomas, offer a note of caution against over-reliance on molecular genetic results to distinguish lipomas from ALT/WDLPS. Nonetheless, because it is also formally possible that lipomas with MDM2 amplification and ring chromosomes are early ALT/WDLPS, these cases should be thoroughly reviewed to exclude a diagnostic error.

The utility of molecular genetic testing in the differential diagnosis of ALT/WDLPS is demonstrated by two case reports. In one case, a 14-year-old girl presented with a soft tissue mass in her right thigh; interphase FISH showed no rearrangement of the 8q11-13 region PLAG1 region, but did show amplification of the MDM2 and CDK4 loci. The molecular findings supported the diagnosis of ALT/WDLPS but not lipoblastoma, a difference of considerable clinical significance (357). In another case, immunohistochemistry for MDM2 expression and semi-quantitative PCR were used to evaluate synchronous inguinal and retroperitoneal fatty tumors in a 60-year-old woman. The patient's inguinal tumor showed a lack of MDM2 amplification and MDM2 protein expression indicative of a lipoma, while her retroperitoneal tumor had a dedifferentiated component and showed MDM2 amplification and MDM2 protein overexpression, indicative of ALT/WDLPS with dedifferentiation (350).

Dedifferentiated Liposarcoma

By definition, dedifferentiated liposarcomas are malignant neoplasms of adipose tissue in which there is a transition from either a primary or recurrent ALT/WDLPS to a nonlipogenic sarcoma of variable histologic grade. Consistent with this morphologic classification, conventional cytogenetic analysis has shown that most dedifferentiated liposarcomas contain ring or giant marker chromosomes with associated amplification of 12q14–15 (313–316,358). The majority of dedifferentiated liposarcomas also overexpress MDM2 protein (314,359,360), although there is some variability in the level of expression that is apparently related to the anatomic site of the tumor (314). The identity of the additional mutations responsible for the transition from ALT/WDLPS to a nonlipogenic sarcoma is unclear, but it may include mutations of TP53 and RB1 (314,359,360).

Comparative genomic hybridization has shown that many malignant fibrous histiocytomas that develop in the retroperitoneum harbor amplification of the 12q13–15 region and overexpress both MDM2 and CDK4 (349). These findings suggest that at least a subset of malignant fibrous histiocytomas of the retroperitoneum actually represent dedifferentiated liposarcomas in which the ALT/WDLPS component is not appreciated.

Myxoid Liposarcoma/Round Cell Liposarcoma

Myxoid liposarcoma is the second most common subtype of liposarcoma. It occurs predominantly in the deep soft tissues of the extremities, and more than two thirds of cases arise within the musculature of the thigh. Myxoid liposarcoma rarely arises in the retroperitoneum or subcutaneous tissue.

Genetics

Approximately 95% of cases of myxoid liposarcoma contain the t(12;16)(q13;p11) translocation that fuses the TLS gene (also known as FUS) at 16p11 with the CHOP gene

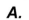

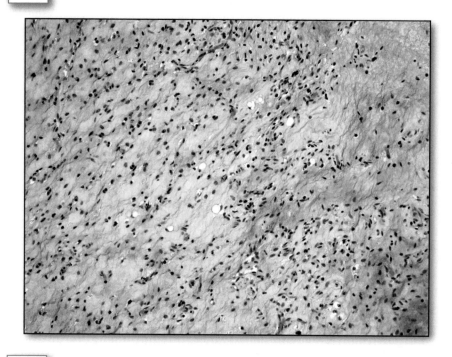

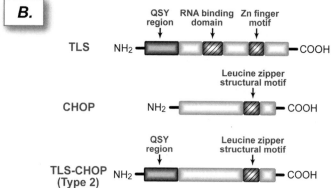

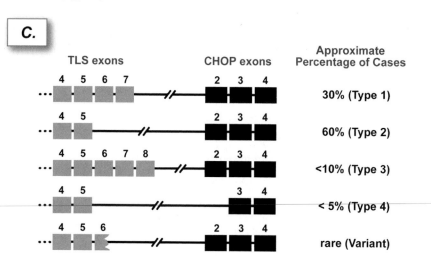

Figure 11.9 The TLS-CHOP fusion protein produced by the t(12;16)(q13;p11) translocation is a hallmark of myxoid liposarcoma. **A**, Photomicrograph of a myxoid liposarcoma from the thigh of a 55-year-old man; signet ring lipoblasts are scattered in a paucicellular myxoid stroma that also contains nonlipidic cells with small uniform nuclei. **B**, Schematic diagram of the TLS-CHOP chimeric protein in which the glutamine-serine-tyrosine rich region (QSY region) of TLS is linked to virtually the full length of the CHOP protein. **C**, Examples of structural heterogeneity in the *TLS-CHOP* fusion genes and fusion transcripts (and chimeric proteins) resulting from differences in the precise site of the translocation break point. (See reference 367 for a complete description of *TLS-CHOP* variants.)

(also known as *DDIT3* and *GADD153*) at 12q13 (317,318,361). Variability in the site of the translocation break point generates structural heterogeneity in the fusion genes (362–366); specifically, the genomic breaks are clustered in introns 5, 7, and 8 of *TLS* and intron 1 of *CHOP* (Fig. 11.9). In the subset of tumors in which the break point is immediately upstream of *CHOP* exon 1 (363), the first *CHOP* exon is systematically spliced out of the initial transcript to maintain the reading frame of the mRNA. Rare variant *TLS-CHOP* fusion genes have been described in which the translocation break point is within a *TLS* exon (367).

The fusion gene encodes a chimeric protein in which the N-terminal region of TLS, which includes a transcriptional activation domain (30,31), is fused to the full length of CHOP, a member of the bZIP family of transcription factors that contains a leucine zipper motif. Because the *TLS* promoter is strongly and broadly activated, the fusion protein is constitutively expressed. Consistent with the normal function of CHOP in adipocyte differentiation and growth arrest (368), the fusion protein has been shown to inhibit the differentiation of preadipocytes (369–371). In addition, in a transgenic mouse model, overexpression of *TLS-CHOP* specifically induces liposarcoma (372).

Given the extensive sequence similarity between *TLS* and *EWS* (30,31), it is not surprising that approximately 5% of cases of myxoid liposarcoma harbor a t(12;22)(q13;q12) translocation in which *EWS* is fused with *CHOP* (319,373,374). In these cases, the chromosomal break point occurs in *EWS* intron 7 or 10, and *CHOP* intron 1 (319,367,373,374). Presumably, EWS-CHOP fusion proteins exert their oncogenic effect through a mechanism analogous to that of TLS-CHOP proteins.

Technical Issues in Molecular Genetic Analysis of Myxoid Liposarcoma

Interphase FISH is a useful method for detecting the translocations characteristic of myxoid liposarcoma, using routinely processed tumor tissue or even cytology samples (68,375,376). Because the translocation break points in the *TLS* (as well as *EWS*) and *CHOP* genes occur within relatively small regions, Southern blot hybridization can also be used to detect the rearrangements characteristic of myxoid liposarcoma. However, as is always the case with Southern blot analysis, the quantity of DNA that is necessary for testing limits the method to those cases for which a relatively large amount of fresh tumor tissue is available, which hinders the utility of the approach in routine clinical practice.

RT-PCR–based testing has been extensively used to demonstrate the presence of *TLS-CHOP* or *EWS-CHOP* fusion transcripts in myxoid liposarcoma and can be especially helpful in cases with an atypical karyotype (377). When fresh tissue is used as the substrate for analysis, studies have shown that a fusion transcript characteristic of the tumor can be detected in up to 95% of cases (59), and RT-PCR testing adapted to analysis of FFPE tissue is not associated with a statistically significant loss of sensitivity (59). Given the limited structural heterogeneity in *TLS-CHOP* and *EWS-CHOP* fusion transcripts, the size of the PCR product as determined by simple gel electrophoresis is usually a reliable guide to its identity. However, DNA sequence analysis may be required to determine whether an atypically sized PCR product represents a variant translocation or merely a PCR artifact.

Diagnostic Issues in Molecular Genetic Analysis of Myxoid Liposarcoma

TLS-CHOP gene fusions are characteristic of both myxoid liposarcoma and round cell liposarcoma, an indication that the two tumor types are etiologically related (365,378), as expected based on the occurrence of cases with mixed histology or histologic progression. *TLS-CHOP* fusions have also been demonstrated in histologic variants of myxoid liposarcoma, such as myxoid liposarcoma with adipocyte maturation (379). Because myxoid liposarcoma harbors distinct cytogenetic abnormalities compared with lipomas and well-differentiated liposarcomas (discussed previously), the latter two tumors are not precursors of myxoid liposarcoma (361,380,381). Similarly, the absence of *TLS-CHOP* and *EWS-CHOP* gene fusions in well-differentiated liposarcoma with secondary myxoid change (382) indicates that these two tumor types are also unrelated.

The rarity of tumors other than myxoid liposarcoma that harbor *TLS-CHOP* rearrangements makes molecular analysis for the fusion very useful in problematic cases, although rare cases of well-differentiated liposarcoma and pleomorphic liposarcoma have been shown to contain *TLS-CHOP* fusions (383). However, given that tumors other than myxoid liposarcoma that harbor *TLS-CHOP* fusions are quite uncommon, the unexpected finding of the rearrangement in a neoplasm other than myxoid liposarcoma should lead to a review of all the clinical and pathologic features of the case to ensure that the tumor is not just a misdiagnosed myxoid liposarcoma.

Prognostic Significance of Transcript Type

Unlike other sarcomas in which specific transcript types are associated with differences in prognosis, different *TLS-CHOP* fusion transcripts do not appear to be directly associated with clinical outcome (367). However, overexpression of *TP53*, which is correlated with decreased survival, has been associated with the expression of the type 2 *TLS-CHOP* fusion (367).

Southern blot analysis, together with RT-PCR, has been used to analyze the genetic structure of tumors from different sites to distinguish metastatic myxoid liposarcoma from synchronous or metachronous multifocal myxoid liposarcoma (384). This result demonstrates that molecular genetic analysis can have a role in providing prognostic information even when testing may not be necessary for diagnosis.

Detection of Minimal Disease

The clinical significance of submicroscopic disease in myxoid liposarcoma remains unclear. In a retrospective study, a variation of standard PCR detected evidence of *TLS-CHOP* or *EWS-CHOP* fusions in the peripheral blood of 20% of patients with myxoid liposarcoma, but the PCR result did not correlate with clinical outcome (385). In a prospective study, RT-PCR analysis detected *TLS-CHOP* fusion transcripts in the bone marrow (two of four cases) and in the peripheral blood (two of five cases) of patients with myxoid liposarcoma, but the prognostic impact of the findings is unknown given the small study size and short duration of follow-up (383).

OTHER SOFT TISSUE TUMORS

Clear Cell Sarcoma

Clear cell sarcoma (CCS) is a rare tumor that predominately occurs in the deep soft tissues of young adults, usually intimately associated with tendons and aponeuroses. Although malignant melanoma of soft parts is often used as a synonym for CCS, CCS differs from conventional malignant melanoma in several important respects: CCS lacks junctional changes in the overlying skin, rarely involves the epidermis, and harbors a translocation that has never been documented in cutaneous melanoma (1–3).

Characterization of the translocation found in CCS (Table 11.8) has broadened the clinicopathologic spectrum of the tumor. Case reports have demonstrated that CCS can involve a wide range of anatomic sites, including the dermis (386), ear (387), penis (388), kidney (389), bone (390,391), and various sites of the gastrointestinal tract, including the stomach, small intestine, and transverse colon (392–395). Despite characterization of the genetic basis of CCS, the identity of the progenitor cell from which the tumor arises remains unknown.

Genetics of CCS

The t(12;22)(q13;q12) translocation is the hallmark of CCS (396–400). The rearrangement results in fusion of the *EWS* gene on chromosome 22 with the *ATF1* gene on chromosome 12 (263–266), yet another example of a oncogenic *EWS* gene fusion (Fig. 11.10). Differences in the position of the translocation break point within the two genes give rise to structural heterogeneity in the resulting *EWS-ATF1* fusion transcripts (Fig. 11.11). A minority of cases of CCS show multiple in-frame fusion transcripts resulting from alternative splicing, and in rare cases in-frame *EWS-ATF1* fusion transcripts are accompanied by

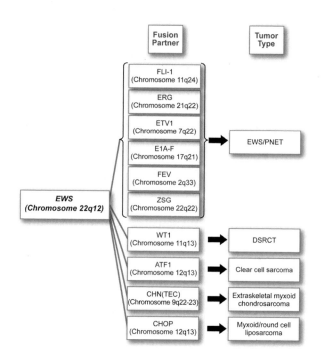

Figure 11.10 Translocations involving the *EWS* gene are characteristic of a number of different tumor types.

out-of-frame transcripts (264). The reciprocal *ATF1-EWS* fusion gene probably does not contribute to the development of CCS, because the encoded fusion transcripts are out of frame.

The EWS-ATF1 chimeric protein consists of the N-terminal region of EWS, which, as noted previously, consists of a strong transcriptional activation domain, fused to the bZIP DNA-binding and dimerization domain of the ATF1 transcription factor. Expression of ATF1 is normally regulated by cAMP (401,402), but the chimeric EWS-ATF1 protein is constitutively expressed because it is under control of the strongly and broadly active *EWS* promoter. Consequently,

---

TABLE 11.8

SUMMARY OF RECURRENT GENETIC ABERRATIONS IN MISCELLANEOUS SOFT TISSUE TUMORS[a]

Tumor	Aberration	Gene(s) Involved	Estimated Prevalence
Clear cell sarcoma	t(12;22)(q13;q12)	*EWS-ATF1*	85%–100%
Extraskeletal myxoid chondrosarcoma	t(9;22)(q22;q12)	*EWS-CHN*	75%
	t(9;17)(q22;q11)	*TAF2N-CHN*	15%–20%
	t(9;15)(q22;q21)	*TCF12-CHN*	Rare
Tenosynovial giant cell tumor	t(1;2)(p11;q35-37)	Not yet identified	Unknown
	t(1;5)(p11;q22-31)		
	t(1;11)(p11;q11-12)		
	t(1;8)(p11;q21-22)		
Alveolar soft part sarcoma	Unbalanced der(17)(X;17)(p11;q25)	*ASPL-TFE3*	Up to 100%
Extrarenal rhabdoid tumor	Biallelic inactivation of 22q11.2	*hSNF5/INI1*	75%–100%

[a]See text for references.

A.

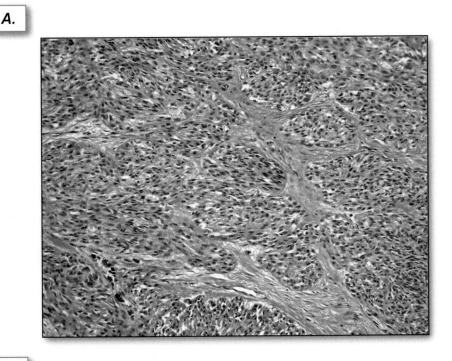

B.

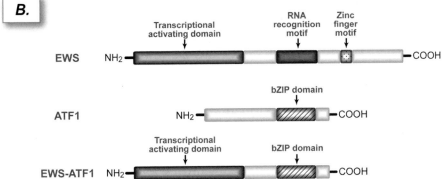

C.

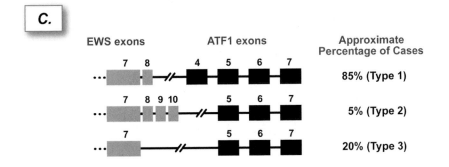

Figure 11.11 The EWS-ATF1 chimeric protein produced by the t(12;22)(q13;q12) is characteristic of clear cell sarcoma (CCS). **A,** Photomicrograph of a CCS from the thigh of a 39-year-old woman; nests of elongated tumor cells with lightly straining cytoplasm are arranged in nests and short fascicles separated by delicate fibrous bands; note the focal pigmentation. **B,** Schematic diagram of the EWS-ATF1 chimeric protein in which the N-terminal transcriptional activation domain of EWS is linked to the bZIP DNA binding and dimerization domain of the ATF1 transcriptional factor. **C,** Differences in the location of the translocation break point cause structural heterogeneity of the fusion gene, fusion transcripts, and chimeric proteins. The designation of the fusion genes is according to reference 266; the percentage of cases with the various transcript types does not add to 100% because some tumors harbor multiple transcript types due to alternative splicing (264).

the EWS-ATF1 protein is thought to lead to dysregulated expression of genes normally controlled by cAMP, although the in vivo targets remain uncertain (401–403).

Additional recurrent cytogenetic changes that have been described in CCS include trisomy 7, trisomy 8, and structural and numerical aberrations of chromosome 22 other than the characteristic translocation (398, 404–406), although the significance of these additional aberrations remains unknown.

Technical Issues in Molecular Genetic Analysis of CCS

Southern blot analysis has been used to demonstrate the presence of the translocation characteristic of CCS (263), but routine use of the method is complicated by the fact that intron 3 of *ATF1*, the intron in which most translocation break points occur, is quite large (approximately 13.5 kb long).

RT-PCR has been widely used to detect the *EWS-ATF1* fusion transcripts that are characteristic of CCS (263–266,407). When fresh tissue is available for testing, a fusion transcript can be demonstrated in virtually 100% of cases (264,266). RT-PCR adapted for use with FFPE tissue demonstrates an *EWS-ATF1* fusion transcript in over 85% of cases (266,408). Because of the structural heterogeneity of *EWS-ATF1* transcripts, maximum test sensitivity is obtained only when multiple primer sets that can detect all fusion transcript variants are employed in the assay.

FISH-based methods can be used to reliably detect the t(12;22) translocation in metaphase chromosomes (389,392), as well as interphase nuclei in tissue sections (265,408).

Diagnostic Issues in Molecular Genetic Analysis of CCS

Because the t(12;22) and the *EWS-ATF1* fusion gene have never been documented in cutaneous melanoma, they are regarded as specific for CCS (266,408). Consequently, the presence of the *EWS-ATF1* fusion gene can be used to differentiate primary CCS from metastatic cutaneous melanoma (408), tumor types that can be indistinguishable by morphologic, histochemical, and electron microscopic features. This result has implications for the diagnostic workup of tumors classified as metastatic melanoma, especially in those patients without a prior history of cutaneous melanoma, because the treatment for patients with CCS is often different than for patients with metastatic melanoma.

A subset of cases of the recently described osteoclast-rich tumor of the gastrointestinal tract also contains the t(12;22)(q13;q12) characteristic of CCS (409). Although this finding suggests a link between osteoclast-rich tumor of the gastrointestinal tract and conventional CCS, analysis of a larger number of cases is required to fully define the relationship.

Prognostic Significance of Transcript Type

Because so few cases of CCS that harbor type 2 or type 3 fusion transcripts have been reported, it is unknown whether fusion transcript type has any clinicopathologic significance.

Alveolar Soft Part Sarcoma

Alveolar soft part sarcoma (ASPS) usually occurs in the second or third decade of life. In children, the tumor preferentially involves the head and neck region, especially the orbit and tongue; in adults the tumor most often involves the deep soft tissues of the extremities, especially the thigh. Morphologically, the tumor is composed of uniform, large epithelioid cells with abundant eosinophilic granular cytoplasm arranged in a characteristic architectural pattern of cell nests separated by delicate sinusoidal vessels.

Genetics

A recurrent nonreciprocal der(17)t(X;17)(p11;q25) translocation has been described in ASPS. The rearrangement results in the formation of an *ASPL-TFE3* fusion gene

(410). Because the der(17)t(X;17)(p11;q25) is nonreciprocal, almost all ASPSs contain a loss of 17q25 sequences telomeric to *ASPL* and a gain of Xp11 sequences telomeric to *TFE3*. It is possible that the resulting losses or gains in the copy number of genes in these regions may also contribute to the pathogenesis of ASPS (410,411).

There is limited variation in the site of the break point in the *ASPL-TFE3* fusion gene (Fig. 11.12). In 75% of cases, the break point occurs within intron 3 of *ASPL*, and in the other 25% of cases the break point occurs within intron 2 of *ASPL* (410). Both of the resulting *ASPL-TFE3* fusion genes encode a chimeric protein in which the N-terminal region of ASPL (also known as RCC17) is linked to the basic helix-loop-helix and leucine zipper DNA-binding and multimerization domains of TFE3 (410,412). Given the apparently constitutive activation of the *ASPL* promoter, high-level expression of ASPL-TFE3 is thought to cause transcriptional deregulation that leads to tumor development (410,411,413). Even though the chimeric protein encoded by so-called type 2 *ASPL-TFE3* fusion transcripts contains an additional TFE3 activation domain not present in the protein encoded by type 1 fusion transcripts (Fig. 11.12), biologically significant differences between the two proteins have yet to be described.

Technical Issues in Molecular Genetic Analysis of ASPS

In most ASPS, the unbalanced der(17)t(X;17)(p11;q25) can be demonstrated by routine cytogenetic analysis. However, in some cases the karyotype can be ambiguous (411) because the translocation is not reciprocal; the der(17)t(X;17) may be described as add(17)(q25) if the quality of the banding does not allow for positive identification of the additional material as originating from Xp (414). Consequently, in some cases the unbalanced translocation is identified only on retrospective review or via advanced cytogenetic techniques such as spectral karyotyping (410,411). Given the difficulty in correctly interpreting the karyotype of some cases of ASPS, FISH can be especially helpful for identifying the unbalanced der(17)t(X;17)(p11;q25) using either metaphase chromosomes or interphase nuclei (410,411).

Because of the limited variability in the position of the translocation break point, Southern blot analysis can be used to demonstrate the presence of the rearrangement that is characteristic of ASPS (410). However, RT-PCR is a less cumbersome method to detect *ASPL-TFE3* fusions. When used to test RNA extracted from frozen tissue, one study showed that RT-PCR can detect *ASPL-TFE3* fusion transcripts in virtually 100% of cases of ASPS (410). The sensitivity of RT-PCR is unknown when FFPE tissue is the substrate for analysis.

Immunohistochemistry

Use of a polyclonal antibody against the C-terminal portion of the native TFE3 protein that is present in the ASPL-TFE3 chimeric protein has been evaluated for its role in diagnosis of ASPS. The immunohistochemical approach has a sensitivity of over 97% and a specificity of a over 99% (415), although the ubiquitous expression of TFE3

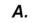

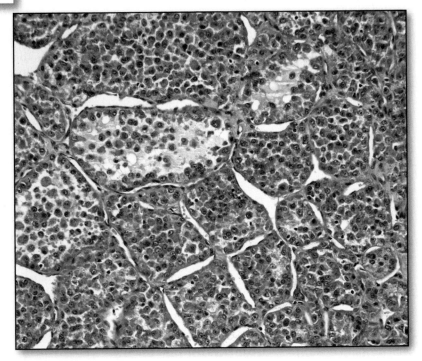

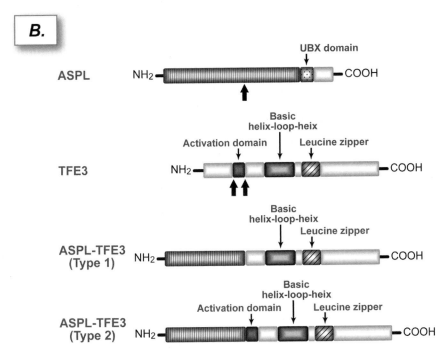

Figure 11.12 The ASPL-TFE3 fusion protein characteristic of alveolar soft part sarcoma (ASPS). **A**, Photomicrograph of an ASPS arising in the posterior axilla of a 14-year-old girl; delicate sinusoidal vessels divide the tumor cells into packets, which assume an alveolar pattern when the cells in the center of the packets become discohesive (*upper left region of micrograph*). **B**, Schematic diagram of the ASPL-TFE3 chimeric protein formed from the nonreciprocal der(17)(X;17)(p11;q25) that is the hallmark of ASPS. Note that type 2 proteins contain a TFE3 activation domain not present in type 1 proteins. *Thick arrows* indicate the sites corresponding to the break points in the underlying *TFE3* and *ASPL* genes.

mandates that the assay sensitivity must first be optimized on known positive and negative cases to minimize false positive results.

Diagnostic Issues in Molecular Genetic Analysis of ASPS

ASPL-TFE3 fusion genes are also characteristic of a distinctive subgroup of primary renal neoplasms in children and young adults (412,416), but the fusion gene is the result of a balanced t(X;17)(p11;q25) translocation in the renal tumors. Together with the distinctive morphologic features of the primary renal neoplasms versus ASPS, the fact that same gene fusion arises through a balanced translocation in the renal tumors versus a nonreciprocal translocation in ASPS has been used to justify classification of the two neoplasms as distinct tumor types (411,416). From a practical point of view, the fact that the two tumor types harbor the same *ASPL-TFE3* fusion usually creates no diagnostic uncertainty because the primary renal neoplasms and ASPS have such different clinicopathologic features. If the diagnosis is in doubt, for example, in the setting of metastatic disease, demonstration of the balanced or unbalanced nature of the associated chromosomal abnormality by cytogenetic analysis or FISH would allow definitive classification (411).

TFE3 is also involved in several fusion genes characteristic of Xp11.2 translocation-associated renal cell carcinomas (417–419) (Chapter 17).

Extraskeletal Myxoid Chondrosarcoma

Despite its name, extraskeletal myxoid chondrosarcoma (EMC) shows no evidence of cartilaginous differentiation, but is instead a multinodular soft tissue tumor with abundant myxoid matrix and chondroblast-like cells arranged in clusters, cords, and delicate networks. Most EMCs arise in deep soft tissues of the proximal extremities, but overall EMC is a rare tumor and accounts for less than 3% of all soft tissue sarcomas (1–3).

Genetics

The translocation t(9;22)(q22;q12) is present in approximately 75% of cases of EMC (Table 11.8). The rearrangement produces a fusion of the *EWS* gene and the *CHN* gene (also known as *TEC*); *CHN* encodes a novel orphan nuclear receptor that belongs to the steroid/thyroid receptor gene superfamily (420,421). Although there is variation in the site of the translocation break point (Fig. 11.13), virtually all *EWS-CHN* fusion genes encode chimeric proteins in which the strong transactivation domain of EWS is linked to the full-length CHN protein.

Approximately 15% to 20% of cases of EMC harbor the t(9;17)(q22;q11) translocation in which the *TAF2N* gene (also known as $TAF_{II}68$ and *RBP56*) is fused with the *CHN* gene (425–428). Given the extensive homology between *EWS* and *TAF2N* (30,31), it is not surprising that *TAF2N-CHN* fusion genes also have a role in the development of EMC. Most of the remaining 10% of cases of EMC appear to result from the t(9;15)(q22;q21) translocation, which creates a *TCF12-CHN* fusion gene (429).

The EWS-CHN fusion protein has been shown to be a much more potent transcriptional activator than native CHN (430), and so both the EWS-CHN and TAF2N-CHN proteins are thought to exert their oncogenic effect by acting as abnormal transcription factors. The recent observation that EWS-CHN also affects pre-mRNA splicing suggests another mechanism by which the EWS-CHN and TAF2N-CHN fusion proteins may dysregulate the normal pattern of gene expression (431). Nonetheless, the three different chimeric proteins are not associated with any particular pattern of morphologic features in individual cases of EMC and are not correlated with any differences in the pattern of disease or prognosis (429,432).

Secondary chromosomal abnormalities are relatively common in EMC. Approximately 50% of cases have trisomy 1q, 7, 8, 12, and 19, either alone or in combination (432), but because of the paucity of data, it remains unknown whether the presence of secondary genetic abnormalities correlates with any of the clinicopathologic features of the tumor.

Technical Issues in Molecular Genetic Analysis of EMC

Cytogenetic analysis, whether by conventional banding techniques or spectral karyotyping, is a reliable and sensitive method for detecting the translocations that are characteristic of EMC (424,425,429,432,433). Conventional cytogenetic analysis alone can be used to identify one of the three characteristic translocations in about 90% of cases (424). Both metaphase FISH (425,432) and interphase FISH (420) have also been used to identify the translocations characteristic of EMC, but no studies have evaluated the FISH approach in routine clinical practice. Because the introns involved in the various break points of the *CHN* gene (and *EWS* gene) are relatively short, Southern blots can be used to detect the translocations associated with EMC (433).

RT-PCR can be used to test for rearrangements that occur in EMC, but there is obviously limited sensitivity to testing that does not employ primer sets designed to detect the fusion transcripts from all three different fusion genes. The sensitivity of RT-PCR–based analysis of fresh tissue in early reports was, in fact, artificially low because the studies were performed before all of the translocations characteristic of EMC had been described. Recent reports show that comprehensive RT-PCR testing of fresh tissue has a sensitivity that is virtually 100% (424,432). RT-PCR has also been adapted for use with FFPE tissue (423,432), but again the reported sensitivity of 78% to 87% may also be artificially low because the analyses were performed before all three of the translocations characteristic of EMC had been described.

Diagnostic Issues in Molecular Genetic Analysis of EMC

The fusion genes produced by the t(9;22), t(9;17), and t(9;15) translocations characteristics of EMC have not been described in any other tumor types and are thus regarded as specific for EMC (422). The lack of all three rearrangements in both chondrosarcoma of skeletal origin (regardless of histology) and extraskeletal mesenchymal chondrosarcoma (433) indicates that there is no etiologic link between EMC and these other two tumor types and highlights the clinical utility of molecular testing in the differential diagnosis of EMC. Whether or not molecular analysis has become the gold standard for the diagnosis of EMC remains controversial (434,435).

Extrarenal Rhabdoid Tumor

Neoplasms with rhabdoid features have been reported in a variety of anatomic sites (436,437). In many tumors, particularly those arising in adults, the rhabdoid phoenotype often represents a poorly differentiated component of an underlying neoplasm that can be easily recognized by routine histopathologic evaluation. In contrast, malignant rhabdoid tumor (MRT) is an extremely aggressive neoplasm

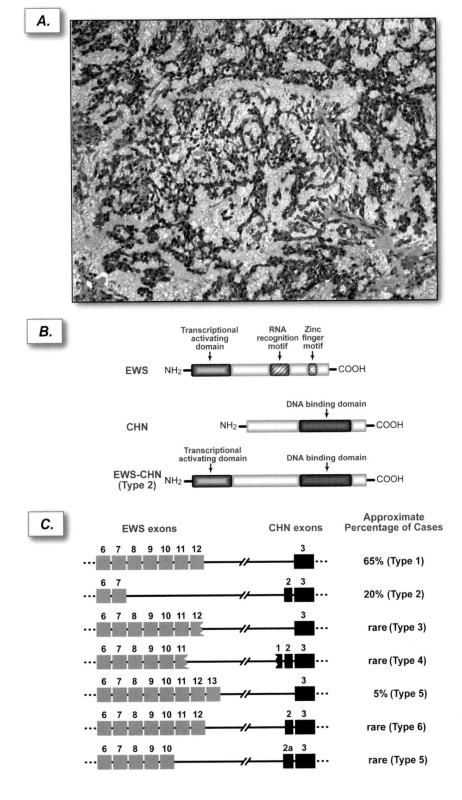

Figure 11.13 EWS-CHN chimeric proteins are present in approximately 75% of cases of extraskeletal myxoid chondrosarcoma (EMC). **A**, Photomicrograph of an EMC; the tumor shows the characteristic linear pattern of uniform small cells in a myxoid matrix. **B**, Schematic diagram of the EWS-CHN chimeric protein that results from the t(9;22)(q22;q12) in which the N-terminal transcriptional activation domain of EWS is linked to the full-length CNH protein. **C**, Differences in the site of the translocation break point result in heterogeneity of the encoded proteins; some rare variants are not shown (420,422,423). Note that different transcript types have been designated type 5 by different authors (422,424).

of infants and young children that has a virtually pure rhabdoid morphology and that characteristically involves the kidney, central nervous system, or, rarely, soft tissue. The following discussion focuses on molecular genetic analysis of soft tissue MRT. Testing for *hSNF5/INI1* mutations in renal and central nervous system MRT is covered in the chapters dealing with those organ systems.

Genetics

The characteristic genetic abnormality in MRT is somatic biallelic alteration of the *hSNF5/INI1/SMARCB1* locus at chromosome band 22q11.2 (438), a pattern of mutation that supports the hypothesis that *hSNF5/INI1* is a tumor suppressor gene. The pattern of alterations includes homozygous deletion; hemizygous deletion with inactivation of the remaining allele by nonsense mutations, frame shift mutations, or other intragenic mutations; and biallelic mutation without evidence of chromosome 22q11.2 deletion (438,439). *hSNF5/INI1* encodes a protein that is a member of the ATP-dependent chromatin-remodeling complex (440–442), although the precise mechanism by which loss-of-function mutations in *hSNF5/INI1* promote oncogenesis remains unknown.

For most MRTs, the alterations of *hSNF5/INI1* are somatic events, and although specific mutations are nonrandomly associated with tumor site, no correlation of individual mutations with prognosis has been described (439). It has recently become clear that germline mutations of *hSNF5/INI1* are responsible for the rhabdoid predisposition syndrome, a hereditary disease predisposing to renal or extrarenal MRT and a variety of tumors of the central nervous system, including central EWS/PNET, medulloblastoma, and choroid plexus carcinoma (443–445).

Technical Issues in Molecular Genetic Analysis of Soft Tissue MRT

Interphase FISH and PCR-based microsatellite loss of heterozygosity (LOH) analysis are currently the most widely used techniques to demonstrate deletions of the long arm of chromosome 22 (439,444,445). By either method, approximately 75% of cases of soft tissue MRT show homozygous deletion of the *hSNF5/INI1* locus. Although a lower percentage of renal or central nervous system MRT show homozygous deletion, the significance of the difference is unclear based on the relatively small number of cases tested (439). Fresh tissue has been used for LOH analysis in most studies, and a potential loss of sensitivity associated with analysis of FFPE tissue has been noted (439).

DNA sequence analysis has been used to demonstrate nonsense or frame shift mutations in the remaining allele in 75% to 100% of cases of MRT without homozygous deletion (438,439,443–445). To detect all inactivating mutations, it is necessary to evaluate all nine exons of the *hSNF5/INI1* gene, or the complete cDNA from the *hSNF5/INI1* transcript (439,443,444). Heteroduplex analysis and single-strand conformational polymorphism analysis have been used to screen for mutations before direct DNA sequence analysis (439,445).

Routine cytogenetic analysis can be used to detect deletions of 22q, often in association with a translocation (438,446–449), but the method lacks the sensitivity to detect the small-scale structural changes or point mutations of *hSNF5/INI1* that are characteristic genetic aberrations in MRT. Southern blot hybridization can be used to demonstrate aberrations in the *hSNF5/INI1* gene, but the method's intrinsic requirement for a relatively large amount of fresh tissue and its inability to detect small scale structural mutations limit its utility in routine practice (438).

So far, biallelic alterations of *hSNF5/INI1* have been present in virtually all MRT of soft tissue that have been comprehensively analyzed by genetic methods (438,439). However, because only slightly more than a dozen cases have been evaluated these results may overestimate the prevalence of mutations. Larger studies of MRT at a variety

of anatomic sites suggest that alterations in the *hSNF5/INI1* gene can be detected in only about 75% of primary rhabdoid tumors (439). Assuming that the mechanisms of oncogenesis are similar in renal, central nervous system, and soft tissue MRTs, this latter figure likely provides a more realistic estimate of the percentage of soft tissue MRTs that can be shown to harbor biallelic loss of function mutations in *hSNF5/INI1* by routine testing.

Immunohistochemistry

Using a monoclonal antibody against the *hSNF5/INI1* gene product, loss of protein expression has been demonstrated in virtually 100% of extrarenal MRTs, including those involving the soft tissue (450). Of note, there was 100% correlation between the molecular demonstration of an *hSNF5/INI1* deletion or mutation and the lack of immunoreactivity. The finding that nuclear immunoreactivity was retained in all tested EWS/PNET, Wilms' tumors, DSRCT, CCS, CMN, SS, and rhabdomyosarcomas suggests that immunohistochemical analysis may be a substitute for molecular analysis.

Diagnostic Issues in Molecular Genetic Analysis of Soft Tissue MRT

Given the wide variety of tumor types that can show rhabdoid features, including carcinomas and sarcomas, the histologic finding of rhabdoid differentiation alone is nonspecific even in infants and children. Because biallelic loss-of-function mutations of *hSNF5/INI1* have not been described as a recurring feature of any soft tissue neoplasm other than MRT, molecular analysis that demonstrates alterations at the locus provides strong support for the diagnosis of soft tissue MRT.

VASCULAR TUMORS

Angiosarcoma

Angiosarcomas are rare malignant tumors that have the phenotypic features of endothelial cells. Many angiosarcomas occur in cutaneous sites, often in association with long-standing lymphedema. However, about 25% develop in the soft tissue, and about 30% arise adjacent to synthetic vascular grafts or other foreign material, following radiation therapy for other malignancies, or in association with benign or malignant nerve sheath tumors (usually in the setting of neurofibromatosis type 1). Angiosarcomas of the liver are correlated with underlying chirosis, exposure to vinyl chloride, thorium dioxide (Thorotrast), or arsenic exposure (1).

Genetics

Conventional cytogenetic analysis shows that angiosarcomas typically contain complex cytogenetic aberrations without a recurring chromosomal abnormality (Table 11.9).

Analysis of sporadic angiosarcomas involving soft tissue or nonhepatic visceral sites shows *TP53* mutations in 11%

TABLE 11.9

SUMMARY OF RECURRENT GENETIC ABERRATIONS IN VASCULAR NEOPLASMS

Tumor	Aberration	Gene(s) Involved	Prevalence	References
Epithelioid hemangioendothelioma	t(1;3)(p36.3;q25)	Not yet identified	—	451
Hemangiopericytoma	Rearrangements of 12q13, 12q24, and 19q13; t(12;19)(p13;q13)	Not yet identified	—	452–454
Angiosarcoma of soft tissue	Complex non-recurring cytogenetic abnormalities	Not yet identified	—	320
	Mutations	TP53	10–50%	455, 456
	Over-expression	MDM2	>65%	456

to 52% of cases by DNA sequence analysis (455,456), and *p53* protein accumulation in 53% of cases evaluated by immunohistochemistry (456). As discussed in more detail in Chapter 15, the incidence of mutations in *TP53* and *K-ras* in hepatic angiosarcomas associated with occupational exposure to vinyl chloride and Thorotrast, respectively, is much higher than in hepatic angiosarcomas not associated with occupational exposure to a known carcinogen (457–460).

Based on the observation that wild-type p53 can be functionally inactivated via binding to the MDM2 protein, and that *MDM2* gene amplification has cellular effects similar to those of *TP53* mutation, deregulation of MDM2 expression is thought to serve as an alternative mechanism for escape from p53-regulated growth control (461). Consistent with this hypothesis, overexpression of MDM2 is present in the majority of angiosarcomas that show no evidence of *TP53* mutation (456). Similarly, increased MDM2 protein expression has been demonstrated in 68% of sporadic nonhepatic angiosarcomas, although the genetic mechanism underlying the overexpression has not been evaluated (456).

Mutated p53 induces expression of vascular endothelial growth factor (VEGF) (462); therefore it was anticipated that escape from *p53*–regulated growth control resulting from genetic alterations of either *TP53* or *MDM2* would be associated with VEGF overexpression. Consistent with this expectation, increased VEGF expression has been demonstrated in nearly 80% of sporadic soft tissue and visceral angiosarcomas (456).

Diagnostic Issues in Molecular Genetic Analysis of Angiosarcoma

Despite the basic science observations that link *TP53*, *K-ras*, and *MDM2* mutations to the pathogenesis of angiosarcoma, molecular genetic assays to detect mutations in these genes have not been evaluated for routine clinical use. The fact that mutations in these genes are present in only a subset of tumors will probably diminish the utility of testing from a diagnostic point of view, and because there is no evidence that the mutations correlate with clinical outcome, there is apparently no value in testing from a prognostic point of view.

TUMORS OF BONE AND CARTILAGE

Adamantinoma

Adamantinoma is a rare, osteolytic, biphasic, low-grade malignant tumor. The tumor involves the diaphysis of the tibia in about 85% to 90% of cases, and about 10% of cases are multifocal, with at least one additional lesion in the ipsilateral fibula. Although most cases of adamantinoma occur in patients in their third or fourth decade, the tumor has been reported in patients from 3 to 86 years of age. Adamantinoma is typically only locally aggressive, but it can metastasize to the lungs, lymph nodes, and abdominal organs, even after long disease-free intervals.

Morphologically, adamantinoma forms a variety of patterns consisting of an epithelioid component and an osteofibrous component in different proportions. The four classic patterns are basaloid, tubular, spindle cell, and squamous (463), but an atypical or EWS/PNET-like subtype and an osteofibrous dysplasia-like subtype have also been described (464–469).

Genetics

Recurrent numerical chromosomal abnormalities, specifically gains of chromosomes 7, 8, 12, 19, and 21, have been described in both classic and osteofibrous dysplasia-like types of adamantinoma (470,471). A subset of classic adamantinoma also shows aneuploidy (472). However, neither aneuploidy nor numerical chromosomal abnormalities have been correlated with disease course.

A few cases of atypical or EWS/PNET-like adamantinoma have been shown to harbor *EWS-FLI1* fusion genes characteristic of conventional EWS/PNET (473), and on the basis of this finding such cases have been reclassified as adamantinoma-like EWS/PNET. However, this reclassification has been somewhat controversial (474), especially because a subsequent larger study failed to detect any evidence of fusion genes characteristic of conventional EWS/PNET in adamantinoma (475).

At a diagnostic level, it is reasonable to argue that the presence of a genetic abnormality characteristic of EWS/PNET in a tumor with Ewing-like features is evidence that the tumor is, in fact, an EWS/PNET with an unusual morphology (473,476). On the other hand, given the lack of absolute specificity of the *EWS-FLI1* fusion gene for EWS/PNET (see the discussion of EWS/PNET in this chapter), it is also reasonable to argue that the presence of the genetic abnormality is not sufficient to classify a tumor as EWS/PNET when the clinical and pathologic features of the neoplasm are otherwise diagnostic of a recognized subtype of adamantinoma (474,475). The rarity of EWS/PNET-like adamantinoma / adamantinoma-like EWS/PNET will make it difficult to collect enough patients for a proper clinical trial to determine the best approach to these problematic cases. However, it is noteworthy that one tumor classified as EWS/PNET-like adamantinoma based on its morphology, but reclassified as adamantinoma-like EWS/PNET because it harbored an *EWS-FLI1* fusion, and showed no response to a chemotherapeutic regimen used to treat conventional EWS/PNET (473).

Aneurysmal Bone Cyst

Aneurysmal bone cyst (ABC) is a benign, rapidly growing and locally aggressive osseous lesion that has a strong tendency to recur (487,488). ABC occurs in all age-groups and can arise in any anatomic location, but the tumor most commonly involves the metaphysis of the long bones of the lower extremities or the vertebrae, most commonly in patients younger than 20 years of age, but rare cases of extraosseous ABC have also been reported (489,490). Histologically, ABC is composed of multiple hemorrhagic cysts separated by fibrous connective tissue septa composed of mitotically active spindle cells, osteoclast-type giant cells, and reactive woven bone. The presence of recurring genetic aberrations (Table 11.10) in ABC has convincingly demonstrated that the lesion is neoplastic and not merely reactive (reviewed in 491).

Genetics

The characteristic genetic abnormalities of ABC involve rearrangements of the *CDH11* gene at 16q22 or the *USP6* gene (also known as *Tre2*) at 17p13 (492,493). Overall, about 70% of cases harbor rearrangements involving these loci. Roughly 44% of cases contain rearrangements of *USP6* alone, about 6% contain rearrangements of *CDH11* alone, and 10% to 19% harbor the translocation t(16;17) (q22;p13), which produces a *CDH11-USP6* fusion gene (491,493). In all cases with t(16;17) thus far reported, the rearrangement produces a fusion gene in which the *CDH11* promoter is juxtaposed to the entire coding sequence of

USP6 (Fig. 11.14), and so the translocation is best characterized as a promoter-swapping event. Rearrangements involving *USP6* and 17p13 are also characteristic of soft tissue ABC, although only a small number of soft tissue cases have been evaluated (489,493).

CDH11 encodes osteoblast cadherin, a cell surface glycoprotein that is involved in cell–cell adhesion (494) and is highly expressed in osteoblasts and osteoblast precursors (495). *USP6* encodes a ubiquitin-specific protease that also contains a domain thought to be involved in GTPase signaling (496). Consequently, the t(16;17) translocation is thought to exert its tumorgenic effect through transcriptional upregulation of *USP6* expression driven by the highly active *CDH11* promoter (492). In this regard, the mechanism of tumorigenesis in ABC parallels the promoter-swapping events that underlie the development of lipoblastoma (discussed in more detail in this chapter) and pleomorphic adenoma of the salivary glands (Chapter 21). It is interesting to note that *CDH11* and *USP6* rearrangements are restricted to the spindle cells of ABC and are not present in the multinucleated giant cells, neoplastic bone-associated osteoblasts, inflammatory cells, and endothelial cells in the lesion. This finding suggests that the spindle cells are the only neoplastic component of the tumor (493).

The identity of the partner genes in cases of ABC with *USP6* rearrangements involving loci other than 16q22, and in cases with *CDH11* rearrangements involving loci other than 17p13, have yet to be described (493). The mechanism of tumorigenesis in these cases is therefore unknown.

Technical Issues in Molecular Genetic Analysis of ABC

In series of unselected cases, conventional cytogenetic evaluation demonstrates rearrangements involving 16q22 or 17p13 in only 19% of ABC (491). Studies that show the presence of rearrangements in a higher percentage of cases invariably analyze only preselected cases, or report only those cases with positive findings, and so do not reflect the sensitivity of conventional cytogenetic analysis in routine practice.

FISH provides a much more sensitive method for detecting the rearrangements associated with ABC. Using metaphase or interphase nuclei by a probe-split or probe-fusion methodology, rearrangements involving 17p13 can be identified in 63% of ABC overall, including over two thirds of specimens that have a normal karyotype by conventional cytogenetic evaluation (491). Interphase FISH by a probe-split methodology can identify rearrangements at the *USP6* and/or *CDH11* loci in 69% of cases (493).

RT-PCR can be used to demonstrate *CDH11-USP6* fusion transcripts (which often show alternative splicing) using either fresh or FFPE tissue, although analysis of FFPE tissue requires a nested approach (492,493). As expected, RT-PCR has a very high technical sensitivity; in fact, several studies have shown that the method can be used to detect *CDH11-USP6* fusion transcripts in virtually 100% of ABCs known to harbor the t(16;17)(q22;p13) translocation by either conventional cytogenetic analysis or FISH (492, 493). Nonetheless, because only 10% to 20% of cases of ABC harbor the t(16;17) translocation, the overall utility of RT-PCR in routine practice is limited (491,493).

TABLE 11.10
SUMMARY OF RECURRENT GENETIC ABERRATIONS IN NONHEMATOPOIETIC TUMORS OF CARTILAGE AND BONE

Tumor	Aberration	Gene(s) Involved	Prevalence	References
Cartilage tumors				
Chondroma	Rearrangements of 12q14-15	HMGA2	50%	497
Osteochondoma	Inactivating mutations	EXT1	45%–65%	3
	Inactivating mutations	EXT2	27%	
Chondromyxoid fibroma	Rearrangements of 6q13 and 6q25	Not yet identified	—	477–479
Chondrosarcoma	Complex nonrecurring	Not yet identified	—	320
Dedifferentiated chondrosarcoma	No recurring aberrations	—	—	320
Mesenchymal chondrosarcoma	Complex nonrecurring	Not yet identified	—	320
Osteogenic Tumors				
Osteoid osteoma	Rearrangements of 22q13; deletions of distal 17q	Not yet identified	—	480
Osteoblastoma	No recurring aberrations	—	—	320
Osteosarcoma	No recurring aberrations	—	—	320
Small cell osteosarcoma	No recurring aberrations	—	—	320
Parosteal osteosarcoma	Supernumerary ring chromosomes; gain of 12q13-15	Amplification of SAS, CDK4, and MDM2	—	481, 482
Fibrohistiocytic tumors				
Malignant fibrous histiocytoma of bone	Loss of 9p21-22	Not yet identified	—	483
Miscellaneous				
EWS/PNET	t(11;22)(q24;q12)	EWS-FLI1	85%–95%	See text
	t(21;22)(q22;q12)	EWS-ERG	5%–10%	
	t(7;22)(p22;q12)	EWS-ETV1	Rare	
	t(17;22)(q21;q12)	EWS-E1AF	Rare	
	t(2;22)(q33;q12)	EWS-FEV	Rare	
	Inversion of 22q	EWS-ZSG	Rare	
	t(16;21)(p11;q22)	TLS-ERG	Rare	
Giant cell tumor	No recurring aberrations	—	—	320
Chordoma	No recurring aberrations	—	—	320
Lipoma of bone	t(3;12)(q28;q14)	HMGA2	—	484, 485
Adamantinoma	Gains of 7,8,12,19,21	—	—	See text
Atypical or EWS/PNET-like adamantinoma	t(11;22)(q24;q12)	EWS/FLI1	Unknown	See text
Aneurysmal bone cyst	Rearrangements of 17p13.2	USP6	45%–65%	See text
	Rearrangements of 16q22	CDH11	6%–25%	See text
Subungual exostosis and bizarre parosteal osteochondromatous proliferation	t(X;6)(q26;q21)	Not yet identified	—	486
Fibrous dysplasia (monostotic, polyostotic, and McCune-Albright syndrome)	Activating mutations	GNAS1	100%	See text

Diagnostic Issues in Molecular Genetic Analysis of ABC

Rearrangements of CDH11 and USP6 are apparently specific for osseous and soft tissue ABC (492,493). FISH analysis has shown that CDH11 and USP6 rearrangements are not present in secondary ABC associated with giant cell tumor, chondroblastoma, osteoblastoma, and fibrous dysplasia (493). Similarly, FISH and RT-PCR testing have shown that CDH11 and USP6 rearrangements are not present in a wide variety of other osseous tumors (including osteosarcoma, osteoblastoma, giant cell tumor, and chondroblastoma), soft tissue malignancies (including EWS/PNET, synovial sarcoma, rhabdomyosarcoma, nodular fasciitis, and leiomyosarcoma), hematolymphoid malignancies, and epithelial malignancies (492).

A.

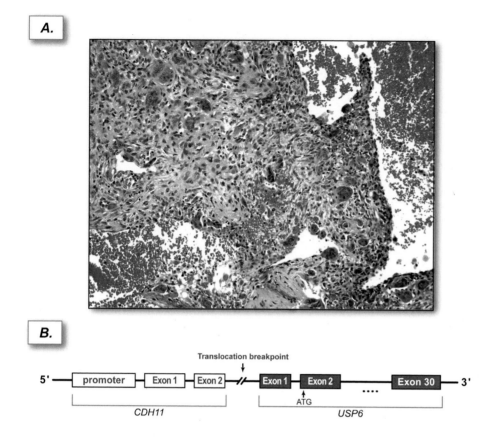

B.

Translocation breakpoint

5' — [promoter] — [Exon 1] — [Exon 2] —//— [Exon 1] — [Exon 2] — · · · · — [Exon 30] — 3'
ATG
CDH11   USP6

Figure 11.14 Rearrangements of *CDH11* and/or *USP6* are characteristic of aneurysmal bone cyst (ABC). **A**, ABC involving the proximal fibula of a 17-year-old boy showing dilated spaces filled with blood; the cysts are delimited by lesional cells and have no endothelial lining. **B**, A subset of ABC harbors the t(16;17)(q22;q13) translocation; the break point occurs in intron 2 of *CDH11* and upstream of exon 1 of *USP6* (schematic diagram is not to scale). The coding regions of *CDH11* begins in exon 3; thus the translocation results in the production of transcripts that encode only the full-length USP6 protein. (The start codon in exon 2 of *USP6* is indicated.)

Prognostic Features of Transcript Type

The presence of *CDH11* and *USP6* rearrangements does not correlate with the clinicopathologic features of ABC (such as patient age, sex, or tumor location) by either univariant or multivariant analysis (493). Similarly, the presence of rearrangements is not statistically associated with local recurrence-free survival (493).

Chondroma

Benign cartilage tumors account for 10% to 25% of primary bone tumors. Chondromas usually occur in the small tubular bones of the hands and feet; periosteal chondromas typically involve the surface of long tubular bones. Soft tissue chondromas, which by definition have no connection to the underlying periosteum or bone, are rare neoplasms that usually involve the fingers.

Genetics

Conventional cytogenetic analysis has shown that rearrangements of 12q14–15 are a recurring abnormality in both skeletal and soft tissue chondromas (335, 497–501); other recurring aberrations include gains of segments from chromosome 5, rearrangements of 6q13, and loss of segments of chromosomes 6, 13, 19, and 22. The aberrations involving 12q14–15 are consistently associated with rearrangements of the *HMGA2* gene, which, as discussed in more detail in the section of this chapter on lipomas, encodes a high mobility group protein that has

an important role during growth and development. Even those chondromas that lack cytogenetic abnormalities of 12q often show altered *HMGA2* transcripts or an abnormal pattern of *HMGA2* expression (335).

Technical Issues in Molecular Genetic Analysis of Chondromas

Rearrangements involving 12q14-15 are present in up to 50% of soft tissue and 50% of skeletal chondromas (335). FISH analysis of metaphase chromosome spreads, using a break-apart methodology with probes that bracket *HMGA2*, has been shown to correlate with the results of cytogenetic analysis in 75% of cases in the small number of cases evaluated (335).

RT-PCR has been used to detect altered *HMGA2* transcripts in chondromas (335). However, given the heterogeneity of the 12q14–15 aberrations in chondromas, PCR is not as well suited for comprehensive clinical testing as break-apart FISH.

Diagnostic Issues in Molecular Genetic Analysis of Chondromas

As shown in Table 11.7, rearrangements involving the 12q14–15 region are characteristic of a wide variety of mesenchymal tumors in many different anatomic sites (301,322). In fact, cases of soft tissue chondroma, lipoma, and pulmonary chondroid hamartoma have even been shown to harbor an identical t(3;12)(q27;q15) translocation that creates an *HMGA2-LPP* fusion gene (323,324,335,336). The fact that *HMGA2* is involved in the development of a number of neoplasms other than chondroma is of little relevance because most of the neoplasms in Table 11.7 do not usually enter into the differential diagnosis of chondroma.

However, rearrangements of 12q14-15 have also been detected in malignant mesenchymal tumors, including approximately 30% of chondrosarcomas (305,314). In addition, there is apparently little correlation between the results of PCR-based *HMGA2* expression analysis and the presence of 12q14-15 rearrangements detected cytogenetically (335). These observations suggest that, from a diagnostic point of view, molecular evaluation of the *HMGA2* locus is not a reliable approach for classifying problematic chondromatous neoplasms.

Fibrous Dysplasia

Fibrous dysplasia (FD), which can involve one or more bones, is characterized by a focal proliferation of fibrous tissue in the bone marrow that leads to an osteolytic lesion with resulting deformity and fractures. There are three forms of FD: monostotic, polyostotic (only one sixth as common as monostotic), and the McCune-Albright syndrome (polyostotic accompanied by endocrinopathies and skin pigmentation) (3).

Genetics

An activating mutation in the guanine nucleotide binding protein encoded by the α-stimulating activity peptide 1 gene (*GNAS1*), located in chromosomal region 20q13, is responsible for McCune-Albright syndrome (502). A single bp substitution in exon 8 at codon 201 results in a constitutively increased intracellular concentration of cAMP, which in turn overactivates the protein kinase A and protein kinase C pathways (503). The same activating point mutation has been identified in nearly all cases of monostotic and polyostotic FD (504,505), and is also responsible for Mazabraud syndrome (polyostotic FD with intramuscular myxomas). The presence of a characteristic activating mutation in FD has led to the suggestion that the disease is a neoplasm rather than a bone disorder (503,506), a classification that is supported by the presence of recurrent structural and numerical chromosomal aberrations in the individual lesions of FD (507).

The *GNAS1* mutations that cause monostotic and polyostotic FD, McCune-Albright syndrome, and Mazabraud syndrome occur sporadically in postzygotic somatic cells and consequently give rise to a mosaic population of cells in affected individuals. The diverse clinical manifestations of the mutations therefore reflect variation during embryogenesis in the size of the cell mass when the mutation occurs and differences in location within the cell mass where the mutation occurs (508).

Technical Issues in Molecular Genetic Analysis of FD

After PCR amplification of *GNAS1* exon 8, activating point mutations at codon 201 in can be identified in 100% of

TABLE 11.11
NEOPLASMS WITH *GNAS1* MUTATIONS

Neoplasm	References
Fibrous dysplasia	502, 504, 505
Thyroid carcinoma	506
Intramuscular myxoma	510
Ovarian and testicular Leydig cell tumor	511
Osteosarcoma	503
Pituitary adenoma[a]	512, 513
Thyroid adenoma	514
Parathyroid adenoma	515
Ovarian cyst	516
Breast carcinoma	515

[a]Mutations in codon 227 of exon 9 have also been described (506).

cases of McCune-Albright syndrome by DNA sequence analysis (504,505). However, analysis must be performed before routine specimen processing because acid decalcification will destroy the nucleic acids in the tissue (504).

Diagnostic Issues in Molecular Genetic Analysis of FD

Activating *GNAS1* mutations at codon 201 have also been described in two cases of liposclerosing myxofibrous tumor, a result that strongly suggests at least a subset of these tumors represent a variant form of FD (509). However, because activating *GNAS1* mutations also occur in osteosarcoma (503), the presence of a mutation at codon 201 of *GNAS1* cannot be used as the sole criterion to classify a bone lesion as FD.

GNAS1 mutations have also been described in a number of other non-osseous neoplasms (Table 11.11). For some tumors (e.g., pituitary adenoma), it is often clear that the neoplasm is a component of McCune-Albright syndrome (506). For other neoplasms (e.g., some Leydig cell tumors and thyroid tumors), it is often uncertain whether the *GNAS1* mutation represents very limited mosaicism as a result of a mutation that occurred during embryogenesis or represents a somatic mutation in mature tissue. In any event, these other tumor types rarely enter into the differential diagnosis of FD; thus the lack of specificity has little impact on testing for *GNAS1* mutations from a practical standpoint.

REFERENCES

1. Weiss SW, Goldblum JR, eds. *Enzinger and Weiss's Soft Tissue Tumors.* 4th ed. St. Louis: Mosby: 2001.
2. Kempson RL, Fletcher CD, Evans HL, et al. eds. *Tumors of the Soft Tissues.* Third Series, Fascicle 30. Washington, DC: Armed Fordes Institute of Pathology; 2001.
3. Fletcher CD, Unni KK, Mertens F, eds. *Pathology and Genetics of Tumours of Soft Tissue and Bone.* IARC Press, Lyon, 2002.
4. Harms D. Soft tissue sarcomas in the Kiel Pediatric Tumor Registry. *Curr Top Pathol* 1995;89:31–45.
5. O'Sullivan MJ, Perlman EJ, Furman J, et al. Visceral primitive peripheral neuroectodermal tumors: a clinicopathologic and molecular study. *Hum Pathol* 2001;32:1109–1115.
6. Lawlor ER, Mathers JA, Bainbridge T, et al. Peripheral primitive neuroectodermal tumors in adults: documentation by molecular analysis. *J Clin Oncol* 1998;16: 1150–1157.
7. Quezado M, Benjamin DR, Tsokos M. *EWS/FLI-1* fusion transcripts in three peripheral primitive neuroectodermal tumors of the kidney. *Hum Pathol* 1997;28:767–771.

8. Marley EF, Liapis H, Humphrey PA, et al. Primitive neuroectodermal tumor of the kidney: another enigma—a pathologic, immunohistochemical, and molecular diagnostic study. *Am J Surg Pathol* 1997;21:354–369.
9. Tsuji S, Hisaoka M, Morimitsu Y, et al. Peripheral primitive neuroectodermal tumour of the lung: report of two cases. *Histopathology* 1998;33:369–374.
10. Kawauchi S, Fukuda T, Miyamoto S, et al. Peripheral primitive neuroectodermal tumor of the ovary confirmed by CD99 immunostaining, karyotypic analysis, and RT-PCR for EWS/FLI-1 chimeric mRNA. *Am J Surg Pathol* 1998;22:1417–1422.
11. Sarangarajan R, Hill DA, Humphrey PA, et al. Primitive neuroectodermal tumors of the biliary and gastrointestinal tracts: clinicopathologic and molecular diagnostic study of two cases. *Pediatr Dev Pathol* 2001;4:185–191.
12. Danner DB, Hruban RH, Pitt HA, et al. Primitive neuroectodermal tumor arising in the pancreas. *Mod Pathol* 1994;7:200–204.
13. Furman J, Murphy WM, Jelsma PF, et al. Primary primitive neuroectodermal tumor of the kidney: case report and review of the literature. *Am J Clin Pathol* 1996;106:339–344.
14. Charney DA, Charney JM, Ghali VS, et al. Primitive neuroectodermal tumor of the myocardium: a case report, review of the literature, immunohistochemical, and ultrastructural study. *Hum Pathol* 1996;27:1365–1369.
15. Hasegawa SL, Davison JM, Rutten A, et al. Primary cutaneous Ewing's sarcoma: immunophenotypic and molecular cytogenetic evaluation of five cases. *Am J Surg Pathol* 1998;22:310–318.
16. Lee CS, Southey MC, Slater H, et al. Primary cutaneous Ewing's sarcoma/peripheral primitive neuroectodermal tumors in childhood: a molecular, cytogenetic, and immunohistochemical study. *Diagn Mol Pathol* 1995;4:174–181.
17. Shek TW, Chan GC, Khong PL, et al. Ewing sarcoma of the small intestine. *J Pediatr Hematol Oncol* 2001;23:530–532.
18. Graham DK, Stork LC, Wei Q, et al. Molecular genetic analysis of a small bowel primitive neuroectodermal tumor. *Pediatr Dev Pathol* 2002;5:86–90.
19. Maesawa C, Iijima S, Sata N, et al. Esophageal extraskeletal Ewing's sarcoma. *Hum Pathol* 2002;33:130–132.
20. Dehner LP. Primitive neuroectodermal tumor and Ewing's sarcoma. *Am J Surg Pathol* 1993;17:1–13.
21. Delattre O, Zucman J, Plougastel B, et al. Gene fusion with an *ETS* DNA-binding domain caused by chromosome translocation in human tumours. *Nature* 1992; 359:162–165.
22. Delattre O, Zucman J, Melot T, et al. The Ewing family of tumors: a subgroup of small-round-cell tumors defined by specific chimeric transcripts. *N Engl J Med* 1994; 331:294–299.
23. Zucman J, Melot T, Desmaze C, et al. Combinatorial generation of variable fusion proteins in the Ewing family of tumours. *EMBO J* 1993;12:4481–4487.
24. Sandberg AA, Bridge JA. Updates on cytogenetics and molecular genetics of bone and soft tissue tumors: Ewing sarcoma and peripheral primitive neuroectodermal tumors. *Cancer Genet Cytogenet* 2000;123:1–26.
25. Sorensen PHB, Lessnick SL, Lopez-Terrada D, et al. A second Ewing's sarcoma translocation, t(21;22), fuses the *EWS* gene to another *ETS*-family transcription factor, *ERG*. *Nat Genet* 1994;6:146–151.
26. Jeon IS, Davis JN, Braun BS, et al. A variant Ewing's sarcoma translocation (7;22) fuses the *EWS* gene to the ETS gene *ETV1*. *Oncogene* 1995;10:1229–1234.
27. Kaneko Y, Yoshida K, Handa M, et al. Fusion of an *ETS*-family gene, *EIAF*, to *EWS* by t(17;22)(q12;q12) chromosome translocation in an undifferentiated sarcoma of infancy. *Genes Chromosomes Cancer* 1996;15:115–121.
28. Urano F, Umezawa A, Hong W, et al. A novel chimera gene between *EWS* and *E1A-F*, encoding the adenovirus E1A enhancer-binding protein, in extraosseous Ewing's sarcoma. *Biochem Biophys Res Commun* 1996;219:608–612.
29. Peter M, Couturier J, Pacquement H, et al. A new member of the *ETS* family fused to *EWS* in Ewing tumors. *Oncogene* 1997;14:1159–1164.
30. Morohoshi F, Arai K, Takahashi EI, et al. Cloning and mapping of a human *RBP56* gene encoding a putative RNA binding protein similar to *FUS/TLS* and *EWS* proteins. *Genomics* 1996;38:51–57.
31. Bertolotti A, Lutz Y, Heard DJ, et al. hTAF(II)68, a novel RNA/ssDNA-binding protein with homology to the pro-oncoproteins *TLS/FUS* and *EWS* is associated with both TFIID and RNA polymerase II. *EMBO J* 1996;15:5022–5031.
32. Shing DC, McMullan DJ, Roberts P, et al. *FUS/ERG* gene fusions in Ewing's tumors. *Cancer Res* 2003;63:4568–4576.
33. Kovar H, Jugovic D, Melot T, et al. Cryptic exons as a source of increased diversity of Ewing tumor-associated *EWS-FLI1* chimeric products. *Genomics* 1999;60:371–374.
34. Giovannini M, Biegel JA, Serra M, et al. *EWS-Erg* and *EWS-Fli1* fusion transcripts in Ewing's sarcoma and primitive neuroectodermal tumors with variant translocations. *J Clin Invest* 1994;94:489–496.
35. Ida K, Kobayashi S, Taki T, et al. *EWS-FLI-1* and *EWS-ERG* chimeric mRNAs in Ewing's sarcoma and primitive neuroectodermal tumor. *Int J Cancer* 1995;63:500–504.
36. Zielenska M, Zhang ZM, Ng K, et al. Acquisition of secondary structural chromosomal changes in pediatric Ewing sarcoma is a probable prognostic factor for tumor response and clinical outcome. *Cancer* 2001;91:2156–2164.
37. Hattinger CM, Zoubek A, Ambros PF. Molecular cytogenetics in Ewing tumors: diagnostic and prognostic information. *Onkologie* 2000;23:416–422.
38. Kullendorff CM, Mertens F, Donner M, et al. Cytogenetic aberrations in Ewing sarcoma: are secondary changes associated with clinical outcome? *Med Pediatr Oncol* 1999; 32:79–83.
39. Graves BJ, Petersen JM. Specificity within the ETS family of transcription factors. *Adv Cancer Res* 1998;75:1–55.
40. Teitell MA, Thompson AD, Sorensen PH, et al. *EWS/ETS* fusion genes induce epithelial and neuroectodermal differentiation in NIH 3T3 fibroblasts. *Lab Invest* 1999; 79:1535–1543.
41. Lin PP, Brody RI, Hamelin AC, et al. Differential transactivation by alternative *EWS-FLI1* fusion proteins correlates with clinical heterogeneity in Ewing's sarcoma. *Cancer Res* 1999;59:1428–1432.
42. de Alava E, Panizo A, Antonescu CR, et al. Association of *EWS-FLI1* type 1 fusion with lower proliferative rate in Ewing's sarcoma. *Am J Pathol* 2000;156:849–855.
43. Ladanyi M. EWS-FLI1 and Ewing's sarcoma: recent molecular data and new insights. *Cancer Biol Ther* 2002;1:330–336.
44. Bennicelli JL, Barr FG. Chromosomal translocations and sarcomas. *Curr Opin Oncol* 2002;14:412–419.
45. May WA, Lessnick SL, Braun BS, et al. The Ewing's sarcoma *EWS/FLI-1* fusion gene encodes a more potent transcriptional activator and is a more powerful transforming gene than *FLI-1*. *Mol Cell Biol* 1993;13:7393–7398.
46. Ohno T, Rao VN, Reddy ES. The *EWS-ATF-1* gene involved in malignant melanoma of soft parts with t(12;22) chromosome translocation, encodes a constitutive transcriptional activator. *Oncogene* 1996;12:159–167.
47. May WA, Gishizky ML, Lessnick SL, et al. Ewing sarcoma 11;22 translocation produces a chimeric transcription factor that requires the DNA-binding domain encoded by *FLI1* for transformation. *Proc Natl Acad Sci USA* 1993;90:5752–5756.
48. Knoop LL, Baker SJ. EWS/FLI alters 5′-splice site selection. *J Biol Chem* 2001; 276:22317–22322.
49. Plougastel B, Zucman J, Peter M, et al. Genomic structure of the *EWS* gene and its relationship to *EWSR1*, a site of tumor-associated chromosome translocation. *Genomics* 1993;18:609–615.
50. Zucman J, Delattre O, Desmaze C, et al. Cloning and characterization of the Ewing's sarcoma and peripheral neuroepithelioma t(11;22) translocation breakpoints. *Genes Chromosomes Cancer* 1992;5:271–277.
51. Ladanyi M, Lewis R, Garin-Chesa P, et al. *EWS* rearrangement in Ewing's sarcoma and peripheral neuroectodermal tumor: molecular detection and correlation with cytogenetic analysis and *MIC2* expression. *Diagn Mol Pathol* 1993;2:141–146.
52. Zucman-Rossi J, Batzer MA, Stoneking M, et al. Interethnic polymorphism of *EWS* intron 6: genome plasticity mediated by *Alu* retroposition and recombination. *Hum Genet* 1997;99:357–363.
53. Peter M, Gilbert E, Delattre O. A multiplex real-time PCR assay for the detection of gene fusions observed in solid tumors. *Lab Invest* 2001;81:905–912.
54. Adams V, Hany MA, Schmid M, et al. Detection of t(11;22)(q24;q12) translocation breakpoint in paraffin-embedded tissue of the Ewing's sarcoma family by nested reverse transcription-polymerase chain reaction. *Diagn Mol Pathol* 1996;5:107–113.
55. Ben-Ezra J, Johnson DA, Rossi J, et al. Effect of fixation on the amplification of nucleic acids from paraffin-embedded material by the polymerase chain reaction. *J Histochem Cytochem* 1991;39:351–354.
56. Foss RD, Guha-Thakurta N, Conran RM, et al. Effects of fixative and fixation time on the extraction and polymerase chain reaction amplification of RNA from paraffin-embedded tissue: comparison of two housekeeping gene mRNA controls. *Diagn Mol Pathol* 1994;3:148–155.
57. Greer CE, Peterson SL, Kiviat NB, et al. PCR amplification from paraffin-embedded tissues: effects of fixative and fixation time. *Am J Clin Pathol* 1991;95:117–124.
58. Ladanyi M, Bridge JA. Contribution of molecular genetic data to the classification of sarcomas. *Hum Pathol* 2000;31:532–538.
59. Hill DA, O'Sullivan MJ, Zhu X, et al. Practical application of molecular genetic testing as an aid to the surgical pathologic diagnosis of sarcomas: a prospective study. *Am J Surg Pathol* 2002;26:965–977.
60. Fritsch MK, Bridge JA, Schuster AE, et al. Performance characteristics of a reverse transcriptase-polymerase chain reaction assay for the detection of tumor-specific fusion transcripts from archival tissue. *Pediatr Dev Pathol* 2003;6:43–53.
61. Krams M, Peters J, Boeckel F, et al. In situ reverse-transcriptase polymerase chain reaction demonstration of the *EWS/FLI-1* fusion transcript in Ewing's sarcomas and peripheral primitive neuroectodermal tumors. *Virchows Arch* 2000;437:234–240.
62. Jin L, Majerus J, Oliveira A, et al. Detection of fusion gene transcripts in fresh-frozen and formalin-fixed paraffin-embedded tissue sections of soft-tissue sarcomas after laser capture microdissection and RT-PCR. *Diagn Mol Pathol* 2003;12:224–230.
63. Giovannini M, Selleri L, Biegel JA, et al. Interphase cytogenetics for the detection of the t(11;22)(q24;q12) in small round cell tumors. *J Clin Invest* 1992;90:1911–1918.
64. Desmaze C, Zucman J, Delattre O, et al. Interphase molecular cytogenetics of Ewing's sarcoma and peripheral neuroepithelioma t(11;22) with flanking and overlapping cosmid probes. *Cancer Genet Cytogenet* 1994;74:13–18.
65. Monforte-Munoz H, Lopez-Terrada D, Affendie H, et al. Documentation of *EWS* gene rearrangements by fluorescence in-situ hybridization (FISH) in frozen sections of Ewing's sarcoma-peripheral primitive neuroectodermal tumor. *Am J Surg Pathol* 1999;23:309–315.
66. Nagao K, Ito H, Yoshida H, et al. Chromosomal rearrangement t(11;22) in extraskeletal Ewing's sarcoma and primitive neuroectodermal tumour analysed by fluorescence in situ hybridization using paraffin-embedded tissue. *J Pathol* 1997;181:62–66.
67. Taylor C, Patel K, Jones T, et al. Diagnosis of Ewing's sarcoma and peripheral neuroectodermal tumour based on the detection of t(11;22) using fluorescence in situ hybridisation. *Br J Cancer* 1993;67:128–133.
68. Yoshida H, Nagao K, Ito H, et al. Chromosomal translocations in human soft tissue sarcomas by interphase fluorescence in situ hybridization. *Pathol Int* 1997;47:222–229.
69. Kumar S, Pack S, Kumar D, et al. Detection of *EWS-FLI-1* fusion in Ewing's sarcoma/peripheral primitive neuroectodermal tumor by fluorescence in situ hybridization using formalin-fixed paraffin-embedded tissue. *Hum Pathol* 1999;30:324–330.
70. Hattinger CM, Rumpler S, Kovar H, et al. Fine-mapping of cytogenetically undetectable *EWS/ERG* fusions on DNA fibers of Ewing tumors. *Cytogenet Cell Genet* 2001;93:29–35.
71. Batanian JR, Bridge JA, Wickert R, et al. *EWS/FLI-1* fusion signal inserted into chromosome 11 in one patient with morphologic features of Ewing sarcoma, but lacking t(11;22). *Cancer Genet Cytogenet* 2002;133:72–75.
72. Gardner LJ, Ayala AG, Monforte HL, Dunphy CH. Ewing sarcoma/peripheral neuroectodermal tumor: adult abdominal tumors with an Ewing sarcoma gene rearrangement demonstrated by fluorescence in situ hybridization in paraffin sections. *Appl Immunohistochem Mol Morphol* 2004;12:160–165.
73. Qian X, Jin L, Shearer BM, et al. Molecular diagnosis of Ewing's sarcoma/primitive neuroectodermal tumor in formalin-fixed paraffin-embedded tissues by RT-PCR and fluorescence in situ hybridization. *Diagn Mol Pathol* 2005;14:23–28.
74. Folpe AL, Hill CE, Parham DM, et al. Immunohistochemical detection of FLI-1 protein expression: a study of 132 round cell tumors with emphasis on CD99-positive mimics of Ewing's sarcoma/primitive neuroectodermal tumor. *Am J Surg Pathol* 2000; 24:1657–1662.
75. Rossi S, Orvieto E, Furlanetto A, et al. Utility of the immunohistochemical detection of *FLI-1* expression in round cell and vascular neoplasm using a monoclonal antibody. *Mod Pathol* 2004;17:547–552.

76. Nilsson G, Wang M, Wejde J, et al. Detection of *EWS/FLI-1* by immunostaining: an adjunctive tool in diagnosis of Ewing's sarcoma and primitive neuroectodermal tumour on cytological samples and paraffin-embedded archival material. *Sarcoma* 1999;3:25–32.
77. Sorensen PH, Shimada H, Liu XF, et al. Biphenotypic sarcomas with myogenic and neural differentiation express the Ewing's sarcoma *EWS/FLI1* fusion gene. *Cancer Res* 1995; 55:1385–1392.
78. Thorner P, Squire J, Chilton-MacNeill S, et al. Is the *EWS/FLI-1* fusion transcript specific for Ewing sarcoma and peripheral primitive neuroectodermal tumor? A report of four cases showing this transcript in a wider range of tumor types. *Am J Pathol* 1996;148:1125–1138.
79. Katz RL, Quezado M, Senderowicz AM, et al. An intra-abdominal small round cell neoplasm with features of primitive neuroectodermal and desmoplastic round cell tumor and a *EWS/FLI-1* fusion transcript. *Hum Pathol* 1997;28:502–509.
80. Thorner P. Intra-abdominal polyphenotypic tumor. *Pediatr Pathol Lab Med* 1996; 16:161–169.
81. de Alava E, Lozano MD, Sola I, et al. Molecular features in a biphenotypic small cell sarcoma with neuroectodermal and muscle differentiation. *Hum Pathol* 1998;29:181–184.
82. Sainati L, Scapinello A, Montaldi A, et al. A mesenchymal chondrosarcoma of a child with the reciprocal translocation (11;22)(q24;q12). *Cancer Genet Cytogenet* 1993;71:144–147.
83. Ordi J, De Alava E, Torne A, et al. Intraabdominal desmoplastic small round cell tumor with *EWS/ERG* fusion transcript. *Am J Surg Pathol* 1998;22:1026–1032.
84. Burchill SA, Wheeldon J, Cullinane C, et al. *EWS-FLI1* fusion transcripts identified in patients with typical neuroblastoma. *Eur J Cancer* 1997;33:239–243.
85. Scotlandi K, Chano T, Benini S, et al. Identification of *EWS/FLI-1* transcripts in giant-cell tumor of bone. *Int J Cancer* 2000;87:328–335.
86. Sandberg AA, Turc-Carel C, Gemmill RM. Chromosomes in solid tumors and beyond. *Cancer Res* 1988;48:1049–1059.
87. Lengauer C, Kinzler KW, Vogelstein B. Genetic instabilities in human cancers. *Nature*. 1998;396:643–649.
88. Michor F, Iwasa Y, Nowak MA. Dynamics of cancer progression. *Nat Rev Cancer* 2004;4:197–205.
89. Pfeifer JD, Hill DA, O'Sullivan MJ, et al. Diagnostic gold standard for soft tissue tumours: morphology or molecular genetics? *Histopathology* 2000;37:485–500.
90. Kilpatrick SE, Garvin AJ. Recent advances in the diagnosis of pediatric soft-tissue tumors. *Med Pediatr Oncol* 1999;32:373–376.
91. Fletcher CD, Fletcher JA, Cin PD, et al. Diagnostic gold standard for soft tissue tumours: morphology or molecular genetics? *Histopathology* 2001;39:100–103.
92. Zoubek A, Dockhorn-Dworniczak B, Delattre O, et al. Does expression of different *EWS* chimeric transcripts define clinically distinct risk groups of Ewing tumor patients? *J Clin Oncol* 1996;14:1245–1251.
93. de Alava E, Kawai A, Healey JH, et al. *EWS-FLI1* fusion transcript structure is an independent determinant of prognosis in Ewing's sarcoma. *J Clin Oncol* 1998; 16:1248–1255.
94. Lin PP, Brody RI, Hamelin A, et al. Differential transactivation by alternative EWS-FLI1 fusion proteins correlates with clinical heterogeneity in Ewing's sarcoma. *Cancer Res* 1999;59:1428–1432.
95. West DC, Grier HE, Swallow MM, et al. Detection of circulating tumor cells in patients with Ewing's sarcoma and peripheral primitive neuroectodermal tumor. *J Clin Oncol* 1997;15:583–588.
96. Zoubek A, Ladenstein R, Windhager R, et al. Predictive potential of testing for bone marrow involvement in Ewing tumor patients by RT-PCR: a preliminary evaluation. *Int J Cancer* 1998;79:56–60.
97. Fagnou C, Michon J, Peter M, et al. Presence of tumor cells in bone marrow but not in blood is associated with adverse prognosis in patients with Ewing's tumor. Societe Francaise d'Oncologie Pediatrique. *J Clin Oncol* 1998;16:1707–1711.
98. de Alava E, Ladanyi M, Rosai J, et al. Detection of chimeric transcripts in desmoplastic small round cell tumor and related developmental tumors by reverse transcriptase polymerase chain reaction: a specific diagnostic assay. *Am J Pathol* 1995;147:1584–1591.
99. Zoubek A, Kovar H, Kronberger M, et al. Mobilization of tumour cells during biopsy in an infant with Ewing sarcoma. *Eur J Pediatr* 1996;155:373–376.
100. Peter M, Magdelenat H, Michon J, et al. Sensitive detection of occult Ewing's cells by the reverse transcriptase-polymerase chain reaction. *Br J Cancer* 1995;72:96–100.
101. Toretsky JA, Neckers L, Wexler LH. Detection of (11;22)(q24;q12) translocation-bearing cells in peripheral blood progenitor cells of patients with Ewing's sarcoma family of tumors. *J Natl Cancer Inst* 1995;87:385–386.
102. Fischmeister G, Zoubek A, Jugovic D, et al. Low incidence of molecular evidence for tumour in PBPC harvests from patients with high risk Ewing tumours. *Bone Marrow Transplant* 1999;24:405–409.
103. Gerald WL, Miller HK, Battifora H, et al. Intra-abdominal desmoplastic small round-cell tumor: report of 19 cases of a distinctive type of high-grade polyphenotypic malignancy affecting young individuals. *Am J Surg Pathol* 1991;15:499–513.
104. Gerald WL, Ladanyi M, de Alava E, et al. Clinical, pathologic, and molecular spectrum of tumors associated with t(11;22)(p13;q12): desmoplastic small round-cell tumor and its variants. *J Clin Oncol* 1998;16:3028–3036.
105. Tison V, Cerasoli S, Morigi F, et al. Intracranial desmoplastic small-cell tumor: report of a case. *Am J Surg Pathol* 1996;20:112–117.
106. Wolf AN, Ladanyi M, Paull G, et al. The expanding clinical spectrum of desmoplastic small round-cell tumor: a report of two cases with molecular confirmation. *Hum Pathol* 1999;30:430–435.
107. Nishio J, Iwasaki H, Ishiguro M, et al. Intra-abdominal small round cell tumour with *EWS-WT1* fusion transcript in an elderly patient. *Histopathology* 2003;42:410–412.
108. Ladanyi M, Gerald W. Fusion of the *EWS* and *WT1* genes in the desmoplastic small round cell tumor. *Cancer Res* 1994;54:2837–2840.
109. Gerald WL, Rasai J, Ladanyi M. Characterization of the genomic breakpoint and chimeric transcripts in the *EWS-WT1* gene fusion of desmoplastic small round cell tumor. *Proc Natl Acad Sci USA* 1995;92:1028–1032.
110. Benjamin LE, Fredericks WJ, Barr FG, et al. Fusion of the *EWS1* and *WT1* genes as a result of the t(11;22)(p13;q12) translocation in desmoplastic small round cell tumors. *Med Pediatr Oncol* 1996;27:434–439.
111. Armstrong JF. The expression of the Wilms' tumour gene, *WT1*, in the developing mammalian embryo. *Mech Dev* 1993;40:85–97.
112. Scharnhorst V, vander Eb AJ, Jochemsen AG, et al. WT1 proteins: functions in growth and differentiation. *Gene* 2001;273:141–161.
113. Carpentieri DF, Nichols K, Chou PM, et al. The expression of WT1 in the differentiation of rhabdomyosarcoma from other pediatric small round blue cell tumors. *Mod Pathol* 2002;15:1080–1086.
114. Charles AK, Moore IE, Berry PJ. Immunohistochemical detection of the Wilms' tumour gene *WT1* in desmoplastic small round cell tumour. *Histopathology* 1997;30:312–314.
115. Ordonez NG. Desmoplastic small round cell tumor. II. An ultrastructural and immunohistochemical study with emphasis on new immunohistochemical markers. *Am J Surg Pathol* 1998;22:1314–1327.
116. Barnoud R, Delattre O, Peoc'h M, et al. Desmoplastic small round cell tumor: RT-PCR analysis and immunohistochemical detection of the Wilm's tumor gene *WT1*. *Pathol Res Pract* 1998;194:693–700.
117. Zhang PJ, Goldblum JR, Pawel BR, et al. Immunophenotype of desmoplastic small round cell tumors as detected in cases with *EWS-WT1* gene fusion product. *Mod Pathol* 2003;16:229–235.
118. Hill DA, Pfeifer JD, Marley EF, et al. *WT1* staining reliably differentiates desmoplastic small round cell tumor from Ewing sarcoma/primitive neuroectodermal tumor: an immunohistochemical and molecular diagnostic study. *Am J Clin Pathol* 2000; 114:345–353.
119. Newton WA, Soule EH, Hamoudi AB, et al. Histopathology of childhood sarcomas, Intergroup Rhabdomyosarcoma Studies I and II: clinicopathologic correlation. *J Clin Oncol* 1988;6:67–75.
120. Caillaud JM, Gerard-Marchant R, Marsden HB, et al. Histopathological classification of childhood rhabdomyosarcoma: a report from the International Society of Pediatric Oncology Pathology Panel. *Med Pediatr Oncol* 1989;17:391–400.
121. Galili N, Davis RJ, Fredericks WJ, et al. Fusion of a fork head domain gene to *PAX3* in the solid tumour alveolar rhabdomyosarcoma. *Nat Genet* 1993;5:230–235.
122. Shapiro D, Sublett JE, Li B, et al. Fusion of *PAX3* to a member of the forkhead family of transcription factors in human alveolar rhabdomyosarcoma. *Cancer Res* 1993;53: 5108–5112.
123. Davis RJ, D'Cruz CM, Lovell MA, et al. Fusion of *PAX7* to *FKHR* by the variant t(1;13)(p36;q14) translocation in alveolar rhabdomyosarcoma. *Cancer Res* 1994; 54:2869–2872.
124. Barr FG, Galili N, Holick J, et al. Rearrangement of the *PAX3* paired box gene in the paediatric solid tumour alveolar rhabdomyosarcoma. *Nat Genet* 1993;3:113–117.
125. Davis RJ, Bennicelli JL, Macina RA, et al. Structural characterization of the *FKHR* gene and its rearrangement in alveolar rhabdomyosarcoma. *Hum Mol Genet* 1995; 4:2355–2362.
126. Fitzgerald JC, Scherr AM, Barr FG. Structural analysis of *PAX7* rearrangements in alveolar rhabdomyosarcoma. *Cancer Genet Cytogenet* 2000;117:37–40.
127. Barr FG, Nauta LE, Davis RJ, et al. In vivo amplification of the *PAX3-FKHR* and *PAX7-FKHR* fusion genes in alveolar rhabdomyosarcoma. *Hum Mol Genet* 1996;5:15–21.
128. Barr FG, Qualman SJ, Macris MH, et al. Genetic heterogeneity in the alveolar rhabdomyosarcoma subset without typical gene fusions. *Cancer Res* 2002;62:4704–4710.
129. Bennicelli JL, Edwards RH, Barr FG. Mechanism for transcriptional gain of function resulting from chromosomal translocation in alveolar rhabdomyosarcoma. *Proc Natl Acad Sci USA* 1996;93:5455–5459.
130. Strachan T, Read AP. *PAX* genes. *Curr Opin Genet Dev* 1994;4:427–438.
131. Barr FG. Gene fusions involving *PAX* and *FOX* family members in alveolar rhabdomyosarcoma. *Oncogene* 2001;20:5736–5746.
132. Anderson MJ, Shelton GD, Cavenee WK, et al. Embryonic expression of the tumor-associated PAX3-FKHR fusion protein interferes with the developmental functions of Pax3. *Proc Natl Acad Sci USA* 2001;98:1589–1594.
133. Gordon AT, Brinkschmidt C, Anderson J. A novel and consistent amplicon at 13q31 associated with alveolar rhabdomyosarcoma. *Genes Chromosomes Cancer* 2000; 28:220–226.
134. Barr FG, Nauta LE, Hollows JC. Structural analysis of *PAX3* genomic rearrangements in alveolar rhabdomyosarcoma. *Cancer Genet Cytogenet* 1998;102:32–39.
135. Barr FG, Chatten J, D'Cruz CM, et al. Molecular assays for chromosomal translocations in the diagnosis of pediatric soft tissue sarcomas. *JAMA* 1995;273:553–557.
136. Downing JR, Khandeker A, Shurtleff SA, et al. Multiplex RT-PCR assay for the differential diagnosis of alveolar rhabdomyosarcoma and Ewing's sarcoma. *Am J Pathol* 1995; 146:626–634.
137. Arden KC, Anderson MJ, Finckenstein FG, et al. Detection of the t(2;13) chromosomal translocation in alveolar rhabdomyosarcoma using the reverse transcriptase-polymerase chain reaction. *Genes Chromosomes Cancer* 1996;16:254–260.
138. Reichmuth C, Markus MA, Hillemanns M, et al. The diagnostic potential of the chromosome translocation t(2;13) in rhabdomyosarcoma: a PCR study of fresh-frozen and paraffin-embedded tumour samples. *J Pathol* 1996;180:50–57.
139. Barr FG, Xiong QB, Kelly K. A consensus polymerase chain reaction-oligonucleotide hybridization approach for the detection of chromosomal translocations in pediatric bone and soft tissue sarcomas. *Am J Clin Pathol* 1995;104:627–633.
140. Edwards RH, Chatten J, Xiong QB, et al. Detection of gene fusions in rhabdomyosarcoma by reverse transcriptase-polymerase chain reaction assay of archival samples. *Diagn Mol Pathol* 1997;6:91–97.
141. Anderson J, Renshaw J, McManus A, et al. Amplification of the t(2; 13) and t(1; 13) translocations of alveolar rhabdomyosarcoma in small formalin-fixed biopsies using a modified reverse transcriptase polymerase chain reaction. *Am J Pathol* 1997;150: 477–482.
142. Biegel JA, Nycum LM, Valentine V, et al. Detection of the t(2;13)(q35;q14) and PAX3-FKHR fusion in alveolar rhabdomyosarcoma by fluorescence in situ hybridization. *Genes Chromosomes Cancer* 1995;12:186–192.
143. McManus AP, O'Reilly MA, Jones KP, et al. Interphase fluorescence in situ hybridization detection of t(2;13)(q35;q14) in alveolar rhabdomyosarcoma: a diagnostic tool in minimally invasive biopsies. *J Pathol* 1996;178:410–414.
144. Dockhorn-Dworniczak B, Schafer KL, Blasius S, et al. Assessment of molecular genetic detection of chromosome translocations in the differential diagnosis of pediatric sarcomas. *Klin Padiatr* 1997;209:156–164.

145. Bridge JA, Liu J, Weibolt V, et al. Novel genomic imbalances in embryonal rhabdomyosarcoma revealed by comparative genomic hybridization and fluorescence in situ hybridization: an intergroup rhabdomyosarcoma study. *Genes Chromosomes Cancer* 2000;27:337–344.

146. de Alava E, Lozano MD, Sola I, et al. Molecular features in a biphenotypic small cell sarcoma with neuroectodermal and muscle differentiation. *Hum Pathol* 1998;29:181–184.

147. Anderson J, Gordon T, McManus A, et al. Detection of the *PAX3-FKHR* fusion gene in paediatric rhabdomyosarcoma: a reproducible predictor of outcome? *Br J Cancer* 2001;85:831–835.

148. Sorensen PH, Lynch JC, Qualman SJ, et al. *PAX3-FKHR* and *PAX7-FKHR* gene fusions are prognostic indicators in alveolar rhabdomyosarcoma: a report from the children's oncology group. *J Clin Oncol* 2002;20:2672–2679.

149. Kelly KM, Womer RB, Sorensen PH, et al. Common and variant gene fusions predict distinct clinical phenotypes in rhabdomyosarcoma. *J Clin Oncol* 1997;15:1831–1836.

150. Kelly KM, Womer RB, Barr FG. Minimal disease detection in patients with alveolar rhabdomyosarcoma using a reverse transcriptase-polymerase chain reaction method. *Cancer* 1996;78:1320–1327.

151. Pawel BR, Hamoudi AB, Asmar L, et al. Undifferentiated sarcomas of children: pathology and clinical behavior—an Intergroup Rhabdomyosarcoma study. *Med Pediatr Oncol* 1997;29:170–180.

152. Kempson RL, Hendrickson MR. An approach to the diagnosis of soft tissue tumors. *Monogr Pathol* 1996;38:1–36.

153. Kushner BH, LaQuaglia MP, Cheung NK, et al. Clinically critical impact of molecular genetic studies in pediatric solid tumors. *Med Pediatr Oncol* 1999;33:530–535.

154. O'Sullivan MJ, Kyriakos M, Zhu X, et al. Malignant peripheral nerve sheath tumors with t(X;18): a pathologic and molecular genetic study. *Mod Pathol* 2000;13:1336–1346.

155. Hisaoka M, Hashimoto H, Iwamasa T, et al. Primary synovial sarcoma of the lung: report of two cases confirmed by molecular detection of *SYT-SSX* fusion gene transcripts. *Histopathology* 1999;34:205–210.

156. Iwasaki H, Ishiguro M, Ohjimi Y, et al. Synovial sarcoma of the prostate with t(X;18)(p11.2;q11.2). *Am J Surg Pathol* 1999;23:220–226.

157. Billings SD, Meisner LF, Cummings OW, et al. Synovial sarcoma of the upper digestive tract: a report of two cases with demonstration of the X;18 translocation by fluorescence in situ hybridization. *Mod Pathol* 2000;13:68–76.

158. Cole P, Ladanyi M, Gerald WL, et al. Synovial sarcoma mimicking desmoplastic small round-cell tumor: critical role for molecular diagnosis. *Med Pediatr Oncol* 1999;32:97–101.

159. Spielmann A, Janzen DL, O'Connell JX, et al. Intraneural synovial sarcoma. *Skeletal Radiol* 1997;26:677–681.

160. O'Connell JX, Browne WL, Gropper PT, et al. Intraneural biphasic synovial sarcoma: an alternative "glandular" tumor of peripheral nerve. *Mod Pathol* 1996;9:738–741.

161. Crew AJ, Clark J, Fisher C, et al. Fusion of SYT to two genes, *SSX1* and *SSX2*, encoding proteins with homology to the Kruppel-associated box in human synovial sarcoma. *EMBO J* 1995;14:2333–2340.

162. De Leeuw B, Balemans M, Olde Weghuis D, et al. Identification of two alternative fusion genes, *SYT-SSX1* and *SYT-SSX2*, in t(X;18)(p11.2;q11.2)-positive synovial sarcomas. *Hum Mol Genet* 1995;4:1097–1099.

163. De Leeuw B, Balemans M, Geurts van Kessel A. novel Kruppel-associated box containing the *SSX* gene (*SSX3*) on the human X chromosome is not implicated in t(X;18)-positive synovial sarcomas. *Cytogenet Cell Genet* 1996;73:179–183.

164. Chand A, Clar J, Cooper CS, et al. Long-range organization of reiterated sequences, including the *SSX1* cDNA at the *OATL1* cluster in Xp11.23. *Genomics* 1995;30:545–552.

165. Kawai A, Woodruff J, Healey JH, et al. *SYT-SSX* gene fusion as a determinant of morphology and prognosis in synovial sarcoma. *N Engl J Med* 1998;338:153–160.

166. De Leeuw B, Suijkerbuijk RF, Olde Weghuis D, et al. Distinct Xp11.2 breakpoint regions in synovial sarcoma revealed by metaphase and interphase FISH: relationship to histologic subtypes. *Cancer Genet Cytogenet* 1994;73:89–94.

167. Antonescu CR, Kawai A, Leung DH, et al. Strong association of *SYT-SSX* fusion type and morphologic epithelial differentiation in synovial sarcoma. *Diagn Mol Pathol* 2000;9:1–8.

168. Skytting B, Nilsson G, Brodin B, et al. A novel fusion gene, *SYT-SSX4*, in synovial sarcoma. *J Natl Cancer Inst* 1999;91:974–975.

169. Brodin B, Haslam K, Yang K, et al. Cloning and characterization of spliced fusion transcript variants of synovial sarcoma: *SYT/SSX4*, *SYT/SSX4v*, and *SYT/SSX2v*: possible regulatory role of the fusion gene product in wild type SYT expression. *Gene* 2001;268:173–182.

170. Tornkvist M, Brodin B, Bartolazzi A, et al. A novel type of *SYT/SSX* fusion: methodological and biological implications. *Mod Pathol* 2002;15:679–685.

171. Nilsson G, Skytting B, Xie Y, et al. The *SYT-SSX1* variant of synovial sarcoma is associated with a high rate of tumor cell proliferation and poor clinical outcome. *Cancer Res* 1999;59:3180–3184.

172. Fligman I, Lonardo F, Jhanwar SC, et al. Molecular diagnosis of synovial sarcoma and characterization of a variant *SYT-SSX2* fusion transcript. *Am J Pathol* 1995;147:1592–1599.

173. Safar A, Wickert R, Nelson M, et al. Characterization of a variant *SYT-SSX1* synovial sarcoma fusion transcript. *Diagn Mol Pathol* 1998;7:283–287.

174. Sanders ME, van de Rijn M, Barr FG. Detection of a variant *SYT-SSX1* fusion in a case of predominantly epithelioid synovial sarcoma. *Mol Diagn* 1999;4:65–70.

175. O'Sullivan MJ, Humphrey PA, Dehner LP, et al. t(X;18) reverse transcriptase-polymerase chain reaction demonstrating a variant transcript. *J Mol Diagn* 2002;4:178–180.

176. Lim FL, Soulez M, Koczan D, et al. A KRAB-related domain and a novel transcription repression domain in proteins encoded by *SSX* genes that are disrupted in human sarcomas. *Oncogene* 1998;17:2013–2018.

177. Margolin JF, Friedman JR, Meyer WK, et al. Kruppel-associated boxes are potent transcriptional repression domains. *Proc Natl Acad Sci USA* 1994;91:4509–4513.

178. Witzgall R, O'Leary E, Leaf A, et al. The Kruppel-associated box-A (KRAB-A) domain of zinc finger proteins mediates transcriptional repression. *Proc Natl Acad Sci USA* 1994;91:4514–4518.

179. Ladanyi M. Fusions of the *SYT* and *SSX* genes in synovial sarcoma. *Oncogene* 2001;20:5755–5762.

180. Sandberg AA, Bridge JA. Updates on the cytogenetics and molecular genetics of bone and soft tissue tumors: osteosarcoma and related tumors. *Cancer Genet Cytogenet* 2003;145:1–30.

181. dos Santos NR, de Bruijn DR, van Kessel AG. Molecular mechanisms underlying human synovial sarcoma development. *Genes Chromosomes Cancer* 2001;30:1–14.

182. van Kessel AG, de Bruijn D, Hermsen L, et al. Masked t(X;18)(p11;q11) in a biphasic synovial sarcoma revealed by FISH and RT-PCR. *Genes Chromosomes Cancer* 1998; 23:198–201.

183. Bijwaard KE, Fetsch JF, Przygodzki, et al. Detection of *SYT-SSX* fusion transcripts in archival synovial sarcomas by real-time reverse transcriptase-polymerase chain reaction. *J Mol Diagn* 2002;4:59–64.

184. Argani P, Zakowski M, Klimstra D, et al. Detection of the *SYT-SSX* chimeric RNA of synovial sarcoma in paraffin-embedded tissue and its application in problematic cases. *Mod Pathol* 1998;11:65–71.

185. Tsuji S, Hisaoka M, Morimitsu Y, et al. Detection of *SYT-SSX* fusion transcripts in synovial sarcoma by reverse transcription-polymerase chain reaction using archival paraffin-embedded tissues. *Am J Pathol* 1998;153:1807–1812.

186. Clark J, Rocques PJ, Crew AJ, et al. Identification of novel genes, *SYT* and *SSX*, involved in the t(X;18)(p11.2;q11.2) translocation found in human synovial sarcoma. *Nat Genet* 1994;7:502–508.

187. Shipley J, Crew J, Birdsall S, et al. Interphase fluorescence in situ hybridization and reverse transcription polymerase chain reaction as a diagnostic aid for synovial sarcoma. *Am J Pathol* 1996;148:559–567.

188. Hill DA, Riedley SE, Patel AR, et al. Real-time polymerase chain reaction as an aid for the detection of *SYT-SSX1* and *SYT-SSX2* transcripts in fresh and archival pediatric synovial sarcoma specimens: report of 25 cases from St. Jude Children's Research Hospital. *Pediatr Dev Pathol* 2003;6:24–34.

189. Yang K, Lui WO, Xie Y, et al. Co-existence of *SYT-SSX1* and *SYT-SSX2* fusions in synovial sarcomas. *Oncogene* 2002;21:4181–4190.

190. Lee W, Han K, Harris CP, et al. Use of FISH to detect chromosomal translocations and deletions: analysis of chromosome rearrangement in synovial sarcoma cells from paraffin-embedded specimens. *Am J Pathol* 1993;143:15–19.

191. Poteat HT, Corson JM, Fletcher JA. Detection of chromosome 18 rearrangement in synovial sarcoma by fluorescence in situ hybridization. *Cancer Genet Cytogenet* 1995; 84:76–81.

192. Yang P, Hirose T, Hasegawa T, et al. Dual-colour fluorescence in situ hybridization analysis of synovial sarcoma. *J Pathol* 1998;184:7–13.

193. Zilmer M, Harris CP, Steiner DS, et al. Use of nonbreakpoint DNA probes to detect the t(X;18) in interphase cells from synovial sarcoma: implications for detection of diagnostic tumor translocations. *Am J Pathol* 1998;152:1171–1177.

194. Surace C, Panagopoulos I, Palsson E, et al. A novel FISH assay for *SS18-SSX* fusion type in synovial sarcoma. *Lab Invest* 2004;84:1185–1192.

195. Tureci O, Chen YT, Sahin U, et al. Expression of *SSX* genes in human tumors. *Int J Cancer* 1998;77:19–23.

196. Coindre JM, Pelmus M, Hostein I, et al. Should molecular testing be required for diagnosing synovial sarcoma? A prospective study of 204 cases. *Cancer* 2003;98:2700–2707.

197. Fuller C, Dalton J, Stewart E, et al. *Mod Pathol* 2005;18(suppl 1):14A.

198. Vang R, Biddle DA, Harrison WR, et al. Malignant peripheral nerve sheath tumor with a t(X;18). *Arch Pathol Lab Med* 2000;124:864–867.

199. Panagopoulos I, Mertens F, Isaksson M, et al. Clinical impact of molecular and cytogenetic findings in synovial sarcoma. *Genes Chromosomes Cancer* 2001;31:362–372.

200. Inagki H, Nagasaka T, Otsuka T, et al. Association of *SYT-SSX* fusion types with proliferative activity and prognosis in synovial sarcoma. *Mod Pathol* 2000;13:482–488.

201. Guillou L, Benhattar J, Bonichon F, et al. Histologic grade, but not *SYT-SSX* fusion type, is an important prognostic factor in patients with synovial sarcoma: a multicenter, retrospective analysis. *J Clin Oncol* 2004;22:4040–4050.

202. Ladanyi M, Antonescu CR, Leung DH, et al. Impact of *SYT-SSX* fusion type on the clinical behavior of synovial sarcoma: a multi-institutional retrospective study of 243 patients. *Cancer Res* 2002;62:135–140.

203. Skytting BT, Szymanska J, Aalto Y, et al. Clinical importance of genomic imbalances in synovial sarcoma evaluated by comparative genomic hybridization. *Cancer Genet Cytogenet* 1999;115:39–46.

204. Hashimoto N, Myoui A, Araki N, et al. Detection of *SYT-SSX* fusion gene in peripheral blood from a patient with synovial sarcoma. *Am J Surg Pathol* 2001;25:406–410.

205. Willeke F, Mechtersheimer G, Schwarzbach M, et al. Detection of *SYT-SSX1/2* fusion transcripts by reverse transcriptase-polymerase chain reaction (RT-PCR) is a valuable diagnostic tool in synovial sarcoma. *Eur J Cancer* 1998;34:2087–2093.

206. Nakasone J, Shimizu T, Gomyo H, et al. Assessment of microinvasion with reverse transcriptase polymerase chain reaction in a case of synovial sarcoma. *J Orthop Sci* 2004; 9:162–165.

207. Hiraga H, Nojima T, Abe S, et al. Diagnosis of synovial sarcoma with the reverse transcriptase-polymerase chain reaction: analyses of 84 soft tissue and bone tumors. *Diagn Mol Pathol* 1998;7:102–110.

208. Naito N, Kawai A, Ouchida M, et al. A reverse transcriptase-polymerase chain reaction assay in the diagnosis of soft tissue sarcomas. *Cancer* 2000;89:1992–1998.

209. Tamborini E, Agus V, Perrone F, et al. Lack of *SYT-SSX* fusion transcripts in malignant peripheral nerve sheath tumors on RT-PCR analysis of 34 archival cases. *Lab Invest* 2002;82:609–618.

210. van de Rijn M, Barr FG, Collins MH, et al. Absence of SYT-SSX fusion products in soft tissue tumors other than synovial sarcoma. *Am J Clin Pathol* 1999;112:43–49.

211. Coindre JM, Hostein I, Benhattar J, et al. Malignant peripheral nerve sheath tumors are t(X;18)-negative sarcomas: molecular analysis of 25 cases occurring in neurofibromatosis type 1 patients, using two different RT-PCR-based methods of detection. *Mod Pathol* 2002;15:589–592.

212. de Alava E. Transcripts, transcripts, everywhere. *Adv Anat Pathol* 2001;8:264–272.

213. Ladanyi M, Woodruff JM, Scheithauer BW, et al. Re: Malignant peripheral nerve sheath tumors with t(X;18): a pathologic and molecular genetic study [Letter]. *Mod Pathol* 2001;14:733–735.

214. O'Sullivan MJ, Wick MR, Kyriakos M, et al. Re: Malignant peripheral nerve sheath tumors with t(X;18): a pathologic and molecular genetic study [Letter]. *Mod Pathol* 2001;14:735–737.

215. O'Sullivan MJ, Pfeifer JD, Dehner LP. Re: Lack of *STY-SSX* fusion transcripts in malignant peripheral nerve sheath tumors on RT-PCR analysis of 34 archival cases, by Tamborini E, et al. [Letter]. *Lab Invest* 2003;83:301–302.

216. Pilotti S, Tamborini E, Pierotti M. Re: Lack of *STY-SSX* fusion transcripts in malignant peripheral nerve sheath tumors on RT-PCR analysis of 34 archival cases, by Tamborini E, et al. [Letter]. *Lab Invest* 2003;83:303.
217. Cessna MH, Zhou H, Sanger WG, et al. Expression of *ALK1* and p80 in inflammatory myofibroblastic tumor and its mesenchymal mimics: a study of 135 cases. *Mod Pathol* 2002;15:931–938.
218. Folpe AL, Schmidt RA, Chapman D, et al. Poorly differentiated synovial sarcoma: immunohistochemical distinction from primitive neuroectodermal tumors and high-grade malignant peripheral nerve sheath tumors. *Am J Surg Pathol* 1998;22:673–682.
219. Van de Rijn M, Barr FG, Xiong QB, et al. Poorly differentiated synovial sarcoma: an analysis of clinical, pathologic, and molecular genetic features. *Am J Surg Pathol* 1999; 23:106–112.
220. Guillou L, Wadden C, Kraus MD, et al. S-100 protein reactivity in synovial sarcomas: a potentially frequent diagnostic pitfall. *Appl Immunohistochem* 1996;4:167–175.
221. Sandberg, AA. "Show me"—Eliza Doolittle in *My Fair Lady*. *Cancer Genet Cytogenet* 2001;128:93–96.
222. Nagayama S, Katagiri T, Tsunoda T, et al. Genome-wide analysis of gene expression in synovial sarcomas using a cDNA microarray. *Cancer Res* 2002;62:5859–5866.
223. Coffin CM, Dehner LP. Fibroblastic-myofibroblastic tumors in children and adolescents: a clinicopathologic study of 108 examples in 103 patients. *Pediatr Pathol* 1991; 11:569–588.
224. Coffin CM, Jaszcz W, O'Shea PA, et al. So-called congenital-infantile fibrosarcoma: does it exist and what is it? *Pediatr Pathol* 1994;14:133–150.
225. Knezevich SR, McFadden DE, Tao W, et al. A novel *ETV6-NTRK3* gene fusion in congenital fibrosarcoma. *Nat Genet* 1998;18:184–187.
226. Schofield DE, Yunis EJ, Fletcher JA. Chromosome aberrations in mesoblastic nephroma. *Am J Pathol* 1993;143:714–724.
227. Lannon CL, Martin MJ, Tognon CE, et al. A highly conserved NTRK3 C-terminal sequence in the ETV6-NTRK3 oncoprotein binds the phosphotyrosine binding domain of insulin receptor substrate-1: an essential interaction for transformation. *J Biol Chem* 2004;279:6225–6234.
228. Ladanyi M. Aberrant ALK tyrosine kinase signaling: different cellular lineages, common oncogenic mechanisms. *Am J Pathol* 2000;157:341–345.
229. Dubus P, Coindre JM, Groppi A, et al. The detection of Tel-TrkC chimeric transcripts is more specific than TrkC immunoreactivity for the diagnosis of congenital fibrosarcoma. *J Pathol* 2001;193:88–94.
230. Wai DH, Snezevich SR, Lucas T, et al. The *ETV6-NTRK3* gene fusion encodes a chimeric protein tyrosine kinase that transforms NIH3T3 cells. *Oncogene* 2000;19:906–915.
231. Rubin BP, Chen CJ, Morgan TW, et al. Congenital mesoblastic nephroma t(12;15) is associated with *ETV6-NTRK3* gene fusion: cytogenetic and molecular relationship to congenital (infantile) fibrosarcoma. *Am J Pathol* 1998;153:1451–1458.
232. Bourgeois JM, Knezevich SR, Mathers JA, et al. Molecular detection of the *ETV6-NTRK3* gene fusion differentiates congenital fibrosarcoma from other childhood spindle cell tumors. *Am J Surg Pathol* 2000;24:937–946.
233. Adem C, Gisselsson D, Dal Cin PD, et al. *ETV6* rearrangements in patients with infantile fibrosarcomas and congenital mesoblastic nephromas by fluorescence in situ hybridization. *Mod Pathol* 2001;14:1246–1251.
234. Knezevich SR, Garnett MJ, Pysher TJ, et al. *ETV6-NTRK3* gene fusions and trisomy 11 establish a histogenetic link between mesoblastic nephroma and congenital fibrosarcoma. *Cancer Res* 1998;58:5046–5048.
235. Argani P, Fritsch M, Kadkol S, et al. Detection of the *ETV6-NTRK3* chimeric RNA of infantile fibrosarcoma/cellular congenital mesoblastic nephroma in paraffin-embedded tissue: application to challenging pediatric renal stromal tumors. *Mod Pathol* 2000;13:29–36.
236. Agrani P, Fritsch MK, Shuster AE, et al. Reduced sensitivity of paraffin-based RT-PCR assays for *ETV6-NTRK3* fusion transcripts in morphologically defined infantile fibrosarcoma [Letter]. *Am J Surg Pathol* 2001;25:1461–1463.
237. Sorensen PH, Mathers J. Reduced sensitivity of paraffin-based RT-PCR assays for *ETV6-NTRK3* fusion transcripts in morphologically defined infantile fibrosarcoma [Letter]. *Am J Surg Pathol* 2001;25:1464.
238. Sheng WQ, Hisaoka M, Okamoto S, et al. Congenital-infantile fibrosarcoma: a clinicopathologic study of 10 cases and molecular detection of the *ETV6-NTRK3* fusion transcripts using paraffin-embedded tissues. *Am J Clin Pathol* 2001;115:348–355.
239. Eguchi M, Eguchi-Ishimae M, Tojo A, et al. Fusion of *ETV6* to neurotrophin-3 receptor TRKC in acute myeloid leukemia with t(12;15)(p13;q25). *Blood* 1999;93:1355–1563.
240. Alessandri AJ, Knezevich SR, Mathers JA, et al. Absence of t(12;15) associated *ETV6-NTRK3* fusion transcripts in pediatric acute leukemias. *Med Pediatr Oncol* 2001; 37:415–416.
241. Tognon C, Knezevich SR, Huntsman D, et al. Expression of the *ETV6-NTRK3* gene fusion as a primary event in human secretory breast carcinoma. *Cancer Cell* 2002; 2:367–376.
242. Eguchi M, Eguchi-Ishimai M. Absence of t(12;15) associated *ETV6-NTRK3* fusion transcripts in pediatric acute leukemias [Letter]. *Med Pediatr Oncol* 2001;37:417.
243. Diallo R, Schaefer KL, Bankfalvi A, et al. Secretory carcinoma of the breast: a distinct variant of invasive ductal carcinoma assessed by comparative genomic hybridization and immunohistochemistry. *Hum Pathol* 2003;34:1299–1305.
244. Griffin CA, Hawkins AL, Dvorak C, et al. Recurrent involvement of 2p23 in inflammatory myofibroblastic tumors. *Cancer Res* 1999;59:2776–2780.
245. Ma Z, Hill DA, Collins MH, et al. Fusion of *ALK* to the Ran-binding protein 2 (*RANBP2*) gene in inflammatory myofibroblastic tumor. *Genes Chromosomes Cancer* 2003; 37:98–105.
246. Lawrence B, Perez-Atayde A, Hibbard MK, et al. *TPM3-ALK* and *TPM4-ALK* oncogenes in inflammatory myofibroblastic tumors. *Am J Pathol* 2000;157:377–384.
247. Bridge JA, Kanamori M, Ma Z. Fusion of the *ALK* gene to the clathrin heavy chain gene, *CLTC*, in inflammatory myofibroblastic tumor. *Am J Pathol* 2001;159:411–415.
248. Cools J, Wlodarska I, Somers R, et al. Identification of novel fusion partners of *ALK*, the anaplastic lymphoma kinase, in anaplastic large-cell lymphoma and inflammatory myofibroblastic tumor. *Genes Chromosomes Cancer* 2002;34:354–362.
249. Debelenko L, Arthur DC, Pack SD, et al. Identification of *CARS-ALK* fusion in primary and metastatic lesions of an inflammatory myofibroblastic tumor. *Lab Invest* 2003; 83:1255–1265.
250. Debiec-Rychter M, Marynen P, Hagemeijer A, et al. *ALK-ATIC* fusion in urinary bladder inflammatory myofibroblastic tumor. *Genes Chromosomes Cancer* 2003;38: 187–190.
251. Lamant L, Gascoyne RD, Duplantier MM, et al. Non-muscle myosin heavy chain (MYH9): a new partner fused to *ALK* in anaplastic large cell lymphoma. *Genes Chromosomes Cancer* 2003;37:427–432.
252. Reading NS, Jenson SD, Smith JK, et al. 5′-(RACE) identification of rare ALK fusion partner in anaplastic large cell lymphoma. *J Mol Diagn* 2003;5:136–140.
253. Coffin CM, Patel A, Perkins S, et al. *ALK1* and *p80* expression and chromosomal rearrangements involving 2p23 in inflammatory myofibroblastic tumor. *Mod Pathol* 2001;14:569–576.
254. Chan JK, Cheuk W, Shimizu M. Anaplastic lymphoma kinase expression in inflammatory pseudotumors. *Am J Surg Pathol* 2001;25:761–768.
255. Cook JR, Dehner LP, Collins MH, et al. Anaplastic lymphoma kinase (ALK) expression in the inflammatory myofibroblastic tumor: a comparative immunohistochemical study. *Am J Surg Pathol* 2001;25:1364–1371.
256. Kazmierczak B, Dal Cin P, Sciot R, et al. Inflammatory myofibroblastic tumor with *HMGIC* rearrangement. *Cancer Genet Cytogenet* 1999;112:156–160.
257. Kapusta LR, Weiss MA, Ramsay J, et al. Inflammatory myofibroblastic tumors of the kidney: a clinicopathologic and immunohistochemical study of 12 cases. *Am J Surg Pathol* 2003;27:658–666.
258. Suzuki R, Seto M, Nakamura S, et al. Sarcomatoid variant of anaplastic large cell lymphoma with cytoplasmic ALK and alpha-smooth muscle actin expression: a mimic of inflammatory myofibroblastic tumor. *Am J Pathol* 2001;159:383–384.
259. Stein H, Foss HD, Durkop H, et al. CD30(+) anaplastic large cell lymphoma: a review of its histopathologic, genetic, and clinical features. *Blood* 2000;96:3681–3695.
260. Chan JK, Buchanan R, Fletcher CD. Sarcomatoid variant of anaplastic large-cell Ki-1 lymphoma. *Am J Surg Pathol* 1990;14:983–988.
261. Waters BL, Panagopoulos I, Allen EF. Genetic characterization of angiomatoid fibrous histiocytoma identifies fusion of the *FUS* and *ATF-1* genes induced by a chromosomal translocation involving bands 12q13 and 16p11. *Cancer Genet Cytogenet* 2000; 121:109–116.
262. Raddaoui E, Donner LR, Panagopoulos I. Fusion of the *FUS* and *ATF1* genes in a large, deep-seated angiomatoid fibrous histiocytoma. *Diagn Mol Pathol* 2002;11:157–162.
263. Zucman J, Delattre O, Desmaze C, et al. *EWS* and *ATF-1* gene fusion induced by t(12;22) translocation in malignant melanoma of soft parts. *Nat Genet* 1993; 4:341–345.
264. Panagopoulos I, Mertens F, Debiec-Rychter M, et al. Molecular genetic characterization of the *EWS/ATF1* fusion gene in clear cell sarcoma of tendons and aponeuroses. *Int J Cancer* 2002;99:560–567.
265. Speleman F, Delattre O, Peter M, et al. Malignant melanoma of the soft parts (clear-cell sarcoma): confirmation of *EWS* and *ATF-1* gene fusion caused by a t(12;22) translocation. *Mod Pathol* 1997;10:496–499.
266. Antonescu CR, Tschernyavsky SJ, Woodruff JM, et al. Molecular diagnosis of clear cell sarcoma: detection of *EWS-ATF1* and *MITF-M* transcripts and histopathological and ultrastructural analysis of 12 cases. *J Mol Diagn* 2002;4:44–52.
267. Evans HL. Low-grade fibromyxoid sarcoma: a report of 12 cases. *Am J Surg Pathol* 1993;17:595–600.
268. Goodlad JR, Mentzel T, Fletcher CD. Low grade fibromyxoid sarcoma: clinicopathological analysis of eleven new cases in support of a distinct entity. *Histopathology* 1995; 26:229–237.
269. Reid R, de Silva MV, Paterson L, et al. Low-grade fibromyxoid sarcoma and hyalinizing spindle cell tumor with giant rosettes share a common t(7;16)(q34;p11) translocation. *Am J Surg Pathol* 2003;27:1229–1236.
270. Folpe AL, Lane KL, Paull G, et al. Low-grade fibromyxoid sarcoma and hyalinizing spindle cell tumor with giant rosettes: a clinicopathologic study of 73 cases supporting their identity and assessing the impact of high-grade areas. *Am J Surg Pathol* 2000; 24:1353–1360.
271. Lane KL, Shannon RJ, Weiss SW. Hyalinizing spindle cell tumor with giant rosettes: a distinctive tumor closely resembling low-grade fibromyxoid sarcoma. *Am J Surg Pathol* 1997;21:1481–1488.
272. Storlazzi CT, Mertens F, Nascimento A, et al. Fusion of the *FUS* and *BBF2H7* genes in low grade fibromyxoid sarcoma. *Hum Mol Genet* 2003;12:2349–2358.
273. Panagopoulos I, Storlazzi CT, Fletcher CD, et al. The chimeric *FUS/CREB3l2* gene is specific for low-grade fibromyxoid sarcoma. *Genes Chromosomes Cancer* 2004;40:218–228.
274. Mertens F, Fletcher CD, Antonescu CR, et al. Clinicopathologic and molecular genetic characterization of low-grade fibromyxoid sarcoma, and cloning of a novel *FUS/CREB3L1* fusion gene. *Lab Invest* 2005;85:408–415.
275. Bejarano PA, Padhya TA, Smith R, et al. Hyalinizing spindle cell tumor with giant rosettes: a soft tissue tumor with mesenchymal and neuroendocrine features—an immunohistochemical, ultrastructural, and cytogenetic analysis. *Arch Pathol Lab Med* 2000;124:1179–1184.
276. Reith JD, Goldblum JR, Lyles RH, et al. Extragastrointestinal (soft tissue) stromal tumors: an analysis of 48 cases with emphasis on histologic predictors of outcome. *Mod Pathol* 2000;13:577–585.
277. Miettinen M, Monihan JM, Sarlomo-Rikala M, et al. Gastrointestinal stromal tumors/smooth muscle tumors (GISTs) primary in the omentum and mesentery: clinicopathologic and immunohistochemical study of 26 cases. *Am J Surg Pathol* 1999; 23:1109–1118.
278. Yamamoto H, Oda Y, Kawaguchi K, et al. *c-kit* and *PDGFRA* mutations in extragastrointestinal stromal tumor (gastrointestinal stromal tumor of the soft tissue). *Am J Surg Pathol* 2004;28:479–488.
279. Medeiros F, Corless CL, Duensing A, et al. *KIT*-negative gastrointestinal stromal tumors: proof of concept and therapeutic implications. *Am J Surg Pathol* 2004;28:889–894.
280. Sakurai S, Hishima T, Takazawa Y, et al. Gastrointestinal stromal tumors and *KIT*-positive mesenchymal cells in the omentum. *Pathol Int* 2001;51:524–531.
281. Hirota S, Isozaki K, Moriyama Y, et al. Gain-of-function mutations of *c-kit* in human gastrointestinal stromal tumors. *Science* 1998;279:577–580.
282. Hirota S, Ohashi A, Nishida T, et al. Gain-of-function mutations of platelet-derived growth factor receptor alpha gene in gastrointestinal stromal tumors. *Gastroenterology* 2003;125:660–667.

283. Heinrich MC, Corless CL, Duensing A, et al. PDGFRA activating mutations in gastrointestinal stromal tumors. *Science* 2003;299:708–710.
284. Lux ML, Rubin BP, Biase TL, et al. *KIT* extracellular and kinase domain mutations in gastrointestinal stromal tumors. *Am J Pathol* 2000;156:791–795.
285. Hirota S, Nishida T, Isozaki K, et al. Gain-of-function mutation at the extracellular domain of KIT in gastrointestinal stromal tumours. *J Pathol* 2001;193:505–510.
286. Lasota J, Wozniak A, Sarloma-Rikala M, et al. Mutations in exons 9 and 13 of *KIT* gene are rare events in gastrointestinal stromal tumors. A study of 200 cases. *Am J Pathol* 2000;157:1091–1095.
287. Nagata H, Worobec AS, Oh CK, et al. Identification of a point mutation in the catalytic domain of the protooncogene *c-kit* in peripheral blood mononuclear cells of patients who have mastocytosis with an associated hematologic disorder. *Proc Natl Acad Sci USA* 1995;92:10560–10564.
288. Furitsu T, Tsujimura T, Tono T, et al. Identification of mutations in the coding sequence of the proto-oncogene *c-kit* in a human mast cell leukemia cell line causing ligand-independent activation of *c-kit* product. *J Clin Invest* 1993;92:1736–1744.
289. Moskaluk CA, Tian Q, Marshall CR, et al. Mutations of c-kit JM domain are found in a minority of human gastrointestinal stromal tumors. *Oncogene* 1999;18: 1897–1902.
290. Wasag B, Debiec-Rychter M, Pauwels P, et al. Differential expression of *KIT/PDGFRA* mutant isoforms in epithelioid and mixed variants of gastrointestinal stromal tumors depends predominantly on the tumor site. *Mod Pathol* 2004;17:889–894.
291. Lasota J, Carlson JA, Miettinen M. Spindle cell tumor of urinary bladder serosa with phenotypic and genotypic features of gastrointestinal stromal tumor. *Arch Pathol Lab Med* 2000;124:894–897.
292. Corless CL, McGreevey L, Haley A, et al. KIT mutations are common in incidental gastrointestinal stromal tumors one centimeter or less in size. *Am J Pathol* 2002;160: 1567–1572.
293. Buchdunger E, Cioffi CL, Law N, et al. Abl protein-tyrosine kinase inhibitor *STI571* inhibits in vitro signal transduction mediated by *c-kit* and platelet-derived growth factor receptors. *J Pharmacol Exp Ther* 2000;295:139–145.
294. Dematteo RP, Heinrich MC, El-Rifai WM, et al. Clinical management of gastrointestinal stromal tumors: before and after *STI-571*. *Hum Pathol* 2002;33:466–477.
295. Tuveson DA, Willis NA, Jacks T, et al. *STI571* inactivation of the gastrointestinal stromal tumor c-KIT oncoprotein: biological and clinical implications. *Oncogene* 2001;20:5054–5058.
296. Ma Y, Zeng S, Metcalfe DD, et al. The c-KIT mutation causing human mastocytosis is resistant to *STI571* and other KIT kinase inhibitors; kinases with enzymatic site mutations show different inhibitor sensitivity profiles than wild-type kinases and those with regulatory-type mutations. *Blood* 2002;99:1741–1744.
297. Sandberg AA. Updates on the cytogenetics and molecular genetics of bone and soft tissue tumors: lipoma. *Cancer Genet Cytogenet* 2004;150:93–115.
298. Sreekantaiah C, Leong SP, Karakousis CP, et al. Cytogenetic profile of 109 lipomas. *Cancer Res* 1991;51:422–433.
299. Willen H, Akerman M, Dal Cin P, et al. Comparison of chromosomal patterns with clinical features in 165 lipomas: a report of the CHAMP study group. *Cancer Genet Cytogenet* 1998;102:46–49.
300. Ashar HR, Fejzo M, Tkachenko A, et al. Disruption of the architectural factor *HMGI-C*: DNA-binding AT hook motifs fused in lipomas to distinct transcriptional regulatory domains. *Cell* 1995;82:57–65.
301. Schoenmakers EF, Wanschura S, Mols R, et al. Recurrent rearrangements in the high mobility group protein gene, *HMGI-C*, in benign mesenchymal tumours. *Nat Genet* 1995;10:436–444.
302. Kazmierczak B, Rosigkeit J, Wanschura S, et al. *HMGI-C* rearrangements as the molecular basis for the majority of pulmonary chondroid hamartomas: a survey of 30 tumors. *Oncogene* 1996;12:515–521.
303. Gisselsson D, Hoglund M, Mertens F, et al. Hibernomas are characterized by homozygous deletions in the multiple endocrine neoplasia type I region: metaphase fluorescence in situ hybridization reveals complex rearrangements not detected by conventional cytogenetics. *Am J Pathol* 1999;155:61–66.
304. Gisselsson D, Domanski HA, Hogland M. Unique cytological features and chromosome aberrations in chondroid lipoma: a case report based on fine-needle aspiration cytology, histopathology, electron microscopy, chromosome banding, and molecular cytogenetics. *Am J Surg Pathol* 1999;23:1300–1304.
305. Thomson TA, Horsman D, Bainbridge TC. Cytogenetic and cytologic features of chondroid lipoma of soft tissue. *Mod Pathol* 1999;12:88–91.
306. Hisaoka M, Sheng WQ, Tanaka A, et al. HMGIC alterations in smooth muscle tumors of soft tissues and other sites. *Cancer Genet Cytogenet* 2002;138:50–55.
307. Hibbard MK, Kozakewich HP, Dal Cin P, et al. *PLAG1* fusion oncogenes in lipoblastoma. *Cancer Res* 2000;60:4869–4872.
308. Astrom A, D'Amore E, Sainati L, et al. Evidence of involvement of the *PLAG1* gene in lipoblastomas. *Int J Oncol* 2000;16:1107–1110.
309. Gisselsson D, Hibbard MK, Dal Cin P, et al. PLAG1 alterations in lipoblastoma: involvement in varied mesenchymal cell types and evidence for alternative oncogenic mechanisms. *Am J Pathol* 2001;159:955–962.
310. Pedeutour F, Forus A, Coindre JM, et al. Structure of the supernumerary ring and giant rod chromosomes in adipose tissue tumors. *Genes Chromosomes Cancer* 1999; 24:30–41.
311. Mandahl N, Hoglund M, Mertens F, et al. Cytogenetic aberrations in 188 benign and borderline adipose tissue tumors. *Genes Chromosomes Cancer* 1994;9:207–215.
312. Pilotti S, Della Torre G, Mezzelani A, et al. The expression of *MDM2/CDK4* gene product in the differential diagnosis of well differentiated liposarcoma and large deep-seated lipoma. *Br J Cancer* 2000;82:1271–1275.
313. Meis-Kindblom JM, Sjogren H, Kindblom LG, et al. Cytogenetic and molecular genetic analyses of liposarcoma and its soft tissue simulators: recognition of new variants and differential diagnosis. *Virchows Arch* 2001;439:141–151.
314. Pilotti S, Della Torre G, Lavarino C, et al. Distinct *mdm2/p53* expression patterns in liposarcoma subgroups: implications for different pathogenetic mechanisms. *J Pathol* 1997;181:14–24.
315. Sirvent N, Forus A, Lescaut W, et al. Characterization of centromere alterations in liposarcomas. *Genes Chromosomes Cancer* 2000;29:117–129.
316. Szymanska J, Tarkkanen M, Wiklund T, et al. Gains and losses of DNA sequences in liposarcomas evaluated by comparative genomic hybridization. *Genes Chromosomes Cancer* 1996;15:89–94.
317. Crozat A, Aman P, Mandahl N, et al. Fusion of *CHOP* to a novel RNA-binding protein in human myxoid liposarcoma. *Nature* 1993;363:640–644.
318. Rabbitts TH, Forster A, Larson R, et al. Fusion of the dominant negative transcription regulator *CHOP* with a novel gene *FUS* by translocation t(12;16) in malignant liposarcoma. *Nat Genet* 1993;4:175–180.
319. Panagopoulos I, Hoglund M, Mertens F, et al. Fusion of the *EWS* and *CHOP* genes in myxoid liposarcoma. *Oncogene* 1996;12:489–494.
320. Mitelman F, Johansson B, Mertens F. Mitelman Database of Chromosome Aberrations in Cancer. http://cgap.nci.nih.gov/Chromsomes/Mitelman.
321. Rubin BP, Dal Cin P. The genetics of lipomatous tumors. *Semin Diagn Pathol* 2001; 18:286–293.
322. Hess J. Chromosomal translocations in benign tumors: the HMGI proteins. *Am J Clin Pathol* 1998;109:251–261.
323. Petit MM, Swarts S, Bridge JA, et al. Expression of reciprocal fusion transcripts of the *HMGIC* and *LPP* genes in parosteal lipoma. *Cancer Genet Cytogenet* 1998;106:18–23.
324. Petit MM, Mols R, Schoenmakers EF, et al. *LPP*, the preferred fusion partner gene of *HMGIC* in lipomas, is a novel member of the *LIM* protein gene family. *Genomics* 1996;36:118–129.
325. Broberg K, Zhang M, Strombeck B, et al. Fusion of *RDC1* with *HMGA2* in lipomas as the result of chromosome aberrations involving 2q35-37 and 12q13-15. *Int J Oncol* 2002;21:321–326.
326. Petit MM, Schoenmakers EF, Huysmans C, et al. LHFP, a novel translocation partner gene of *HMGIC* in a lipoma, is a member of a new family of *LHFP*-like genes. *Genomics* 1999;57:438–4341.
327. Kazmierczak B, Dal Cin P, Wanschura S, et al. Cloning and molecular characterization of part of a new gene fused to *HMGIC* in mesenchymal tumors. *Am J Pathol* 1998; 152:431–435.
328. Geurts JM, Schoenmakers EF, Roijer E, et al. Expression of reciprocal hybrid transcripts of *HMGIC* and *FHIT* in a pleomorphic adenoma of the parotid gland. *Cancer Res* 1997;57:13–17.
329. Merscher S, Marondel I, Pedeutour F, et al. Identification of new translocation breakpoints at 12q13 in lipomas. *Genomics* 1997;46:70–77.
330. Reeves R. Molecular biology of HMGA proteins: hubs of nuclear function. *Gene* 2001;277:63–81.
331. Tallini G, Vanni R, Manfioletti G, et al. HMGI-C and HMGI(Y) immunoreactivity correlates with cytogenetic abnormalities in lipomas, pulmonary chondroid hamartomas, endometrial polyps, and uterine leiomyomas and is compatible with rearrangement of the *HMGI-C* and *HMGI(Y)* genes. *Lab Invest* 2000;80:359–369.
332. Rogalla P, Drechsler K, Frey G, et al. HMGI-C expression patterns in human tissues: implications for the genesis of frequent mesenchymal tumors. *Am J Pathol* 1996;149:775–779.
333. Tallini G, Dal Cin P, Rhoden KJ, et al. Expression of *HMGI-C* and *HMGI(Y)* in ordinary lipoma and atypical lipomatous tumors: immunohistochemical reactivity correlates with karyotypic alterations. *Am J Pathol* 1997;151:37–43.
334. Dei Tos AP, Doglioni C, Piccinin S, et al. Coordinated expression and amplification of the *MDM2*, *CDK4*, and *HMGI-C* genes in atypical lipomatous tumours. *J Pathol* 2000;190:531–536.
335. Dahlen A, Mertens F, Rydholm A, et al. Fusion, disruption, and expression of *HMGA2* in bone and soft tissue chondromas. *Mod Pathol* 2003;16:1132–1140.
336. Rogalla P, Lemke I, Kazmierczak B, et al. An identical *HMGIC-LPP* fusion transcript is consistently expressed in pulmonary chondroid hamartomas with t(3;12)(q27-28; q14-15). *Genes Chromosomes Cancer* 2000;29:363–366.
337. Mine N, Kurose K, Konishi H, et al. Fusion of a sequence from HEI10 (14q11) to the *HMGIC* gene at 12q15 in a uterine leiomyoma. *Jpn J Cancer Res* 2001;92:135–139.
338. Mine N, Kurose K, Nagai H, et al. Gene fusion involving *HMGIC* is a frequent aberration in uterine leiomyomas. *J Hum Genet* 2001;46:408–412.
339. Sciot R, De Wever I, Debiec-Rychter M. Lipoblastoma in a 23-year-old male: distinction from atypical lipomatous tumor using cytogenetic and fluorescence in-situ hybridization analysis. *Virchows Arch* 2003;442:468–471.
340. Astrom A, Voz ML, Kas K, et al. Conserved mechanism of *PLAG1* activation in salivary gland tumors with and without chromosome 8q12 abnormalities: identification of *SII* as a new fusion partner gene. *Cancer Res* 1999;59:918–923.
341. Kas K, Voz M, Roijer E, et al. Promoter swapping between the genes for a novel zinc finger protein and beta-catenin in pleiomorphic adenomas with t(3;8)(p21;q12) translocations. *Nat Genet* 1997;15:170–174.
342. Voz ML, Astrom A, Kas K, et al. The recurrent translocation t(5;8)(p13;q12) in pleomorphic adenomas results in upregulation of *PLAG1* gene expression under control of the LIFR promoter. *Oncogene* 1998;16:1409–1416.
343. Dal Cin P, Kools P, Sciot R, et al. Cytogenetic and fluorescence in situ hybridization investigation of ring chromosomes characterizing a specific pathologic subgroup of adipose tissue tumors. *Cancer Genet Cytogenet* 1993;68:85–90.
344. Forus A, Bjerkehagen B, Sirvent N, et al. A well-differentiated liposarcoma with a new type of chromosome 12-derived markers. *Cancer Genet Cytogenet* 2001;131:13–18.
345. Nilsson M, Meza-Zepeda LA, Mertens F, et al. Amplification of chromosome 1 sequences in lipomatous tumors and other sarcomas. *Int J Cancer* 2004;109:363–369.
346. Storlazzi CT, Mertens F, Domanski H, et al. Ring chromosomes and low-grade gene amplification in an atypical lipomatous tumor with minimal nuclear atypia. *Int J Oncol* 2003;23:67–71.
347. Hostein I, Pelmus M, Aurias A, et al. Evaluation of *MDM2* and *CDK4* amplification by real-time PCR on paraffin wax-embedded material: a potential tool for the diagnosis of atypical lipomatous tumours/well-differentiated liposarcomas. *J Pathol* 2004; 202:95–102.
348. Miyajima K, Tamiya S, Oda Y, et al. Relative quantitation of *p53* and *MDM2* gene expression in leiomyosarcoma; real-time semi-quantitative reverse transcription-polymerase chain reaction. *Cancer Lett* 2001;164:177–188.
349. Coindre JM, Mariani O, Chibon F, et al. Most malignant fibrous histiocytomas developed in the retroperitoneum are dedifferentiated liposarcomas: a review of 25 cases initially diagnosed as malignant fibrous histiocytoma. *Mod Pathol* 2003;16:256–262.

350. Boltze C, Schneider-Stock R, Jager V, et al. Distinction between lipoma and liposarcoma by *MDM2* alterations: a case report of simultaneously occurring tumors and review of the literature. *Pathol Res Pract* 2001;197:563–568.
351. Reid AH, Tsai MM, Venzon DJ, et al. *MDM2* amplification, *P53* mutation, and accumulation of the p53 gene product in malignant fibrous histiocytoma. *Diagn Mol Pathol* 1996;5:65–73.
352. Cordon-Cardo C, Latres E, Drobnjak M. Molecular abnormalities of *mdm2* and *p53* genes in adult soft tissue sarcomas. *Cancer Res* 1994;54:794–799.
353. Oliner JD, Kinzler KW, Meltzer PS, et al. Amplification of a gene encoding a p53-associated protein in human sarcomas. *Nature* 1992;358:80–83.
354. Nilbert M, Rydholm A, Willen H, et al. *MDM2* gene amplification correlates with ring chromosome in soft tissue tumors. *Genes Chromosomes Cancer* 1994;9:261–265.
355. Nakayama T, Toguchida J, Wadayama B, et al. MDM2 gene amplification in bone and soft-tissue tumors: association with tumor progression in differentiated adipose-tissue tumors. *Int J Cancer* 1995;64:342–346.
356. Nilbert M, Rydholm A, Mitelman F, et al. Characterization of the 12q13-15 amplicon in soft tissue tumors. *Cancer Genet Cytogenet* 1995;83:32–36.
357. Kuhnen C, Mentzel T, Fisseler-Eckhoff A, et al. Atypical lipomatous tumor in a 14-year-old patient: distinction from lipoblastoma using FISH analysis. *Virchows Arch* 2002;441:299–302.
358. Adachi T, Oda Y, Sakamoto A, et al. Immunoreactivity of p53, mdm2, and p21WAF1 in dedifferentiated liposarcoma: special emphasis on the distinct immunophenotype of the well-differentiated component. *Int J Surg Pathol* 2001;9:99–109.
359. Schneider-Stock R, Walter H, Radig K, et al. *MDM2* amplification and loss of heterozygosity at *Rb* and *p53* genes: no simultaneous alterations in the oncogenesis of liposarcomas. *J Cancer Res Clin Oncol* 1998;124:532–540.
360. Dei Tos AP, Doglioni C, Piccinin S, et al. Molecular abnormalities of the *p53* pathway in dedifferentiated liposarcoma. *J Pathol* 1997;181:8–13.
361. Tallini G, Akerman M, Dal Cin P, et al. Combined morphologic and karyotypic study of 28 myxoid liposarcomas: implications for a revised morphologic typing, (a report from the CHAMP Group). *Am J Surg Pathol* 1996;20:1047–1055.
362. Panagopoulos I, Mandahl N, Mitelman F, et al. Two distinct *FUS* breakpoint clusters in myxoid liposarcoma and acute myeloid leukemia with the translocations t(12;16) and t(16;21). *Oncogene* 1995;11:1133–1137.
363. Kanoe H, Nakayama T, Hosaka T, et al. Characteristics of genomic breakpoints in *TLS-CHOP* translocations in liposarcomas suggest the involvement of Translin and topoisomerase II in the process of translocation. *Oncogene* 1999;18:721–729.
364. Panagopoulos I, Mandahl N, Ron D, et al. Characterization of the *CHOP* breakpoints and fusion transcripts in myxoid liposarcomas with the 12;16 translocation. *Cancer Res* 1994;54:6500–6503.
365. Kuroda M, Ishida T, Horiuchi H, et al. Chimeric *TLS/FUS-CHOP* gene expression and the heterogeneity of its junction in human myxoid and round cell liposarcoma. *Am J Pathol* 1995;147:1221–1227.
366. Hisaoka M, Tsuji S, Morimitsu Y, et al. Detection of *TLS/FUS-CHOP* fusion transcripts in myxoid and round cell liposarcomas by nested reverse transcription-polymerase chain reaction using archival paraffin-embedded tissues. *Diagn Mol Pathol* 1998;7:96–101.
367. Antonescu CR, Tschernyavsky SJ, Decuseara R, et al. Prognostic impact of p53 status, *TLS-CHOP* fusion transcript structure, and histological grade in myxoid liposarcoma: a molecular and clinicopathologic study of 82 cases. *Clin Cancer Res* 2001;7:3977–3987.
368. Ron D, Habener JF. CHOP, a novel developmentally regulated nuclear protein that dimerizes with transcription factors C/EBP and LAP and functions as a dominant-negative inhibitor of gene transcription. *Genes Dev* 1992;6:439–453.
369. Kuroda M, Ishida T, Takanashi M, et al. Oncogenic transformation and inhibition of adipocytic conversion of preadipocytes by TLS/FUS-CHOP type II chimeric protein. *Am J Pathol* 1997;151:735–744.
370. Adelmant G, Gilbert JD, Freytag SO. Human translocation liposarcoma-CCAAT/enhancer binding protein (C/EBP) homologous protein (TLS-CHOP) oncoprotein prevents adipocyte differentiation by directly interfering with C/EBP β function. *J Biol Chem* 1998;273:15574–15581.
371. Ron D. TLS-CHOP and the role of RNA-binding proteins in oncogenic transformation. *Curr Top Microbiol Immunol* 1997;220:131–142.
372. Perez-Losada J, Pintado B, Gutierrez-Adan A, et al. The chimeric FUS/TLS-CHOP fusion protein specifically induces liposarcomas in transgenic mice. *Oncogene* 2000;19:2413–2422.
373. Dal Cin P, Sciot R, Panagopoulos I, et al. Additional evidence of a variant translocation t(12;22) with *EWS/CHOP* fusion in myxoid liposarcoma: clinicopathological features. *J Pathol* 1997;182:437–441.
374. Hosaka T, Nakashima Y, Kusuzaki K, et al. A novel type of *EWS-CHOP* fusion gene in two cases of myxoid liposarcoma. *J Mol Diagn* 2002;4:164–171.
375. Aoki T, Hisaoka M, Kouho H, et al. Interphase cytogenetic analysis of myxoid soft tissue tumors by fluorescence in situ hybridization and DNA flow cytometry using paraffin-embedded tissue. *Cancer* 1997;79:284–293.
376. Mezzelani A, Sozzi G, Pierotti MA, et al. Rapid differential diagnosis of myxoid liposarcoma by fluorescence in situ hybridization on cytological preparations. *J Clin Pathol* 1996;49:M308.
377. Birch NC, Antonescu CR, Nelson M, et al. Inconspicuous insertion 22;12 in myxoid/round cell liposarcoma accompanied by the secondary structural abnormality der(16)t(1;16). *J Mol Diagn* 2003;5:191–194.
378. Knight JC, Renwick PJ, Dal Cin P, et al. Two categories of synovial sarcoma defined by divergent chromosome translocation breakpoints in Xp11.2, with implications for the histologic sub-classification of synovial sarcoma. *Cytogenet Cell Genet* 1995;70:58–63.
379. Nakanishi H, Araki N, Joyama S, et al. Myxoid liposarcoma with adipocytic maturation: detection of *TLS/CHOP* fusion gene transcript. *Diagn Mol Pathol* 2004;13:92–96.
380. Rosai J, Akerman M, Dal Cin P, et al. Combined morphologic and karyotypic study of 59 atypical lipomatous tumors: evaluation of their relationship and differential diagnosis with other adipose tissue tumors (a report of the CHAMP Study Group). *Am J Surg Pathol* 1996;20:1182–1189.
381. Fletcher CD, Akerman M, Dal Cin P, et al. Correlation between clinicopathological features and karyotype in lipomatous tumors: a report of 178 cases from the Chromosomes and Morphology (CHAMP) Collaborative Study Group. *Am J Pathol* 1996;148:623–630.
382. Antonescu CR, Elahi A, Humphrey M, et al. Specificity of TLS-CHOP rearrangement for classic myxoid/round cell liposarcoma: absence in predominantly myxoid well-differentiated liposarcomas. *J Mol Diagn* 2000;2:132–138.
383. Willeke F, Ridder R, Mechtersheimer G, et al. Analysis of FUS-CHOP fusion transcripts in different types of soft tissue liposarcoma and their diagnostic implications. *Clin Cancer Res* 1998;4:1779–1784.
384. Antonescu CR, Elahi A, Healey JH, et al. Monoclonality of multifocal myxoid liposarcoma: confirmation by analysis of TLS-CHOP or EWS-CHOP rearrangements. *Clin Cancer Res* 2000;6:2788–2793.
385. Panagopoulos I, Aman P, Mertens F, et al. Genomic PCR detects tumor cells in peripheral blood from patients with myxoid liposarcoma. *Genes Chromosomes Cancer* 1996;17:102–107.
386. Scott GA, Trepeta R. Clear cell sarcoma of tendons and aponeuroses and malignant blue nevus arising in prepubescent children: report of two cases and review of the literature. *Am J Dermatopathol* 1993;15:139–145.
387. Kindblom LG, Lodding P, Angervall L. Clear-cell sarcoma of tendons and aponeuroses: an immunohistochemical and electron microscopic analysis indicating neural crest origin. *Virchows Arch A Pathol Anat Histopathol* 1983;401:109–128.
388. Saw D, Tse CH, Chan J, et al. Clear cell sarcoma of the penis. *Hum Pathol* 1986;17:423–425.
389. Rubin BP, Fletcher JA, Renshaw AA. Clear cell sarcoma of soft parts: report of a case primary in the kidney with cytogenetic confirmation. *Am J Surg Pathol* 1999;23:589–594.
390. Gelczer RK, Wenger DE, Wold LE. Primary clear cell sarcoma of bone: a unique site of origin. *Skeletal Radiol* 1999;28:240–243.
391. Yokoyama R, Mukai K, Hirota T, et al. Primary malignant melanoma (clear cell sarcoma) of bone: report of a case arising in the ulna. *Cancer* 1996;77:2471–2475.
392. Pauwels P, Debiec-Rychter M, Sciot R, et al. Clear cell sarcoma of the stomach. *Histopathology* 2002;41:526–530.
393. Ekfors TO, Kujari H, Isomaki M. Clear cell sarcoma of tendons and aponeuroses (malignant melanoma of soft parts) in the duodenum: the first visceral case. *Histopathology* 1993;22:255–259.
394. Donner LR, Tromler RA, Dobin S. Clear cell sarcoma of the ileum: the crucial role of cytogenetics for the diagnosis. *Am J Surg Pathol* 1998;22:121–124.
395. Fukuda T, Kakihara T, Baba K, et al. Clear cell sarcoma arising in the transverse colon. *Pathol Int* 2000;50:412–416.
396. Bridge JA, Borek DA, Neff JR, et al. Chromosomal abnormalities in clear cell sarcoma: implications for histogenesis. *Am J Clin Pathol* 1990;93:26–31.
397. Reeves BR, Fletcher CD, Gusterson BA. Translocation t(12;22)(q13;q13) is a nonrandom rearrangement in clear cell sarcoma. *Cancer Genet Cytogenet* 1992;64:101–103.
398. Rodriguez E, Sreekantaiah C, Reuter VE, et al. (12;22)(q13;q13) and trisomy 8 are nonrandom aberrations in clear-cell sarcoma. *Cancer Genet Cytogenet* 1992;64:107–110.
399. Stenman G, Kindblom LG, Angervall L. Reciprocal translocation t(12;22)(q13;q13) in clear-cell sarcoma of tendons and aponeuroses. *Genes Chromosomes Cancer* 1992;4:122–127.
400. Sandberg AA, Bridge JA. Updates on the cytogenetics and molecular genetics of bone and soft tissue tumors: clear cell sarcoma (malignant melanoma of soft parts). *Cancer Genet Cytogenet* 2001;130:1–7.
401. Brown AD, Lopez-Terrada D, Denny CT, et al. Promoters containing ATF-binding sites are de-regulated in cells that express the EWS/ATF1 oncogene. *Oncogene* 1995;10:1749–1756.
402. Fujimura Y, Ohno T, Siddique H, et al. The EWS-ATF-1 gene involved in malignant melanoma of soft parts with t(12;22) chromosome translocation, encodes a constitutive transcriptional activator. *Oncogene* 1996;12:159–167.
403. Li KK, Lee KA. MMSP tumor cells expressing the EWS/ATF1 oncogene do not support cAMP-inducible transcription. *Oncogene* 1998;16:1325–1331.
404. Travis JA, Bridge JA. Significance of both numerical and structural chromosomal abnormalities in clear cell sarcoma. *Cancer Genet Cytogenet* 1992;64:104–106.
405. Speleman F, Colpaert C, Goovaerts G, et al. Malignant melanoma of soft parts: further cytogenetic characterization. *Cancer Genet Cytogenet* 1992;60:176–179.
406. Limon J, Debiec-Rychter M, Nedoszytko B, et al. Aberrations of chromosome 22 and polysomy of chromosome 8 as non-random changes in clear cell sarcoma. *Cancer Genet Cytogenet* 1994;72:141–145.
407. Pellin A, Monteagudo C, Lopez-Gines C, et al. New type of chimeric fusion product between the *EWS* and *ATF1* genes in clear cell sarcoma (malignant melanoma of soft parts). *Genes Chromosomes Cancer* 1998;23:358–360.
408. Covinsky M, Gong S, Rajaram V, et al. EWS-ATF1 fusion transcripts in gastrointestinal tumors previously diagnosed as malignant melanoma. *Hum Pathol* 2005;36:74–81.
409. Zambrano E, Reyes-Mugica M, Franchi A, et al. An osteoclast-rich tumor of the gastrointestinal tract with features resembling clear cell sarcoma of soft parts: reports of 6 cases of a GIST simulator. *Int J Surg Pathol* 2003;11:75–81.
410. Ladanyi M, Lui MY, Antonescu CR, et al. The der(17)t(X;17)(p11;q25) of human alveolar soft part sarcoma fuses the *TFE3* transcription factor gene to *ASPL*, a novel gene at 17q25. *Oncogene* 2001;20:48–57.
411. Sandberg AA, Bridge JA. Updates on the cytogenetics and molecular genetics of bone and soft tissue tumors: alveolar soft part sarcoma. *Cancer Genet Cytogenet* 2002;136:1–9.
412. Heimann P, El Housni H, Ogur G, et al. Fusion of a novel gene, *RCC17*, to the *TFE3* gene in t(X;17)(p11.2;q25.3)-bearing papillary renal cell carcinomas. *Cancer Res* 2001;61:4130–4135.
413. Weterman MA, van Groningen JJ, Jansen A, et al. Nuclear localization and transactivating capacities of the papillary renal cell carcinoma-associated TFE3 and PRCC (fusion) proteins. *Oncogene* 2000;19:69–74.
414. Sciot R, Dal Cin P, de Vos R, et al. Alveolar soft-part sarcoma: evidence for its myogenic origin and for the involvement of 17q25. *Histopathology* 1993;23:439–444.
415. Argani P, Lal P, Hutchinson B, et al. Aberrant nuclear immunoreactivity for TFE3 in neoplasms with *TFE3* gene fusions: a sensitive and specific immunohistochemical assay. *Am J Surg Pathol* 2003;27:750–761.
416. Argani P, Antonescu CR, Illei PB, et al. Primary renal neoplasms with the *ASPL-TFE3* gene fusion of alveolar soft part sarcoma: a distinctive tumor entity previously included among renal cell carcinomas of children and adolescents. *Am J Pathol* 2001;159:179–192.

417. Sidhar SK, Clark J, Gill S, et al. The t(X;1)(p11.2;q21.2) translocation in papillary renal cell carcinoma fuses a novel gene *PRCC* to the *TFE3* transcription factor gene. *Hum Mol Genet* 1996;5:1333–1338.
418. Weterman MA, Wilbrink M, Geurts van Kessel A. Fusion of the transcription factor *TFE3* gene to a novel gene, *PRCC*, in t(X;1)(p11;q21)-positive papillary renal cell carcinomas. *Proc Natl Acad Sci USA* 1996;93:15294–15298.
419. Clark J, Lu YJ, Sidhar SK, et al. Fusion of splicing factor genes *PSF* and *NonO* (*p54nrb*) to the *TFE3* gene in papillary renal cell carcinoma. *Oncogene* 1997;15:2233–2239.
420. Labelle Y, Zucman J, Stenman G, et al. Oncogenic conversion of a novel orphan nuclear receptor by chromosome translocation. *Hum Mol Genet* 1995;4:2219–2226.
421. Clark J, Benjamin H, Gill S, et al. Fusion of the *EWS* gene to *CHN*, a member of the steroid/thyroid receptor gene superfamily, in a human myxoid chondrosarcoma. *Oncogene* 1996;12:229–235.
422. Sjogren H, Meis-Kindblom JM, Orndal C, et al. Studies on the molecular pathogenesis of extraskeletal myxoid chondrosarcoma-cytogenetic, molecular genetic, and cDNA microarray analyses. *Am J Pathol* 2003;162:781–792.
423. Antonescu CR, Argani P, Erlandson RA, et al. Skeletal and extraskeletal myxoid chondrosarcoma: a comparative clinicopathologic, ultrastructural, and molecular study. *Cancer* 1998;83:1504–1521.
424. Panagopoulos I, Mertens F, Isaksson M, et al. Molecular genetic characterization of the *EWS/CHN* and *RBP56/CHN* fusion genes in extraskeletal myxoid chondrosarcoma. *Genes Chromosomes Cancer* 2002;35:340–352.
425. Sjogren H, Meis-Kindblom J, Kindblom LG, et al. Fusion of the *EWS*-related gene *TAF2N* to TEC in extraskeletal myxoid chondrosarcoma. *Cancer Res* 1999;59:5064–5067.
426. Panagopoulos I, Mencinger M, Dietrich CU, et al. Fusion of the *RBP56* and *CHN* genes in extraskeletal myxoid chondrosarcomas with translocation t(9;17)(q22;q11). *Oncogene* 1999;18:7594–7598.
427. Attwooll C, Tariq M, Harris M, et al. Identification of a novel fusion gene involving *hTAFII68* and *CHN* from a t(9;17)(q22;q11.2) translocation in an extraskeletal myxoid chondrosarcoma. *Oncogene* 1999;18:7599–7601.
428. Bjerkehagen B, Dietrich C, Reed W, et al. Extraskeletal myxoid chondrosarcoma: multimodal diagnosis and identification of a new cytogenetic subgroup characterized by t(9;17)(q22;q11). *Virchows Arch* 1999;435:524–530.
429. Sjogren H, Wedell B, Meis-Kindblom J, et al. Fusion of the NH2-terminal domain of the basic helix-loop-helix protein TCF12 to TEC in extraskeletal myxoid chondrosarcoma with translocation t(9;15)(q22;q21). *Cancer Res* 2000;60:6832–6835.
430. Labelle Y, Bussieres J, Courjal F, et al. The EWS/TEC fusion protein encoded by the t(9;22) chromosomal translocation in human chondrosarcomas is a highly potent transcriptional activator. *Oncogene* 1999;18:3303–3308.
431. Ohkura N, Yaguchi H, Tsukada T, et al. The *EWS/NOR1* fusion gene product gains a novel activity affecting pre-mRNA splicing. *J Biol Chem* 2002;277:535–543.
432. Okamoto S, Hisaoka M, Ishida T, et al. Extraskeletal myxoid chondrosarcoma: a clinicopathologic, immunohistochemical, and molecular analysis of 18 cases. *Hum Pathol* 2001;32:1116–1124.
433. Brody RI, Ueda T, Hamelin A, et al. Molecular analysis of the fusion of *EWS* to an orphan nuclear receptor gene in extraskeletal myxoid chondrosarcoma. *Am J Pathol* 1997;150:1049–1058.
434. Healey JH. Extraskeletal myxoid chondrosarcoma of the knee [Letter]. *Skeletal Radiol* 2000;29:302–303.
435. Gebhardt MC, Parekh SG, Rosenberg AE, et al. Reply to Letter: Extraskeletal myxoid chondrosarcoma of the knee. *Skeletal Radiol* 2000;29:303.
436. Parham DM, Weeks DA, Beckwith JB. The clinicopathologic spectrum of putative extrarenal rhabdoid tumors: an analysis of 42 cases studied with immunohistochemistry or electron microscopy. *Am J Surg Pathol* 1994;18:1010–1029.
437. Wick MR, Ritter JH, Dehner LP. Malignant rhabdoid tumors: a clinicopathologic review and conceptual discussion. *Semin Diagn Pathol* 1995;12:233–248.
438. Versteege I, Sevenet N, Lange J, et al. Truncating mutations of *hSNF5/INI1* in aggressive paediatric cancer. *Nature* 1998;394:203–206.
439. Biegel JA, Tan L, Zhang F, et al. Alterations of the *hSNF5/INI1* gene in central nervous system atypical teratoid/rhabdoid tumors and renal and extrarenal rhabdoid tumors. *Clin Cancer Res* 2002;8:3461–3467.
440. Kalpana GV, Marmon S, Wang W, et al. Binding and stimulation of HIV-1 integrase by a human homolog of yeast transcription factor *SNF5*. *Science* 1994;266:2002–2006.
441. Muchardt C, Sardet C, Bourachot B, et al. A human protein with homology to *Saccharomyces cerevisiae SNF5* interacts with the potential helicase hbrm. *Nucleic Acids Res* 1995;23:1127–1132.
442. Roberts CW, Orkin SH. The *SWI/SNF* complex: chromatin and cancer. *Nat Rev Cancer* 2004;4:133–142.
443. Lee HY, Yoon CS, Sevenet N, et al. Rhabdoid tumor of the kidney is a component of the rhabdoid predisposition syndrome. *Pediatr Dev Pathol* 2002;5:395–399.
444. Sevenet N, Sheridan E, Amram D, et al. Constitutional mutations of the *hSNF5/INI1* gene predispose to a variety of cancers. *Am J Hum Genet* 1999;65:1342–1348.
445. Kusafuka T, Miao J, Yoneda A, et al. Novel germ-line deletion of *SNF5/INI1/SMARCB1* gene in neonate presenting with congenital malignant rhabdoid tumor of kidney and brain primitive neuroectodermal tumor. *Genes Chromosomes Cancer* 2004;40:133–139.
446. Shashi V, Lovell MA, von Kap-herr C, et al. Malignant rhabdoid tumor of the kidney: involvement of chromosome 22. *Genes Chromosomes Cancer* 1994;10:49–54.
447. Biegel JA, Allen CS, Kawasaki K, et al. Narrowing the critical region for a rhabdoid tumor locus in 22q11. *Genes Chromosomes Cancer* 1996;16:94–105.
448. Rosty C, Peter M, Zucman J, et al. Cytogenetic and molecular analysis of a t(1;22)(p36;q11.2) in a rhabdoid tumor with a putative homozygous deletion of chromosome 22. *Genes Chromosomes Cancer* 1998;21:82–89.
449. Rousseau-Merck MF, Versteege I, Legrand I, et al. *hSNF5/INI1* inactivation is mainly associated with homozygous deletions and mitotic recombinations in rhabdoid tumors. *Cancer Res* 1999;59:3152–3156.
450. Hoot AC, Russo P, Judkins AR, et al. Immunohistochemical analysis of *hSNF5/INI1* distinguishes renal and extra-renal malignant rhabdoid tumors from other pediatric soft tissue tumors. *Am J Surg Pathol* 2004;28:1485–1485.
451. Mendlick MR, Nelson M, Pickering D, et al. Translocation t(1;3)(p36.3;q25) is a nonrandom aberration in epithelioid hemangioendothelioma. *Am J Surg Pathol* 2001;25:684–687.
452. Perez-Atayde AR, Kozakewich HW, McGill T, et al. Hemangiopericytoma of the tongue in a 12-year-old child: ultrastructural and cytogenetic observations. *Hum Pathol* 1994;25:425–429.
453. Hallen M, Parada LA, Gorunova L, et al. Cytogenetic abnormalities in a hemangiopericytoma of the spleen. *Cancer Genet Cytogenet* 2002;136:62–65.
454. Sreekantaiah C, Bridge JA, Rao UN, et al. Clonal chromosomal abnormalities in hemangiopericytoma. *Cancer Genet Cytogenet* 1991;54:173–181.
455. Naka N, Tomita Y, Nakanishi H, et al. Mutations of *p53* tumor-suppressor gene in angiosarcoma. *Int J Cancer* 1997;71:952–955.
456. Zietz C, Rössle M, Haas C, et al. MDM-2 oncoprotein overexpression, *p53* gene mutation, and VEGF up-regulation in angiosarcomas. *Am J Pathol* 1998;153:1425–1433.
457. Hollstein M, Marion MJ, Lehman T, et al. *p53* mutations at A:T base pairs in angiosarcomas of vinyl chloride-exposed factory workers. *Carcinogenesis* 1994;15:1–3.
458. Marion MJ, Froment O, Trépo C. Activation of Ki-*ras* gene by point mutation in human liver angiosarcoma associated with vinyl chloride exposure. *Mol Carcinog* 1991;4:450–454.
459. Przygodzki RM, Finkelstein SD, Keohavong P, et al. Sporadic and Thorotrast-induced angiosarcomas of the liver manifest frequent and multiple point mutations in K-*ras*-2. *Lab Invest* 1997;76:153–159.
460. Soini Y, Welsh JA, Ishak KG, et al. *p53* mutations in primary hepatic angiosarcomas not associated with vinyl chloride exposure. *Carcinogenesis* 1995;16:2879–2881.
461. Momand J, Zambetti GP. *Mdm-2*: "big brother" of *p53*. *J Cell Biochem* 1997;64:343–352.
462. Gospodarowicz D, Abraham JA, Schilling J. Isolation and characterization of a vascular endothelial cell mitogen produced by pituitary-derived folliculo stellate cells. *Proc Natl Acad Sci USA* 1989;86:7311–7315.
463. Weiss SW, Dorfman HD. Adamantinoma of long bone: an analysis of nine new cases with emphasis on metastasizing lesions and fibrous dysplasia-like changes. *Hum Pathol* 1977;8:141–153.
464. Fukunaga M, Ushigome S. Periosteal Ewing-like adamantinoma. *Virchows Arch* 1998;433:385–389.
465. Ishida T, Kikuchi F, Oka T, et al. Case report 727: juxtacortical adamantinoma of humerus (simulating Ewing tumor). *Skeletal Radiol* 1992;21:205–209.
466. Lipper S, Kahn LB. Case report 235: Ewing-like adamantinoma of the left radial head and neck. *Skeletal Radiol* 1983;10:61–66.
467. Meister P, Konrad E, Hubner G. Malignant tumor of humerus with features of "adamantinoma" and Ewing's sarcoma. *Pathol Res Pract* 1979;166:112–122.
468. van Haelst UJ, de Haas van Dorsser AH. A perplexing malignant bone tumor: highly malignant so-called adamantinoma or non-typical Ewing's sarcoma. *Virchows Arch A Pathol Anat Histol* 1975;365:63–74.
469. Czerniak B, Rojas-Corona RR, Dorfman HD. Morphologic diversity of long bone adamantinoma: the concept of differentiated (regressing) adamantinoma and its relationship to osteofibrous dysplasia. *Cancer* 1989;64:2319–2334.
470. Kanamori M, Antonescu CR, Scott M, et al. Extra copies of chromosomes 7, 8, 12, 19, and 21 are recurrent in adamantinoma. *J Mol Diagn* 2001;3:16–21.
471. Hazelbag HM, Wessels JW, Mollevangers P, et al. Cytogenetic analysis of adamantinoma of long bones: further indications for a common histogenesis with osteofibrous dysplasia. *Cancer Genet Cytogenet* 1997;97:5–11.
472. Hazelbag HM, Fleuren GJ, Cornelisse CJ, et al. DNA aberrations in the epithelial cell component of adamantinoma of long bones. *Am J Pathol* 1995;147:1770–1779.
473. Bridge JA, Fidler ME, Neff JR, et al. Adamantinoma-like Ewing's sarcoma: genomic confirmation, phenotypic drift. *Am J Surg Pathol* 1999;23:159–165.
474. Gaffney EF. 'Like—but oh, how different!'. *Am J Surg Pathol* 2000;24:322–323.
475. Hauben E, van den Broek LC, van Marck EV, et al. Adamantinoma-like Ewing's sarcoma and Ewing's-like adamantinoma: the t(11;22), t(21;22) status. *J Pathol* 2001;195:218–221.
476. Bridge JA, Fidler ME, Seemayer TA, et al. 'Like–but oh, how different!' [Letter]. *Am J Surg Pathol* 2000;24:323.
477. Granter SR, Renshaw AA, Kozakewich HP, et al. The pericentromeric inversion, inv (6)(p25q13), is a novel diagnostic marker in chondromyxoid fibroma. *Mod Pathol* 1998;11:1071–1074.
478. Safar A, Nelson M, Neff JR, et al. Recurrent anomalies of 6q25 in chondromyxoid fibroma. *Hum Pathol* 2000;31:306–311.
479. Tallini G, Dorfman H, Brys P, et al. Correlation between clinicopathological features and karyotype in 100 cartilaginous and chordoid tumours: a report from the Chromosomes and Morphology (CHAMP) Collaborative Study Group. *J Pathol* 2002;196:194–203.
480. Baruffi MR, Volpon JB, Neto JB, et al. Osteoid osteomas with chromosome alterations involving 22q. *Cancer Genet Cytogenet* 2001;124:127–131.
481. Sinovic JF, Bridge JA, Neff JR. Ring chromosome in parosteal osteosarcoma: clinical and diagnostic significance. *Cancer Genet Cytogenet* 1992;62:50–52.
482. Szymanska J, Mandahl N, Mertens F, et al. Ring chromosomes in parosteal osteosarcoma contain sequences from 12q13-15: a combined cytogenetic and comparative genomic hybridization study. *Genes Chromosomes Cancer* 1996;16:31–34.
483. Martignetti JA, Gelb BD, Pierce H, et al. Malignant fibrous histiocytoma: inherited and sporadic forms have loss of heterozygosity at chromosome bands 9p21-22: evidence for a common genetic defect. *Genes Chromosomes Cancer* 2000;27:191–195.
484. Bridge JA, DeBoer J, Walker CW, et al. Translocation t(3;12)(q28;q14) in parosteal lipoma. *Genes Chromosomes Cancer* 1995;12:70–72.
485. Petit MM, Swarts S, Bridge JA, et al. Expression of reciprocal fusion transcripts of the HMGIC and LPP genes in parosteal lipoma. *Cancer Genet Cytogenet* 1998;106:18–23.
486. Zambrano E, Nose V, Perez-Atayde AR, et al. Distinct chromosomal rearrangements in subungual (Dupuytren) exostosis and bizarre parosteal osteochondromatous proliferation (Nora lesion). *Am J Surg Pathol* 2004;28:1033–1039.
487. Martinez V, Sissons HA. Aneurysmal bone cyst: a review of 123 cases including primary lesions and those secondary to other bone pathology. *Cancer* 1988;61:2291–2304.
488. Vergel De Dios AM, Bond JR, Shives TC, et al. Aneurysmal bone cyst: a clinicopathologic study of 238 cases. *Cancer* 1992;69:2921–231.
489. Nielsen GP, Fletcher CD, Smith MA, et al. Soft tissue aneurysmal bone cyst: a clinicopathologic study of five cases. *Am J Surg Pathol* 2002;26:64–69.
490. Dal Cin P, Kozakewich HP, Goumnerova L, et al. Variant translocations involving 16q22 and 17p13 in solid variant and extraosseous forms of aneurysmal bone cyst. *Genes Chromosomes Cancer* 2000;28:233–234.

491. Althof PA, Ohmori K, Zhou M, et al. Cytogenetic and molecular cytogenetic findings in 43 aneurysmal bone cysts: aberrations of 17p mapped to 17p13.2 by fluorescence in situ hybridization. *Mod Pathol* 2004;17:518–525.

492. Oliveira AM, Hsi BL, Weremowicz S, et al. *USP6 (Tre2)* fusion oncogenes in aneurysmal bone cyst. *Cancer Res* 2004;64:1920–1923.

493. Oliveira AM, Perez-Atayde AR, Inwards CY, et al. *USP6* and *CDH11* oncogenes identify the neoplastic cell in primary aneurysmal bone cysts and are absent in so-called secondary aneurysmal bone cysts. *Am J Pathol* 2004;165:1773–1780.

494. Nollet F, Kools P, van Roy F. Phylogenetic analysis of the cadherin superfamily allows identification of six major subfamilies besides several solitary members. *J Mol Biol* 2000;299:551–72.

495. Okazaki M, Takeshita S, Kawai S, et al. Molecular cloning and characterization of OB-cadherin, a new member of cadherin family expressed in osteoblasts. *J Biol Chem* 1994;269:12092–12098.

496. Paulding CA, Ruvolo M, Haber DA. The *Tre2 (USP6)* oncogene is a hominoid-specific gene. *Proc Natl Acad Sci USA* 2003;100:2507–2511.

497. Tallini G, Dorfman H, Brys P, et al. Correlation between clinicopathological features and karyotype in 100 cartilaginous and chordoid tumours: a report from the Chromosomes and Morphology (CHAMP) Collaborative Study Group. *J Pathol* 2002;196:194–203.

498. Mandahl N, Heim S, Arheden K, et al. Chromosomal rearrangements in chondromatous tumors. *Cancer* 1990;65:242–248.

499. Bridge JA, Bhatia PS, Anderson JR, et al. Biologic and clinical significance of cytogenetic and molecular cytogenetic abnormalities in benign and malignant cartilaginous lesions. *Cancer Genet Cytogenet* 1993;69:79–90.

500. Mandahl N, Willen H, Rydholm A, et al. Rearrangement of band q13 on both chromosomes 12 in a periosteal chondroma. *Genes Chromosomes Cancer* 1993;6:121–123.

501. Mertens F, Jonsson K, Willen H, et al. Chromosome rearrangements in synovial chondromatous lesions. *Br J Cancer* 1996;74:251–254.

502. Weinstein LS, Shenker A, German PV, et al. Activating mutations of the stimulatory G protein in the McCune-Albright syndrome. *N Engl J Med* 1991;325:1688–1695.

503. Cohen MM Jr, Howell RE. Etiology of fibrous dysplasia and McCune-Albright syndrome. *Int J Oral Maxillofac Surg* 1999;28:366–371.

504. Shenker A, Weinstein LS, Sweet DE, et al. An activating Gs α mutation is present in fibrous dysplasia of bone in the McCune-Albright syndrome. *J Clin Endocrinol Metab* 1994;79:750–755.

505. Alman BA, Greel DA, Wolfe HJ. Activating mutations of Gs protein in monostotic fibrous lesions of bone. *J Orthop Res* 1996;14:311–315.

506. Cohen MM Jr. Fibrous dysplasia is a neoplasm. *Am J Med Genet* 2001;98:290–293.

507. Dal Cin P, Sciot R, Brys P, et al. Recurrent chromosome aberrations in fibrous dysplasia of the bone: a report of the CHAMP study group. *Cancer Genet Cytogenet* 2000;122:30–32.

508. Happle R. The McCune-Albright syndrome: a lethal gene surviving by mosaicism. *Clin Genet* 1986;29:321–324.

509. Matsuba A, Ogose A, Tokunaga K, et al. Activating Gs α mutation at the Arg[201] codon in liposclerosing myxofibrous tumor. *Hum Pathol* 2003;34:1204–1209.

510. Cabral CE, Guedes P, Fonseca T, et al. Polyostotic fibrous dysplasia associated with intramuscular myxomas: Mazabraud's syndrome. *Skeletal Radiol* 1998;27:278–282.

511. Fragoso MC, Latronico AC, Carvalho FM, et al. Activating mutation of the stimulatory G protein (gsp) as a putative cause of ovarian and testicular human stromal Leydig cell tumors. *J Clin Endocrinol Metab* 1998;83:2074–2078.

512. Faglia G, Arosio M, Spada A. GS protein mutations and pituitary tumors: functional correlates and possible therapeutic implications. *Metabolism* 1996;45:117–119.

513. Williamson EA, Ince PG, Harrison D, et al. G-protein mutations in human pituitary adrenocorticotrophic hormone-secreting adenomas. *Eur J Clin Invest* 1995;25:128–131.

514. Russo D, Arturi F, Wicker R, et al. Genetic alterations in thyroid hyperfunctioning adenomas. *J Clin Endocrinol Metab* 1995;80:1347–1351.

515. Collins MT, Shenker A. McCune-Albright syndrome: new insights. *Endocrinol Diabetes* 6:119–125.

516. Pienkowski C, Lumbroso S, Bieth E, et al. Recurrent ovarian cyst and mutation of the Gs alpha gene in ovarian cyst fluid cells: what is the link with McCune-Albright syndrome? *Acta Paediatr* 1997;86:1019–1021.

Endocrine System

THYROID

Conventional Papillary Thyroid Carcinoma

Papillary thyroid carcinoma (PTC) accounts for about 80% of all thyroid malignancies. Conventional PTC is characterized by two general types of mutations, chromosomal rearrangements of the tyrosine kinase proto-oncogenes *RET* (located at 10q11.2) and *NTRK* (located at 1q22) and point mutations of the serine-thronine kinase *BRAF* (located at 7q34). The morphologic variants of PTC share the same pattern of cytologic features as conventional PTC, including nuclear clearing, elongation, overlapping, and pseudo-inclusions (1,2), thus, it is not surprising that the variants harbor some of the same genetic aberrations as conventional PTC.

Genetics of *RET* and *NTRK1* Mutations

The *RET* tyrosine kinase is involved in rearrangements with a number of different partner genes in PTC, as shown in Table 12.1. Only *RET/PTC1* (and its variant *RET/PTCIL*), *RET/PTC2*, *RET/PTC3*, and *RET/ELKS* have been detected in non–radiation associated PTC. The rest of the rearrangements have been identified from PTC that developed in individuals from zones contaminated by the Chernobyl nuclear power plant accident, which emphasizes the link between *RET* and radiation-induced thyroid carcinogenesis. It is interesting to note that *RET* and its partner loci show a high level of spatial contiguity in normal interphase nuclei; this proximity may contribute some specificity to the rearrangements found in PTC by allowing a single radiation track to produce double-strand breaks in both of the involved genes (3,19).

All of the proteins encoded by the genes involved in *RET* fusions in PTC share two features: they are expressed in thyroid follicular cells and they contain putative dimerization domains (Fig. 12.1). The dimerization domains are

thought to mediate ligand-independent association of two chimeric protein molecules; the subsequent constitutive activation of the intracellular tyrosine kinase of RET is responsible for tumor development (20).

A much smaller subset of PTC shows rearrangements in the *NTRK1* gene (21), and the percentage of tumors that harbor *NTRK1* rearrangements does not seem to be increased in Chernobyl-associated tumors (18). Native *NTRK1* encodes a transmembrane tyrosine kinase receptor that is activated by binding nerve growth factor, but in *NTRK1* proteins the extracellular N-terminal region of *NTRK1* is replaced by a dimerization domain (22,23). As with *RET* fusions, the dimerization domain contributed by the fusion partner is thought to mediate ligand-independent association of two chimeric protein molecules with resulting constitutive activation of the *NTRK1* tyrosine kinase (20), an oncogenic mechanism that is supported by a mouse model of *TRK-T1* overexpression (24).

Technical Issues in Molecular Genetic Analysis of *RET* and *NTRK1*

Conventional cytogenetic analysis was used to identify many of the rearrangements that are associated with PTC (11,25), but because most studies only report positive cases, the sensitivity of the method in routine use is unknown. The fact that cytogenetic analysis requires fresh tissue limits the utility of the technique in routine use because many PTCs only become apparent during microscopic evaluation of fixed tissue.

The genetic aberrations characteristic of PTC are readily detected by reverse transcriptase polymerase chain reaction (RT-PCR) and interphase fluorescence in situ hybridization (FISH); these two approaches are the most widely used methods for molecular evaluation of PTC. However, it is difficult to determine the sensitivity of RT-PCR and FISH for detecting *RET* and *NTRK1* rearrangements in PTC for three reasons. First, the frequency of genetic aberrations at the two loci varies by the geographic origin of the patient

TABLE 12.1
RET AND *NTRK1* FUSION PARTNERS IN PAPILLARY THYROID CARCINOMA

Fusion Gene	Activating Gene	Activating Gene Function	Activating Gene Location	References
***RET* proto-oncogene fusions**				
RET/PTC1[a]	H4/D10S170	Unknown	10q21	3–5
RET/PTC2	PRKAR1A	Protein kinase regulatory subunit	17q24.2	3
RET/PTC3	ELE1	Androgen receptor–associated protein	10q11.2	6
RET/PTC4[b]	ELE1 (alternative break point)	Androgen receptor–associated protein	10q11.2	7, 8
RET/PTC5	GOLGA5/RFG5	Golgi autoantigen	14q22.1	9
RET/PTC6	TIF1α	Transcription intermediary factor	7q33–34	10
RET/PTC7	TIF1γ / RFG7	Transcription intermediary factor	1p13.2	10
RET/PTC8	KTN1	Vesicle membrane anchored protein	14q22.1	11
RET/PTC9	RFG9	Unknown	18q21.3	12
RET/PCM1	PCM1	Centrosomal protein	8p22	13
RET/ELKS	ELKS	Unknown	12p13.3	14
RET/ΔRFP	RFP	RET finger protein	6p21.3	15
***NTRK1* proto-oncogene fusions**				
TRK-TPM3	TPM3	Cytoskeletal tropomyosin involved in stabilization of cytoskeleton actin filaments	1q21.3	16
TRK-T1	TPR	Nuclear protein transport	1q25	17
TRK-T2	TPR (alternative break point)	Nuclear protein transport	1q25	18
TRK-T3	TFG	Unknown	3q11–q12	17

[a]The partner genes were originally referred to as "PTC" for "papillary thyroid carcinoma," a nomenclature that persists for the more common gene fusions.
[b]Also known as *RET/PTC3r2*.

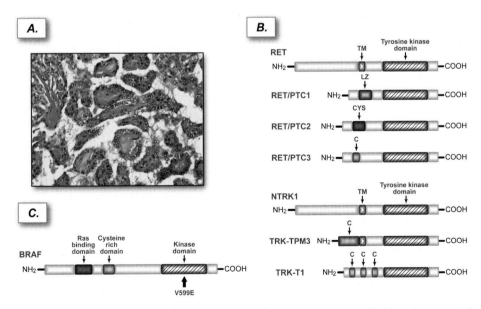

Figure 12.1 **A**, Papillary thyroid carcinoma, a neoplasm that is associated with a characateristic pattern of genetic aberrations. **B**, Schematic diagram of representative RET fusion proteins and NTRK1 fusion proteins in papillary thyroid carcinoma. All the fusion proteins consist of a dimerization domain from the amino terminal region of the fusion partner linked to the tyrosine kinase domain of native RET or NTRK1. LZ, leucine zipper dimerization domain; CYS, dimerization region with adjacent cysteine residues; C, coiled-coil dimerization domain; TM, transmembrane region. **C**, Schematic diagram of the BRAF protein indicating the location of the V599E missense mutation responsible for a subset of papillary thyroid carcinomas.

population, the age of the patient population, and exposure to ionizing radiation (22,26–29). Second, given the number of genes that can form fusions with *RET* or *NTRK1*, the sensitivity of testing depends on the comprehensiveness of the testing protocol; published RT-PCR and probe-fusion FISH studies differ in the number of fusion genes that are evaluated (25,29–31). Third, there is variability in the level of expression of the different fusion genes, and so different RT-PCR reaction conditions have different detection rates (32). With these provisos in mind, studies from North America, western Europe, and Asia show that rearrangements of the *RET* tyrosine kinase gene can be detected in 9% to 61% of sporadic PTC by RT-PCR (29,31,33,34), and about three times as many tumors harbor the *RET/PTC1* fusion gene compared with the *RET/PTC3* fusion (29,35,36). However, the *RET/PTC3* fusion is the most common rearrangement in radiation-induced tumors, with a prevalence of approximately 25% to 60% in patients exposed to the radioactivity of the Chernobyl nuclear power plant accident (23,25,30). Other genes are involved in *RET* rearrangements in PTC much less frequently. The relatively low prevalence of *RET* and *NTRK1* rearrangements in PTC constrains the utility of molecular testing in routine clinical practice because the predictive value of a negative result is so low (37,38).

Immunohistochemistry

Because the RET and NTRK1 chimeric proteins are overexpressed, they can be detected by routine immunohistochemistry, unlike native RET and NTRK1 proteins, which are not detectable in normal adult thyroid follicular or parafollicular cells (39). Consistent with the molecular biology of the rearrangements of *RET* in PTC, immunoreactivity for the tyrosine kinase domain of RET (which is conserved in the chimeric protein regardless of the fusion partner) is consistently associated with a lack of immunoreactivity for the juxtamembrane domain of RET (which is lost in the chimeric protein) in cases of PTC (40). In tumors for which parallel immunohistochemical and genetic analysis has been performed, the results from the two methods have been in complete concordance (26,40).

Diagnostic Issues in Molecular Genetic Analysis of *RET* and *NTRK1*

Although *RET* and *NTRK1* rearrangements are characteristically associated with PTC and its variants (the genetics of PTC variants is discussed more fully below), the same rearrangements have occasionally been detected in other types of follicular lesions. *RET* rearrangements have been detected in 57% of Hurthle cell adenomas (41), but not in non-oncocytic hyperplastic lesions or adenomas (40,42). At most, 13% of poorly differentiated carcinomas harbor *RET* or *NTRK1* fusions when evaluated by a combined RT-PCR and immunohistochemical approach (26,40), a finding that suggests only a subset of poorly differentiated thyroid carcinomas evolves from ordinary PTC that harbor *RET* or *NTRK1* rearrangements. The *RET* locus is virtually never rearranged in follicular thyroid carcinoma or undifferentiated (anaplastic) thyroid carcinoma (40). However, *RET* rearrangements have been detected in a subset of cases of Hashimoto's thyroiditis, as is discussed more fully later (43–45).

Analysis of thyroid nodules that show at least focal cytologic features of PTC has shown that about 70% harbor *RET/PTC1* or *RET/PTC3* fusion transcripts when tested by nested RT-PCR, and that about 65% show immunoreactivity for the tyrosine kinase domain of RET (46). Although *RET* activation closely paralleled the cytologic changes associated with PTC in this study, clonality analysis demonstrated that the regions containing *RET/PTC* fusion genes were polyclonal in about half of the cases and that *RET/PTC* fusion transcripts were not present in areas of the same nodules that lacked the cytologic features suggestive of PTC. Consequently, although it is possible that microscopic foci with the cytologic features of PTC may represent precursors of invasive PTC, the foci do not justify interpretation of the entire lesion as PTC (46). These findings emphasize that molecular genetic analysis of a problematic thyroid nodule should not be performed in a vacuum, but should be coupled with a careful morphologic evaluation of the lesion (46).

Prognostic Implications of *RET* and *NTRK1* Rearrangements

Although *RET* or *NTRK1* activation has been shown to correlate with locally advanced stage at presentation in one study (21), the type of *RET* rearrangement does not correlate with tumor size or long-term prognosis (29,33,40,47) in patients with non–radiation-associated PTC. In contrast, in patients with radiation-induced PTC, different *RET* gene fusions do correlate with the clinical features of disease; *RET/PTC3* rearrangements, independent of the age at irradiation, are associated with a shorter period of latency and a more advanced clinical stage at presentation than tumors that harbor other *RET/PTC* rearrangements (30).

Genetics of *BRAF* Mutations

BRAF is a serine-threonine kinase and is one of three isoforms of RAF encoded by the human genome. In all cases of PTC evaluated thus far, the *BRAF* mutation is a unique missense T to A transversion at nucleotide 1796 of codon 599 in exon 15, in the region of the gene that encodes the activation segment of the kinase domain. The mutation causes a valine to glutamic acid substitution (V599E) that is thought to result in a protein with constitutive maximal kinase activity (48). However, the limited mutational profile of *BRAF* in PTC may be a reflection of the small number of cases that has been tested. The lack of overlap between *RET/PTC*, *ras*, and *BRAF* mutations in PTC (49–53) implies that mutations in *BRAF* and *RET* are alternative events in the development of PTC and that constitutive activation of any component of the *RET-ras-BRAF-MAPK* signaling pathway is sufficient for the initiation of sporadic PTC (51,53,54). Although the *BRAF* V599E mutation appears to be a more common genetic event in sporadic PTC than rearrangement of *RET*, combined analysis of *RET* and *BRAF* still detects a genetic abnormality characteristic of conventional PTC in only 55% to 64% of cases (50,51).

Technical Issues in Molecular Genetic Analysis of *BRAF*

In studies in which fresh tissue was used for mutation analysis, either predominantly or exclusively, 38% to 53% of cases of PTC harbor the V599E missense mutation in exon 15 of *BRAF* (50–52,54). In these studies, PCR was used to amplify *BRAF* mutation hotspots and then DNA sequence analysis was either performed on all the PCR products (52) or only on those PCR products that had an altered pattern of electrophoretic mobility by single-strand conformational polymorphism (SSCP) analysis (50,51) (in fact, the two approaches have been shown to provide similar sensitivity for the detection of *BFAF* mutations [54]). A real-time PCR approach that takes advantage of the fact that all *BRAF* mutations thus far identified in PTC are restricted to nucleotide 1796 has been used to screen PTC and has been shown to have a sensitivity that is indistinguishable from direct DNA sequencing with or without prior SSCP analysis (54).

When formalin-fixed, paraffin-embedded (FFPE) tissue is used exclusively as the substrate for testing, V599E mutations of *BRAF* are detected in only 29% of cases of PTC (55), a level of sensitivity that is statistically significantly lower than for testing performed using predominantly or exclusively fresh tissue.

Diagnostic Issues in Molecular Genetic Analysis of BRAF

V599E mutations have not been observed in follicular adenomas, nodular goiters, follicular thyroid carcinomas, medullary thyroid carcinomas, Hurthle cell carcinomas, or Hurthle cell adenomas (49,51,52,54–56). However, the missense mutation has been detected in 14% of poorly differentiated thyroid carcinomas and in 10% to 50% of anaplastic carcinomas (54–56), findings that suggest at least a subset of these two tumor types evolve from ordinary PTC.

A number of tumor types other than PTC also harbor *BRAF* mutations, including melanoma, and carcinomas of the lung, colon, and ovary (48). In these other tumor types, there are two mutational hotspots in *BRAF*; 89% of mutations occur in the activation segment of the kinase domain encoded by exon 15, while 11% occur in the glycine-rich loop of the kinase domain encoded by exon 11.

Prognostic Implications of BRAF Mutations

Presence of the V599E mutation has been shown to significantly correlate with an advanced clinical stage at presentation in two series (54,55), although a more recent study failed to confirm the association (51).

It is worthwhile to note that several new drugs have recently been described that are RAF kinase inhibitors, some of which are currently undergoing clinical evaluation as potential therapeutic agents in a wide variety of malignancies (57,58). Assuming that a link between *BRAF* V599E and clinical outcome does exist or that some of the new drugs have a therapeutic effect, *BRAF* mutational analysis may become a routine part of the evaluation of conventional PTC and anaplastic thyroid carcinoma for prognostic or therapeutic purposes, even if mutational analysis has little role in diagnosis.

Genetics of Other Mutations in PTC

The contribution of other oncogenes to the development of PTC is uncertain (59–63). For example, the role of *ras* mutations is unclear because there is significant variation in the prevalence of *ras* mutations in conventional PTC, the follicular variant of PTC, and PTC arising in iodide-deficient areas (28,59,64,65), and the prevalence of mutations does not seem to be increased in victims of the Chernobyl accident (60,61). For other oncogenes, the rate of mutations is quite low; for example, less than 10% of PTC harbors *TP53* mutations (50,66) and only about 6% of PTC contains mutations in the MET receptor tyrosine kinase (67). Loss of heterozygosity (LOH) of chromosomal regions linked to a number of different tumor suppressor genes has been related to a poor prognosis in some studies (62), but the identity of the specific loci within these regions that are responsible for the poor clinical outcome has not been definitively established.

Morphologic Variants of Papillary Thyroid Carcinoma

Between 3% and 25% of cases of the follicular variant of PTC contain *RET/PTC1* or *RET/PTEC3* rearrangements (34,68), although 20% to 43% of cases harbor *ras* mutations (68,69). The tall cell variant of PTC typically harbors the *RET/PTC3* fusion gene, which apparently is present in virtually 100% of cases (34). The solid variant of PTC also preferentially harbors *RET/PTC3* fusions, especially in radiation-induced carcinomas (70,71). *RET* fusion genes have been shown to be present in 100% of cases of the diffuse sclerosing variant of PTC and in 100% of cases of the mixed variant of PTC, although the number of cases that has been evaluated is quite small (70).

The prevalence of *BRAF* mutations in the morphologic variants of PTC has recently been evaluated. About 40% of cases of the oncocytic variant of PTC harbor V599E mutations, as do about 75% of cases of Warthin-like PTC (72). A case of the tall cell variant of PTC that harbors the V599E mutation has also been documented (72). Of particular interest, 9% of cases of the follicular variant of PTC harbor a K600E missense mutation in exon 15 of *BRAF* (72).

The cribriform-morular variant of PTC is classically associated with either germline or, rarely, sporadic mutations in the *APC* gene (73), although *RET/PTC1* fusion genes have also been reported in patients with germline *APC* mutations (74).

Follicular Thyroid Carcinoma

Follicular thyroid carcinoma (FTC) accounts for 5% to 15% of malignant thyroid neoplasms, depending on the criteria used for diagnosis. Follicular carcinomas that show invasion only into or through the tumor capsule without angioinvasion have an excellent prognosis; therefore a three-tier classification for FTC has been proposed: minimally invasive (tumors that invade only into or through the tumor capsule), grossly encapsulated angioinvasive (tumors with identifiable vascular invasion of medium to large vessels at the level of the tumor capsule), and widely invasive (tumors that are multifocal or extend beyond the thyroid capsule) (2,75).

Genetics

A characteristic feature of FTC is the t(2;3)(q13;p25) translocation that produces a *PAX8-PPARγ1* fusion gene (76,77). The *PAX8* gene at 2q13 encodes a transcription factor that is essential for development of the thyroid follicular epithelial cell lineage (78), and the *PPARγ1* gene at 3p25 encodes a ligand-dependent nuclear transcription factor that is a member of the perioxisome proliferator-activated receptor family (79). The fusion gene encodes a chimeric protein in which the paired and partial homeobox DNA binding domains of PAX8 are fused with virtually the entire length of PPARγ1 (Fig. 12.2). The precise boundary of the translocation break point varies between individual follicular carcinomas, and the heterogeneity of fusion transcripts (and thus chimeric proteins) is further augmented by alternative splicing (76,77,80).

Functionally, the PAX8-PPARγ1 protein is a dominant negative suppressor of wild-type PPARγ1 function (76), but the mechanism by which suppression of PPARγ promotes follicular carcinoma formation is not well characterized. Genetic analysis of follicular carcinomas that show a rearrangement at 3p25 but not 2q13 suggests that some follicular carcinomas harbor fusions between *PPARγ1* and a different partner gene (76), and the presence of PPARγ1 proteins of altered size in these tumors is consistent with this hypothesis (81).

Thus far, the presence or absence of *PAX8-PPARγ1* rearrangements has not been associated with prognostic differences in cases of FTC. Similarly, the position of the

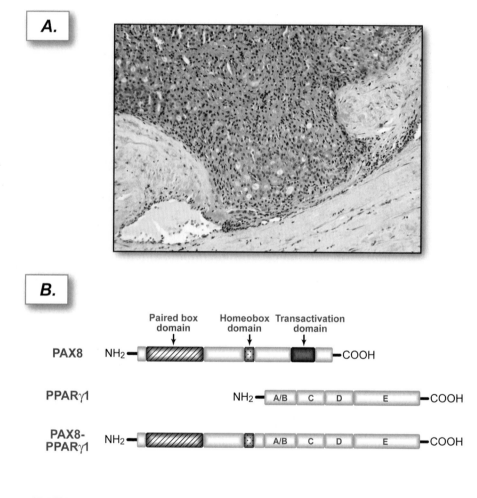

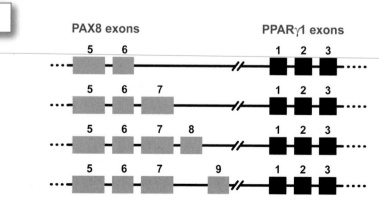

Figure 12.2 A, Well-differentiated follicular carcinoma, a tumor that characteristically harbors a *PAX8-PPARγ1* fusion. **B**, Schematic diagram of the PAX8-PPARγ1 chimeric protein; the paired box and partial homeobox domains of PAX8 are fused to the ligand-independent transcriptional activation domain (A/B), DNA binding domain (C), nuclear localization domain (D), and ligand binding domain (E) of PPARγ1. **C**, An example of the heterogeneity of *PAX8-PPARγ1* transcripts (and thus chimeric proteins) within an individual tumor that results from alternative splicing (from reference 80).

break point within the *PAX8-PPARγ1* fusion gene, or the presence of alternatively spliced transcripts, has not been associated with differences in prognosis.

Technical Issues in Molecular Genetic Analysis of FTC

As the studies that characterized the t(2;3)(q13;p25) translocation demonstrate, the rearrangement is readily detected by conventional cytogenetic analysis (76,77). However, given the bias associated with selective reporting of positive cases, the sensitivity of cytogenetic analysis in routine practice is unknown.

Interphase FISH using the probe-fusion approach has also been used to detect the t(2;3) translocation and has a high concordance with the results of RT-PCR–based testing of frozen tissue (76,81). Interphase FISH using the probe-split approach also can be used to detect rearrangements of the 3p25 *PPARγ1* locus that are suggestive of variant *PPARγ1* fusion genes in those FTC without the conventional t(2;3) (76).

PAX8-PPARγ1 fusion transcripts can be detected in 12% to 63% of FTC by RT-PCR when frozen tissue is used as the substrate for testing (76,77,80,81), and RT-PCR modified for use with FFPE tissue is not associated with a significant decrease in sensitivity (82). A nested approach tends to achieve a higher sensitivity with both fresh and FFPE tissue (76,77,80–82), and given the heterogeneity in the precise translocation break point in *PAX8-PPARγ1* rearrangements, optimum sensitivity in PCR-based assays requires multiple primer pairs. Many studies do not subcategorize the follicular carcinomas as minimally invasive or widely invasive, thus it is unknown whether or not there is a difference in the prevalence of *PAX8-PPARγ1* fusions in these different tumor groups.

Immunohistochemistry

From 53% to 88% of cases of FTC show strong diffuse nuclear immunostaining using antibodies against wild-type PPARγ as opposed to the faint focal nuclear staining that is due to expression of native PPARγ (76,77,80,82). Strong diffuse nuclear reactivity is highly correlated with the presence of underlying *PAX8-PPARγ1* fusion genes detected by RT-PCR (76,77). The small number of cases in which strong diffuse nuclear staining is present despite a negative RT-PCR result is another indication that *PPARγ1* rearrangements with as yet unidentified genes may underlie the development of a subset of FTC (76,77).

Diagnostic Issues in Molecular Genetic Analysis of FTC

The *PAX8-PPARγ1* fusion has not been detected in PTC (including the follicular variant of papillary carcinoma), anaplastic thyroid carcinoma, nodular hyperplasia, and Hurthle cell carcinoma (76,77,81,82). The *PAX8-PPARγ1* rearrangement also has not been detected in poorly differentiated thyroid carcinoma (82) or anaplastic thyroid carcinoma (77,81,82), a result that suggests FTC harboring the *PAX8-PPARγ1* fusions infrequently, if ever, progress to poorly differentiated or anaplastic carcinoma.

However, there is uncertainty as to whether or not the *PAX8-PPARγ1* fusion gene is present in follicular adenomas. Initial reports found no evidence of the rearrangement outside of FTC (76), but *PAX8-PPARγ1* fusion transcripts have been detected by RT-PCR in 8% to 55% of follicular thyroid adenomas in more recent studies (77,80,82). *PAX8-PPARγ1* rearrangements have also been demonstrated in 5% of atypical follicular thyroid adenomas by RT-PCR, interphase FISH, and western blot analysis (81). The presence of a *PAX8-PPARγ1* fusion gene in at least a subset of follicular adenomas supports the hypothesis that the rearrangement may be related to progression from an adenoma to a carcinoma (83). The hypothesis that FTC can arise from malignant transformation of a preexisting adenoma is consistent with mutational genotyping assays that show an increasing frequency of allelic loss in the adenoma to minimally invasive/angioinvasive FTC sequence (84). Alternatively, neoplasms expressing PAX8-PPARγ1 that are classified as follicular adenomas based on their morphologic features may actually represent FTC in which areas of capsular penetration or angioinvasion are not identified in the areas sampled for microscopic evaluation (27,80). Either way, the current data suggest that demonstration of *PAX8-PPARγ1* rearrangements by RT-PCR is not a reliable method to differentiate FTCs from follicular thyroid adenomas, in either excision specimens or fine-needle aspiration biopsies.

Genetics of Other Mutations in FTC

Single point mutations in the *ras* oncogene, usually detected by RT-PCR–based assays, are most frequently found in codons 12 and 13 that encode the GTP binding domain and in codon 16 that encodes the GTPase domain (85). Although mutations in *ras* have been reported in up to 50% of follicular adenomas and in up to 53% of follicular carcinomas (86–88), the presence of mutations does not separate benign from malignant lesions and is not associated with differences in prognosis. Consequently, molecular genetic analysis of *ras* mutations in FTC has little diagnostic or prognostic utility.

LOH has been demonstrated in FTC at numerous loci encoding known as well as putative tumor suppressor genes, including *PTEN* (discussed more fully in the section on Cowden syndrome below), *TP53*, and *VHL*. Although the presence of LOH at tumor suppressor loci has been shown to correlate with tumor aggressiveness in some studies (89), a diagnostic role for LOH analysis has not been established.

Medullary Thyroid Carcinoma

Medullary thyroid carcinoma (MTC) originates from the C-cells, or parafollicular cells, of the thyroid and accounts for 5% to 10% of primary thyroid malignancies. Approximately 20% of cases of MTC are familial and can be classified into three well-defined syndromes: multiple endocrine neoplasia (MEN) 2A, MEN2B, and familial medullary carcinoma. The remaining 80% of cases occur as sporadic tumors.

Genetics

MEN2A

The MEN2A syndrome is characterized by medullary carcinoma, pheochromocytoma, and hyperparathyroidism and is the result of missense mutations in the cysteine-rich extracellular domain of *RET* (Fig. 12.3). Missense mutations in cysteine residues in exons 10 or 11 account for approximately 95% of MEN2A families (22,27); of these, a base pair (bp) substitution in codon 634 that results in the substitution of cysteine by arginine in the encoded amino acid (C634R) is found in over 80% of cases. Because the cysteine residues participate in intramolecular disulfide bonds in the native RET protein, missense mutations leave unpaired cysteine residues that form intermolecular disulfide bonds between two mutant RET receptor molecules. The intermolecular disulfide bonds result in ligand-independent RET dimerization, with subsequent constitutive activation of RET tyrosine kinase activity (90). Nine bp and 12 bp duplications in the critical cysteine-rich domain (both of which maintain the RET open reading frame) have also been described (91,92).

MEN2B

The MEN2B syndrome is characterized by medullary thyroid carcinoma, pheochromocytoma, Marfanoid body habitus, and ganglioneuromas of the mucosal surfaces and gastrointestinal tract. About 95% of MEN2B cases are the result of a codon 918 mutation in exon 16 of RET (Fig. 12.3), which results in the substitution of a threonine for a methionine in the tyrosine kinase domain of the protein (22,27). The M918T mutation does not cause constitutive activation of the receptor as a result of aberrant dimerization, but instead results in a shift in the substrate specificity of RET, altering the pattern of RET autophosphorylation and RET-mediated phosphorylation of intracellular proteins (22,90). Other rare mutations also occur in exon 15 or exon 16.

Familial Medullary Thyroid Carcinoma

Familial medullary thyroid carcinoma (FMTC) is characterized by MTC without other clinical features of the MEN2A and MEN2B syndromes. In addition, MTC usually develops in patients of an older age and has a more benign course. Some RET mutations that are responsible for FMTC alter the cysteine-rich extracellular domain of the protein and occur in the same cysteine encoding codons as in MEN2A (Fig. 12.3). The missense mutations are thought to have different functional consequences in FMTC because they cause a significantly lower activation of RET (90), although the underlying mechanism is unknown.

Other RET mutations responsible for FMTC alter the tyrosine kinase domain. Most are single bp substitutions (Fig. 12.3), although a rare nine bp duplication in exon 8 (which retains the RET open reading frame) has recently been described (93). As with mutations that alter the cysteine-rich domain of RET, the mechanism by which identical mutations of the RET tyrosine kinase domain cause a different pattern of disease in FMTC versus MEN2B is unknown (20,27,90).

Sporadic MTC

From 40% to 80% of sporadic MTC harbor somatic RET mutations in the cysteine-rich extracellular domain or the tyrosine kinase domain (94–96) (Fig. 12.3). Attempts to more precisely define the prevalence of RET mutations in sporadic MTC are complicated by the fact that multiple different mutations can be found in different cell populations of the same tumor and its metastases (95,96).

Syndromes with MTC and PTC

Several recent reports have documented germline RET mutations that are associated with PTC. A V804M missense mutation in two kindreds with FMTC of variable expressivity is associated with papillary microcarcinomas in about 25% of family members (97). Germline mutations in codons 790, 791, and 804 associated with MTC are linked with an increased incidence of papillary microcarcinomas (98), and a novel germline RET mutation at codon 603 cosegregates with both MTC and PTC (99). The association of both MTC and PTC with specific germline RET mutations suggests that there is some overlap in the oncogenic pathways of the two tumor types (22), a hypothesis that is consistent with the coexistence of both MTC and PTC and one transgenic mouse model of thyroid carcinoma (100).

Technical Issues in Molecular Genetic Analysis of RET Mutations

From a practical standpoint, testing for RET mutations is straightforward. After PCR amplification of the regions of the gene most likely to be altered, mutations are detected by SSCP analysis or, most often, by direct DNA sequence analysis. Testing can be performed on either fresh or FFPE tissue (27). However, as noted above, analysis of RET in sporadic MTC is complicated by the heterogeneous distribution of mutations, and therefore test sensitivity is dependent on the number of tumor samples evaluated and even on the number of microdissected regions from each tumor sample (95,96). Guidelines for standardized testing have yet to be proposed, which complicates the interpretation of the results from analysis of sporadic MTC from different laboratories.

Diagnostic Issues in Molecular Genetic Analysis of RET Mutations

Although there is little need for genetic analysis of RET mutations in sporadic MTC from a diagnostic standpoint, a role for testing from a prognostic standpoint is suggested by the finding that mutations of codon 918 are associated with a poor clinical outcome (95,101). Separate from analysis of the RET gene, evaluation of the frequency of allelic loss at a panel of tumor suppressor genes may also identify a group of patients with MTC that are at high risk for tumor recurrence (102).

However, the demonstration that approximately 6% of patients with presumed sporadic MTC actually harbor a germline RET mutation (103) indicates that the role of molecular genetic testing extends beyond analysis of tumor tissue for somatic mutations that may be of prognostic significance. Although controversial, some groups recommend genetic screening for germline RET mutations in all patients with MTC, especially because a late tumor onset is still consistent with a familial syndrome (104). Mutations in exons 13, 14, and 15 appear to be over-represented in individuals who present with presumed sporadic MTC; therefore an extended mutational panel should be used for genetic analysis of this group of patients (105).

Familial Nonmedullary Thyroid Cancer

Approximately 5% of nonmedullary thyroid cancers are familial. Three well-characterized syndromes that are

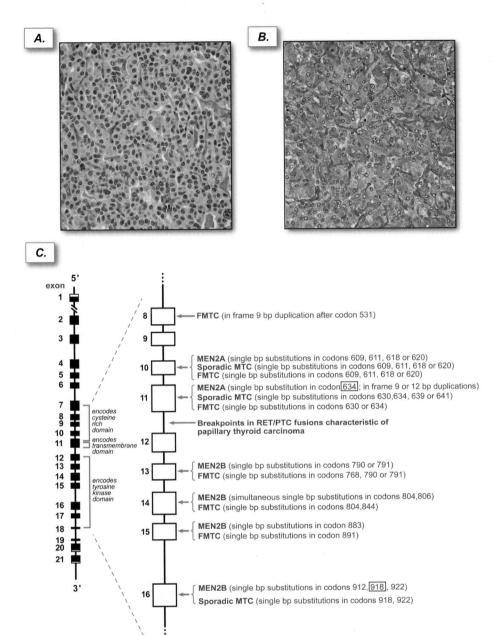

Figure 12.3 Mutations in *RET* are associated with medullary thyroid carcinoma. **A**, Medullary thyroid carcinoma from a patient with MEN2A known to have a mutation in codon 634; she also has a history of bilateral pheochromocytomas (**B**). **C**, Schematic illustration of the spectrum of mutations in the *RET* gene associated with medullary thyroid carcinoma in various hereditary cancer syndromes. MTC, medullary thyroid carcinoma; FMTC, familial MTC; MEN, multiple endocrine neoplasia. The boxed 634 and 918 indicate the site of the most common mutations in *MEN2A* and *MEN2B*, respectively.

associated with a hereditary predisposition to nonmedullary carcinoma are familial adenomatous polyposis (FAP), Cowden syndrome, and familial multinodular goiter (106,107). The thyroid carcinomas in these syndromes tend to behave more aggressively and have an earlier age of onset.

Familial Adenomatous Polyposis

As noted above, the cribriform-morular variant of PTC is often, but not always, associated with FAP (72,73,108). Two features of the cribriform-morular variant support the hypothesis that biallelic inactivation of the *APC* gene is involved in the oncogenesis of this rare tumor type: first, patients with FAP often have multiple tumors, each of which shows a different somatic mutation of the *APC* gene and, second, tumors that arise in patients without a family history of FAP also harbor somatic mutations in the *APC* gene (72). Nonetheless, the association between

APC mutations and PTC remains somewhat uncertain because some of the thyroid tumors that arise in patients with FAP are conventional PTC that harbor *PTC/RET* rearrangements (74,109), often without LOH at the *APC* locus (109).

Cowden Syndrome

Germline mutations in the *PTEN* gene are responsible for Cowden syndrome, an autosomal dominant cancer predisposition syndrome characterized by multiple hamartomas of the skin, intestine, breast, and thyroid and associated with an elevated risk of carcinomas of the breast and thyroid (110). About 67% of patients have benign thyroid abnormalities (including follicular adenomas, multinodular goiter, and thyroiditis), and about 10% of patients develop thyroid carcinomas, usually FTC.

Mutations in *PTEN* are also present in sporadic, nonsyndromic thyroid lesions. In sporadic cases, direct sequence analysis of all nine exons of *PTEN* performed on frozen or FFPE tissue shows that mutations are present in less than 10% of FTC and less than 5% of PTC, although LOH of *PTEN* is present in up to 27% of informative FTC and 26% of benign tumors, including follicular adenomas and Hurthle cell adenomas (111,112). Increased *PTEN* expression may be a more characteristic feature of thyroid carcinomas than *PTEN* coding mutations (113,114), but the utility of immunohistochemistry and quantitative RT-PCR for *PTEN* expression in the clinical evaluation of sporadic thyroid neoplasms remains unknown.

Other Syndromes

A few other rare hereditary syndromes are also associated with nonmedullary carcinoma. Familial Hurthle cell carcinoma has been linked to the *TCO* locus at 19p13.2 and the *NMTC1* locus at 2q21, although additional genetic heterogeneity is present (107,115,116). Familial follicular thyroid cancer is caused by mutations in the thyroid-stimulating hormone receptor (106). However, a role for molecular analysis in routine diagnostic pathology to detect mutations associated with these syndromes has not been established.

Poorly-Differentiated Thyroid Carcinoma and Anaplastic Thyroid Carcinoma

Although anaplastic thyroid carcinoma (ATC) accounts for less than 5% of thyroid malignancies, many patients have known benign thyroid disease, and 20% to 90% of patients have either a coexisting well-differentiated PTC or FTC, or a history of well-differentiated thyroid carcinoma (54,117,118). These clinical features of ATC suggest that at least some cases arise through the progression of well-differentiated carcinoma to poorly differentiated carcinoma to anaplastic carcinoma, a model that is supported by several facts that have emerged from genetic analysis of ATC. First, case reports have shown a pattern of mutations consistent with clonal evolution of follicular lesions or conventional papillary carcinoma to ATC (119,120). Second, the pattern of allelic loss at tumor suppressor loci in coexisting well-differentiated thyroid carcinoma and ATC is consistent with evolution of the anaplastic carcinoma from the preexisting well-differentiated tumor (121). Third, *BRAF* mutations or rearrangements of *RET* or *NTRK1* that are characteristic of well-differentiated papillary carcinoma have been demonstrated in a subset of poorly-differentiated thyroid carcinomas and *BRAF* mutations are present in a subset of ATC.

Genetics

At most 13% of poorly differentiated carcinomas harbor *RET* rearrangements based on RT-PCR or immunoreactivity with antibodies specific for the tyrosine kinase domain of RET (26,40). *RET* rearrangements are more common in cases with coexisting PTC, or that show at least focal cytologic features suggestive of PTC, but the presence of rearrangements does not correlate with any other clinicopathologic parameters. Rearrangements of *RET* have not

been detected in anaplastic (undifferentiated) thyroid carcinoma (40).

The V599E *BRAF* mutation has been identified in a subset of poorly differentiated thyroid carcinomas and ATC. In a series that evaluated fresh and FFPE tissue, 14% of poorly differentiated carcinomas and 10% anaplastic carcinomas showed the V599E mutation, and all the positive tumors contained areas of preexisting PTC that also harbored the *BRAF* mutation (54). In smaller series that evaluated only FFPE tissue, 33% to 50% of anaplastic carcinomas were shown to harbor *BRAF* mutations (55,56). *PAX8-PPARγ1* fusions have not been detected in ATC (77,81,82).

Despite that fact that mutations characteristic of well-differentiated thyroid carcinoma can be identified in a subset of poorly differentiated thyroid carcinomas and ATC, genetic testing is of little diagnostic utility for several reasons. First, even though the morphologic appearance of poorly differentiated carcinoma and ATC can be variable, the gross and microscopic features of both tumors are nonetheless usually diagnostic. Second, the prevalence of *BRAF* mutations and *RET*, *NTRK1*, or *PAX8-PPARγ* rearrangements is relatively low, and so from a diagnostic perspective, testing has a limited sensitivity. Third, genetic analysis does not provide any prognostic information because the presence or type of mutation does not appear to correlate with clinical outcome for poorly differentiated carcinoma or ATC. However, if clinical trials demonstrate that RAF kinase inhibitors have activity against tumors with *BRAF* mutations (57,58), it is possible that genetic analysis of poorly differentiated or ATC will be necessary to direct appropriate therapy.

Finally, it is worth noting that activating mutations in exon 3 of the *CTNNB1* gene (which encodes β-catenin) are present in about 25% of poorly differentiated thyroid carcinomas and in about 66% of ATC, and are associated with abnormalities in β-catenin expression and localization by immunohistochemical analysis (122). Well-differentiated PTC and FTC do not harbor *CTNNB1* mutations (122). However, β-catenin aberrations are a feature of a wide variety of tumor types and the role of analysis of the *CTNNB1* locus in the evaluation of thyroid neoplasms in routine clinical practice has not been demonstrated (123,124).

Hyalinizing Trabecular Tumors

As originally described, hyalinizing trabecular adenoma is composed of elongated tumor cells with cytologic features that overlap those of PTC arranged in a trabecular growth pattern surrounded by a dense hyaline material sometimes accompanied by stromal calcifications resembling psammoma bodies (125). Cytoplasmic and cell membrane staining for Ki-67 with the MIB-1 antibody and the presence of cytoplasmic yellow bodies have been recently proposed as additional characteristic features of hyalinizing trabecular adenoma (126,127). Although all of the cases in the initial series were benign, subsequent reports described cases classified as hyalinizing trabecular carcinoma because of the presence of vascular invasion, invasive growth into the surrounding thyroid, and even metastasis (128,129). In addition, a relationship between hyalinizing trabecular adenoma and PTC has been suggested because approximately one third of cases harbor a conventional

PTC (reviewed in 128,129). However, different criteria have been used to classify the neoplasms in these studies, and therefore the relationship between hyalinizing trabecular adenoma and other hyalinizing trabecular tumors remains unclear (129).

Technical Issues in Molecular Genetic Analysis of Hyalinizing Trabecular Tumors

Based on two studies of hyalinizing trabecular tumors (HTT), RT-PCR analysis of FFPE tissue using primers for the most common *RET* fusion partners (including at least *PTC1*, *PTC2*, and *PTC3*) will detect rearrangements in 25% to 63% of cases, and immunohistochemistry using a polyclonal antibody directed against the tyrosine kinase domain of RET will detect increased expression in 30% to 75% of cases (130,131). The disparate estimates of the prevalence of aberrations is likely due, at least in part, to the small size of the studies. Thus far, the prevalence of *BRAF* mutations in HTT has not been evaluated.

Diagnostic Issues in Molecular Genetic Analysis of Hyalinizing Trabecular Tumors

Some authors have suggested that the presence of *RET* rearrangements in HTT is evidence that the neoplasms represent a morphologic variant of PTC (130,131), although this suggestion has been somewhat controversial (128,129) for two main reasons. First, given the uncertainly in the classification of HTT noted above, it is not entirely clear that all the study cases represent the same lesions originally described as hyalinizing trabecular adenomas. Second, because *RET* fusion genes can be detected in benign thyroid lesions such as Hurthle cell adenomas and even Hashimoto's thyroiditis (discussed below), the presence of *RET* rearrangements in an HTT is not a specific indication that the lesion is malignant. Because the therapy for a lesion 1 cm or larger in diameter classified as a hyalinizing trabecular variant of papillary carcinoma would include total thyroidectomy, usually accompanied by postoperative radioiodine therapy, these issues are not moot points (128,129). Until long-term follow-up data are available on HTT that harbor *RET* rearrangements and that additionally do or do not meet strict criteria for the diagnosis of hyalinizing trabecular adenoma, it seems premature to classify the neoplasms based purely on the molecular genetic findings. Instead, it seems most prudent to integrate the molecular genetic findings with all the other clinical and pathologic features of the neoplasm (128,129).

Hurthle Cell Tumors

Hurthle cell tumors are composed of large polygonal oncocytes that have abundant eosinophilic granular cytoplasm (resulting from an abnormal accumulation of mitochondria) and hyperchromatic nuclei that are often atypical.

Genetics

Two studies have shown that *RET* activation is a characteristic feature of Hurthle cell tumors. RT-PCR analysis of fresh and FFPE tissue has demonstrated that 54% to 58% of Hurthle cell adenomas and 57% to 79% of Hurthle cell carcinomas harbor *RET/PCT1*, *RET/PTC2*, or *RET/PTC3* fusions (42,132). Consistent with these molecular genetic results, immunohistochemistry using antibodies specific for the RET tyrosine-kinase domain has shown *RET* activation in 38% to 60% of Hurthle cell adenomas and 47% to 68% of Hurthle cell carcinomas (42,132). In these studies, hyperplastic nodules with Hurthle cell change did not show evidence of *RET* activation by either immunohistochemistry or RT-PCR for *RET* gene rearrangements.

Somatic mitochondrial mutations, including point mutations and large deletions, occur at a significantly higher rate in Hurthle cell tumors compared with non-Hurthle cell neoplasms (133–135). Consequently, it has been hypothesized that the mitochondrial proliferation that occurs in oncocytes may be a compensatory response to decreased oxidative phosphorylation as a result of mtDNA damage (134).

Diagnostic Issues in Molecular Genetic Analysis of Hurthle Cell Tumors

Because *RET* rearrangements are present in both Hurthle cell adenomas and carcinomas, mutational analysis of *RET* cannot be used to distinguish benign from malignant lesions. Furthermore, because it has yet to be established that the presence of *RET* aberrations correlates with clinical outcome for patients with Hurthle cell carcinomas, there is also no prognostic role for mutational or immunohistochemical analysis of *RET* activation.

The mtDNA mutations that have been described in Hurthle cell tumors are also not a specific finding. A subset of the same mtDNA mutations has also been demonstrated in other thyroid neoplasms, including conventional PTC, thyroid adenomas, and Hashimoto's thyroiditis (133,135,136). Some of the same mtDNA mutations have even been detected in neoplasms at other anatomic sites, including Warthin's tumor of the salivary gland (134) and oncocytic lesions of the parathyroid and kidney (137,138). Given this lack of specificity, there is currently no role for mtDNA mutation analysis in routine practice.

Hashimoto's Thyroiditis

There are conflicting reports as to whether or not *RET* rearrangements are a feature of Hashimoto's thyroiditis. Two studies have shown that 94% to 95% of histologically benign thyroid glands affected by Hashimoto's thyroiditis contain *RET/PTC* rearrangements when evaluated by RT-PCR (44,45), and that an additional 43% of benign thyroid glands with lymphocytic thyroiditis harbor *RET* rearrangements (45). In contrast, a more recent RT-PCR–based study failed to detect any *RET/PTC* rearrangements in 26 cases of Hashimoto's thyroiditis (43), a result more consistent with prospective case control studies that have failed to detect any increase in thyroid cancer in patients with Hashimoto's thyroiditis despite a 67-fold increased relative risk for lymphoma (139).

Differences in methodology may explain the markedly different findings. The two studies that found a high prevalence of *RET* rearrangements tested FFPE tissue by nested

PCR, with an unusually high number of amplification cycles, an approach that increases the risk of false positive results due to cross-contamination or amplification of nonspecific sequences (43,140). In contrast, the study that found a lack of *RET* rearrangements tested primarily frozen tissue, used a single PCR amplification, and confirmed the identity of the PCR products by Southern blot hybridization. Study of Hashimoto's thyroiditis by independent molecular genetic methodologies such as interphase FISH should help to clarify the prevalence of *RET* (and *NTRK1*) rearrangements. In the meantime, given the disparity in the molecular results reported thus far, it seems premature to use molecular results to alter established treatment regimens of patients with Hashimoto's thyroiditis.

PARATHYROID GLANDS

Parathyroid Adenomas and Hyperparathyroidism

Nonfamilial primary hyperthyroidism resulting from sporadic parathyroid adenomas is associated with mutations of the *MEN1* gene (which encodes menin) or the *cyclinD1/PRAD1* gene (which encodes a key regulator of the cell cycle). In particular, somatic mutation or deletion of both *MEN1* alleles is responsible for about 20% of sporadic adenomas and activating mutations of *cyclinD1* with associated overexpression of the gene product are present in 5% to 40% of adenomas (141,142). Recurring numerical chromosomal abnormalities are also present in up to 73% of adenomas (143–145).

Familial primary hyperparathyroidism is caused by germline mutations in several genes. Mutations in *MEN1* are responsible for MEN1 syndrome, mutations in *RET* are responsible for MEN2A syndrome, and mutations in *HRPT2* are associated with the hyperparathyroidism–jaw tumor syndrome (HPT-JT syndrome, consisting of primary hyperparathyroidism, ossifying fibromas of the maxilla and mandible, and assorted cystic and neoplastic renal abnormalities).

With the exception of the *HRPT2* gene linked to HPT-JT syndrome (discussed below), the mutations in the genes responsible for familial primary hyperthyroidism and sporadic parathyroid adenomas, as well as numerical chromosome abnormalities, are not associated with an increased incidence of parathyroid carcinoma.

Parathyroid Carcinoma

Parathyroid carcinoma is responsible for only about 1% to 2% of cases of primary hyperparathyroidism. Because the tumor usually presents as an ill-defined mass that is densely adherent to the surrounding soft tissues, parathyroid carcinoma has a propensity for local recurrence even after en bloc resection, with associated metastasis to regional lymph nodes and distant sites.

Genetics

A germline mutation that inactivates the *HRPT2* tumor suppressor gene is present in about half of the kindreds

with HPT-JT syndrome (126). The *HRPT2* gene maps to the 1q25 region and encodes the novel protein known as parafibromin, which has an unknown function (146,147). Consistent with the observation that the HPT-JT syndrome is associated with a high incidence of parathyroid carcinoma, *HRPT2* mutations are also present in the majority of patients with apparently sporadic parathyroid carcinoma (146,148,149).

Up to 78% of parathyroid carcinomas show recurring numerical chromosomal abnormalities (143,150), and 33% of carcinomas have been shown to harbor allelic loss of *TP53* (151). Overexpression of other oncogenes has been demonstrated in parathyroid carcinoma; for example, over 90% of tumors overexpress cyclin D1 (152).

Technical Issues in Molecular Genetic Analysis of Parathyroid Carcinoma

Inactivating mutations can be demonstrated in the *HRPT2* gene in 67% to 100% of cases of presumed sporadic parathyroid carcinoma when fresh tissue is the substrate for analysis (148,153). The clonal distribution of the mutations, together with the concordance of mutations between the primary tumor and metastasis in individual patients, supports the hypothesis that *HRPT2* mutations contribute to the oncogenesis of parathyroid carcinomas at an early stage in tumor development. DNA sequence analysis of exons 1, 2, and 7 of *HRPT2* will detect about 80% of mutations. However, because the remaining mutations are not clustered in any specific region, higher sensitivity testing requires analysis of all 17 exons, the flanking intronic sequences, and the 3' and 5' untranslated regions of the gene.

Diagnostic Issues in Molecular Genetic Analysis of Parathyroid Carcinoma

In patients without HPT-JT syndrome, somatic inactivating mutations have been detected in rare cases of parathyroid adenomas, some of which also harbor LOH at the 1q24–32 region (147). Similarly, mutations in *HRPT2* with associated LOH of 1q24–32 have been demonstrated in rare adenomas in patients from kindreds with familial isolated hyperparathyroidism (153). PCR-based microsatellite analysis has also demonstrated LOH of the 1q24–32 region in 9% to 13% of sporadic parathyroid adenomas (154–156). These findings indicate that molecular evidence of an *HRPT2* mutation, LOH at 1q24–32, or even biallelic inactivation of *HRPT2*, is not diagnostic of malignancy in parathyroid neoplasms.

Another complicating feature of mutational analysis of *HRPT2* is the observation that in approximately 30% of cases of presumed sporadic parathyroid carcinoma, the patient actually harbors a germline mutation of the gene (148). This unexpected finding suggests that many sporadic cases of parathyroid carcinoma are actually occult forms of HPT-JT syndrome, a result that has significant implications for the workup of patients diagnosed with parathyroid carcinoma (146,148). It has been suggested that, at the very least, all patients with parathyroid carcinoma should undergo jaw and renal imaging studies, and that, if the additional workup leads to a diagnosis of

HPT-JT syndrome, family members should also undergo detailed screening (146). Mutational analysis of *HRPT2* in all patients with parathyroid carcinoma has also been proposed (146); although analysis of the entire *HRPT2* gene is admittedly quite laborious, identification of a mutation not only establishes the diagnosis of HPT-JP, but also simplifies screening of the patient's family members. For family members shown to be at high risk, periodic testing for hypercalcemia potentially offers the opportunity to detect parathyroid carcinoma at an early stage, but the role of more aggressive prophylaxis, such as subtotal or even total parathyroidectomy, remains unknown (146).

The frequency and pattern of numerical chromosomal abnormalities in parathyroid adenomas and parathyroid hyperplasia shows significant overlap with the frequency and pattern in parathyroid carcinoma (143); therefore, analysis of numerical chromosomal abnormalities cannot be used to distinguish benign from malignant parathyroid proliferations. And although allelic loss of *TP53* or other tumor suppressor genes is present in almost two thirds of parathyroid carcinomas, up to 15% of adenomas and cases of parathyroid hyperplasia also show allelic loss (151,157), findings that suggest that evaluation of allelic loss is also of limited clinical utility for the diagnosis of parathyroid carcinoma.

ADRENAL GLAND

Pheochromocytoma

Pheochromocytoma is often referred to as the "10% tumor" because 10% of cases are malignant, 10% are extra-adrenal, and 10% are hereditary. However, these percentages vary widely in different studies depending on the characteristics of the population evaluated.

Genetics

Although most pheochromocytomas are sporadic, the tumor is a characteristic feature of several cancer syndromes (Table 12.2) that have an autosomal dominate pattern of inheritance, including MEN2A and MEN2B (caused by gain of function mutations in *RET*, as discussed above; Fig. 12.3), von Hippel-Lindau disease (caused by loss of function mutations in *VHL*), neurofibromatosis type 1 (caused by loss of function mutations in *NF1*), and the recently described paraganglioma syndrome type 1 (PGL-1, caused by loss of function mutations in *SDHD* encoding succinate dehydrogenase subunit D) and type 4 (PGL-4, caused by mutations in *SDHB* coding succinate dehydrogenase subunit B) (158–161). The loss of function mutations in *VHL*, *SDHD*, and *SDHB* are thought to promote tumor development through a mechanism that involves activation of hypoxic signaling pathways (162–164).

Technical Issues in Molecular Genetic Analysis of Pheochromocytoma

Molecular analysis shows that approximately 24% of patients who present with a presumed sporadic pheochromocytoma actually harbor a germline mutation in *RET*,

VHL, *SDHD*, or *SDHB*. A recent large study demonstrated that 5% of these patients harbor germline mutations in *RET*, 11% harbor germline mutations in *VHL*, 4% harbor germline mutations in *SDHD*, and 4% harbor germline mutations in *SDHB* (165), results that are in agreement with frequency estimates provided by several earlier smaller studies (158,166,167). Even more astonishing, for patients who present with presumed sporadic disease and a negative family history, up to 84% of multifocal pheochromocytomas (including bilateral tumors), 59% of pheochromocytomas in children 18 years old or younger, and 47% of extra-adrenal tumors are actually hereditary (161,165).

Somatic mutations in the genes responsible for syndromic pheochromocytomas are also present in a minority of true sporadic pheochromocytomas (as confirmed by molecular analysis of germline DNA). Specifically, up to 21% of sporadic pheochromocytomas have a *RET* mutation, about 4% have a *VHL* mutation, and about 6% have an *SDHD* mutation based on analysis of fresh (158,166,168–171) or FFPE tissue (170).

Diagnostic Issues in Molecular Genetic Analysis of Pheochromocytoma

Because the prevalence of mutations in *RET, VHL, SDHD,* and *SDHB* in apparently sporadic pheochromocytomas is so low, DNA sequence analysis of tumor tissue is of little utility from a diagnostic perspective. The analysis of tumor tissue also seems to be unwarranted from a prognostic perspective because specific mutations have not been associated with any clinicopathologic features of disease in true sporadic cases.

Instead, the most useful clinical information is actually obtained from testing somatic tissue, usually peripheral blood (165), because testing for germline mutations can address the question of whether a presumed sporadic pheochromocytoma is actually a manifestation of an occult familial cancer syndrome resulting from a germline mutation in *RET, VHL, SDHD,* or *SDHB* (161,165). Because recent data suggest that distinct clinical features are associated with *SDHD* mutation carriers (e.g., more frequent multifocal head and neck paragangliomas) and *SDHB* mutation carriers (increased frequency of malignant disease, and possibly of extraparaganglial neoplasms) (161), testing for germline mutations can also stratify patients into different prognostic groups.

The fact that almost one quarter of patients who present with apparently sporadic adrenal, extra-adrenal, or thoracic pheochromocytomas or head and neck paragangliomas are carriers of a germline mutation associated with a familial cancer syndrome suggests that there may be a role for genetic screening of all patients with newly diagnosed pheochromocytoma, especially if the tumor is multifocal, if the patient is 18 years old or younger, or if the tumor is extra-adrenal (161,162). From a practical perspective, analysis of *RET* is straightforward because activating mutations cluster within exons 10, 11, and 13–16. However, analysis of *VHL* is more involved because loss of function mutations occur in all three exons of the gene, as well as in splice donor or acceptor sequences (Chapter 17). And, based on the cases that have been described so far,

TABLE 12.2

HEREDITARY SYNDROMES ASSOCIATED WITH PHEOCHROMOCYTOMA

Syndrome	Mutated Gene	Function of Gene	Clinical Components	Risk of Pheochromocytoma (or Paraganglioma)
MEN2A	RET	Receptor tyrosine kinase	Medullary thyroid carcinoma; pheochromocytoma; hyperparathyroidism	50%
MEN2B	RET	Receptor tyrosine kinase	Medullary thyroid carcinoma; pheochromocytoma; hyperparathyroidism; mucosal neuromas; Marfanoid habitus	50%
Familial paraganglioma syndrome type 1	SDHD	Succinate dehydrogenase subunit D	Pheochromocytoma; multifocal paragangliomas	20%–53%[a]
Familial paraganglioma syndrome type 4	SDHB	Succinate dehydrogenase subunit B	Pheochromocytoma; multifocal paragangliomas; increased frequency of malignant paragangliomas	20%–28%[b]
von Hippel-Lindau disease	VHL	Control of cell cycle; targeting of proteins for breakdown; control of expression of genes regulated by cellular oxygen tension	Cerebellar hemangioblastoma; retinal angioma; renal cell carcinoma; renal, pancreatic, and epididymal cysts	14%[c]
Neurofibromatosis-1	NF1	Regulation of RAS/MAPK pathway; regulation of cAMP/PKA pathway? Control of Ca^{++} regulated signaling?	Neurofibromas; café au lait spots	1%

[a]Risk of head and neck paraganglioma is almost 80% (161,165).
[b]Risk of head and neck paraganglioma is over 30% (161,165).
[c]Frequency varies markedly depending on the specific mutation, ranging from 0 to greater than 90%; 14% is the mean (158).

there is no clustering of the mutations in *SDHD* or *SDHB*, and so mutation testing would require analysis of the entire coding region of both (161,165). Consequently, despite the obvious clinical utility, genetic screening for mutations in *RET, VHL, SDHD,* and *SDHB* is not currently feasible.

Adrenocortical Tumors

Genetics

Adrenocortical tumorigenesis is a multistep process in which a number of genetic changes are associated with the progression from normal adrenal tissue to adrenocortical hyperplasia (which is polyclonal) to adrenocortical adenoma (which is usually monoclonal) to adrenocortical carcinoma (ACC, which are mostly monoclonal) (172). However, the fact that so few benign lesions progress to ACC indicates that oncogenesis in adrenocortical cells does not strictly parallel tumor development at other epithelial sites (172).

Mutations in a number of specific proteins have been shown to be involved in adrenocortical tumorigenesis, including p53, insulin-like growth factor type II (IGF2), and endothelin 1 (172). However, the missense mutation R337H in *TP53* that contributes to an inheritable pediatric ACC syndrome (173) is the only specific alteration that has thus far been shown to have independent clinicopathologic significance.

Technical and Diagnostic Issues in Molecular Genetic Analysis of Adrenocortical Tumors

LOH analysis of microsatellites linked to punitive tumor suppressor genes (including *TP53*, the neuroblastoma candidate gene at 1p, *p16, VHL,* and the retinoblastoma gene *RB1*) has shown that LOH of at least one locus is present in about 60% of ACC, but is extremely rare in cortical adenomas or benign cortical tissue (174–176). Because FFPE tissue can be used as the substrate for analysis and there is apparently a 100% concordance rate in the molecular results from paired cytology and FFPE tissue specimens, LOH analysis seems to be well suited for use in routine clinical practice. Nonetheless, the utility of LOH analysis of adrenocortical neoplasms remains unknown for several reasons (177). First, fewer than a dozen adrenal cortical adenomas and cases of adrenal cortical hyperplasia have been evaluated, and thus the accuracy of the estimates of LOH test performance is unclear. Second, the relatively low sensitivity of only 60% for detecting ACC makes the test of questionable diagnostic utility, although it is possible that LOH analysis of additional loci may increase the sensitivity of testing without a significant negative impact on the specificity of testing. Third, as discussed in Chapter 8, the utility of a test also depends on the prevalence of disease in the patient population; an appraisal of the usefulness of LOH analysis must address the fact that the incidence of malignancy is very low in incidental nonfunctioning adrenal nodules commonly discovered during imaging studies. Until these issues are resolved, it is probably premature to rely on LOH analysis to distinguish adrenocortical adenomas from adrenocortical carcinomas (177).

Evaluation of numerical chromosomal aberrations has been shown to be an insensitive method for distinguishing benign from malignant cortical neoplasms (178). Similarly, even though comparative genomic hybridization (CGH) has demonstrated genetic changes that are associated with benign and malignant tumors in both pediatric and adult populations, there is little correlation in the pattern of gains and losses between studies (178,180). CGH may have a basic science role for identifying chromosomal regions that are important for development of ACC, but does not yet have a role in routine clinical practice.

Neuroblastoma

Neuroblastoma is the most common malignancy of children under 5 years old and overall accounts for 8% to 10% of all pediatric malignancies (181). Clinical outcome is associated with the pathologic subtype of the tumor, patient age at diagnosis, clinical stage, and mitosis-karyorrhexis index measure of cellular turnover (182,183), but current morphologic categories and prognostic groupings alone are insufficient to account for the diversity in clinical outcome. Consequently, molecular genetic analysis has a role at the time of diagnosis for stratifying patients into appropriate treatment groupings, as well as for providing additional tumor-specific prognostic information. Current standard of care molecular testing includes DNA index and *MYCN* amplification status (182,184), but a number of additional markers are under evaluation to see if they can provide additional clinically relevant information (185,187).

Technical Issues in Molecular Genetic Analysis of Neuroblastoma

MYCN

Amplification of *MYCN* is present in about 25% of neuroblastomas and is associated with an aggressive clinical course (188,189). *MYCN* amplification can be detected cytogenetically as extrachromosomal double-minute and homogenously staining regions (190,191), although analysis of tumor specimens is usually performed on fresh or frozen tissue by Southern blot hybridization, FISH (Fig. 12.4), or PCR (192–197). In many cases, chromosomal segments adjacent to *MYCN* are also amplified, but it remains unclear whether any of these other genes contribute to the oncogenesis of neuroblastoma, the maintenance of the amplified DNA, or prognosis (185,198). Parenthetically, from a diagnostic perspective, it is important to recognize that *MYCN* amplification is not specific for neuroblastoma but has been also described in rare cases of alveolar rhabdomyosarcoma, another malignant round cell tumor of children (199,200).

DNA Index

The nuclear DNA content (ploidy) of tumor cells correlates with outcome (201–203). Diploid tumors tend to have a high proliferative activity (201), while tumors with an aneuploid (hyperdiploid) stem line and low percentage of cells in the S, G2, and M phases of the cell cycle tend to be associated with a favorable prognosis.

Cytogenetic Aberrations

Several cytogenetic aberrations other than those associated with *MYCN* amplification have also been shown to have prognostic implications. Allelic loss of the short arm of chromosome 1 is associated with an unfavorable outcome (204), but there is considerable diversity in the 1p regions that are deleted, which suggests that a single gene is not responsible for the adverse clinical effect (185).

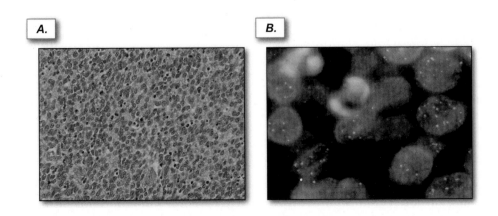

A.   **B.**

Figure 12.4 Example of *MYCN* amplification in neuroblastoma. **A,** A poorly differentiated neuroblastoma from a 4-year-old girl who presented with an adrenal mass. The tumor had a high mitosis-karyorrhexis index. **B,** FISH analysis using a probe for *MYCN* demonstrates high-level amplification of the gene. (Courtesy Drs. Ashley Hill and Arie Perry, Washington University School of Medicine, St. Louis, MO.) (See color insert.)

Unbalanced gain of the long arm of chromosome 17 is also common in neuroblastomas, often as an unbalanced translocation. Gain of 17q is associated with an unfavorable outcome independent of disease stage, patient age at diagnosis, and *MYCN* amplification (205); the segmental gains usually span about 20 mb, but the specific loci that are responsible for the adverse prognosis have not been identified. Interphase FISH is a sensitive and specific method for evaluating 17q allelic status, and spectral karyotyping (SKY) has also been used to identify gain of 17q (206). Recently, quantitative PCR has been shown to be an extremely sensitive and specific method for detecting even single copy chromosome 17 gain, although tumor heterogeneity and inherit complexity in the rearrangements that cause unbalanced gain of 17q may limit analysis of individual neuroblastomas (207).

Other cytogenetic abnormalities that have been associated with a worse prognosis include deletion of the short arm of chromosome 11 in tumors without *MYCN* amplification, and loss of heterozygosity of the long arm of chromosome 2. Loss of heterozygosity of 3p, 11q, and 14q has been associated with an intermediate prognosis, while loss of heterozygosity for the 19q13 region has been shown in multivariate analysis to be associated with tumor recurrence. Nonetheless, a clinical role for testing directed at demonstrating the presence of any of these gross structural aberrations has yet to be established, and the specific genetic loci responsible for the differences in prognosis remain to be identified (186,206).

TrkA Expression

Development of the synpathoadrenal cell lineage depends on the interaction of a number of different neurotrophins with cell receptors that have tyrosine kinase activity including TrkA, TrkB, and TrkC, and the TrkA receptor is normally also found on most mature neurons in sympathetic ganglia (208). Lack of expression of functional TrkA by neuroblastoma tumor cells is an independent predictor of a poor prognosis (209–212), and high expression is associated with a favorable outcome (212). However, neuroblastoma classification schemes that incorporate the expression status of neurotrophin receptors still do not adequately account for the wide diversity in natural history and treatment outcome (185).

Other Markers

Expression of a number of other tumor markers is correlated with the natural history of neuroblastoma and treatment outcome. For example, telomerase activity and telomerase subunit gene expression patterns are correlated with a poor outcome (213). Expression of bcl-2 (which suppresses apoptosis) is associated with *MYCN* amplification, unfavorable tumor histology, and poor prognosis (214). RT-PCR–based analysis of tissue-specific gene expression of tyrosine hydroxylase and doublecortin has been used to detect submicroscopic disease dissemination and minimal residual disease in patients with neuroblastoma (215–217), which, in at least one study, has been shown to be an independent poor prognostic indicator in a subgroup of patients (218). However, molecular genetic analysis of any of these markers is not a routine part of the pathologic eval-

uation of tumor specimens because none have a well-established role in the classification of neuroblastoma into clinically and biologically relevant subtypes.

Because multiple pathways are likely to be involved in the oncogenesis of neuroblastoma, surveys of gene expression profiles may ultimately identify patterns of transcription that can be used to optimize patient classification (185). Similarly, mutational analysis of groups of genes, rather than analysis of individual loci, may prove to be more highly correlated with clinical outcome. However, at present, these methods are experimental and have no role in the routine evaluation of neuroblastoma.

REFERENCES

1. Rosai J, Carcangiu ML, Delellis RA, eds. *Tumors of the Thyroid Gland*, Third Series, Fascicle 5. Washington, DC: Armed Forces Institute of Pathology, 1992.
2. LiVolsi VA. *Surgical Pathology of the Thyroid*. Philadelphia, W.B. Saunders, 1990.
3. Smanik PA, Furminger TL, Mazzaferri EL, et al. Breakpoint characterization of the ret/PTC oncogene in human papillary thyroid carcinoma. *Hum Mol Genet* 1995;4:2313–2318.
4. Giannini R, Salvatore G, Monaco C, et al. Identification of a novel subtype of H4-RET rearrangement in a thyroid papillary carcinoma and lymph node metastasis. *Int J Oncol* 2000;16:485–489.
5. Elisei R, Romei C, Soldatenko P, et al. New breakpoints in both the H4 and RET genes create a variant of PTC-1 in a post-Chernobyl papillary thyroid carcinoma. *Clin Endocrinol (Oxf)* 2000;53:131–136.
6. Santoro M, Dathan NA, Berlingieri MT, et al. Molecular characterization of RET/PTC3; a novel rearranged version of the RET proto-oncogene in a human thyroid papillary carcinoma. *Oncogene* 1994;9:509–516.
7. Fugazzola L, Pierotti MA, Vigano E, et al. Molecular and biochemical analysis of RET/PTC4, a novel oncogenic rearrangement between RET and ELE1 genes, in a post-Chernobyl papillary thyroid cancer. *Oncogene* 1996;13:1093–1097.
8. Klugbauer S, Demidchik EP, Lengfelder E, et al. Molecular analysis of new subtypes of ELE/RET rearrangements, their reciprocal transcripts and breakpoints in papillary thyroid carcinomas of children after Chernobyl. *Oncogene* 1998;16:671–675.
9. Klugbauer S, Demidchik EP, Lengfelder E, et al. Detection of a novel type of RET rearrangement (PTC5) in thyroid carcinomas after Chernobyl and analysis of the involved RET-fused gene RFG5. *Cancer Res* 1998;58:198–203.
10. Klugbauer S, Rabes HM. The transcription coactivator HTIF1 and a related protein are fused to the RET receptor tyrosine kinase in childhood papillary thyroid carcinomas. *Oncogene* 1999;18:4388–4393.
11. Salassidis K, Bruch J, Zitzelsberger H, et al. Translocation t(10;14)(q11.2:q22.1) fusing the kinetin to the RET gene creates a novel rearranged form (PTC8) of the RET proto-oncogene in radiation-induced childhood papillary thyroid carcinoma. *Cancer Res* 2000;60:2786–2789.
12. Klugbauer S, Jauch A, Lengfelder E, et al. A novel type of RET rearrangement (PTC8) in childhood papillary thyroid carcinomas and characterization of the involved gene (RFG8). *Cancer Res* 2000;60:7028–7032.
13. Corvi R, Berger N, Balczon R, et al. RET/PCM-1: a novel fusion gene in papillary thyroid carcinoma. *Oncogene* 2000;19:4236–4242.
14. Yokota T, Nakata T, Minami S, et al. Genomic organization and chromosomal mapping of ELKS, a gene rearranged in a papillary thyroid carcinoma. *J Hum Genet* 2000;45:6–11.
15. Saenko V, Rogounovitch T, Shimizu-Yoshida Y, et al. Novel tumorigenic rearrangement, Delta rfp/ret, in a papillary thyroid carcinoma from externally irradiated patient. *Mutat Res* 2003;527:81–90.
16. Butti MG, Bongarzone I, Ferraresi G, et al. A sequence analysis of the genomic regions involved in the rearrangements between TPM3 and NTRK1 genes producing TRK oncogenes in papillary thyroid carcinomas. *Genomics* 1995;28:15–24.
17. Greco A, Mariani C, Miranda C, et al. The DNA rearrangement that generates the TRK-T3 oncogene involves a novel gene on chromosome 3 whose product has a potential coiled-coil domain. *Mol Cell Biol* 1995;15:6118–6127.
18. Beimfohr C, Klugbauer S, Demidchik EP, et al. NTRK1 re-arrangement in papillary thyroid carcinomas of children after the Chernobyl reactor accident. *Int J Cancer* 1999;80:842–847.
19. Nikiforova MN, Stringer JR, Blough R, et al. Proximity of chromosomal loci that participate in radiation-induced rearrangements in human cells. *Science* 2000;290:138–141.
20. Pierotti MA. Chromosomal rearrangements in thyroid carcinomas: a recombination or death dilemma. *Cancer Lett* 2001;166:1–7.
21. Bongarzone I, Vigneri P, Mariani L, et al. RET/NTRK1 rearrangements in thyroid gland tumors of the papillary carcinoma family: correlation with clinicopathological features. *Clin Cancer Res* 1998;4:223–228.
22. Alberti L, Carniti C, Miranda C, et al. RET and NTRK1 proto-oncogenes in human diseases. *J Cell Physiol* 2003;195:168–186.
23. Rabes HM. Gene rearrangements in radiation-induced thyroid carcinogenesis. *Med Pediatr Oncol* 2001;36:574–582.
24. Russell JP, Powell DJ, Cunnane M, et al. The TRK-T1 fusion protein induces neoplastic transformation of thyroid epithelium. *Oncogene* 2000;19:5729–5735.
25. Santoro M, Thomas GA, Vecchio G, et al. Gene rearrangement and Chernobyl related thyroid cancers. *Br J Cancer* 2000;82:315–322.
26. Santoro M, Papotti M, Chiappetta G, et al. RET activation and clinicopathologic features in poorly differentiated thyroid tumors: RET activation and clinicopathologic features in poorly differentiated thyroid tumors. *J Clin Endocrinol Metab* 2002;87:370–379.

27. Hunt JL. Molecular mutations in thyroid carcinogenesis. *Am J Clin Pathol* 2002;118(suppl):S116–S127.
28. Tallini G. Molecular pathobiology of thyroid neoplasms. *Endocr Pathol* 2002;13:271–288.
29. Tallini G, Asa SL. *RET* oncogene activation in papillary thyroid carcinoma. *Adv Anat Pathol* 2001;8:345–354.
30. Rabes HM, Demidchik EP, Sidorow JD, et al. Pattern of radiation-induced *RET* and *NTRK1* rearrangements in 191 post-chernobyl papillary thyroid carcinomas: biological, phenotypic, and clinical implications. *Clin Cancer Res* 2000;6:1093–1103.
31. Cinti R, Yin L, Ilc K, et al. RET rearrangements in papillary thyroid carcinomas and adenomas detected by interphase FISH. *Cytogenet Cell Genet* 2000;88:56–61.
32. Rhoden KJ, Johnson C, Brandao G, et al. Real-time quantitative RT-PCR identifies distinct *c-RET*, *RET/PTC1* and *RET/PTC3* expression patterns in papillary thyroid carcinoma. *Lab Invest* 2004;84:1557–1570.
33. Basolo F, Molinaro E, Agate L, et al. RET protein expression has no prognostic impact on the long-term outcome of papillary thyroid carcinoma. *Eur J Endocrinol* 2001; 145:599–604.
34. Basolo F, Giannini R, Monaco C, et al. Potent mitogenicity of the *RET/PTC3* oncogene correlates with its prevalence in tall-cell variant of papillary thyroid carcinoma. *Am J Pathol* 2002;160:247–254.
35. Chung JH, Hahm JR, Min YK, et al. Detection of *RET/PTC* oncogene rearrangements in Korean papillary thyroid carcinomas. *Thyroid* 1999;9:1237–1243.
36. Sugg SL, Ezzat S, Rosen IB, et al. Distinct multiple *RET/PTC* gene rearrangements in multifocal papillary thyroid neoplasia. *J Clin Endocrinol Metab* 1998;83:4116–4122.
37. Puxeddu E, Fagin JA. Genetic markers in thyroid neoplasia. *Endocrinol Metab Clin North Am* 2001;30:493–513.
38. Bongarzone I, Pierotti MA. The molecular basis of thyroid epithelial tumorigenesis. *Tumori* 2003;89:514–516.
39. Japon MA, Urbano AG, Saez C, et al. Glial-derived neurotropic factor and *RET* gene expression in normal human anterior pituitary cell types and in pituitary tumors. *J Clin Endocrinol Metab* 2002;87:1879–1884.
40. Tallini G, Santoro M, Helie M, et al. *RET/PTC* oncogene activation defines a subset of papillary thyroid carcinomas lacking evidence of progression to poorly differentiated or undifferentiated tumor phenotypes. *Clin Cancer Res* 1998;4:287–294.
41. Miyaki M, Iijima T, Ishii R, et al. Molecular evidence for multicentric development of thyroid carcinomas in patients with familial adenomatous polyposis. *Am J Pathol* 2000;157:1825–1827.
42. Chiappetta G, Toti P, Cetta F, et al. The *RET/PTC* oncogene is frequently activated in oncocytic thyroid tumors (Hurthle cell adenomas and carcinomas), but not in oncocytic hyperplastic lesions. *J Clin Endocrinol Metab* 2002;87:364–369.
43. Nikiforova MN, Caudill CM, Biddinger P, et al. Prevalence of *RET/PTC* rearrangements in Hashimoto's thyroiditis and papillary thyroid carcinomas. *Int J Surg Pathol* 2002;10:15–22.
44. Wirtschafter A, Schmidt R, Rosen D, et al. Expression of the *RET/PTC* fusion gene as a marker for papillary carcinoma in Hashimoto's thyroiditis. *Laryngoscope* 1997; 107:95–100.
45. Sheils OM, O'Leary JJ, Uhlmann V, et al. *ret/PTC-1* activation in Hashimoto thyroiditis. *Int J Surg Pathol* 2000;8:185–189.
46. Fusco A, Chiappetta G, Hui P, et al. Assessment of *RET/PTC* oncogene activation and clonality in thyroid nodules with incomplete morphological evidence of papillary carcinoma: a search for the early precursors of papillary cancer. *Am J Pathol* 2002;160:2157–2167.
47. Kjellman P, Learoyd DL, Messina M, et al. Expression of the *RET* proto-oncogene in papillary thyroid carcinoma and its correlation with clinical outcome. *Br J Surg* 2001;88:557–563.
48. Davies H, Bignell GR, Cox C, et al. Mutations of the *BRAF* gene in human cancer. *Nature* 2002;417:949–954.
49. Soares P, Trovisco V, Rocha AS, et al. *BRAF* mutations and *RET/PTC* rearrangements are alternative events in the etiopathogenesis of PTC. *Oncogene* 2003;22:4578–4580.
50. Sugg SL, Ezzat S, Zheng L, et al. Oncogene profile of papillary thyroid carcinoma. *Surgery* 1999;125:46–452.
51. Puxeddu E, Moretti S, Elisei R, et al. *BRAF(V599E)* mutation is the leading genetic event in adult sporadic papillary thyroid carcinomas. *J Clin Endocrinol Metab* 2004; 89:2414–2420.
52. Fukushima T, Suzuki S, Mashiko M, et al. *BRAF* mutations in papillary carcinomas of the thyroid. *Oncogene* 2003;22:6455–6457.
53. Kimura ET, Nikiforova MN, Zhu Z, et al. High prevalence of *BRAF* mutations in thyroid cancer: genetic evidence for constitutive activation of the RET/PTC-RAS-BRAF signaling pathway in papillary thyroid carcinoma. *Cancer Res* 2003;63:1454–1457.
54. Nikiforova MN, Kimura ET, Gahndhi M, et al. BRAF mutations in thyroid tumors are restricted to papillary carcinomas and anaplastic or poorly differentiated carcinomas arising from papillary carcinomas. *J Clin Endocrinol Metab* 2003;88:5399–5404.
55. Namba H, Nakashima M, Hayashi T, et al. Clinical implication of hot spot *BRAF* mutation, *V599E*, in papillary thyroid cancers. *J Clin Endocrinol Metab* 2003;88:4393–4397.
56. Begum S, Rosenbaum E, Henrique R, et al. *BRAF* mutations in anaplastic thyroid carcinoma: implications for tumor origin, diagnosis and treatment. *Mod Pathol* 2004; 17:1359–1363.
57. Tuveson DA, Weber BL, Herlyn M. *BRAF* as a potential therapeutic target in melanoma and other malignancies. *Cancer Cell* 2003;4:95–98.
58. Bollag G, Freeman S, Lyons JF, et al. Raf pathway inhibitors in oncology. *Curr Opin Investig Drugs* 2003;4:1436–1441.
59. Salvatore D, Celetti A, Fabien N, et al. Low frequency of *p53* mutations in human thyroid tumours; *p53* and *Ras* mutation in two out of fifty-six thyroid tumours. *Eur J Endocrinol* 1996;134:177–183.
60. Nikiforov YE, Nikiforova MN, Gnepp Dr, et al. Prevalence of mutations of *ras* and *p53* in benign and malignant thyroid tumors from children exposed to radiation after the Chernobyl nuclear accident. *Oncogene* 1996;13:687–693.
61. Suchy B, Waldmann V, Klugbauer S, et al. Absence of *RAS* and *p53* mutations in thyroid carcinomas of children after Chernobyl in contrast to adult thyroid tumours. *Br J Cancer* 1998;77:952–955.
62. Kitamura Y, Shimizu K, Tanaka S, et al. Association of allelic loss on 1q, 4p, 7q, 9p, 9q, and 16q with postoperative death in papillary thyroid carcinoma. *Clin Cancer Res* 2000;6:1819–1825.
63. Gillespie JW, Nasir A, Kaiser HE. Loss of heterozygosity in papillary and follicular thyroid carcinoma: a mini review. *In Vivo* 2000;14:139–140.
64. Esapa CT, Johnson SJ, Kendall-Taylor P, et al. Prevalence of Ras mutations in thyroid neoplasia. *Clin Endocrinol (Oxf)* 1999;50:529–535.
65. Shi YF, Zou MJ, Schmidt H, et al. High rates of ras codon 61 mutation in thyroid tumors in an iodide-deficient area. *Cancer Res* 1991;51:2690–2693.
66. Ho YS, Tseng SC, Chin TY, et al. *p53* gene mutation in thyroid carcinoma. *Cancer Lett* 1996;103:57–63.
67. Wasenius VM, Hemmer S, Karjalainen-Lindsberg ML, et al. MET receptor tyrosine kinase sequence alterations in differentiated thyroid carcinoma. *Am J Surg Pathol* 2005;29:544–549.
68. Zhu Z, Gandhi M, Nikiforova MN, et al. Molecular profile and clinical-pathologic features of the follicular variant of papillary thyroid carcinoma: an unusually high prevalence of *ras* mutations. *Am J Clin Pathol* 2003;120:71–77.
69. De Micco C, Vasko V, Ferrand M, et al. N-*ras* oncogene mutations in the follicular variant of papillary thyroid carcinomas. *Cancer Detect Prev* 2000;24(S1):S74.
70. Nikiforov YE, Rowland JM, Bove KE, et al. Distinct pattern of *ret* oncogene rearrangements in morphological variants of radiation-induced and sporadic thyroid papillary carcinomas in children. *Cancer Res* 1997;57:1690–1694.
71. Thomas GA, Bunnell H, Cook HA, et al. High prevalence of *RET/PTC* rearrangements in Ukrainian and Belarussian post-Chernobyl thyroid papillary carcinomas: a strong correlation between *RET/PTC3* and the solid-follicular variant. *J Clin Endocrinol Metab*; 84:4232–4238.
72. Trovisco V, de Castro IV, Soares P, et al. *BRAF* mutations are associated with some histological types of papillary thyroid carcinoma. *J Pathol* 2004; 202: 247–251.
73. Harach HR, Williams GT, Williams ED. Familial adenomatous polyposis associated thyroid carcinoma: a distinct type of follicular cell neoplasm. *Histopathology* 1994; 25:549–561.
74. Cetta F, Toti P, Petracci M, et al. Thyroid carcinoma associated with familial adenomatous polyposis. *Histopathology* 1997;31:231–236.
75. Baloch ZW, LiVolsi VA. Follicular-patterned lesions of the thyroid: the bane of the pathologist. *Am J Clin Pathol* 2002;117:143–150.
76. Kroll TG, Sarraf P, Pecciarini L, et al. *PAX8-PPARγ1* fusion oncogene in human thyroid carcinoma. *Science* 2000;289:1357–1360.
77. Marques AR, Espadinha C, Catarino AL, et al. Expression of *PAX8-PPARγ1* rearrangements in both follicular thyroid carcinomas and adenomas. *J Clin Endocrinol Metab* 2002;87:3947–3952.
78. Mansouri A, Chowdhury K, Gruss P. Follicular cells of the thyroid gland require *Pax8* gene function. *Nat Genet* 1998;19:87–90.
79. Fajas L, Auboeuf D, Raspe E. The organization, promoter analysis, and expression of the human *PPARγ gene*. *J Biol Chem* 1997;272:18779–18789.
80. Cheung L, Messina M, Gill A, et al. Detection of the *PAX8-PPARγ* fusion oncogene in both follicular thyroid carcinomas and adenomas. *J Clin Endocrinol Metab* 2003; 88:354–357.
81. Dwight T, Thoppe SR, Foukakis T, et al. Involvement of the PAX8/peroxisome proliferator-activated receptor gamma rearrangement in follicular thyroid tumors. *J Clin Endocrinol Metab* 2003;88:4440–4445.
82. Nikiforova MN, Biddinger PW, Caudill CM, et al. *PAX8-PPARγ* rearrangement in thyroid tumors: RT-PCR and immunohistochemical analyses. *Am J Surg Pathol* 2002; 26:1016–1023.
83. Gimm O. Thyroid cancer. *Cancer Lett* 2001;163:143–156.
84. Hunt JL, Livolsi VA, Baloch ZW, et al. A novel microdissection and genotyping of follicular-derived thyroid tumors to predict aggressiveness. *Hum Pathol* 2003;34: 375–380.
85. Capella G, Matias-Guiu X, Ampudia X, et al. *Ras* oncogene mutations in thyroid tumors: polymerase chain reaction-restriction-fragment-length polymorphism analysis from paraffin-embedded tissues. *Diagn Mol Pathol* 1996;5:45–52.
86. Ezzat S, Zheng L, Kolenda J, et al. Prevalence of activating *ras* mutations in morphologically characterized thyroid nodules. *Thyroid* 1996;6:409–416.
87. Esapa CT, Johnson SJ, Kendall-Taylor P, et al. Prevalence of *RAS* mutations in thyroid neoplasia. *Clin Endocrinol (Oxf)* 1999;50:529–535.
88. Vasko V, Ferrand M, Di Cristofaro J, et al. Specific pattern of *RAS* oncogene mutations in follicular thyroid tumors. *J Clin Endocrinol Metab* 2003;88:2745–2752.
89. Hunt JL, Yim JH, Tometsko M, et al. Loss of heterozygosity of the *VHL* gene identifies malignancy and predicts death in follicular thyroid tumors. *Surgery* 2003;134: 1043–1047.
90. Santoro M, Melillo RM, Carlomagno F, et al. Molecular biology of the *MEN2* gene. *J Intern Med* 1998;243:505–508.
91. Hoppner W, Ritter MM. A duplication of 12 bp in the critical cysteine rich domain of the *RET* proto-oncogene results in a distinct phenotype of multiple endocrine neoplasia type 2A. *Hum Mol Genet* 1997;6:587–590.
92. Hoppner W, Dralle H, Brabant G. Duplication of 9 base pairs in the critical cysteine-rich domain of the *RET* proto-oncogene causes multiple endocrine neoplasia type 2A. *Hum Mutat* 1998;Suppl 1:S128–SS130.
93. Pigny P, Bauters C, Wemeau JL, et al. A novel 9-base pair duplication in *RET* exon 8 in familial medullary thyroid carcinoma. *J Clin Endocrinol Metab* 1999;84:1700–1704.
94. van der Harst E, de Krijger RR, Bruining HA, et al. Prognostic value of p53, bcl-2, and c-erbB-2 protein expression in phaeochromocytomas. *J Pathol* 1999;188:51–55.
95. Schilling T, Burck J, Sinn HP, et al. Prognostic value of codon 918 (ATG→ACG) *RET* proto-oncogene mutations in sporadic medullary thyroid carcinoma. *Int J Cancer* 2001;95:62–66.
96. Eng C, Mulligan LM, Healey CS, et al. Heterogeneous mutation of the *RET* proto-oncogene in subpopulations of medullary thyroid carcinoma. *Cancer Res* 1996;56:2167–2170.
97. Feldman GL, Edmonds MW, Ainsworth PJ, et al. Variable expressivity of familial medullary thyroid carcinoma (FMTC) due to a *RET V804M* (GTGSATG) mutation. *Surgery* 2000;128:93–98.
98. Brauckhoff M, Gimm O, Hinze R, et al. Papillary thyroid carcinoma in patients with *RET* proto-oncogene germline mutation. *Thyroid* 2002;12:557–561.
99. Rey JM, Brouillet JP, Fonteneau-Allaire J, et al. Novel germline *RET* mutation segregating with papillary thyroid carcinomas. *Genes Chromosomes Cancer* 2001;32:390–391.

100. Reynolds L, Jones K, Winton DJ, et al. C-cell and thyroid epithelial tumours and altered follicular development in transgenic mice expressing the long isoform of *MEN 2A RET*. *Oncogene* 2001;20:3986–3994.
101. Zedenius J, Larsson C, Bergholm U, et al. Mutations of codon 918 in the *RET* proto-oncogene correlate to poor prognosis in sporadic medullary thyroid carcinomas. *J Clin Endocrinol Metab* 1995;80:3088–3090.
102. Sheikh HA, Tometsko M, Niehouse L, et al. Molecular genotyping of medullary thyroid carcinoma can predict tumor recurrence. *Am J Surg Pathol* 2004;28:101–106.
103. Learoyd DL, Messina M, Zedenius J, et al. Molecular genetics of thyroid tumors and surgical decision-making. *World J Surg* 2000;24:923–933.
104. Gimm O, Sutter T, Dralle H. Diagnosis and therapy of sporadic and familial medullary thyroid carcinoma. *J Cancer Res Clin Oncol* 2001;127:156–165.
105. Niccoli-sire P, Murat A, Rohmer V, et al. Familial medullary thyroid carcinoma with noncysteine *ret* mutations: phenotype-genotype relationship in a large series of patients. *J Clin Endocrinol Metab* 2001;86:3746–3753.
106. Alsanea O, Clark OH. Familial thyroid cancer. *Curr Opin Oncol* 2001;13:44–51.
107. Canzian F, Amati P, Harach R, et al. A gene predisposing to familial thyroid tumors with cell oxyphilia maps to chromosome 19p13.2. *Am J Hum Genet* 1998;63:1743–1748.
108. Cameselle-Teijeiro J, Chan JK. Cribriform-morular variant of papillary carcinoma: a distinctive variant representing the sporadic counterpart of familial adenomatous polyposis-associated thyroid carcinoma? *Mod Pathol* 1999;12:400–411.
109. Cetta F, Curia MC, Montalto G, et al. Thyroid carcinoma usually occurs in patients with familial adenomatous polyposis in the absence of biallelic inactivation of the adenomatous polyposis coli gene. *J Clin Endocrinol Metab* 2001;86:427–432.
110. Liaw D, Marsh DJ, Li J, et al. Germline mutations of the *PTEN* gene in Cowden disease, an inherited breast and thyroid cancer syndrome. *Nat Genet* 1997;16:64–67.
111. Halachmi N, Halachmi S, Evron E, et al. Somatic mutations of the *PTEN* tumor suppressor gene in sporadic follicular thyroid tumors. *Genes Chromosomes Cancer* 1998; 23:239–243.
112. Dahia PL, Marsh DJ, Zheng Z, et al. Somatic deletions and mutations in the Cowden disease gene, *PTEN*, in sporadic thyroid tumors. *Cancer Res* 1997;57:4710–4713.
113. Bruni P, Boccia A, Baldassarre G, et al. *PTEN* expression is reduced in a subset of sporadic thyroid carcinomas: evidence that *PTEN*-growth suppressing activity in thyroid cancer cells mediated by p27kip1. *Oncogene* 2000;19:3146–3155.
114. Gimm O, Perren A, Weng LP, et al. Differential nuclear and cytoplasmic expression of *PTEN* in normal thyroid tissue, and benign and malignant epithelial thyroid tumors. *Am J Pathol* 2000;156:1693–1700.
115. Stankov K, Pastore A, Toschi L, et al. Allelic loss on chromosomes 2q21 and 19p 13.2 in oxyphilic thyroid tumors. *Int J Cancer* 2004;111:463–467.
116. Bevan S, Pal T, Greenberg CR, et al. A comprehensive analysis of MNG1, TCO1, fPTC, PTEN, TSHR, and TRKA in familial nonmedullary thyroid cancer: confirmation of linkage to TCO1. *J Clin Endocrinol Metab* 2001;86:3701–3704.
117. Wiseman SM, Loree TR, Rigual NR, et al. Anaplastic transformation of thyroid cancer: review of clinical, pathologic, and molecular evidence provides new insights into disease biology and future therapy. *Head Neck* 2003;25:662–670.
118. Pasieka JL. Anaplastic thyroid cancer. *Curr Opin Oncol* 2003;15:78–83.
119. Asakawa H, Kobayashi T. Multistep carcinogenesis in anaplastic thyroid carcinoma: a case report. *Pathology* 2002;34:94–97.
120. Wiseman SM, Loree TR, Hicks WL Jr., et al. Anaplastic thyroid cancer evolved from papillary carcinoma: demonstration of anaplastic transformation by means of the inter-simple sequence repeat polymerase chain reaction. *Arch Otolaryngol Head Neck Surg* 2003; 129:96–100.
121. Hunt JL, Tometsko M, LiVolsi VA, et al. Molecular evidence of anaplastic transformation in coexisting well-differentiated and anaplastic carcinomas of the thyroid. *Am J Surg Pathol* 2003;27:1559–1564.
122. Garcia-Rostan G, Camp RL, Herrero A, et al. Beta-catenin dysregulation in thyroid neoplasms: down-regulation, aberrant nuclear expression, and CTNNB1 exon 3 mutations are markers for aggressive tumor phenotypes and poor prognosis. *Am J Pathol* 2001;158:987–996.
123. Sparks AB, Morin PJ, Vogelstein B, et al. Mutational analysis of the APC/beta-catenin/Tcf pathway in colorectal cancer. *Cancer Res* 1998;58:1130–1134.
124. Miller JR, Hocking AM, Brown JD, et al. Mechanism and function of signal transduction by the Wnt/beta-catenin and Wnt/Ca2+ pathways. *Oncogene* 1999;18:7860–7872.
125. Carney JA, Ryan J, Goellner JR. Hyalinizing trabecular adenoma of the thyroid gland. *Am J Surg Pathol* 1987;11:583–591.
126. Rothenberg JN, Goellner JR, Carney JA. Hyalinizing trabecular adenoma of the thyroid gland: recognition and characterization of its cytoplasmic yellow body. *Am J Surg Pathol* 1999;23:118–125.
127. Hirokawa M, Carney JA. Cell membrane and cytoplasmic staining for MIB-1 in hyalinizing trabecular adenoma of the thyroid gland. *Am J Surg Pathol* 2000; 24:575–578.
128. Lloyd RV. Hyalinizing trabecular tumors of the thyroid: a variant of papillary carcinoma? *Adv Anat Pathol* 2002;9:7–11.
129. LiVolsi VA. Hyalinizing trabecular tumor of the thyroid: adenoma, carcinoma, or neoplasm of uncertain malignant potential? *Am J Surg Pathol* 2000;24:1683–1684.
130. Papotti M, Volante M, Giuliano A, et al. *RET/PTC* activation in hyalinizing trabecular tumors of the thyroid. *Am J Surg Pathol* 2000;24:1615–1621.
131. Cheung CC, Boerner SL, MacMillan CM, et al. Hyalinizing trabecular tumor of the thyroid: a variant of papillary carcinoma proved by molecular genetics. *Am J Surg Pathol* 2000;24:1622–1626.
132. Cheung CC, Ezzat S, Ramyar L, et al. Molecular basis of Hurthle cell papillary thyroid carcinoma. *J Clin Endocrinol Metab* 2000;85:878–882.
133. Maximo V, Soares P, Lima J, et al. Mitochondrial DNA somatic mutations (point mutations and large deletions) and mitochondrial DNA variants in human thyroid pathology: a study with emphasis on Hurthle cell tumors. *Am J Pathol* 2002;160:1857–1865.
134. Lewis PD, Baxter P, Griffiths A, et al. Detection of damage to the mitochondrial genome in the oncocytic cells of Warthin's tumour. *J Pathol* 2000;191:274–281.
135. Maximo V, Soares P, Rocha AS, et al. The common deletion of mitochondrial DNA is found in goiters and thyroid tumors with and without oxyphil cell change. *Ultrastruct Pathol* 1998;22:271–273.
136. Muller-Hocker J, Jacob U, Seibel P. Hashimoto thyroiditis is associated with defects of cytochrome-c oxidase in oxyphil Askanazy cells and with the common deletion (4,977) of mitochondrial DNA. *Ultrastruct Pathol* 1998;22:91–100.
137. Muller-Hocker J. Random cytochrome-C-oxidase deficiency of oxyphil cell nodules in the parathyroid gland: A mitochondrial cytopathy related to cell ageing? *Pathol Res Pract* 1992;188:701–706.
138. Tallini G, Ladanyi M, Rosai J, et al. Analysis of nuclear and mitochondrial DNA alterations in thyroid and renal oncocytic tumors. *Cytogenet Cell Genet* 1994;66:253–259.
139. Holm LE, Blomgren H, Lowhagen T. Cancer risks in patients with chronic lymphocytic thyroiditis. *N Engl J Med* 1985;312:601–604.
140. Hill DA, O'Sullivan MJ, Zhu X, et al. Practical application of molecular genetic testing as an aid to the surgical pathologic diagnosis of sarcomas: a prospective study. *Am J Surg Pathol* 2002;26:965–977.
141. Arnold A, Shattuck TM, Mallya SM, et al. Molecular pathogenesis of primary hyperparathyroidism. *J Bone Miner Res* 2002;17(suppl 2):N30–N36.
142. Harach HR. Chapter 7. The parathyroid gland. In: Stefaneanu L, Sasano H, Kovacs K, eds. *Molecular and Cellular Endocrine Pathology*. New York: Oxford University Press; 2000.
143. Erickson LA, Jalal SM, Harwood A, et al. Analysis of parathyroid neoplasms by interphase fluorescence in situ hybridization. *Am J Surg Pathol* 2004;28:578–584.
144. Garcia JL, Tardio JC, Gutierrez NC, et al. Chromosomal imbalances identified by comparative genomic hybridization in sporadic parathyroid adenomas. *Eur J Endocrinol* 2002;146:209–213.
145. Palanisamy N, Imanishi Y, Rao PH, et al. Novel chromosomal abnormalities identified by comparative genomic hybridization in parathyroid adenomas. *J Clin Endocrinol Metab* 1998;83:1766–1770.
146. Weinstein LS, Simonds WF. *HRPT2*, a marker of parathyroid cancer. *N Engl J Med* 2003;349:1691–1692.
147. Carpten JD, Robbins CM, Villablanca A, et al. *HRPT2*, encoding parafibromin, is mutated in hyperparathyroidism-jaw tumor syndrome. *Nat Genet* 2002;32:676–680.
148. Shattuck TM, Valimaki S, Obara T, et al. Somatic and germ-line mutations of the *HRPT2* gene in sporadic parathyroid carcinoma. *N Engl J Med* 2003;349:1722–1729.
149. Cavaco BM, Guerra L, Bradley KJ, et al. Hyperparathyroidism-jaw tumor syndrome in Roma families from Portugal is due to a founder mutation of the *HRPT2* gene. *J Clin Endocrinol Metab* 2004;89:1747–1752.
150. Kytola S, Farnebo F, Obara T, et al. Patterns of chromosomal imbalances in parathyroid carcinomas. *Am J Pathol* 2000;157:579–586.
151. Cryns VL, Rubio MP, Thor AD, et al. *p53* abnormalities in human parathyroid carcinoma. *J Clin Endocrinol Metab* 1994;78:1320–1324.
152. Vasef MA, Brynes RK, Sturm M, et al. Expression of cyclin D1 in parathyroid carcinomas, adenomas, and hyperplasias: a paraffin immunohistochemical study. *Mod Pathol* 1999;12:412–416.
153. Howell VM, Haven CJ, Kahnoski K, et al. *HRPT2* mutations are associated with malignancy in sporadic parathyroid tumours. *J Med Genet* 2003;40:657–663.
154. Dwight T, Twigg, S, Delbridge L, et al. Loss of heterozygosity in sporadic parathyroid tumours: involvement of chromosome 1 and the *MEN1* gene locus in 11q13. *Clin Endocrinol (Oxf)* 2000;53:85–92.
155. Villablanca A, Farnebo F, Teh BT, et al. Genetic and clinical characterization of sporadic cystic parathyroid tumours. *Clin Endocrinol (Oxf)* 2002;56:261–269.
156. Farnebo F, Teh BT, Dotzenrath C, et al. Differential loss of heterozygosity in familial, sporadic, and uremic hyperparathyroidism. *Hum Genet* 1997;99:342–349.
157. Hunt JL. Carty SE, Yim JH, et al. Allelic loss in parathyroid neoplasia can help characterize malignancy. *Am J Surg Pathol* 2005;29:1049–1055.
158. Eng C, Crossey PA, Mulligan LM, et al. Mutations in the *RET* proto-oncogene and the von Hippel-Lindau disease tumour suppressor gene in sporadic and syndromic phaeochromocytomas. *J Med Genet* 1995;32:934–937.
159. Baysal BE, Ferrell RE, Willett-Brozick JE, et al. Mutations in *SDHD*, a mitochondrial complex II gene, in hereditary paraganglioma. *Science* 2000;287:848–851.
160. Astuti D, Latif F, Dallol A, et al. Gene mutations in the succinate dehydrogenase subunit SDHB cause susceptibility to familial pheochromocytoma and to familial paraganglioma. *Am J Hum Genet* 2001;69:49–54.
161. Neumann HP, Pawlu C, Peczkowska M, et al. Distinct clinical features of paraganglioma syndromes associated with *SDHB* and *SDHD* gene mutations. *JAMA* 2004; 292:943–951.
162. Dluhy RG. Pheochromocytoma: death of an axiom. *N Engl J Med* 2002;346:1486–1488.
163. Maxwell PH, Wiesener MS, Chang GW, et al. The tumour suppressor protein VHL targets hypoxia-inducible factors for oxygen-dependent proteolysis. *Nature* 1999; 399:271–275.
164. Ackrell BA. Progress in understanding structure-function relationships in respiratory chain complex II. *FEBS Lett* 2000;466:1–5.
165. Neumann H, Bausch B, McWhinney SR, et al. Germ-line mutations in nonsyndromic pheochromocytoma. *N Engl J Med* 2002;346:1459–1466.
166. Gimm O, Armanios M, Dziema H, et al. Somatic and occult germ-line mutations in SDHD, a mitochondrial complex II gene, in nonfamilial pheochromocytoma. *Cancer Res* 2000;60:6822–6825.
167. Aguiar RC, Cox G, Pomeroy SL, et al. Analysis of the *SDHD* gene, the susceptibility gene for familial paraganglioma syndrome (PGL1), in pheochromocytomas. *J Clin Endocrinol Metab* 2001;86:2890–2894.
168. Lindor NM, Honchel R, Khosla S, et al. Mutations in the *RET* protooncogene in sporadic pheochromocytomas. *J Clin Endocrinol Metab* 1995;80:627–629.
169. Beldjord C, Desclaux-Arramond F, Raffin-Sanson M, et al. The *RET* protooncogene in sporadic pheochromocytomas: frequent *MEN* 2-like mutations and new molecular defects. *J Clin Endocrinol Metab* 1995;80:2063–2068.
170. Komminoth P, Kunz E, Hiort O, et al. Detection of *RET* proto-oncogene point mutations in paraffin-embedded pheochromocytoma specimens by nonradioactive single-strand conformation polymorphism analysis and direct sequencing. *Am J Pathol* 1994;145:922–929.
171. Rodien P, Jeunemaitre X, Dumont C, et al. Genetic alterations of the *RET* proto-oncogene in familial and sporadic pheochromocytomas. *Horm Res* 1997;47:263–268.
172. Stratakis CA. Genetics of adrenocortical tumors: gatekeepers, landscapers and conductors in symphony. *Trends Endocrinol Metab* 2003;14:404–410.

173. Ribeiro RC, Sandrini F, Figueiredo B, et al. An inherited *p53* mutation that contributes in a tissue-specific manner to pediatric adrenal cortical carcinoma. *Proc Natl Acad Sci USA* 2001;98:9330–9335.

174. Fogt F, Vargas MP, Zhuang Z, et al. Utilization of molecular genetics in the differentiation between adrenal cortical adenomas and carcinomas. *Hum Pathol* 1998;29:518–521.

175. Abati A, Sanjuan X, Wilder A, et al. Utilization of microdissection and the polymerase chain reaction for the diagnosis of adrenal cortical carcinoma in fine-needle aspiration cytology. *Cancer* 1999;87:231–237.

176. Reincke M, Wachenfeld C, Mora P, et al. *p53* mutations in adrenal tumors: Caucasian patients do not show the exon 4 "hot spot" found in Taiwan. *J Clin Endocrinol Metab* 1996;81:3636–3638.

177. Mansukhani MM, Greenebaum E. Loss of heterozygosity analysis to diagnose adrenal cortical carcinoma: are we there yet? *Cancer* 1999;87:173–177.

178. Shono T, Sakai H, Takehara K, et al. Analysis of numerical chromosomal aberrations in adrenal cortical neoplasms by fluorescence in situ hybridization. *J Urol* 2002; 168:1370–1373.

179. Kjellman M, Kallioniemi OP, Karhu R, et al. Genetic aberrations in adrenocortical tumors detected using comparative genomic hybridization correlate with tumor size and malignancy. *Cancer Res* 1996;56:4219–4223.

180. Figueiredo BC, Stratakis CA, Sandrini R, et al. Comparative genomic hybridization analysis of adrenocortical tumors of childhood. *J Clin Endocrinol Metab* 1999; 84:1116–1121.

181. Conran RM, Askin FB, Dehner LP. Chapter 22. The pineal, pituitary, parathyroid, thyroid, and adrenal glands. In: Stocker JT, Dehner LP, eds. *Pediatric Pathology*, 2nd ed. Philadelphia: Lippincott Williams & Wilkins; 2001:1017–1093.

182. Shimada H, Ambros IM, Dehner LP, et al. The International Neuroblastoma Pathology Classification (the Shimada system). *Cancer* 1999;86:364–372.

183. Shimada H, Ambros IM, Dehner LP, et al. Terminology and morphologic criteria of neuroblastic tumors: recommendations by the International Neuroblastoma Pathology Committee. *Cancer* 1999;86:349–363.

184. Brodeur GM, Maris JM. Neuroblastoma. In: Pizzo PA, Paplack DG, ed. *Principles and Practice of Pediatric Oncology*, 4th ed. Philadelphia: Lippincott; 2002:895–938.

185. Schwab M, Westermann F, Hero B, et al. Neuroblastoma: biology and molecular and chromosomal pathology. *Lancet Oncol* 2003;4:472–480.

186. Tonini G, Romani M. Genetic and epigenetic alterations in neuroblastoma. *Cancer Lett* 2003;197:69–73.

187. van Noesel MM, Versteeg R. Pediatric neuroblastomas: genetic and epigenetic 'danse macabre.' *Gene* 2004;325:1–15.

188. Seeger RC, Brodeur GM, Sather H, et al. Association of multiple copies of the *N-myc* oncogene with rapid progression of neuroblastomas. *N Engl J Med* 1985;313:1111–1116.

189. Tsuda T, Obara M, Hirano H, et al. Analysis of *N-myc* amplification in relation to disease stage and histologic types in human neuroblastomas. *Cancer* 1987;60:820–826.

190. Brodeur GM, Maris JM, Yamashiro DJ, et al. Biology and genetics of human neuroblastomas. *J Pediatr Hematol Oncol* 1997;19:93–101.

191. Gilbert F, Chattopadhyay S. Neuroblastoma: chromosome abnormalities and their possible significance. In: Slyser M, Voute A, eds. *Molecular Biology and Genetics of Childhood Cancers: Approaches to Neuroblastoma*. New York: John Wiley & Sons; 1992:56–71.

192. Crabbe DC, Peters J, Seeger RC. Rapid detection of *MYCN* gene amplification in neuroblastomas using the polymerase chain reaction. *Diagn Mol Pathol* 1992;1:229–234.

193. Shapiro DN, Valentine MB, Rowe ST, et al. Detection of *N-myc* gene amplification by fluorescence in situ hybridization: diagnostic utility for neuroblastoma. *Am J Pathol* 1993;142:1339–1346.

194. Cohen PS, Seeger RC, Triche TJ, et al. Detection of *N-myc* gene expression in neuroblastoma tumors by in situ hybridization. *Am J Pathol* 1988;131:391–397.

195. Komuro H, Valentine MB, Rowe ST, et al. Fluorescence in situ hybridization analysis of chromosome 1p36 deletions in human *MYCN* amplified neuroblastoma. *J Pediatr Surg* 1998;33:1695–1698.

196. Squire JA, Thorner P, Marrano P, et al. Identification of *MYCN* copy number heterogeneity by direct FISH analysis of neuroblastoma preparations. *Mol Diagn* 1996; 1:281–289.

197. Tajiri T, Shono K, Fujii Y, et al. Highly sensitive analysis for *N-myc* amplification in neuroblastoma based on fluorescence in situ hybridization. *J Pediatr Surg* 1999; 34:1615–1619.

198. Scott D, Elsden J, Pearson A, et al. Genes co-amplified with MYCN in neuroblastoma: silent passengers or co-determinants of phenotype? *Cancer Lett* 2003;197:81–86.

199. Driman D, Thorner PS, Greenberg ML, et al. *MYCN* gene amplification in rhabdomyosarcoma. *Cancer* 1994;73:2231–2237.

200. Hachitanda Y, Toyoshima S, Akazzawa K, et al. *N-myc* gene amplification in rhabdomyosarcoma detected by fluorescence in situ hybridization: its correlation with histologic features. *Mod Pathol* 1998;11:1222–1227.

201. Cohn SL, Rademaker AW, Salwen HR, et al. Analysis of DNA ploidy and proliferative activity in relation to histology and *N-myc* amplification in neuroblastoma. *Am J Pathol* 1990;136:1043–1052.

202. Bourhis J, De Vathaire F, Wilson GD. Combined analysis of DNA ploidy index and *N-myc* genomic content in neuroblastoma. *Cancer Res* 1991;51:33–36.

203. Carlsen NL, Ornvold K, Chrisensen IJ, et al. Prognostic importance of DNA flow cytometrical, histopathological parameters in neuroblastomas. *Virchows Arch A Pathol Anat Histopathol* 1992;420:411–418.

204. Caron H, van Sluis P, de Kraker J, et al. Allelic loss of chromosome 1p as a predictor of unfavorable outcome in patients with neuroblastoma. *N Engl J Med* 1996;334: 225–230.

205. Bown N, Cotterill S, Lastowska M, et al. Gain of chromosome arm 17q and adverse outcome in patients with neuroblastoma. *N Engl J Med* 1999;340:1954–1961.

206. Stark B, Jeison M, Glaser-Gabay L, et al. der(11)t(11;17): a distinct cytogenetic pathway of advanced stage neuroblastoma (NBL)—detected by spectral karyotyping (SKY). *Cancer Lett* 2003;197:75–79.

207. Morowitz M, Shusterman S, Mosse Y, et al. Detection of single-copy chromosome 17q gain in human neuroblastomas using real-time quantitative polymerase chain reaction. *Mod Pathol* 2003;16:1248–1256.

208. Snider WD. Functions of the neurotrophins during nervous system development: what the knockouts are teaching us. *Cell* 1994;77:627–638.

209. Nakagawara A. The NGF story and neuroblastoma. *Med Pediatr Oncol* 1998;31: 113–115.

210. Eggert A, Ikegaki N, Liu S, et al. MYC messenger RNA expression predicts survival outcome in childhood primitive neuroectodermal tumor/medulloblastoma. *Clin Cancer Res* 2001;7:2425–2433.

211. Kramer K, Gerald W, LeSauteur L, et al. Prognostic value of TrkA protein detection by monoclonal antibody 5C3 in neuroblastoma. *Clin Cancer Res* 1996;2:1361–1367.

212. Nakagawara A, Arima-Nakagawara M, Scavarda NJ, et al. Association between high levels of expression of the *TRK* gene and favorable outcome in human neuroblastoma. *N Engl J Med* 1993;328:847–854.

213. Poremba C, Scheel C, Hero B, et al. Telomerase activity and telomerase subunits gene expression patterns in neuroblastoma: a molecular and immunohistochemical study establishing prognostic tools for fresh-frozen and paraffin-embedded tissues. *J Clin Oncol* 2000;18:2582–2592.

214. Castle VP, Heidelberger KP, Bromberg J, et al. Expression of the apoptosis-suppressing protein bcl-2, in neuroblastoma is associated with unfavorable histology and *N-myc* amplification. *Am J Pathol* 1993;143:1543–1550.

215. Oltra S, Martinez F, Orellana C, et al. The doublecortin gene, a new molecular marker to detect minimal residual disease in neuroblastoma. *Diagn Mol Pathol* 2005;14: 53–57.

216. Lambooy LH, Gidding CE, van den Heuvel LP, et al. Real-time analysis of tyrosine hydroxylase gene expression: a sensitive and semiquantitative marker for minimal residual disease detection of neuroblastoma. *Clin Cancer Res* 2003;9:812–819.

217. Trager C, Kogner P, Lindskog M, et al. Quantitative analysis of tyrosine hydroxylase mRNA for sensitive detection of neuroblastoma cells in blood and bone marrow. *Clin Chem* 2003;49:104–112.

218. Burchill SA, Lewis IJ, Abrams KR, et al. Circulating neuroblastoma cells detected by reverse transcriptase polymerase chain reaction of tyrosine hydroxylase mRNA are an independent poor prognostic indicator in stage 4 neuroblastoma in children over 1 year. *J Clin Oncol* 2001;19:1795–1801.

Molecular Diagnostics in Hematopathology

M. Rajan Mariappan   *Daniel A. Arber*

Tremendous advances in the past two decades have advanced the application of molecular biology techniques in the initial diagnosis and management of patients with hematopoietic neoplasms. Recent expression microarray data have added to the prognostic and diagnostic markers, and utilization of molecular techniques has become an essential step for the hematopathologist and hematologist.

Historically, the Philadelphia chromosome, eventually shown to represent t(9;22), was the first chromosomal translocation identified in hematologic neoplasms (1,2). Following this, the search for chromosomal abnormalities in leukemias and lymphomas introduced the application of the Southern blot technique in the diagnostic laboratory (3–5). With the introduction of amplification methods, particularly the polymerase chain reaction (PCR), the sensitivity of detection increased tremendously and quantitative reverse transcriptase PCR (qRT-PCR) methods are now commonly used for minimal residual disease detection.

Hematopoietic neoplasms constitute over 40% of malignancies in children and 3% to 8% of adult-onset malignancies (6). These represent a wide range of disorders that include acute and chronic leukemias, lymphomas, and histiocytic malignancies (7). This chapter focuses on the role of molecular methods in the diagnosis and prognosis of common hematopoietic neoplasms and their pathologic subclassification. The current World Health Organization (WHO) classification of hematopoietic neoplasms is extensively influenced by the detection of molecular and cytogenetic abnormalities (8).

The chapter is organized to address diseases in the two broad groups of hematopoietic neoplasms: leukemias and lymphomas. Molecular changes and biologic aspects underlying most hematopoietic neoplasms are discussed. To provide practical insight to the clinician, emphasis is placed on the more commonly used tests, rather than uncommonly performed tests or tests that to date have limited clinical utility.

ROLE OF MOLECULAR TESTING IN THE MANAGEMENT OF HEMATOPOIETIC DISORDERS

The primary diagnosis of hematopoietic neoplasms is usually made by morphologic (H&E) examination of peripheral blood, bone marrow, or tissue and is usually supplemented by immunohistochemistry or immunophenotyping by flow cytometry (6,9). In a large number of cases of lymphoma, additional molecular studies are not needed. However, many acute leukemias, in addition to immunophenotyping, require chromosomal analysis or nucleic acid–based molecular testing. Such additional tests for lymphomas and leukemias include conventional karyotyping, fluorescence in situ hybridization (FISH) analysis, and amplification-based molecular studies.

Molecular tests performed in the laboratory can be categorized into three broad types: (a) detection of physiologic rearrangements (e.g., B- and T-cell–associated gene rearrangements), (b) detection of disease-specific translocations (such as t(9;22)), and (c) detection of mutations (such as *FLT3*). From a clinical perspective, molecular tests can be used for three different purposes: (a) initial diagnosis and categorization of disease, (b) prognostication by disease specific-markers, and (c) follow-up by minimal residual disease detection.

MOLECULAR EVALUATION OF LEUKEMIA

Chronic Myelogenous Leukemia

Chronic myelogenous leukemia (CML) is prototypical of the chronic myeloproliferative disorders. The detection of the Philadelphia chromosome or molecular evidence of t(9;22)/*BCR-ABL* is, by definition, a diagnostic requirement for CML (8). The translocation t(9;22)(q34;q11), or

Philadelphia chromosome, results in a fusion of *BCR* on chromosome 22 and *ABL* on chromosome 9. Cases that are Philadelphia chromosome–negative are now considered to represent other diseases, such as atypical chronic myeloid leukemia and chronic myelomonocytic leukemia (10–12). The detection of a *BCR-ABL* fusion by molecular methods is useful in the exclusion of other chronic myeloproliferative disorders or reactive causes of leukocytosis.

The translocation t(9;22)(q34;q11) can result in three different-sized variants of the *BCR-ABL* fusion product (Fig. 13.1) (13,14). The p190 results from what is termed an e1a2 junction and is most commonly associated with precursor B–acute lymphoblastic leukemia (ALL). The p210 variant is usually formed from a splicing of b2a2, b3a2 or a mixture of the two and is most often associated with CML. A less common variant, p230, is formed from an e19a2 junction and is associated with a rare neutrophilic type of CML (15).

The *BCR-ABL* fusion product results in unregulated tyrosine kinase activity and activates a number of pathways, including those in which RAS, JUN-kinase, and PI-3 have a central role. This results in an increase in cell proliferation and a decrease in apoptosis. Successful blockage of tyrosine kinase activity by imatinib mesylate (Gleevec) causes hematologic and cytogenetic remission and in a few cases has been shown to induce molecular remission at the detection level of most diagnostic laboratory testing (Fig. 13.2).

A combination of cytogenetics (karyotype/FISH) with qualitative RT-PCR is employed in the first-line detection of patients suspected to have CML (16). Although karyotype alone is sufficient for a diagnosis, knowledge of the specific break point by molecular methods is necessary for future monitoring by these methods. Molecular methods alone, however, are not optimal for diagnosis, because karyotype analysis allows for the detection of abnormalities other than t(9;22), which may also have clinical significance. Once the translocation and specific break point are determined, quantitative RT-PCR is used to establish baseline transcript levels before the institution of imatinib mesylate therapy (17). An algorithm for testing that is generally accepted is given in Figure 13.3. Table 13.1 lists some general recommendations for the use of *BCR-ABL* testing in CML.

A practical issue related to *BCR-ABL* qRT-PCR testing is interlaboratory variation in methods used and reporting of quantitative results. This is especially problematic in patients who are initially treated in one institution and later are followed in another. Because the laboratory methodologies may differ, quantitative *BCR-ABL* transcript levels among laboratories may not be comparable. A log-reduction method for reporting *BCR-ABL* transcript levels may be the best way to compare test results between laboratories (18), but this method of reporting is not currently used by most institutions. If a laboratory encounters a follow-up sample from a patient who was originally tested at another institution, the best way to compare the results between the institutions is to obtain an archived specimen from the previous laboratory to establish transcript equivalence.

Molecular testing is also used to monitor the treatment response to imatinib mesylate therapy (19,20). Most hematologists initiate imatinib mesylate therapy soon after

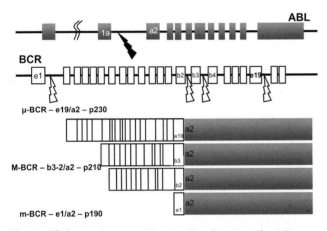

Figure 13.1 *BCR-ABL* translocation break points. The *ABL* gene break point is fairly constant between exons 1a and a2, whereas the *BCR* break points vary (e19, b3, b2, or e1), resulting in three different fusion products (p230, p210, and p190, respectively).

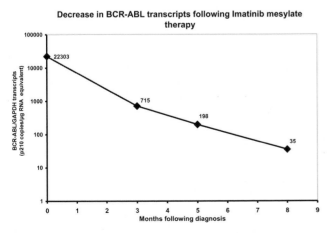

Figure 13.2 Decrease in *BCR-ABL* transcripts following imatinib mesylate therapy. Graph shows major molecular response following imatinib mesylate therapy. The transcript level decreased by more than 3 logarithms from pretreatment levels, in 8 months following therapy.

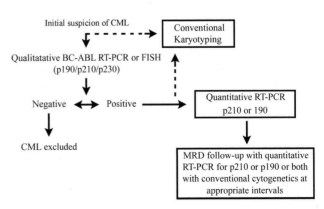

Figure 13.3 Suggested algorithm for molecular testing in chronic myelogenous leukemia.

TABLE 13.1

PROPOSED GUIDELINES FOR MINIMAL RESIDUAL TESTING IN CHRONIC MYELOGENOUS LEUKEMIA

1. MRD testing is appropriate following stem-cell transplant (to allow early detection of relapse) and following IFN-α and imatinib mesylate therapy (to gauge response and detect relapse).
2. Peripheral blood and bone marrow specimen provide equivalent *BCR-ABL* transcript levels. Because bone marrow aspiration is an invasive procedure, peripheral blood is probably sufficient for monitoring MRD.
3. Serial quantitative determinations are necessary to predict response or relapse. A single quantitative value should not be used to guide therapy or predict relapse.
4. Post-transplant positivity of *BCR-ABL* transcripts is inconsequential in the first 6 months, but after 6 months is predictive of high risk for relapse.
5. RT-PCR relapse occurs earlier than cytogenetic or hematologic relapse.
6. MRD in IFN-α or imatinib mesylate–treated patients should be tested by quantitative methods and not qualitative RT-PCR.
7. Generally, regardless of methodology, transcript level differences of 1-logarithm or more are significant.
8. MRD testing should be done every 3 to 6 months initially; following molecular remission, testing can be done once a year.
9. In imatinib mesylate–treated patients, only 5% of cases achieve true molecular remission, whereas >70% of these patients are karyotype negative.
10. A three log reduction in *BCR-ABL* transcripts within 1 year following imatinib mesylate treatment is generally accepted as good predictor.

From references 19,20.
MRD; IFN-α, interferon-alpha; RT-PCR, reverse transcriptase polymerase chain reaction.

a diagnosis of CML. Patients who respond to this drug have been shown to achieve complete hematologic response quite early, followed by major cytogenetic response and complete cytogenetic remission; 81% have a complete cytogenetic response at 30 months (21). In patients with a complete cytogenetic response, serial quantitative RT-PCR can identify those patients who are responding to therapy or who will develop imatinib mesylate resistance and relapse or progress to blast crisis (17,22). Falling levels of *BCR-ABL* messenger ribonucleic acid (mRNA) compared to pretherapeutic levels correlate well with risk of disease progression; more specifically, if *BCR-ABL* mRNA transcripts decrease by at least three orders of magnitude (3 logarithmic scale units) in 12 months, progression-free survival is predicted to be 100%, a state termed a major molecular response (21). A recent study (23) of 246 patients showed that 26.4% of patients with complete cytogenetic response relapse at 4 years; it also identified three general patterns of outcome among patients who initially had a complete cytogenetic response: initial responders with eventual relapse, "continuing to decline," and "reach a plateau." However, given that the median follow-up was only 30.3 months, the results could not be used to predict which of the patients in the latter two groups would relapse.

Patients who secondarily develop resistance to a tyrosine kinase inhibitor and relapse, or who relapse after stem cell transplantation, show early increases in *BCR-ABL* transcripts (17,23–25). Three possible mechanisms are thought to play a role in the development of imatinib mesylate resistance (26): (a) amplification and overexpression of *BCR-ABL*, (b) development of *BCR-ABL* point mutations, and (c) clonal evolution of a distinct leukemic population that typically exhibit additional karyotypic abnormalities, even at the time of initial diagnosis. Mutations in the *ABL* kinase domain (KD) are found in 50% to 90% of patients with secondary resistance and commonly involve four distinct clusters in *ABL-KD*, specifically the ATP-binding loop (P-loop—~40%), T315 (~30%), M351 (15%), and A-loop (15%). Currently, few laboratories perform sequencing to identify mutations associated with imatinib mesylate resistance, but such testing is expected to become more common in the future.

Other Chronic Myeloproliferative Disorders

There is a growing list of related kinases linking tumorigenesis in chronic myeloproliferative disorders (CMPDs), which have been elucidated by recent "kinomic" studies (27). Tyrosines comprise one group of related kinases, of which Abl is perhaps the most well-known. A few other members of the group include PDGFR-α, PDGFR-β, and JAK2, all of which are involved in the pathogenesis of a subset of CMPDs. FLT3 is another kinase that is associated with AML (see later discussion).

Other than CML, the CMPDs of the WHO classification include chronic neutrophilic leukemia, chronic eosinophilic leukemia, polycythemia vera, chronic idiopathic myelofibrosis, and essential thrombocythemia (8). Although often confusing, cases with neutrophilia and a p230 *BCR-ABL* fusion are considered neutrophilic variants of CML rather than chronic neutrophilic leukemia (15). The latter term should be reserved for truly t(9;22)/*BCR-ABL*–negative CMPDs with neutrophilia. All patients with a suspected

TABLE 13.2

EXAMPLES OF NONRANDOM GENETIC ABNORMALITIES IN LEUKEMIAS[a]

Disease	Genetic Aberration	Genes
Chronic Myeloproliferative Diseases		
Chronic myelogenous leukemia	t(9;22)(q34;q11)	BCR-ABL
Chronic eosinophilic leukemia/ hypereosinophilic syndrome	t(5;12)(q33;p13) variant 5q33 translocations rearrangements of 4q12	TEL-PGFRβ other PDGFRβ fusions FIP1L1-PDGFRα
Polycythemia vera	Missense mutations	JAK2
Myelodysplastic/myelo- proliferative diseases		
Chronic myelomonocytic leukemia	t(5;12)(q33;p13) variant 5q33 translocations mutations	TEL-PDGFRβ other PDGRFβ fusions RAS
Myelodysplastic syndrome	Activating mutations or internal tandem duplications	FLT3
Acute Myeloid Leukemia		
Acute promyelocytic leukemia	t(15;17)(q22;q21) variant 17q21 translocations	PML-RARα other RARα fusions
Acute myeloid leukemia with t(8;21)	t(8;21)(q22;q22)	AML1-ETO
Acute myeloid leukemia with inv(16) or t(16;16)	inv(16)(p13q22) t(16;16)(p13;q22)	CBFB-MYH11 CBFB-MYH11
Acute myeloid leukemia with 11q23 abnormalities	11q23 abnormalities	MLL

[a]See also Tables 13.3 and 13.4.

CMPD should have routine karyotyping and RT-PCR for *BCR-ABL* to exclude CML (28). Once a diagnosis of CML is excluded, a specific diagnosis of one of the other chronic myeloproliferative disorders is made by a combination of morphology, clinical features, and other laboratory data. Trisomy 8 is often noted as a recurring, nonspecific abnormality in these patients, especially with progression of disease.

A specific t(5;12)(q33;p13) translocation that involves the *PDGFβ* receptor and *TEL* (Table 13.2) is seen in at least a subset of cases of chronic eosinophilic leukemia (29,30). The fusion protein TEL-PDGFRβ results in constitutive activation of the kinase domain in PDGFRβ. Another recently identified rearrangement involves the *FIP1-like1* (*FIP1L1*) and *PDGFRα* genes (31,32). The FIP1L1-PDGFRα fusion protein transforms hematopoietic cells, and this fusion product is inhibited by therapeutic levels of imatinib mesylate, but conventional karyotyping does not detect this aberration. Amplification-based testing is not yet offered in most diagnostic laboratories, but a surrogate FISH assay is available that detects deletions of *CHIC2* located centromeric to *PDGFRα* (31).

Recently, studies associating mutations of the *JAK* (Janus kinase) genes (members of the tyrosine kinase family) with CMPDs were made almost simultaneously by four different institutions (33–36). The identified point mutation in *JAK2* is located in the pseudo-kinase domain and is associated with polycythemia vera. This mutation (G>T; V617F) is also seen in a subset of patients with

myelofibrosis and essential thrombocythemia. Testing for this point mutation is now available in some diagnostic laboratories.

Mixed Myelodysplastic Syndrome/ Myeloproliferative Diseases

The four categories of diseases included under this class (chronic myelomonocytic leukemia [CMML], juvenile myelomonocytic leukemia [JMML], atypical chronic myeloid leukemia [aCML], and myelodysplastic syndrome/ myeloproliferative disease [MDS/MPD] unclassifiable) are diagnosed by morphologic, laboratory, and clinical criteria (8). Although all four disorders may have karyotypic abnormalities, especially −7, +8, 12p abnormalities, +13, i(17p), and del(20q), they are not used for diagnosis or categorization. Like other CMPDs, routine karyotyping and *BCR-ABL* testing are done to exclude an unusual presentation of chronic myelogenous leukemia (37). A relatively high frequency of *RAS* mutations has been described in CMML and JMML, and these mutations are thought to be the primary dysregulatory genetic event in those cases. Abnormalities of *NF1* are also reported in a subset of JMML cases.

Two specific chromosomal translocations, t(5;10) and t(5;12), result in fusion products that increase tyrosine kinase activity of the PDGFβ receptor (29). The t(5;12)(q31;p12) involving *PDGFβ* and *TEL* is most commonly associated with CMML with eosinophilia, but this unusual type of

CMML is also reported to occur with other *TEL* translocations (38). Monosomy 7 occurs in a subset of JMML cases that were previously termed monosomy 7 syndrome (39–42).

Myelodysplastic Syndromes

With the exception of FISH studies to follow some patients with monosomies or trisomies, molecular studies are of limited utility in the myelodysplastic syndromes (MDS). Patients with myelodysplasia may show abnormalities of chromosomes 5 or 7 or complex karyotypes (43,44), but recurring balanced translocations are uncommon in this disease. One distinct disease group, the 5q-minus syndrome, is included in the WHO classification and is best detected by karyotype analysis (45). In general, 5q-minus syndrome is associated with a better prognosis. Other than the cytogenetic abnormalities, point mutations are also seen in MDS. A recent study showed that 3.4% of MDS patients were positive for activating *FLT3* gene mutations involving D835 (46), and in a separate study 2.5% were positive for an internal tandem duplication (ITD) of FLT3 (47). Although the clinical relevance of the D835 mutation is not clearly known, it is thought to forebode a poor prognosis. On the other hand, progression to AML was rapid in the *FLT3*-ITD–positive patients (47). These studies highlight the fact that *FLT3* mutations may be of prognostic significance in patients with MDS.

Acute Myeloid Leukemia

The WHO classification of acute myeloid leukemia (AML) recognizes four leukemias with recurrent cytogenetic abnormalities (8). These include acute promyelocytic leukemia with t(15;17)(q22;q21) or *PML-RARα* and variants, AML with t(8;21)(q22;q22) or *AML1-ETO*, AML with inv(16)(p13q22)/t(16;16)(p13;q22) or *CBFβ-MYH11*, and AML with 11q23 (*MLL*) abnormalities. Confirmation of these abnormalities by karyotype or molecular genetic analysis is required for these disease types, and cases with these abnormalities are considered acute leukemias without regard to the blast cell count.

Acute Promyelocytic Leukemia

Acute promyelocytic leukemia results from abnormalities of the *RARα* gene at chromosome region 17q21 (48). In most cases of acute promyelocytic leukemia, the *RARα* gene fuses with the *PML* gene on chromosome 15q22 (49,50). RARα is a nuclear hormone receptor that forms a heterodimeric complex with retinoic-X receptors (RXRα), and these RARα /RXRα complexes bind to specific DNA sequences (referred to as retinoic acid response elements) and repress transcription through a variety of mechanisms. Physiologic concentrations of retinoic acid control this activity, allowing for normal activation of gene transcription (51). With the *PML-RARα* fusion, physiologic levels of retinoic acid are no longer sufficient to control the effects of RARα and gene transcription is blocked. The drug all-*trans* retinoic acid (ATRA) provides pharmacologic concentrations of retinoic acid that allow for the return of normal transcription, and consequently this

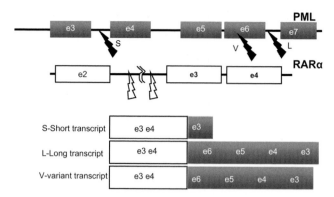

Figure 13.4 *PML-RARα* translocation break points. The break point at the *RARα* gene is fairly constant in intron 2, whereas the *PML* break points vary (intron 3, intron 6 or within exon 6, overlapping e6 in figure), resulting in three different fusion products (S,V, and L, respectively).

leukemia type has a generally good prognosis when treated with ATRA-containing regimens. Arsenic trioxide has also been shown to be effective in the treatment of acute promyelocytic leukemia (52); this drug is thought to cause post-translational degradation of the fusion transcript, NADPH oxidase-mediated reactive oxygen species production, and cytotoxicity of tumor cells.

The t(15;17) is usually detectable by karyotype analysis at diagnosis. Molecular detection of *PML-RARα* may be performed by RT-PCR or FISH analysis (48,53). Three different isoforms of the fusion may occur, and RT-PCR assays should be designed to detect all of these forms. They vary by differences in break points within the *PML* gene, with breaks in intron 6 termed bcr-1, long, or L forms; breaks in exon 6 termed bcr-2, variable, or V forms; and breaks in intron 3 termed bcr-3, short, or S forms (Fig. 13.4). Subtle differences in clinical presentation occur with the different forms, including an association between the S-form and the microgranular morphologic variant. V-form disease may have a lower disease-free survival (51). Despite this, most laboratories do not distinguish between the different break point types, and either a FISH- or an RT-PCR–based strategy may be adequate for primary diagnosis.

The *PML-RARα* RT-PCR test has an advantage over FISH methods because it can detect lower levels of residual or recurrent disease, is useful in the early detection of residual disease, and has utility as a predictor of relapse in acute promyelocytic leukemia (53,54). Most assays for *PML-RARα* can detect one translocated cell in 10^4 to 10^5 cells, and nested PCR with two rounds of amplification is capable of detecting even lower transcript levels (55). The clinical utility of more sensitive assays capable of detecting 1 in 10^6 cells is probably low, given that patients who are in long-term remission are persistently positive by these highly sensitive tests, but relapse occurs only in a small minority of patients (55,56). Despite this, serial quantitative assays are used to follow patients with very low levels of disease.

Although *PML-RARα* is the most common fusion in this disease, other translocations of *RARα* on chromosome 17 with *PLZF* at 11q23, *NuMA* at 11q13, *NPM* at 5q35, and *STAT5b* at 17q11 occur in less than 1% of patients with promyelocytic leukemia (49,50,53,57). Cases that lack an

RARα translocation or have a translocation involving *PLZF* or *STAT5b* do not respond to all-*trans* retinoic acid and require a different therapeutic approach (49,57). Detection of these variant translocations is frequently aided by FISH break-apart probes targeting *RARα*. Given the other variant translocations that are usually not detected by PCR targeting *PML-RARα*, a diagnosis of promyelocytic leukemia should not be excluded based solely on PCR testing.

Core Binding Factor Leukemias [AMLs with t(8;21) and inv(16)]

The disruption of normal transcription factor activity is one molecular aberration that commonly occurs in acute leukemia. The core-enhancer DNA sequence TGT/cGGT was identified in the early 1990s as a transcriptional regulatory sequence that controls expression of many viral and hematopoietic specific genes (58–60). The core binding factor is a protein complex that includes elements encoded by the *AML1* (also known as *RUNX1* or *CBFα2*) gene on chromosome 21q22 and the *CBFβ* gene at 16q22. Recurring translocations of these genes are some of the most common in acute leukemia (58,61). The core binding factor is critical in normal hematopoietic development (62), and so translocations involving these genes result in disruption of hematopoiesis by a variety of mechanisms and are characteristic of acute leukemias (63). Establishment of murine models of this translocation has helped make possible significant progress in the understanding of the pathogenesis of these leukemias (58).

The t(8;21)(q22;q22) results in an *AML1-ETO* fusion (also known as *RUNX1-MTG8*) that eliminates the transcriptional activating domain of the core binding factor (64–66). This abnormality is associated with 12% of all de novo acute myeloid leukemias and 40% of M2 AMLs in the French-American-British (FAB) classification; it is a distinct AML type in the acute leukemias with recurrent cytogenetic abnormalities of the WHO classification. Another distinct type of AML in the WHO classification commonly has admixed abnormal eosinophils and is termed M4Eo in the FAB classification. It is associated with inv(16)(p13q22) or t(16;16)(p13;q22), these abnormalities that result in a fusion of the *CBFβ* and *MYH11* gene of chromosome 16 that encodes the smooth muscle myosin heavy chain (67). Although this fusion does not directly affect the transcriptional activating domain of the core binding factor, it still acts as a suppressor of *AML1* function and may sequester *AML1* from transcriptionally active sites. Both of these leukemia types show a good to intermediate response to current therapy (63,68).

The core binding factor, and specifically the *AML1* gene, is also involved in other types of leukemia. The *AML1* gene is associated with chromosome 3 translocations that involve the *EVI1* and *MDS1* genes in association with myelodysplasia and blast transformation of CML. Point mutations in *CBFα2* and *AML1* are seen in MDS with a high risk of progression (69) and have been shown to block myeloid differentiation (70). In addition, *AML1* fuses with the *TEL* gene in the t(12;21)(p13;q22) translocation characteristic of pediatric ALL (see later discussion).

Most of the translocations that involve the core binding factor proteins can be detected by karyotype analysis, but the inv(16) of *CBFβ-MYH11* may be more difficult to identify (25) and the t(12;21) of *TEL-AML1* is not usually detectable by routine karyotype. For these abnormalities, molecular studies are often needed at the time of the original diagnosis. RT-PCR and FISH assays are most commonly performed (71). RT-PCR for *AML1-ETO* and *CBFβ-MYH11* may be used for minimal residual disease detection (72), but the significance of a qualitative positive result for *AML1-ETO* is controversial, with some studies suggesting that low levels of this transcript after therapy may not be clinically significant (73,74), whereas more recent studies suggest complete eradication of this fusion is necessary for long-term survival (75,76). Other genetic aberrations, which may not be detectable by karyotype analysis, are probably necessary for these types of leukemia to develop (77). Quantitative RT-PCR methods, however, are now more commonly used for residual disease testing of both translocations, and this approach has been shown to be of clinical significance in more recent studies (60,78,79).

Acute Myeloid Leukemia with 11q23/MLL Abnormalities

AML with 11q23 (*MLL*) abnormalities is a specific subtype of AML in the WHO classification (8). Abnormalities involving *MLL* are found in 5% to 6% of patients with AML, 7% to 10% of patients with ALL, and 60% to 70% of infants with acute leukemias. *MLL* abnormalities are also found in more than 80% of acute leukemias that develop after treatment with topoisomerase II inhibitors. These *MLL*-related leukemias fall into several categories of the WHO classification. Although the category of AML with 11q23 abnormalities generally confers a poor prognosis, it represents a fairly heterogenous group of diseases with as many as 40 different translocation partners being reported with the *MLL* gene. In addition, abnormalities that are not associated with balanced translocations may occur with *MLL*, a large 90-kb gene that contains 36 exons and codes for a 431-kDa protein (80,81). The protein contains AT-hooks, which recognize specific DNA structures and are known to regulate transcription by inducing changes in DNA conformation that permit the association of other proteins that contain regulatory regions. Other regions of *MLL* repress transcription from reporter constructs, mediate homodimerization, mediate interactions with nuclear proteins, activate transcription, and are involved with ATP-dependent chromatin remodeling. Recent gene expression profiling data showed lineage-specific differences, the most significant of which were *PAX5* and *EBF* expression in B-cell committed *MLL* leukemias (82).

The most common translocation partners in AML with 11q23 abnormalities are chromosomes 6q27 (*AF6* gene), 9p22 (*AF9* gene), 19p13.3 (*ENL* gene), 19p13.1 (*ELL* gene), 19p13.3 (*EEN* gene), 16p13 (*CBP* gene) and 22q13 (*p300* gene). The t(4;11) involving the *AF4* gene is more common in infant ALL and adult therapy-related ALL than in AML. *MLL* abnormalities are common in therapy-related AML, particularly after therapy with topoisomerase II inhibitors, as noted previously. Partial tandem duplications of *MLL* also occur in AML and are more common in patients with normal karyotypes or trisomy 11 (83–85). In general, the presence of *MLL* translocations and partial tandem duplications indicates an unfavorable prognosis, but the t(9;11) in childhood AML has been shown to confer a good prognosis (86).

Abnormalities of 11q23 may be missed by karyotype analysis, and this method cannot detect partial tandem duplications of the *MLL* gene. Because of the multitude of possible *MLL* translocation partners, PCR-based tests are of limited value and so most laboratories use FISH-based testing to detect *MLL* translocations, even though FISH will not detect internal tandem duplications. RT-PCR for *MLL* internal tandem duplications is not performed in most laboratories, and reports of such duplications in healthy donors (84) suggest that only a quantitative assay for this abnormality would be useful as a diagnostic test. Recently, a commercial product, (MLL FusionChip, Ipsogen) has become available that can detect 32 partner genes, as well the partial duplication. Analysis utilizing this gene chip requires RT-PCR followed by hybridization of the amplicons to long fusion-specific oligonucleotides spotted on the chip, which produces a visual read-out that can be used to identify the fusion partner (Fig. 13.5). Given the high incidence of *MLL*-related leukemia, this chip could prove useful in the diagnosis of *MLL*-related leukemia.

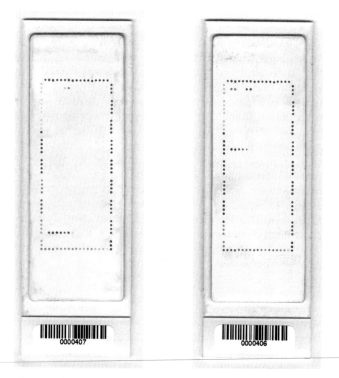

Figure 13.5 *MLL* FusionChip (Ipsogen, Marseille, France). The chip enables visual readout without the need of specialized scanners. In the two examples, the *MLL* gene is translocated and the fusion partner can be identified by amplification and hybridization. The hybridization signals from the slide are read out by comparing them to the interpretation chart provided by the manufacturer. The outer circumferential spots are controls, showing that there was optimal hybridization for test interpretation.

Nucleoporin Protein Fusions in AML

Nucleoporins represent one of several components of nuclear pore complexes, structures that allow macromolecules to cross the cell nuclear membrane. A number of chromosomal rearrangements in de novo AML, therapy-related AML, and myelodysplasia involve nucleoporins (87,88). The most commonly involved genes are *NUP98* on chromosome 11p15 and *CAN* (as known as *NUP214*) on chromosome 9q34. Nucleoporin fusion proteins not only alter nuclear transport by binding to soluble transport factors, but also apparently act as aberrant transcription factors. *NUP98* usually fuses with one of the homeobox genes, such as *HOXA9* (on chromosome 7p15), *PMX1* (at 1q24), and *HOXD13* (at 2q31), but other gene fusions have been described. *CAN* most commonly fuses with the *DEK* gene in the t(6;9)(p23;q34), a translocation characteristic of a de novo AML type that is associated with erythroid hyperplasia, dysplasia, and bone marrow basophilia (87,89). Although RT-PCR or FISH can be performed to test for all of these abnormalities, such testing is not offered in most molecular diagnostic laboratories.

Other Genetic Abnormalities in AML

In acute myeloid leukemia, genetic abnormalities of transcriptional control elements lead to uncontrolled cellular proliferation or maturation arrest. As discussed above, abnormalities in some members of the kinase family, specifically cell surface receptor tyrosine kinases involved in signal transduction and ligand binding (90), have been linked to pathogenesis and progression of acute leukemia. Genes that encode receptor tyrosine kinases include c-*kit*, *PDGFRβ*, c-*fms*, and *FLT3*, and mutations, internal duplications, and tyrosine kinase fusion proteins involving these genes occur in several different leukemia types. One tyrosine kinase gene of interest in a variety of diseases is c-*kit*, and c-kit protein (CD117) is often expressed in AML. This gene is mutated in gastrointestinal stromal tumors and mast cell disease, but is relatively infrequently mutated in AML. *FLT3* (also known as *STK1* and *flk2*), is another tyrosine kinase gene that frequently undergoes length mutations in AML and is currently the subject of much study (91,92).

The FLT3 protein is expressed in early hematopoietic progenitor cells and is involved in early stem cell survival and myeloid differentiation (93). *FLT3* mutations occur in 20% to 28% of adult AML and 11.5% of all de novo pediatric AML. They occur with almost any FAB type of AML and in association with any of the recurring cytogenetic abnormalities, but are most common in acute promyelocytic leukemia and in AMLs that have a normal karyotype and are associated with decreased disease-free survival in adult AML. Because of the relatively high frequency and clinical significance of these mutations in AML, *FLT3* mutation testing has become an essential component in AML prognostication (94–97).

The fms-like tyrosine kinase 3 (*FLT3*) gene encodes a receptor tyrosine kinase that regulates proliferation and differentiation. *FLT3* mutations are of two types: an ITD has been reported in nearly 25% of patients with AML, and a substitution mutation termed D835 at the aspartic acid

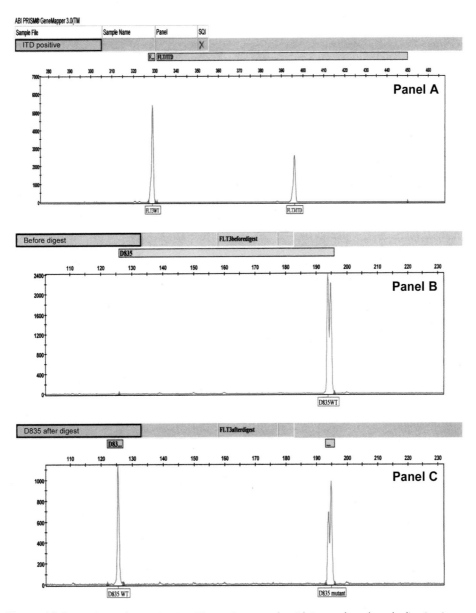

Figure 13.6 **A** shows the *FLT3*—ITD. The patient sample with internal tandem duplication in one allele (*FLT3*/ITD-peak at 395 base pairs [bp]) is 66 bp larger than the wild-type (*FLT3*/WT-peak at 329 bp). **B** and **C** show the D835 mutation. The mutation is resistant to restriction enzyme digestion by *Eco*RV (**C** shows the D835 mutant), whereas the normal allele is digested to a smaller fragment (D835WT). (See color insert.)

residue encoded by codon 835 of *FLT3* in 7% of patients with AML. The ITD and D835 mutations can be detected by PCR of the juxtamembrane region and activation loop encoded by exons 11 and 12, respectively, of the *FLT3* gene (98). The D835 mutation can be easily detected by its resistance to digestion by the restriction enzyme *Eco*RV. ITDs (which are always in multiples of 3 bases, usually from approximately 15 to 180 bp long) can be easily detected by simple agarose gel electrophoresis, although very rarely occurring small-length ITDs (of 3 bp length) cannot be resolved in an agarose gel and are more reliably detected by capillary electrophoresis analysis (Fig. 13.6). The ITD and D835 mutations usually occur alone, but rare

instances of concurrent double mutations have been reported. D835 mutations are also known to occur in approximately 3% of MDS, as discussed previously, and 3% of acute lymphoblastic leukemias. Clinical trials that include targeted drug therapy by *FLT3*-specific tyrosine kinase inhibitors are currently underway.

In cells undergoing hematopoiesis, the basic zipper (B-ZIP) transcription factor CCAAT/enhancer binding protein α (C/EBPα) is exclusively expressed in myelomonocytic cells and is required for granulocytic differentiation (99,100). Mutations of the gene coding C/EBPα (*CEBPA*) result in inactivation of differentiation and occur in 7% to 11% of AML (101). Mutations may occur in both the C- and

N-terminal of the gene; C-terminal mutations of *CEBPA* disrupt the B-ZIP region that contains both DNA-binding and dimerization domains, while N-terminal mutations disrupt the reading frame and result in premature termination and truncation of the normal 42-kDa protein and enhanced translation of a 30-kDa protein initiated downstream. Acute myeloid leukemias with *CEPBA* mutations are associated with intermediate-risk cytogenetics and are more commonly associated with FAB M1 or M2 morphology (although virtually all FAB types are reported). Detection of a *CEPBA* mutation is generally associated with a favorable prognosis, although patients with both *FLT3* and *CEPBA* mutations have an intermediate prognosis (102).

MOLECULAR EVALUATION OF ACUTE LYMPHOBLASTIC LEUKEMIA/LYMPHOMA

Acute lymphoblastic leukemias and lymphomas (ALLs) are usually initially separated into precursor B and precursor T-cell lineages. The designations of leukemia and lymphoma are somewhat arbitrary, with the "lymphomas" defined by the presence of less than 25% bone marrow involvement at the time of diagnosis and the "leukemias" showing 25% or more marrow disease at diagnosis. Cases with a leukemic presentation are most commonly of the precursor B-cell type. These tumors may be subdivided into prognostically significant groups by the detection of recurring cytogenetic or molecular genetic subgroups. About 70% of ALLs show molecular/cytogenetic abnormalities (103,104). A comprehensive list of molecular abnormalities and their relative frequencies is shown in Table 13.3.

Precursor B-Cell Lymphoblastic Leukemia/Lymphoma

ALL with t(12;21) and the Associated TEL-RUNX1 Fusion

Precursor B cell ALL with the translocation t(12;21) (p13;q22) is the most common genetic subtype of ALL in children and constitutes at least 20% to 30% of childhood ALL (104–107). This disease is most common in children between 2 and 5 years of age and is extremely uncommon in adults (108). The disease is associated with relatively low peripheral white blood cell counts and nonhyperdiploidy. The leukemic blasts characteristically lack expression of CD9 and CD20, while often showing aberrant expression of the myeloid-associated antigen CD13 (109–111). This type of ALL is generally considered to have a good prognosis, but very late relapses may occur.

The t(12;21) results in a fusion of the core binding factor gene *AML1* (also known as *RUNX1*) on chromosome 21 and the *TEL (ETV6)* gene on chromosome 12 (105,106). *TEL* is normally a transcriptional repressor and consequently the *TEL-AML1* fusion redirects this repressor function to *AML1* targets. Although the t(12;21) aberration is not detectable by routine karyotype analysis, both FISH and RT-PCR methods can detect the translocation (109,112) and several reports using quantitative PCR have shown this to be a reliable method of following patients for residual disease (113,114).

ALL with t(4;11) and the Associated AF4-MLL, and Other MLL Abnormalities

Precursor B-cell ALL with *MLL* abnormalities, particularly t(4;11)(q21;q23), are the most common ALL type in infants and represent approximately 6% of ALLs in older children or adults (80,115–119). This disease has an unfavorable prognosis and is usually associated with a characteristic pro–B-cell immunophenotype that is CD10 negative with aberrant expression of myeloid-associated antigens CD15 or CD65 (120,121). Although this ALL phenotype in an infant is characteristic of an underlying *MLL* genetic abnormality, molecular testing is warranted in all infant ALL to confirm its presence, which is relatively frequent in this age-group. A disease with essentially identical immunophenotypic and molecular genetic features may also occur in adults with therapy-related ALL (122). Recently, *FLT3* mutations, which are generally uncommon in ALL, have been described in association with infant ALL with *MLL* aberrations, as well as in hyperdiploid ALL (123,124).

ALL with *E2A* Abnormalities

Several translocations involving the *E2A* gene on chromosome 19q23 occur in ALL, but t(1;19)(q23;p13.3) is the most common (125). These abnormalities are most common in childhood and occur in approximately 6% of pediatric ALL, but they may occur at any age (126,127). These *E2A* abnormalities in ALL are associated with expression of cytoplasmic μ and lack of CD34 (often termed pre-B) (128–130). *E2A* is a helix-loop-helix protein-coding gene involved in B-cell development (131,132), and it most commonly fuses with the *PBX1* gene on chromosome 1q23, which is a homeodomain-containing HOX cofactor. This fusion results in the synthesis of a homeobox fusion mRNA that codes for an apparent chimeric transcription factor (133). Less often, *E2A* fuses with the *HLF* gene on chromosome 17q21-22, and the resulting protein activates antiapoptotic pathways (134). Karyotype, FISH, or RT-PCR can usually detect both abnormalities, but up to 25% of cases with underlying *E2A-PBX1* fusions detected by

TABLE 13.3

INCIDENCE OF MOLECULAR ABNORMALITIES IN PEDIATRIC PRECURSOR AND MATURE B-ALL AND THEIR RELATIVE FREQUENCIES

Type	Relative Frequency (%)
Hyperdiploid (>50 chromosomes)	50
TEL-AML1	20
MLL t(4:11), t(11;19)	6
E2A-PBX1 t(1;19)	5
BCR-ABL t(9;22)ᵃ	4
E2A-HLF	1
MYC t(8;14), t(2;8), t(8;22)	2
Unknown	30

From reference 104.
ᵃt(9;22) *BCR-ABL* is also found in 20% to 25% of adult ALL.

TABLE 13.4

NONRANDOM MOLECULAR ABNORMALITIES IN T-ALL

TAL1 disruption		
TAL-1 (SCL; TCL-5)	t(1;14)	1%–3%
SIL-TAL fusion		9%–26%
HOX11 (TLX1; TCL3) overexpression	t(10;14)(q24;q11) or t(7;10)	5%
HOX11L2 (RNX; TLX3)	t(5:14)(q35;q32)	23%

From reference 103.

molecular genetic studies may have normal karyotypes. Thus, molecular methods may be preferable when immunophenotypic studies suggest this abnormality. This genetic subtype of ALL is generally considered to have an unfavorable prognosis, which may be overcome by more intensive therapy regimens.

ALL with t(9;22) and the Associated *BCR-ABL* Fusion

The Philadelphia chromosome resulting from the t(9;22)(q34;q11.2) translocation is most commonly associated with chronic myelogenous leukemia (discussed in more detail previously). This abnormality, however, also occurs in 20% to 25% of adult and 2% to 3% of pediatric precursor B-cell ALLs (135,136). ALLs with t(9;22) are of precursor B-cell lineage (CD10, CD19, and TdT positive) and are often associated with aberrant expression of the myeloid-associated antigens CD13 and CD33, as well as CD38. As noted above, three BCR-ABL fusion proteins occur (137–139), but the p190 (also known as p185) variant is most commonly associated with acute lymphoblastic leukemia (139,140). Some adult Ph+ ALL cases will demonstrate the p210 variant, rather than p190, and both types of Ph+ ALL in adults are generally considered to have a poor prognosis. Approximately 5% to 10% of cases display normal karyotypes with a *BCR-ABL* fusion product only detectable by molecular methods.

Precursor T Lymphoblastic Leukemia/Lymphoma

Precursor T lymphoblastic tumors are less frequent than precursor B-cell neoplasms, but constitute 85% to 90% of cases that present as lymphoblastic lymphoma (141). Recurring cytogenetic subgroups of T-ALL are not as well recognized as those for precursor B-cell ALL, but improved survival is associated with an abnormal karyotype or with t(10;14)(p13;q11) (142). A variety of molecular genetic aberrations are associated with the T-cell lymphoblastic malignancies (Table 13.4), and many of these involve loci encoding T-cell receptor genes or various transcription factors. Detection of these aberrations at diagnosis may be useful for disease monitoring, but in contrast to precursor B-cell tumors, distinct prognostic disease groups defined by recurring cytogenetic abnormalities are not yet part of any major classification scheme.

Gene expression profiling studies of T-ALL have identified genetically distinct subgroups. These subgroups appear to correspond to specific stages of intrathymic maturational arrest but are independent of specific chromosomal translocations (143,144). These studies suggest that expression of *HOX11* is associated with a favorable prognosis, whereas expression of *TAL1*, *LYL1*, or *HOX11L2* is associated with a worse response to therapy. Most diagnostic laboratories, however, do not test for these T-ALL markers at this time.

Other Prognostic Groups in ALL

Additional clinically significant disease subtypes of ALL exist, and more are likely to emerge from future studies. One prognostic subgroup of clinical significance consists of cases of ALL with a diploid or near diploid karyotype (50 or fewer chromosomes) that lack the abnormalities described previously, and these cases are associated with a worse prognosis compared to that in patients with hyperdiploid ALL (defined as over 50 chromosomes) (145,146). Hypodiploidy is present in only approximately 5% of cases of ALL; however, patients with less than 40 chromosomes have a poorer outcome compared to those with "high hypodipoidy" of 42 to 45 chromosomes (147). Gene expression profiling has confirmed the biologic significance of the ALL subgroups listed previously, as well as hyperdiploid ALL and T-cell ALL (148,149). In addition, these studies identified cases in which recurring abnormalities were missed on initial screening, as well as a novel subgroup of precursor B-cell ALLs. Although this latter group represents only 4% of pediatric ALLs studied, further analyses may determine key markers of this new ALL disease subgroup.

MOLECULAR EVALUATION OF MALIGNANT LYMPHOMAS

Common molecular techniques useful in the diagnosis of lymphomas include establishment of clonality and detection of chromosomal translocations. Virtually all B- and T-cell lymphomas present with clonal rearrangements of antigen receptor genes, and, in 25% to 30% of cases, well-defined translocations are also present (9).

Clonality Studies Targeting Physiologic Rearrangements

For most patients with a clinical suspicion of a lymphoproliferative disorder (LPD), morphology supplemented with immunohistochemistry or flow-cytometric immunophenotyping can discriminate between a malignant and reactive lymphoproliferation. In 5% to 10% of cases, a definite diagnosis by these means cannot be made and molecular methods are essential. Clonality assessment lends support to the diagnosis of lymphoma, because in principle all cells in a LPD have a common clonal origin, whereas a reactive process will usually be polyclonal. Most lymphoid malignancies are of B-cell origin (90% to 95%), with the rest being of T-cell (5% to 7%) or NK-cell lineage (<2%).

Molecular methods are the gold standard to establish clonality in T- and B-cell lymphoma, and the assays focus on immunoglobulin (IG) and T-cell receptors (TCR), both of which are heterodimers composed of two disulfide-linked chains (150–153). The *IG* and *TCR* gene loci contain many different variable (V) and joining (J) segments, and some of these genes also contain diversity (D) segments. One gene segment each from the V, D, and J loci rearranges to form a unique gene sequence (Fig. 13.7), which is then transcribed and translated into peptide components of IG and TCR heterodimeric complexes. V-D-J rearrangements are sequential; a D-J rearrangement is followed by V to D-J in the case of *IGH*, *TCRβ*, and *TCRδ* genes, while direct V to J rearrangement is seen in *IGκ*, *IGλ*, *TCRα*, and *TCRγ*. Because the chromosomal regions for immunoglobulin and the T-cell antigen receptor contain 38 to 200 functional and nonfunctional variable (V) regions, 23 diversity (D) and 6 joining (J) regions, the rearrangements produce a large combinatorial repertoire, which is estimated to be approximately 2×10^6 for the IG molecules, 3×10^6 for TCRαβ, and 5×10^3 for the TCRγδ molecules. Additional diversity is created by the random addition of so-called N-nucleotides between V, D, and J segments by terminal deoxynucleotidyl transferase, which further varies the size of the rearrangement.

Following rearrangement of the immunoglobulin heavy chain gene, the immunoglobulin kappa light chain region

of chromosome 2p11 rearranges in a similar fashion, with the exception that it does not contain diversity (D) regions. If this rearrangement is not productive in either allele (approximately one third of cases), the kappa light chain constant region locus is deleted and the immunoglobulin lambda light chain region on chromosome 22q11 undergoes rearrangement (154,155). B-lymphocytes further extend the variability via the process of maturation that occurs in the germinal centers of lymph nodes upon antigenic stimulation. This maturation results in somatic hypermutation, the process by which single-nucleotide mutations or deletions/insertions of short segments occur in the V(D)J exonic regions of *IGH* and *IGκ/λ*. The importance of detecting B-cell somatic hypermutation is important for prognostication of outcome in CLL patients, as discussed later.

The T-cell receptor (*TCR*) genes undergo VDJ or VJ rearrangements similar to the immunoglobulin heavy and kappa light chain genes in the sequential order of *TCRδ* (chromosome 14q11), *TCRγ* (7q15), *TCRβ* (7q34), and *TCRα* (14q11). Approximately 95% of circulating T-cells are of the α/β type, but a small population are γ/δ T-cells, some of which do not undergo *TCRβ* and *TCRα* rearrangements.

Scenarios for performing clonality studies in lymphoid proliferations would include atypical B-cell proliferations, including post-transplant and immunodeficiency-related proliferations in which immunophenotyping studies for clonality are inconclusive or not available; atypical T-cell proliferations; disorders for which no immunophenotypic markers for clonality are usually available; and comparison of clones from lymphomas involving more than one site to determine if the second site represents a recurrence versus a new neoplasm. Less commonly, clonality studies are used to evaluate specimens for evidence of minimal residual disease.

Current Techniques for Clonality Studies

Diagnostic laboratories generally use Southern blot analysis and PCR-based methods for clonality assessment (156,157). PCR-based methods usually employ multiple primer sets and most commonly test for the *TCRγ*, *TCRβ*, and *IGH* rearrangements. These PCR-based methods have become the method of choice for most laboratories because they are easy to perform and detect lower levels of disease than Southern blot analysis. Southern blotting methods, despite their labor-intensive methods and low sensitivity, are still considered the gold standard for clonality analysis, but they are currently offered by fewer laboratories than in the past.

Southern Blot Analysis

The Southern blot method is described in more detail in Chapter 6, but some key points will be reiterated. Southern blot analysis requires high molecular weight, good-quality DNA from freshly frozen material. The DNA is subjected to restriction enzyme digestion, and clonal rearrangements result in restriction fragment length alterations different from the germline DNA configuration, alterations that are manifested as extra bands after the digested DNA is hybridized to a labeled probe. Other than the requirement

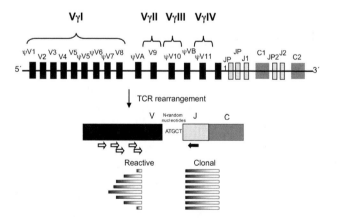

Figure 13.7 T-cell gamma receptor gene (chromosome 7p15). The *V* and *J* region break and rearrange with random multiple N-nucleotides added by TdT. Both the random breakage and nucleotide insertions cause rearranged *TCR*. Amplification with a fixed primer targeting *J* and a set of primers targeting multiple regions of the *V* locus would result in different-sized products, if the rearrangement is random as in reactive proliferations. Clonally rearranged lymphocytes result in identical-sized products that can be detected by a bright band in an agarose gel or dominant peak in electropherogram (see Fig. 13.8).

of high-quality, high molecular weight DNA, Southern blot techniques require that at least 5%, and usually 10% or more, of the sample represent the clonal population. Therefore, this method is not adequate for fixed specimens or samples with only a small percentage of tumor cells. A sensitivity control in which a control population of clonal cells is diluted to 5% to 10% in a background of normal cells is usually run in parallel.

Southern blot assays for B-cell clonality usually use probes directed against the joining (J) regions of the immunoglobulin heavy chain or the immunoglobulin kappa light chain genes, probes that together should detect all clonal B-cell disorders if sufficient clonal cells are present in the sample. Southern blot analysis of the T-cell receptor β gene (*TCRβ*) will detect over 90% of T-cell malignancies, but will not generally detect gene rearrangements in malignancies of γ/δ T-cells or natural killer cells. Southern blot analysis for T-cell clonality uses probes directed against the *TCRβ* constant region (Cβ) or a cocktail of probes directed against *TCRβ* joining regions 1 and 2 (Jβ1 and 2).

PCR-based Clonality Studies

Southern blot analysis is a labor-intensive technique; thus many laboratories are now routinely performing PCR-based tests for clonality. PCR-based methods usually employ multiple primer sets targeting different gene segments that are potentially rearranged. Primers for the antigen receptor genes are generally designed to anneal with families of variable and joining regions, and are termed consensus primers because they are not perfect matches to any one gene region. Because of variations in the primer sequences, these consensus primers do not anneal as tightly to the target as more specific primers that are designed against a single target area and thus do not amplify as efficiently.

Because these methods amplify both clonal and background polyclonal cells, they often show a smear or ladder with gel-based detection systems. Fluorochrome-labeled primers, however, result in a product that can be separated on the basis of size using a capillary sequencing polymer by capillary electrophoresis (Fig. 13.8). This approach allows for more clear separation of PCR products and makes it possible to more easily discriminate clonal populations from polyclonal background populations.

PCR testing for rearrangements of the immunoglobulin heavy chain gene is one of the most common tests performed in diagnostic molecular hematopathology laboratories. The VDJ rearrangement of this locus can be further subdivided based on which framework region (FR) is involved. Although there are three FRs in the V_H region of the *IGH* gene, all of which sequence similarly, assays with the highest detection rate for the immunoglobulin heavy chain gene rearrangements employ primers directed against the FRIII region of the various V_H genes and a less variable J_H region. Assays that employ FRIII and J_H primers detect 60% to 70% of clonal B-cell malignancies. The

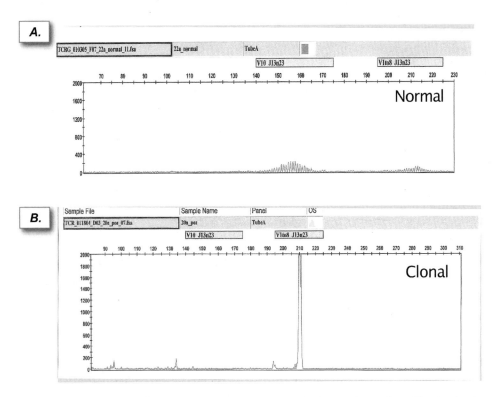

Figure 13.8 Electropherogram of TCRγ rearrangement. **A,** The products of amplification by the primers targeting *V10-J13* (BIOMED-2) show a Gaussian distribution, confirming that the rearrangements were random. **B,** shows one dominant peak, revealing that the amplification product was of one size, which could originate only in the presence of a clonal rearrangement. (See color insert.)

addition of primers to other framework regions, such as FRI or FRII, will increase the detection rate of this test. FRI, however, is composed of multiple families of regions, and so multiple PCR reactions are required to reliably detect rearrangements. Also, the products from FRI are often too large to be reproducibly amplified from paraffin-embedded tissues. Consequently, a combination of primers is most suitable for analysis of all specimen types, and most noncommercial methods of *IGH* PCR that use multiple primer sets detect 70% to 80% of B-cell neoplasms (158), depending on the type of disease. More extensive primer sets that have been recently studied as part of the BIOMED-2 project (159) appear to detect an even higher percentage of B-cell clones, and these primer sets are now commercially available for clinical use.

It should be stressed, however, that PCR-based methods will fail to detect some B-cell clones. False negative results most commonly occur in lymphoma types that are associated with somatic hypermutation of the immunoglobulin heavy chain gene. This phenomenon occurs with chronic lymphocytic leukemia (see below), but is most problematic with follicular lymphomas and plasma cell malignancies. Therefore, alternative methods of testing clonality, including detection of disease-specific translocations, should be considered in specimens suspected of these types of lymphoid neoplasms in the face of a negative *IGH* PCR test. Alternatively, samples with frozen tissue and a negative PCR result can be tested by Southern blot analysis for B-cell clonality.

PCR tests directed against rearrangement of the kappa light chain gene (*IGκ*) or the kappa deleting segment are also useful in the detection of B-cell clonality in mature B-cell proliferations and are reported to successfully detect clonality in 50% to 72% of B-cell lymphomas (154,160). This test can therefore be useful as a second-line test to exclude a false negative *IGH* PCR result.

PCR-based assays for T-cell clonality are usually directed against either *TCRβ* or *TCRγ*. Because of the complexity of the *TCRβ* locus, with 65 V regions, 2 D regions and 13 J regions, PCR for these rearrangements requires a large number of primers. The *TCRγ* gene is less complex, with only 4 V region families containing 11 loci and 5 J regions, and because the *TCRγ* locus is consistently rearranged before the *TCRβ* locus, PCR analysis with primers directed against the four V region families (Vγ1-8, Vγ9, Vγ10, and Vγ11) coupled with a multiplex of J region primers will detect over 90% of clonal T-cell neoplasms (161–163). In addition, *TCRγ* rearrangements can be detected in lymphomas of γ/δ T-cells that may not demonstrate evidence of clonality on Southern blot analysis for *TCRβ*. In contrast to the PCR for *IGH* gene rearrangements, if all of the *TCRγ* variable and joining regions sequences are covered by the PCR reactions, this test will result in few false negative reactions when compared to Southern blot analysis.

Because the PCR-based assays for antigen receptors (*IGH*, *IGκ*, and *TCRγ*) are directed against genomic DNA, they can be performed on paraffin-embedded tissue, a tissue substrate that is not amenable to Southern blot analysis. Furthermore, the limit of detection using *IGH* and *TCRγ* consensus primers can be as sensitive as 1% (e.g., 10 clonal cells present in a background of 990 polyclonal

cells). This certainly can be useful for initial diagnosis and is more sensitive than Southern blot methods.

For minimal residual disease testing, more sensitive methods are often required. Recent studies have shown that patient-specific primers are especially useful for minimal residual disease testing and can be used to detect as low as 1 tumor cell in 10^5 normal cells. However, this approach requires amplifying the original tumor sample clone using consensus primers, followed by sequencing of the PCR product in order to design the patient-specific primers. Because patient-specific primers anneal much better to the tumor DNA than consensus primers, they can be used to detect a lower level of disease (164). However, the primers are obviously useful only for samples from the same patient and will not detect development of new clones or second clones that were not identified in the initial sequencing. This labor-intensive approach is not offered by most diagnostic laboratories at this time, but is a powerful method for minimal residual disease detection (165,166).

Limitations to antigen receptor testing, other than the disorder-specific false negative results already described, include false negative results related to three other causes, specifically, DNA degradation, lineage infidelity, and presence of clonal populations in non-neoplastic conditions.

As far as DNA degradation is concerned, false negative rates are higher in paraffin samples compared with frozen samples (158,167). Although detection of an internal control gene is useful in confirming DNA integrity in a sample, it will not completely eliminate false negative results, especially if the amount of target DNA in a sample is less than that of the internal control gene. Whenever the clinical suspicion is high and not concordant with clonality studies, analysis should be performed on fresh or frozen tissue from a new biopsy of the lesion.

Lineage infidelity refers to the detection of clonal rearrangement in a different cell type from that supported by other methods, especially immunophenotyping (e.g., a *TCR* gene rearrangement in a B-cell lymphoma). This may occur with any type of lymphoma, but is most common in the lymphoblastic malignancies (168), and in fact, detection of both *IGH* and *TCRβ* gene rearrangements is a common finding in precursor B-cell acute lymphoblastic leukemia. Detection of these aberrant molecular rearrangements is often still helpful in confirming the clonal nature of a lymphoid infiltrate, but molecular studies should clearly not be used alone to assign cell lineage (159). Instead, immunophenotyping studies should be the primary method used to define cell lineage in cases with evidence of both T- and B-cell clonality.

Detection of "clonal" rearrangements in non-neoplastic conditions is also a well-recognized source of erroneous test results (169–172), and oligoclones are more commonly detected by capillary electrophoresis detection methods that achieve better separation of DNA fragments than standard gel-based methods. Some putative clonal populations actually represent oligoclonal proliferations, which are most common with viral infections such as infectious mononucleosis. Clonal rearrangements also have been reported in some preneoplastic conditions, such as angioimmunoblastic lymphadenopathy with dysproteinemia (AILD, which is now considered a type of T-cell lymphoma), and lymphomatoid papulosis. Pseudo-clones may also be detected from very small biopsy specimens containing small numbers of the targeted lymphoid cells; these pseudo-clones most often represent selective amplification of a sparse cell population and are not usually reproducible on repeat analysis. Therefore, PCR clonality studies of small samples should demonstrate an identical abnormality on repeat testing before being considered as supporting clonality in a sample (173).

Molecular Abnormalities Unique to Specific B-Cell Lymphoma Types

The immunoglobulin genes (*IGH*, *IGκ*, and *IGλ*) and the T-cell receptor genes (α, β, δ, or γ) are commonly involved as fusion partners in chromosomal translocations (Table 13.5). Some of these translocations are relatively disease specific. Genes commonly juxtaposed to the antigen receptor genes are putative oncogenes, which turn on the cell cycle and presumably trigger a clonal lymphoid proliferation. These translocations may be detectable by conventional karyotype analysis, but this method is often negative because of problems with cell growth in culture that are especially common for many of the low-grade lymphomas. Consequently, FISH analysis is more sensitive than karyotyping, although FISH will not detect secondary abnormalities. FISH techniques employing break-apart probes

have the advantage of being able to detect translocations involving a given common partner gene, but require additional studies to confirm the identity of the fusion partner. Amplification-based molecular methods, such as PCR, are employed in many clinical laboratories and can be more sensitive than FISH for detecting very low levels of a specific translocation. However, PCR methods will not detect all the variant break points that are usually detectable by FISH analysis with break-apart probes, or even by karyotype analysis. Therefore, there are advantages and disadvantages to the different methods of detection, and the method of choice for a given abnormality can vary (see later discussion).

Follicular Lymphoma

The translocation t(14;18)(q32;q21) was one of the earliest translocations described in lymphomas, and it most commonly characterizes follicular center cell lymphoma (174). The t(14;18) juxtaposes *IGH* (or J_H) gene on chromosome 14 and *BCL2* gene on chromosome 18 (175–177). *BCL2* expression is associated with inhibition of apoptosis, and the translocation results in an increased proliferation of B-lymphocytes of follicular center cell origin; 70% to 80% of follicular lymphomas carry t(14;18), which is also seen in 17% to 38% of diffuse large B-cell lymphomas (178). There

TABLE 13.5
EXAMPLES OF NONRANDOM ABNORMALITIES CHARACTERISTIC OF LYMPHOMAS

Disease	Genetic Aberration	Genes	Frequency (%)
B-cell neoplasms			
Follicular center cell lymphoma	t(14;18)(q32;q21)	IGH-BCL2	70–80
	t(2;18)(p12;q21)	IGλ-BCL2	Rare
Mantle cell lymphoma	t(11;14)(q13;q32)	IGH-BCL1	>95
	deletions of 11q22-23	ATM	30
Marginal zone lymphoma	t(11;18)(q21;q21)	API2-MALT1	14
	t(14;18)(q32;q21)	IGH-MALT1	11
	t(3;14)(p14.1;q32)	IGH-FOXP1	10
	t(1;14)(q21-22;q32)	IGH-BCL10	Rare
B-cell small lymphomatic lymphoma/chronic lymphocytic leukemia	Deletions of 13q14, 11q22-23, 17p13, 6q21; trisomy 12	Unknown	80
Diffuse large B-cell lymphoma	t(14;18)(q32;q21)	IGH-BLC2	17–38
	rearrangements of 3q27	BCL6	33
Burkitt's lymphoma/Burkitt's-like lymphoma	t(8;14)(q24;q32)	IGH-CMYC	80
	t(8;22)(q24;q11)	IGκ-CMYC	
	t(2;8)(p12;q24)	IGλ-CMYC	
T-cell neoplasms			
Anaplastic large cell lymphoma	t(2;5)(p23;q35)	NPM-ALK	70–80[a]
	t(1;2)(q21;q23)	TPM3-ALK	10–20
	t(2;3)(p23;p21)	TFG-ALK	2–5
	t(2;2)(p23;q35)	ATIC-ALK	2–5
	t(2;17)(p23;q23)	CTLC-ALK	1–5
	t(X;2)(q11-12;p23)	MSN-ALK	<1
T-cell prolymphocytic leukemia	Abnormalities of 14q, 8q, 11q	Unknown	

[a]Of cases with an ALK rearrangement; overall, only about 40% of anaplastic large cell lymphomas harbor an ALK rearrangement.

are five common *BCL2* break points involved in the t(14;18), specifically major breakpoint region (MBR), minor (mcr) and intermediate (icr) cluster regions, 3'*BCL2*, and 5'MCR (179,180), and different PCR primer sets are needed to detect all the individual *BCL2* break points. Most laboratories only use primer sets to detect the MBR and mcr break points which will detect the t(14;18) in approximately 70% of cases (181,182). However, given recent data that suggest that some of the less commonly tested break points may be more frequent than previously appreciated, and even more frequent than the mcr break point (180,183), the MBR and mcr PCR–based tests that are offered in most laboratories may not provide for sensitive detection of t(14;18). In contrast, FISH-based assays using either fusion or break-apart probes will detect these cases (184).

As a result of somatic hypermutation of the immunoglobulin heavy chain gene in follicular center cells, only 35% to 50% of follicular lymphomas will have a detectable immunoglobulin heavy chain rearrangement by PCR analysis using a single FRIII primer set (185,186). However, because these mutations do not affect the overall gene rearrangement, virtually all follicular lymphomas will show a rearrangement by Southern blot analysis (187). Despite the relatively high false negative rate for immunoglobulin heavy chain gene rearrangement by PCR analysis, 70% to 80% of follicular lymphomas will nonetheless demonstrate t(14;18)(q32;q21) involving the immunoglobulin heavy chain gene on chromosome 14 and the *BCL2* gene on chromosome 18 by either PCR or FISH (188). Although most translocations can be detected from paraffin-embedded tissues, some minor break points result in PCR products that are very large and that therefore are not reliably detected after formalin fixation (189).

The t(14;18) has been reported to be detected by J_H/*BCL2* PCR analysis in normal peripheral blood and in reactive lymph nodes (190–192). These reports suggest that the translocation can occur in small numbers of cells without the development of malignant lymphoma. Nonnested PCR tests for J_H/*BCL2* that do not employ more than 45 cycles do not usually detect these false positive cases (186).

Detection of t(14;18) by molecular methods is not necessary for the diagnosis of most cases of follicular lymphoma (193–195). However, such testing may be valuable in the detection of minimal residual disease, such as in bone marrow aspirate material following chemotherapy or bone marrow transplantation for follicular lymphoma. Because the PCR-based assays are directed against specific break points, they can detect much lower levels of residual disease (1 in 100,000 cells) than the consensus primers used for *IGH* PCR (196,197).

Mantle Cell Lymphoma

The t(11;14)(q13;q32), which involves the immunoglobulin heavy chain gene of chromosome 14 and the *BCL1/PRAD1* gene of chromosome 11, is present in the majority of cases of mantle cell lymphoma (MCL) (198–200). The *BCL1* gene encodes a cell cycle protein (termed cyclin D1), and overexpression is associated with the aggressive behavior of this tumor. The major translocation cluster (MTC) region is involved in 40% of cases, but the remaining translocations involve a multitude of different *BCL1* sites that are not easily detectable by PCR analysis (201). Methods that target *BCL1* mRNA detect over 95% of cases of MCL, and the mRNA expression presumably occurs with translocations that involve the MTC, as well as other break points. However, assays that target *BCLI* mRNA require a quantitative RT-PCR procedure that is not readily available in most laboratories (202,203).

MCLs also demonstrate nuclear overexpression of BCL1/cyclin D1 protein that is a result of the translocation involving *BCL1/PRAD1*. As mentioned above, BCL1 cyclinD1 mRNA can be detected by PCR (204–206), but identification of cyclin D1 protein expression by immunohistochemistry is more sensitive than direct PCR for the MTC break point of J_H/*BCL1* (207,208). Weak expression of cyclin D1 has been described in other lymphoid tumors, including hairy cell leukemia and multiple myeloma (207).

FISH detection of t(11;14) is more sensitive than PCR and is particularly useful on peripheral blood specimens that are not optimal for immunohistochemistry (209). In a comparative study of 35 cases of MCL, 97% of cases were detected by FISH, whereas PCR tested positive in only 37% of cases (208). Recent gene expression studies have confirmed the existence of BCL1-negative MCL, which correlates with decreased proliferation and improved survival (210). These cases have an otherwise similar gene expression profile to cyclin D1-positive cases.

About 30% of MCL patients (209) show a deletion of chromosome 11q22-23 (211), and the putative gene in this deleted locus is *ATM* (ataxia telangiectasia mutated) in at least 75% of patients. Defects in DNA double-strand breakage repair, together with the resulting chromosomal translocations during VDJ rearrangements, are thought to be the underlying genetic event in *ATM* deletions leading to MCL (211–213).

Marginal Zone Lymphomas

Translocations involving the *MALT1* (also referred to as *MLT*) gene on chromosome 11q21 are present in approximately one quarter of marginal zone lymphomas (214, 215). The t(11;18)(q21;q21) is the most common translocation, seen in 13.5% of cases, especially in the lung and gastrointestinal tract; the t(11;18) involves the apoptosis inhibitor gene (*API2*) on chromosome 11 (215,216). The t(14;18)(q32;q21) involves *IGH* and *MALT1* and occurs in 10.8% of cases, especially in ocular adnexa, cutaneous, and salivary gland marginal zone lymphomas.

MALT1 translocations appear to be specific for only the nonsplenic, extranodal marginal zone lymphomas and are not detected in splenic marginal zone lymphomas and the primary nodal marginal zone lymphomas previously termed monocytoid B-cell lymphomas (217–219). In addition, extranodal marginal zone lymphomas with increased large cells or evidence of large cell transformation do not demonstrate these translocations, even in the accompanying low-grade component (215,220), and the presence of t(11;18) in gastric marginal zone lymphoma is associated with a lack of response to *Helicobacter pylori* therapy (221). More recently, a t(3;14)(p14.1;q32) involving *IGH* and *FOXP1* has been described, and is reported to occur in 9.9% of marginal zone lymphomas with a predilection for the ocular adnexa, skin, and thyroid (222). Rare cases (<2%) have a t(1;14) translocation involving *BCL10* on chromosome 1q21-22 and *IGH*, a translocation that results in overexpression of nuclear BCL10 protein, which also appears to occur in cases with *MALT1* translocations (223,224). Finally, trisomies of chromosomes 3 and 18 are also common in marginal zone lymphomas, although the relevant genes have not been identified.

Multiple break point sites have been described for *API2-MALT1* translocations, and RT-PCR or FISH analyses are usually needed to detect the abnormality (215,225). Because most marginal zone lymphomas are now diagnosed based on small tissue biopsies for which frozen tissue is not available, FISH analysis on paraffin-embedded tissue is often the best method to detect this translocation (Fig. 13.9). Although the use of break-apart *MALT1* probes by FISH analysis allows for the identification of cases with either *API2-MALT1* or *IGH-MALT1*, the method does not confirm the translocation partner.

Amplification-based methods have also been used and are more sensitive than cytogenetic methods, but RNA extraction and RT-PCR–based amplification are difficult to perform from small FFPE tissue biopsy samples (226).

B-cell Small Lymphocytic Lymphoma/Chronic Lymphocytic Leukemia

Molecular studies are usually not necessary for the diagnosis of B-cell small lymphocytic lymphoma/chronic lymphocytic leukemia (CLL) (227). All cases show immunoglobulin

heavy chain gene rearrangements, and these gene rearrangements are usually detectable by PCR. Characteristic cytogenetic abnormalities in CLL include deletions of 13q14, 11q22-23, 17p13, and 6q21, as well as trisomy 12; 13q deletions have the best prognosis, 17p deletions the worst. Trisomy 12, originally thought to be common in CLL, is more commonly associated with cases that have atypical features or are undergoing transformation to a higher-grade process. Because the genetic abnormalities in CLL do not represent recurring balanced translocations, they cannot be routinely tested for using PCR. The most common deletions and trisomies are usually evaluated by FISH (228,229).

Generally, CLL is an indolent disease. Most patients have a protracted course, and only a minority succumb to rapid progression. Recent study of *IGH* mutational status in CLL and its correlation with long-term outcome has evoked interest in identifying the subset of patients who are at risk for progression (230,231). *IGH* undergoes somatic hypermutation in some B-cells, and this most commonly occurs in postgerminal center B-cells; and lack of hypermutation of this gene in CLL is associated with more aggressive disease. However, this type of testing is labor intensive, and so it is offered by few diagnostic laboratories. The test requires amplification of the CLL *IGH* gene rearrangement followed by DNA sequence of the PCR product; the sequence of the immunoglobulin variable region is then compared to consensus sequence data for the region to determine the mutational status.

Gene expression studies on CLL patients have also identified surrogate markers that correlate with mutational

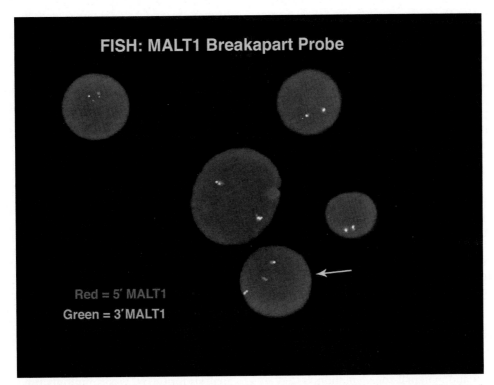

Figure 13.9 Break-apart FISH targeting 3′ and 5′ regions of *MALT1* shows a fusion of red and green (*yellow signal*) in the normal allele. In the presence of a translocation (indicated by the *arrow*), the targets are spliced apart, resulting in two different signals (*red* and *green*). The nucleus also shows one normal allele. (Courtesy Mr. Charles Dana Bangs, Cytogenetics Laboratory, Stanford University Medical Center.) (See color insert.)

status. These surrogate markers include CD38 and ZAP-70. ZAP-70 expression is considered more consistent with the lack of *IGH* mutations and can be evaluated by immuno-histochemistry and flow cytometry (232,233).

Lymphoplasmacytic Lymphoma

The t(9;14)(p13;q32) translocation was originally reported to occur in up to half of lymphoplasmacytic lymphomas, as well as in rare cases of marginal zone lymphoma (234) and diffuse large B-cell lymphoma (235,236). This transloca-tion involves the *PAX5* gene on chromosome 9 and the immunoglobulin heavy chain gene on chromosome 14. The translocation occurs 3' to the constant region of the immunoglobulin heavy chain locus in the switch μ region, different from the region involved in the $J_H/BCL1$ and $J_H/BCL2$ translocations. *PAX5* normally encodes a B-cell–specific transcription factor known as B-cell–specific activator protein (BSAP), which regulates B-cell prolifera-tion and differentiation (237). Although molecular analysis for *PAX5-IGH* is not offered in most diagnostic laboratories, several investigators have developed FISH probes to this translocation. Those studies have not been able to confirm an association of this translocation with lymphoplasma-cytic lymphoma (225,238), and this abnormality actually appears to be fairly uncommon.

Diffuse Large B-cell Lymphoma

The t(14;18)(q32;q21), identical to the translocation char-acteristic of follicular lymphomas, is identified in 17% to 38% of diffuse large B-cell lymphomas using detection methods identical to those described above (178). Some studies have suggested that the presence of t(14;18) in large cell lymphoma is a poor prognostic indicator (239,240), which appears to contradict the findings of gene array studies (see later discussion) (241). In both fol-licular lymphomas and diffuse large B-cell lymphomas, detection of the t(14;18) translocation does not correlate with the level of BCL2 protein expression.

Up to one third of diffuse large B-cell lymphomas, including some with t(14;18), have abnormalities involv-ing the *BCL6* gene on chromosome region 3q27 (242–244). *BCL6* abnormalities are also found in higher-grade (grade 3) follicular lymphoma with a diffuse large B-cell component, which correlates somewhat with pro-gression (245). The most common abnormalities of *BCL6* are translocations involving the immunoglobulin heavy chain region of 14q32, the kappa light chain region of 2p11, or the lambda light chain region of 22q11 as fusion partners. Translocations involving *BCL6* are more com-monly associated with extranodal disease than nodal lym-phomas (246), and translocations involving *BCL6* and chromosomes 1, 9, 11, and 12 have also been reported and are apparently correlated with a relatively worse outcome (246). Rearrangements of *BCL6* have been reported to occur in other types of B-cell lymphoma, particularly fol-licular lymphomas and marginal zone lymphomas (247).

The clinical significance of the detection of *BCL6* rearrangements in large cell lymphoma is controversial. PCR-based detection methods are limited by the large number of translocations that occur with the *BCL6* gene,

the high frequency of somatic mutations of the *BCL6* gene, and the fact that the translocations usually take place within an intron adjacent to the coding regions of the gene (248). Consequently, long-range PCR, RT-PCR, or FISH methods are needed for analysis (249), most of which require fresh or frozen tissue, although FISH can be per-formed on paraffin-embedded tissue. Quantitative detec-tion of *BCL6* mRNA has been shown to have prognostic significance, but has not found popular usage (250).

Although *BCL6* expression and t(14;18) are both mark-ers of a possible germinal center cell origin in diffuse large B-cell lymphoma, gene array studies have identified a more comprehensive set of markers for identifying a germinal center cell phenotype (251–256). There are differences in the methods and conclusions of the various gene array studies in diffuse large B-cell lymphoma; these studies have identified distinct gene-expression subgroups of dif-fuse large B-cell lymphoma. The *germinal center B-cell–like* lymphomas express genes characteristic of normal germi-nal centers. Detection of c-*rel* amplification and t(14;18) are the most specific abnormalities in the germinal center B-cell–like group, but in contrast to previous studies on the prognostic significance of t(14;18), this lymphoma group is reported to be associated with a more favorable progno-sis. The *activated B-cell–like* group expresses genes charac-teristic of mitogenically activated peripheral blood B-cells and are associated with a worse prognosis. *Type 3* lym-phomas do not express either germinal center or activated B-cell genes at a high level. Although these subgroups are prognostically significant, gene array methods are not cur-rently offered for diagnostic use. However, expression pro-filing has identified candidate markers (252,254) such as human germinal-center–associated lymphoma (HGAL), which may be useful for prognostication (257).

Burkitt's Lymphoma/Burkitt's-like Lymphoma

Burkitt's lymphoma is associated with translocations involving the *CMYC* gene of chromosome region 8q24 (258–260). The most common translocation is t(8;14) (q24;q32), which involves *IGH* and occurs in approxi-mately 80% of cases. The remaining cases demonstrate t(8;22)(q24;q11), involving the kappa light chain gene, or t(2;8)(p11;q24), involving the lambda light chain gene. It is noteworthy that the site of translocation differs between endemic and sporadic Burkitt's lymphoma; in endemic disease, the t(8;14) occurs up to 300 kb 5' from the coding region of *CMYC*, while in sporadic Burkitt's lymphoma the translocation characteristically involves a break point that is within in *CMYC* (261,262). The same translocations may also occur in the Burkitt's-like lym-phomas and in a small number of diffuse large B-cell lymphomas.

Variations in the translocation break points, including translocations involving the constant regions rather than joining regions of 14q32, make them poor targets for detection by routine PCR (263). In the past, Southern blot analysis for *CMYC* was commonly used, but FISH studies with break-apart probes are now more commonly used, especially because they can be used on paraffin-embedded tissues (264). Cases of atypical Burkitt's lymphoma arising from follicular lymphoma often have both *CMYC* translocations and the t(14;18) and are thought to have an aggressive course (265).

Molecular Abnormalities Unique to Specific T-Cell Lymphoma Types

T-cell Lymphomas

Other than T-cell gene rearrangements, abnormalities of *ALK* on chromosome 2p23 are the most commonly targeted aberrations and are associated with noncutaneous types of anaplastic large cell lymphoma (ALCL) (266–269). The t(2;5)(p23;q35) is the most common translocation, with a reported frequency of 40% in ALCL (270), and results in a fusion of the nucleolar phosphoprotein (*NPM*) gene of chromosome 5 and *ALK*; this fusion is present in 70% to 80% of all *ALK*-positive ALCLs. Other reported *ALK* gene fusion partners are *TPM3* at 1q21 (10% to 20%), *TFG* at 3q21 (2% to 5%), *ATIC* at 2q35 (2% to 5%), *CTLC* at 17q23 (1% to 5%), and *MSN* at Xq11-12 (<1%) (271–275). All the rearrangements cause overexpression of ALK protein, which is a leukocyte tyrosine kinase, driven by the fusion partner.

The t(2;5) fusion product can be detected by RT-PCR via amplification of a fairly small cDNA fragment (276). Because the fusion product is small, it may also be detected from FFPE tissue in some cases. The abnormality may also be detected by FISH analysis, a more sensitive approach than RT-PCR.

Because all of the *ALK* abnormalities result in expression of the ALK protein in varying patterns and ALK expression does not normally occur in lymphoid cells (277,278), ALK expression can be detected by immunohistochemistry and correlates well with FISH and other tests for *ALK* gene abnormalities (278–280). ALK expression has also been shown to correlate with improved survival, compared with ALK-negative ALCL (270,281). ALK expression may be nuclear, cytoplasmic, or both, depending on the *ALK* fusion partner.

The improved survival of ALK-positive lymphomas is independent of the translocation partner. Nevertheless, because all *ALK* translocations, including many *NPM-ALK* translocations, are not detectable by RT-PCR analysis, and because protein expression has such clinical relevance, ALK immunohistochemistry or *ALK* FISH with break-apart probes are the preferred tests for this disease, although RT-PCR may still have utility in monitoring for minimal residual disease.

Finally, it is worth noting that although ALK protein expression and gene abnormalities occur most commonly in ALCL, they are not restricted to this T-cell neoplasm. These are also described in normal nonhematopoietic tissues, rare types of B-cell lymphoma (282), and some soft tissue tumors, including inflammatory myofibroblastic tumor (283,284) (Chapter 11).

T-cell prolymphocytic leukemia is associated with cytogenetic abnormalities of chromosome regions 14q, 8q, and 11q (285–287). The most common abnormality is inv(14)(q11q32), and the chromosome 8 abnormalities include iso(8q) or trisomy 8. The chromosome 11 abnormalities involve 11q23, but do not appear to include the *MLL* gene. Several reports have identified the combined cytogenetic abnormality of isochromosome 7q and trisomy 8 in hepatosplenic T cell lymphoma (286,288). Even though FISH or karyotype analyses are the best methods for detecting many of the changes, none of these abnormalities are routinely evaluated for diagnostic purposes.

Viruses in Lymphoma

Several lymphoma types are associated with clonal viral integration of the lymphoma cells. Detection of the associated virus is often helpful in the classification of the neoplastic process.

Epstein-Barr Virus

The Epstein-Barr virus (EBV) is probably the most commonly studied virus in malignant lymphomas (289). In B-cell neoplasms, it is associated with Burkitt's lymphoma and the large B-cells of lymphomatoid granulomatosis (290,291). EBV RNA is detectable by molecular methods in 90% of endemic cases of Burkitt's lymphoma, compared to 20% to 30% in sporadic cases (291). Cases of EBV-positive Burkitt's lymphoma, however, are usually negative for EBV latent membrane protein (LMP) by immunohistochemistry, and in situ hybridization testing for EBER RNA is the preferred method for detecting EBV in this disease. EBV is also associated with most cases of post-transplant lymphoproliferative disorder (PTLD), which is usually a B-cell proliferation that occurs after solid organ transplantation and less commonly after hematopoietic stem cell transplantation (292,293). PTLD usually has evidence of B-cell clonality by *IGH* PCR and also shows EBV infection in virtually all of the tumor cells. EBV infection is also associated with the rare plasmablastic lymphomas and primary effusion lymphomas, both of which are also associated with infection with human immunodeficiency virus.

Nasal-type NK/T cell lymphoma has a high association with clonal EBV in the tumor cells (294,295). In situ hybridization detection of the virus may be diagnostically useful in the (usually) small biopsy specimens obtained to evaluate this disease. Because many of these cases are true NK neoplasms, they do not demonstrate T-cell receptor gene rearrangements, and so detection of EBV by in situ hybridization in the tumor cells is often the only diagnostic molecular test that is helpful. However, it is worth noting that these tumors often will not express EBV LMP by immunohistochemistry.

Angioimmunoblastic T-cell lymphoma is also associated with EBV infection (296–298). The EBV-infected cells in this proliferation, however, are admixed B-cell immunoblasts, and a subset of these patients will develop associated B-cell lymphomas (298).

EBV is detectable in the neoplastic cells of approximately 40% of cases of classical Hodgkin's lymphoma (299). The virus is most commonly detected in cases of the mixed cellularity type and may be detected by either in situ hybridization or EBV LMP immunohistochemistry. EBV infects only the neoplastic Reed-Sternberg cells, and most of the background cells are negative, and EBV testing represents one of the few settings in which molecular testing is useful for the diagnosis of Hodgkin's lymphoma. Although classic Hodgkin's lymphoma is now recognized to be a neoplasm of clonal B-cells, most cases do not have enough neoplastic cells to detect a B-cell gene rearrangement; consequently, only microdissected specimens or samples with very large numbers of Reed-Sternberg cells show evidence of B-cell clonality.

Finally, EBV positivity has also been observed in cases of inflammatory pseudo-tumor of the liver and spleen (300,301), although the significance of this observation remains uncertain.

EBV testing is often helpful in the diagnosis of a lymph node or tonsil biopsy from a patient with infectious mononucleosis, a sample that may be mistaken for Hodgkin's lymphoma or large B-cell lymphoma by histology alone. Infectious mononucleosis shows a large number of EBV-infected cells that have a wide variation in cell size, both features that are useful for differentiating infectious mononucleosis from Hodgkin's lymphoma (302,303).

Hepatitis C

Hepatitis C virus (HCV) is reported to be associated with a variety of types of B-cell lymphomas (304,305). Most of the reported cases occur in patients with mixed cryoglobulinemia, a disease with a known association with lymphoplasmacytic lymphoma. An association between hepatitis C and splenic marginal zone lymphoma has also been suggested (306,307). Because most studies of HCV and lymphoma use serologic or PCR methodologies, definite infection of the lymphoma cells with the virus has not been clearly demonstrated for most cases. However, because persistent antigen-driven stimulation of B-cells is thought to be an inciting event for the development of lymphoma, the fact that the B-cell surface receptor CD81 binds to HCV envelope-specific proteins and stimulates proliferation (308) suggests one mechanism by which HCV infection may contribute to lymphomagenesis.

Human Herpesvirus-8

Infection with the Kaposi's sarcoma herpesvirus/human herpes virus-8 (KSHV/HHV-8) is associated with primary effusion lymphomas, plasmablastic lymphoma, and multicentric Castleman's disease (309–311). KSHV/HHV-8 is usually detected by direct PCR (312), but recently described antibodies directed against the latent nuclear antigen (LANA) of KSHV are suitable for use in paraffin section and offer an alternative to PCR testing (313). Detection of KSHV/HHV-8 is particularly useful in the rare primary effusion lymphomas, a disease with pleomorphic cells that are not usually immunoreactive with T- or B-cell antibodies.

Human T-cell Leukemia Virus-1

There is a strong association between human T-cell leukemia virus-1 (HTLV-1) infection and adult T-cell leukemia/lymphoma (ATLL) (314–316). Clonal integration of the virus occurs in almost all ATLL patients, but in situ hybridization studies for this virus are difficult to perform and are not routinely offered. The virus may be detectable by serologic studies or quantified by RT-PCR analysis (317).

PRACTICAL ISSUES IN HEMATOPATHOLOGY RELATED TO MOLECULAR DIAGNOSTICS

The quantity and quality of genomic DNA or mRNA, together with the assay type, are major limiting factors in the performance of the various types of molecular tests used to evaluate LPDs. Paraffin-embedded tissues constitute the primary specimens available for testing in most cases, but, as discussed in detail in Chapter 5, the type of fixative and duration of fixation influence the maximum size of amplicons in PCR-based testing (318). Most fixatives in general use in hematopathology, such as B5 and Bouin's, yield very poor DNA (319), although Carnoy's and Zenker's yield a better quality of DNA. Acetone, alcohol, or 10% neutral-buffered formalin (159) yield the best-quality DNA and should be used whenever possible. The BIOMED-2 study (159) also suggested that a concentration of 50 to 100 ng of extracted DNA was ideal in amplification-based assays and that a higher concentration may be inhibitory.

The use of eosin stain for tissue visibility in paraffin embedding and processing may introduce an artifactual peak (Fig. 13.10) of about 71 bp in capillary electrophoresis analysis (320). This eosin peak seems to arise from autofluorescence of eosin and is seen most in the green region but

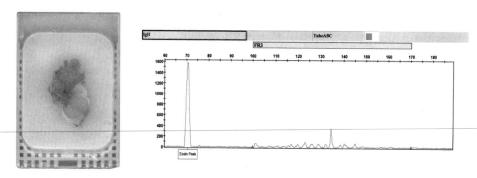

Figure 13.10 Eosin peak. Tissue marked with eosin (paraffin block) for visibility during processing, retain minute amounts of eosin during DNA extraction. Electropherogram tracings in the 71 base pair (bp) region shows a very bright signal, resulting from autofluorescence of eosin. In this particular specimen, which was tested for *IGH* rearrangements, this eosin peak did not fall within the clonal region. A clonal peak about 133 bp is also seen in this patient with a B-cell non-Hodgkin lymphoma. (See color insert.)

is also present in the yellow and blue spectral regions. This artifact will not occur in conventional gel-based testing.

When Is FISH Better Than Amplification-based Testing?

In general, PCR-based amplification testing permits faster, more specific, and more sensitive results, especially when the target genetic defect is very well characterized (321,322). In a few instances, however, PCR may not be an ideal test and instead in-situ hybridization is of higher utility.

When the cytogenetic aberration is known, but the specific genes involved have not been characterized, conventional cytogenetics or FISH are useful, for example, for detection of trisomy 8 or trisomy 12 or for detection of complex karyotypic abnormalities. For genetic abnormalities involving chromosomal translocations, rearrangements that involve multiple fusion partners are less amenable to PCR-based testing because this requires multiple primer sets. In this situation, FISH testing employing break-apart probes is extremely useful to screen for the characteristic chromosomal abnormalities, a strategy typically employed in testing for Burkitt's lymphoma, marginal zone lymphoma, and promyelocytic leukemia with cryptic translocations. However, FISH is not as sensitive as PCR-based methods, and so PCR is the most suitable for minimal residual disease detection.

FUTURE DIRECTIONS IN MOLECULAR DIAGNOSTICS OF HEMATOPOIETIC NEOPLASMS

The rapid expansion in new technologies for molecular analysis creates an overwhelming potential for future testing. The most visible new technology over the last few years has been chip-based gene microarrays (323–326) (Chapter 9). Gene arrays allow for the evaluation of the pattern of expression of thousands of genes from a single sample, but they usually generate too much data for use in diagnostic laboratories. The development of disease-specific arrays may make testing more amenable to routine diagnostic testing, and the recent availability of an array that allows detection of fusion partners of *MLL* translocations (*MLL* FusionChip, Ipsogen), illustrates that this technology is not far from being practically applied in routine clinical diagnosis. However, research studies with arrays have identified disease markers that are useful for clinical testing; for example, immunophenotypic analysis of ZAP-70 expression is a test that evolved from gene array studies (232,233).

With the development of more commercially available break-apart FISH probes, as well as multicolor FISH methods such as spectral karyotyping (327,328), FISH-based testing will continue to be even more widely applied in the diagnostic laboratory. Similarly, the increasing use of quantitative methods will contribute to increases in PCR-based testing, and the development of commercially available PCR primers and probes will allow for more standardization of PCR-based testing (329).

Finally, research in protein expression and identification of novel proteins (proteomics) will result in the identification of new disease markers and molecular targets. Despite significant technologic advances, technical challenges still limit the current use of proteome-based diagnostic testing in the molecular laboratory (330,331), although these methods have the advantage of high throughput and low test costs once uniform platforms and methods have been established. Taken together, these types of advances point to a bright future and continued growth of molecular diagnostics in hematopathology.

REFERENCES

1. Hungerford DA, Nowell PC. Chromosome studies in human leukemia. III. Acute granulocytic leukemia. *J Natl Cancer Inst* 1962;29:545–565.
2. Rowley JD. Letter: A new consistent chromosomal abnormality in chronic myelogenous leukaemia identified by quinacrine fluorescence and Giemsa staining. *Nature* 1973;243:290–293.
3. Seidman JG, Leder P. The arrangement and rearrangement of antibody genes. *Nature* 1978;276:790–795.
4. Arnold A, Cossman J, Bakhshi A, et al. Immunoglobulin-gene rearrangements as unique clonal markers in human lymphoid neoplasms. *N Engl J Med* 1983;309:1593–1599.
5. Cleary ML, Chao J, Warnke R, et al. Immunoglobulin gene rearrangement as a diagnostic criterion of B-cell lymphoma. *Proc Natl Acad Sci USA* 1984;81:593–597.
6. Arber DA, Downing J, and Cleary M. Pathology and molecular diagnosis of leukemias and lymphomas. In: Pizzo PA, Polack DG, eds. *Principles and Practice of Pediatric Oncology.* Philadelphia: Lippincott Williams & Wilkins; 2006 (In press).
7. U.S. Cancer Statistics Working Group. United States Cancer Statistics: 1999–2001 Incidence and Mortality Web-based Report Version. Atlanta (GA): Department of Health and Human Services, Centers for Disease Control and Prevention, and National Cancer Institute; 2004. Available at: www.cdc.gov/cancer/npcr/uses. Accessed 3/10/2005.
8. Jaffe ES, Harris NL, Stein H, et al., eds. *World Health Organization Classification of Tumours: Pathology and Genetics of Tumours of Haematopoietic and Lymphoid Tissues.* Lyon: IARC Press; 2001.
9. Arber DA. *Cancer Diagnostics: Current and Future Trends.* Totawa, NJ: Humana Press Inc. 2004; 233–259.
10. Kurzrock R, Bueso-Ramos CE, Kantarjian H, et al. BCR rearrangement-negative chronic myelogenous leukemia revisited. *J Clin Oncol* 2001;19:2915–2926.
11. Costello R, Sainty D, Lafage-Pochitaloff M, et al. Clinical and biological aspects of Philadelphia-negative/BCR-negative chronic myeloid leukemia. *Leuk Lymphoma* 1997;25:225–232.
12. Costello R, Lafage M, Toiron Y, et al. Philadelphia chromosome-negative chronic myeloid leukaemia: a report of 14 new cases. *Br J Haematol* 1995;90:346–352.
13. Melo JA. BCR-ABL gene variants. *Baillieres Clin Haematol* 2002;10:203–222.
14. Advani AS, Pendergast AM. Bcr-Abl variants: biological and clinical aspects. *Leuk Res* 2002;26:713–720.
15. Pane F, Frigeri F, Sindona M, et al. Neutrophilic-chronic myeloid leukemia: a distinct disease with a specific molecular marker (BCR/ABL with C3/A2 junction). *Blood* 1996;88:2410–2414.
16. Raanani P, Ben Bassat I, Gan S, et al. Assessment of the response to imatinib in chronic myeloid leukemia patients: comparison between the FISH, multiplex and RT-PCR methods. *Eur J Haematol* 2004;73:243–250.
17. Goldman J. Monitoring minimal residual disease in BCR-ABL-positive chronic myeloid leukemia in the imatinib era. *Curr Opin Hematol* 2005;12:33–39.
18. van Dongen JJ, Macintyre EA, Gabert JA, et al. Standardized RT-PCR analysis of fusion gene transcripts from chromosome aberrations in acute leukemia for detection of minimal residual disease: Report of the BIOMED-1 Concerted Action—investigation of minimal residual disease in acute leukemia. *Leukemia* 1999;13:1901–1928.
19. Radich JP, Gooley T, Bryant E, et al. The significance of bcr-abl molecular detection in chronic myeloid leukemia patients "late," 18 months or more after transplantation. *Blood* 2001;98:1701–1707.
20. Hardling M, Wei Y, Palmqvist L, et al. Serial monitoring of BCR-ABL transcripts in chronic myelogenous leukemia (CML) treated with imatinib mesylate. *Med Oncol* 2004;21:349–358.
21. Deininger M, Buchdunger E, Druker BJ. The development of imatinib as a therapeutic agent for chronic myeloid leukemia. *Blood* 2005;105:2640–2653.
22. Goldman J. CML resistance to tyrosine kinase inhibitors: how is the laboratory to tell? *Lab Hematol* 2004;10:181–184.
23. Marin D, Kaeda J, Szydlo R, et al. Monitoring patients in complete cytogenetic remission after treatment of CML in chronic phase with imatinib: patterns of residual leukaemia and prognostic factors for cytogenetic relapse. *Leukemia* 2005;19:507–512.
24. Lange T, Bumm T, Otto S, et al. Quantitative reverse transcription polymerase chain reaction should not replace conventional cytogenetics for monitoring patients with chronic myeloid leukemia during early phase of imatinib therapy. *Haematologica* 2004;89:49–57.
25. Lahaye T, Riehm B, Berger U, et al. Response and resistance in 300 patients with BCR-ABL-positive leukemias treated with imatinib in a single center: a 4.5-year follow-up. *Cancer* 2005;103:1659–1669.
26. Goldman JM. A unifying mutation in chronic myeloproliferative disorders. *N Engl J Med* 2005;352:1744–1746.
27. Manning G, Whyte DB, Martinez R, et al. The protein kinase complement of the human genome. *Science* 2002;298:1912–1934.
28. Bacher U, Haferlach T, Kern W et al. Conventional cytogenetics of myeloproliferative diseases other than CML contribute valid information. *Ann Hematol* 2005;84:250–257.
29. Baxter EJ, Kulkarni S, Vizmanos JL, et al. Novel translocations that disrupt the platelet-derived growth factor receptor beta (PDGFRB) gene in BCR-ABL-negative chronic myeloproliferative disorders. *Br J Haematol* 2003;120:251–256.

30. Golub TR, Barker GF, Lovett M, et al. Fusion of PDGF receptor b to a novel *ets*-like gene, *tel*, in chronic myelomonocytic leukemia with t(5;12) chromosomal translocation. *Cell* 1994;77:307–316.

31. Gotlib J, Cools J, Malone JM, III, et al. The FIP1L1-PDGFRalpha fusion tyrosine kinase in hypereosinophilic syndrome and chronic eosinophilic leukemia: implications for diagnosis, classification, and management. *Blood* 2004;103:2879–2891.

32. Cools J, DeAngelo DJ, Gotlib J, et al. A tyrosine kinase created by fusion of the *PDGFRA* and *FIP1L1* genes as a therapeutic target of imatinib in idiopathic hypereosinophilic syndrome. *N Engl J Med* 2003;348:1201–1214.

33. Levine RL, Wadleigh M, Cools J, et al. Activating mutation in the tyrosine kinase *JAK2* in polycythemia vera, essential thrombocythemia, and myeloid metaplasia with myelofibrosis. *Cancer Cell* 2005;7:387–397.

34. Kralovics R, Passamonti F, Buser AS, et al. A gain-of-function mutation of *JAK2* in myeloproliferative disorders. *N Engl J Med* 2005;352:1779–1790.

35. James C, Ugo V, Le Couedic JP, et al. A unique clonal *JAK2* mutation leading to constitutive signalling causes polycythaemia vera. *Nature* 2005;434:1144–1148.

36. Baxter EJ, Scott LM, Campbell PJ, et al. Acquired mutation of the tyrosine kinase JAK2 in human myeloproliferative disorders. *Lancet* 2005;365:1054–1061.

37. Bacher U, Haferlach T, Kern W, et al. Conventional cytogenetics of myeloproliferative diseases other than CML contribute valid information. *Ann Hematol* 2005;84:250–257.

38. Wlodarska I, Mecucci C, Marynen P, et al. *TEL* gene is involved in myelodysplastic syndromes with either the typical t(5;12)(q33;p13) translocation or its variant t(10;12)(q24;p13). *Blood* 1995;85:2848–2852.

39. McKenna RW. Myelodysplasia and myeloproliferative disorders in children. *Am J Clin Pathol* 2004;122:S58–S69.

40. Passmore SJ, Chessells JM, Kempski H, et al. Paediatric myelodysplastic syndromes and juvenile myelomonocytic *leukaemia* in the UK: a population-based study of incidence and survival. *Br J Haematol* 2003;121:758–767.

41. Hasle H, Arico M, Basso G, et al. Myelodysplastic syndrome, juvenile myelomonocytic leukemia, and acute myeloid leukemia associated with complete or partial monosomy 7. European Working Group on MDS in Childhood (EWOG-MDS). *Leukemia* 1999; 13:376–385.

42. Woods WG, Barnard DR, Alonzo TA, et al. Prospective study of 90 children requiring treatment for juvenile myelomonocytic leukemia or myelodysplastic syndrome: a report from the Children's Cancer Group. *J Clin Oncol* 2002;20:434–440.

43. Fidler C, Watkins F, Bowen DT, et al. *NRAS*, *FLT3* and *TP53* mutations in patients with myelodysplastic syndrome and a del(5q). *Haematologica* 2004;89:865–866.

44. Fenaux P. Chromosome and molecular abnormalities in myelodysplastic syndromes. *Int J Hematol* 2001;73:429–437.

45. Giagounidis AA, Germing U, Wainscoat JS, et al. The 5q- syndrome. *Hematology* 2004;9:271–277.

46. Yamamoto Y, Kiyoi H, Nakano Y, et al. Activating mutation of D835 within the activation loop of FLT3 in human hematologic malignancies. *Blood* 2001;97: 2434–2439.

47. Shih LY, Lin TL, Wang PN, et al. Internal tandem duplication of fms-like tyrosine kinase 3 is associated with poor outcome in patients with myelodysplastic syndrome. *Cancer* 2004;101:989–998.

48. Grimwade D. The pathogenesis of acute promyelocytic leukaemia: evaluation of the role of molecular diagnosis and monitoring in the management of the disease. *Br J Haematol* 1999;106:591–613.

49. Zelent A, Guidez F, Melnick A, et al. Translocations of the *RARalpha* gene in acute promyelocytic leukemia. *Oncogene* 2001;20:7186–7203.

50. Melnick A, Licht JD. Deconstructing a disease: *RARalpha*, its fusion partners, and their roles in the pathogenesis of acute promyelocytic leukemia. *Blood* 1999;93: 3167–3215.

51. Gonzalez M, Barragan E, Bolufer P, et al. Pretreatment characteristics and clinical outcome of acute promyelocytic leukaemia patients according to the PML-RAR alpha isoforms: a study of the PETHEMA group. *Br J Haematol* 2001;114:99–103.

52. Chou WC, Dang CV. Acute promyelocytic leukemia: recent advances in therapy and molecular basis of response to arsenic therapies. *Curr Opin Hematol* 2005; 12:1–6.

53. Reiter A, Lengfelder E, Grimwade D. Pathogenesis, diagnosis and monitoring of residual disease in acute promyelocytic leukaemia. *Acta Haematol* 2004;112:55–67.

54. Miller WH, Jr, Levine K, DeBlasio A, et al. Detection of minimal residual disease in acute promyelocytic leukemia by a reverse transcription polymerase chain reaction assay for the PML/RAR-alpha fusion mRNA. *Blood* 1993;82:1689–1694.

55. Tobal K, Liu Yin JA. RT-PCR method with increased sensitivity shows persistence of PML-RARA fusion transcripts in patients in long-term remission of APL. *Leukemia* 1998;12:1349–1354.

56. Tobal K, Moore H, Macheta M et al. Monitoring minimal residual disease and predicting relapse in APL by quantitating PML-RARalpha transcripts with a sensitive competitive RT-PCR method. *Leukemia* 2001;15:1060–1065.

57. Nicci C, Ottaviani E, Luatti S, et al. Molecular and cytogenetic characterization of a new case of t(5;17)(q35;q21) variant acute promyelocytic leukemia. *Leukemia* 2005; 19:470–472.

58. Downing JR. The core-binding factor leukemias: lessons learned from murine models. *Curr Opin Genet Dev* 2003;13:48–54.

59. Guidez F, Petrie K, Ford AM, et al. Recruitment of the nuclear receptor corepressor N-CoR by the TEL moiety of the childhood leukemia-associated TEL-AML1 oncoprotein. *Blood* 2000;96:2557–2561.

60. Krauter J, Gorlich K, Ottmann O, et al. Prognostic value of minimal residual disease quantification by real-time reverse transcriptase polymerase chain reaction in patients with core binding factor leukemias. *J Clin Oncol* 2003;21:4413–4422.

61. Dann EJ, Fears S, Arad-Dann H, et al. Lineage specificity of CBFA2 fusion transcripts. *Leuk Res* 2000;24:11–17.

62. Downing JR. AML1/CBFbeta transcription complex: its role in normal hematopoiesis and leukemia. *Leukemia* 2001;15:664–665.

63. Peterson LF, Zhang DE. The 8;21 translocation in leukemogenesis. *Oncogene* 2004; 23:4255–4262.

64. Downing JR. The AML1-ETO chimaeric transcription factor in acute myeloid leukaemia: biology and clinical significance. *Br J Haematol* 1999;106:296–308.

65. Downing JR, Higuchi M, Lenny N, et al. Alterations of the AML1 transcription factor in human leukemia. *Semin Cell Dev Biol* 2000;11:347–360.

66. Licht JD. AML1 and the AML1-ETO fusion protein in the pathogenesis of t(8;21) AML. *Oncogene* 2001;20:5660–5679.

67. Liu PP, Hajra A, Wijmenga C, et al. Molecular pathogenesis of the chromosome 16 inversion in the M4Eo subtype of acute myeloid leukemia. *Blood* 1995;85:2289–2302.

68. Chan NP, Wong WS, Ng MH, et al. Childhood acute myeloid leukemia with CBFbeta-MYH11 rearrangement: study of incidence, morphology, cytogenetics, and clinical outcomes of Chinese in Hong Kong. *Am J Hematol* 2004;76:300–303.

69. Steensma DP, Gibbons RJ, Mesa RA, et al. Somatic point mutations in RUNX1/CBFA2/AML1 are common in high-risk myelodysplastic syndrome, but not in myelofibrosis with myeloid metaplasia. *Eur J Haematol* 2005;74:47–53.

70. Vradii D, Zaidi SK, Lian JB, et al. Point mutation in AML1 disrupts subnuclear targeting, prevents myeloid differentiation, and effects a transformation-like phenotype. *Proc Natl Acad Sci USA* 2005;102:7174–7179.

71. Merchant SH, Haines S, Hall B, et al. Fluorescence in situ hybridization identifies cryptic t(16;16)(p13;q22) masked by del(16)(q22) in a case of AML-M4 Eo. *J Mol Diagn* 2004;6:271–274.

72. Saal RJ, Marlton PV, Timson G, et al. A rapid RT-PCR screening assay incorporating multiplexed validated control genes for CBF rearrangements at diagnosis in AML. *Pathology* 2004;36:335–342.

73. Jurlander J, Caligiuri MA, Ruutu T, et al. Persistence of the *AML1/ETO* fusion transcript in patients treated with allogeneic bone marrow transplantation for t(8;21) leukemia. *Blood* 1996;88:2183–2191.

74. Tobal K, Johnson PR, Saunders MJ, et al. Detection of *CBFB/MYH11* transcripts in patients with inversion and other abnormalities of chromosome 16 at presentation and remission. *Br J Haematol* 1995;91:104–108.

75. Leroy H, de Botton S, Grardel-Duflos N, et al. Prognostic value of real-time quantitative PCR (RQ-PCR) in AML with t(8;21). *Leukemia* 2005;19:367–372.

76. Mitterbauer M, Mitterbauer-Hohendanner G, Sperr WR, et al. Molecular disease eradication is a prerequisite for long-term remission in patients with t(8;21) positive acute myeloid leukemia: a single center study. *Leuk Lymphoma* 2004;45:971–977.

77. Higuchi M, O'Brien D, Kumaravelu P, et al. Expression of a conditional *AML1-ETO* oncogene bypasses embryonic lethality and establishes a murine model of human t(8;21) acute myeloid leukemia. *Cancer Cell* 2002;1:63–74.

78. Buonamici S, Ottaviani E, Testoni N, et al. Real-time quantitation of minimal residual disease in inv(16)-positive acute myeloid leukemia may indicate risk for clinical relapse and may identify patients in a curable state. *Blood* 2002;99:443–449.

79. Guerrasio A, Pilatrino C, De Micheli D, et al. Assessment of minimal residual disease (MRD) in *CBFbeta/MYH11*-positive acute myeloid leukemias by qualitative and quantitative RT-PCR amplification of fusion transcripts. *Leukemia* 2002;16:1176–1181.

80. DiMartino JF, Cleary ML. *MLL* rearrangements in haematological malignancies: lessons from clinical and biological studies. *Br J Haematol* 1999;106:614–626.

81. Ayton PM, Cleary ML. Molecular mechanisms of leukemogenesis mediated by MLL fusion proteins. *Oncogene* 2001;20:5695–5707.

82. Kohlmann A, Schoch C, Dugas M, et al. New insights into *MLL* gene rearranged acute leukemias using gene expression profiling: shared pathways, lineage commitment, and partner genes. *Leukemia* 2005;19:953–964.

83. Schnittger S, Kinkelin U, Schoch C, et al. Screening for MLL tandem duplication in 387 unselected patients with AML identify a prognostically unfavorable subset of AML. *Leukemia* 2000;14:796–804.

84. Schnittger S, Wormann B, Hiddemann W, et al. Partial tandem duplications of the *MLL* gene are detectable in peripheral blood and bone marrow of nearly all healthy donors. *Blood* 1998;92:1728–1734.

85. Dohner K, Tobis K, Ulrich R, et al. Prognostic significance of partial tandem duplications of the *MLL* gene in adult patients 16 to 60 years old with acute myeloid leukemia and normal cytogenetics: a study of the Acute Myeloid Leukemia Study Group Ulm. *J Clin Oncol* 2002;20:3254–3261.

86. Rubnitz JE, Raimondi SC, Tong X et al. Favorable impact of the t(9;11) in childhood acute myeloid leukemia. *J Clin Oncol* 2002;20:2302–2309.

87. Alsabeh R, Brynes RK, Slovak ML, et al. Acute myeloid leukemia with t(6;9) (p23;q34): association with myelodysplasia, basophilia, and initial CD34 negative immunophenotype. *Am J Clin Pathol* 1997;107:430–437.

88. Scandura JM, Boccuni P, Cammenga J, et al. Transcription factor fusions in acute leukemia: variations on a theme. *Oncogene* 2002;21:3422–3444.

89. Oyarzo MP, Lin P, Glassman A, et al. Acute myeloid leukemia with t(6;9)(p23;q34) is associated with dysplasia and a high frequency of *flt3* gene mutations. *Am J Clin Pathol* 2004;122:348–358.

90. Gupta R, Knight CL, Bain BJ. Receptor tyrosine kinase mutations in myeloid neoplasms. *Br J Haematol* 2002;117:489–508.

91. Schnittger S, Schoch C, Dugas M, et al. Analysis of *FLT3* length mutations in 1003 patients with acute myeloid leukemia: correlation to cytogenetics, FAB subtype, and prognosis in the AMLCG study and usefulness as a marker for the detection of minimal residual disease. *Blood* 2002;100:59–66.

92. Kottaridis PD, Gale RE, Linch DC. Flt3 mutations and leukaemia. *Br J Haematol* 2003;122:523–538.

93. Naoe T, Kiyoi H. Normal and oncogenic *FLT3*. *Cell Mol Life Sci* 2004;61:2932–2938.

94. Thiede C, Steudel C, Mohr B, et al. Analysis of *FLT3*-activating mutations in 979 patients with acute myelogenous leukemia: association with FAB subtypes and identification of subgroups with poor prognosis. *Blood* 2002;99:4326–4335.

95. Kottaridis PD, Gale RE, Frew ME, et al. The presence of a *FLT3* internal tandem duplication in patients with acute myeloid leukemia (AML) adds important prognostic information to cytogenetic risk group and response to the first cycle of chemotherapy: analysis of 854 patients from the United Kingdom Medical Research Council AML 10 and 12 trials. *Blood* 2001;98:1752–1759.

96. Kottaridis PD, Gale RE, Linch DC. Prognostic implications of the presence of *FLT3* mutations in patients with acute myeloid leukemia. *Leuk Lymphoma* 2003;44:905–913.

97. Kottaridis PD, Gale RE, Langabeer SE, et al. Studies of FLT3 mutations in paired presentation and relapse samples from patients with acute myeloid leukemia: implications for the role of *FLT3* mutations in leukemogenesis, minimal residual disease detection, and possible therapy with *FLT3* inhibitors. *Blood* 2002;100:2393–2398.

98. Murphy KM, Levis M, Hafez MJ, et al. Detection of *FLT3* internal tandem duplication and D835 mutations by a multiplex polymerase chain reaction and capillary electrophoresis assay. *J Mol Diagn* 2003;5:96–102.
99. Leroy H, Roumier C, Huyghe P, et al. CEBPA point mutations in hematological malignancies. *Leukemia* 2005;19:329–334.
100. Pabst T, Mueller BU, Zhang P, et al. Dominant-negative mutations of CEBPA, encoding CCAAT/enhancer binding protein-alpha (C/EBPalpha), in acute myeloid leukemia. *Nat Genet* 2001;27:263–270.
101. Preudhomme C, Sagot C, Boissel N, *et al.* Favorable prognostic significance of CEBPA mutations in patients with de novo acute myeloid leukemia: a study from the Acute Leukemia French Association (ALFA). *Blood* 2002;100:2717–2723.
102. Barjesteh van Waalwijk van Doorn-Khosrovani, Erpelinck C, Meijer J, et al. Biallelic mutations in the CEBPA gene and low CEBPA expression levels as prognostic markers in intermediate-risk AML. *Hematol J* 2003;4:31–40.
103. Schneider NR, Carroll AJ, Shuster JJ, et al. New recurring cytogenetic abnormalities and association of blast cell karyotypes with prognosis in childhood T-cell acute lymphoblastic leukemia: a pediatric oncology group report of 343 cases. *Blood* 2000; 96:2543–2549.
104. Borkhardt A, Cazzaniga G, Viehmann S, et al. Incidence and clinical relevance of *TEL/AML1* fusion genes in children with acute lymphoblastic leukemia enrolled in the German and Italian multicenter therapy trials. Associazione Italiana Ematologia Oncologia Pediatrica and the Berlin-Frankfurt-Munster Study Group. *Blood* 1997; 90:571–577.
105. Golub TR, Barker GF, Bohlander SK, et al. Fusion of the *TEL* gene on 12p13 to the *AML1* gene on 21q22 in acute lymphoblastic leukemia. *Proc Natl Acad Sci USA* 1995; 92:4917–4921.
106. Romana SP, Mauchauffe M, Le Coniat M, et al. The t(12;21) of acute lymphoblastic leukemia results in a *tel-AML1* gene fusion. *Blood* 1995;85:3662–3670.
107. Shurtleff SA, Buijs A, Behm FG, et al. *TEL/AML1* fusion resulting from a cryptic t(12;21) is the most common genetic lesion in pediatric ALL and defines a subgroup of patients with an excellent prognosis. *Leukemia* 1995;9:1985–1989.
108. Raynaud S, Mauvieux L, Cayuela JM, et al. *TEL/AML1* fusion gene is a rare event in adult acute lymphoblastic leukemia. *Leukemia* 1996;10:1529–1530.
109. Zelent A, Greaves M, Enver T. Role of the *TEL-AML1* fusion gene in the molecular pathogenesis of childhood acute lymphoblastic leukaemia. *Oncogene* 2004;23:4275–4283.
110. Borowitz MJ, Rubnitz J, Nash M, et al. Surface antigen phenotype can predict *TEL-AML1* rearrangement in childhood B-precursor ALL: a Pediatric Oncology Group study. *Leukemia* 1998;12:1764–1770.
111. De Zen L, Orfao A, Cazzaniga G, et al. Quantitative multiparametric immunophenotyping in acute lymphoblastic leukemia: correlation with specific genotype. I. *ETV6/AML1* ALLs identification. *Leukemia* 2000;14:1225–1231.
112. Kempski H, Chalker J, Chessells J, et al. An investigation of the t(12;21) rearrangement in children with B-precursor acute lymphoblastic leukaemia using cytogenetic and molecular methods. *Br J Haematol* 1999;105:684–689.
113. Drunat S, Olivi M, Brunie G, et al. Quantification of *TEL-AML1* transcript for minimal residual disease assessment in childhood acute lymphoblastic leukaemia. *Br J Haematol* 2001;114:281–289.
114. de Haas V, Breunis WB, Dee R, et al. The *TEL-AML1* real-time quantitative polymerase chain reaction (PCR) might replace the antigen receptor-based genomic PCR in clinical minimal residual disease studies in children with acute lymphoblastic leukaemia. *Br J Haematol* 2002;116:87–93.
115. Heerema NA, Sather HN, Ge J, et al. Cytogenetic studies of infant acute lymphoblastic leukemia: poor prognosis of infants with t(4;11): a report of the Children's Cancer Group. *Leukemia* 1999;13:679–686.
116. Heerema NA, Sather HN, Sensel MG, et al. Frequency and clinical significance of cytogenetic abnormalities in pediatric T-lineage acute lymphoblastic leukemia: a report from the Children's Cancer Group. *J Clin Oncol* 1998;16:1270–1278.
117. Pui CH, Chessells JM, Camitta B, et al. Clinical heterogeneity in childhood acute lymphoblastic leukemia with 11q23 rearrangements. *Leukemia* 2003;17:700–706.
118. Rubnitz JE, Link MP, Shuster JJ, et al. Frequency and prognostic significance of *HRX* rearrangements in infant acute lymphoblastic leukemia: a Pediatric Oncology Group study. *Blood* 1994;84:570–573.
119. Taki T, Ida K, Bessho F, et al. Frequency and clinical significance of the *MLL* gene rearrangements in infant acute leukemia. *Leukemia* 1996;10:1303–1307.
120. Pui CH, Rubnitz JE, Hancock ML, et al. Reappraisal of the clinical and biologic significance of myeloid-associated antigen expression in childhood acute lymphoblastic leukemia. *J Clin Oncol* 1998;16:3768–3773.
121. Lenormand B, Bene MC, Lesesve JF, et al. PreB1 (CD10-) acute lymphoblastic leukemia: immunophenotypic and genomic characteristics, clinical features and outcome in 38 adults and 26 children. The Groupe dEtude Immunologique des Leucemies. *Leuk Lymphoma* 1998;28:329–342.
122. Ishizawa S, Slovak ML, Popplewell L, et al. High frequency of pro-B acute lymphoblastic leukemia in adults with secondary leukemia with 11q23 abnormalities. *Leukemia* 2003;17:1091–1095.
123. Armstrong SA, Mabon ME, Silverman LB, et al. *FLT3* mutations in childhood acute lymphoblastic leukemia. *Blood* 2004;103:3544–3546.
124. Taketani T, Taki T, Sugita K, et al. *FLT3* mutations in the activation loop of tyrosine kinase domain are frequently found in infant ALL with *MLL* rearrangements and pediatric ALL with hyperdiploidy. *Blood* 2004;103:1085–1088.
125. Crist WM, Carroll AJ, Shuster JJ, et al. Poor prognosis of children with pre-B acute lymphoblastic leukemia is associated with the t(1;19)(q23;p13): a Pediatric Oncology Group study. *Blood* 1990;76:117–122.
126. Khalidi HS, O'Donnell MR, Slovak ML, et al. Adult precursor-B acute lymphoblastic leukemia with translocations involving chromosme band 19p13 is associated with poor prognosis. *Cancer Genet Cytogenet* 1999;109:58–65.
127. Secker-Walker LM, Berger R, Fenaux P, et al. Prognostic significance of the balanced t(1;19) and unbalanced der(19)t(1;19) translocations in acute lymphoblastic leukemia. *Leukemia* 1992;6:363–369.
128. Crist WM, Carroll AJ, Shuster JJ, et al. Poor prognosis of children with pre-B acute lymphoblastic leukemia is associated with the t(1;19)(q23;p13): a Pediatric Oncology Group study. *Blood* 1990;76:117–122.
129. Secker-Walker LM, Berger R, Fenaux P, et al. Prognostic significance of the balanced t(1;19) and unbalanced der(19)t(1;19) translocations in acute lymphoblastic leukemia. *Leukemia* 1992;6:363–369.
130. Borowitz MJ, Hunger SP, Carroll AJ, et al. Predictability of the t(1;19)(q23;p13) from surface antigen phenotype: implications for screening cases of childhood acute lymphoblastic leukemia for molecular analysis: a Pediatric Oncology Group study. *Blood* 1993;82:1086–1091.
131. Kee BL, Quong MW, Murre C. E2A proteins: essential regulators at multiple stages of B-cell development. *Immunol Rev* 2000;175:138–149.
132. Aspland SE, Bendall HH, Murre C. The role of E2A-PBX1 in leukemogenesis. *Oncogene* 2001;20:5708–5717.
133. Nourse J, Mellentin JD, Galili N, et al. Chromosomal translocation t(1;19) results in synthesis of a homeobox fusion mRNA that codes for a potential chimeric transcription factor. *Cell* 1990;60:535–545.
134. Seidel MG, Look AT. *E2A-HLF* usurps control of evolutionarily conserved survival pathways. *Oncogene* 2001;20:5718–5725.
135. Uckun FM, Nachman JB, Sather HN, et al. Clinical significance of Philadelphia chromosome positive pediatric acute lymphoblastic leukemia in the context of contemporary intensive therapies: a report from the Children's Cancer Group. *Cancer* 1998; 83:2030–2039.
136. Uckun FM, Nachman JB, Sather HN, et al. Poor treatment outcome of Philadelphia chromosome-positive pediatric acute lymphoblastic leukemia despite intensive chemotherapy. *Leuk Lymphoma* 1999;33:101–106.
137. Melo JA. *BCR-ABL* gene variants. *Baillieres Clin Haematol* 1997;10:203–222.
138. Advani AS, Pendergast AM. *Bcr-Abl* variants: biological and clinical aspects. *Leuk Res* 2002;26:713–720.
139. Holyoake TL. Recent advances in the molecular and cellular biology of chronic myeloid leukaemia: lessons to be learned from the laboratory. *Br J Haematol* 2001;113:11–23.
140. Advani AS, Pendergast AM. *Bcr-Abl* variants: biological and clinical aspects. *Leuk Res* 2002;26:713–720.
141. Uckun FM, Sensel MG, Sun L, et al. Biology and treatment of childhood T-lineage acute lymphoblastic leukemia. *Blood* 1998;91:735–746.
142. Schneider NR, Carroll AJ, Shuster JJ, et al. New recurring cytogenetic abnormalities and association of blast cell karyotypes with prognosis in childhood T-cell acute lymphoblastic leukemia: a pediatric oncology group report of 343 cases. *Blood* 2000;96:2543–2549.
143. Ferrando AA, Neuberg DS, Staunton J, et al. Gene expression signatures define novel oncogenic pathways in T cell acute lymphoblastic leukemia. *Cancer Cell* 2002;1:75–87.
144. Cave H, Suciu S, Preudhomme C, et al. Clinical significance of HOX11L2 expression linked to t(5;14)(q35;q32), of HOX11 expression, and of SIL-TAL fusion in childhood T-cell malignancies: results of EORTC studies 58881 and 58951. *Blood* 2004;103:442–450.
145. Trueworthy R, Shuster J, Crist W, et al. Ploidy of lymphoblasts is the strongest predictor of treatment outcome in B-progenitor cell acute lymphoblastic leukemia of childhood: a Pediatric Oncology Group study. *J Clin Oncol* 1992;10:606–613.
146. Ito C, Kumagai M, Manabe A, et al. Hyperdiploid acute lymphoblastic leukemia with 51 to 65 chromosomes: a distinct biological entity with a marked propensity to undergo apoptosis. *Blood* 1999;93:315–320.
147. Harrison CJ, Moorman AV, Broadfield ZJ, et al. Three distinct subgroups of hypodiploidy in acute lymphoblastic leukaemia. *Br J Haematol* 2004;125:552–559.
148. Yeoh EJ, Ross ME, Shurtleff SA, et al. Classification, subtype discovery, and prediction of outcome in pediatric acute lymphoblastic leukemia by gene expression profiling. *Cancer Cell* 2002;1:133–143.
149. Ross ME, Zhou X, Song G, et al. Classification of pediatric acute lymphoblastic leukemia by gene expression profiling. *Blood* 2003;102:2951–2959.
150. Arber DA. Molecular diagnostic approach to non-Hodgkin's lymphoma. *J Mol Diag* 2000;2:178–190.
151. Korsmeyer SJ, Hieter PA, Revetch JV, et al. Developmental hierarchy of immunoglobulin gene rearrangements in human leukemic pre-B-cells. *Proc Natl Acad Sci USA* 1981; 78:7096–7100.
152. Cossman J, Uppenkamp M, Sundeen J, et al. Molecular genetics and the diagnosis of lymphoma. *Arch Pathol Lab Med* 1988;112:117–127.
153. Pascual V, Capra JD. Human immunoglobulin heavy-chain variable region genes: organization, polymorphism, and expression. *Adv Immunol* 1991;49:1–74.
154. Gong JZ, Zheng S, Chiarle R, et al. Detection of immnoglobulin k light chain rearrangements by polymerase chain reaction: an improved method for detecting clonal B-cell lymphoproliferative disorders. *Am J Pathol* 1999;155:355–363.
155. Seriu T, Hansen-Hagge TE, Stark Y, et al. Immunoglobulin k gene rearrangements between the k deleting element and Jk recombination signal sequences in acute lymphoblastic leukemia and normal hematopoiesis. *Leukemia* 2000;14:671–674.
156. Aisenberg AC. Utility of gene rearrangements in lymphoid malignancies. *Annu Rev Med* 1993;44:75–84.
157. Sklar J, Weiss LM. Applications of antigen receptor gene rearrangements to the diagnosis and characterization of lymphoid neoplasms. *Annu Rev Med* 1988;39:315–334.
158. Bagg A, Braziel RM, Arber DA, et al. Immunoglobulin heavy chain gene analysis in lymphomas: a multi-center study demonstrating the heterogeneity of performance of polymerase chain reaction assays. *J Mol Diagn* 2002;4:81–89.
159. van Dongen JJ, Langerak AW, Bruggemann M, et al. Design and standardization of PCR primers and protocols for detection of clonal immunoglobulin and T-cell receptor gene recombinations in suspect lymphoproliferations: report of the BIOMED-2 Concerted Action BMH4-CT98-3936. *Leukemia* 2003;17:2257–2317.
160. Pai RK, Chakerian AE, Binder JM, et al. B-cell clonality determination using an immunoglobulin kappa light chain polymerase chain reaction method. *J Mol Diagn* 2005;7:300–307.
161. Greiner TC, Raffeld M, Lutz C, et al. Analysis of T cell receptor-g gene rearrangements by denaturing gradient gel electrophoresis of GC-clamped polymerase chain reaction products: correlation with tumor-specific sequences. *Am J Pathol* 1995;146:46–55.
162. Theodorou J, Bigorgne C, Delfau M-H, et al. VJ rearrangements of the *TCRg* locus in peripheral T-cell lymphomas: analysis by polymerase chain reaction and denaturing gradient gel electrophoresis. *J Pathol* 1996;178:303–310.
163. Greiner TC, Rubocki RJ. Effectiveness of capillary electrophoresis using fluorescent-labeled primers in detecting T-cell receptor gamma gene rearrangements. *J Mol Diagn* 2002;4:137–143.

164. Tarusawa M, Yashima A, Endo M, et al. Quantitative assessment of minimal residual disease in childhood lymphoid malignancies using an allele-specific oligonucleotide real-time quantitative polymerase chain reaction. *Int J Hematol* 2002;75:166–173.
165. Sabesan V, Cairo MS, Lones MA, et al. Assessment of minimal residual disease in childhood non-Hodgkin lymphoma by polymerase chain reaction using patient-specific primers. *J Pediatr Hematol Oncol* 2003;25:109–113.
166. van der Velden, V, Bruggemann M, Hoogeveen PG, et al. *TCRB* gene rearrangements in childhood and adult precursor-B-ALL: frequency, applicability as MRD-PCR target, and stability between diagnosis and relapse. *Leukemia* 2004;18:1971–1980.
167. Arber DA, Braziel RM, Bagg A, et al. Evaluation of T cell receptor testing in lymphoid neoplasms: results of a multicenter study of 29 extracted DNA and paraffin-embedded samples. *J Mol Diagn* 2001;3:133–140.
168. Szczepanski T, Beishuizen A, Pongers-Willemse MJ, et al. Cross-lineage T cell receptor gene rearrangements occur in more than ninety percent of childhood precursor-B acute lymphoblastic leukemias: alternative PCR targets for detection of minimal residual disease. *Leukemia* 1999;13:196–205.
169. McClain KL, Natkunam Y, Swerdlow SH. Atypical cellular disorders. *Hematology (Am Soc Hematol Educ Prog)* 2004;283–296.
170. Vallat L, Benhamou Y, Gutierrez M, et al. Clonal B cell populations in the blood and liver of patients with chronic hepatitis C virus infection. *Arthritis Rheum* 2004;50:3668–3678.
171. Tindle BH. The pathology of immunoblastic proliferations: reaction, prelymphoma, lymphoma. *Pathol Annu* 1991;26(Pt 2):145–186.
172. Dadej K, Gaboury L, Lamarre L, et al. The value of clonality in the diagnosis and follow-up of patients with cutaneous T-cell infiltrates. *Diagn Mol Pathol* 2001;10:78–88.
173. Vega F, Luthra R, Medeiros LJ, et al. Clonal heterogeneity in mycosis fungoides and its relationship to clinical course. *Blood* 2002;100:3369–3373.
174. Weiss LM, Warnke RA, Sklar J, et al. Molecular analysis of the t(14;18) chromosomal translocation in malignant lymphomas. *N Engl J Med* 1987;317:1185–1189.
175. Wei MC. *Bcl-2*-related genes in lymphoid neoplasia. *Int J Hematol* 2004;80:205–209.
176. Ngan BY, Chen-Levy Z, Weiss LM, et al. Expression in non-Hodgkin's lymphoma of the bcl-2 protein associated with the t(14;18) chromosomal translocation. *N Engl J Med* 1988;318:1638–1644.
177. Ngan BY, Nourse J, Cleary ML. Detection of chromosomal translocation t(14;18) within the minor cluster region of bcl-2 by polymerase chain reaction and direct genomic sequencing of the enzymatically amplified DNA in follicular lymphomas. *Blood* 1989;73:1759–1762.
178. Skinnider BF, Horsman DE, Dupuis B, et al. Bcl-6 and Bcl-2 protein expression in diffuse large B-cell lymphoma and follicular lymphoma: correlation with 3q27 and 18q21 chromosomal abnormalities. *Hum Pathol* 1999;30:803–808.
179. Buchonnet G, Jardin F, Jean N, et al. Distribution of *BCL2* breakpoints in follicular lymphoma and correlation with clinical features: specific subtypes or same disease? *Leukemia* 2002;16:1852–1856.
180. Shum C, Arber DA. Frequency of "minor" *JH/BCL2* breakpoints in follicular lymphoma. *J Mol Diagn* 2004;6:418.
181. Horsman DE, Gascoyne RD, Coupland RW, et al. Comparison of cytogenetic analysis, southern analysis, and polymerase chain reaction for the detection of t(14;18) in follicular lymphoma. *Am J Clin Pathol* 1995;103:472–478.
182. Aiello A, Delia D, Giardini R, et al. PCR analysis of IgH and *BCL2* gene rearrangement in the diagnosis of follicular lymphoma in lymph node fine-needle aspiration: a critical appraisal. *Diagn Mol Pathol* 1997;6:154–160.
183. Batstone PJ, Goodlad JR. Efficacy of screening the intermediate cluster region of the *bcl2* gene in follicular lymphomas by PCR. *J Clin Pathol* 2005;58:81–82.
184. Shaminie J, Peh SC, Tan MJ. Improvement in the detection rate of t(14;18) translocation on paraffin-embedded tissue: a combination approach using PCR and FISH. *Pathology* 2003;35:414–421.
185. Segal GH, Jorgensen T, Scott M, et al. Optimal primer selection for clonality assessment by polymerase chain reaction analysis. II. Follicular lymphomas. *Hum Pathol* 1994; 25:1276–1282.
186. Segal GH, Scott M, Jorgensen T, et al. Standard polymerase chain reaction analysis does not detect t(14;18) in reactive lymphoid hyperplasia. *Arch Pathol Lab Med* 1994; 118:791–794.
187. Ladanyi M, Wang S. Detection of rearrangements of the *BCL2* major breakpoint region in follicular lymphomas: correlation of polymerase chain reaction results with Southern blot analysis. *Diagn Mol Pathol* 1992;1:31–35.
188. Matsumoto Y, Nomura K, Matsumoto S, et al. Detection of t(14;18) in follicular lymphoma by dual-color fluorescence in situ hybridization on paraffin-embedded tissue sections. *Cancer Genet Cytogenet* 2004;150:22–26.
189. Wang YL, Addya K, Edwards RH, et al. Novel *bcl-2* breakpoints in patients with follicular lymphoma. *Diagn Mol Pathol* 1998;7:85–89.
190. Limpens J, de Jong D, van Krieken JH, et al. *Bcl-2/JH* rearrangements in benign lymphoid tissues with follicular hyperplasia. *Oncogene* 1991;6:2271–2276.
191. Limpens J, Stad R, Vos C, et al. Lymphoma-associated translocation t(14;18) in blood B cells of normal individuals. *Blood* 1995;85:2528–2536.
192. Ohshima K, Kikuchi M, Kobari S, et al. Amplified *bcl-2/JH* rearrangements in reactive lymphadenopathy. *Virchows Arch B Cell Pathol Incl Mol Pathol* 1993;63:197–198.
193. Swerdlow SH. Small B-cell lymphomas of the lymph nodes and spleen: practical insights to diagnosis and pathogenesis. *Mod Pathol* 1999;12:125–140.
194. Turner GE, Ross FM, Krajewski AS. Detection of t(14;18) in British follicular lymphoma using cytogenetics: Southern blotting and the polymerase chain reaction. *Br J Haematol* 1995;89:223–225.
195. Ashton-Key M, Diss TC, Isaacson PG, et al. A comparative study of the value of immunohistochemistry and the polymerase chain reaction in the diagnosis of follicular lymphoma. *Histopathology* 1995;27:501–508.
196. Rambaldi A, Lazzari M, Manzoni C, et al. Monitoring of minimal residual disease after CHOP and rituximab in previously untreated patients with follicular lymphoma. *Blood* 2002;99:856–862.
197. Galoin S, al Saati T, Schlaifer D, et al. Oligonucleotide clonospecific probes directed against the junctional sequence of t(14;18): a new tool for the assessment of minimal residual disease in follicular lymphomas. *Br J Haematol* 1996;94:676–684.
198. Rosenberg CL, Wong E, Petty EM, et al. *PRAD1*, a candidate *BCL1* oncogene: mapping and expression in centrocytic lymphoma. *Proc Natl Acad Sci USA* 1991;88:9638–9642.
199. Rimokh R, Berger F, Delsol G, et al. Detection of the chromosomal translocation t(11;14) by polymerase chain reaction in mantle cell lymphomas. *Blood* 1994;83:1871–1875.
200. Bertoni F, Zucca E, Cotter FE. Molecular basis of mantle cell lymphoma. *Br J Haematol* 2004;124:130–140.
201. Raynaud SD, Bekri S, Leroux D, et al. Expanded range of 11q13 breakpoints with differing patterns of cyclin D1 expression in B-cell malignancies. *Genes Chromosomes Cancer* 1993;8:80–87.
202. de Boer CJ, van Krieken JH, Kluin-Nelemans HC, et al. Cyclin D1 messenger RNA overexpression as a marker for mantle cell lymphoma. *Oncogene* 1995;10:1833–1840.
203. Jones CD, Darnell KH, Warnke RA, et al. *CyclinD1/CyclinD3* ratio by real-time PCR improves specificity for the diagnosis of mantle cell lymphoma. *J Mol Diagn* 2004; 6:84–89.
204. Bosch F, Jares P, Campo E, et al. *PRAD-1/cyclin D1* gene overexpression in chronic lymphoproliferative disorders: a highly specific marker of mantle cell lymphoma. *Blood* 1994;84:2726–2732.
205. Campo E, Raffeld M, Jaffe ES. Mantle-cell lymphoma. *Semin Hematol* 1999;36:115–127.
206. Aguilera NS, Bijwaard KE, Duncan B, et al. Differential expression of *cyclin D1* in mantle cell lymphoma and other non-Hodgkin's lymphomas. *Am J Pathol* 1998; 153:1969–1976.
207. de Boer CJ, van Krieken JH, Schuuring E, et al. *Bcl-1/cyclin D1* in malignant lymphoma. *Ann Oncol* 1997;8(suppl 2):109–117.
208. Belaud-Rotureau MA, Parrens M, Dubus P, et al. A comparative analysis of FISH, RT-PCR, PCR, and immunohistochemistry for the diagnosis of mantle cell lymphomas. *Mod Pathol* 2002;15:517–525.
209. Li JY, Gaillard F, Moreau A, et al. Detection of translocation t(11;14)(q13;q32) in mantle cell lymphoma by fluorescence in situ hybridization. *Am J Pathol* 1999; 154:1449–1452.
210. Rosenwald A, Wright G, Wiestner A, et al. The proliferation gene expression signature is a quantitative integrator of oncogenic events that predicts survival in mantle cell lymphoma. *Cancer Cell* 2003;3:185–197.
211. Bertoni F, Conconi A, Cogliatti SB, et al. Immunoglobulin heavy chain genes somatic hypermutations and chromosome 11q22–23 deletion in classic mantle cell lymphoma: a study of the Swiss Group for Clinical Cancer Research. *Br J Haematol* 2004; 124:289–298.
212. Camacho E, Hernandez L, Hernandez S, et al. *ATM* gene inactivation in mantle cell lymphoma mainly occurs by truncating mutations and missense mutations involving the phosphatidylinositol-3 kinase domain and is associated with increasing numbers of chromosomal imbalances. *Blood* 2002;99:238–244.
213. Camacho FI, Algara P, Rodriguez A, et al. Molecular heterogeneity in MCL defined by the use of specific *VH* genes and the frequency of somatic mutations. *Blood* 2003;101:4042–4046.
214. Auer IA, Gascoyne RD, Connors JM, et al. t(11;18)(q21;q21) is the most common translocation in MALT lymphomas. *Ann Oncol* 1997;8:979–985.
215. Streubel B, Simonitsch-Klupp I, Mullauer L, et al. Variable frequencies of MALT lymphoma-associated genetic aberrations in MALT lymphomas of different sites. *Leukemia* 2004;18:1722–1726.
216. Dierlamm J, Baens M, Wlodarska I, et al. The apoptosis inhibitor gene *API2* and a novel 18q gene, *MLT*, are recurrently rearranged in the t(11;18)(q21;q21) associated with mucosa-associated lymphoid tissue lymphomas. *Blood* 1999;93:3601–3609.
217. Remstein ED, James CD, Kurtin PJ. Incidence and subtype specificity of *API2-MALT1* fusion translocations in extranodal, nodal, and splenic marginal zone lymphomas. *Am J Pathol* 2000;156:1183–1188.
218. Motegi M, Yonezumi M, Suzuki H, et al. *API2-MALT1* chimeric transcripts involved in mucosa-associated lymphoid tissue type lymphoma predict heterogeneous products. *Am J Pathol* 2000;156:807–812.
219. Rosenwald A, Ott G, Stilgenbauer S, et al. Exclusive detection of the t(11;18)(q21;q21) in extranodal marginal zone B cell lymphomas (MZBL) of MALT type in contrast to other MZBL and extranodal large B cell lymphomas. *Am J Pathol* 1999;155:1817–1821.
220. Schreuder MI, Hoefnagel JJ, Jansen PM, et al. FISH analysis of MALT lymphoma-specific translocations and aneuploidy in primary cutaneous marginal zone lymphoma. *J Pathol* 2005;205:302–310.
221. Liu H, Ruskon-Fourmestraux A, Lavergne-Slove A, et al. Resistance of t(11;18) positive gastric mucosa-associated lymphoid tissue lymphoma to *Helicobacter pylori* eradication therapy. *Lancet* 2001;357:39–40.
222. Streubel B, Vinatzer U, Lamprecht A, et al. T(3;14)(p14.1;q32) involving IGH and FOXP1 is a novel recurrent chromosomal aberration in MALT lymphoma. *Leukemia* 2005;19:652–658.
223. Ye H, Gong L, Liu H, et al. MALT lymphoma with t(14;18)(q32;q21)/IGH-MALT1 is characterized by strong cytoplasmic MALT1 and BCL10 expression. *J Pathol* 2005; 205:293–301.
224. Liu H, Ye H, Dogan A, et al. T(11;18)(q21;q21) is associated with advanced mucosa-associated lymphoid tissue lymphoma that expresses nuclear BCL10. *Blood* 2001; 98:1182–1187.
225. Cook JR, Aguilera NI, Reshmi-Skarja S, et al. Lack of *PAX5* rearrangements in lymphoplasmacytic lymphomas: reassessing the reported association with t(9;14). *Hum Pathol* 2004;35:447–454.
226. Paternoster SF, Brockman SR, McClure RF, et al. A new method to extract nuclei from paraffin-embedded tissue to study lymphomas using interphase fluorescence in situ hybridization. *Am J Pathol* 2002;160:1967–1972.
227. Montillo M, Hamblin T, Hallek M, et al. Chronic lymphocytic leukemia: novel prognostic factors and their relevance for risk-adapted therapeutic strategies. *Haematologica* 2005;90:391–399.
228. Dohner H, Stilgenbauer S, Benner A, et al. Genomic aberrations and survival in chronic lymphocytic leukemia. *N Engl J Med* 2000;343:1910–1916.
229. Glassman AB, Hayes KJ. The value of fluorescence in situ hybridization in the diagnosis and prognosis of chronic lymphocytic leukemia. *Cancer Genet Cytogenet* 2005; 158:88–91.
230. Damle RN, Wasil T, Fais F, et al. Ig *V* gene mutation status and CD38 expression as novel prognostic indicators in chronic lymphocytic leukemia. *Blood* 1999;94:1840–1847.
231. Hamblin TJ, Davis Z, Gardiner A, et al. Unmutated Ig *V(H)* genes are associated with a more aggressive form of chronic lymphocytic leukemia. *Blood* 1999;94:1848–1854.

232. Crespo M, Bosch F, Villamor N, et al. ZAP-70 expression as a surrogate for immunoglobulin-variable-region mutations in chronic lymphocytic leukemia. *N Engl J Med* 2003;348:1764–1775.
233. Orchard JA, Ibbotson RE, Davis Z, et al. ZAP-70 expression and prognosis in chronic lymphocytic leukaemia. *Lancet* 2004;363:105–111.
234. Morrison AM, Jager U, Chott A, et al. Deregulated *PAX-5* transcription from a translocated IgH promoter in marginal zone lymphoma. *Blood* 1998;92:3865–3878.
235. Offit K, Parsa NZ, Filippa D, et al. t(9;14)(p13;q32) denotes a subset of low-grade non-Hodgkin's lymphoma with plasmacytoid differentiation. *Blood* 1992;80:2594–2599.
236. Iida S, Rao PH, Nallasivam P, et al. The t(9;14)(p13;q32) chromosomal translocation associated with lymphoplasmacytoid lymphoma involves the *PAX-5* gene. *Blood* 1996; 88:4110–4117.
237. Hagman J, Wheat W, Fitzsimmons D, et al. *Pax-5/BSAP*: regulator of specific gene expression and differentiation in B lymphocytes. *Curr Top Microbiol Immunol* 2000; 245:169–194.
238. George TI, Wrede JE, Bangs D, et al. Low grade B-cell lymphomas with plasmacytic differentiation lack *PAX5* gene rearrangements. *J Mol Diagn* 2005;7:346–351.
239. Yunis JJ, Mayer MG, Arnesen MA, et al. *bcl-2* and other genomic alterations in the prognosis of large-cell lymphoma. *N Engl J Med* 1989;320:1047–1054.
240. Hill ME, MacLennan KA, Cunningham DC, et al. Prognostic significance of *BCL-2* expression and *bcl-2* major breakpoint region rearrangement in diffuse large cell non-Hodgkin's lymphoma: a British National Lymphoma Investigation Study. *Blood* 1996; 88:1046–1051.
241. Dybkaer K, Iqbal J, Zhou G, et al. Molecular diagnosis and outcome prediction in diffuse large B-cell lymphoma and other subtypes of lymphoma. *Clin Lymphoma* 2004; 5:19–28.
242. Bastard C, Tilly H, Lenormand B, et al. Translocations involving band 3q27 and Ig gene regions in non-Hodgkin's lymphoma. *Blood* 1992;79:2527–2531.
243. Ye BH, Lista F, Lo CF, et al. Alterations of a zinc finger-encoding gene, *BCL-6*, in diffuse large-cell lymphoma. *Science* 1993;262:747–750.
244. Lo CF, Ye BH, Lista F, et al. Rearrangements of the *BCL6* gene in diffuse large cell non-Hodgkin's lymphoma. *Blood* 1994;83:1757–1759.
245. Katzenberger T, Ott G, Klein T, et al. Cytogenetic alterations affecting *BCL6* are predominantly found in follicular lymphomas grade 3B with a diffuse large B-cell component. *Am J Pathol* 2004;165:481–490.
246. Ueda C, Akasaka T, Ohno H. Non-immunoglobulin/*BCL6* gene fusion in diffuse large B-cell lymphoma: prognostic implications. *Leuk Lymphoma* 2002;43:1375–1381.
247. Muramatsu M, Akasaka T, Kadowaki N, et al. Rearrangement of the *BCL6* gene in B-cell lymphoid neoplasms. *Leukemia* 1997;11:318–320.
248. Akasaka H, Akasaka T, Kurata M, et al. Molecular anatomy of *BCL6* translocations revealed by long-distance polymerase chain reaction-based assays. *Cancer Res* 2000; 60:2335–2341.
249. Sonoki T, Willis TG, Oscier DG, et al. Rapid amplification of immunoglobulin heavy chain switch (IGHS) translocation breakpoints using long-distance inverse PCR. *Leukemia* 2004;18:2026–2031.
250. Kawamata N, Nakamura Y, Miki T, et al. Detection of chimaeric transcripts of the immunoglobulin heavy chain and *BCL6* genes by reverse-transcriptase polymerase chain reaction in B-cell non-Hodgkin's lymphomas. *Br J Haematol* 1998;100:484–489.
251. Rimsza LM, Roberts RA, Miller TP, et al. Loss of MHC class II gene and protein expression in diffuse large B-cell lymphoma is related to decreased tumor immunosurveillance and poor patient survival regardless of other prognostic factors: a follow-up study from the Leukemia and Lymphoma Molecular Profiling Project. *Blood* 2004; 103:4251–4258.
252. Lossos IS, Czerwinski DK, Alizadeh AA, et al. Prediction of survival in diffuse large-B-cell lymphoma based on the expression of six genes. *N Engl J Med* 2004; 350:1828–1837.
253. Alizadeh AA, Eisen MB, Davis RE, et al. Distinct types of diffuse large B-cell lymphoma identified by gene expression profiling. *Nature* 2000;403:503–511.
254. Rosenwald A, Wright G, Chan WC, et al. The use of molecular profiling to predict survival after chemotherapy for diffuse large-B-cell lymphoma. *N Engl J Med* 2002; 346:1937–1947.
255. Lossos IS, Jones CD, Warnke R, et al. Expression of a single gene, *BCL-6*, strongly predicts survival in patients with diffuse large B-cell lymphoma. *Blood* 2001;98:945–951.
256. Iqbal J, Sanger WG, Horsman DE, et al. BCL2 translocation defines a unique tumor subset within the germinal center B-cell-like diffuse large B-cell lymphoma. *Am J Pathol* 2004;165:159–166.
257. Natkunam Y, Lossos IS, Taidi B, et al. Expression of the human germinal center-associated lymphoma (HGAL) protein, a new marker of germinal center B-cell derivation. *Blood* 2005;105:3979–3986.
258. Dalla-Favera R, Bregni M, Erikson J, et al. Human c-*myc* onc gene is located on the region of chromosome 8 that is translocated in Burkitt lymphoma cells. *Proc Natl Acad Sci USA* 1982;79:7824–7827.
259. Battey J, Moulding C, Taub R, et al. The human c-*myc* oncogene: structural consequences of translocation into the IgH locus in Burkitt lymphoma. *Cell* 1983; 34:779–787.
260. Hecht JL, Aster JC. Molecular biology of Burkitt's lymphoma. *J Clin Oncol* 2000; 18:3707–3721.
261. Neri A, Barriga F, Knowles DM, et al. Different regions of the immunoglobulin heavy-chain locus are involved in chromosomal translocations in distinct pathogenetic forms of Burkitt lymphoma. *Proc Natl Acad Sci USA* 1988;85:2748–2752.
262. Pelicci PG, Knowles DM, Magrath I, et al. Chromosomal breakpoints and structural alterations of the c-*myc* locus differ in endemic and sporadic forms of Burkitt lymphoma. *Proc Natl Acad Sci USA* 1986;83:2984–2988.
263. Joos S, Falk MH, Lichter P, et al. Variable breakpoints in Burkitt lymphoma cells with chromosomal t(8;14) translocation separate c-*myc* and the *IgH* locus up to several hundred kb. *Hum Mol Genet* 1992;1:625–632.
264. Haralambieva E, Schuuring E, Rosati S, et al. Interphase fluorescence in situ hybridization for detection of 8q24/*MYC* breakpoints on routine histologic sections: validation in Burkitt lymphomas from three geographic regions. *Genes Chromosomes Cancer* 2004; 40:10–18.
265. Voorhees PM, Carder KA, Smith SV, et al. Follicular lymphoma with a Burkitt translocation: predictor of an aggressive clinical course—a case report and review of the literature. *Arch Pathol Lab Med* 2004;128:210–213.
266. Le Beau MM, Bitter MA, Larson RA, et al. The t(2;5)(p23;q35): a recurring chromosomal abnormality in Ki-1-positive anaplastic large cell lymphoma. *Leukemia* 1989; 3:866–870.
267. Kutok JL, Aster JC. Molecular biology of anaplastic lymphoma kinase-positive anaplastic large-cell lymphoma. *J Clin Oncol* 2002;20:3691–3702.
268. Sarris AH, Luthra R, Papadimitracopoulou V, et al. Amplification of genomic DNA demonstrates the presence of the t(2;5) (p23;q35) in anaplastic large cell lymphoma, but not in other non-Hodgkin's lymphomas, Hodgkin's disease, or lymphomatoid papulosis. *Blood* 1996;88:1771–1779.
269. Morris SW, Kirstein MN, Valentine MB, et al. Fusion of a kinase gene, *ALK*, to a nucleolar protein gene, *NPM*, in non-Hodgkin's lymphoma. *Science* 1994;263:1281–1284.
270. Escalon MP, Liu NS, Yang Y, et al. Prognostic factors and treatment of patients with T-cell non-Hodgkin lymphoma. *Cancer* 2005;103:2091–2098.
271. Drexler HG, Gignac SM, von Wasielewski R, et al. Pathobiology of *NPM-ALK* and variant fusion genes in anaplastic large cell lymphoma and other lymphomas. *Leukemia* 2000;14:1533–1559.
272. Duyster J, Bai RY, Morris SW. Translocations involving anaplastic lymphoma kinase (ALK). *Oncogene* 2001;20:5623–5637.
273. Rosenwald A, Ott G, Pulford K, et al. t(1;2)(q21;p23) and t(2;3)(p23;q21): two novel variant translocations of the t(2;5)(p23;q35) in anaplastic large cell lymphoma. *Blood* 1999;94:362–364.
274. Falini B, Pulford K, Pucciarini A, et al. Lymphomas expressing ALK fusion protein(s) other than NPM-ALK. *Blood* 1999;94:3509–3515.
275. Krause JR, Shahidi-Asl M. Molecular pathology in the diagnosis and treatment of non-Hodgkin's lymphomas. *J Cell Mol Med* 2003;7:494–512.
276. Beylot-Barry M, Lamant L, Vergier B, et al. Detection of t(2;5)(p23;q35) translocation by reverse transcriptase polymerase chain reaction and in situ hybridization in CD30-positive primary cutaneous lymphoma and lymphomatoid papulosis. *Am J Pathol* 1996;149:483–492.
277. Schumacher JA, Jenson SD, Elenitoba-Johnson KS, et al. Utility of linearly amplified RNA for RT-PCR detection of chromosomal translocations: validation using the t(2;5)(p23;q35) *NPM-ALK* chromosomal translocation. *J Mol Diagn* 2004;6:16–21.
278. Cataldo KA, Jalal SM, Law ME, et al. Detection of t(2;5) in anaplastic large cell lymphoma: comparison of immunohistochemical studies, FISH, and RT-PCR in paraffin-embedded tissue. *Am J Surg Pathol* 1999;23:1386–1392.
279. Pulford K, Lamant L, Morris SW, et al. Detection of anaplastic lymphoma kinase (ALK) and nucleolar protein nucleophosmin (NPM)-ALK proteins in normal and neoplastic cells with the monoclonal antibody ALK1. *Blood* 1997;89:1394–1404.
280. Liang X, Meech SJ, Odom LF, et al. Assessment of t(2;5)(p23;q35) translocation and variants in pediatric ALK+ anaplastic large cell lymphoma. *Am J Clin Pathol* 2004; 121:496–506.
281. Gascoyne RD, Aoun P, Wu D, et al. Prognostic significance of anaplastic lymphoma kinase (ALK) protein expression in adults with anaplastic large cell lymphoma. *Blood* 1999;93:3913–3921.
282. Ladanyi M, Cavalchire G, Morris SW, et al. Reverse transcriptase polymerase chain reaction for the Ki-1 anaplastic large cell lymphoma-associated t(2;5) translocation in Hodgkin's disease. *Am J Pathol* 1994;145:1296–1300.
283. Li XQ, Hisaoka M, Shi DR, et al. Expression of anaplastic lymphoma kinase in soft tissue tumors: an immunohistochemical and molecular study of 249 cases. *Hum Pathol* 2004;35:711–721.
284. Shabrawi-Caelen L, Kerl K, Cerroni L, et al. Cutaneous inflammatory pseudotumor:a spectrum of various diseases? *J Cutan Pathol* 2004;31:605–611.
285. Kadin ME. Genetic and molecular genetic studies in the diagnosis of T-cell malignancies. *Hum Pathol* 2003;34:322–329.
286. Belhadj K, Reyes F, Farcet JP, et al. Hepatosplenic gammadelta T-cell lymphoma is a rare clinicopathologic entity with poor outcome: report on a series of 21 patients. *Blood* 2003;102:4261–4269.
287. Brito-Babapulle V, Pomfret M, Matutes E, et al. Cytogenetic studies on prolymphocytic leukemia. II. T cell prolymphocytic leukemia. *Blood* 1987;70:926–931.
288. Jonveaux P, Daniel MT, Martel V, et al. Isochromosome 7q and trisomy 8 are consistent primary, non-random chromosomal abnormalities associated with hepatosplenic T gamma/delta lymphoma. *Leukemia* 1996;10:1453–1455.
289. Young LS, Rickinson AB. Epstein-Barr virus: 40 years on. *Nat Rev Cancer* 2004; 4:757–768.
290. Chang KL, Weiss LM. The association of the Epstein-Barr virus with malignant lymphoma. *Biomed Pharmacother* 1996;50:459–467.
291. Cohen JI. Epstein-Barr virus infection. *N Engl J Med* 2000;343:481–492.
292. Stevens SJ, Verschuuren EA, Verkuujlen SA, et al. Role of Epstein-Barr virus DNA load monitoring in prevention and early detection of post-transplant lymphoproliferative disease. *Leuk Lymphoma* 2002;43:831–840.
293. George TI, Jeng M, Berquist W, et al. Epstein-Barr virus-associated peripheral T-cell lymphoma and hemophagocytic syndrome arising after liver transplantation: case report and review of the literature. *Pediatr Blood Cancer* 2005;44:270–276.
294. Gaal K, Weiss LM, Chen WG, et al. Epstein-Barr virus nuclear antigen (EBNA)-1 carboxy-terminal and EBNA-4 sequence polymorphisms in nasal natural killer/T-cell lymphoma in the United States. *Lab Invest* 2002;82:957–962.
295. Gaal K, Sun NC, Hernandez AM, et al. Sinonasal NK/T-cell lymphomas in the United States. *Am J Surg Pathol* 2000;24:1511–1517.
296. White AC, Jr, Katz BZ, Silbert JA. Association of Epstein-Barr virus with an angioimmunoblastic lymphadenopathy-like lymphoproliferative syndrome. *Yale J Biol Med* 1989;62:263–269.
297. Luzzatto F, Pruneri G, Benini E, et al. Angioimmunoblastic T-cell lymphoma with hyperplastic germinal centres and a high content of EBV-infected large B-cells carrying IgH chain gene monoclonal rearrangement. *Histopathology* 2005;46:464–466.
298. Ohshima K, Takeo H, Kikuchi M, et al. Heterogeneity of Epstein-Barr virus infection in angioimmunoblastic lymphadenopathy type T-cell lymphoma. *Histopathology* 1994; 25:569–579.

299. Jarrett RF. Risk factors for Hodgkin's lymphoma by EBV status and significance of detection of EBV genomes in serum of patients with EBV-associated Hodgkin's lymphoma. *Leuk Lymphoma* 2003;44(suppl 3):S27–S32.

300. Arber DA, Weiss LM, Chang KL. Detection of Epstein-Barr Virus in inflammatory pseudotumor. *Semin Diagn Pathol* 1998;15:155–160.

301. Cook JR, Dehner LP, Collins MH, et al. Anaplastic lymphoma kinase (ALK) expression in the inflammatory myofibroblastic tumor: a comparative immunohistochemical study. *Am J Surg Pathol* 2001;25:1364–1371.

302. Ohshima K, Suzumiya J, Kanda M, et al. Genotypic and phenotypic alterations in Epstein-Barr virus-associated lymphoma. *Histopathology* 1999;35:539–550.

303. Kojima M, Nakamura S, Itoh H, et al. Occurrence of monocytoid B-cells in reactive lymph node lesions. *Pathol Res Pract* 1998;194:559–565.

304. Fisher SG, Fisher RI. The epidemiology of non-Hodgkin's lymphoma. *Oncogene* 2004;23:6524–6534.

305. Lai R, Weiss LM. Hepatitis C virus and non-Hodgkin's lymphoma. *Am J Clin Pathol* 1998;109:508–510.

306. Fiorilli M, Mecucci C, Farci P, et al. HCV-associated lymphomas. *Rev Clin Exp Hematol* 2003;7:406–423.

307. Negri E, Little D, Boiocchi M, et al. B-cell non-Hodgkin's lymphoma and hepatitis C virus infection: a systematic review. *Int J Cancer* 2004;111:1–8.

308. Weng WK, Levy S. Hepatitis C virus (HCV) and lymphomagenesis. *Leuk Lymphoma* 2003;44:1113–1120.

309. Dupin N, Fisher C, Kellam P, et al. Distribution of human herpesvirus-8 latently infected cells in Kaposi's sarcoma, multicentric Castleman's disease, and primary effusion lymphoma. *Proc Natl Acad Sci USA* 1999;96:4546–4551.

310. Hengge UR, Ruzicka T, Tyring SK, et al. Update on Kaposi's sarcoma and other HHV8 associated diseases. II. Pathogenesis, Castleman's disease, and pleural effusion lymphoma. *Lancet Infect. Dis* 2002;2:344–352.

311. Hengge UR, Ruzicka T, Tyring SK, et al. Update on Kaposi's sarcoma and other HHV8 associated diseases. I. Epidemiology, environmental predispositions, clinical manifestations, and therapy. *Lancet Infect Dis* 2002;2:281–292.

312. Pan L, Milligan L, Michaeli J, et al. Polymerase chain reaction detection of Kaposi's sarcoma-associated herpesvirus-optimized protocols and their application to myeloma. *J Mol Diagn* 2001;3:32–38.

313. Hong A, Davies S, Lee CS. Immunohistochemical detection of the human herpes virus 8 (HHV8) latent nuclear antigen-1 in Kaposi's sarcoma. *Pathology* 2003;35:448–450.

314. Minamoto GY, Gold JW, Scheinberg DA, et al. Infection with human T-cell leukemia virus type I in patients with leukemia. *N Engl J Med* 1988;318:219–222.

315. Nicot C. Current views in HTLV-I-associated adult T-cell leukemia/lymphoma. *Am J Hematol* 2005;78:232–239.

316. Muller AM, Ihorst G, Mertelsmann R, et al. Epidemiology of non-Hodgkin's lymphoma (NHL): trends, geographic distribution, and etiology. *Ann Hematol* 2005; 84:1–12.

317. Lee TH, Chafets DM, Busch MP, et al. Quantitation of HTLV-I and II proviral load using real-time quantitative PCR with SYBR Green chemistry. *J Clin Virol* 2004; 31:275–282.

318. Macabeo-Ong M, Ginzinger DG, Dekker N, et al. Effect of duration of fixation on quantitative reverse transcription polymerase chain reaction analyses. *Mod Pathol* 2002; 15:979–987.

319. Greer CE, Wheeler CM, and Manos MM. PCR amplification from paraffin-embedded tissues: sample preparation and the effects of fixation. In: Dieffenbach CW, Dveksler GS, eds. *PCR Primer*. Plainview, NY: Cold Spring Harbor Laboratory Press; 1995:99–112.

320. Murphy KM, Berg KD, Geiger T, et al. Capillary electrophoresis artifact due to eosin: implications for the interpretation of molecular diagnostic assays. *J Mol Diagn* 2005; 7:143–148.

321. Spagnolo DV, Ellis DW, Juneja S, et al. The role of molecular studies in lymphoma diagnosis: a review. *Pathology* 2004;36:19–44.

322. Cook JR. Paraffin section interphase fluorescence in situ hybridization in the diagnosis and classification of non-hodgkin lymphomas. *Diagn Mol Pathol* 2004;13:197–206.

323. Going JJ, Gusterson BA. Molecular pathology and future developments. *Eur J Cancer* 1999;35:1895–1904.

324. Zitzelsberger H, Lehmann L, Werner M, et al. Comparative genomic hybridisation for the analysis of chromosomal imbalances in solid tumours and haematological malignancies. *Histochem Cell Biol* 1997;108:403–417.

325. Yeoh EJ, Ross ME, Shurtleff SA, et al. Classification, subtype discovery, and prediction of outcome in pediatric acute lymphoblastic leukemia by gene expression profiling. *Cancer Cell* 2002;1:133–143.

326. Ferrando AA, Neuberg DS, Staunton J, et al. Gene expression signatures define novel oncogenic pathways in T cell acute lymphoblastic leukemia. *Cancer Cell* 2002;1:75–87.

327. Rao PH, Cigudosa JC, Ning Y, et al. Multicolor spectral karyotyping identifies new recurring breakpoints and translocations in multiple myeloma. *Blood* 1998;92:1743–1748.

328. Bayani JM, Squire JA. Applications of *SKY* in cancer cytogenetics. *Cancer Invest* 2002; 20:373–386.

329. Bernard PS, Wittwer CT. Real-time PCR technology for cancer diagnostics. *Clin Chem* 2002;48:1178–1185.

330. Lin Z, Jenson SD, Lim MS, et al. Application of SELDI-TOF mass spectrometry for the identification of differentially expressed proteins in transformed follicular lymphoma. *Mod Pathol* 2004;17:670–678.

331. Lim MS, Elenitoba-Johnson KS. Proteomics in pathology research. *Lab Invest* 2004; 84:1227–1244.

Molecular Diagnostics of CNS Tumors and Neurodegenerative Diseases

Pang-hsien Tu   Christine Fuller   Arie Perry

With the advent of both conventional and high-throughput research tools, such as DNA and tissue microarrays, the genetic underpinnings of numerous sporadic and hereditary diseases of the central nervous system (CNS) are rapidly being discovered, ranging from primary CNS neoplasia to neurodegenerative diseases to developmental malformations. Often, these important findings quickly lead to the development of practical tools that allow genetic testing and screening of these diseases on the individual level or at a larger scale. The results of molecular diagnostics may in turn enhance our understanding of these disease processes, help reclassify or subclassify certain groups of diseases and more precisely differentiate many diseases from their mimics.

Genetic testing can be broadly classified based on the purpose of the test itself. The first category is confirmatory testing, which likely constitutes an overwhelming percentage of the tests conducted clinically. The purpose of these tests is to establish or confirm a clinically suspected diagnosis, for example, to perform genetic testing to determine the numbers of the CAG repeats in a patient manifesting signs of Huntington's disease. The second is therapeutic predictive testing in which the results can be used to guide therapeutic strategies and predict the outcomes of specific interventions. An excellent example is the co-deletion of chromosomes 1p and 19q in oligodendrioglioma, which serves as a marker of a "genetically favorable" variant that carries a better overall prognosis and a higher response rate to a variety of therapeutic modalities than that encountered in gliomas without this co-deletion. The third is a predictive testing for disease in which the tests are performed in asymptomatic or presymptomatic individuals at risk for developing familial diseases.

Numerous molecular diagnostic techniques are available and used to varying degrees in pathology departments at major medical centers. These include western, Southern, and northern blots, reverse transcriptase polymerase chain reaction (RT-PCR), various forms of quantitative PCR, methylation-specific PCR, mutation analysis by single-strand conformation polymorphism (SSCP) and DNA sequencing, loss of heterozygosity (LOH) by microsatellite analysis, fluorescence in situ hybridization (FISH), comparative genomic hybridization (CGH), array CGH [also known as bacterial artificial chromosome (BAC) arrays], single nucleotide polymorphism (SNP) arrays, expression profiling with oligonucleotide or cDNA microarrays, and serial analysis of gene expression (SAGE) (see previous chapters). Some of these are global genomic screening techniques, whereas others assess specific alterations. Each of these techniques provides information at the DNA, RNA, or protein levels and has distinct advantages and disadvantages.

The common reasons for pursuing genetic testing are to provide an explanation for symptoms, emotional relief, and information for future planning (1). Many of the diseases that are being tested do not yet have a cure, and the test results may pose a significant psychologic impact on tested subjects. However, previous studies looking into this important issue have produced conflicting results. Some supported (2,3), but others refuted (4,5), the negative effects on individuals with positive test results. Given the conflicting data on the benefits and harms genetic testing may have in combination with technique and interpretation issues, it is prudent to follow strict guidelines for genetic testing, such as those published to avoid potentially detrimental effects. Information on guidelines for different genetic tests can be found at the website of the National Guideline Clearinghouse* (NGC), a public resource for evidence-based clinical practice guidelines. NGC is an initiative of the Agency for Healthcare Research and Quality (AHRQ), U.S. Department of Health and Human Services. NGC was originally created by AHRQ in partnership with the American Medical Association and America's Health Insurance Plans (AHIP). More information on specific guidelines can be found on the websites of other organizations such as the American College of Medical Genetics.† The information on the commercial laboratories that perform specific genetic tests can be found at the GeneTests website,‡ which is sponsored by the National Institutes of Health.

PRIMARY CENTRAL NERVOUS SYSTEM TUMORS

The complementary roles of morphology and tumor genetics are aptly highlighted in the current World Health Organization (WHO) "blue book" of CNS tumors, which includes both pathology and genetics in its title (6). The most common utilization of molecular diagnostics is testing for co-deletion of chromosomes 1p and 19q (1p/19q co-deletion) as an ancillary diagnostic, prognostic, and predictive aid in oligodendrogliomas. At Washington University, this is most often achieved using FISH, though LOH is also popular in some centers. Technical aspects of such testing and illustrations of FISH examples can be found in Chapter 4. Rapid progress in the elucidation of genetic alterations in subsets in all of the major classes of brain tumors will surely increase the list of clinically useful assays over the next few years.

Unfortunately, brain tumors are not characterized by signature translocations and fusion products as encountered in hematologic and soft tissue tumors. Therefore, the alterations of interest consist predominantly of gains in oncogene function and tumor suppressor losses, through a variety of genetic and epigenetic mechanisms. The major genetic alerations of CNS tumors have been summarized in Table 14.1.

Astrocytomas

Diffusely infiltrative astrocytomas are among the most common and deadly of all CNS tumors. Although patients with these lesions are still currently stratified predominantly by age and histologic grade, these parameters alone do not fully account for the broad biologic spectrum encountered clinically. In addition, conventional therapeutic options are limited. Therefore, there is great interest in finding useful biomarkers and astrocytomas are the most thoroughly studied of all CNS tumors in terms of molecular pathogenesis. Most of our current knowledge of molecular alterations is derived from studies of adult patients with diffuse astrocytomas. Considerably less is known about pediatric and circumscribed (favorable)

astrocytoma variants (i.e., pilocytic astrocytoma and pleomorphic xanthoastrocytoma).

In adults, at least two distinct pathogenetic variants of glioblastoma (also known as WHO grade IV astrocytoma) have been identified. Primary (de novo) glioblastomas are defined by a short (<3 months) clinical presentation with no evidence of a lower grade precursor lesion identified. They frequently harbor amplification of the epidermal growth factor receptor gene (EGFR; 7p12) and are associated with an older age of onset and a particularly aggressive clinical course. In contrast, secondary glioblastomas arise from lower grade precursors (e.g., diffuse astrocytoma, WHO grade II or anaplastic astrocytoma, and WHO grade III) and are characterized by frequent alterations of the p53 gene (17p13.1) and a more protracted clinical course (7–9). Although p53 mutation and EGFR amplification are generally mutually exclusive alterations, occasional glioblastomas harbor both (6). There is conflicting evidence in the literature as to whether or not these alterations independently correlate with patient survival (10–14), although they may indirectly affect prognosis within specific subsets of glioblastoma patients. For example, a significant association between EGFR and shortened survival was identified by Simmons et al. (15) in their younger patients (<55 years old), but only in tumors that simultaneously lacked p53 alterations. Although detected with much less frequency than in their grade IV counterparts, EGFR gains or gains of chromosome 7 in low-grade (WHO II) and anaplastic astrocytomas (WHO III) have also been linked with shortened survival, with some such cases potentially representing undersampled glioblastomas (16–18).

Of particular interest is the frequent finding of EGFR amplification in malignant astrocytomas exhibiting a small cell phenotype (19–21). Small cell astrocytoma is notable for its deceptively bland monomorphous cellularity, which may closely mimic that of anaplastic oligodendroglioma (19). Discriminating between these lesions is clinically important, because even in the absence of endothelial hyperplasia and necrosis necessary for a WHO grade IV designation, small cell astrocytomas have been shown to behave as aggressively as primary glioblastoma (20). FISH analyses may be especially useful for this diagnostic consideration in that the 1p and 19q codeletion commonly encountered in anaplastic oligodendragliom as is not a feature of small cell astrocytoma, whereas EGFR amplification and chromosome 10q deletions are common (see discussion of FISH examples in Chapter 4). Immunohistochemical detection of EGFR protein overexpression, both wild-type and the constitutively activated EGFRvIII variant, is likewise more frequent in small cell as opposed to conventional fibrillary astrocytomas (20). EGFRvIII overexpression itself has been associated with decreased survival times in patients with malignant astrocytomas in some studies (22,23). It is important to emphasize that in the workup of malignant gliomas with bland monotonous nuclei, positive staining with EGFR immunohistochemistry alone should be viewed with caution because this may occur in the absence of gene amplification in other glioma subtypes, including oligodendrogliomas; EGFRvIII immunopositivity or detection of EGFR amplification and 10q deletion by FISH analysis

---

*National Guideline Clearinghouse, http://www.ngc.gov.
†American College of Medical Genetics, http://www.acmg.net.
‡GeneTests, www.genetests.org.

TABLE 14.1

SUMMARY OF GENETIC ABNORMALITIES OF CNS TUMORS

Tumor Category	Genetic Changes	Tumor/Grade	Detection Methods	Significance
Astrocytoma	*p53* alterations	Low and high grades Secondary GBM	SSCP, sequencing, IHC	Diagnostic marker
	10q deletion (*PTEN* deletion)	High grade	FISH, LOH	Poor prognosis
	EGFR amplification	Primary GBM Small cell variant GBM	FISH, qPCR	Diagnostic and ?predictive marker
	Hypermethylation of *MGMT* promoter	25% of GBM	Methylation-specific PCR	Sensitivity to temozolomide
	p16 (9p21) deletion	High grade	FISH, qPCR	Chemosensitive?
	Deletion of chromosome 19q	High grade	FISH, LOH	Good prognosis?
Oligodendroglioma	1p/19q co-deletion	Low and high grades	FISH, LOH, qPCR	Diagnostic marker Good prognosis Increased therapeutic sensitivity
	p16 (9p21) deletion	High grade	FISH, qPCR	Poor prognosis
Mixed oligoastrocytoma	Deletion of chromosome 19q	Low and high grades	FISH, LOH	Good prognosis?
	Co-deletion of chromosome 1p/19q	Low and high grades	FISH, LOH	Good prognosis
	p16 (9p21) deletion	High grade	FISH, qPCR	Poor prognosis
	10q deletion (*PTEN* deletion)	High grade	FISH, LOH	Poor prognosis
Ependymoma	*NF2* (22q12) deletion/mutation	Spinal variant	FISH, LOH, SSCP	Diagnostic marker
	Protein 4.1B loss/*4.1B* deletion	Intracranial variant	FISH, IHC	Diagnostic marker
Medulloblastoma sporadic	Isochromosome 17q	Anaplastic/large cell variant	FISH	Poor prognosis
	Loss of chromosome 17p	Anaplastic/large cell variant	FISH, LOH	Poor prognosis
	Erb B2 overexpression	Any variant	IHC	Poor prognosis
	c-myc/N-*myc* amplification	Anaplastic/large cell variant	FISH, qPCR	Poor prognosis
	Loss of chromosome 10q	Anaplastic/large cell variant	FISH, LOH	Poor prognosis
	Trk C overexpression	Nodular/desmoplastic variant	mRNA ISH	Favorable prognosis?
Atypical teratoid/ rhabdoid tumor	*INI1/hSNF5* (22q) deletion *INI1/hSNF5* mutations Loss of expression		FISH, LOH SSCP/Sequencing IHC	Diagnostic marker
Meningioma	*NF2* deletion/merlin loss	Low and high grades	FISH, LOH, IHC	Diagnostic marker
	Protein 4.1B loss/*4.1B* deletion	Low and high grades	FISH, IHC	Diagnostic marker
	Chromosome 14q deletion	Recurrent, high grade	FISH, LOH	Diagnostic marker
	Chromosome 1p deletion	High grade	FISH, LOH	Diagnostic marker
	p16 (9p21) deletion	High grade	FISH	Diagnostic marker, poor prognosis
	pS6K (17q23) amplification	High grade	FISH	Diagnostic marker, poor prognosis
Familial syndromes				
Gorlin	*PTCH* germline mutations	Medulloblastoma	Sequencing	Heritability
Turcot	*APC* germline mutations	Medulloblastoma	Sequencing	Heritability
Turcot	*Mismatch* repair genes germline mutations	Glioblastoma	Sequencing	Heritability
Li-Fraumeni	*p53* germline mutations	Astrocytomas/glioblastoma	Sequencing	Heritability

FISH, fluorescence *in situ* hybridization; GBM, glioblastoma; IHC, immunohistochemistry; LOH, loss of heterozygosity; mRNA, messenger ribonucleic acid; SSCP, single-strand conformational polymorphism; PCR, polymerase chain reaction.

provide the strongest molecular evidence in support of a small cell astrocytoma diagnosis (20,24,25).

Second only to gains on chromosome 7, losses involving chromosome 10 are quite frequent in astrocytomas, limited mainly to high-grade examples (26,27). The majority of CGH and FISH studies to date have identified 10q loss/monosomy 10 as an independent predictor of shorter patient survival (26–32). Several candidate tumor suppressor genes have been mapped to 10q, including *PTEN* (10q23), *DMBT1* (10q25.3-26.1), and more recently, *annexinVII* (*ANX7*; 10q21). Loss of *PTEN* function by way of deletion or inactivating mutations may be seen in association with both primary and secondary glioblastoma variants; though similar to chromosome 10 losses in general, this finding is relatively limited to high-grade astrocytomas (33,34). Although codeletion of *PTEN* and *DMBT1* by FISH analysis is most common (35), biallelic inactivation of *DMBT1* has not been found and only *PTEN* alterations have been specifically associated with a negative prognosis in high-grade astrocytomas (36–38). However, in a recent study of 99 glioblastomas, immunohistochemical detection of *ANX7* was found to be a strong predictor of prolonged patient survival, independent of other clinical variables (39). Additional validation of this finding will be necessary to determine whether *ANX7* is truly an effective clinical prognosticator, independent of *PTEN* or 10q loss in general.

In addition to *p53*, alterations in a variety of other genes regulating the G_1 checkpoint of the cell cycle are involved in the malignant progression of astrocytomas, some of which show potential in serving as molecular prognostic indicators (40–43). The p16/RB/CDK4 pathway is disrupted in the majority of high-grade astrocytomas, with homozygous deletion of *p16* representing the most common mechanism of pathway inactivation (40,44–46). Although a number of reports show *p16* gene deletion or decreased p16 protein expression as independent predictors of poor patient survival (41,47), these same findings failed to reach significance on multivariate analysis in others, possibly because of the close association of *p16* alterations and high-grade histology in general (38,45). Nonetheless, Iwadate et al. (48) found an association between mutations and homozygous deletions of *p16* and increased sensitivity to antimetabolite chemotherapeutic agents, suggesting that *p16* status may be helpful in predicting chemosensitivity in individual patients. MDM2 is a regulator of *p53* that is overexpressed and to a lesser extent amplified in high-grade astrocytomas; its overexpression was found to be a negative prognostic indicator in some studies (43,49,50). The p27/CDK2/cyclinE pathway also influences the G_1 checkpoint, and several independent studies have shown decreased *p27* expression to be related to high astrocytoma grade and poor patient outcome (42,51–53).

There are a few molecular alterations in adult astrocytomas that deserve further consideration. For example, chromosome 19 alteration is a feature shared by all three diffuse glioma subtypes; although 19q deletion has been associated with malignant progression in astrocytic lesions, there is also evidence to suggest that this may be a marker of long-term survival (28,29,32,54–56). Both *VEGF* and *ErbB2* expression are likewise more common in high-grade lesions, although data on prognostic usefulness are conflicting (13,24,57–66). In summary, *EGFR* amplification/*EGFRvIII* overexpression and losses involving 10q, p16, 19q, and *p27* are alterations that all have shown strong promise as prognostic markers in astrocytoma in adults, several additionally serving as potential targets for novel therapies (67–69). It is likely that some of these will eventually get incorporated into developing clinical and molecular patient stratification schemes, necessitating their detection by FISH or other means on a routine basis.

In contrast to their adult counterparts, much less is known about the molecular events involved in the pathogenesis and progression of pediatric astrocytomas. Whereas glioblastomas predominate in adults, low-grade lesions are more prevalent in children and include both diffuse infiltrative astrocytomas and "circumscribed" or clinically favorable variants, such as pilocytic astrocytoma

and pleomorphic xanthoastrocytoma (PXA). The anatomic distribution also differs from that in adults, with the majority of childhood tumors arising within the subcortical deep gray matter, brain stem, and posterior fossa (6). Despite these differences, some studies have confirmed that several of the molecular alterations common in astrocytomas in adults may be found in the diffuse pediatric astrocytomas, though in most cases at a much lower incidence (6,70–73). Interestingly, children harboring malignant astrocytomas tend to have a more favorable outcome than adults with similar tumors. Also, in contrast to their adult counterparts, in children *EGFR* amplifications are encountered only rarely (73–79). Similarly, *PTEN* mutations are seen in only a minority of such cases, but nonetheless are associated with shortened survival (75). On the other hand, chromosome 17p LOH and *p53* alterations are fairly common in high-grade astrocytomas (73,76,79–81). Pollack's group (80,81) reported a correlation between *p53* alterations and adverse patient outcome, although this has not been a consistent finding in other studies.

The majority of pilocytic astrocytomas have no detectable chromosomal abnormalities, although gains of chromosomes 5 to 9 have been infrequently observed (70,82,83). When these lesions arise in the setting of neurofibromatosis type 1 (NF1), however, alterations of the *NF1* gene with associated loss of neurofibromin expression are frequently encountered (84,85). Similarly, PXAs tend to lack most alterations seen in astrocytomas in adults, though a handful of studies have documented occasional gains on chromosome 7, losses on 8p, and *p53* mutations (86–88).

In spite of the numerous genetic alterations known to occur in astrocytomas, their incorporation into molecular diagnostic testing has not been associated with obvious clinical utility in most cases. However, epidermal growth factor receptor (EGFR) tyrosine kinase inhibitors (TKIs), gefitinib (Iressa) and erlotinib (Tarceva), have been successfully used in subsets of lung cancer patients (most often nonsmokers, of East Asian descent, female, and with adenocarcinoma histology) (89–91), likely as a result of mutations in the EGFR kinase domain (92). Such mutations are rare in gliomas. Nevertheless, erlotinib with or without temozolomide has been used to treat 41 gliomas in a phase I study and showed some benefit in approximately 25% of cases, more frequently than not in cases with *EGFR* expression or *EGFR* amplification (93). These findings indicate a potential for *EGFR* testing if similar results are reproduced in subsequent larger studies.

Epigenetic silencing of the *MGMT* (O6-methylguanine–DNA methyltransferase) DNA-repair gene by promoter methylation is identified in approximately 45% of glioblastomas, and this alteration is detected by methylation-specific PCR analysis. In a recent large international clinical study, *MGMT* promoter methylation was found to be an independent favorable prognostic factor, and a survival benefit was particularly observed in patients treated with temozolomide and radiotherapy, with a median survival of 21.7 months compared with 15.3 months for nonmethylated cases (94). These findings have ignited a great deal of excitement in the neurooncology community because it provides the first convincing result using genetic testing for targeted drug therapy in the highly lethal brain tumor GBM. This type of testing is expected to become a standardized care procedure for GBM if similar benefit can be reproduced in subsequent studies.

Oligodendroglial Tumors

In no other area of brain tumor pathology has genotyping proven more clinically valuable than in the genetic profiling of oligodendroglial tumors. Comprising 15% to 25% of adult gliomas, oligodendrogliomas tend to behave in a less aggressive fashion than astrocytomas, with slower progression and longer patient survival (6,30,95,96). Likewise, the dramatic therapeutic responses to PCV (procarbazine, CCNU, vincristine) chemotherapy reported in subsets of patients with anaplastic oligodendroglioma is a noteworthy finding compared to the usual lack of response in astrocytomas (97–99). LOH and FISH studies have reported 1p/19q codeletion in 60% to 90% of oligodendrogliomas (100–105). The landmark study of Cairncross et al. (106) was the first to establish an association between anaplastic oligodendrogliomas with this molecular signature and both favorable therapeutic response and prolonged survival. Similarly, Smith et al. (107) reported that combined 1p/19q deletions were associated with prolonged survival in oligodendrogliomas, including low-grade examples. Studies have further suggested that these genetically favorable oligodendrogliomas are also more sensitive to other forms of therapy, including radiation and less toxic chemotherapeutic agents, such as temozolomide (108,109). Although 1p/19q co-deletion has been found to be highly associated with classic oligodendroglioma histology (107,110,111), some authors have suggested that 1p/19q status alone may correlate with chemoresponsiveness, independent of tumor morphology (112,113). There has been tremendous interest within the neurooncology community for incorporating 1p/19q testing into routine glioma diagnosis, especially those with obvious or even subtle oligodendroglial features.

In oligodendrogliomas with 1p/19q codeletion, typically one entire 1p and one entire 19q chromosomal arm is lost, making the localization of relevant tumor suppressor genes difficult, if not impossible. Mapping of occasional tumors with partial LOH have yielded regions of minimal deletion on 1p36 and 19q13.3, though many of the deletion-defining tumors have not been oligodendrogliomas (56, 105,114,115). In line with that hypothesis is the general observation that in contrast to those with whole arm losses, tumors harboring small interstitial deletions tend to have a more astrocytic morphology (116) and are often biologically aggressive. Thus, it is unclear that these regions truly harbor oligodendroglioma-specific genes. Although the precise mechanism(s) relating whole chromosome arm loss of 1p and 19q to tumorigenesis remains a mystery, it is possible that (a) haploinsufficiency of multiple genes is somehow sufficient without the need for a "second hit," (b) epigenetic events such as hypermethylation of CpG islands are inactivating genes on the remaining copies of 1p and 19q, or (c) this cytogenetic signature is simply a marker of a specific glioma type, mechanistically unrelated to other, yet to be identified tumorigenic events.

Given the prognostic and therapeutic implications, 1p/19q testing in all oligodendrogliomas and tumors with suspected oligodendroglial features has become relatively routine. We have reported our initial observations in detail (103) and they have remained valid over time, with over 1,300 gliomas tested thus far. Dual-color FISH is our method of choice, based primarily on our laboratories' familiarity with this approach, its applicability to paraffin-embedded tissue, the lack of matching normal blood or tissue requirements, its basis in morphology, and a rapid turnaround time (2 to 3 working days for two batches per week). Other commonly used techniques in clinical laboratories include LOH and QuMA (100). As in a number of retrospective series, we have found 1p/19q codeletion to be highly associated with morphology: 84% in pure oligodendrogliomas, 15% in mixed oligoastrocytomas (MOAs), and less than 1% in astrocytomas ($p < 0.001$). Loss of 19q alone has been described in a smaller subset and in our experience is particularly common in MOAs, often associated with a favorable biology (103,117). With respect to patient survival, our results have been similar to those of retrospective studies in that the genetically favorable (1p/19q codeletion) pattern is over-represented in long-term survivors (103). However, there have been notable exceptions: many with nondeleted tumors enjoyed long survival times, particularly younger patients with low-grade tumors, whereas a few patients with 1p/19q codeleted tumors died shortly after biopsy, mostly older individuals with large ring-enhancing high-grade gliomas. The latter patients may well have had oligodendrogliomas that remained asymptomatic for many years, finally coming to clinical attention when advanced progression-associated changes had occurred. Nonetheless, these exceptions reinforce the continued relevance of other well-established prognostic variables, rather than relying solely on genetic features.

Apart from the obvious prognostic implication discussed above, identification of 1p/19q codeletions may also be helpful in daily pathology, because there are a number of lesions that pose formidable diagnostic challenges. For example, dysembryoplastic neuroepithelial tumors (DNTs), central neurocytomas, extraventricular neurocytomas, and clear cell ependymomas may closely resemble oligodendrogliomas; however, no deletions have been identified in any of these, with the exception of extraventricular neurocytomas (EVNs) (118–120). Two of 12 EVNs harbored 1p/19q codeletion, suggesting that either this genetic signature is not entirely specific or that these rare tumors may be histogenetically related to oligodendrogliomas. Reports of oligodendrogliomas with neurocytic differentiation support the latter theory (121). An even more common differential diagnostic consideration is small cell glioblastoma, also discussed in the previously astrocytoma section. A highly aggressive tumor with monomorphic bland nuclei, the occasional presence of clear haloes, delicate capillaries, and microcalcifications overlaps considerably with anaplastic oligodendroglioma or GBM with oligodendroglial elements (19,20). To date, none of these cases have shown 1p/19q codeletions. Instead, EGFR amplification is found in approximately 70% and 10q deletions are nearly universal (20).

Alterations of chromosomes 9p and 10q have been encountered in anaplastic oligodendrogliomas, albeit at a lower frequency than is typical of high-grade astrocytic lesions (104,122–126). Likewise, deletions of *p16* and loss or mutation of *PTEN* have both been associated with anaplasia and short survival, the latter occurring preferentially in tumors with intact 1p and 19q (37,41,106,125,127–129). Of interest, Sasaki et al. (129) found that allelic loss of chromosome 10q was negatively associated with 1p loss and that *PTEN* gene alterations were independently predictive of poor survival in patients with anaplastic oligodendrogliomas, even those with initially favorable chemotherapeutic response.

Although the majority of published data correlating survival and molecular alterations in oligodendrogliomas is based on the initial diagnostic sample, a common request is for genetic testing of oligodendrogliomas at the time of recurrence. Therefore, we recently assayed 138 primary and recurrent oligodendroglial tumors from 80 patients with a variety of FISH probes (130). Our data suggest that the enhanced survival in 1p/19q-deleted cases is partially retained after recurrence, with a postrecurrence median survival of 3.5 years in genetically favorable cases versus 1.5 years in the nondeleted group (*p* < 0.001). Additionally, *p16* deletion was a common progression-associated event, correlating with reduced progression-free survivals in both the 1p/19q-deleted and nondeleted cases. Last, we found both *EGFR* amplifications and 10q deletions to be extremely uncommon in pure oligodendrogliomas, suggesting that some of the previously reported cases with these alterations may in fact be small cell glioblastomas or other astrocytic tumors.

Compared to their adult counterparts, pediatric oligodendroglial tumors are far less common, with little published data regarding their clinicopathologic or molecular characterization. In their review of 26 cases by Raghavan et al., 1p/19q deletions were rare and not obviously associated with clinical outcome (131). We have recently looked at a larger collection of samples from patients treated for oligodendroglial tumor at St. Jude (132). Following histologic review, 21 of these samples were reclassified as various other entities (infiltrative astrocytoma, pilocytic astrocytoma, DNET, and clear cell ependymoma), underscoring the need for careful evaluation of these oligodendroglioma mimics in the pediatric population. The remaining 47 specimens were evaluated by FISH for copy number alterations of 1p, 19q, and a variety of other glioma-associated markers. We too encountered 1p/19q codeletion at a lower incidence (27% of cases) than is typical of oligodendroglioma in adults, and similar to the findings of Raghavan et al., the vast majority of these patients were more than 9 years old. Deletions of p16 and 10q were seen in 45% and 18% respectively; the 9% of cases with detectable *EGFR* amplification were quite reminiscent of those with small cell astrocytoma (131). At present there is no clear correlation between these molecular alterations and prognosis, and thus it would appear that genetic testing may be of limited clinical value in children with oligodendrogliomas.

As alluded to previously, gliomas showing ambiguous morphologic features pose a significant diagnostic problem in neuropathology. Despite their histologic heterogeneity, multiple studies have indicated that they are in fact predominantly monoclonal tumors, harboring alterations more typical of either pure oligodendroglioma or astrocytoma (101,133–136). The majority of studies have found 1p/19q co-deletion at an incidence of approximately 33%; however, these mainly focused on biphasic MOAs with geographic zones of clear-cut oligodendroglial and astrocytic components (104,105,123). Recently, we retrospectively studied 90 morphologically ambiguous gliomas, including those with vague oligodendroglial features and diffuse MOAs (95). Only 9% showed 1p/19q co-deletion, consistent with the opinion that such deletions are primarily encountered in the most classic-appearing oligodendrogliomas. Interestingly, approximately 30% had p16 deletion, 10q deletion, or *EGFR* amplification and these patients had significantly shortened survival times, whereas those with 1p/19q co-deletion, solitary 19q deletion (22%), or no detectable alterations (41%) generally had favorable outcomes. Bissola et al. (137) likewise found LOH 1p and 10q to hold similar prognostic significance in their analysis. There are also some data to suggest that the solitary 19q deletion pattern in MOAs may additionally be genetically favorable (103,117), though further analysis is needed to address the above issues.

Ependymomas

Although they constitute only a small proportion of neuroepithelial tumors overall, ependymomas represent the third most common brain tumor in children and account for at least half of all spinal gliomas (6). The vast majority of pediatric examples are intracranial, whereas those arising in adults are evenly distributed between the brain and spinal cord. There is increasing evidence that spinal and intracranial ependymomas represent two distinct tumor subsets, not only relative to age of occurrence and biologic potential, but in terms of genetic alterations as well.

Loss of chromosome 22q is a common finding in adult ependymomas and is strongly associated with a spinal location (138–146). Although many of these spinal tumors will have a concomitant mutation of *NF2*, the same cannot be said of intracranial ependymomas that harbor 22q deletions (147–151). In a comparative IHC/FISH study by Singh et al. (152), deletions/loss of *NF2* (22q12) were likewise encountered primarily in spinal ependymomas, whereas loss of *4.1B* (formerly known as *DAL-1*: differentially expressed in adenocarcinoma of the lung 1) (153,154), a second protein 4.1 family member and structurally homologous tumor suppressor gene on chromosome 18p11.3, was more frequent in intracranial examples (152). Recent evidence suggests that a third protein 4.1 gene, *4.1R* on 1p32-33, may also play an important role (155). Additional age- and site-related differences documented by CGH include gain of 1q and losses involving chromosomes 6q, 9,13, and 17p in pediatric intracranial and gain of chromosome 7 in spinal ependymomas (143,144,146,148,156,157).

Unfortunately, there is no one unifying genetic signature for ependymomas, and, in fact, up to 40% will have no detectable alterations (143,146,156). Molecular analysis may nonetheless be of benefit when applied to specific diagnostic dilemmas. For example, clear cell ependymoma (CCE) may resemble a variety of tumors, including oligodendroglioma, central neurocytoma, hemangioblastoma, and metastatic renal cell carcinoma (158). Differentiation of these lesions, all containing sheets of uniform rounded cells with clear perinuclear halo/cytoplasm, is imperative because the prognosis and treatment of each may differ significantly. When the differential diagnosis is between CCE and oligodendroglioma, FISH determination of chromosome 1p, 19q, and 18 copy number and DAL-1 gene dosage may prove helpful: deletions involving DAL-1 and/or monosomy 18 have been detected in up to 67% of CCE, whereas the 1p/19q co-deletions typical of oligodendrogliomas are absent in these tumors (103,120). Because a 1q reference probe is often paired with 1p, gain of 1q may also be detected in a subset of these ependymoma cases.

Regarding prognosis, the predictive value of histologic grading of ependymomas remains unresolved (159–163). Many series have been unable to demonstrate a definite association with either overall or recurrence-free survival times, though objective grading criteria have yet to be universally applied and accepted. A statistically significant association was recently reported by Korshunov et al. (164), who examined 258 cases. Although extent of resection remains the most meaningful prognostic determinant (159,161), several studies have offered encouraging data to suggest that the detection of specific patterns of genetic imbalances may also be helpful in predicting clinical outcome. Using CGH, Dyer et al. (157) defined three genetic patterns within their cohort of 52 pediatric intracranial ependymomas based on the absence ("balanced") or presence of partial ("structural") or whole chromosome ("numerical") gain or loss. They found that their "structural" group correlated with a significantly worse clinical outcome compared to the other two genetic groups. This series and others have also established that not only is gain of chromosome 1q quite frequently encountered in intracranial ependymomas, particularly within the pediatric age-group, but it also tends to correlate with histologic anaplasia and may be a marker of aggressive biologic potential (144,146,157). ErbB2 and ErbB4 receptor status was evaluated in another large cohort of pediatric ependymomas by Gilbertson et al. (165). Using IHC, western blotting, and quantitative PCR, they demonstrated a strong positive correlation between elevated ErbB2/4 coexpression levels and high Ki-67 proliferation index, as well as a clear trend toward worse clinical outcome. When this molecular risk factor was combined with proliferation index and extent of surgical excision, a significantly greater degree of survival discrimination was obtained than by any of these individual factors alone (165). Additional prospective studies on contemporarily treated patients will allow the importance of the above findings to be assessed. At the moment, there are no ancillary molecular diagnostic tests routinely applied to ependymomas.

Embryonal Neoplasms

Embryonal tumors represent the largest group of malignant brain tumors in children, and it is therefore not surprising that the bulk of pediatric brain tumor research has focused on these lesions. The current WHO classification of tumors of the nervous system recognizes five main histologic subtypes, all of which contain a population of primitive cells with a variable capacity for divergent differentiation (6). At one end of the spectrum, medulloblastomas and supratentorial primitive neuroectodermal tumors (sPNET) represent prototypical small blue cell tumors, with generally monotonous cell populations showing variable degrees of neuronal and, less commonly, glial differentiation. Situated in the cerebellum, medulloblastoma is by far the most frequently encountered CNS embryonal tumor; sPNET may appear morphologically identical, though it is much less common, more biologically aggressive, and genetically distinct (166–168). Three additional subtypes (atypical teratoid/rhabdoid tumor [ATRT], ependymoblastoma, and medulloepithelioma) harbor distinguishing microscopic features in addition to areas resembling PNET (6,169,170). Although all are more clinically aggressive than medulloblastoma, only ATRT is encountered with sufficient frequency to have been studied at the molecular level.

As a group, medulloblastomas not only demonstrate a broad range of histomorphologic patterns, but are also notable for variable therapeutic responsiveness and biologic behavior. Current treatment strategies center on the stratification of patients into average-risk and high-risk categories based on age at diagnosis, presence of metastatic disease, and volume of residual tumor on postresection imaging studies (171,172). Unfortunately, clinical staging alone is unable to account for the numerous outliers that exist within these risk groups, and there is increasing evidence that patient stratification strategies that include histologic subclassification and molecular markers may provide a more accurate and individualized risk assessment (171,173–178).

Apart from medulloblastoma arising in the context of rare familial syndromes in which specific genetic mutations have been identified (Shh/PTCH/SMOH in Gorlin syndrome, APC/β-catenin in Turcot syndrome, and p53 in Li-Fraumeni syndrome) (171,179), a variety of nonrandom genetic alterations have been detected in sporadic tumors. Abnormalities of chromosome 17, particularly isochromosome 17q [i(17q)], were the most frequent findings of early cytogenetic studies, with subsequent data from modern molecular techniques documenting i(17q) or deletions involving 17p in 30% to 60% of medulloblastoma (166,167,177,180–190). Although 17p loss frequently involves the majority of the chromosomal arm, the centromere is often not the break point site and smaller deletions involving only the most telomeric region have been encountered (191–193). Several putative tumor suppressors mapping to this region have been identified, though their roles in medulloblastoma tumorigenesis remains to be elucidated (191,194,195).

Recent evidence suggests that abnormalities of 17p may be associated with a more clinically aggressive subset of medulloblastoma. Similar to findings by Eberhart et al. (196), we have detected 17p loss by FISH analysis almost exclusively in the context of large cell/anaplastic morphology (unpublished data), a histologic phenotype repeatedly shown to be associated with highly aggressive clinical behavior (175,178,197,198). Several independent investigators have similarly linked deletions of 17p (particularly those arising in the absence of isochromosome 17q) with more aggressive biologic potential and poor prognosis (177,187,188,199); others have not been able to confirm this association (185,186,189). Although *p53* mutations in medulloblastoma are fairly uncommon (193,200), Frank et al. have shown that the p53-ARF tumor suppressor pathway is frequently disrupted in large cell/anaplastic medulloblastoma, and other investigators have reported an association between immunohistochemical detection of *p53* overexpression in medulloblastoma and poor survival (201,202). Until a more concrete association between these 17p alterations and clinical outcome is established, detection of i(17q) or 17p loss may nonetheless be useful in the diagnostic realm in differentiating histologically ambiguous medulloblastoma from ATRT, the latter harboring deletions and mutations involving the *INI1* gene on 22q11.23 instead (see later discussion).

A variety of oncogenes appear to be involved in medulloblastomas, providing possible targets for novel therapeutic interventions. Of these, *ErbB2* has shown the most promise as a potential molecular marker of patient outcome. In contrast to breast carcinomas, in which gene amplification accounts for the vast majority of ErbB2 protein overexpression, *ErbB2* amplification is not prevalent in medulloblastomas. Expression of ErbB2 at the protein level, however, has been detected by immunohistochemical methods in up to 80% of cases, suggesting genetic or epigenetic mechanisms other than gene amplification. The presence of high-level expression (>50% of tumor cells immunopositive for anti-ErbB2) has been consistently associated with a statistically significant decrease in patient survival (177,203–205). Like *ErbB2* overexpression, c-*myc* and more recently N-*myc* amplifications have been regularly encountered in the large cell/anaplastic subtype, although the latter have been reported in only a small percentage of medulloblastomas overall (174,175,178,196, 198,206). Although some studies have indicated a significant association between these amplifications and poor prognosis (199,207,208), this has not been a universal finding (177). Several independent investigators using quantitative PCR methods or ISH have detected a much higher incidence of c-*myc* mRNA overexpression in medulloblastoma than can be accounted for by amplification alone, all but one likewise showing a close association between elevated c-*myc* mRNA and poor prognosis (173,174,209,210). In contrast, elevated TrkC expression, more frequently encountered in the desmoplastic or nodular variant of medulloblastoma, has been shown by some to portend a favorable prognosis (209,211). More recent studies have unfortunately not been able to substantiate this association (173,174,212). In a recent multi-institutional study, 97 fresh-frozen primary childhood medulloblastoma samples were assayed for ErbB2 protein and c-*myc*, N-*myc*, and TrkC mRNA levels; only *ErbB2* overexpression proved to be a strong predictor of poor prognosis, independent of established clinical risk factors and histologic subtype (174). Whereas *ErbB2* status will likely be included in upcoming clinical protocols for patient stratification purposes, additional prospective studies are needed to determine the prognostic significance of other potential biomarkers discussed previously.

Several microsatellite analysis and CGH studies have indicated LOH or deletions of chromosome 10q in up to 40% of medulloblastomas (190,199,213). *PTEN* (10q23) and *DMBT1* (deleted in malignant brain tumors 1; 10q25) are putative tumor suppressor genes mapping to this region. Mutations in the former have been associated with tumor progression and poor clinical outcome in diffuse astrocytomas (37,75,117,129,214,215). However, studies of these genes in CNS embryonal tumors are limited. Nonetheless, a recent study by Yin et al. (213) indicates LOH frequencies of 24% and 47%, respectively, for *PTEN* and *DMBT1* in medulloblastomas. We have recently looked at c-*myc* amplification and 10q dosage via FISH analysis in a group of 79 medulloblastomas at Saint Jude Children's Research Hospital. Using probes targeting multiple sites along 10q (TNKS2) (10q23.32), *PTEN* (10q23.31), and *DMBT1* (10q25.3-26.1), detectable 10q loss was present in 8% of cases overall, with all three of the targeted loci codeleted in each case, consistent with a large region of chromosomal loss. Similar to c-*myc* amplification, 10q loss appeared to correlate with the large cell/anaplastic morphology, the latter alteration encountered twice as often as the former in our series (unpublished data). This association with an aggressive medulloblastoma phenotype is intriguing, requiring further correlation with clinical variables and outcomes to determine whether 10q loss will be of prognostic relevance.

Arising most frequently in infants less than 2 years of age, ATRTs exhibit extremely aggressive behavior with early metastases throughout the CNS and resistance to conventional medulloblastoma treatment protocols (169, 216–218). As opposed to their relative biologic uniformity, these tumors are notable for a diverse histomorphologic spectrum, resulting in frequent confusion with a variety of other CNS neoplasms, especially medulloblastoma and PNET. ATRTs are typically polyphenotypic (i.e., display expression of markers associated with multiple lines of differentiation) and contain varying numbers of the diagnostic rhabdoid cells with eosinophilic paranuclear filamentous inclusions, eccentric nuclei, and prominent nucleoli. However, these cells are scarce in some examples and they may also display epithelial, mesenchymal, or immature round blue cell elements. Similar to their presumed counterparts situated outside the CNS (renal and extrarenal malignant rhabdoid tumors [MRT]), the majority of ATRTs have been found to harbor alterations of chromosome 22, particularly involving 22q11.2 (169,218,219). Recently, the *INI1/hSNF5* gene (also known as *SMARCB1* or *BAF47*) was mapped to this region, and subsequently deletions or mutation of *INI1* have been detected in the majority of these rhabdoid lesions (220–226). Constitutional mutations and deletions of *INI1* are also the hallmark of rhabdoid predisposition syndrome, a hereditary syndrome in which the afflicted are more prone to develop renal or extrarenal MRT and a variety of CNS tumors, including ATRT and choroid plexus carcinoma (227,228).

Whereas up to 75% of ATRT will have demonstrable monosomy 22 or 22q deletion by FISH analysis, these alterations are generally not detected in PNETs and medulloblastomas (71,221,222,228–231). From a diagnostic standpoint, this difference is clearly helpful in separating ATRT from PNET and medulloblastoma, particularly in tumors with ambiguous morphologic and immunohistochemical features. It is therefore not surprising that assessment of 22q dosage in pediatric embryonal tumors has become commonplace, second only to 1p/19q analysis in gliomas with respect to the frequency of FISH testing performed on CNS tumors. A commercially available LSI probe directed against the nearby *bcr* gene also displays excellent hybridization efficiency and sensitivity for detecting these 22q11.2 deletions (221,222).

FISH analysis provides for a rapid assessment of 22q dosage and is applicable to formalin-fixed, paraffin-embedded (FFPE) tissue; however, this assay is not without its limitations, because it is not yet widely available and up to 30% of ATRTs and MRTs will have no detectable deletions. Unfortunately *INI1* mutational analysis is not practical for real-time diagnostic situations. A recently released commercial antibody for the INI1/BAF47 protein shows promise in addressing these issues. Preliminary testing has demonstrated a universal loss of nuclear expression for BAF47 protein in ATRT and MRT, but not in the majority of other pediatric CNS and soft tissue tumors; there was likewise close correlation between these immunohistochemical findings and other molecular techniques in these studies (232,233). To complicate matters, composite rhabdoid tumors (CRTs) deriving from a variety of primary tumors may also involve the CNS, and although they too contain rhabdoid cells and are biologically aggressive, their distinction from ATRT remains important because of therapeutic implications. FISH analysis for 22q dosage is useful in separating ATRT and MRT from CRT in most cases (221); however, FISH alone is unable to make this distinction when the parent tumor of a CRT also has frequent 22q deletions, as do meningiomas, for example. We recently employed both immunohistochemistry and FISH to study BAF47 protein expression and 22q dosages in 40 CRTs in an attempt to address these problematic cases. Although rare in most other CRTs, 22q deletion was detected in 71% of rhabdoid meningiomas; however, nuclear BAF47 expression was retained in all of these cases, including the meningiomas with 22q deletion (234). These preliminary studies indicate that immunohistochemistry for INI1/BAF47 shows great promise as a sensitive and specific methods for distinguishing ATRTs from other CNS tumors and CRTs, though further validation is clearly indicated before employing this technique as a diagnostic gold standard.

MENINGIOMAS

Significant advances have been made recently in our understanding of meningioma biology. Based on two large clinicopathologic studies, the most recent version of the WHO classification has adopted more stringent and objective histologic criteria for grading, allowing for enhanced diagnostic reproducibility and prognostic predictability for benign (WHO grade I), atypical (grade II), and anaplastic (grade III) meningiomas (6,234,235). At the same time, a number of characteristic cytogenetic and molecular genetic aberrations have been associated with meningioma tumorigenesis and progression. Although extent of tumor resection and histologic grade are the two strongest predictors of tumor recurrence, there remains significant clinical variability and additional biomarkers

(i.e., hormone receptor status, telomerase activity, proliferation index), including a number of genetic alterations, may also play a significant role in determining which tumors will behave in a biologically aggressive fashion (236–239). For a more comprehensive summary on meningioma pathology, genetics, and biology, the reader is directed to a recent review (240).

Inactivation of the neurofibromatosis 2 (*NF2*) gene on 22q12 and loss of its protein product merlin is seen in roughly half of sporadic and virtually all *NF2*-associated meningiomas (237,241–245). Merlin belongs to the protein 4.1 family of membrane-associated proteins, a group of tumor suppressors to which two additional members implicated in meningioma tumorigenesis have recently been added: protein 4.1B (previously called DAL-1 or "differentially expressed in adenocarcinoma of the lung") and protein 4.1R (246–248). In an immunoprofiling study of 175 meningiomas, Perry et al. (237,241) identified loss of merlin or protein 4.1B expression in the vast majority of cases (92%), and in a subsequent analysis of 53 cases of pediatric and *NF2*-associated meningiomas detected a similarly high frequency of deletion of *NF2* or *4.1B* genes (82% for each) by FISH. Protein 4.1R interacts with surface cell signaling–associated molecules, such as CD44 and βII-spectrin and reduces cellular growth when reintroduced into meningioma cell lines, similar to merlin and protein 4.1B (247). Lastly, *TSLC1* ("tumor suppressor in lung cancer-1"), one of the major protein 4.1B interactors, has itself been implicated in meningioma tumor progression (249). The data further suggest that loss of *TSLC1* expression may be associated with decreased patient survival, particularly in the group of atypical meningiomas, though larger series are needed to confirm or refute this possibility.

Although these protein 4.1–associated alterations have not been shown to have any prognostic relevance independent of histologic grading (with the possible exception of *TSLC1*), their detection may be helpful from a diagnostic standpoint in selected cases. Because the histologic spectrum of meningiomas is quite broad in terms of both cytomorphology (e.g., spindled versus epithelioid) and degree of pleomorphism and anaplasia, the differential diagnosis can be wide. Considerations such as solitary fibrous tumor, hemangiopericytoma, other sarcomas, dural invasion by gliomas, and metastatic carcinomas and melanomas would not often be expected to show deletions of 22q12 (*NF2*), 18p11.3 (*4.1B*), or 1p36 (*4.1R*) by FISH or losses of merlin, protein 4.1B, or protein 4.1R expression by immunohistochemistry.

Several additional progression-associated sites of chromosomal loss and gain have been identified in meningiomas, and the responsible oncogenes or tumor suppressors have been established in only rare instances. A great deal of interest has centered on chromosomes 1p and 14q, because a significant association has been established between deletions involving one or both of these sites and histologic progression to WHO grades II or III (239,241,250–257). In one FISH study of 180 meningiomas, Cai et al. (250) found combined 1p/14q deletions to be highly associated with increasing histologic grade; of interest, 14q deletions were more common in their histologically benign meningiomas that recurred despite prior gross total resection. More recently, Maillo et al. (253) have provided further evidence that 14q status together with tumor grade and patient age are independent variables for predicting progression-free survival, and, likewise, deletions of 1p have been found to correlate with increased risk of recurrence and shorter progression-free survival in two independent studies (239,257). Most recently, *NDRG2* has been identified as a likely meningioma-associated tumor suppressor gene on 14q11.2, implicated in malignant progression (258). These chromosomal alterations are also frequent in pediatric and *NF2*-associated meningiomas, often accompanying other aggressive features such has high tumor grade, elevated mitotic rate, brain invasion, and frequent recurrence (241). As in the previous discussion, we have used FISH for 22q (*NF2*), 18p (*4.1B*), 1p, and 14q status in selected cases to support the diagnosis of anaplastic meningioma and rule out other malignancies in the differential. For example, we recently found that losses of these markers were highly sensitive and specific in distinguishing anaplastic meningiomas from meningeal hemangiopericytomas (259).

Multiple investigators using CGH, immunoblotting, and PCR-based techniques have demonstrated inactivation of the cell cycle regulators p16^{INK4A}, p14^{ARF}, and p15^{INK4B} (all three on 9p21) in a large proportion of anaplastic meningiomas, in most instances secondary to hemi or homozygous deletions (251,252,260). In another study using archival tissue from 117 tumor samples, FISH-detectable deletions of p16 were similarly associated with malignant progression, but, more importantly, identified a subset of anaplastic meningioma patients with a significantly worse prognosis and shortened survival (261). CGH and FISH studies have also documented amplifications involving 17q23, and a putative oncogene, *PS6K*, has been implicated in a small subset of anaplastic meningiomas (251,262–264). Other genes within the region are likely to be targeted in other tumors, and it remains unclear which 17q23 gene is most critical to tumor progression. LOH of several regions of chromosome 10 have also been shown to correlate with grade, patient survival, and recurrence (239,251,265). All of these markers deserve further consideration in large correlative studies to determine their statistical power as prognostic indicators for meningioma patients and in the potential development of a useful molecular classification and stratification schema.

NEURODEGENERATIVE DISEASES

Alzheimer's Disease

Alzheimer's disease (AD) is the most common neurodegenerative disease that leads to dementia, defined clinically as a progressive decline in two or more cognitive functions from previous higher levels by different but highly concordant criteria including DSM-IV and NINCDS-ADRDA (266,267). Its prevalence increases with age, and the incidence doubles every 5 years after 65 years of age (268). The patients usually first notice a gradual decline in their cognitive function in the anterograde component of short-term memory without much deterioration in retrieving the long-term memory. With progression, disturbances in verbal, visuospatial, and executive functions are also affected.

The pathologic hallmarks of AD include amyloid plaques and neurofibrillary tangles (NFTs) (269). The amyloid plaques are extracellular accumulations of fibrillar materials predominantly composed of amyloid peptide generated from the full-length amyloid precursor protein (APP) after two cleavages by β- and γ-secretases (270). In contrast, the NFTs are intracellular neuronal inclusions of paired helical filaments composed of hyperphosphorylated τ protein (271). Several kinases, including cyclin-dependent kinase 5, glycogen synthase kinase-3β, calmodulin kinase, and phosphatases have been implicated to have a role in the hyperphosphorylation of τ protein (272). However, the culprit in vivo remains to be defined.

Extensive research efforts have been applied to identifying specific biomarkers, using a wide array of techniques. For example, alterations in the levels of synaptic proteins (273), the hyperphosphorylated τ protein (274), and the amyloid β (Aβ) peptide (275) in the cerebrospinal fluid of AD patients by enzyme-linked immunosorbent assay (ELISA) have been reported by several studies. Unfortunately, lack of sufficient sensitivity and specificity limits their use as in vivo markers to differentiate AD from other dementias or controls (276). Currently, the diagnosis of AD still requires postmortem tissue examination because of lack of specific biomarkers. Recently, positron emission tomography (PET) and magnetic resonance imaging (MRI) neuroimaging with newly developed molecules targeting amyloid plaques (see later discussion) (277–279) offer a potential means of accurate antemortem diagnosis of AD, with the hope of early diagnosis and treatment.

The etiology of AD remains unknown. Many studies suggest that both environmental (280,281) and genetic factors (282) have important pathogenic roles. Familial cases provide important insights into this issue. Heritable mutations in several genes have been identified, and subsequent studies have confirmed their causative role in the pathogenesis of AD subsets (Table 14.2). For example, mutations in the *PSEN1* gene, encoding presenilin (PS) protein, *PSEN2*, a homologue of *PSEN1*, and the *APP* gene have all been identified in cases of early-onset (onset <60 years of age) familial AD (283–285). In contrast, a common ε4 allele encoded by the *APOE* gene (286) is linked to late-onset AD. *PSEN1* mutations account for more than 50% of early-onset familial ADs, and they are inherited in an autosomal dominant fashion. The PS protein is an essential part of the γ-secretase enzyme. Mutant protein promotes the formation of amyloid plaques by tilting the production of Aβ peptide toward a longer form that has enhanced fibrillogenic properties. *PSEN2* and *APP* mutations are both inherited in autosomal dominant fashion. Several *APP* mutations also favor the production of the longer form of Aβ peptide. The APOE protein binds Aβ peptide. Although the ε4 allele is neither necessary nor sufficient to cause AD, it may act as a risk modifier of AD. Genetic testing for *PSEN1* mutations and *APOE* genotyping are available through multiple commercial sources and are also done at several National Institutes of Health–funded AD research centers. However, it should be noted that only a small percentage (<10%) of AD cases are hereditary and carry mutations in *PSEN1*, *PSEN2*, or *APP* genes. Many familial cases do not have detectable mutations in any of these three genes. Furthermore,

TABLE 14.2
TABLE 14.2
SUMMARY OF THE GENETIC ABNORMALITIES OF THE NEURODEGENERATIVE DISEASES

Disease	Gene Affected	Protein Product	Inheritance	Biomarker	Genetic Testing
Alzheimer's disease				CSF τ and Aβ peptide	
Sporadic					
Familial					
AD1	APP	Amyloid precursor protein	AD		T, P©
AD2	APOE e4	Apolipoprotein ϵ4	AD		T
AD3	PSEN1	Presenilin 1	AD		T, P©
AD4	PSEN2	Presenilin 2	AD		T, P©
AD5	12p11.23-q13.12		AD		R
Parkinson's disease					
Sporadic					
Familial					
PARK1	SNCA	α-Synuclein	AD		
PARK2	Parkin	Parkin	AR		T
PARK3	2p13		AD		
PARK4	SNCA	α-Synuclein	AD		
PARK5	UCH-L1	Ubiquitin carboxyl-terminal esterase L1	AD		
PARK6	PINK1	PTEN-induced putative kinase 1	AR/AD		
PARK7	DJ1	Oncogene DJ1 protein	AR		
PARK8	LRRK2	dardarin	AD		**
PARK9	1p36		AR		
PARK10	1p36				
PARK11	2q36-37		AD		
Frontotemporal dementia with parkinsonism-	MAPT	τ Protein	AD		T, P
Motor neuron disease					
Amyotrophic lateral sclerosis					
Sporadic					
Familial					
ALS1	SOD1	Cu/Zn superoxide dismutase	AD		T, P
ALS2	ALS2	Alsin	AR		R, P©
ALS3	18q21		AD		
ALS4	SETX	Senataxin	AD		
ALS5	15q15.1-q21.1		AR		
ALS6	16q12.1-q12.2		AD		
ALS7	20ptel		AD		
ALS8	VAPB	Vesicle-associated membrane protein	AD		
Progressive lower motor neuron disease without sensory symptoms	DCTN1	Dynactin	AD		
Spinal muscular atrophy					
SMN1-related SMA					
Type I	SMN1	Survival of motor neurons	AR		T, P
Type II	SMN1		AR		T, P
Type III	SMN1		AR		T, P
non–SMN1-related SMA					
Trinucleotide repeat diseases					
CAG/CTG repeat diseases					
Huntington's disease	HD	Huntingtin	AD		T, P
Huntington's disease-like 2	JPH3	Junctophilin 3	AD		T, P©
Spinocerebellar atrophy					
SCA1	ATXN1	Ataxin 1	AD		T, P
SCA2	ATXN2	Ataxin 2	AD		T, P
SCA3	ATXN3	Ataxin 3	AD		T, P
SCA6	CACNA1A	Alpha-1A-voltage-dependent Ca^{2+} channel	AD		T, P

(continued)

TABLE 14.2
(continued)

SCA7	*ATXN7*	Ataxin 7	AD	T, P
SCA8	*ATXN8*	Ataxin 8	AD	T, P
SCA12	PPP2R2B	Regulatory subunit of the protein phosphatase PP2A	AD	T, P
SCA17	*TBP*	TATA box-binding protein	AD	T, P
Dentatorubral-pallidoluysian atrophy	*DRPLA*	Atrophin-1	AD	T, P
CCG repeat diseases				
Fragile X syndrome	*FMR1*	Fragile X mental retardation 1 protein	X-linked	T, P
GAA repeat diseases				
Friedreich ataxia	*FRDA1* *FRDA2*	Frataxin	AR	T, P
Pentanucleotide (ATTCT) repeat				
SCA10	*ATXN10*	Ataxin 10	AD	T, P
Others				
SCA4	16q22.1		AD	
SCA5	11q13		AD	
SCA11	15q14-q21.3		AD	
SCA13	19q13.3-q13.4		AD	
SCA14	*PRKCG*	Protein kinase C-gamma	AD	T, P
SCA15	3p24.2-3pter		AD	
SCA16	8q22.1-24.1		AD	
SCA18	7q22-q32		AD	
SCA19	1p21-q21		AD	
SCA20	11p13-q11		AD	
SCA21	7p21.3-p15.1		AD	

T, clinical genetic testing available.
P, prenatal testing available.
P©, prenatal testing for the family at risk available at research laboratories.
**, clinical testing expected to be available in the near future.

multiple studies have been conducted to evaluate the predictive utility of *APOE* genotype in the conversion or development of AD from previously mild cognitive impairment or controls (287–289). The results remain controversial, with evidence both supporting and refuting its potential applicability. Therefore, the American Geriatrics Society* currently cautions against the use of these genetic tests in the clinical settings. Specific recommendations for genetic testing of AD were also made by the Stanford Program in Genomics, Ethics, and Society (290), which should also be useful to interested readers.

Parkinson's Disease

Parkinson's disease (PD) is the most common neurodegenerative disease presenting as a movement disorder in aged individuals. Its prevalence is estimated to be as high as 1 or 2 per 1,000 population, with regional variation (291). It is characterized clinically by rigidity, bradykinesia and akinesia, resting tremor, and postural instability caused by progressive loss of the dopaminergic nigrostri-

atal system (292). Histopathologically, pallor of the substantia nigra and locus ceruleus are readily appreciated. Lewy bodies, intraneuronal eosinophilic inclusions with peripheral clear halos, and Lewy neurites, seen in the vulnerable neuronal populations, are the hallmark lesions of PD (293). α-Synuclein has been identified as the major proteinaceous component of the filamentous building blocks of Lewy bodies and Lewy neurites (294,295). Lewy bodies are also found in the neocortical neurons in a related neurodegenerative disease, dementia with Lewy bodies, which is the second most common neurodegenerative disease that causes dementia and is encountered as a coexisting pathology in approximately 25% of AD. Interestingly, α-synuclein–containing neuronal or glial inclusions are also found in other diseases, including neurodegeneration with brain iron accumulation, type I (NBIA-1), and multiple system atrophy (MSA), collectively classified under the term synucleinopathy (296). Several neurodegenerative diseases, such as progressive supranuclear palsy, corticobasal degeneration, and others, produce PD-like symptoms or parkinsonism, but Lewy bodies are not seen. In view of these recent molecular biologic innovations, a need to redefine PD has been proposed (297).

Recent advances in the identification of genetic mutations in familial PD demonstrate that PD represents a

*American Geriatrics society, http://www.americangeriatrics.org/products/positionpapers/gentest.shtml.

genetically heterogeneous group of diseases, which share common clinical phenotypes (Table 14.2). To this date, at least 11 chromosomal loci have been linked to PD (298), and several disease-causative mutations in the responsible genes have recently been identified, including α-synuclein (*SNCA*) (299), *parkin* (300), *UCH-L1* (301), *neurofilament M* (302), *DJ1* (303), *PINK1* (304), and *LRRK2* (305). However, it remains to be determined if these familial PDs also develop Lewy pathology similar to that in sporadic PDs. Some of the familial PARK8 patients with mutations in the *LRRK2* gene develop Lewy bodies (305), but others, such as the autosomal recessive familial juvenile PD with mutations in the gene *PARKIN*, do not (306). Most of the mutations are found in only a few characterized families, with a strong racial preference (298). They account for only a minute fraction of all PD cases and thus have very limited value in clinical practice. On the other hand, the heterozygous mutations in the *LRRK2* gene appear to be relatively common in familial cases across the world (307–309) and are estimated to account for up to 1% to 5% of the late-onset familial cases of PD. Therefore, this mutation is expected to become a component of genetic testing (targeted DNA sequencing) for familial PD in the near future.

Motor Neuron Diseases

Motor neuron diseases (MNDs) are a heterogeneous group of neurodegenerative diseases that affect predominantly motor neurons in the precentral gyrus, brain stem, and anterior horns of the spinal cord (310). The clinical presentations are further classified as amyotrophic lateral sclerosis (ALS), when both upper and lower motor neurons are affected; primary lateral sclerosis (PLS), when only upper motor neurons affected; and spinal muscular atrophy (SMA), when the disease is limited to lower motor neurons. This classification is not only useful clinically, but also correlates with different etiologies.

ALS has an incidence of approximately 1 to 3 cases per 100,000 (311,312), and typically presents as progressive muscular weakness or stiffness, predominantly in adults, although inherited juvenile forms are also encountered (313). A small fraction of patients present with difficulties in respiration or swallowing (bulbar form) because of the early involvement with motor neurons in the brain stem. The great majority of these patients are sporadic, although familial forms are encountered in 5% to 10% (314). The identity of PLS is a little unclear. It may represent a variant of ALS with prominent loss of upper motor neurons. However, variants of SMA are principally MNDs of childhood (315), with an incidence that may be as high as 7.8 in 100,000 live births (316).The death of lower motor neurons leads to reduced fetal movement, delay of motor development, contractures, and paralysis in infants or young children.

The etiology of ALS remains incompletely understood. Both environmental (317) and genetic factors (314) are considered to have important roles (Table 14.2). Mutations in the copper/zinc superoxide dismutase (*SOD1*) gene were first identified in several families and account for approximately 20% of all familial cases (318). Although SOD1 protein functions as an important enzyme to reduce oxidative stress by converting superoxide to peroxide, the mutant

SOD1 is believed to cause disease through a gain of toxic property (319). Several other genes encoding neurofilament H (*NEFH*) (320), *alsin* (321,322), *DCTN1* (323), *SETX* (324), and peripherin (325) were recently identified in familial ALS, indicating etiologic heterogeneity. PLS is almost always reported as a sporadic disorder; no mutant genes have been identified. The three common forms of SMA are all linked to the same survival motor neuron (*SMN*) gene on chromosome 5 (326,327). Other genes such as the neuronal apoptosis inhibitory protein (NAIP) (328) and SMN2 (329) may act as modifiers of the mutant *SMN* gene. Genetic testing for *SOD1* mutation–related ALS and SMA types are available at different laboratories. However, testing for other ALS-causing mutations are not readily available because of the rarity of such cases. Prenatal screening for SMA is also available and is important for those families at risk.

Trinucleotide Repeat Disorders

Trinucleotide repeat disorders (TRDs) are a heterogeneous group of neurodegenerative diseases characterized by expansion of various trinucleotide repeats, each involving a distinct disease-associated gene (Table 14.2) (330). The clinical phenotypes correlate with the neuronal populations that are selectively targeted in each disease. For example, choreiform movement and dementia in Huntington's disease (HD) are explained by the preferential losses of neurons in the basal ganglia and neocortex (331); gait disturbance, ataxia nystagmus, and other motor problems characteristic of spinocerebellar ataxias are mainly caused by the demise of cerebellar Purkinje neurons and neurons in spinal cord and brain stem (332). It is interesting to note that all of the TRDs present as neurologic disorders. However, Friedreich's ataxia (FA) also has cardiomyopathy in addition to ataxia and proprioceptive sensory disturbances. It has long been observed that within a family, these hereditary TRDs develop a progressively earlier age of onset or increased severity with successive generations. This stereotyped phenomenon, or genetic anticipation, is characteristic of these TRDs. However, similar phenomena have also been observed in other non-neurological diseases such as rheumatoid arthritis (333), Crohn's disease (334), Graves' disease (335), and diabetes mellitus (336) and neuropsychiatric diseases, such as schizophrenia and bipolar disorder (337) suggesting that trinucleotide repeat may also serve as a possible genetic abnormality of these diseases. If this is true, the TRDs will be further expanded. Genetic anticipation is caused by further increases in the number of trinucleotide repeats in successive generations, through germline expansion resulting from several mechanisms (338). Collectively, the longer mutant alleles correlate with earlier onset and more severe disease, but the age of onset cannot be precisely predicted solely based on the length of expanded alleles.

Although expansion of the trinucleotide repeats underlies all of the TRDs, at least three different types of TRDs exist.

1. CAG repeats. Expansion of the CAG repeats are identified in several TRDs, including HD (339), SCA types 1 (340), 2 (341), 3 (342), 6 (343), 7 (344), 12 (345),

and 17 (346), as well as dentatorubropallidoluysian atrophy (DRPLA) (347). Typically, the expanded CAG repeats are found in the coding exons and these diseases are inherited in an autosomal dominant fashion. For each disease, the expanded alleles are located at different genes and the number of repeats appears to be disease specific.

2. *GAA repeats.* The GAA expansion is found in FA, the most common autosomal recessive ataxia (348). The expanded GAA repeats are located in intron 1 of the gene *FRDA1*, which encodes a mitochondrial protein, frataxin, involved in iron metabolism (349). The homozygosity of the expanded GAA alleles leads to a reduction in the frataxin level and the disease. More than 95% of cases are caused by homozygous GAA expansion. Truncating and missense mutations account for only a small percentage of FA.

3. Other trinucleotide and pentanucleotide repeats. The expanded CTG and CTG/CAG repeats are found in the SCA type8 (350) and HD-like 2 disease (351), respectively. Another recently described expanded GCG repeat encodes a polyalanine expansion that causes several diseases predominantly presenting as congenital malformation syndromes (352). The expansion of the rare ATTCT pentanucleotide repeat underlies the SCA type 10 (353).

The mechanisms leading to the TRD diseases remain incompletely understood. The similarities of the clinical presentations between HD and DRPLA and among the different entities of SCAs and also the autosomal dominant inheritance argue that gains of novel toxic properties resulting from the expanded alleles rather than losses of the function are important for the pathogenesis of these diseases. Consistent with this concept, the expanded CAG repeats have been shown to encode a polyglutamine stretch in the affected gene products, which in turn results in formation of ubiquitinated polyglutamine-containing intranuclear inclusions common to all of these CAG repeats diseases (354,355). These inclusions can be recognized by a mouse monoclonal antibody 1C2 raised against an expanded polyglutamine moiety (Chemicon, CA), indicating the presence of the affected gene sequences within these inclusions. These findings demonstrate an aberrant localization or process of the affected cytoplasmic proteins such as huntingtin protein in HD. More importantly, inhibition of the formation of these inclusions rescues the neurodegeneration in the animal model (356). This result clearly establishes the essential role of the neuronal inclusions in cell death. In addition, expanded repeats form DNA secondary structures, confer genetic instability, and most likely contribute to altered chromatin configuration, leading to transcriptional silencing (357). Recently, CAG expansion was found to interfere with fast axonal transport, which leads to subsequent neurodegeneration (358). In summary, the expanded trinucleotide or pentanucleotide repeats cause neurodegeneration, most likely through multiple different mechanisms.

With the identification of the trinucleotide repeats, direct genetic testing and screening becomes available for this group of diseases (Table 14.2). In fact, HD is the archetypal neurodegenerative disease to which genetic testing is applied, and it remains one of the best characterized entities in terms of the psychosocial impact of the test results on tested individuals. Expansion of CAG trinucleotide accounts for more than 99% of cases of HD; therefore, tests that effectively measure the CAG-repeat region of the HD or *IT-15* gene provide a sensitivity greater than 99%. The positive results (at least one allele of 40 CAG repeats or more) are 100% specific for HD, and negative results (allele sizes of 26 CAG repeats and lower) have never been associated with a HD phenotype. However, allele sizes of 36 to 39 CAG repeats have been reported in both clinically affected and unaffected individuals and do not correlate with clinical outcomes. It is advisable for an individual to read the techinal and ethical guidelines for genetic testings for HD developed by the American College of Medical Genetics (359). Furthermore, the allele sizes in each TRDs vary significantly. The reader should refer to the specific guidelines of each disease.

REFERENCES

1. Smith CO, Lipe HP, Bird TD. Impact of presymptomatic genetic testing for hereditary ataxia and neuromuscular disorders. *Arch Neurol* 2004;61:875–880.
2. Tibben A, Duivenvoorden HJ, Niermeijer MF, et al. Psychological effects of presymptomatic DNA testing for Huntington's disease in the Dutch program. *Psychosom Med* 1994;56:526–532.
3. Codori AM, Slavney PR, Rosenblatt A, et al. Prevalence of major depression one year after predictive testing for Huntington's disease. *Genet Test* 2004;8:114–119.
4. Wiggins S, Whyte P, Huggins M, et al. The psychological consequences of predictive testing for Huntington's disease. Canadian Collaborative Study of Predictive Testing. *N Engl J Med* 1992;327:1401–1405.
5. Decruyenaere M, Evers-Kiebooms G, Boogaerts A, et al. Prediction of psychological functioning one year after the predictive test for Huntington's disease and impact of the test result on reproductive decision making. *J Med Genet* 1996;33:737–743.
6. Kleihues P, Cavenee WK. *World Health Organization Classification of Tumours: Pathology and Genetics of Tumours of the Nervous System.* Lyon: IARC Press; 2000.
7. Lang FF, Miller DC, Kislow M, et al. Pathways leading to glioblastoma multiforme: a molecular analysis of genetic alterations in 65 astrocytic tumors. *J Neurosurg* 1994; 81:427–436.
8. von Deimling A, Louis DN, Wiestler OD. Molecular pathways in the formation of gliomas. *Glia* 1995;15:328–338.
9. Watanabe K, Tachibana O, Sata K, et al. Overexpression of the EGF receptor and *p53* mutations are mutually exclusive in the evolution of primary and secondary glioblastomas. *Brain Pathol* 1996;6:216–223.
10. Schmidt MC, Antweiler S, Urban N, et al. Impact of genotype and morphology on the prognosis of glioblastoma. *J Neuropathol Exp Neurol* 2002;61:321–328.
11. Burton EC, Lamborn K, Forsyth P, et al. Aberrant *p53, mdm2,* and proliferation differ in glioblastomas from long-term compared with typical survivors. *Clin Cancer Res* 2002; 8:180–187.
12. Stander M, Peraud A, Leroch B, et al. Prognostic impact of *TP53* mutation status for adult patients with supratentorial World Health Organization grade II astrocytoma or oligoastrocytoma. *Cancer* 2004;101:1028–1035.
13. Hwang SL, Hong YR, Chai CY, et al. Prognostic evaluation in supratentorial astrocytic tumors using *p53,* epidermal growth factor receptor, *c-erbB-2* immunostaining. *Kaohsiung J Med Sci* 1998;14:607–615.
14. Newcomb EW, Cohen H, Lee SR, et al. Survival of patients with glioblastoma multiforme is not influenced by altered expression of *p16, p53, EGFR, MDM2* or *Bcl-2* genes. *Brain Pathol* 1998;8:655–667.
15. Simmons ML, Lamborn K, Takahashi MA, et al. Analysis of complex relationships between age, *p53,* epidermal growth factor receptor, and survival in glioblastoma patients. *Cancer Res* 2001;61:1122–1128.
16. Wessels PH, Twijnstra A, Kessels AGH, et al. Gain of chromosome 7, as detected by in situ hybridization, strongly correlates with shorter survival in astrocytoma grade 2. *Genes Chromosomes Cancer* 2002;33:279–284.
17. Kunwar S, Mohapatra G, Bollen A, et al. Genetic subgroups of anaplastic astrocytomas correlate with patient age and survival. *Cancer Res* 2001;61:7683–7688.
18. Varela M, Ranuncolo SM, Morandi A, et al. *EGF-R* and *PDGF-R,* but not *bcl-2,* overexpression predict overall survival in patients with low-grade astrocytomas. *J Surg Oncol* 2004;86:34–40.
19. Burger PC, Pearl DK, Aldape K, et al. Small cell architecture: a histological equivalent of *EGFR* amplification in glioblastoma multiforme? *J Neuropathol Exp Neurol* 2001; 60:1099–1104.
20. Perry A, Aldape K, George DH, et al. Small cell astrocytoma: an aggressive variant that is clinicopathologically and genetically distinct from anaplastic oligodendroglioma. *Cancer* 2004;101:2318–2326.
21. Korshunov A, Golanov A, Sycheva R. Immunohistochemical markers for prognosis of cerebral glioblastoma. *J Neurooncol* 2002;58:217–236.
22. Aldape K, Ballman K, Furth A, et al. Immunohistochemical detection of *EGFRvIII* in high malignancy grade astrocytomas and evaluation of prognostic significance. *J Neuropathol Exp Neurol* 2004;63:700–707.

23. Shinojima WD N, Tada K, Shiraishi S, et al. Prognostic value of epidermal growth factor receptor in patients with glioblastoma multiforme. *Cancer Res* 2993;63:6962–6970.
24. Andersson U, Guo D, Malmer B, et al. Epidermal growth factor receptor family (EGFR, ErbB2-4) in gliomas and meningiomas. *Acta Neuropathol (Berl)* 2004;108:135–142.
25. Smith JS, Jenkins RB. Genetic alterations in adult diffuse glioma: occurrence, significance, and prognostic implications. *Front Biosci* 2000;5:213–231.
26. Cianciulli AM, Morace E, Coletta AM, et al. Investigation of genetic alterations associated with development and adverse outcome in patients with astrocytic tumor. *J Neurooncol* 2000;48:95–101.
27. Perry A, Tonk V, McIntire DD, et al. Interphase cytogenetics (in situ hybridization) analysis of astrocytomas using archival, formalin-fixed, paraffin-embedded tissue and nonfluorescent light microscopy. *Am J Clin Pathol* 1997;108:166–174.
28. Burton EC, Lamborn KR, Feuerstein BG, et al. Genetic aberrations defined by comparative genomic hybridization distinguish long-term from typical survivors of glioblastoma. *Cancer Res* 2002;62:6205–6210.
29. Arslantas A, Artan S, Oner U, et al. The importance of genomic copy number changes in the prognosis of glioblastoma multiforme. *Neurosurg Rev* 2004;27:58–64.
30. Ganju V, Jenkins RB, O'Fallon JR, et al. Prognostic factors in gliomas: A multivariate analysis of clinical, pathologic, flow cytometric, cytogenetic, and molecular markers. *Cancer* 1994;74:920–927.
31. Horiguchi H, Hirose T, Sano T, et al. Loss of chromosome 10 in glioblastoma: relation to proliferation and angiogenesis. *Pathol Int* 1999;49:681–686.
32. Brat D, Seiferheld WF, Perry A, et al. Analysis of 1p, 19q, 9p, and 10q as prognostic markers for high-grade astrocytomas using fluorescence in situ hybridization on tissue microarrays from Radiation Therapy Oncology Group trials. *Neuro-oncol* 2004;6:96–103.
33. Schmidt EE, Ichimura K, Gioke HM, et al. Mutational profile of the *PTEN* gene in primary human astrocytic tumors and cultivated xenografts. *J Neuropathol Exp Neurol* 1999;58:1170–1183.
34. Zhou XP, Li YJ, Hoang-Xuan K, et al. Mutational analysis of the *PTEN* gene in gliomas: molecular and pathological correlations. *Int J Cancer* 1999;84:150–154.
35. Fuller CE, Wang H, Zhang W, et al. High-throughput molecular profiling of high-grade astrocytomas: the utility of fluorescence in situ hybridization on tissue microarrays (TMA-FISH). *J Neuropathol Exp Neurol* 2002;61:1078–1084.
36. Sasaki H, Betensky RA, Cairncross JG, et al. *DMBT1* polymorphisms: relationship to malignant glioma tumorigenesis. *Cancer Res* 2002;62:1790–1796.
37. Lin H, Bondy ML, Langford LA, et al. Allelic deletion analyses of *MMAC/PTEN* and *DMBT1* loci in gliomas: relationship to prognostic significance. *Clin Cancer Res* 1998; 4:2447–2454.
38. Korshunov A, Golanov A, Sycheva R. Immunohistochemical markers for prognosis of anaplastic astrocytomas. *J Neurooncol* 2002;58:203–215.
39. Hung KS, Howng SL. Prognostic significance of annexin VII expression in glioblastomas multiforme in humans. *J Neurosurg* 2003;99:886–892.
40. Schmidt EE, Ichimura K, Reifenberger G, et al. *CDKN2 (p16/MTS1)* gene deletion of CDK4 amplification occurs in the majority of glioblastomas. *Cancer Res* 1994; 54:6321–6324.
41. Miettinen H, Kononen J, Sallinen PK, et al. *CDKN2/p16* predicts survival in oligodendrogliomas: comparison with astrocytomas. *J Neurooncol* 1999;41:205–211.
42. Mizumatsu S, Tamiya T, Ono Y, et al. Expression of cell cycle regulator p27Kip1 is correlated with survival of patients with astrocytoma. *Clin Cancer Res* 1999;5:551–557.
43. Biernat W, Kleihues P, Yonekawa T, et al. Amplification and overexpression of MDM2 in primary (de novo) glioblastomas. *J Neuropathol Exp Neurol* 1997;56:180–185.
44. Biernat W, Tohma Y, Yonekawa Y, et al. Alteration of cell cycle regulatory genes in primary (de novo) and secondary glioblastomas. *Acta Neuropathol (Berl)* 1997;94: 303–309.
45. Perry A, Anderl K, Borell TJ, et al. Detection of *p16*, *RB*, *CDK4*, and *p53* gene deletion and amplification by fluorescence in situ hybridization in 96 gliomas. *Am J Clin Pathol* 1999;112:801–809.
46. Ueki K, Ono Y, Henson JW, et al. *CDKN2/p16* or *RB* alterations occur in the majority of glioblastomas and are inversely correlated. *Cancer Res* 1996;56:150–153.
47. Kirla R, Salminen E, Huhtala S, et al. Prognostic value of the expression of tumor suppressor genes *p53*, *p21*, *p16* and *pRB*, and Ki-67 labeling in high grade astrocytomas treated with radiotherapy. *J Neurooncol* 2000;46:71–80.
48. Iwadate Y, Mochizuki S, Fujimoto S, et al. Alteration of *CDKN2/p16* in human astrocytic tumors is related with increased susceptibility to antimetabolite anticancer agents. *Int J Oncol* 2000;17:501–505.
49. Korkolopoulou P, Christodoulou P, Kouzelis K, et al. MDM2 and *p53* expression in gliomas: a multivariate survival analysis including proliferation markers and epidermal growth factor receptor. *Br J Cancer* 1997;75:1269–1278.
50. Rainov NG, Dobberstein KU, Bahn H, et al. Prognostic factors in malignant glioma: influence of the overexpression of oncogene and tumor-suppressor gene products on survival. *J Neurooncol* 1997;35:13–28.
51. Kirla R, Haapasalo HK, Kalimo H, et al. Low expression of *p27* indicates a poor prognosis in patients with high-grade astrocytomas. *Cancer* 2003;97:644–648.
52. Piva R, Cavalla P, Bortolotto S, et al. *p27/kip1* expression in human astrocytic gliomas. *Neurosci Lett* 1997;234:127–130.
53. Tamiya T, Mizumatsu S, Ono Y, et al. High cyclin E/low *p27Kip1* expression is associated with poor prognosis in astrocytomas. *Acta Neuropathol (Berl)* 2001;101:334–340.
54. von Deimling A, Louis DN, von Ammon K, et al. Evidence for a tumor suppressor gene on chromosome 19q associated with human astrocytomas, oligodendrogliomas, and mixed gliomas. *Cancer Res* 1992;52:4277–4279.
55. von Deimling A, Bender B, Jahnke R, et al. Loci associated with malignant progression in astrocytomas: a candidate on chromosome 19q. *Cancer Res* 1992;54:1397–1401.
56. Smith JS, Tachibana I, Lee HK, et al. Mapping of the chromosome 19q-arm glioma tumor suppressor gene using fluorescence in situ hybridization and novel microsatellite markers. *Genes Chromosomes Cancer* 2000;29:16–25.
57. Abdulrauf SI, Edvardsen K, Ho KL, et al. Vascular endothelial growth factor expression and vascular density as prognostic markers of survival in patients with low grade astrocytoma. *J Neurosurg* 1998;88:513–520.
58. Dietzmann K, vonBossanyi P. Coexpression of epidermal growth factor receptor protein and c-erbB-2 oncoprotein in human astrocytic tumors: an immunohistochemical study. *Zentralbl Pathol* 1994;140:335–341.
59. Haapasalo H, Hyytinen E, Sallinen P, et al. *c-erbB-2* in astrocytomas: infrequent overexpression by immunohistochemistry and absence of gene amplification by fluorescence in situ hybridization. *Br J Cancer* 1996;73:620–623.
60. Hiesiger EM, Hayes RL, Pierz DM, et al. Prognostic relevance of epidermal growth factor receptor (EGF-R) and *c-neu/erbB2* expression in glioblastomas (GBMs). *J Neurooncol* 1993;16:93–104.
61. Hwang SL, Chai CY, Lin H, et al. Expression of epidermal growth factor receptors and c-erbB-2 proteins in human astrocytic tumors. *Kaohsiung J Med Sci* 1997;13:417–424.
62. Koka V, Potti A, Forseen SE, et al. Role of *her-2/neu* overexpression and clinical determinants of early mortality in glioblastoma multiforme. *Am J Clin Oncol* 2003; 26:332–335.
63. Lafuente JV, Adan B, Alkiza K, et al. Expression of vascular endothelial growth factor (VEGF) and platelet-derived growth factor receptor-beta (PDGFR-beta) in human gliomas. *J Mol Neurosci* 1999;13:177–185.
64. Nam DH, Park K, Suh YL, et al. Expression of VEGF and brain specific angiogenesis inhibitor-1 in glioblastoma: prognostic significance. *Oncol Rep* 2004;11:863–869.
65. Oehring RD, Miletic M, Valter MM, et al. Vascular endothelial growth factor (VEGF) in astrocytic gliomas: a prognostic factor? *J Neurooncol* 1999;45:117–125.
66. Yao Y, Kubota T, Sato K, et al. Prognostic value of vascular endothelial growth factor and its receptors Flt-1 and Flk-1 in astrocytic tumours. *Acta Neurochir (Wien)* 2001;143:159–166.
67. Eller JL, Longo SL, Hicklin DJ, et al. Activity of anti-epidermal growth factor receptor monoclonal antibody C225 against glioblastoma multiforme. *Neurosurgery* 2002;51:1005–1013.
68. Mamot C, Drummond DC, Greiser U, et al. Epidermal growth factor receptor (EGFR)-targeted immunoliposomes mediate specific and efficient drug delivery to *EGFR*- and *EGFRvIII*-overexpressing tumor cells. *Cancer Res* 2003;63:3154–3161.
69. Park KH, Lee J, Yoo CG, et al. Application of *p27* gene therapy for human malignant glioma potentiated by using mutant *p27*. *J Neurosurg* 2004;101:505–510.
70. Agamanolis DP, Malone JM. Chromosomal abnormalities in 47 pediatric brain tumors. *Cancer Genet Cytogenet* 1995;81:125–134.
71. Biegel JA. Genetics of pediatric central nervous system tumors. *J Pediatr Hematol Oncol* 1997;19:492–501.
72. Sure U, Ruedi D, Tachibana O, et al. Determination of *p53* mutations, *EGFR* overexpression, and loss of *p16* expression in pediatric glioblastomas. *J Neuropathol Exp Neurol* 1997;56:782–789.
73. Cheng Y, Ng HK, Zhang SF, et al. Genetic alterations in pediatric high-grade astrocytomas. *Hum Pathol* 1999;30:1284–1290.
74. Raffel C. Molecular biology of pediatric gliomas. *J Neurooncol* 1996;28:121–128.
75. Raffel C, Frederick L, O'Fallon JR, et al. Analysis of oncogene and tumor suppressor gene alterations in pediatric malignant astrocytomas reveals reduced survival for patients with *PTEN* mutations. *Clin Cancer Res* 1999;5:4085–4090.
76. Sung T, Miller DC, Hayes RL, et al. Preferential inactivation of the *p53* tumor suppressor pathway and lack of *EGFR* amplification distinguish de novo high grade pediatric astrocytomas from de novo adult astrocytomas. *Brain Pathol* 2000;10:249–259.
77. Bredel M, Pollack IF, Hamilton RL, et al. Epidermal growth factor receptor expression and gene amplification in high-grade non-brainstem gliomas of childhood. *Clin Cancer Res* 1999;5:1786–1792.
78. DiSapio A, Morra I, Pradotto L, et al. Molecular genetic changes in a series of neuroepithelial tumors of childhood. *J Neurooncol* 2002;59:117–122.
79. Kraus JA, Felsberg J, Tonn J, et al. Molecular genetic analysis of the *TP53*, *PTEN*, *CDKN2A*, *EGFR*, *CDK4*, and *MDM2* tumour-associated genes in supratentorial primitive neuroectodermal tumours and glioblastomas of childhood. *Neuropathol Appl Neurobiol* 2002;28:325–333.
80. Pollack IF, Hamilton RL, Finkelstein SD, et al. The relationship between *TP53* mutations and overexpression of *p53* and prognosis in malignant gliomas of childhood. *Cancer Res* 1997;57:304–309.
81. Pollack IF, Finkelstein SD, Woods J, et al. Expression of *p53* and prognosis in children with malignant gliomas. *N Engl J Med* 2002;346:420–427.
82. Cheng Y, Pang JC, Ng HK, et al. Pilocytic astrocytomas do not show most of the genetic changes commonly seen in diffuse astrocytomas. *Histopathology* 2000;37: 437–444.
83. Sanoudou D, Tingby O, Ferguson-Smith MA, et al. Analysis of pilocytic astrocytoma by comparative genomic hybridization. *Br J Cancer* 2000;82:1218–1222.
84. Gutmann DH, Donahoe J, Brown T, et al. Loss of neurofibromatosis 1 (*NF1*) gene expression in *NF1*-associated pilocytic astrocytomas. *Neuropathol Appl Neurobiol* 2000; 26:361–367.
85. Li J, Perry A, James CD, et al. Cancer-related gene expression profiles in *NF1*-associated pilocytic astrocytomas. *Neurology* 2001:56:885–890.
86. Giannini C, Hebrink D, Scheithauer BW, et al. Analysis of *p53* mutation and expression in pleomorphic xanthoastrocytoma. *Neurogenetics* 2001;3:159–162.
87. Yin XL, Bik-Yu A, Liong EC, et al. Genetic imbalances in pleomorphic xanthoastrocytoma detected by comparative genomic hybridization and literature review. *Cancer Genet Cytogenet* 2002;132:14–19.
88. Paulus W, Lisle DK, Tonn J, et al. Molecular genetic alterations in pleomorphic xanthoastrocytoma. *Acta Neuropathol (Berl)* 1996;91:293–297.
89. Fukuoka M, Yano S, Giaccone G, et al. Multi-institutional randomized phase II trial of gefitinib for previously treated patients with advanced non-small-cell lung cancer (the IDEAL 1 Trial). *J Clin Oncol* 2003;21:2237–2246.
90. Kris MG, Natale RB, Herbst RS, et al. Efficacy of gefitinib, an inhibitor of the epidermal growth factor receptor tyrosine kinase, in symptomatic patients with non-small cell lung cancer: a randomized trial. *JAMA* 2003;290:2149–2158.
91. Perez-Soler R, Chachoua A, Hammond L, et al. Determinants of tumor response and survival with erlotinib in patients with non-small cell lung cancer (NSCLC). *J Clin Oncol* 2004;22:3238–3247.
92. Sordella R, Bell DW, Haber DA, et al. Gefitinib-sensitizing *EGFR* mutations in lung cancer activate anti-apoptotic pathways. *Science* 2004;305:1163–1167.
93. Haas-Kogan DA, Prados MD, Tihan T, et al. Epidermal growth factor receptor, protein kinase B/Akt, and glioma response to erlotinib. *J Natl Cancer Inst* 2005;97:880–887.
94. Hegi ME, Diserens AC, Gorlia T, et al. *MGMT* gene silencing and benefit from temozolomide in glioblastoma. *N Engl J Med* 2005;352:997–1003.
95. Fuller CE, Perry A. Pathology of low- and intermediate-grade gliomas. *Semin Rad Oncol* 2001;11:95–102.

96. Shaw EG, Scheithauer BW, O'Fallon JR. Supratentorial gliomas: a comparative study by grade and histologic type. *J Neurooncol* 1997;31:273–278.
97. Cairncross JG, Macdonald DR. Successful chemotherapy for recurrent malignant oligodendroglioma. *Ann Neurol* 1988;23:360–364.
98. Fortin D, Cairncross JG, Hammond RR. Oligodendroglioma: an appraisal of recent data pertaining to diagnosis and treatment. *Neurosurgery* 1999;45:1279–1291.
99. Glass J, Hochberg FH, Gruber ML, et al. The treatment of oligodendrogliomas and mixed oligodendroglioma-astrocytomas with PCV chemotherapy. *J Neurosurg* 1992; 76:741–745.
100. Nigro JM, Takahashi MA, Ginzinger DG, et al. Detection of 1p and 19q loss in oligodendroglioma by quantitative microsatellite analysis, a real-time quantitative polymerase chain reaction assay. *Am J Pathol* 2001;158:1253–1262.
101. Kraus JA, Koopmann J, Kaskel P, et al. Shared allelic losses on chromosomes 1p and 19q suggest a common origin of oligodendroglioma and oligoastrocytoma. *J Neuropathol Exp Neurol* 1995;54:91–95.
102. Perry A. Oligodendroglial neoplasms: current concepts, misconceptions, and folklore. *Adv Anat Pathol* 2001;8:183–199.
103. Perry A, Fuller CE, Banerjee R, et al. Ancillary FISH analysis for 1p and 19q status: preliminary observations in 287 gliomas and oligodendroglioma mimics. *Front Biosci* 2003;8:a1–9.
104. Reifenberger J, Reifenberger G, Liu L, et al. Molecular genetic analysis of oligodendroglial tumors shows preferential allelic deletions on 19q and 1p. *Am J Pathol* 1994; 145:1175–1190.
105. Smith JS, Alderete B, Minn Y, et al. Localization of common deletion regions on 1p and 19q in human gliomas and their association with histological subtype. *Oncogene* 1999;18:4144–4152.
106. Cairncross JG, Ueki K, Zlatescu MC, et al. Specific genetic predictors of chemotherapeutic response and survival in patients with anaplastic oligodendrogliomas. *J Natl Cancer Inst* 1998;90:1473–1479.
107. Smith JS, Perry A, Borell TJ, et al. Alterations of chromosome arms 1p and 19q as predictors of survival in oligodendrogliomas, astrocytomas, and mixed oligoastrocytomas. *J Clin Oncol* 2000;18:636–645.
108. Bauman GS, Ino Y, Ueki K, et al. Allelic loss of chromosome 1p and radiotherapy plus chemotherapy in patients with oligodendrogliomas. *Int J Radiat Oncol Biol Phys* 2000; 48:825–830.
109. Chahlavi A, Kanner A, Peereboom D, et al. Impact of chromosome 1p status in response of oligodendroglioma to temozolomide: preliminary results. *J Neurooncol* 2003;61: 267–273.
110. Ueki K, Nishikawa R, Nakazato Y, et al. Correlation of histology and molecular genetic analysis of 1p, 19q, 10q, TP53, EGFR, CDK4, and CDKN2A in 91 astrocytic and oligodendroglial tumors. *Clin Cancer Res* 2002;8:196–201.
111. Watanabe T, Nakamura M, Kros JM, et al. Phenotype versus genotype correlation in oligodendrogliomas and low-grade diffuse astrocytomas. *Acta Neuropathol (Berl)* 2004; 103:267–275.
112. Sasaki H, Zlatescu MC, Betensky RA, et al. Histopathological-molecular genetic correlations in referral pathologist-diagnosed low-grade "oligodendroglioma." *J Neuropathol Exp Neurol* 2002;61:58–63.
113. van den Bent MJ, Looijenga LHJ, Langenberg K, et al. Chromosomal anomalies in oligodendroglial tumors are correlated with clinical features. *Cancer* 2003;97:1276–1284.
114. Felsberg J, Erkwoh A, Sabel M, et al. Oligodendroglial tumors: refinement of candidate regions on chromosome arm 1p and correlation of 1p/19q status with survival. *Brain Pathol* 2004;14:121–130.
115. Hashimoto N, Murakami M, Takahashi Y, et al. Correlation between genetic alteration and long-term clinical outcome of patients with oligodendroglial tumors, with identification of a consistent region of deletion on chromosome arm 1p. *Cancer* 2003; 97:2254–2261.
116. Ritland SR, Ganju V, Jenkins RB. Region-specific loss of heterozygosity on chromosome 19 is related to the morphologic type of human glioma. *Genes Chromosomes Cancer* 1995;12:277–282.
117. Fuller CE, Schmidt RS, Roth KA, et al. Clinical utility of fluorescence in situ hybridization (FISH) in morphologically ambiguous gliomas with hybrid oligodendroglial/astrocytic features. *J Neuropathol Exp Neurol* 2003;62:1118–1128.
118. Johnson MD, Vnencak-Jones CL, Toms SA, et al. Allelic losses in oligodendroglial and oligodendroglioma-like neoplasms. *Arch Pathol Lab Med* 2003;127:1573–1579.
119. Prayson RA, Castilla EA, Hartke M, et al. Chromosome 1p allelic loss by fluorescence in situ hybridization is not observed in dysembryoplastic neuroepithelial tumors. *Am J Clin Pathol* 2002;118:512–517.
120. Fouladi M, Helton K, Dalton J, et al. Clear cell ependymoma: a clinicopathologic and radiographic analysis of 10 patients. *Cancer* 2003;98:2232–2244.
121. Perry A, Scheithauer BW, Macaulau RJ, et al. Oligodendrogliomas with neurocytic differentiation: a report of 4 cases with diagnostic and histogenetic implications. *J Neuropathol Exp Neurol* 2002;61:947–955.
122. Bello MJ, de Campos JM, Vaquero J, et al. Molecular and cytogenetic analysis of chromosome 9 deletions in 75 malignant gliomas. *Genes Chromosomes Cancer* 1994;9: 33–41.
123. Bigner SH, Matthews MR, Rasheed BK, et al. Molecular genetic aspects of oligodendrogliomas including analysis by comparative genomic hybridization. *Am J Pathol* 1999;155:375–386.
124. Hoang-Xuan K, He J, Huguet S, et al. Molecular heterogeneity of oligodendrogliomas suggests alternative pathways in tumor progression. *Neurology* 2001;57:1278–1281.
125. Sanson M, Leuraud P, Aguirre-Cruz L, et al. Analysis of loss of chromosome 10q, *DMBT1* homozygous deletions and *PTEN* mutations in oligodendrogliomas. *J Neurosurg* 2002;97:1397–1401.
126. Thiessen B, Maguire J, McNeil K, et al. Loss of heterozygosity for loci on chromosome arms 1p and 10q in oligodendroglial tumors: relationship to outcome and chemosensitivity. *J Neurooncol* 2003;64:271–278.
127. Bortolotto S, Chiado-Piat L, Cavalla P, et al. *CDKN2A/p16* inactivation in the prognosis of oligodendrogliomas. *Int J Cancer* 2000;88:554–557.
128. Jeuken JWM, Nelen MR, Vermeer H, et al. *PTEN* mutation analysis in two genetic subtypes of high-grade oligodendroglial tumors: *PTEN* is only occasionally mutated in one of the two genetic subtypes. *Cancer Genet Cytogenet* 2000;119:42–46.
129. Sasaki H, Zlatescu MC, Betensky RA, et al. *PTEN* is a target of chromosome 10q loss in anaplastic oligodendrogliomas and *PTEN* alterations are associated with poor prognosis. *Am J Pathol* 2001;159:359–367.
130. Fallon KB, Palmer CA, Roth KA, et al. Prognostic value of 1p, 19q, 9p, 10q, and EGFR-FISH analyses in recurrent oligodendrogliomas. *J Neuropathol Exp Neurol* 2004; 63:314–322.
131. Raghavan R, Balani J, Perry A, et al. Pediatric oligodendrogliomas: a study of molecular alterations on 1p and 19q using fluorescence in situ hybridization. *J Neuropathol Exp Neurol* 2003;62:530–537.
132. Fuller CE, Dalton J, Fouladi M, et al. Molecular characterization of pediatric oligodendroglial neoplasms: the St. Jude experience. *J Neuropathol Exp Neurol* 2004;63:552.
133. Jeuken JWM, Sprenger SHE, Boerman RH, et al. Subtyping of oligo-astrocytic tumours by comparative genomic hybridization. *J Pathol* 2001;194:81–87.
134. Maintz D, Fiedler K, Koopmann J, et al. Molecular genetic evidence for subtypes of oligoastrocytomas. *J Neuropathol Exp Neurol* 1997;56:1098–1104.
135. Mueller W, Hartmann C, Abbas F, et al. Genetic signature of oligoastrocytomas correlates with tumor location and denotes distinct molecular subsets. *Am J Pathol* 2002; 161:313–319.
136. Dong Z-Q, Pang JC, Tong CY, et al. Clonality of oligoastrocytomas. *Hum Pathol* 2002;33:528–535.
137. Bissola L, Eoli M, Pollo B, et al. Association of chromosome 10 losses and negative prognosis in oligoastrocytomas. *Ann Neuro* 2002;52:842–845.
138. Jenkins RB, Kimmel DW, Moertel CA, et al. A cytogenetic study of 53 human gliomas. *Cancer Genet Cytogenet* 1989;39:253–279.
139. Weremowicz S, Kupsky WJ, Morton CC, et al. Cytogenetic evidence for a chromosome 22 tumor suppressor gene in ependymoma. *Cancer Genet Cytogenet* 1992;61:193–196.
140. Bijlsma EK, Voesten AM, Bijleveld EH, et al. Molecular analysis of genetic changes in ependymomas. *Genes Chromosomes Cancer* 1995;13:272–277.
141. Wernicke C, Thiel G, Lozanova T, et al. Involvement of chromosome 22 in ependymomas. *Cancer Genet Cytogenet* 1995;79:173–176.
142. Zheng PP, Pang JC, Hui AB, et al. Comparative genomic hybridization detects losses of chromosomes 22 and 16 as the most common recurrent genetic alterations in primary ependymomas. *Cancer Genet Cytogenet* 2000;122:18–25.
143. Ward S, Harding B, Wilkins P, et al. Gain of 1q and loss of 22 are the most common changes detected by comparative genomic hybridization in paediatric ependymoma. *Genes Chromosomes Cancer* 2001;32:59–66.
144. Hirose T, Aldape K, Bollen A, et al. Chromosomal abnormalities subdivide ependymal tumors into clinically relevant groups. *Am J Pathol* 2001;158:1137–1143.
145. Jeuken JWM, Sprenger SHE, Gilhuis J, et al. Correlation between localization, age, and chromosomal imbalances in ependymal tumours as detected by CGH. *J Pathol* 2002;197:238–244.
146. Carter M, Nicholson J, Ross F, et al. Genetic abnormalities detected in ependymomas by comparative genomic hybridization. *Br J Cancer* 2002;83:929–939.
147. Birch BD, Johnson JP, Parsa A, et al. Frequent type 2 neurofibromatosis gene transcript mutations in sporadic intramedullary spinal cord ependymomas. *Neurosurgery* 1996; 39:135–140.
148. von Haken MS, White EC, Daneshvar-Shyesther L, et al. Molecular genetic analysis of chromosome arm 17p and chromosome arm 22q DNA sequences in sporadic pediatric ependymomas. *Genes Chromosomes Cancer* 1996;17:37–44.
149. Ebert C, von Haken MS, Meyer-Puttlitz B, et al. Molecular genetic analysis of ependymal tumors: *NF2* mutations and chromosome 22q loss occur preferentially in intramedullary spinal ependymomas. *Am J Pathol* 1999;155:627–632.
150. Rosseau-Merck MF, Versteege I, Zattara-Cannoni H, et al. Fluorescence in situ hybridization determination of 22q12-q13 deletion in two intracerebral ependymomas. *Cancer Genet Cytogenet* 2000;121:223–227.
151. Lamszus K, Lachenmayer LK, Heinemann U, et al. Molecular genetic alterations on chromosomes 11 and 22 in ependymomas. *Int J Cancer* 2001;91:803–808.
152. Singh PK, Gutmann DH, Fuller CE, et al. Differential involvement of protein 4.1 family members DAL-1 and NF2 in intracranial and intraspinal ependymomas. *Mod Pathol* 2002;15:526–531.
153. Tran Y, Benbatoul K, Gorse K, et al. Novel regions of allelic deletion on chromosome 18p in tumors of the lung, brain, and breast. *Oncogene* 1998;17:3499–3505.
154. Tran YK, Bogler O, Gorse K, et al. A novel member of the FN2/ERM/4.1 superfamily with growth suppressing properties in lung cancer. *Cancer Res* 1999;59:35–43.
155. Rajaram V, Gutmann DH, Conboy JG, et al. Deletion testing of protein 4.1 family members by fluorescence in-situ hybridization (FISH) in ependymomas. *J Neuropathol Exp Neurol* 2003;62:545.
156. Reardon DA, Entrekin RE, Sublett J, et al. Chromosome arm 6q loss is the most common recurrent autosomal alteration detected in primary pediatric ependymoma. *Genes Chromosomes Cancer* 1999;24:230–237.
157. Dyer, S Prebble E, Davison V, et al. Genomic imbalances in pediatric intracranial ependymomas define clinically relevant groups. *Am J Pathol* 2002;161:2133–2141.
158. Min K-W, Scheithauer BW. Clear cell ependymoma: a mimic of oligodendroglioma: clinicopathologic and ultrastructural considerations. *Am J Surg Pathol* 1997;21:820–826.
159. Figarella-Branger D, Civatte M, Bouvier-Labit C, et al. Prognostic factors in intracranial ependymomas in children. *J Neurosurg* 2000;93:605–613.
160. Merchant TE, Jenkins JJ, Burger PC, et al. Influence of tumor grade on time to progression after irradiation for localized ependymoma in children. *Int J Radiat Oncol Biol Phys* 2002;53:52–57.
161. Perilongo G, Massimino M, Sotti G, et al. Analyses of prognostic factors in a retrospective review of 92 children with ependymoma: Italian Pediatric Neuro-Oncology Group. *Med Pediatr Oncol* 1997;29:79–85.
162. Teo C Nakaji P, Symons P, et al. Ependymoma. *Child's Nerv Syst* 2003;19:270–285.
163. Schwartz TH, Kim S, Glick RS, et al. Supratentorial ependymomas in adult patients. *Neurosurgery* 1999;44:721–731.
164. Korshunov A, Golanov A, Sycheva R, et al. The histologic grade is a main prognostic factor for patients with intracranial ependymomas treated in the microneurosurgical era: an analysis of 258 patients. *Cancer* 2003;100:1230–1237.
165. Gilbertson R, Bentley L, Hernan R, et al. ERBB receptor signaling promotes ependymoma cell proliferation and represents a potential novel therapeutic target for this disease. *Clin Cancer Res* 2002;8:3054–3064.

166. Burnett ME, White EC, Sih S, et al. Chromosome arm 17p deletion analysis reveals molecular genetic heterogeneity in supratentorial and infratentorial primitive neuroectodermal tumors of the central nervous system. *Cancer Genet Cytogenet* 1997;97:25–31.
167. Russo C, Pellarin M, Tingby O, et al. Comparative genomic hybridization in patients with supratentorial and infratentorial primitive neuroectodermal tumors. *Cancer* 1999; 86:331–339.
168. Nicholson JC, Ross F, Kohler JA, et al. Comparative genomic hybridization and histologic variation in primitive neuroectodermal tumours. *Br J Cancer* 1999;80:1322–1331.
169. Burger PC, Yu IT, Tihan T, et al. Atypical teratoid/rhabdoid tumor of the central nervous system: a highly malignant tumor of infancy and childhood frequently mistaken for medulloblastoma. *Am J Surg Pathol* 1998;22:1083–1092.
170. Rorke LB, Packer RJ, Biegel JA. Central nervous system atypical teratoid/rhabdoid tumors of infancy and childhood: definition of an entity. *J Neurosurg* 1996;85:56–65.
171. Ellison D. Classifying the medulloblastoma: insights from morphology and molecular genetics. *Neuropathol Appl Neurobiol* 2002;28:247–282.
172. Packer RJ, Rood BR, MacDonald TJ. Medulloblastoma: present concepts of stratification into risk groups. *Pediatr Neurosurg* 2003;39:60–67.
173. Eberhart CG, Kratz JE, Wang Y, et al. Histopathological and molecular prognostic markers in medulloblastoma: *c-myc, N-myc, TrkC,* and anaplasia. *J Neuropathol Exp Neurol* 2004;63:441–449.
174. Gajjar A, Hernan R, Kocak M, et al. Clinical, histopathologic, and molecular markers of prognosis: toward a new disease risk stratification system for medulloblastoma. *J Clin Oncol* 2004;22:971–974.
175. Giangaspero F, Rigobello L, Badiali M, et al. Large-cell medulloblastomas: a distinct variant with highly aggressive behavior. *Am J Surg Pathol* 1992;16:687–693.
176. Giangaspero F, Perilongo G, Fondelli MP, et al. Medulloblastoma with extensive nodularity: a variant with favorable prognosis. *J Neurosurg* 1999;91:971–977.
177. Gilbertson R, Wickramasinghe C, Hernan R, et al. Clinical and molecular stratification of disease risk in medulloblastoma. *Br J Cancer* 2001;85:705–712.
178. Brown HG, Kepner JL, Perlman EJ, et al. "Large cell/anaplastic" medulloblastomas: a Pediatric Oncology Group study. *J Neuropathol Exp Neurol* 2000;59:857–865.
179. Taylor MD, Mainprize TG, Rutka J. Molecular insight into medulloblastoma and central nervous system primitive neuroectodermal tumor biology from hereditary syndromes: a review. *Neurosurgery* 2000;47:888–901.
180. Biegel JA, Rorke LB, Packer RJ, et al. Isochromosome 17q in primitive neuroectodermal tumors of the central nervous system. *Genes Chromosomes Cancer* 1989;1:139–147.
181. Bigner SH, Vogelstein B. Cytogenetics and molecular genetics of malignant gliomas and medulloblastoma. *Brain Pathol* 1990;1:12–18.
182. DeChiara C, Borghese A, Fiorillo A, et al. Cytogenetic evaluation of isochromosome 17q in posterior fossa tumors of children and correlation with clinical outcome in medulloblastoma. *Child's Nerv Syst* 2002;18:380–384.
183. Karnes PS, Tran TN, Cui MY, et al. Cytogenetic analysis of 39 pediatric central nervous system tumors. *Cancer Genet Cytogenet* 1992;59:12–19.
184. Nam DH, Wang KC, Kim YM, et al. The effect of isochromosome 17q presence, proliferative and apoptotic indices, expression of c-erbB-2, bcl-2 and p53 proteins on the prognosis of medulloblastoma. *J Korean Med Sci* 2000;15:452–456.
185. Biegel JA, Janss AJ, Raffel C, et al. Prognostic significance of chromosome 17p deletions in childhood primitive neuroectodermal tumors (medulloblastomas) of the central nervous system. *Clin Cancer Res* 1997;3:473–478.
186. Emandian SM, McDonald JD, Gerken SC, et al. Correlation of chromosome 17p loss with clinical outcome in medulloblastoma. *Clin Cancer Res* 1996; 2:1559–1564.
187. Cogen PH. Prognostic significance of molecular genetic markers in childhood brain tumors. *Pediatr Neurosurg* 1991;17:245–250.
188. Batra SK, McLendon RE, Koo JS, et al. Prognostic implications of chromosome 17p deletions in human medulloblastomas. *J Neurooncol* 1995;24:39–45.
189. Jung HL, Wang K-C, Kim S-K, et al. Loss of heterozygosity analysis of chromosome 17p13.1-13.3 and its correlation with clinical outcome in medulloblastomas. *J Neurooncol* 2004;67:41–46.
190. Reardon DA, Michalkiewixz E, Boyett J, et al. Extensive genomic abnormalities in childhood medulloblastoma by comparative genomic hybridization. *Cancer Res* 1997; 57:4042–4047.
191. McDonald JD, Daneshvar L, Willert JR, et al. Physical mapping of chromosome 17p13.3 in the region of a putative tumor suppressor gene important in medulloblastoma. *Genomics* 1994;23:229–232.
192. Scheurlen WG, Seranski P, Mincheva A, et al. High-resolution deletion mapping of chromosome arm 17p in childhood primitive neuroectodermal tumors reveals a common chromosomal disruption within the Smith-Magenis region, an unstable region in chromosome band 17p11.2. *Genes Chromosomes Cancer* 1997;18:50–58.
193. Biegel JA, Burk CD, Barr RG, et al. Evidence for a 17p tumor related locus distinct from *p53* in pediatric primitive neuroectodermal tumors. *Cancer Res* 1992;52:3391–3395.
194. Rood BR, Zhang H, Weitman DM, et al. Hypermethylation of HIC-1 and 17p allelic loss in medulloblastoma. *Cancer Res* 2002;62:3794–3797.
195. Smith JS, Tachibana I, Allen C, et al. Cloning of a human ortholog (RPH3AL) of (RNO)Rph3al from a candidate 17p13.3 medulloblastoma tumor suppressor locus. *Genomics* 1999;59:97–101.
196. Eberhart CG, Kratz JE, Schuster A, et al. Comparative genomic hybridization detects an increased number of chromosomal alterations in large cell/anaplastic medulloblastomas. *Brain Pathol* 2002;12:36–44.
197. Eberhart CG, Kepner JL, Goldthwaite PT, et al. Histopathologic grading of medulloblastomas: a Pediatric Oncology Group study. *Cancer* 2002;94:552–460.
198. Leonard JR, Cai DX, Rivet DJ, et al. Large cell/anaplastic medulloblastomas and medullomyoblastomas: clinicopathological and genetic features. *J Neurosurg* 2001;95:82–88.
199. Scheurlen W, Schwabe GC, Joos S, et al. Molecular analysis of childhood primitive neuroectodermal tumors defines markers associated with poor outcome. *J Clin Oncol* 1998;16:2478–2485.
200. Adesina AM, Nalbantoglu J, Cavenee WK. *p53* gene mutations and *mdm2* gene amplification are uncommon in medulloblastoma. *Cancer Res* 1994;54:5649–5651.
201. Adesina A, Dunn ST, Moore WE, et al. Expression of *p27kip1* and *p53* in medulloblastoma: relationship with cell proliferation and survival. *Pathol Res Pract* 2000;196: 243–250.
202. Jaros E, Lunec J, Perry RH, et al. p53 protein overexpression identifies a group of central primitive neuroectodermal tumours with poor prognosis. *Br J Cancer* 1993; 68:801–807.
203. Gilbertson R, Perry RH, Kelly PJ, et al. Prognostic significance of *HER2* and *HER4* coexpression in childhood medulloblastoma. *Cancer Res* 1997;57:3272–3280.
204. Gilbertson R, Pearson A, Perry R, et al. Prognostic significance of the *c-erbB-2* oncogene product in childhood medulloblastoma. *Br J Cancer* 1995;71:473–477.
205. Herms J, Behnke J, Bergmann M, et al. Potential prognostic value of *c-erbB-2* expression in medulloblastomas in very young children. *J Pediatr Hematol Oncol* 1997;19:510–515.
206. Reardon DA, Jenkins JJ, Sublett J, et al. Multiple genomic alterations including *N-myc* amplification in a primary large cell medulloblastoma. *Pediatr Neurosurg* 2000; 32:187–191.
207. Aldosari N, Bigner SH, Burger PC, et al. *MYCC* and *MYCN* oncogene amplification in medulloblastoma: a fluorescence in situ hybridization study on paraffin sections from the Children's Oncology Group. *Arch Pathol Lab Med* 2003;126:540–544.
208. Badiali M, Pession A, Basso G, et al. N-*myc* and c-*myc* oncogenes amplification in medulloblastomas: evidence of particularly aggressive behavior of a tumor with c-*myc* amplification. *Tumori* 1991;77:118–121.
209. Grotzer MA, Hogarty MD, Janss AJ, et al. *MYC* messenger RNA expression predicts survival outcome in childhood primitive neuroectodermal tumor/medulloblastoma. *Clin Cancer Res* 2001;7:2425–2433.
210. Herms J, Neidt I, Luscher B, et al. *C-myc* expression in medulloblastoma and its prognostic value. *Int J Cancer* 2000;89:395–402.
211. Grotzer MA, Janss AJ, Fung JA, et al. *TrkC* expression predicts good clinical outcome in primitive neuroectodermal brain tumors. *J Clin Oncol* 2000;18:1027–1035.
212. Korshunov A, Savostikova M, Ozerov S. Immunohistochemical markers for prognosis of average-risk pediatric medulloblastomas: the effect of apoptotic index, *TrkC*, and *c-myc* expression. *J Neurooncol* 2002;58:271–279.
213. Yin XL, Pang JC, Liu YH, et al. Analysis of loss of heterozygosity on chromosomes 10q, 11, and 16 in medulloblastomas. *J Neurosurg* 2001;94:799–805.
214. Smith JS, Tachibana I, Passe SM, et al. *PTEN* mutation, *EGFR* amplification and outcome in patients with anaplastic astrocytoma and glioblastoma multiforme. *J Natl Cancer Inst* 2001;93:1246–1256.
215. Mollenhauer J, Wiemann S, Scheurlen W, et al. DMBT1, a new member of the SRCR superfamily, on chromosome 10q25.3–26.1 is deleted in malignant brain tumours. *Nat Genet* 1997;17:32–39.
216. Bambakidis NC, Robinson S, Cohen M, et al. Atypical teratoid/rhabdoid tumors of the central nervous system: clinical, radiographic and pathologic features. *Pediatr Neurosurg* 2002;37:64–70.
217. Packer RJ, Biegel JA, Blaney S, et al. Atypical teratoid/rhabdoid tumor of the central nervous system: report on workshop. *J Pediatr Hematol Oncol* 2002; 24:337–342.
218. Rorke LB, Packer RJ, Biegel JA. Central nervous system atypical teratoid/rhabdoid tumors of infancy and childhood. *J Neurooncol* 1995;24:21–28.
219. Biegel JA, Allen CS, Kawasaki K, et al. Narrowing the critical region for a rhabdoid tumor locus in 22q11. *Genes Chromosomes Cancer* 1996;16:94–105.
220. Sevenet N, Lellouch-Tubiana A, Schofield D, et al. Spectrum of *hSNF5/INI1* somatic mutations in human cancer and genotype-phenotype correlations. *Hum Mol Genet* 1999;8:2359–2368.
221. Fuller CE, Pfeifer J, Humphrey P, et al. Chromosome 22q dosage in composite extrarenal rhabdoid tumors: clonal evolution or a phenotypic mimic? *Hum Pathol* 2001;32:1102–1108.
222. Bruch LA, Hill DA, Cai DX, et al. A role for fluorescence in situ hybridization detection of chromosome 22q dosage in distinguishing atypical teratoid/rhabdoid tumors from medulloblastoma/central primitive neuroectodermal tumors. *Hum Pathol* 2001; 32:156–162.
223. Versteege I, Sevenet N, Lange J, et al. Truncating mutations of *hSNF5/INI1* in aggressive paediatric cancer. *Nature* 1998;394:203–206.
224. Biegel JA, Tan L, Zhang F, et al. Alterations of the *hSNF5/INI1* gene in central nervous system atypical teratoid/rhabdoid tumors and renal and extrarenal rhabdoid tumors. *Clin Cancer Res* 2002;8:3461–3467.
225. Versteege I, Medjkane S, Rouillard D, et al. A key role of the *hSNF5/INI1* tumor suppressor in the control of the G1-S transition of the cell cycle. *Oncogene* 2002; 21:6403–6412.
226. Rousseau-Merck MF, Versteege I, Legrand I, et al. *hSNF5/INI1* inactivation is mainly associated with homozygous deletions and mitotic recombinations in rhabdoid tumors. *Cancer Res* 1999;59:3152–3156.
227. Sevenet N, Sheridan E, Amram D, et al. Constitutional mutations of the *hSNF5/INI1* gene predispose to a variety of cancers. *Am J Hum Genet* 1999;65:1342–1348.
228. Biegel JA, Zhou JY, Rorke LB, et al. Germ-line and acquired mutations of *INI1* in atypical teratoid and rhabdoid tumors. *Cancer Res* 1999;59:74–79.
229. Kraus JA, Oster C, Sorensen N, et al. Human medulloblastomas lack point mutations and homozygous deletions of the *hSNF5/INI1* tumour suppressor gene. *Neuropathol Appl Neurobiol* 2002;28:136–141.
230. Biegel JA, Fogelgren B, Zhou JY, et al. Mutations of the *INI1* rhabdoid tumor suppressor gene in medulloblastomas and primitive neuroectodermal tumors of the central nervous system. *Clin Cancer Res* 2000;6:2759–2763.
231. Weber M, Stockhammer F, Schmitz U, et al. Mutational analysis if *INI1* in sporadic human brain tumors. *Acta Neuropathol (Berl)* 2001;101:479–482.
232. Judkins AR, Mauger J, Rorke LB, et al. Immunohistochemical analysis of *hSNF5/INI1* in pediatric CNS neoplasms. *Am J Surg Pathol* 2004;28:644–650.
233. Hoot AC, Russo P, Judkins AR, et al. Immunohistochemical analysis of *hSNF5/INI1* distinguishes renal and extra-renal malignant rhabdoid tumors from other pediatric soft tissue tumors. *Am J Surg Pathol* 2004;28:1485–1491.
234. Perry A, Fuller CE, Judkins AR, et al. *INI1* expression is retained in composite rhabdoid tumors, including rhabdoid meningiomas. *Mod Pathol* 2005;18:951–958.
235. Perry A, Stafford SL, Scheithauer BW, et al. Meningioma grading: an analysis of histologic parameters. *Am J Surg Pathol* 1997;21:1455–1465.
236. Perry A, Scheithauer BW, Stafford SL, et al. "Malignancy" in meningiomas: a clinicopathologic study of 116 patients, with grading implications. *Cancer* 1999;85: 2046–2056.

237. Perry A, Cai DX, Scheithauer BW, et al. Merlin, DAL-1, and progesterone receptor expression in clinicopathologic subsets of meningioma: a correlative immunohisto-chemical study of 175 cases. *J Neuropathol Exp Neurol* 2000;59:872–879.

238. Lanzafame S, Torrisi A, Barbagallo G, et al. Correlation between histologic grade, MIB-1, p53, and recurrence in 69 completely resected primary intracranial menin-giomas with a 6 year mean follow-up. *Pathol Res Pract* 2000;196:483–488.

239. Leuraud P, Dezamis E, Aguirre-Cruz L, et al. Prognostic value of allelic losses and telom-erase activity in meningiomas. *J Neurosurg* 2004;100:303–309.

240. Perry A, Gutmann DH, Reifenberger G. Molecular pathogenesis of meningiomas. *J Neurooncol* 2004;70:183–202.

241. Perry A, Giannini C, Raghavan R, et al. Aggressive phenotypic and genotypic features in pediatric and NF2-associated meningiomas: a clinocopathologic study of 53 cases. *J Neuropathol Exp Neurol* 2001;60:994–1003.

242. Ruttledge MH, Sarrazin J, Rangaratnam S, et al. Evidence for the complete inactivation of the *NF2* gene in the majority of sporadic meningiomas. *Nat Genet* 1994;6:180–184.

243. Ueki K, Wen-Bin C, Narita Y, et al. Tight association of loss of Merlin expression with loss of heterozygosity at chromosome 22q in sporadic meningiomas. *Cancer Res* 1999;59:5995–5998.

244. Lamszus K, Vahldiek F, Mautner VF, et al. Allelic losses in neurofibromatosis 2-associated meningiomas. *J Neuropathol Exp Neurol* 2000;59:504–512.

245. Gutmann DH, Giovannini M, Fishback AS, et al. Loss of Merlin expression in sporadic meningiomas, ependymomas, and schwannomas. *Neurology* 1997;49:267–270.

246. Gutmann DH, Hirbe A, Huang ZY, et al. The protein 4.1 tumor suppressor, DAL-1, impairs cell motility, but regulates proliferation in a cell-type-specific fashion. *Neurobiol Dis* 2001;8:266–278.

247. Robb VA, Li W, Gascard P, et al. Identification of a third protein 4.1 tumor suppressor, protein 4.1R, in meningioma pathogenesis. *Neurobiol Dis* 2003;13:191–202.

248. Gutmann DH, Donahoe J, Perry A, et al. Loss of DAL-1, a protein 4.1-related tumor suppressor, is an important early event in the pathogenesis of meningiomas. *Hum Mol Genet* 2000;9:1495–1500.

249. Surace EI, Lusis E, Murakami Y, et al. Loss of tumor suppressor in lung cancer-1 (TSLC1) expression in meningioma correlates with increased malignancy grade and reduced patient survival. *J Neuropathol Exp Neurol* 2004;63:1015–1027.

250. Cai DX, Banerjee R, Scheithauer BW, et al. Chromosome 1p and 14 q FISH analysis in clinicopathologic subsets of meningioma: diagnostic and prognostic implications. *J Neuropathol Exp Neurol* 2001;60:628–636.

251. Weber RG, Bostrom J, Wolters M, et al. Analysis of genomic alterations in benign, atyp-ical, and anaplastic meningiomas: towards a genetic model of meningioma progres-sion. *Proc Natl Acad Sci USA* 1997;94:14719–14725.

252. Bostrom J, Meyer-Puttlitz B, Wolter M, et al. Alterations of the tumor suppressor genes *CDKN2A (p16^{INK4a})*, *p14^{ARF}*, *CDKN2B (p15^{INK4b})*, and *CDKN2C (p18^{INK4c})* in atypical and anaplastic meningiomas. *Am J Pathol* 2001;159:661–669.

253. Maillo A, Orfao A, Sayagues JM, et al. New classification scheme for the prognostic strat-ification of meningioma on the basis of chromosome 14 abnormalities, patient age, and tumor histopathology. *J Clin Oncol* 2003;21:3285–3295.

254. Tse JY, Ng HK, Lau KM, et al. Loss of heterozygosity of chromosome 14q in low-and high-grade meningiomas. *Hum Pathol* 1997;28:779–785.

255. Arslantas A, Artan S, Oner U, et al. comparative genomic hybridization analysis of genomic alterations in benign, atypical, and anaplastic meningiomas. *Acta Neurol Belg* 2002;102:53–62.

256. Lopez-Gines C, Cerda-Nicolas M, Gil-Benso R, et al. Association of loss of 1p and alter-ations of chromosome 14 in meningioma progression. *Cancer Genet Cytogenet* 2004; 148:123–128.

257. Murakami M, Hashimoto N, Takahashi Y, et al. A consistent region of deletion on 1p36 in meningiomas: identification and relation to malignant progression. *Cancer Genet Cytogenet* 2003;140:99–106.

258. Lusis EA, Watson MA, Chicoine MR, et al. Integrative genomic analysis identifies *NDRG2* as a candidate tumor suppressor gene frequently inactivated in clinically aggressive meningioma. *Cancer Res* 2005;65:7121–7126.

259. Rajaram V, Brat D, Perry A. Anaplastic meningioma vs. meningeal hemangiopericy-toma: immunohistochemical and genetic markers. *Hum Pathol* 2004;35:1413–1418.

260. Simon M, Park T-W, Koster G, et al. Alterations of *INK4a^{p16-p14/ARF}* /*INK4b^{p15}* expression and telomerase activation in meningioma progression. *J Neurooncol* 2001;55:149–158.

261. Perry A, Banerjee R, Lohse CM, et al. A role for chromosome 9p21 deletions in the malignant progression of meningiomas and the prognosis of anaplastic meningiomas. *Brain Pathol* 2002;12:183–190.

262. Cai DX, James CD, Scheithauer BW, et al. *PS6K* amplification characterizes a small sub-set of anaplastic meningiomas. *Am J Clin Pathol* 2001;115:213–218.

263. Buschges R, Ichimura K, Weber RG, et al. Allelic gain and amplification on the long arm of chromosome 17 in anaplastic meningiomas. *Brain Pathol* 2002;12:145–153.

264. Surace EI, Lusis E, Haipek CA, et al. Functional significance of *S6K* overexpression in meningioma progression. *Ann Neurol* 2004;56:295–298.

265. Mihaila D, Jankowski M, Gutierrez JA, et al. Meningiomas: loss of heterozygosity on chromosome 10 and marker-specific correlations with grade, recurrence, and survival. *Clin Cancer Res* 2003;9:4443–4451.

266. McKhann G, Drachman D, Folstein M, et al. Clinical diagnosis of Alzheimer's disease: report of the NINCDS-ADRDA Work Group under the auspices of Department of Health and Human Services Task Force on Alzheimer's Disease. *Neurol* 1984; 34:939–944.

267. Morris JC. Dementia update 2003. *Alzheimer Dis Assoc Disord* 2003;17:245–258.

268. Jorm AF, Korten AE, Henderson AS. The prevalence of dementia: a quantitative integra-tion of the literature. *Acta Psychiatr Scand* 1987;76:465–479.

269. Duyckaerts C, Dickson DW. Neuropathology of Alzheimer's disease. In: Dickson DW, ed. *Neurodegeneration: The Molecular Pathology of Dementia and Movement Disorders.* Basel, Switzerland: ISN Neuropath Press; 2003:47–65.

270. Wilquet V, De Strooper B. Amyloid-beta precursor protein processing in neurodegener-ation. *Curr Opin Neurobiol* 2004;14:582–588.

271. Binder LI, Guillozet-Bongaarts AL, Garcia-Sierra F, et al. Tau, tangles, and Alzheimer's disease. *Biochem Biophys Acta* 2005;1739:216–223.

272. Stoothoff WH, Johnson GV. Tau phosphorylation: physiological and pathological con-sequences. *Biochim Biophys Acta* 2005;1739:280–297.

273. Ho L, Sharma N, Blackman L, et al. From proteomics to biomarker discovery in Alzheimer's disease. *Brain Res Brain Res Rev* 2005;48:360–369.

274. Andreasen N, Minthon L, Clarberg A, et al. Sensitivity, specificity and stability of CSF t-tau in AD in a community-based patient sample. *Neurol* 1999;53:1488–1494.

275. Blennow K, Hampel H. CSF markers for incipient Alzheimer's disease. *Lancet Neurol* 2003;2:605–613.

276. Andreasen N, Blennow K. CSF biomarkers for mild cognitive impairment and early Alzheimer's disease. *Clin Neurol Neurosurg* 2005;107:165–173.

277. Klunk WE, Engler H, Nordberg A, et al. Imaging brain amyloid in Alzheimer's disease with Pittsburgh Compound-B. *Ann Neurol* 2004;55:306–319.

278. Hintersteiner M, Enz A, Frey P, et al. In vivo detection of amyloid-beta deposits by near-infrared imaging using an oxazine-derivative probe. *Nat Biotechnol* 2005;23:577–583.

279. Higuchi M, Iwata N, Matsuba Y, et al. 19F and 1H MRI detection of amyloid beta plaques in vivo. *Nat Neurosci* 2005;8:527–533.

280. Lazarov O, Robinson J, Tang YP, et al. Environmental enrichment reduces A beta levels and amyloid deposition in transgenic mice. *Cell* 2005;120:701–713.

281. Spires TL, Hannan AJ. Nature, nurture and neurology: gene-environment interactions in neurodegenerative disease. FEBS Anniversary Prize Lecture delivered on 27 June 2005. *FEBS J* 2005;272:2347–2361.

282. St George-Hyslop PH, Petit A. Molecular biology and genetics of Alzheimer's disease. *C R Biol* 2005;328:119–130.

283. Sherrington R, Rogaev EI, Liang Y, et al. Cloning of a gene bearing mis-sense mutations in early-onset familial Alzheimer's disease. *Nature* 1995;375:754–760.

284. Levy-Lahad E, Wasco W, Poorkaj P, et al. Candidate gene for the chromosome 1 famil-ial Alzheimer's disease locus. *Science* 1995;269:973–977.

285. Goate A, Chartier-Harlin MC, Mullan M, et al. Segregation of a missense mutation in the amyloid precursor protein gene with familial Alzheimer's disease. *Nature* 1991; 349:704–706.

286. Corder EH, Saunders AM, Strittmatter WJ, et al. Gene dose of apolipoprotein E type 4 allele and the risk of Alzheimer's disease in late onset families. *Science* 1993; 261:921–923.

287. O'Hara R, Yesavage JA, Kraemer HC. The apoE epsilon4 allele is associated with decline on delayed recall performance in community-dwelling older adults. *J Am Geriatr Soc* 1998;46:1493–1498.

288. Hirono N, Hashimoto M, Yasuda M. Accelerated memory decline in Alzheimer's disease with apolipoprotein epsilon4 allele. *J Neuropsych. Clin Neurosci* 2003;15:354–358.

289. Devanand DP, Pelton GH, Zamora D, et al. Predictive utility of apolipoprotein E geno-type for Alzheimer disease in outpatients with mild cognitive impairment. *Arch Neurol* 2005;62:975–980.

290. McConnell LM, Koenig BA, Greely HT, et al. Genetic testing and Alzheimer disease: recommendations of the Stanford Program. *Genet Test* 1999;3:3–12.

291. Twelves D, Perkins KS, Counsell C. Systematic review of incidence studies of Parkinson's disease. *Mov Disord* 2003;18:19–31.

292. Widnell K. Pathophysiology of motor fluctuation in Parkinson's disease. *Mov Disord* 2005;20:S17–S22.

293. Jellinger KA, Mizuno Y. Parkinson's disease. In: Dickson DW, ed. *Neurodegeneration: The Molecular Pathology of Dementia and Movement Disorders.* Basel, Switzerland: ISN Neuropath Press; 2003:159–187.

294. Spillantini MG, Schmidt ML, Lee VM, et al. Alpha-synuclein in Lewy bodies. *Nature* 1997;388:839–840.

295. Baba M, Nakajo S, Tu PH, et al. Aggregation of alpha-synuclein in Lewy bodies of spo-radic Parkinson's disease and dementia with Lewy bodies. *Am J Pathol* 1998; 152:879–884.

296. Tu PH, Galvin JE, Baba M, et al. Glial cytoplasmic inclusions in white matter oligoden-drocytes of multiple system atrophy brains contain insoluble alpha-synuclein. *Ann Neurol* 1998;44:415–22.

297. Calne D. A definition of Parkinson's disease. *Parkinsonism Relat Disord* 2005;11:S39–S40.

298. McInerney-Leo A, Hadley DW, Gwinn-Hardy K, et al. Genetic testing in Parkinson's dis-ease. *Mov Disord* 2005;20:1–10.

299. Polymeropoulos MH, Lavedan C, Leroy E, et al. Mutation in the alpha-synuclein gene identified in families with Parkinson's disease. *Science* 1997;276:2045–2047.

300. Kitada T, Asakawa S, Hattori N, et al. Mutations in the parkin gene cause autosomal recessive juvenile parkinsonism. *Nature* 1998;392:605–608.

301. Leroy E, Boyer R, Auburger G, et al. The ubiquitin pathway in Parkinson's disease [Letter]. *Nature* 1998;395:451–452.

302. Kruger R, Fischer C, Schulte T, et al. Mutation analysis of the neurofilament M gene in Parkinson's disease. *Neurosci Lett* 2003;351:125–129.

303. Bonifati V, Rizzu P, van Baren MJ, et al. Mutations in the *DJ-1* gene associated with auto-somal recessive early-onset parkinsonism. *Science* 2003;299:256–259.

304. Valente EM, Abou-Sleiman PM, Caputo V, et al. Hereditary early-onset Parkinson's dis-ease caused by mutations in *PINK1*. *Science* 2004;304:1158–1160.

305. Paisan-Ruiz C, Jain S, Evans EW, et al. Cloning of the gene containing mutations that cause *PARK8*-linked Parkinson's disease. *Neuron* 2004;44:595–600.

306. Hayashi S, Wakabayashi K, Ishikawa A, et al. An autopsy case of autosomal-recessive juvenile parkinsonism with a homozygous exon 4 deletion on the parkin gene. *Mov Disord* 2000;15:884–888.

307. Aasly JO, Toft M, Fernandez-Mata I, et al. Clinical features of *LRRK2*-associated Parkinson's disease in central Norway. *Ann Neurol* 2005;57:762–765.

308. Funayama M, Hasegawa K, Ohta E, et al. An *LRRK2* mutation as a cause for the parkin-sonism in the original *PARK8* family. *Ann Neurol* 2005;57:918–921.

309. Kachergus J, Mata IF, Hulihan M, et al. Identification of a novel *LRRK2* mutation linked to autosomal dominant parkinsonism: evidence of a common founder across European populations. *Am J Hum Genet* 2005;76:672–680.

310. Swash M, Desai J. Motor neuron disease: classification and nomenclature. *Amyotroph Lateral Scler Other Motor Neuron Disord* 2000;1:105–112.

311. Jackson CE, Bryan WW. Amyotrophic lateral sclerosis. *Semin Neurol* 1998;18:27–39.

312. Traynor BJ, Codd MB, Corr B, et al. Incidence and prevalence of ALS in Ireland, 1995–1997: a population-based study. *Neurol* 1999;52:504–509.

313. Hadano W, Nichol K, Brinkman RR, et al. A yeast artificial chromosome-based physical map of the juvenile amyotrophic lateral sclerosis (ALS2) critical region on human chro-mosome 2q33-q34. *Genomics* 1999;55:106–112.

314. Veldink JH, Van den Berg LH, Wokke JH. The future of motor neuron disease: the challenge is in the genes. *J Neurol* 2004;251:491–500.

315. Pearn JH, Gardner-Medwin D, Wilson J. A clinical study of chronic childhood spinal muscular atrophy: a review of 141 cases. *J Neurol Sci* 1978;38:23–37.

316. Mostacciuolo ML, Danieli GA, Trevisan C, et al. Epidemiology of spinal muscular atrophies in a sample of the Italian population. *Neuroepidemiology* 1992;11:34–38.

317. Wicklund MP. Amyotrophic lateral sclerosis: possible role of environmental influences. *Neurol Clin* 2005;23:461–484.

318. Rosen DR Siddique T, Patterson D, et al. Mutations in Cu/Zn superoxide dismutase gene are associated with familial amyotrophic lateral sclerosis. *Nature* 1994;362:59–62.

319. Bruijn LI, Houseweart MK, Kato S, et al. Aggregation and motor neuron toxicity of an ALS-linked *SOD1* mutant independent from wild-type *SOD1*. *Science* 1998; 281:1851–1854.

320. Al-Chalabi A, Andersen PM, Nilsson P, et al. Deletions of the heavy neurofilament subunit tail in amyotrophic lateral sclerosis. *Hum Mol Genet* 1999;8:157–164.

321. Hadano S, Hand CK, Osuga H, et al. A gene encoding a putative GTPase regulator is mutated in familial amyotrophic lateral sclerosis 2. *Nat Genet* 2001;29:166–173.

322. Yang Y, Hentati A, Deng HX, et al. The gene encoding alsin, a protein with three guanine-nucleotide exchange factor domains, is mutated in a form of recessive amyotrophic lateral sclerosis. *Nat Genet* 2001;29:160–165.

323. Munch C, Sedlmeier R, Meyer T, et al. Point mutations of the *p150* subunit of dynactin (*DCTN1*) gene in ALS. *Neurol* 2004;63:724–726.

324. Chen YZ, Bennett CL, Huynh HM, et al. DNA/RNA helicase gene mutations in a form of juvenile amyotrophic lateral sclerosis (ALS4). *Am J Hum Genet* 2004;74:1128–1135.

325. Gros-Louis F, Lariviere R, Gowing G, et al. A frameshift deletion in peripherin gene associated with amyotrophic lateral sclerosis. *J Biol Chem* 2004;279:45951–45956.

326. Lefebvre S, Burglen L, Reboullet S, et al. Identification and characterization of a spinal muscular atrophy-determining gene. *Cell* 1995;80:155–165.

327. Samilchuk E, D'Souza B, Bastaki L. Deletion analysis of the *SMN* and *NAIP* genes in Kuwaiti patients with spinal muscular atrophy. *Hum Genet* 1996;98:524–527.

328. Roy N, Mahadevan MS, McLean M, et al. The gene for neuronal apoptosis inhibitory protein is partially deleted in individuals with spinal muscular atrophy. *Cell* 1995; 80:167–178.

329. Hahnen E, Schonling J, Rudnik-Schoneborn S, et al. Hybrid survival motor neuron genes in patients with autosomal recessive spinal muscular atrophy: new insights into molecular mechanisms responsible for the disease. *Am J Hum Genet* 1996; 59:1057–1065.

330. Everett CM, Wood NW. Trinucleotide repeats and neurodegenerative disease. *Brain* 2004;27:2385–2405.

331. Grove M, Vonsattel JP, Mazzoni P, et al. Huntington's disease. *Sci Aging Knowledge Environ* 2003;43:dn3.

332. Koeppen AH. The pathogenesis of spinocerebellar ataxia. *Cerebellum* 2005;4:62–73.

333. Radstake TR, Barrera P, Albers MJ, et al. Genetic anticipation in rheumatoid arthritis in Europe. European Consortium on Rheumatoid Arthritis Families. *J Rheumatol* 2001;28:962–967.

334. Polito JM 2nd, Rees RC, Childs B, et al. Preliminary evidence for genetic anticipation in Crohn's disease. *Lancet* 1996;347:798–800.

335. Brix TH, Petersen HC, Iachine I, et al. Preliminary evidence of genetic anticipation in Graves' disease. *Thyroid* 2003;13:447–451.

336. Yaturu S, Bridges JF, Dhanireddy RR. Preliminary evidence of genetic anticipation in type 2 diabetes mellitus. *Med Sci Monit* 2005;11:CR262–CR265.

337. Saleem Q, Dash D, Gandhi C, et al. Association of CAG repeat loci on chromosome 22 with schizophrenia and bipolar disorder. *Mol Psychiatry* 2001;6:694–700.

338. Wells RD, Dere R, Hebert ML, et al. Advances in mechanisms of genetic instability related to hereditary neurological diseases. *Nucl Acids Res* 2005;33:3785–3798.

339. McDonald ME, Ambrose CM, Duyao MP, et al. A novel gene containing a trinucleotide repeat that is expanded and unstable on Huntington's disease chromosomes. *Cell* 1993;72:971–983.

340. Orr HT, Chung M, Banfi S, et al. Expansion of an unstable trinucleotide CAG repeat in spinocerebellar ataxia type 1. *Nature Genet* 1993;4:221–226.

341. Pulst SM, Nechiporuk A, Nechiporuk T, et al. Moderate expansion of a normally biallelic trinucleotide repeat in spinocerebellar ataxia type 2. *Nature Genet* 1996; 14:269–276.

342. Kawaguchi Y, Okamoto T, Taniwaki M, et al. CAG expansions in a novel gene for Machado-Joseph disease at chromosome 14q32.1. *Nature Genet* 1994;8:221–228.

343. Zhuchenko O, Bailey J, Bonnen P, et al. Autosomal dominant cerebellar ataxia (SCA6) associated with small polyglutamine expansions in the alpha(1A)-voltage-dependent calcium channel. *Nature Genet* 1997;15:62–69.

344. David G, Abbas N, Stevanin G, et al. Cloning of the *SCA7* gene reveals a highly unstable CAG repeat expansion. *Nature Genet* 1997;17:65–70.

345. Holmes SE, O'Hearn EE, McInnis MG, et al. Expansion of a novel CAG trinucleotide repeat in the 5-prime region of PPP2R2B is associated with *SCA12* [Letter]. *Nature Genet* 1999;23:391–392.

346. Nakamura K, Jeong SY, Uchihara T, et al. SCA17, a novel autosomal dominant cerebellar ataxia caused by an expanded polyglutamine in TATA-binding protein. *Hum Mol Genet* 2001;10:1441–1448.

347. Koide R, Ikeuchi T, Onodera O, et al. Unstable expansion of CAG repeat in hereditary dentatorubral-pallidoluysian atrophy. *Nature Genet* 1994;6:9–13.

348. Campuzano V, Montermini L, Molto MD, et al. Friedreich's ataxia: autosomal recessive disease caused by an intronic GAA triplet repeat expansion. *Science* 1996;271: 1423–1427.

349. Campuzano V, Montermini L, Lutz Y, et al. Frataxin is reduced in Friedreich ataxia patients and is associated with mitochondrial membranes. *Hum Mol Genet* 1997; 6:1771–1780.

350. Koob MD, Moseley ML, Schut LJ, et al. An untranslated CTG expansion causes a novel form of spinocerebellar ataxia (SCA8). *Nature Genet* 1999;21:379–384.

351. Holmes SE, O'Hearn E, Rosenblatt A, et al. A repeat expansion in the gene encoding junctophilin-3 is associated with Huntington disease-like 2. *Nature Genet* 2001;29:377–378.

352. Amiel J, Trochet D, Clement-Ziza M, et al. Polyalanine expansions in human. *Hum Mol Genet* 2004;13:R235–R243.

353. Matsuura T, Yamagata T, Burgess DL, et al. Large expansion of the ATTCT pentanucleotide repeat in spinocerebellar ataxia type 10. *Nature Genet* 2000;26:191–194.

354. Davies SW, Turmaine M, Cozens BA, et al. Formation of neuronal intranuclear inclusions underlies the neurological dysfunction in mice transgenic for the HD mutation. *Cell* 1997;90:537–548.

355. Yamada M, Tsuji S, Takahashi H. Pathology of CAG repeat diseases. *Neuropathology* 2000;20:319–325.

356. Zhang X, Smith DL, Meriin AB, et al. A potent small molecule inhibits polyglutamine aggregation in Huntington's disease neurons and suppresses neurodegeneration in vivo. *Proc Natl Acad Sci USA* 2005;102:892–897.

357. Galvao R, Mendes-Soares L, Camara J, et al. Triplet repeats, RNA secondary structure and toxic gain-of-function models for pathogenesis. *Brain Res Bull* 2001;56:191–201.

358. Szebenyi G, Morfini GA, Babcock A, et al. Neuropathogenic forms of huntingtin and androgen receptor inhibit fast axonal transport. *Neuron* 2003;40:41–52.

359. Potter NT, Spector EB, Prior TW. Technical standards and guidelines for Huntington disease testing. *Genet Med* 2004;6:61–65.

Gastrointestinal Tract

ADENOCARCINOMA

Large Intestine

In the United States, colorectal adenocarcinoma is the fourth leading cause of cancer death (1). There are approximately 150,000 new cases per year, roughly equally distributed between women and men; in the general population, the lifetime risk of colorectal adenocarcinoma is about 5%. About 75% of cases are sporadic, about 5% to 10% occur in the setting of a well-defined hereditary colorectal cancer syndrome (Table 15.1), and about 20% are familial (defined as occurring in patients who have two or more first- or second-degree relatives with colorectal cancer without an identified hereditary syndrome) (2–4).

Genetics

The familiar model proposed by Vogelstein et al. (5,6) describes the process of colorectal tumor evolution as the sequential acquisition of mutations at a number of different

TABLE 15.1

GENETIC SYNDROMES ASSOCIATED WITH AN INCREASED RISK OF COLORECTAL ADENOCARCINOMA

Syndrome	Gene	Mode of Inheritance	Function of Gene Product
Familial adenomatous polyposis (FAP)	APC	Autosomal dominant	Transcriptional control
Multiple adenomatous polyposis	MYH	Autosomal recessive	Repair of oxidative DNA damage
Hereditary nonpolyposis colorectal cancer (HNPCC)	MSH2, MLHI, and others (see Table 15.4)	Autosomal dominant	DNA mismatch repair
Familial colorectal cancer type X	Unknown	Unknown	
Juvenile polyposis	SMAD4/DPC4	Autosomal dominant	TGFβ signaling
Cowden	PTEN	Autosomal dominant	Phosphatase
Li-Fraumeni	TP53	Autosomal dominant	Control of apoptosis
Familial breast cancer	BRCA1	Autosomal dominant	DNA damage repair; others?
Peutz-Jeghers	LKB1/STK11	Autosomal dominant	Serine/threonine kinase

loci (Fig. 15.1). An initial mutation in a single cell generates a clone of cells with a selective growth advantage; within this clone, a single cell acquires an additional mutation that provides a further growth advantage, and so on, until a fully developed invasive adenocarcinoma emerges. Even in syndromes in which there is an inherited predisposition to colorectal adenocarcinoma, tumorigenesis still requires somatic mutations in the same dozen or so genes. Alterations of APC

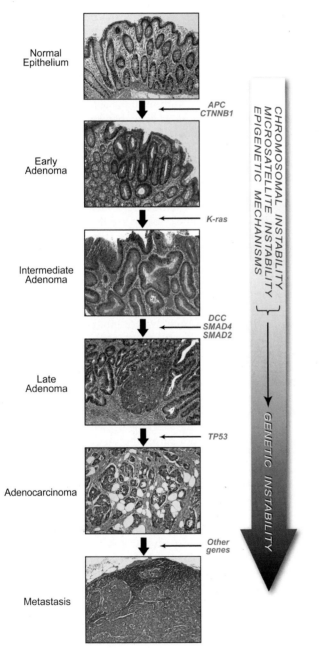

Figure 15.1 The genetic model for the molecular pathogenesis of colorectal adenocarcinoma. The left side of the diagram emphasizes the role of genes in which mutations or epigenetic modifications are known to contribute directly to tumorigenesis (from references 2, 5, 6). The right side of the diagram emphasizes the indirect role of three general pathways of genetic instability in the development of the genetic aberrations that underlie tumorigenesis.

(present in over 80% of sporadic colorectal adenocarcinomas) are an early event in the formation of adenomas. Progression to a fully malignant tumor occurs via mutations in other genes, most importantly the K-ras oncogene (present in about 50% of colorectal adenocarcinomas), the tumor suppressor gene TP53 (inactivated in at least 85% of tumors), and the tumor suppressor genes DCC, SMAD2, and SMAD4 (all three are located on chromosome 18q, and a mutation in at least one of them is present in over 40% of adenocarcinomas, mutations of SMAD4 being the most frequent).

Several features of the model are important because they have implications for molecular genetic analysis of colorectal neoplasms. First, the range of mutations is extremely variable, and so every tumor does not harbor the same mutations in the same set of genes. Although mutations in APC, K-ras, TP53, and the 18q tumor suppressor genes are the most common, alterations of other genes can substitute in the tumorigenic pathway, including PTEN, CTNNB1 (encodes β-catenin), HER2/neu, MYC, and SRC (7–11). For example, because the protein encoded by the APC gene is responsible for inhibition of β-catenin–mediated transcription of growth promoting genes, β-catenin mutations can substitute for mutations in APC (12). Second, different tumors accumulate mutations in a different sequence. Nonetheless, the sequence in which mutations are acquired can have a significant impact on tumorigenesis, as shown by the fact that patients with germline mutations in TP53 do not develop colonic polyposis even though TP53 mutations are present in 85% of colorectal adenocarcinomas (2,5,6).

At a mechanistic level, three different pathways are responsible for the genetic aberrations that underlie tumorigenesis. The first and most frequent mechanism (present in about 85% of colorectal adenocarcinomas) is the chromosomal-instability pathway or characterized by widespread loss of heterozygosity (LOH), chromosomal amplifications, and translocations (13–15). The genetic loci responsible for the generalized chromosomal instability are not well characterized, but mutations in the CDC4 gene involved in the execution of metaphase may be important (16,17).

The second mechanism involves frame shift mutations and base pair (bp) substitutions characteristic of the type of alterations that result from defective DNA mismatch repair (Chapter 2), without aneuploidy and other gross structural aberrations. This pattern of mutagenesis, referred to as the microsatellite-instability phenotype, is characteristic of hereditary nonpolyposis colon cancer and also underlies about 15% of sporadic colorectal adenocarcinomas (13,15,18). In these tumors, mismatch repair genes are inactivated by mutations (most often MSH2 or MLH1, but sometimes MSH6, MSH3, PMS1, or PMS2) or show markedly decreased expression resulting from methylation of their promoter sequences (19,20). Defective mismatch repair facilitates malignant transformation by allowing mutations to accumulate in genes with critical cellular functions (21,22), and, not unexpectedly, genes that harbor coding microsatellites are frequently mutated. For example, approximately 35% of tumors with defective mismatch repair contain mutations in the BAX gene (involved in control of apoptosis), which has a $(G)_8$ microsatellite within its coding region (23,24). Similarly, many tumors with defective mismatch repair harbor frame shift mutations in the TGFβRII gene (which encodes the tumor suppressor transforming growth factor β receptor II) that contains an $(A)_{10}$ repeat (25) or *IGFIIR* (which encodes the insulin-like growth factor II receptor) that contains a $(G)_8$ repeat (26). Even other mismatch repair genes themselves, specifically *MSH6*, *PMS1*, and *PMS2*, often harbor frame shift mutations.

The third pathway responsible for the genetic aberrations that underlie tumorigenesis involves epigenetic mechanisms, primarily alterations in the pattern of methylation at CpG islands (Chapter 1). The altered methylation alters the expression of many of the genes involved in malignant transformation, including cell cycle control genes, DNA repair genes, and mismatch-repair genes (27–29).

Familial Adenomatous Polyposis

Mutations in the *APC* gene are responsible for the autosomal dominant familial adenomatous polyposis (FAP) inherited cancer syndrome, which accounts for about 1% of colorectal adenocarcinomas overall. Patients with FAP develop thousands of adenomas and have a lifetime risk of almost 100% of developing adenocarcinoma unless treated by prophylactic colectomy (30). Although FAP has an autosomal dominant pattern of inheritance, 10% to 30% of mutations arise de novo (2,30). Intragenic *APC* mutations, the vast majority of which are predicted to result in truncation of the APC protein, are present in about 80% of FAP kindreds (31). Most of the remaining kindreds harbor deletions or mutations that reduce gene expression (32), although kindreds with disease resulting from chromosome rearrangements have also been described (33). As is shown in Figure 15.2, both the colonic and extracolonic manifestations of disease (which include congenital hypertrophy of the retinal pigment epithelium [CHRPE] and Gardner's syndrome [colonic polyps, epidermoid skin cysts, benign osteomas of the mandible and long bones, desmoid tumors, and

hepatoblastoma]) vary with the position of the truncating mutation (34–39). It is interesting to note that a missense mutation of *APC* (specifically, I1307K) is associated with a 1.5- to 2-fold increased risk of colorectal adenocarcinoma through a novel genetic mechanism; the mutation does not directly affect function of the APC protein, but instead functions as a premutation that predisposes the adjacent regions of the gene to somatic mutations (40).

Multiple Adenomatous Polyposis

Classic FAP is traditionally defined as greater than 100 colonic polyps; the pattern of disease referred to as multiple colorectal adenomas is usually defined as 15 to 100 adenomas. About 5% to 10% of patients with multiple colorectal adenomas actually represent cases of attenuated FAP that result from a specific pattern of truncating *APC* mutations (Fig. 15.2).

However, it has recently become clear that perhaps as many as 30% of patients with multiple colorectal adenomas harbor mutations in the *MYH* gene that is involved in repair of oxidative DNA damage (41–44). Multiple adenomatous polyposis caused by biallelic inactivation of the *MYH* gene has an autosomal recessive pattern of inheritance, and the underlying missense mutations seem to differ among ethnic groups (41–43). As expected, the pattern of *APC* mutations in patients with biallelic germline *MYH* mutations is primarily a transversion of a guanine:cytosine to a thymine:adenine bp (G:C→T:A), a pattern that results from replication of DNA templates containing 8-oxodeoxyguanine mispairs (Chapter 2).

Hereditary Nonpolyposis Colorectal Cancer

Hereditary nonpolyposis colorectal cancer (HNPCC), also known as Lynch syndrome, was originally defined based on clinical and pedigree criteria (45,46), the most recent versions of which are presented in Tables 15.2 and 15.3. Because there are ethnic differences in the pattern of mutations, different diagnostic guidelines have been developed for patients from Japan, Korea, and China (47).

Mutations in DNA mismatch repair genes are present in 5% to 80% of families that meet the Bethesda or Amsterdam criteria, although it is not surprising that differences in the criteria used to define HNPCC are associated with differences in the prevalence of underlying mismatch repair gene mutations (47–49). Genetic heterogeneity in families that meet the Amsterdam criteria is underscored by the demonstration that one group of families (group A families) develops tumors with microsatellite instability and shows all the other clinical features of Lynch syndrome, whereas another group of families (group B families) develops tumors without microsatellite instability and does not show the other clinical features of Lynch syndrome (50). Although the clinicopathologic features of group B families indicate that they have a different disease, which is at present referred to as familial colorectal cancer type X, the genetic basis for the disorder is as yet unknown.

As shown in Table 15.4, within kindreds that harbor mismatch repair gene mutations, about 90% occur in *MLH1* or *MSH2* and about 10% occur in *MSH6* (53,54). Hundreds of different germline mutations in the mismatch repair genes have been identified (55), although in the 15% to 40% of cases in which the sequence change is a missense mutation,

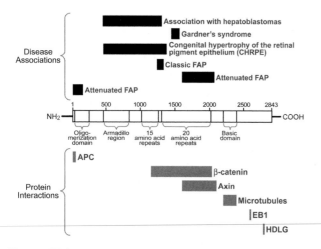

Figure 15.2 Schematic diagram of the APC protein. The upper part of the figure shows the regions of the protein associated with various diseases. The lower part of the figure shows the domains that interact with other proteins (APC indicates the domain involved in APC homodimerization; axin is a scaffold protein that is a negative regulator of signaling; EB1 may be involved in the checkpoint control of the cell cycle; HDLG is a tumor suppressor protein). (Modified from references 69 and 70.)

TABLE 15.2

THE REVISED BETHESDA GUIDELINES FOR TESTING COLORECTAL TUMORS FOR MICROSATELLITE INSTABILITY (MSI)

Tumors from individuals should be tested for MSI in the following situations:
1. Colorectal cancer diagnosed in a patient under age 50
2. Presence of synchromous or metachronous colorectal or other HNPCC-associated tumors[a], regardless of age
3. Colorectal cancer with MSI-H histology[b] diagnosed in patient less than age 60
4. Colorectal cancer diagnosed in one or more first-degree relatives who also have an HNPCC-related tumor, with the first cancer diagnosed when the relative was under age 50
5. Colorectal cancer diagnosed in two or more first- or second-degree relatives with HNPCC-related tumors, regardless of the relatives' ages at diagnosis

From reference 46.
[a]HNPCC-related tumors include colorectal, endometrial, gastric, ovarian, pancreatic, ureteral and renal pelvic, and biliary tract carcinomas; CNS tumors (usually glioblastomas as seen in Turcot syndrome); sebaceous gland adenoma and keratoacanthoma; and adenocarcinoma of the small bowel (see reference 48).
[b]Presence of tumor infiltrating lymphocytes, Crohn's-like lymphocytic reaction, mucinous/signet ring differentiation, or medullary growth pattern.

TABLE 15.3

THE REVISED INTERNATIONAL COLLABORATIVE GROUP ON HEREDITARY NONPOLYPOSIS COLORECTAL CANCER CRITERIA (AMSTERDAM CRITERIA II)

There should be at least three relatives with an HNPCC-associated cancer (colorectal carcinoma, or carcinoma of the endometrium, small bowel, ureter, or renal pelvis).
One individual should be a first-degree relative of the other two.
At least two successive generations should be affected.
At least one indivudal should be diagnosed before age 50.
Familial adenomatous polyposis should be excluded in the colorectal carcinoma case(s).
Tumors should be verified by pathologic examination.

From reference 45.

TABLE 15.4

DNA MISMATCH REPAIR GENES

Gene	Chromosomal Location	Prevalence of Mutations[a] (%)
MSH2	2p21	25–60 } together, about 90%[b]
MLH1	3p21	17–65
PMS1	2p31	<10
PMS2	7p22	<5
MSH6	2p21	5–10[c]
MSH3	5q14	Rare

[a]In families with mismatch repair mutations.
[b]The prevalence of MSH2 and MLH1 vary widely, but together account for about 90% of cases in most studies (references 48, 51, 52).
[c]In cases of atypical HNPCC, the prevalence is 70% (reference 53).

interpretation of the genetic data is complicated by the fact that it is often unclear whether the mutation is pathogenic or merely a polymorphism (48). Large structural changes involving the mismatch repair genes also occur (56,57). Although admittedly rare, epigenetic silencing of the *MLH1* gene via hypermethylation can also underlie the development of HNPCC (58), which raises the possibility of unconventional patterns of inheritance in some cases of HNPCC, especially because the epigenic alteration can be present in the germline (58).

The colonic adenocarcinomas that arise in patients with HNPCC have characteristic clinical and pathologic features. Typically, the tumors arise proximal to the splenic flexure, and about one third occur in the cecum. They are associated with an excess of synchronous (within 6 months) or metachronous (occurring after more than 6 months) colorectal adenocarcinomas (48,49,59,60). And finally, the tumors have distinct histologic features (but not necessarily pathognomonic, as discussed later); they are poorly differentiated with a mucinous, solid-cribriform, or solid-medullary pattern, and have a prominent peritumoral lymphocytic infiltrate (60,61).

It is important to emphasize that defects in the DNA mismatch repair system are not limited to HNPCC, but are present in about 15% of colorectal adenocarcinomas overall. However, in many sporadic tumors that show microsatellite instability, the deficiency of mismatch repair is due to epigenetic silencing of the genes by methylation of promoter CpG sites rather than mutation of the genes themselves (19,62–66).

Technical and Diagnostic Issues in Molecular Genetic Analysis of Colorectal Adenocarcinoma

Sporadic Tumors

Mutational Analysis. As noted previously, even though the progression from normal mucosa to adenoma to invasive adenocarcinoma involves an accumulation of mutations in colonic epithelial cells, there is significant variability in the range of mutations of each gene, every tumor does not harbor mutations in the same set of genes, and different tumors acquire mutations in a different sequence. Consequently, mutational analysis of the genes involved in the adenocarcinoma sequence, either individually or in aggregate, does not have high enough sensitivity or specificity to be useful in diagnostic testing for colorectal adenocarcinoma (67,68). For example, because mutations in the *APC* gene are present in adenomas and carcinomas, and in sporadic neoplasms as well as familial syndromes, including hereditary multiple colorectal adenomas, FAP, and even HNPCC, analysis of tumor tissue does not provide definitive evidence of malignancy or even of a hereditary cancer syndrome.

Prognostic Testing. The role of mutational analysis in providing prognostic information has been explored (reviewed in 60,71). Some genetic changes, for example, loss of chromosome 17p and 18q, are associated with an increased rate of metastasis and a worse clinical outcome (72,73). Other markers, including mutations in the DNA mismatch repair genes, especially *MLH1*, are apparently associated with increased patient survival (74,75). However, many of the studies that have shown prognostic significance have only assessed an individual marker, and in most studies the clinical impact of the findings in terms of patient management has not been established. Consequently, whether or not mutational analysis of marker genes provides clinically relevant prognostic information in routine use has not been established (76,77).

Although expression analysis of individual genes does not reliably identify those patients who will have a poor outcome, microarray analysis of thousands of genes has successfully been used not only to identify gene clusters that can discriminate normal versus tumor tissue, but also to identify patterns of messenger ribonucleic acid (mRNA) expression that can consistently predict prognosis and response to established chemotherapy regimens. Microarray analysis has been used to identify a panel of 23 genes that accurately predicts recurrence in 78% of patients with stage II tumors (78); and a panel of 194 genes and 41 expressed sequence tags (ESTs) that can separate patients that present with stage III or IV disease into groups that have a 100% 5-year survival versus only 40% 5-year survival (79). Although these studies involved only a limited number of cases, and even though the ability to predict patient groups with a poor prognosis does not imply that the high-risk patients will benefit from additional therapy (80), the results are important because the management of patients with stage II or III colorectal adenocarcinoma is an area of debate (the combined 5-year survival for patients with stage II or III disease is about 60%, but only about 20% of stage III patients treated with 5-fluorouracil [5-FU] show improved disease-free and overall survival, and adjuvant chemotherapy is associated with even less of a survival benefit in patients with stage II disease [80,81]). At the very least, the findings suggest the potential of microarray analysis for identifying patients whose risk of recurrence is so low that they can be spared the toxicity and expense associated with chemotherapy.

Therapeutic Testing. Microarray analysis has also been used to correlate the expression profile of colorectal adenocarcinoma cell lines with the response of the tumors to treatment with specific chemotherapeutic drugs. A panel of 50 genes predicts tumor response to 5-FU more accurately than the status of any of the markers that are established determinants of 5-FU response, including thymidylate synthase, thymidine phosphorylase, p53, and DNA mismatch repair status (81). The expression levels of a panel of 15 genes and 9 ESTs correlates with tumor response to cisplatin (82). A panel of 149 genes has been shown to predict response to camptothecin, an alternative chemotherapeutic agent for treatment of colorectal adenocarcinoma (81). Although the pattern of gene expression in cell lines in vitro does not always mimic the pattern of expression of primary tumors in vivo, these results suggest that microarray analysis may eventually be used to predict whether or not an individual patient's tumor will respond to specific chemotherapeutic regimens. In addition, microarray analysis may prove useful for identifying the characteristics of tumors that respond to novel chemotherapy agents, making it possible to identify small patient groups that will have a significant response even though the same drugs might not have a significant therapeutic effect on larger unselected cohorts of patients.

Hereditary Tumors

Mutational analysis clearly has a role for excluding hereditary cancer syndromes, but analysis in this setting should be performed only with appropriate consent in association with detailed pre-test and post-test genetic counseling (30,82,83).

Familial Adenomatous Polyposis. Testing for mutations in the *APC* gene was traditionally performed by the protein truncation test (Chapter 7). However, because the protein truncation test methodology is so cumbersome, most mutational analysis is currently performed by direct genomic DNA sequence analysis (84).

Multiple Colorectal Adenomas. As noted above, mutations in *APC* or *MYH* have been shown to give rise to the pattern of disease classified as multiple colorectal adenomas. The protein truncation test can be used to identify the 5% to 10% of patients whose disease actually represents attenuated FAP resulting from a specific pattern of *APC* mutations (Fig. 15.2).

Since inactivation of *MYH* produces a characteristic pattern of mutations consisting of transversions of G:C bp to T:A bp (Chapter 2), a screen for somatic *APC* mutations can be used to identify those patients whose disease is likely due to the presence of biallelic germline inactivating mutations of *MYH* (41). Although this indirect approach can be used to test formalin-fixed, paraffin-embedded (FFPE) tissue specimens (41), the method has not been clinically validated for either the exclusion of FAP resulting from *APC* mutations or the diagnosis of hereditary multiple colorectal adenomas caused by *MYH* mutations.

Hereditary Nonpolyposis Colorectal Cancer. Several factors make mutational analysis of the DNA mismatch repair system difficult. First, the proteins involved in the DNA mismatch repair system are encoded by a number of different genes (Table 15.4). Second, there are no specific mutation hot spots in the genes (55), and pathogenic mutations include splice site alterations and large deletions. Third, mismatch repair genes may be inactive as a result of epigenetic silencing from promoter methylation rather than mutation (85,86). Therefore, even though direct DNA sequence analysis (48,87), indirect methods such as single-strand conformational polymorphism (SSCP) analysis or denaturing gradient-gel electrophoresis (DGGE) (88,89), or even modified complementation analysis (56) can be used to screen for mutations in DNA mismatch repair genes, mutational analysis is a time-consuming and inefficient approach for detecting mutations. Consequently, in the recommended approach for molecular evaluation of patients identified as being at risk for HNPCC (Table 15.5), DNA sequence analysis is performed only if other indirect tests are positive.

A more straightforward, though indirect, method uses PCR amplification to detect short increases or decreases in the length of known microsatellites. This approach is based on the fact that microsatellite instability (MSI) is a hallmark of DNA mismatch repair defects (Chapter 2). In the context of colorectal cancer, a National Cancer Institute (NCI) working group has recommended evaluation of five specific microsatellites for the analysis of MSI (46,90), which has become the standard panel in the United States and most other countries. The panel includes two mononucleotide repeats (*BAT25* and *BAT26*) and three dinucleotide repeats (*D2S123*, *D5S346*, and *D17S250*). For all five loci, MSI is defined as a change of any length because of insertion or deletion of a repeating unit in the microsatellite when compared with normal tissue (Fig. 15.3). Although analysis of a smaller subset of microsatellite loci has been shown to identify a cohort of patients who have more homogeneous clinical features and a favorable prognosis (92,93), and

---

TABLE 15.5

RECOMMENDATIONS FOR THE PROCESS OF MOLECULAR EVALUATION OF PATIENTS IDENTIFIED AS BEING AT RISK BASED ON THE BETHESDA GUIDELINES

1. The optimal approach is microsatellite instability analysis (using the NCI recommended panel of markers) or immunohistochemical analysis, followed by germline *MSH2/MLH1* testing of patients whose tumors are MSI-H or show a loss of expression of one of the mismatch repair genes.[a,b]
2. If a mutation is identified, at-risk relatives should be referred for genetic counseling.
3. Direct germline analysis of the *MSH2/MLH1* genes is an alternative approach in cases in which tissue testing is not feasible.
4. If no mismatch repair gene mutation is found in a proband with an MSI-H tumor or a clinical history of HNPCC, the genetic test result is noninformative; in these cases, the patient and relatives should be counseled as if HNPCC were confirmed and high-risk surveillance should be undertaken.
5. Patients should be assured of confidentiality to allay fears related to discrimination based on genetic status.

From reference 46.
[a]Mutation detection techniques include single-strand conformational polymorphism analysis, denaturing gradient-gel electrophoresis analysis, DNA sequencing, monoallelic expression analysis, Southern blot analysis, and quantitative polymerase chain reaction.
[b]For families with a strong suspicion of HNPCC, germline testing should be considered even if the MSI or immunohistochemical results indicate MSI-L, MSS, or normal expression. Admittedly, the likelihood of finding a germline mutation in the *MSH2/MLH1* genes of patients with colorectal tumors that are not MSI-H is expected to be low, but this likelihood has not been thoroughly studied.

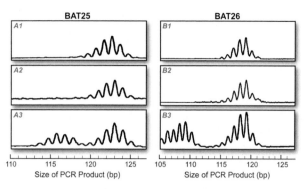

Figure 15.3 Microsatellite instability (MSI) analysis via fluorophore-labeled PCR products. The mononucleotide repeat *BAT25* is shown on the left, the mononucleotide repeat *BAT26* on the right. **A1** and **B1** are from analysis of normal mucosa. Each tracing shows a single central peak (with stuttering caused by the gain or loss of a few nucleotides as a result of slippage of the thermostable polymerase during PCR), indicating that the patient is homozygous for both markers. It is noteworthy that the stuttering is a technical artifact that mirrors the errors at short repeats by replication polymerases that are the fundamental cause of MSI to begin with (Chapter 2). **A2** and **B2** are from a crude manual dissection of adenomatous mucosa that contains a microscopic focus of invasive adenocarcinoma. There is no evidence of MSI because for each marker there is still only one central peak of the same size as in normal mucosa. **A3** and **B3** are from the invasive adenocarcinoma collected by laser microdissection. The presence of a new *BAT25* allele about 7 base pairs (bp) smaller than the normal allele is indicative of MSI. The presence of a new *BAT26* allele about 10 bp smaller than the normal allele is indicative of MSI at this locus as well. (Modified from *J Mol Diagn* 2004;6:308–315 with permission from the American Society for Investigative Pathology and the Association for Molecular Pathology.)

even though alternative panels have been suggested to simplify testing (94), routine clinical analysis still relies on the NCI panel.

For diagnostic MSI analysis, polymerase chain reaction (PCR) amplification of each of the microsatellites in the panel is performed on DNA isolated from tumor tissue and from paired normal tissue; the assay can be performed in a multiplex format, which greatly simplifies testing (92,95). When instability is present at two or more of the five markers (i.e., the markers show insertion or deletion mutations), the tumor is defined as MSI–high frequency (MSI-H). When one reference marker shows instability, the tumor is defined as low-frequency MSI (MSI-L), although it remains uncertain whether MSI-L tumors represent a distinct phenotype or merely a technical artifact of highly sensitive PCR assays (47). When a tumor is classified is MSI-L based on evaluation of the initial panel of markers, analysis of an additional panel of five secondary microsatellites is recommended to definitively determine the status of the tumor (when a total of 10 markers is used for evaluation, MSI is defined as instability at three or more markers and MSI-L is defined as instability at one or two markers). Tumors that show no mutations are considered to be microsatellite stable (MSS). MSI testing based on patients selected according to the revised Bethesda guidelines has been shown to be an effective approach for identifying patients that carry *MSH2* or *MLH1* gene mutations (96), and high-throughput methods that facilitate clinical testing have been developed (97).

As discussed in more detail in Chapter 5, several technical features of MSI analysis can complicate its use in routine practice. First, as shown in Figure 15.3, reliable results require microdissection of the area of most advanced tumor from surrounding normal tissue (90,98). Second, even though the analysis can be performed on fresh or FFPE tissue, reproducible results require a minimum DNA input so that the test outcome is not influenced by artifactual dropout resulting from limiting DNA template concentrations (90,99). Third, although in most cases the profile of the PCR product permits straightforward determination of whether or not MSI is present at that microsatellite locus, there are no uniform criteria for interpretation of marginal test results, although standards have been proposed (90,100).

Immunohistochemistry using antibodies specific for the mismatch repair enzymes has been shown to be a very reliable method for detecting tumors that are classified as MSI-H by standard microsatellite stability testing. [In fact, immunohistochemical testing based on selection of patients according to the revised Bethesda guidelines has been shown to be an effective approach for identifying patients that carry *MSH2* or *MLH1* mutations (96).] Using antibodies for *MLH1* and *MSH2*, immunohistochemistry has a sensitivity of 80% to 100% for detecting MSI-H tumors with a specificity that approaches 100% (93, 101–111), and use of antibodies to additional mismatch repair enzymes, specifically MSH6, may increase test sensitivity even further (98,110–113). Nonetheless, testing can achieve this level performance only if it is carried out using standardized conditions and interpreted by trained pathologists (96,110). Immunohistochemistry identifies the gene most likely to be mutated, and thus the result can be used to guide DNA sequence analysis if required (90,98). However, immunohistochemical analysis will always produce some false negative results because a subset of mutations in the genes encoding mismatch repair enzymes result in nonfunctional proteins that are nonetheless expressed at normal levels.

Finally, given that the colorectal adenocarcinomas that occur in HNPCC have a characteristic histologic appearance (48,49,59–61), it has been suggested that morphology alone may be sufficient for identifying those cases with defects in the mismatch repair pathway that should be subjected to further genetic analysis (114). In fact, some studies (115), although not all (116), have demonstrated that histologic features can be used to distinguish sporadic colorectal adenocarcinomas from those with MSI-H that arise in the setting of HNPCC and that there may even be reproducible morphologic differences between tumors that harbor mutations in *MLH1* versus *MSH2* (91). Although poor differentiation, medullary morphology, a signet ring cell component, and a high number of tumor-infiltrating lymphocytes are histologic features that have a specificity approaching 100% for tumors that have an MSI-H genotype, the overall sensitivity of tumor morphology for identifying MSI-H tumors may be as low as 15% (91,116). Even if the clinical utility of routine histology alone remains unproven, the high specificity of the characteristic morphologic pattern indicates that the HNPCC syndrome should be considered whenever a colorectal adenocarcinoma has the corresponding histologic features. The appropriate follow-up in these cases should include a discussion with the patient's physician regarding the pathologic findings and the need for a medical genetics consult. In this context, it is worth noting that there is general agreement that sequence analysis of the genes encoding the DNA mismatch repair enzymes constitutes genetic testing, and that MSI analysis and immunohistochemical evaluation of the mismatch repair enzymes could also be considered genetic tests because both methods yield results that are so highly correlated with the presence of germline mutation in the underlying genes (47).

Molecular Genetic Analysis for Screening, Staging, and Treatment Planning

Screening

Current guidelines for colorectal cancer screening include colonoscopy and fecal occult blood assessment. Although colonoscopy is a very sensitive test, its invasiveness is a major barrier to large scale-screening. Fecal occult blood testing is not invasive, but it has a low sensitivity, especially for early-stage tumors. Consequently, there has been interest in the use of molecular genetic techniques to screen for colorectal adenocarcinoma by detecting mutations associated with cancer in stool (117).

Technically, stool-based methods must overcome several obstacles. First, although the total DNA that can be recovered from feces is quite high because of bacterial contamination, DNA from sloughed epithelial cells usually represents only 0.01% to 0.1% of the total. Second, even in the presence of a tumor, neoplastic cells contribute at most 1% of the sloughed epithelial cells. Third, the recovered DNA is often fragmented, although several methods can be used to retrieve DNA fragments large enough for analysis, including oligonucleotide-based hybridization capture and acrylamide gel purification before PCR analysis (118,119).

Various different genes have been employed as targets in fecal screening assays. Use of the *APC* gene has the advantage of a high theoretical sensitivity, because as noted earlier, *APC* is mutated in over 80% of sporadic carcinomas and is often one of the first genes mutated in the adenoma to adenocarcinoma sequence. However, testing is cumbersome because there are no mutational hot spots in the gene; even though most mutations result in a stop codon, which makes it possible to use the protein truncation test (PTT) for the analysis, the PTT itself is technically demanding (Chapter 7). In one recent large study, fecal screening that employed the PTT to detect *APC* mutations had a sensitivity of 61% for patients with Duke's stage B2 adenocarcinomas and a sensitivity of 50% for patients with adenomas at least 1 cm in diameter, and a specificity of virtually 100% (119). Nonetheless, the methodology required 144 separate PCR reactions on each stool sample, which obviously limits the utility of the approach for screening large patient populations.

Analysis of K-*ras* mutations in fecal DNA has also been used to screen for colorectal adenocarcinoma. Although testing is simplified by the fact that mutations cluster in codons 12, 13, and 16 of the gene, the maximum sensitivity of analysis is limited because the prevalence of K-*ras* mutations in colorectal adenomas and adenocarcinomas is

only 30% to 40% (120–122). Consequently, even though mutations can be detected in the stool of 47% to 53% of patients whose tumors harbor K-*ras* mutations, testing has only an 18% to 21% overall sensitivity for detecting colorectal adenocarcinomas (121,122) and only an 8% overall sensitivity for detecting colorectal adenomas (122).

Because mutational analysis of individual genes has such limited sensitivity, a number of groups have evaluated the use of multiple genetic targets in fecal DNA screening. One testing approach includes mutational analysis of several genes, such as *TP53*, K-*ras*, and *APC*, as well as microsatellite instability analysis of the *BAT26* locus. This approach has a sensitivity of 52% to 71% for invasive adenocarcinoma (which is not surprising because an aberration of at least one of these four markers is present in 76% to 83% of colorectal adenocarcinomas), with a specificity of 94% to 100% (118,121,123). The finding that there is no significant correlation of the test result with either the location of the tumor or disease stage is consistent with the fact that mutations of these markers in the primary tumor are not associated with lymph node metastases or patient survival (68). Nonetheless, the extensive molecular analysis that is required to achieve these results constrains the utility of the approach for screening large patient populations (117).

Staging

Whether or not molecular genetic analysis can provide more accurate staging information in patients with colorectal adenocarcinoma has been evaluated in a number of settings, including detection of tumor cells in peripheral blood, bone marrow, or lymph nodes. In practice, most assays use reverse transcriptase PCR (RT-PCR) to detect the mRNA transcripts of marker genes whose expression is presumed to be limited to the malignant epithelial cells. Although the clinical significance of malignant cells that can be detected only by molecular genetic techniques (often referred to as submicroscopic disease) remains to be clarified from a clinical perspective, there are two issues that confound the utility of analysis from a purely technical perspective—the lack of specificity of the marker genes and the lack of morphologic correlation.

Lack of Specificity. Transcripts of marker genes that were presumed to be specifically expressed by the malignant epithelial cells of colorectal adenocarcinoma based on early reports have been subsequently shown to be more ubiquitously expressed. For example, transcripts encoding cytokeratin-19 (CK-19), CK-20, carcinoembryonic antigen (CEA), and guanylyl cyclase C (GCC) can be detected by RT-PCR in a significant percentage of control peripheral blood samples, bone marrow specimens, and lymph nodes obtained from patients with no history of malignancy. Specifically, using sensitive assays, CEA transcripts can be detected in the peripheral blood, bone marrow, and lymph nodes of up to 64%, 26%, and 100%, respectively, of patients without colorectal adenocarcinoma (124–129); CK-19 transcripts in the blood and lymph nodes of up to 77% and 100%, respectively, of patients without adenocarcinoma (124–127); CK-20 transcripts in the blood, bone marrow, and lymph nodes of up to 100%,

40%, and 100%, respectively, of patients without adenocarcinoma (129–132); and GCC transcripts in the blood and lymph nodes of 82% and 13%, respectively, of patients with no history of malignancy (128,132,133). The same lack of specificity has been demonstrated for other putative tumor markers, including the genes encoding epithelial glycoprotein-40 and -2 (125,134) and the mucin gene *MUC1* (135).

There are several explanations for these high false positive rates, including the fact that some genes are expressed at low levels by the endothelial cells and fibroblasts in lymph nodes, either physiologically or as the result of illegitimate transcription (126,128,136). Furthermore, RT-PCR is so sensitive that it can detect nucleic acids within cellular debris that has drained to lymph nodes, even in the absence of viable tumor cells. In fact, in one well-controlled model system, a marker gene was detected in draining and systemic lymph nodes by PCR for up to 4 days following injection of purified cell-free DNA (137).

Quantitative RT-PCR can theoretically be used to establish the minimum level of expression that correlates with the presence of viable malignant cells (131,138). However, in practice it may still be difficult to distinguish between physiologic expression of a marker gene by a very small number of viable tumor cells, low expression of the marker resulting from illegitimate transcription by nonmalignant cells, and cell free nucleic acids in debris that has drained to lymph nodes. Attempts to use RT-PCR analysis of a panel of markers to increase test specificity have met with only limited success (127,132).

Lack of Morphologic Correlation.

The specificity of imunohistochemical evaluation of lymph nodes and bone marrow is optimized by the fact that the architectural and cytologic features of the immunopositive cells can be used as a guide to their diagnostic significance. However, it is impossible to directly evaluate the morphologic features of the cells that are responsible for a positive PCR result because the tissue sample is destroyed during nucleic acid extraction. Given that the lack of specificity of many of the markers used for RT-PCR analysis of lymph nodes can lead to false positive RT-PCR results, the fact that the RT-PCR results cannot be confirmed by direct morphologic correlation is not a moot point.

Testing for Submicroscopic Disease.

Despite these limitations, RT-PCR has been used in many studies to detect disseminated tumor cells in peripheral blood, bone marrow, or lymph nodes of patients who have colorectal adenocarcinoma (127,139,140), and in some reports a positive RT-PCR result has been shown to have a statistically significant association with a worse clinical outcome, even among patients with known metastatic disease (126,129, 141,142). However, because multivariant analysis was not performed in these studies, it is still unclear whether molecular analysis provides any independent clinical information (126,137,140,142).

In some studies, PCR-based analysis has focused on detection of marker genes that are often mutated in colorectal adenocarcinoma. Although there is no doubt

that this approach increases the specificity of testing, the fact that only a subset of colorectal tumors harbors mutations in the marker genes limits maximal test sensitivity. For example, RT-PCR has been used to detect K-*ras* mutations in the serum of patients with colorectal adenocarcinoma, but even though the test has 100% specificity, its sensitivity is only 39% to 43% (143,144). Similarly, methylation-specific PCR has been used to detect altered patterns of promoter methylation of the marker gene *p16* in the serum of patients with colorectal adenocarcinoma with 100% specificity but only 27% sensitivity (145). However, in most studies of this type, detection of the altered marker in blood or bone marrow correlates with disease stage, and in the absence of multivariant analysis it is difficult to know whether molecular analysis provides any independent clinically relevant information.

Sentinel Lymph Nodes.

Identification of sentinel nodes (SN) is thought to improve the accuracy of disease staging for patients with colorectal adenocarcinoma (146,147). SN mapping is rarely used to plan the surgical management of colorectal adenocarcinoma because aberrant lymphatic drainage beyond the normal margins of resection is identified in only about 8% of patients (148,149). Instead, SN mapping is used to identify those lymph nodes more likely to harbor metastases so that they can be subject to more intensive histopathologic evaluation, which in many studies includes RT-PCR for expression of tumor marker genes.

An early study that focused on the detection of mRNA encoding CEA showed a markedly decreased 5-year survival rate for patients with submicroscopic nodal metastatses (150). However, the nodes were subjected to only limited conventional histopathologic evaluation, which together with the lack of specificity of CEA and the small number of nodes evaluated makes it difficult to determine the significance of the result (151,152). Subsequent RT-PCR analysis of SN using a panel of markers has been shown to increase test specificity (148,153), but whether the molecular results correlate with patient outcome was not evaluated.

These issues contribute to the general uncertainty regarding the role of SN biopsy in the management of patients with colorectal adenocarcinoma. The prognostic significance of occult metastases in pericolonic SN detected only by RT-PCR remains unknown; although the 5-year survival for stage I disease is 90%, and for stage II is only 75% to 80%, it has not been demonstrated that patients with occult metastases detected only by RT-PCR–based testing represent a subgroup of patients with a poor outcome. Similarly, it is unclear whether the presence of only submicroscopic metastatic disease indicates a need for additional treatment in patients who otherwise would not have received adjuvant therapy. Until prospective randomized clinical trials with long-term follow-up define the clinical significance of submicroscopic disease, molecular analysis of pericolic SN is best considered experimental.

Treatment Planning

Several recent reports suggest that molecular genetic analysis will likely assume a significant role in guiding therapy based on the profile of mutations present in each individual patient's tumor (154). For example, for patients with colorectal adenocarcinoma, the benefit of treatment using a fluorouracil-based adjuvant chemotherapy regimen is significantly associated with the microsatellite stability status of the patient's tumor. The overall survival among patients with MSS or MSI-L tumors is improved by adjuvant chemotherapy, although there is no benefit (and maybe even decreased overall survival) among patients whose tumors are MSI-H (155). In patients whose tumors harbor mismatch repair deficiencies, other drugs such as topoisomerase-1 inhibitors may provide a better therapeutic option (156). Similarly, the resistance to adjuvant chemotherapy with fluorouracil has been shown to correlate with high thymidylate synthase mRNA levels (157–159) (fluorouracil inhibits DNA replication by irreversibly blocking the thymidylate synthase enzyme; tumors with low expression of thymidylate synthase therefore show a better response to the drug). Since the level of thymidylate synthase mRNA can be measured by quantitative RT-PCR using fresh or FFPE tissue, molecular genetic analysis may provide an approach to identify those patients who are unlikely to respond to adjuvant therapy involving fluorouracil but who may benefit from earlier treatment by alternative protocols (157). Finally, a small molecule termed RITA has been shown to restore the apoptosis-inducing function of p53 in tumor cells that retain the wild-type gene (160); although the results are very preliminary, they suggest that there may eventually be a role for mutational analysis of TP53 (as well as other genes that regulate p53 function) to identity patients most likely to benefit from therapy with this class of compounds.

Small Intestine

Malignant epithelial tumors of the small intestine are only about 2% as common as malignant epithelial tumors of the large intestine, a remarkably low incidence given that the combined surface area of the duodenum, jejunum, and ileum is approximately 10 times that of the large intestine. Although rare, adenocarcinoma of the small intestine shares many of the risk factors associated with adenocarcinoma of the colorectum (161–163). An increased risk is associated with several hereditary syndromes (including FAP, HNPCC, and Peutz-Jeghers syndrome), chronic inflammation (including Crohn's disease and celiac disease), prior surgical procedures (including cholecystectomy, or creation of an ileostomy, ileal conduit, or ileal reservoir), and lifestyle choices (including cigarette smoking and excessive alcohol consumption) (3,162).

On a molecular level, many of the same genes that are involved in the adenoma-carcinoma sequence of colorectal adenocarcinoma have also been implicated in the tumorigenesis of small intestinal epithelial malignancies, including K-ras, TP53, APC, CTNNB1, the genes involved in the TGF-β signaling pathway, and genes encoding proteins involved in the DNA mismatch repair system (3,164). Nonetheless, there are some significant differences in the tumorigenesis of small intestinal versus colorectal adenocarcinomas. For example, disruption of the TGF-β signaling pathway appears to play a more important role in the tumorigenesis of small intestinal versus colorectal adenocarcinomas (165). Similarly, β-catenin abnormalities apparently serve as an alternative to APC mutations for

activation of the tumorigenic pathway in small intestinal carcinomas (166) because mutations of CTNNB1 are a common finding, whereas mutations of the APC gene occur at a much lower frequency (165,167,168). The molecular pathway for small bowel adenocarcinomas that develop in the setting of long-standing inflammation (such as Crohn's-associated tumors) seems to be similar to that for sporadic adenocarcinomas (168), and, in general, the pattern of mutations in ampullary adenocarcinomas is more similar to that of other small intestinal adenocarcinomas than to pancreatic ductal adenocarcinomas (169–171).

Molecular Genetic Analysis for Diagnosis and Prognostic Evaluation of Small Intestinal Adenocarcinomas

As with molecular genetic analysis of colorectal adenocarcinomas, the low sensitivity and specificity of mutational analysis of the individual genes associated with epithelial tumorigenesis precludes a role for diagnostic genetic testing of sporadic tumors. However, in those cases in which the clinical setting of the tumor suggests the possibility of an underlying familial cancer syndrome, it is appropriate to suggest a genetics consultation to exclude a defined hereditary cancer syndrome. The presence of a hereditary syndrome not only has obvious implications for the patient's follow-up, but also can have an impact on the patient's prognosis. For example, patients who develop small bowel adenocarcinoma in the setting of HNPCC apparently have a better prognosis than the general population (172).

The role of molecular genetic analysis in the evaluation of endoscopic biopsies taken from adenocarcinomas of the head of the pancreas that merge with periampullary adenocarcinomas is covered in the section of this chapter on tumors of the exocrine pancreas.

Stomach

Gastric carcinomas are often divided into two general categories, intestinal type carcinomas and diffuse type carcinomas (173). The two categories (Figure 15.4) have different epidemiologic and clinicopathologic features and, not surprisingly, also have different underlying mechanisms of tumorigenesis (174–177). MSI is present in about 15% to 50% of intestinal type carcinomas (178,179), often associated with frame shift mutations in TGFβRII, IGFIIR, BAX, MSH6, MSH3, and E2F4 (180,181). Intestinal type carcinomas also have a higher prevalence of TP53 mutations (182) and a higher level of hTERT expression (183). Diffuse type carcinomas show microsatellite instability much less frequently. Instead, diffuse type tumors harbor functionally relevant mutations in the CDH1 gene encoding E-cadherin in up to 50% of cases, often with associated downregulation of expression resulting from hypermethylation of the gene's promoter; they also show an altered pattern of expression of genes encoding extracellular matrix components and proteins involved in cell–matrix interactions (174,175,181,184–186).

Technical and Diagnostic Issues in Molecular Genetic Analysis of Gastric Carcinoma
Microsatellite Instability. The role of MSI analysis in the evaluation of gastric carcinomas is less well established

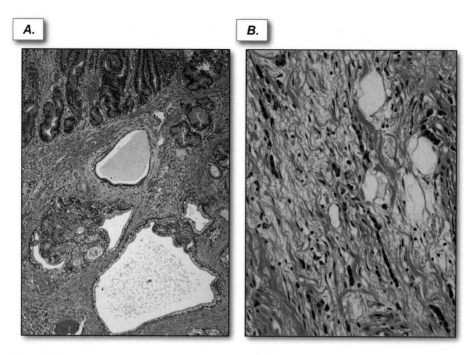

Figure 15.4 The two general categories of gastric adenocarcinoma are associated with different underlying mechanisms of tumorigenesis. Intestinal type adenocarcinomas (**A**, in which the tumor forms glands) frequently show microsatellite instability, *TP53* mutations, and a high level of *hTERT* expression. In contrast, diffuse type carcinomas (**B**, in which the malignant cells do not form glands, but instead invade as linear aggregates of cells, so-called Indian-files) harbor mutations in the *CDH1* gene encoding E-cadherin, often associated with hypermethylation of the gene's promoter. Diffuse type carcinomas also typically show an altered pattern of expression of genes encoding extracellular matrix components and proteins involved in cell-matrix interactions.

than for colorectal adenocarcinomas, primarily because no consensus approach has been developed for testing gastric tumors. In some studies of gastric tumors, unique panels of microsatellite markers (in terms of both the number and chromosomal location of the markers) and nonstandard rules have been used to classify tumors as positive for MSI. In other studies, the criteria developed for the diagnosis of MSI in colorectal adenocarcinoms have been applied to carcinomas arising in the stomach (176). Given the lack of uniform criteria for classifying tumors as MSI positive, it is not surprising that consistent correlations between protein expression by immunohistochemistry, mismatch repair gene promoter hypermethylation, and MSI classification have not been observed (176,187), which has obviously further hindered evaluation of the clinical utility of MSI analysis. A standardized method for MSI detection in gastric carcinomas has recently been proposed (176), but whether this approach will become the consensus method remains to be seen.

Mutational Analysis of E-Cadherin. The mature E-cadherin protein is a cell–cell adhesion molecule that has an important role in the maintenance of cell differentiation and normal architecture of epithelial tissues (reviewed in 184). *CDH1* mutations are detectable in up to 50% of cases of sporadic diffuse gastric cancer and are the hallmark of the hereditary diffuse gastric cancer (HDGC) syndrome (Table 15.6), an autosomal dominant syndrome with incomplete penetrance that is characterized by

early-onset poorly differentiated diffuse gastric cancer (184,188). In HDGC syndrome, one of the *CDH1* alleles is inactivated by a germline mutation, but loss of expression of the second *CDH1* allele is typically due to epigenetic inactivation by hypermethylation rather than mutation or deletion. Consistent with this finding, 40% to 80% of sporadic diffuse gastric cancers also show *CDH1* promoter hypermethylation (186).

From a technical perspective, mutational analysis of *CDH1* is complicated by the fact that the gene can be inactivated by several different mechanisms. Missense mutations and frameshift mutations occur in most of the coding sequence, without defined hot spots, and so virtually the entire gene must be screened (189). Because single bp substitutions that alter splice slice site consensus sequences have also been described, mutational analysis must also include evaluation of intron-exon boundaries. Since epigenetic changes can affect the level of gene expression, the promoter region must be tested for an altered pattern of methylation. Recently, a set of antibodies that recognize CDH1 proteins with specific mutations has been described (190) that may simplify testing for individual mutations.

From a diagnostic perspective, mutational analysis of *CDH1* does not seem to have a role in the routine evaluation of sporadic cases of diffuse gastric cancer because the diagnosis is usually straightforward by routine histopathologic evaluation. However, the observation that specific mutations are associated with clinical outcome offers the

TABLE 15.6

GENETIC SYNDROMES ASSOCIATED WITH AN INCREASE RISK OF GASTRIC CANCER[a]

Syndrome	Gene	Mode of Inheritance	Function of Gene Product
Hereditary diffuse gastric carcinoma	CDH1	Autosomal dominant	Cell–cell adhesion
Hereditary nonpolyposis colon cancer (HNPCC)	MSH2, MLH1, and others (see Table 15.4)	Autosomal dominant	DNA mismatch repair
Familial adenomatous polyposis (FAP)	APC	Autosomal dominant	Transcriptional control
Peutz-Jeghers	LKB1/STK11	Autosomal dominant	Serine/threonine kinase
Li-Fraumeni	TP53	Autosomal dominant	Control of apoptosis
Familial breast cancer	BRCA2	Autosomal dominant	DNA damage repair; others?

[a]Overall, only about 8% to 10% of gastric carcinomas have an inherited component reference (3).

first hint that mutational analysis may assume a prognostic role. Specifically, *CDH1* exon 8 or exon 9 deletions are associated with poor survival (190), but the fact that the mutations can be detected using mutation-specific antibodies (192) suggests that immunohistochemical approaches may supplant genetic testing once the molecular basis of tumorigenesis is more well defined.

Since novel DNA methyltransferase inhibitors are under development (191,192), molecular genetic analysis of the pattern of epigenetic changes of the *CDH1* promoter may assume a role in the pathologic workup of gastric carcinoma by identifying those patients most likely to respond to the new drugs. However, analysis of the methylation status of the *CDH1* promoter will likely not be limited to cases of diffuse gastric carcinoma because a subset of intestinal type carcinomas also show decreased expression of E-cadherin resulting from promoter hypermethylation (186).

Gene Expression Analysis. Several studies have shown that gene expression analysis of gastric carcinoma has potential for providing diagnostic information that cannot be obtained from mutational analysis of individual genes. For example, gene expression analysis has identified a set of genes that can reliably distinguish nonmalignant disease of the stomach (including gastritis and intestinal metaplasia) from carcinoma (193,194), although it has not yet been established that gene expression profiles have a role for evaluation of patients with intestinal metaplasia who are at a high risk for the presence of malignancy.

Molecular Genetic Analysis for Staging and Determination of Prognosis

Staging. Molecular genetic analysis can potentially provide more accurate staging information for patients with gastric cancer and has specifically been used to detect tumor cells in peripheral blood, bone marrow, or lymph nodes. As noted in the discussion of molecular genetic analysis for staging colorectal adenocarcinomas, there are several issues that confound the utility of analysis from a purely technical perspective, primarily the lack of specificity of the presumed tumor markers and the fact that the molecular results cannot be correlated with the morphologic features of the positive cells.

Whether SN biopsy itself has a role in the management of patients with gastric carcinoma is still a matter of debate (195,196). Nonetheless, PCR-based methods have been used to supplement the histopathologic evaluation of excised SN. In one study (196), RT-PCR of a panel of four markers (encoding CK-18, CEA, hTERT, and MUC1) detected metastases in 8% of SN without histologically evident metastatic disease. However, because all the RT-PCR–positive nodes were from patients who had metastatic disease in other lymph nodes that was detected by routine microscopy or immunohistochemistry, the clinical utility of the testing is unclear.

RT-PCR has also been used to detect disseminated tumor cells in peripheral blood and bone marrow of patients with gastric carcinoma, although, again, it has not been established that submicroscopic disease detected only by molecular genetic techniques should be incorporated into the traditional staging classification. For example, in patients with gastric carcinoma, the presence of mRNA encoding CK-20 has been associated with statistically significant shorter survival when detected in both peripheral blood and bone marrow or bone marrow alone (129). However, because the positive RT-PCR result also is related to the clinical stage of disease, it is not clear whether molecular analysis provides any independent information.

Determination of Prognosis. For patients with gastric carcinoma, the most frequent mode of metastasis and recurrence after surgery is peritoneal dissemination, although the tumor T-stage assigned by the traditional TMN classification is not a reliable method for predicting peritoneal recurrence (197). However, the presence of tumor cells in the peritoneal cavity does correlate with peritoneal recurrence (198,199), and consequently molecular genetic demonstration of free tumor cells in the peritoneal cavity has been used to identify high-risk patients most likely to benefit from adjuvant chemotherapy.

In most studies, RT-PCR for a presumed tumor-specific mRNA is performed on peritoneal lavage specimens. Notwithstanding technical considerations regarding the specificity of various mRNA markers for viable tumor cells, quantitative RT-PCR for mRNA encoding CEA has a 77% and 68% sensitivity and specificity, respectively, for predicting peritoneal recurrence compared with a 23% and 98% sensitivity and specificity, respectively, for conventional cytologic evaluation (200). A combination of cytology and RT-PCR may provide for optimal sensitivity and specificity (201). Transcription-mediated amplification (Chapter 22; Figure 22.3) has also been used to demonstrate the presence of metastatic disease in peritoneal lavage specimens (202). The advantage of the TRC reaction is the method's quick turnaround time, as short as 1 hour, which makes it possible to incorporate the test result into decisions regarding the need for interperitoneal chemotherapy at the time of the primary surgery (203).

Quantitative RT-PCR has been used to show that changes in the level of CEA mRNA over time correlate with the clinical response to chemotherapy in patients with advanced gastric carcinoma (201).

Gene Expression Analysis. Genomewide analysis of gene expression patterns has been used to provide prognostic information on patients with gastric cancer. In particular, a set of 12 to17 genes has been described that can identify a subgroup of patients who exhibit significantly better overall survival (204), and a panel of 5 genes can be used to reliability predict the lymph node status at the time of excision (205). Nonetheless, the clinical utility of microarray gene expression analysis remains somewhat unclear because there is little overlap between the panels of genes shown to correlate with specific clinicopathologic features in different studies (204–206).

Separate from any role in prognostic testing, gene expression analysis of gastric carcinoma may prove to be useful for identifying the patients most likely to benefit from specific therapeutic regimens. In a basic science setting, microarray analysis has been used to characterize changes in gene expression in gastric carcinoma cell lines that are sensitive versus resistant to 5-FU (207). In a clinical setting, quantitative RT-PCR measurement of the level of expression of a panel of 7 markers has been used to individualize chemotherapy to achieve markedly better clinical outcomes than would have been possible based on routine regimens (208). The fact that most of the genes in the marker panel are not thought to be directly involved in the development of gastric carcinomas emphasizes the fact that optimum treatment may not rely solely on the identification of somatic mutations in the tumor. These studies highlight the potential role of gene expression analysis for tailoring chemotherapeutic regimens to individual patients, but at present expression analysis is not a part of the routine pathologic evaluation of gastric carcinomas.

Esophagus

Adenocarcinoma

The incidence of adenocarcinoma of the esophagus has risen dramatically in the United States and other western countries in the last three decades (1). Although the etiology and epidemiology of adenocarcinoma differs from that of squamous cell carcinoma of the esophagus in several ways, the most significant difference is the association of adenocarcinoma with Barrett's esophagus. Barrett's esophagus is the single most important precursor lesion for esophageal adenocarcinoma and, in fact, can be detected in more than 80% of patients who develop esophageal adenocarcinoma (209,210).

The most common underlying cause of Barrett's esophagus is chronic gastroesophageal reflux, which causes mucosal injury by repetitively exposing the esophageal epithelium to gastric acids and duodenal contents (including bile acids and pancreatic enzymes). The resulting chronic injury drives the progression from Barrett's metaplasia to dysplasia to adenocarcinoma (Fig. 15.5), which is thought to result from the stepwise accumulation of a series of genetic abnormalities in a number of different tumor suppressor genes, oncogenes, growth factor receptors, cell adhesion molecules, and extracellular poetesses analogous to the stepwise progression characteristic of tumorigenesis of colorectal adenocarcinoma (reviewed in 211-213). However, there is significant variability among different studies regarding the prevalence of individual genetic alterations, which likely reflects the fact that the genetic and epigenetic alterations responsible for the progression from normal mucosa to adenocarcinoma occur in a variable pattern and sequence, as well as the fact that the various techniques used to evaluate the molecular pathogenesis of adenocarcinoma do not have the same sensitivity and specificity.

Squamous Cell Carcinoma

There is an almost 10-fold difference in the incidence of squamous cell carcinoma of the esophagus depending on geographic location (3). Some of difference is accounted for by environmental or lifestyle risk factors. In western countries, cigarette smoking and alcohol use together account for nearly 90% of the risk. Worldwide, dietary deficiencies in trace elements or regular consumption of extremely hot beverages are significant predisposing factors. The extent to which genetic differences among various ethnic groups contribute to the risk of squamous cell carcinoma has not been well characterized. Three large families with tylosis (focal nonepidermolytic palmoplantar keratoderma) have been associated with early-onset squamous cell carcinoma, but the genetic basis of disease in these families has yet to be described (214).

As with adenocarcinoma, squamous cell carcinoma develops through the accumulation of somatic mutations and epigenetic changes in the genome of esophageal epithelial cells that alter the structure or expression of a

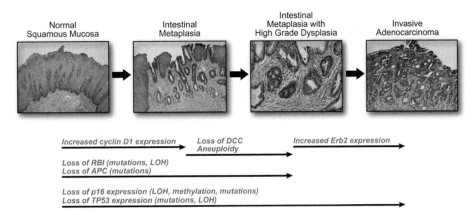

Figure 15.5 Schematic diagram of a genetic model for the molecular pathogenesis of esophageal adenocarcinoma from Barrett's esophagus. The model shows that progression is associated with changes in gene expression, mutations, and epigenetic modifications. The model also emphasizes that the exact sequence of events is unknown and probably variable; multiple pathways likely interact during progression. (For more detail, see references 211–213.)

number of oncogenes, tumor suppressor genes, and cell adhesion molecules (reviewed in 175,211). However, there is significant variability among different studies regarding the prevalence of the various genetic alterations and the role, if any, of diagnostic or prognostic testing in clinical practice. These differences reflect the fact that the numerous techniques used to evaluate the molecular pathogenesis of squamous cell carcinoma do not have the same sensitivity and specificity, and that there are variations in the molecular pathogenesis of squamous cell carcinoma in different areas of the world (3,175,211).

Molecular Genetic Analysis for Diagnosis and Prognosis

Although many individual markers have been evaluated for their role in providing diagnostic and prognostic information in epithelial malignancies of the esophagus, none has shown the sensitivity or specificity required for routine use. Consequently, as with other sites in the gastrointestinal tract, microarray analysis has been used to identify patterns of gene expression that can provide either diagnostic or prognostic information. For example, microarray analysis has demonstrated different patterns of gene expression between Barrett's esophagus and esophageal carcinoma (215) and has been used to predict the sensitivity of esophageal carcinomas to adjuvant chemotherapy. In one study, a group of 52 genes was identified that were highly correlated with patient response to cisplatin and 5-FU (216); even though the study involved only patients with advanced-stage disease and a limited panel of chemotherapy agents, the result nonetheless suggests that gene expression profiling may prove useful for directing the choice of adjuvant chemotherapy.

Molecular Genetic Analysis for Tumor Staging

Esophageal carcinomas frequently metastasize to lymph nodes distant from the primary tumor, including abdominal and cervical lymph nodes (217), but there is ongoing debate regarding the efficacy of extended three-field lymphadenectomy (which includes aggressive dissection of mediastinal, abdominal, and cervical lymph nodes) in patient management (218–220). A rapid quantitative RT-PCR method has recently been evaluated for its role in guiding surgical therapy in this setting (221); the assay can be completed in only 2½ hours from the time of tissue sampling (a turnaround time short enough that the results can be used intraoperatively to direct the extent of the surgical excision), and, of equal if not greater importance, the assay employes three different markers to increase test sensitivity and specificity. In one study, the method detected metastatic disease in 30% of patients whose lymph nodes were negative by conventional intraoperative frozen sections, and the PCR results showed 100% correlation with the presence or absence of metastasis in the permanent sections of the nodes (221). This result suggests that rapid molecular assays may well have a role in directing the intraoperative surgical management of patients, despite the limitations that are inherent in RT-PCR analysis of lymph nodes (discussed previously).

Evaluation of Composite Versus Collision Tumors

A molecular genetic approach that includes mutational analysis of *TP53* and LOH analysis of several microsatellite loci has been used to show that traditional morphologic and immunohistochemical criteria do not accurately differentiate collision tumors (two independent tumors that are coincidently juxtaposed) from composite tumors (single tumors with divergent lineages of differentiation) of the gastroesophageal junction (222). This finding mirrors the demonstration that conventional morphologic and immunohistochemical criteria often do not accurately distinguish between recurrent tumors and independent second primary tumors at other anatomic sites (223,224). Molecular genetic analysis therefore seems warranted in those cases in which the distinction between a collision tumor and a composite tumor would have a significant impact on patient therapy or prognosis.

TABLE 15.7

GENETIC SYNDROMES WITH AN INCREASED RISK OF PANCREATIC CANCER

Syndrome	Mode of Inheritance	Gene	Lifetime Risk of Pancreatic Cancer
Hereditary pancreatitis	Autosomal dominant	Cationic trypsinogen	30% (50-fold increased risk of pancreatic cancer)
Familial pancreatic cancer	Autosomal dominant	Unknown	5- to10-fold increased risk if a first-degree relative has pancreatic cancer
Familial atypical mole and melanoma (FAMMM)	Autosomal dominant	p16/CMM2	10%
Familial breast cancer	Autosomal dominant	BRCA2	5% to 10%
Ataxia-telangiectasia	Autosomal dominant	ATM	Increased[a]
Peutz-Jeghers	Autosomal dominant	STK11/LKB1	Increased[a]
Hereditary nonpolyposis colorectal cancer (HNPCC)	Autosomal dominant	MSH2, MLH1, and others (see Table 15.4)	Unknown; somewhat increased

Modified from reference 3.
[a]Magnitude of increase is unknown.

Pancreas

Pancreatic adenocarcinomas develop through a multistep pathway of carcinogenesis analogous to the oncogenic pathway in colorectal adenocarcinomas, although the general pattern of mutations is different (225). In sporadic pancreatic adenocarcinomas, activating point mutations in K-ras are present in more than 90% of tumors, and inactivation of the tumor suppressor genes TP53 and p16 is present in 50% to 75% and more than 90% of tumors, respectively. Genes involved in cell signaling that are most commonly disrupted include DPC4 and SMAD4 of the TGF-β pathway, SHH of the Hedgehog signaling pathway, and HER2/neu (reviewed in 225–228).

The importance of these genes in the tumorigenesis of pancreatic adenocarcinoma is emphasized by the fact that germline mutations at many of the same loci are responsible for genetic syndromes that have a predisposition for pancreatic adenocarcinoma (Table 15.7) including Li-Fraumeni syndrome, Puetz-Jeghers syndrome, familial breast cancer associated with BRCA-2 mutations, familial atypical mole and melanoma syndrome, hereditary pancreatitis, and ataxia telangiectasia (227,229). Overall, about 10% of pancreatic adenocarcinomas show familial clustering.

Technical and Diagnostic Issues in Molecular Genetic Analysis of Pancreatic Adenocarcinoma

A number of different molecular genetic methods have been used to evaluate a wide variety of markers for their role in providing diagnostic or prognostic information in pancreatic adenocarcinoma. However, given the multistep mechanism of tumorigenesis for pancreatic adenocarcinoma, it is not surprising that molecular analysis of most, if not all,

individual markers lacks the sensitivity and specificity required for diagnostic testing in routine clinical practice. For example, mutations in K-ras in pancreatic adenocarcinoma are restricted to codon 12 in the vast majority of cases (230,231), but the same pattern of activating point mutations in codon 12 is also seen in benign hyperplastic duct cells in patients without associated pancreatic disease, in reactive ductal epithelium in a background of chronic inflammation, and in patients with intraductal papillary neoplasms (232–235). Similarly, because only 50% to 75% of adenocarcinomas harbor TP53 mutations, mutational analysis of the gene is not a component of the routine diagnostic evaluation of pancreatic adenocarcinomas (225–227).

Pancreatic adenocarcinomas that arise in the setting of HNPCC have a characteristic medullary phenotype that includes poor differentiation, pushing borders, and a syncytial growth pattern (236,237) and can be used as a clue to the presence of the underlying defect in DNA mismatch repair. However, the role of MSI analysis in the evaluation of pancreatic adenocarcinomas is less well established than for adenocarcinomas at other sites in the gastrointestinal tract. No consensus approach has been developed for testing, in terms of either the number or chromosomal location of the microsatellite markers in the test panel, and there are no standardized criteria for classifying tumors as positive for MSI based on the profile of microsatellite alterations. Similarly, the correlations between immunohistochemical demonstration of the loss of DNA repair enzymes and MSI classification are also not well established.

Telomere Metabolism

Abnormalities of telomere metabolism are a characteristic feature of pancreatic neoplasms. When assessed by the telomerase repeat amplification protocol (TRAP; Chapter 5), abnormal telomerase activity is present in over 80% of pancreatic adenocarcinomas (including malignant intraductal papillary mucinous neoplasms and adenosquamous carcinomas), 63% of ampullary carcinomas, 79% of periampullary adenocarcinomas, and 100% of cholangiocarcinomas, but is present in less than 5% of pancreatic adenomas, and only 0 to 3% of cases of chronic pancreatitis; it is virtually never present in serous cystadenomas, benign cystic mucinous neoplasms, neuroendocrine carcinomas, or acinar cell carcinomas (238,239). The TRAP assay also has been used as an adjunct to the cytologic diagnosis of pancreatic adenocarcinoma. Abnormal telomerase activity is present in virtually 100% of fine needle aspiration (FNA) specimens from patients with adenocarcinoma and shows 100% correlation with the results of traditional cytopathologic evaluation, but because testing has been performed on so few cases that are not positive for malignancy the specificity of the assay is unknown (240). On the other hand, because a high level of telomerase mRNA is present in normal and inflamed pancreatic tissue, quantitative RT-PCR is required for highly sensitive and specific differentiation of benign from malignant disease in assays based on analysis of telomerase mRNA expression (238).

Gene Expression Analysis

Genomewide analysis of gene expression profiles has potential utility in the diagnostic and prognostic evaluation of pancreatic adenocarcinomas, although the approach is still experimental. For example, gene expression profiling using oligonucleotide microarrays has identified a panel of four genes that has a sensitivity of 73% and a specificity of 100% for identifying intraductal papillary mucinous neoplasms (IPMNs) that have an associated invasive component (241).

Molecular Genetic Testing for Prognosis

Some studies have shown that mutational analysis of individual genes has the potential to provide therapeutically useful information for patients with pancreatic adenocarcinoma. For example, FISH-based testing to detect amplification of *Her2/neu* and the *TOP2A* gene that encodes topoisomerase IIα may prove useful for identifying patients who would benefit from therapy with trastuzumab, topoisomerase inhibitors, or both (242).

Molecular Genetic Analysis for Screening for Pancreatic Adenocarcinoma

Because telomerase activity as measured by the TRAP protocol has a high sensitivity and specificity for pancreatic adenocarcinoma, the method has been used to diagnose malignancy in pancreatic juice samples obtained by endoscopic retrograde pancreatography (243–246). In this setting, telomerase activity can be detected in 80% to 83% of patients with adenocarcinoma, but in less than 5% of patients with pancreatic adenomas, and in virtually none of patients who have chronic pancreatitis or no primary pancreatic disease (243,244). In parallel analysis, the sensitivity and specificity of the TRAP assay are superior to mutational analysis of K-*ras* (243). The TRAP assay has also

been used to diagnose malignant IPMN based on analysis of pancreatic juice (245).

The vast majority of mutations in K-*ras* and pancreatic adenocarcinoma occur in codon 12 (231) and mutations in K-*ras* are early events in the development of pancreatic neoplasia; therefore, testing for K-*ras* mutations would seem to be a straightforward method for detecting early and potentially curable tumors. However, the method has only limited sensitivity, as demonstrated by one study in which RT-PCR testing designed to detect K-*ras* mutations in stool samples that match those of the primary pancreatic lesion was positive in only 45% of cases of adenocarcinoma (247). The fact that K-*ras* mutations are also present in non-neoplastic lesions of the pancreas further limits the usefulness of the method, as noted above. In fact, 9% of patients with adenocarcinoma and 33% of patients with chronic pancreatitis harbor mutations in their stool samples that are not present in the primary lesion itself but rather in the pancreatic ductal mucinous cell hyperplasia adjacent to the primary lesion (247).

Molecular Genetic Testing for Staging Pancreatic Adenocarcinoma

RT-PCR has been used to detect disseminated tumor cells in the bone marrow, peripheral blood, and lymph nodes of patients who have pancreatic adenocarcinoma, using several different markers including CK-20 and K-*ras* (129,248), although the technical issues discussed previously that confound the utility of molecular genetic analysis for staging colorectal adenocarcinomas also confound molecular staging of pancreatic adenocarcinoma. Furthermore, from a clinical perspective, the significance of submicroscopic disease remains to be clarified because it is not yet established that malignant cells detected only by extremely sensitive molecular genetic techniques carry the same prognostic and therapeutic implications of metastases detected by conventional histopathologic examination.

Nonetheless, RT-PCR–based testing has shown that 19% of bone marrow samples and 9% of peripheral blood samples from patients with pancreatic adenocarcinoma yield a positive result when tested for mRNA encoding CK-20, and that all positive results occur in patients with advanced disease when staged by standard criteria (129). Similarly, PCR designed to detect mutations in codon 12 of K-*ras* demonstrates circulating tumor cells in blood samples from 33% of patients with adenocarcinoma (248); however, although based on the limited number of patients evaluated, it is impossible to correlate the molecular results with disease stage as assessed by standard criteria.

PCR-based assays have also been used to detect cells harboring mutations in codon 12 of K-*ras* in para-aortic lymph nodes in patients with adenocarcinoma, and have shown that metastases can be detected in 29% to 53% of patients by PCR compared with only 0 to 19% by standard histopathologic evaluation with or without immunohistochemical staining (249,250). Similarly, PCR-based analysis, restriction fragment length polymorphism (RFLP) analysis, and SSCP analysis of regional lymph nodes detect submicroscopic disease that would upstage the TNM grouping in 68%, 73%, and 60%, respectively, of patients (251–253). Patients with submicroscopic disease detected by molecular testing show a statistically significant decrease in survival (249–253), and the potential utility of detection of submicroscopic disease by molecular analysis is emphasized by the observation that patients with stage I adenocarcinoma and submicroscopic regional lymph node metastases detected by analysis of K-*ras* have an improved survival when treated with adjuvant chemoradiation (251).

Evaluation of Composite Versus Collision Tumors

LOH analysis of a panel of six microsatellite markers, together with mutational analysis of K-*ras* codon 12, has been used to demonstrate that pancreatic mucinous cystic neoplasms with sarcomatous stroma have a monoclonal origin (254), which indicates that these neoplasms represent tumors with divergent differentiation rather than collision tumors.

NEUROENDOCRINE TUMORS

Carcinoid tumor (well-differentiated neuroendocrine carcinoma) not only has a different molecular pathogenesis than enteric adenocarcinoma, but also harbors a different pattern of genetic changes depending on where it arises in the gastrointestinal tract (255,256). Foregut neuroendocrine tumors (those involving the esophagus, stomach, pancreas, and duodenum proximal to ampulla of Vater, as well as the lower respiratory tract) are frequently associated with deletions and mutations of the *MEN1* gene and loss of LOH of 11q, but only rarely harbor *TP53* or K-*ras* mutations (257–260). Midgut tumors (involving the duodenum distal to the ampulla of Vater, jejunum, ileum, cecum, appendix, and proximal portion of the transverse colon) show an increased frequency of chromosome 18 and 16q loss, but less frequently show mutations of *MEN1* or LOH of 11q, and rarely harbor *TP53* or K-*ras* mutations (255,256,259–261). Hindgut neuroendocrine tumors (involving the distal transverse colon, descending colon, sigmoid, rectum, and superior portion of the anal canal) frequently develop through an autocrine mechanism that involves transforming growth factor-α and the epidermal growth factor receptor (255,256). Different patterns of altered expression of β-catenin, E-cadherin, and other proteins resulting from epigenetic modifications rather than mutations are also characteristic of the different groups of carcinoid tumors (256,262,263).

Genetics

MEN1 gene

Multiple endocrine neoplasia type 1 (MEN1) syndrome is characterized by foregut neuroendocrine tumors, parathyroid hyperplasia, and pituitary adenomas and is due to mutations in the *MEN1* gene at 11q13 (264). Germline mutations in *MEN1* are present in about 80% of MEN1 families, and are also present in about 80% of patients who present with clinical features diagnostic of MEN1 but who do not have a family history of the syndrome (sporadic MEN1). The *MEN1* gene encodes the protein menin,

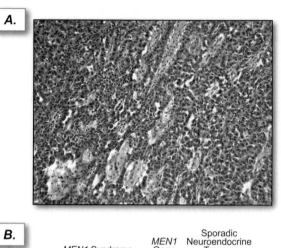

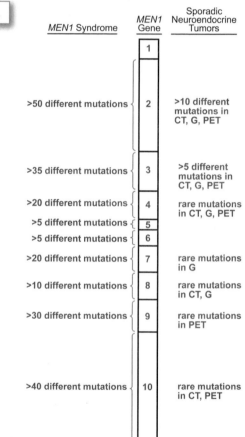

Figure 15.6 Mutations in the *MEN1* gene are associated with foregut neuroendocrine tumors. **A**, A well-differentiated neuroendocrine neoplasm (islet cell tumor) arising in the tail of the pancreas in a man with *MEN1* syndrome. Panel **B**, Schematic diagram of the *MEN1* gene; the 10 exons are labeled. The location of germline mutations associated with the MEN1 syndrome is shown on the left of the figure; the location of somatic mutations associated with sporadic tumors is shown on the right. CT, carcinoid tumor; G, gastinoma; PET, pancreatic endocrine tumor. The types of mutations in sporadic tumors include truncating mutations (frame shift, splice site, and nonsense mutations), missense mutations, and in-frame insertions and deletions. (Compiled from references 264–266.)

which has no significant homology to any other protein but is thought to function as a tumor suppressor. As shown in Figure 15.6, hundreds of unique germline mutations have been identified in hereditary cases and sporadic cases of the MEN1 syndrome, including missense mutations, in-frame deletions, and truncating mutations resulting from nonsense mutations, frameshift mutations, or splice site mutations.

Somatic *MEN1* mutations are also present in a significant percentage of sporadic foregut and midgut neuroendocrine tumors. Overall, about 17% of sporadic foregut tumors and about 15% of sporadic midgut tumors harbor *MEN1* mutations (267). Among foregut tumors, about 33% of gastrinomas (268,269) and about 17% of insulinomas (268) harbor *MEN1* mutations, and in most cases the mutations are associated with LOH of 11q13 (267). However, because up to 2 to 3 times as many sporadic tumors harbor 11q13 LOH as *MEN1* gene mutations, other tumor-suppressor genes in the vicinity of *MEN1*, undetected *MEN1* mutations, or epigenetic inactivation of intact *MEN1* alleles must also play a role in tumorigenesis (264,267).

Other Predisposing Loci

Mutations in the *NF1* gene, which encodes the protein neurofibromin, are responsible for neurofibromatosis type 1 (NF1, or von Recklinghausen disease), and patients who suffer from NF1 have an increased risk of periampullary neoplasms, most commonly somatostatinoma (3,270,271). Mutations in the *VHL* gene cause von Hippel-Lindau syndrome, in which about 10% of patients develop pancreatic islet cell tumors (272). There are still other familial neuroendocrine tumor syndromes in which the underlying molecular abnormality has not been characterized, including familial insulinoma (273), as well as familial carcinoid involving the duodomen, terminal ileum, or appendix (274–276).

Role of Molecular Genetic Analysis of Neuroendocrine Tumors

The morphology and immunoprofile of neuroendocrine tumors are pathognomonic, and so there is no established role for molecular genetic analysis in their diagnosis. In addition, phenotypic features such as invasiveness do not seem to correlate with specific mutations, at least for tumors associated with germline or somatic *MEN1* mutations (264,277). Even though oligonucleotide microarrays have been used to identify a number of different genes whose expression is altered in neuroendocrine neoplasms of the pancreas versus normal islet cells, no clinical role for such analysis has yet been demonstrated (278).

Although there is no role for mutational analysis of individual loci in the diagnosis of neuroendocrine tumor, there may be a role for testing to exclude hereditary disease in the setting of sporadic MEN1 syndrome because as noted previously, up to 80% of patients with sporadic MEN1 syndrome harbor germline mutations in *MEN1*. However, testing in this scenario does not have the urgency of germline testing in other multiple endocrine neoplasia syndromes such as MEN2A or MEN2B because a positive test result, even though it has significant health implications for both the patient and the patient's family, does not mandate a specific intervention (264).

Evaluation of Composite Versus Collision Tumors

Mixed endocrine-exocrine tumors have been described in several locations of the gut, including the stomach, small intestine, and large intestine. Mutational analysis of *TP53* and LOH analysis of microsatellite loci can be used to ascertain whether such tumors represent composite or collision tumors, if clinically required. It is interesting to note that virtually all mixed endocrine-exocrine tumors thus far evaluated represent monoclonal neoplasms with divergent differentiation (279,280).

LYMPHOMA

Primary lymphomas of the gastrointestinal tract make up only about 1% to 4% of all gastrointestinal malignancies, although the gastrointestinal tract is the site of 15% to 20% of all extranodal lymphomas (281). Molecular analysis of lymphoid infiltrates has historically been performed by Southern hybridization using probes for the immunoglobulin heavy-chain genes or T-cell antigen receptor genes. However, the utility of Southern hybridization in routine clinical practice is limited by the requirement for a relatively large sample of unfixed tissue; by one estimate, a tissue fragment 30-fold larger than the standard gastrointestinal biopsy would be required to yield the quantity of DNA required for analysis (282). Most analysis of lymphoid infiltrates performed on gastrointestinal biopsy specimens is therefore performed by PCR.

B-Cell Lymphomas

PCR-based testing is performed using a nested or seminested approach with consensus primers to the V and J regions of the *IgH* locus. Several factors limit test performance on a purely technical level. First, even when amplifiable DNA is present, sensitivity is critically dependent on primer design. Individual primer pairs can detect only about 95% of V and J regions, so multiple primer sets are required to achieve optimum test sensitivity (Chapter 13). The lack of standardized primer sets often complicates interpretation of the experimental results reported by different investigators (283,284). Second, because there are no standard criteria to determine whether or not a dominant amplicon represents a monoclonal population, there is interobserver variability in the interpretation of the electrophoretic profiles even when evaluated by quantitative methods (283,285). Third, as a result of dilutional effects, analysis based on a very low quantity of input DNA is more likely to yield pseudo-clonal bands (286,287) and is also more likely to miss true clonal B-cell populations (283,284).

The biologic features of lymphoid infiltrates limit the diagnostic specificity of the assay even when a monoclonal B-cell population is identified because demonstration of a monoclonal population is not synonymous with the presence of a malignant B-cell population (288,289). Monoclonal infiltrates have been documented in cases of chronic active gastritis (290), in the lymphoid infiltrates associated with carcinoma (291,292), and even in benign lymphoid tissues (293,294). Normal physiologic antigen-specific responses can also generate small clonal B-cell populations (283,284).

The ways in which these sensitivity and specificity issues affect routine testing are illustrated by the application of PCR analysis to the evaluation of gastric lymphoid infiltrates in either gastric biopsies or gastric washings (283,295). Monoclonal B-cell clones can be detected by PCR in 63% to 88% of patients with histologically proven mucosa-associated lymphoid tissue (MALT) lymphoma (283,296,297) as well as 1% to 85% of gastric biopsies from patients without B-cell lymphoma (reviewed in reference 285). Some studies have also demonstrated that monoclonal B-cell populations remain detectable for several years by PCR in follow-up biopsies of patients with MALT lymphoma who are histologically in complete remission after successful eradication of *Helicobacter pylori* infection (285,298) (it is unknown whether or not patients with persistent evidence of a monoclonal population are at a higher risk for disease relapse). Consequently, most, but not all, authors agree that the presence of B-cell monoclonality based on PCR analysis alone is insufficient to assign a diagnosis of malignancy, and that although PCR results may raise the index of suspicion, a definitive diagnosis requires clear histologic proof of lymphoma (283–285).

T-cell Lymphomas

T-cell lymphomas of the gastrointestinal tract occur less frequently than B-cell lymphomas, but have a worse prognosis (299); the most common subtype is enteropathy-type intestinal T-cell lymphoma (EITCL). Histologically, EITCL shows an increased number of intraepithelial T lymphocytes (IEL), with villous atrophy, crypt hyperplasia, and an increased number of IEL adjacent to or even distant from the primary tumor site (300). Consequently, it is often difficult to distinguish villous atrophy that results from a number of other unrelated disorders from EITCL (300,301).

PCR-based testing using consensus primers to the V and J regions of the T-cell receptor γ (TCRγ) chain gene has been used to detect the presence of clonal rearrangements as an aid in the diagnosis of EITCL. This approach is subject to many of the same technical limitations discussed previously for PCR-based B-cell clonality assays, and so it is not surprising that test sensitivity is as low as 54%, although detection of a clonal T-cell population is apparently virtually 100% specific for the presence of EITCL (300). In fact, the high test specificity has been used to support the view that the presence of clonal T-cell populations in refractory celiac sprue (defined as celiac disease–like enteropathy that does not respond to a gluten-free diet) is an indication that the disease represents a cryptic stage of EITCL in which the neoplastic cell population is spread diffusely throughout the gastrointestinal tract and peripheral blood (302).

MESENCHYMAL TUMORS

Gastrointestinal Stromal Tumor

Gastrointestinal stromal tumor (GIST) is the most common nonepithelial tumor of the gastrointestinal tract. The tumor is of mesenchymal origin, and is thought to be

derived from the interstitial cells of Cajal. The stomach is the most common site for GIST, followed by the small intestine, rectum, and colon. Tumor size and mitotic rate are used to assess the risk of metastasis, but it is notoriously difficult to predict the behavior of GIST based on pathologic features (303–305).

Approximately 85% of GIST harbor a gain-of-function mutation in the c-*kit* gene. C-*kit* encodes the KIT receptor tyrosine kinase that is normally activated when it binds stem cell factor (306). In GIST, the activating mutations in c-*kit* occur in exons 9, 11, 13, and 17, which encode the extracellular, juxtamembrane, tyrosine kinase I, and tyrosine kinase II domains, respectively, of the kit protein (Fig. 15.7). The role of c-*kit* mutations in the tumorigenesis of GIST is emphasized by the observation that individuals from kindreds with germline c-*kit* mutations are at high risk for developing multiple GISTs (307–312).

About 30% to 40% of GISTs that do not have mutations in c-*kit* harbor gain-of-function mutations in the related *PDGFRA* gene that encodes the platelet-derived growth factor receptor α tyrosine kinase (313,314). The activating mutations in *PDGFRA* occur in exons 12, 14, and 18, which encode the juxtamembrane, tyrosine kinase I, and tyrosine kinase II domains, respectively, of the PDGFRA protein (313–316) (Fig. 15.7).

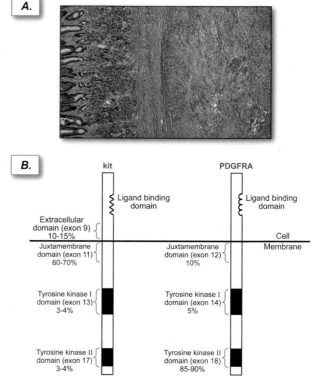

Figure 15.7 Mutations of c-*kit* and *PDGFRA* are characteristic of gastrointestinal stromal tumor (GIST). **A**, A GIST arising in the wall of the stomach of a 57-year-old woman; the tumor showed strong, diffuse kit (CD117) immunoreactivity. **B**, Schematic diagram of the distribution of gain-of-function mutations in the kit and PDGFRA cell surface receptors. About 85% of GIST harbor gain-of-functions mutations in c-*kit*; about 30% to 40% of the remainder harbor gain-of-function mutations in *PDGFRA*. Note that mutations in c-*kit* and *PDGFRA* occur in exons that encode analogous regions of the receptors.

Technical Issues in Molecular Genetic Analysis of GIST

Because the activating mutations in c-kit and PDGFRA include missense mutations, small in-frame insertions and deletions, and small deletions at intron and exon boundaries (303,313–319), the mutations can only be efficiently detected by DNA sequence analysis. For mutational analysis, individual exons are amplified by PCR from genomic DNA, followed either by direct DNA sequence analysis of the PCR products (Fig. 7.3) (320), or of only those samples shown to harbor mutations by screening SSCP or denaturing high-pressure liquid chromatography (315,316,321–323). Several studies have shown that mutational analysis can easily be performed on DNA extracted from FFPE tissue.

Diagnostic and Prognostic Issues in Molecular Genetic Analysis of GIST

The phenotypic and immunohistochemical features of GIST, together with the clinical setting of the tumor, are usually sufficient for diagnosis without the need for molecular genetic analysis. Recent data suggest that specific mutations correlate with tumor phenotype; for example, GISTs with PDGFRA mutations typically have an epithelial morphology, are more likely to involve the stomach, and often show a lack of c-kit expression by immunohistochemical staining (315,316,321–323), whereas GISTs with internal tandem duplications at the 3' end of exon 11 of c-kit are more likely to involve the stomach (317,325). However, mutations in c-kit or PDGFRA are not strongly correlated with the biologic potential of individual GISTs. The accumulated data show that c-kit mutations are not preferentially present in high-grade tumors, but can also be found in small incidental tumors and tumors that have a benign course (318,320,323,326). Similarly, mutational analysis of PDGFRA cannot be used to predict the behavior of individual GISTs, although, as a group, tumors with PDGFRA mutations may be associated with a better clinical outcome (322,324).

Recent studies suggest that telomere metabolism may be a more reliable indicator of the biologic potential of GIST than the pattern of mutations in c-kit or PDGFRA. Expression of human telomerase reverse transcriptase (hTERT) measured by immunohistochemistry or RT-PCR is correlated with malignant behavior (327,328), as is expression of human telomerase RNA component (hTR) as measured by RT-PCR (328), and telomerase activity as measured by the TRAP assay (329). However, whether or not molecular evaluation of telomere metabolism offers independent, clinically relevant prognostic or therapeutic information that should be incorporated into patient management remains to be evaluated in formal prospective trials.

Therapeutic Issues in Molecular Genetic Analysis of GIST

Even though mutational analysis of c-kit and PDGFRA does not provide prognostic information, it may still be important from a therapeutic standpoint. Imatinib mesylate (Gleevec), an inhibitor of both the kit and PDGFRA receptor tyrosine kinases (330), has been shown to be effective for treating patients with GIST (331–334). However, consistent with in vitro studies that have shown that the degree of receptor inhibition depends on which functional domain is mutated (335,336), the clinical response to the drug differs among patients. Based on the results of recent phase I and phase II trials of the drug in both the United States and Europe (337,338), patients whose tumor harbors a c-kit mutation in exon 11 have a higher clinical response rate and better overall survival than patients whose tumor harbors either wild-type c-kit or c-kit mutated in exon 9 or exon 17. Similarly, different mutations in PDGFRA are associated with different responses to imatimib therapy (313,337,338); although only a small number of patients have thus far been evaluated, GISTs with mutations in exon 18 (including the most common missense mutation, D842V) seem to be intrinsically imatimib resistant. Consequently, mutational analysis of GIST may become a routine part of the pathologic evaluation of GIST to determine whether a patient is likely to benefit from imatinib chemotherapy or should instead be treated with a tyrosine kinase inhibitor that has a different profile of target enzyme inhibition (339).

Other Mesenchymal Tumors

A number of other spindle cell neoplasms that characteristically involve the soft tissue also occur as primary neoplasms of the gastrointestinal tract. For example, synovial sarcoma has been described as a primary malignancy of the esophagus, stomach, and jejunum (340–342), and inflammatory myofibroblastic tumor has been described as a primary neoplasm of the gastroesophageal junction, stomach, small intestine, pancreas, and hepatobiliary system (343–347). Malignant round cell tumors also occur as primary malignancies of the gastrointestinal tract. Ewing sarcoma/peripheral neuroectodermal tumor has been described in the duodenum, ileum, rectum, hepatobiliary tract, and pancreas (348–354). Primary desmoplastic small round cell tumor of the stomach and pancreas has been reported (355,356), as has primary alveolar soft part sarcoma of the stomach (357). Even primary clear cell sarcomas of the gastrointestinal tract have been described (reviewed in 358). The issues involved in the molecular genetic evaluation of these neoplasms are the same regardless of whether they occur primarily in the gastrointestinal tract or soft tissue (Chapter 11).

DISEASES OF THE LIVER

Hepatocellular Carcinoma

The etiologic risk factors for hepatocellular carcinoma (HCC) include hepatitis B or hepatitis C viral infection, dietary aflatoxin B_1 exposure, and chronic alcohol consumption. As with other gastrointestinal malignancies, HCC has a multistep pattern of oncogenesis (3,359,360), and although the early molecular steps in the development of HCC are not well defined, the genetic mechanisms by which the different etiologic risk factors contribute to oncogenesis are beginning to emerge.

Etiology

Hepatitis B Infection

Hepatitis B virus (HBV) is thought to have a direct oncogenic effect via structural aberrations that are associated with integration of the viral DNA into chromosomal DNA, including translocations, deletions, and inverted duplications (359,361). For some of the chromosomal rearrangements, the oncogenic link is evident, as for example aberrations that produce LOH of 17p (the location of the tumor suppressor gene *TP53*), although the mechanism by which many other rearrangements promote tumor development is not as clear. HBV also has a direct oncogenic effect through some of its encoded proteins. For example, the hepatitis B virus X protein not only inhibits nucleotide excision repair (362) but also inhibits *TP53* regulation of transcriptional activity and apoptosis, thereby increasing genomic instability and disrupting control of the cell cycle (359,363,364).

Hepatitis C Infection

There is no evidence that hepatitis C virus (HCV) integrates into the cellular DNA or has any other direct role in the development of the genetic abnormalities that lead to HCC. Instead, the chronic liver injury that results from HCV infection is thought to lead to increased cellular proliferation with selective clonal expansion of cells that contain growth-promoting mutations, with progression through fibrosis and cirrhosis to HCC (359,360).

Alcohol

Although there is significant individual variability, regular daily consumption of ethanol (>50 grams for women, >80 for men) induces liver cirrhosis and is the most important risk factor for HCC among Western populations (365). Even though ethanol does not apparently have a direct role in the molecular pathogenesis of HCC, abuse promotes the development of HCC through chronic liver injury that progresses to cirrhosis. It is therefore not surprising that patients who abuse alcohol and have coexisting liver disease, especially HCV, have the highest risk for developing HCC (366,367).

Aflatoxin B1

Aflatoxin B1(AFB1) is produced by *Aspergillus parasiticus* and *Aspergillus flavus*, both of which typically contaminate grain (particularly peanuts) under hot and humid conditions, usually in tropical countries. Cytochrome P450 metabolism converts AFB1 to a reactive intermediate, which preferentially reacts with guanine (Fig. 2.5). In the liver, the end result is a selective G→T transversion in codon 249 of the *TP53* gene that results in an arginine to serine substitution in p53 (368,369), a mutation that provides hepatocytes with a selective growth advantage (364,370). The risk of developing HCC is markedly increased in patients who have a high dietary exposure to AFB1 and coexisting chronic HCV infection.

Genetics

In patients with HBV infection, cirrhotic nodules have clonal patterns of viral DNA integration (371). Analysis of HCC that emerges as a so-called nodule-in-nodule has shown that the early and advanced components of the tumor usually harbor an identical integration pattern of HBV (372,373), as well as a pattern of *TP53* mutations indicative of tumor progression (374,375). Genomewide gene expression profiles show that HCC harbors a set of genetic changes that seem to overlie the pattern found in cirrhotic nodules (360). Taken together, these experimental observations support a multistep model of HCC oncogenesis in which liver injury resulting from viral hepatitis, environmental carcinogens, or alcohol causes chronic injury and regeneration, producing cirrhotic nodules and eventually HCC. During regeneration, hepatocytes that have accumulated inactivating mutations in tumor suppressor genes or activating mutations in oncogenes have a selective growth advantage, producing expanded clones of cells which are at risk for acquisition of additional mutations that provide further growth advantages, and so on, until a fully development HCC emerges (3,359).

Diagnostic and Prognostic Issues in Molecular Genetic Analysis of HCC

Given that the oncogenesis of HCC is a multistep process, it is not surprising that genetic analysis of individual genes cannot be used to reliably differentiate cirrhotic or displastic nodules from early well-differentiated hepatocellular carcinoma. However, molecular testing does have diagnostic applications in some settings. For example, both comparative genomic hybridization (Chapter 6) and identity determination based on analysis of highly polymorphic short tandem repeat loci (Chapter 23) have been used to differentiate primary from recurrent HCC (376–378), a difference that has therapeutic implications.

Molecular testing may also have a role for predicting prognosis. For example, high levels of mRNA encoding the $VEGF_{165}$ isoform correlate with a significant risk of HCC recurrence-related mortality (379), RT-PCR–based detection of transcripts encoding survivin mRNA is significantly associated with a worse clinical outcome (380), and the presence of *TP53* mutations is associated with a statistically significantly decrease in patient survival (381). However, the sensitivity of all these tests is limited because a significant percentage of HCC lacks mutations at the target loci.

Oligonucleotide microarray analysis of the genomewide profile of gene expression has great potential from both a diagnostic and prognostic perspective. Gene-expression profiling has identified patterns of gene expression that are associated with progression of precancerous lesions (382), HCC metastasis (383,384), and HCC recurrence (385). In one study, a group of 406 genes was identified that predicted faster tumor progression and decreased survival regardless of whether HBV, HCV, or nonviral causes were associated with the tumor's development (386). It is interesting to note that the identity of the genes in the predictive group suggests that it is the underlying proliferative and apoptotic rates of HCC that are critical for predicting prognosis, a finding consistent with the fact that traditional histopathologic evaluation of the number of apoptotic cells (as determined by direct counting) and rate of cell proliferation (as measured by Ki-67 immunohistochemistry) can be used to predict prognosis (386–388).

Gene expression analysis has been used to identify cohorts of genes that are associated with the response of HCC to specific chemotherapeutic regimens such as 5-FU and cisplatin (389,390). This result implies that microarray profiling may eventually be of use for optimizing the chemotherapeutic regimen of individual patients, although gene expression analysis is not yet a routine part of the pathologic evaluation of HCC.

Molecular Genetic Analysis for Detection of Submicroscopic Disease

Genetic analysis of individual markers in peripheral blood has been evaluated for its role in diagnostic or prognostic testing of HCC, with mixed results. For example, the presence of transcripts encoding alpha fetoprotein (AFP) detected by RT-PCR cannot be used to reliably predict which patients with compensated cirrhosis will develop HCC (391), but may have a role for predicting tumor recurrence in patients who have undergone curative resection for HCC (392–395). Similarly, RT-PCR detection of mRNA encoding VEGF$_{165}$ in preoperative peripheral blood has been shown to correlate with the risk of HCC recurrence and recurrence-related mortality (396), although the low predictive value of either a positive or negative result limits the utility of the analysis.

Hepatocellular Lymphoepithelial-Like Carcinoma

Lymphoepithelial-like carcinoma (LELC) is a rare hepatic tumor. The tumor is an undifferentiated carcinoma accompanied by an intense lymphocytic infiltrate that is morphologically similar to nasopharyngeal carcinoma and LELCs that arise in other visceral sites and are typically associated with Epstein-Barr virus (EBV) (Fig. 22.7) (397–401). However, EBV has been convincingly demonstrated in only a single case of hepatocellular LELC (397); this EBV-positive case had a rapidly fatal course, in contrast to the improved 5-year survival and higher rates of spontaneous regression that are characteristic of hepatocellular carcinomas with abundant lymphoid stroma that lack EBV association (402). Analysis of additional cases is required to determine whether the presence of EBV is, in fact, a marker for worse prognosis in hepatocellular LELC or HCC with an abundant lymphoid stroma, but the analysis should be straightforward because in situ hybridization or PCR-based testing for EBV can be easily performed on both FFPE and fresh tissue.

Angiosarcoma

Hepatic angiosarcoma is a rare tumor, and approximately 75% of cases cannot be associated with a specific underlying etiology (403). However, about 25% of cases arise in a background of cirrhosis or in patients who have a history of exposure to vinyl chloride, thorium dioxide (Thorotrast), or arsenic.

Approximately half of hepatic angiosarcomas associated with occupational exposure to vinyl chloride harbor TP53 mutations and over 80% harbor K-ras mutations; in both genes, the mutations are transitions as well as transversions consistent with the fact that vinyl chloride exerts its mutagenic effect through adduct formation (404–406). K-ras point mutations are present in 40% to 83% of thorium dioxide–induced hepatic angiosarcomas, primarily single bp transitions consistent with the fact that thorium dioxide produces oxidative DNA damage (405,406). Hepatic angiosarcomas not associated with occupational exposure to a known carcinogen show a P53 mutation in only 9% of cases, and a K-ras mutation in only 26% of cases (405,407). Whether deregulation of MDM2 expression can serve as an alternative mechanism for escape from p53-regulated growth control in hepatic angiosarcomas, as has been demonstrated for angiosarcomas of soft tissue and visceral sites, remains to be determined (408). Similarly, the role of increased VEGF expression in the genesis of hepatic angiosarcoma also remains to be determined, although it has been demonstrated in nearly 80% of sporadic soft tissue and visceral angiosarcomas (408).

Despite the basic science observations that link TP53, K-ras, MDM2, and VEGF aberrations to the pathogenesis of angiosarcoma, the role of molecular genetic analysis to detect mutations or altered expression of these genes has not been established. From a diagnostic point of view, testing has limited sensitivity because mutations in these genes are present in only a subset of tumors. Similarly, there is no evidence that specific mutations correlate with clinical outcome, so testing also seems to be of little value prognostically.

Viral Hepatitis

In routine practice, acute or chronic HCV infection is diagnosed by elevated serum aspartate aminotransferase and alanine aminotransferase levels, enzyme-linked immunosorbent assay (ELISA) for antiviral antibodies, and the presence of HCV RNA in serum. Although a liver biopsy is required to grade and stage the hepatitis, a biopsy is usually not obtained for diagnosis. Nonetheless, ambiguous or negative serum test results occasionally make it necessary to evaluate a liver biopsy to provide definitive evidence of ongoing HCV infection. For example, immunocompromised liver transplant recipients may be unable to mount an immune response, and analysis of a liver biopsy specimen from these patients can confirm reinfection of the allograft. Likewise, a subset of immunocompetent patients who are seropositive for anti-HCV antibody show no evidence of HCV RNA in their serum, and although some of these patients may have cleared the infection, in others the viral RNA may simply be below the level of detection (409).

Both RT-PCR and ISH methods have been used to detect HCV in liver biopsy specimens. Both methods focus on the 5'-noncoding region of the virus which is highly conserved between the (at least) 6 genotypes and more than 90 subtypes of HCV that have been described worldwide (410). Direct comparison of the RT-PCR and ISH has shown excellent agreement between the two approaches (411).

To achieve maximal sensitivity, testing for HCV via RT-PCR typically employs either a nested RT-PCR approach or RT-PCR followed by Southern hybridization to detect the PCR products. By either method, HCV can be detected in 70% to 100% of excised liver tissue or needle biopsy specimens from patients who are serum antibody positive (409,411,412) and in about 50% of patients who are serum antibody negative (411). Both RT-PCR approaches can be performed on FFPE tissue (409), but the nested RT-PCR method is more clinically useful because it avoids the extra time and expense of Southern blotting. Although an in situ RT-PCR approach has been described (413), the technique has too low a sensitivity to be of diagnostic use.

In patients with suspected HCV infection, ISH using a riboprobe (Chapter 6) against the genomic RNA strand of the virus is positive in 95% of liver biopsy specimens from patients who are serum antibody positive and in 50% of biopsy specimens from patients who are serum antibody negative (411). Although production of the riboprobe adds an additional step to this testing approach, two technical factors increase the method's utility in routine practice. First, the analysis is performed using probes that can be detected via a chromogenic reaction (eliminating the cumbersome and expensive safety procedures associated with the use of probes labeled with a radioisotope), and second, the analysis can be performed on FFPE tissue.

Although diagnostic testing for HCV infection relies on detection of the virus's highly conserved 5'-noncoding region, analysis of viral sequences specific for individual genotypes and subtypes can also be performed (414). This more detailed analysis has a role in some specialized settings, for example, establishing the provenance of liver biopsy specimens (415), but has no role in routine testing.

REFERENCES

1. http://www.cancer.org/docroot/HOME/pro/pro_0.asp?level=0.
2. Kinzler KW, Vogelstein B. Colorectal tumors. In: Vogelstein B, Kinzler KW, eds. *The Genetic Basis of Human Cancer*, 2nd ed. New York: McGraw Hill; 2002:583–612.
3. Hamilton SR, Aaltonen LA, eds. *Pathology and Genetics of Tumours of the Digestive System.* Lyon: IARC Press; 2000.
4. de la Chapelle A. Genetic predisposition to colorectal cancer. *Nat Rev Cancer* 2004;4:769–780.
5. Feron ER, Vogelstein B. A genetic model for colorectal tumorigenesis. *Cell* 1990;61:759–767.
6. Vogelstein B, Kinzler KW. The multistep nature of cancer. *Trends Genet* 1993;9:138–141.
7. Guanti G, Resta N, Simone C, et al. Involvement of PTEN mutations in the genetic pathways of colorectal cancerogenesis. *Hum Mol Genet* 2000;9:283–287.
8. Osako T, Miyahara M, Uchino S, et al. Immunohistochemical study of c-erbB-2 protein in colorectal cancer and the correlation with patient survival. *Oncology* 1998;55:548–555.
9. Kakisako K, Miyahara M, Uchino S, et al. Prognostic significance of c-myc mRNA expression assessed by semi-quantitative RT-PCR in patients with colorectal cancer. *Oncol Rep* 1998;5:441–445.
10. Iravani S, Mao W, Fu L, et al. Elevated c-Src protein expression is an early event in colonic neoplasia. *Lab Invest* 1998;78:365–371.
11. Polakis P, Hart M, Rubinfeld B. Defects in the regulation of beta-catenin in colorectal cancer. *Adv Exp Med Biol* 1999;470:23–32.
12. Klymkowsky MW. Beta-catenin and its regulatory network. *Hum Pathol* 2005;36:225–227.
13. Kinzler KW, Vogelstein B. Lessons from hereditary colorectal cancer. *Cell* 1996;87:159–170.
14. Lengauer C, Kinzler KW, Vogelstein B. Genetic instabilities in human cancers. *Nature* 1998;396:643–649.
15. Lothe RA, Peltomaki P, Meling GI, et al. Genomic instability in colorectal cancer: relationship to clinicopathological variables and family history. *Cancer Res* 1993;53:5849–5852.
16. Rajagopalan H, Jallepalli PV, Rago C, et al. Inactivation of hCDC4 can cause chromosomal instability. *Nature* 2004;428:77–81.
17. Rajagopalan H, Lengauer C. Aneuploidy and cancer. *Nature* 2004;432:338–341.
18. Gryfe R, Kim H, Hsieh ET, et al. Tumor microsatellite instability and clinical outcome in young patients with colorectal cancer. *N Engl J Med* 2000;342:69–77.
19. Xiong Z, Wu AH, Bender CM, et al. Mismatch repair deficiency and CpG island hypermethylation in sporadic colon adenocarcinomas. *Cancer Epidemiol Biomarkers Prev* 2001;10:799–803.
20. Yuen ST, Chan TL, Ho JW, et al. Germline, somatic and epigenetic events underlying mismatch repair deficiency in colorectal and HNPCC-related cancers. *Oncogene* 2002;21:7585–7592.
21. de la Chapelle A. Microsatellite instability. *N Engl J Med* 2003;349:209–210.
22. Jass JR, Whitehall VL, Young J, et al. Emerging concepts in colorectal neoplasia. *Gastroenterology* 2002;123:862–876.
23. Yamamoto H, Sawai H, Weber TK, et al. Somatic frameshift mutations in DNA mismatch repair and proapoptosis genes in hereditary nonpolyposis colorectal cancer. *Cancer Res* 1998;58:997–1003.
24. Miquel C, Borrini F, Grandjouan S, et al. Role of bax mutations in apoptosis in colorectal cancers with microsatellite instability. *Am J Clin Pathol* 2005;123:562–570.
25. Markowitz S, Wang J, Myeroff L, et al. Inactivation of the type II TGF-beta receptor in colon cancer cells with microsatellite instability. *Science* 1995;268:1336–1338.
26. Souza RF, Appel R, Yin J, et al. Microsatellite instability in the insulin-like growth factor II receptor gene in gastrointestinal tumours. *Nat Genet* 1996;14:255–257.
27. Lee S, Hwang KS, Lee HJ, et al. Aberrant CpG island hypermethylation of multiple genes in colorectal neoplasia. *Lab Invest* 2004;84:884–893.
28. Jubb AM, Bell SM, Quirke P. Methylation and colorectal cancer. *J Pathol* 2001;195:111–134.
29. Chiriac LR, Shen L, Catalano PJ, et al. Phenotype of microsatellite-stable colorectal carcinomas with CpG island methylation. *Am J Surg Pathol* 2005;29:429–436.
30. Sifri R, Gangadharappa S, Acheson LS. Identifying and testing for hereditary susceptibility to common cancers. *CA Cancer J Clin* 2004;54:309–326.
31. Nagase H, Nakamura Y. Mutations of the APC (adenomatous polyposis coli) gene. *Hum Mutat* 1993;2:425–434.
32. Laken SJ, Papadopoulos N, Petersen GM, et al. Analysis of masked mutations in familial adenomatous polyposis. *Proc Natl Acad Sci USA* 1999;96:2322–2326.
33. de Chadarevian JP, Dunn S, Malatack JJ, et al. Chromosome rearrangement with no apparent gene mutation in familial adenomatous polyposis and hepatocellular neoplasia. *Pediatr Dev Pathol* 2002;5:69–75.
34. Olschwant S, Tiret A, Laurent-Puig P, et al. Restriction of ocular fundus lesions to a specific subgroup of APC mutations in adenomatous polyposis coli patients. *Cell* 1993;75:959–968.
35. Wallis YL, Macdonald F, Hulten M, et al. Genotype-phenotype correlation between position of constitutional APC gene mutation and CHRPE expression in familial adenomatous polyposis. *Hum Genet* 1994;94:543–548.
36. Caspari R, Olschwang S, Friedl W, et al. Familial adenomatous polyposis: desmoid tumours and lack of ophthalmic lesions (CHRPE) associated with APC mutations beyond codon 1444. *Hum Mol Genet* 1995;4:337–340.
37. Friedl W, Meuschel S, Caspari R, et al. Attenuated familial adenomatous polyposis due to a mutation in the 3' part of the APC gene: a clue for understanding the function of the APC protein. *Hum Genet* 1996;97:579–584.
38. Soravia C, Berk T, Madlensky L, et al. Genotype-phenotype correlations in attenuated adenomatous polyposis coli. *Am J Hum Genet* 1998;62:1290–1301.
39. Brensinger JD, Laken SJ, Luce MC, et al. Variable phenotype of familial adenomatous polyposis in pedigrees with 3' mutation in the APC gene. *Gut* 1998;43:548–552.
40. Laken SJ, Petersen GM, Gruber SB, et al. Familial colorectal cancer in Ashkenazim due to a hypermutable tract in APC. *Nat Genet* 1997;17:79–83.
41. Sieber OM, Lipton L, Crabtree M, et al. Multiple colorectal adenomas, classic adenomatous polyposis, and germ-line mutations in MYH. *N Engl J Med* 2003;348:791–799.
42. Al-Tassan N, Chmiel NH, Maynard J, et al. Inherited variants of MYH associated with somatic G:C—> T:A mutations in colorectal tumors. *Nat Genet* 2002;30:227–232.
43. Jones S, Emmerson P, Maynard J, et al. Biallelic germline mutations in MYH predispose to multiple colorectal adenoma and somatic G:C—>T:A mutations. *Hum Mol Genet* 2002;11:2961–2967.
44. Marra G, Jiricny J. Multiple colorectal adenomas: is their number up? *N Engl J Med* 2003;348:845–847.
45. Vasen HF, Watson P, Mecklin JP, et al. New clinical criteria for hereditary nonpolyposis colorectal cancer (HNPCC, Lynch syndrome) proposed by the International Collaborative group on HNPCC. *Gastroenterology* 1999;116:1453–1456.
46. Umar A, Boland CR, Terdiman JP, et al. Revised Bethesda Guidelines for hereditary nonpolyposis colorectal cancer (Lynch syndrome) and microsatellite instability. *Natl Cancer Inst* 2004;96:261–268.
47. Umar A, Risinger JI, Hawk ET, et al. Testing guidelines for hereditary non-polyposis colorectal cancer. *Nat Rev Cancer* 2004;4:153–158.
48. Lynch HT, de la Chapelle A. Hereditary colorectal cancer. *N Engl J Med* 2003;348:919–932.
49. Hanna NN, Mentzer RM Jr. Molecular genetics and management strategies in hereditary cancer syndromes. *J Ky Med Assoc* 2003;101:100–107.
50. Lindor NM, Rabe K, Petersen GM, et al. Lower cancer incidence in Amsterdam-I criteria families without mismatch repair deficiency: familial colorectal cancer type X. *JAMA* 2005;293:1979–1985.
51. Liu B, Parsons R, Papadopoulos N, et al. Analysis of mismatch repair genes in hereditary non-polyposis colorectal cancer patients. *Nat Med* 1996;2:169–174.
52. Wang Q, Lasset C, Desseigne F, et al. Prevalence of germline mutations of hMLH1, hMSH2, hPMS1, hPMS2, and hMSH6 genes in 75 French kindreds with nonpolyposis colorectal cancer. *Hum Genet* 1999;105:79–85.
53. Wijnen J, de Leeuw W, Vasen H, et al. Familial endometrial cancer in female carriers of MSH6 germline mutations. *Nat Genet* 1999;23:142–144.
54. Miyaki M, Konishi M, Tanaka K, et al. Germline mutation of MSH6 as the cause of hereditary nonpolyposis colorectal cancer. *Nat Genet* 1997;17:271–272.
55. http://www.insight-group.org/.
56. Casey G, Lindor NM, Papadopoulos N, et al. Conversion analysis for mutation detection in MLH1 and MSH2 in patients with colorectal cancer. *JAMA* 2005;293:799–809.
57. Wagner A, van der Klift H, Franken P, et al. A 10-mb paracentric inversion of chromosome arm 2p inactivates MSH2 and is responsible for hereditary nonpolyposis colorectal cancer in a North-American kindred. *Genes Chromosomes Cancer* 2002;35:49–57.
58. Suter CM, Martin DI, Ward RL. Germline epimutation of MLH1 in individuals with multiple cancers. *Nat Genet* 2004;36:497–501.
59. Müller A, Fishel R. Mismatch repair and the hereditary non-polyposis colorectal cancer syndrome (HNPCC). *Cancer Invest* 2002;20:102–109.
60. Compton CC. Colorectal carcinoma: diagnostic, prognostic, and molecular features. *Mod Pathol* 2003;16:376–388.
61. Greenson JK, Bonner JD, Ben-Yzhak O, et al. Phenotype of microsatellite unstable colorectal carcinomas: Well-differentiated and focally mucinous tumors and the absence of dirty necrosis correlate with microsatellite instability. *Am J Surg Pathol* 2003;27:563–570.

62. Kane MF, Loda M, Gaida GM, et al. Methylation of the *hMLH1* promoter correlates with lack of expression of *hMLH1* in sporadic colon tumors and mismatch repair-defective human tumor cell lines. *Cancer Res* 1997;57:808–811.
63. Herman JG, Umar A, Polyak K, et al. Incidence and functional consequences of *hMLH1* promoter hypermethylation in colorectal carcinoma. *Proc Natl Acad Sci USA* 1998;95: 6870–6875.
64. Cunningham JM, Christensen ER, Tester DJ, et al. Hypermethylation of the *hMLH1* promoter in colon cancer with microsatellite instability. *Cancer Res* 1998;58: 3455–3460.
65. Veigl ML, Kasturi L, Olechnowicz J, et al. Biallelic inactivation of *hMLH1* by epigenetic gene silencing, a novel mechanism causing human MSI cancers. *Proc Natl Acad Sci USA* 1998;95:8698–8702.
66. Roh SA, Kim HC, Kim JS, et al. Characterization of mutator pathway in younger-age-onset colorectal adenocarcinomas. *J Korean Med Sci* 2003;18:387–391.
67. Sugai T, Habano W, Uesugi N, et al. Molecular validation of the modified Vienna classification of colorectal tumors. *J Mol Diagn* 2002;4:191–200.
68. Zauber NP, Wang C, Lee PS, et al. Ki-ras gene mutations, LOH of the *APC* and *DCC* genes, and microsatellite instability in primary colorectal carcinoma are not associated with micrometastases in pericolonic lymph nodes or with patients' survival. *J Clin Pathol* 2004;57:938–942.
69. Fearnhead NS, Britton MP, Bodmer WF. The ABC of *APC*. *Hum Mol Genet* 2001;10:721–733.
70. Kolligs FT, Bommer G, Goke B. Wnt/beta-catenin/tcf signaling: a critical pathway in gastrointestinal tumorigenesis. *Digestion* 2002;66:131–144.
71. McLeod HL, Murray GI. Tumour markers of prognosis in colorectal cancer. *Br J Cancer* 1999;79:191–203.
72. Shibata D, Reale MA, Lavin P, et al. The DCC protein and prognosis in colorectal cancer. *N Engl J Med* 1996;335:1727–1732.
73. Ogunbiyi OA, Goodfellow PJ, Hergarth K, et al. Confirmation that chromosome 18q allelic loss in colon cancer is a prognostic indicator. *J Clin Oncol* 1998;16:427–433.
74. Sankila R, Aaltonen LA, Jarvinen HJ, et al. Better survival rates in patients with *MLH1*-associated hereditary colorectal cancer. *Gastroenterology* 1996;110:682–687.
75. Samowitz WS, Curtin K, Ma KN, et al. Microsatellite instability in sporadic colon cancer is associated with an improved prognosis at the population level. *Cancer Epidemiol Biomarkers Prev* 2001;10:917–923.
76. Compton CC, Fielding LP, Burgart LJ. Prognostic factors in colorectal cancer. College of American Pathologists Consensus Statement 1999. *Arch Pathol Lab Med* 2000;124: 979–994.
77. Compton CC, Fenoglio-Preiser CM, Pettigrew N, et al. American Joint Committee on Cancer Prognostic Factors Consensus Conference: Colorectal Working Group. *Cancer* 2000;88:1739–1757.
78. Wang Y, Jatkoe T, Zhang Y, et al. Gene expression profiles and molecular markers to predict recurrence of Dukes' B colon cancer. *J Clin Oncol* 2004;22:1564–1571.
79. Bertucci F, Salas S, Eysteries S, et al. Gene expression profiling of colon cancer by DNA microarrays and correlation with histoclinical parameters. *Oncogene* 2004;23: 1377–1391.
80. Johnston PG. Of what value genomics in colorectal cancer? Opportunities and challenges. *J Clin Oncol* 2004;22:1538–1539.
81. Mariadason JM, Arango D, Shi Q, et al. Gene expression profiling-based prediction of response of colon carcinoma cells to 5-fluorouracil and camptothecin. *Cancer Res* 2003;63:8791–8812.
82. Huerta S, Harris DM, Jazierehi A, et al. Gene expression profile of metastatic colon cancer cells resistant to cisplatin-induced apoptosis. *Int J Oncol* 2003;22:663–670.
83. American Society of Clinical Oncology. American Society of Clinical Oncology policy statement update: genetic testing for cancer susceptibility. *J Clin Oncol* 2003;21:2397–2406.
84. http://www.genetests.org/servlet/access?id.
85. Veigl ML, Kasturi L, Olechnowicz J, et al. Biallelic inactivation of hMLH1 by epigenetic gene silencing, a novel mechanism causing human MSI cancers. Proc *Natl Acad Sci USA* 1998;95:8698–8702.
86. Herman JG, Umar A, Polyak K, et al. Incidence and functional consequences of *hMLH1* promoter hypermethylation in colorectal carcinoma. *Proc Natl Acad Sci USA* 1998;95:6870–6875.
87. Peltomaki P, Vasen HF. Mutations predisposing to hereditary nonpolyposis colorectal cancer: database and results of a collaborative study. The International Collaborative Group on Hereditary Nonpolyposis Colorectal Cancer. *Gastroenterology* 1997;113:1146–1158.
88. Wijnen J, Vasen H, Meera Khan P, et al. Seven new mutations in *hMSH2*, an HNPCC gene, identified by denaturing gradient-gel electrophoresis. *Am J Hum Genet* 1995;56; 1060–1066.
89. Beck N, Tomlinson I, Homfray T. Use of SSCP analysis to identify germline mutations in HNPCC families fulfilling the Amsterdam criteria. *Hum Genet* 1997;99: 219–224.
90. Boland CR, Thibodeau SN, Hamilton SR, et al. A National Cancer Institute Workshop on microsatellite instability for cancer detection and familial predisposition: development of international criteria for the determination of microsatellite instability in colorectal cancer. *Cancer Res* 1998;58:5248–5257.
91. Wright CL, Stewart ID. Histopathology and mismatch repair status of 458 consecutive colorectal carcinomas. *Am J Surg Pathol* 2003;27:1393–1406.
92. Nash GM, Gimbel M, Shia J, et al. Automated, multiplex assay for high-frequency microsatellite instability in colorectal cancer. *J Clin Oncol* 2003;21:3105–3112.
93. Jover R, Paya A, Alenda C, et al. Defective mismatch-repair colorectal cancer: clinicopathologic characteristics and usefulness of immunohistochemical analysis for diagnosis. *Am J Clin Pathol* 2004;122:389–394.
94. Suraweera N, Duval A, Reperant M, et al. Evaluation of tumor microsatellite instability using five quasimonomorphic mononucleotide repeats and pentaplex PCR. *Gastroenterology* 2002;123:1804–1811.
95. Berg KD, Glaser CL, Thompson RE, et al. Detection of microsatellite instability by fluorescence multiplex polymerase chain reaction. *J Mol Diagn* 2000;2:20–28.
96. Pinol V, Castells A, Andreu M, et al. Accuracy of revised Bethesda guidelines, microsatellite instability, and immunohistochemistry for the identification of patients with hereditary nonpolyposis colorectal cancer. *JAMA* 2005;293:1986–1994.
97. Pan KF, Liu W, Lu YY, et al. High throughput detection of microsatellite instability by denaturing high-performance liquid chromatography. *Hum Mutat* 2003;22:388–394.
98. Muller A, Giuffre G, Bocker Edmonston TB. Challenges and pitfalls in HNPCC screening by microsatellite analysis and immunohistochemistry. *J Mol Diagn* 2004;6:308–3015.
99. Sieben NL, ter Haar NT, Cornelisse CJ, et al. PCR artifacts in LOH and MSI analysis of microdissected tumor cells. *Hum Pathol* 2000;31:1414–1419.
100. Maehara Y, Oda S, Sugimachi K. The instability within: problems in current analyses of microsatellite instability. *Mutat Res* 2001;461:249–263.
101. Lindor NM, Burgart LJ, Leontovich O, et al. Immunohistochemistry versus microsatellite instability testing in phenotyping colorectal tumors. *J Clin Oncol* 2002;20:1043–1048.
102. Cawkwell L, Gray S, Murgatroyd H, et al. Choice of management strategy for colorectal cancer based on a diagnostic immunohistochemical test for defective mismatch repair. *Gut* 1999;45:409–415.
103. Gafa R, Maestri I, Matteuzzi M, et al. Sporadic colorectal adenocarcinomas with high-frequency microsatellite instability. *Cancer* 2000;89:2025–2037.
104. Lanza G, Gafa R, Maestri I, et al. Immunohistochemical pattern of *MLH1/MSH2* expression is related to clinical and pathological features in colorectal adenocarcinomas with microsatellite instability. *Mod Pathol* 2002;15:741–749.
105. Michael-Robinson JM, Biemer-Huttmann A, Purdie DM, et al. Tumour infiltrating lymphocytes and apoptosis are independent features in colorectal cancer stratified according to microsatellite instability status. *Gut* 2001;48:360–366.
106. Stone JG, Robertson D, Houlston RS, et al. Immunohistochemistry for *MSH2* and *MHL1*: a method for identifying mismatch repair deficient colorectal cancer. *J Clin Pathol* 2001;54:484–487.
107. Wahlberg SS, Schmeits J, Thomas G, et al. Evaluation of microsatellite instability and immunohistochemistry for the prediction of germ-line *MSH2* and *MLH1* mutations in hereditary nonpolyposis colon cancer families. *Cancer Res* 2002;62:3485–3492.
108. Paraf F, Gilquin M, Longy M, et al. MLH1 and MSH2 protein immunohistochemistry is useful for detection of hereditary non-polyposis colorectal cancer in young patients. *Histopathology* 2001;39:250–258.
109. Salahshor S, Koelble K, Rubio C, et al. Microsatellite Instability and *hMLH1* and *hMSH2* expression analysis in familial and sporadic colorectal cancer. *Lab Invest* 2001;81:535–541.
110. Chapusot C, Martin L, Puig PL, et al. What is the best way to assess microsatellite instability status in colorectal cancer? Study on a population base of 462 colorectal cancers. *Am J Surg Pathol* 2004;28:1553–1559.
111. Shia J, Klimstra DS, Nafa K, et al. Value of immunohistochemical detection of DNA mismatch repair proteins in predicting germline mutation in hereditary colorectal neoplasms. *Am J Surg Pathol* 2005;29:96–104.
112. Plaschke J, Kruger S, Pistorius S, et al. Involvement of *hMSH6* in the development of hereditary and sporadic colorectal cancer revealed by immunostaining is based on germline mutations, but rarely on somatic inactivation. *Int J Cancer* 2002;97: 643–648.
113. Kakar S, Aksoy S, Burgart L, et al. Mucinous carcinoma of the colon: correlation of loss of mismatch repair enzymes with clinicopathologic features and survival. *Mod Pathol* 2004;17:696–700.
114. Alexander J, Watanabe T, Wu TT, et al. Histopathological identification of colon cancer with microsatellite instability. *Am J Pathol* 2001;158:527–535.
115. Young J, Simms LA, Biden KG, et al. Features of colorectal cancers with high-level microsatellite instability occurring in familial and sporadic settings: parallel pathways of tumorigenesis. *Am J Pathol* 2001;159:2107–2116.
116. Shia J, Ellis NA, Paty PB, et al. Value of histopathology in predicting microsatellite instability in hereditary nonpolyposis colorectal cancer and sporadic colorectal cancer. *Am J Surg Pathol* 2003;27:1407–1417.
117. Woolf SH. Smarter strategy? Reflections on fecal DNA screening for colorectal cancer. *N Engl J Med* 2004;351:2755–2758.
118. Whitney D, Skoletsky J, Moore K, et al. Enhanced retrieval of DNA from human fecal samples results in improved performance of colorectal cancer screening test. *J Mol Diagn* 2004;6:386–395.
119. Traverso G, Shuber A, Levin B, et al. Detection of *APC* mutations in fecal DNA from patients with colorectal tumors. *N Engl J Med* 2002;346:311–320.
120. Berger BM, Robison L, Glickman J. Colon cancer-associated DNA mutations: marker selection for the detection of proximal colon cancer. *Diagn Mol Pathol* 2003;12:187–192.
121. Dong SM, Traverso G, Johnson C, et al. Detecting colorectal cancer in stool with the use of multiple genetic targets. *J Natl Cancer Inst* 2001;93:858–865.
122. Hasegawa Y, Takeda S, Ichii S, et al. Detection of *K-ras* mutations in DNAs isolated from feces of patients with colorectal tumors by mutant-allele-specific amplification (MASA). *Oncogene* 1995;10:1441–1445.
123. Imperiale TF, Ransohoff DF, Itzkowitz SH, et al. Fecal DNA versus fecal occult blood for colorectal-cancer screening in an average-risk population. *N Engl J Med* 2004;351:2704–2714.
124. Bostick PJ, Chatterjee S, Chi DD, et al. Limitations of specific reverse-transcriptase polymerase chain reaction markers in the detection of metastases in the lymph nodes and blood of breast cancer patients. *J Clin Oncol* 1998;16:2632–2640.
125. Zippelius A, Kufer P, Honold G, et al. Limitations of reverse-transcriptase polymerase chain reaction analyses for detection of micrometastatic epithelial cancer cells in bone marrow. *J Clin Oncol* 1997;15:2701–2708.
126. Dingemans A-MC, Brakenhoff RH, Postmus PE, et al. Detection of cytokeratin-19 transcripts by reverse transcriptase-polymerase chain reaction in lung cancer cell lines and blood of lung cancer patients. *Lab Invest* 1997;77:213–220.
127. Burchill SA, Bradbury MF, Pittman K, et al. Detection of epithelial cancer cells in peripheral blood by reverse transcriptase-polymerase chain reaction. *Br J Cancer* 1995;71:278–281.
128. Vlems FA, Diepstra JH, Cornelissen IM, et al. Investigations for a multi-marker RT-PCR to improve sensitivity of disseminated tumor cell detection. *Anticancer Res* 2003;23:179–186.
129. Jung R, Petersen K, Kruger W, et al. Detection of micrometastasis by cytokeratin 20 RT-PCR is limited due to stable background transcription in granulocytes. *Br J Cancer* 1999;81:870–873.
130. Soeth E, Vogel I, Roder C, et al. Comparative analysis of bone marrow and venous blood isolates from gastrointestinal cancer patients for the detection of disseminated tumor cells using reverse transcription PCR. *Cancer Res* 1997;57:3106–3110.

131. Bustin SA, Gyselman VG, Siddiqi S, et al. Cytokeratin 20 is not a tissue-specific marker for the detection of malignant epithelial cells in the blood of colorectal cancer patients. *Int J Surg Investig* 2000;2:49–57.
132. Bustin SAV, Siddiqi S, Ahmed S, et al. Quantification of cytokeratin 20, carcinoembryonic antigen and guanylyl cyclase C mRNA levels in lymph nodes may not predict treatment failure in colorectal cancer patients. *Int J Cancer* 2004;108:412–417.
133. Chen G, McIver CM, Texler M, et al. Detection of occult metastasis in lymph nodes from colorectal cancer patients: a multiple-marker reverse transcriptase-polymerase chain reaction study. *Dis Colon Rectum* 2004;47:679–686.
134. de Graaf H, Maelandsmo GM, Ruud P, et al. Ectopic expression of target genes may represent an inherent limitation of RT-PCR assays used for micrometastasis detection: studies on the epithelial glycoprotein gene *EGP-2*. *Int J Cancer* 1997;72:191–196.
135. Dent GA, Civalier CJ, Brecher ME, et al. *MUC1* expression in hematopoietic tissues. *Am J Clin Pathol* 1999;111:741–747.
136. Traweek ST, Liu J, Battifora H. Keratin gene expression in non-epithelial tissues: detection with polymerase chain reaction. *Am J Pathol* 1993;142:1111–1118.
137. Yamamoto N, Kato Y, Yanagisawa A, et al. Predictive value of genetic diagnosis for cancer micrometastasis: histologic and experimental appraisal. *Cancer* 1997;80:1393–1398.
138. Hampton R, Walker M, Marshall J, et al. Differential expression of carcinoembryonic antigen (CEA) splice variants in whole blood of colon cancer patients and healthy volunteers: implication for the detection of circulating colon cancer cells. *Oncogene* 2002;21:7817–7823.
139. Weitz J, Kienle P, Lacroix J, et al. Dissemination of tumor cells in patients undergoing surgery for colorectal cancer. *Clin Cancer Res* 1998;4:343–348.
140. Carrithers SL, Barber MT, Biswas S, et al. Guanylyl cyclase C is a selective marker for metastatic colorectal tumors in human extraintestinal tissues. *Proc Natl Acad Sci USA* 1996;93:14827–14832.
141. Uchikura K, Ueno S, Takao S, et al. Perioperative detection of circulating cancer cells in patients with colorectal hepatic metastases. *Hepatogastroenterology* 2002;49:1611–1614.
142. Soeth E, Roder C, Juhl H, et al. The detection of disseminated tumor cells in bone marrow from colorectal-cancer patients by a cytokeratin-20-specific nested reverse-transcriptase-polymerase-chain reaction is related to the stage of disease. *Int J Cancer* 1996;69:278–282.
143. Kopreski MS, Benko FA, Kwee C, et al. Detection of mutant *K-ras* DNA in plasma or serum of patients with colorectal cancer. *Br J Cancer* 1997;76:1293–1299.
144. Anker P, Lefort F, Vasioukhin V, et al. *K-ras* mutations are found in DNA extracted from the plasma of patients with colorectal cancer. *Gastroenterology* 1997;112:1114–1120.
145. Zou HZ, Yu BM, Wang ZW, et al. Detection of aberrant p16 methylation in the serum of colorectal cancer patients. *Clin Cancer Res* 2002;8:188–191.
146. Saha S, Dan AG, Bilchik AJ, et al. Historical review of lymphatic mapping in gastrointestinal malignancies. *Ann Surg Oncol* 2004;11:245S-249S.
147. Johnson DS, Wong JH. The impact on nodal staging of lymphatic mapping in carcinoma of the colon and rectum. *Semin Oncol* 2004;31:403–408.
148. Bilchik AJ, Nora D, Tollenaar RA, et al. Ultrastaging of early colon cancer using lymphatic mapping and molecular analysis. *Eur J Cancer* 2002;38:977–985.
149. Bilchik AJ, Saha S, Tsioulias GJ, et al. Aberrant drainage and missed micrometastases: the value of lymphatic mapping and focused analysis of sentinel lymph nodes in gastrointestinal neoplasms. *Ann Surg Oncol* 2001;8:82S–85S.
150. Liefers GJ, Cleton-Jansen AM, van de Velde CJ, et al. Micrometastases and survival in stage II colorectal cancer. *N Engl J Med* 1998;339:223–228.
151. Merrie AE, Yun K, McCall JL. Detection of carcinoembryonic antigen messenger RNA in lymph nodes from patients with colorectal cancer [Letter]. *N Engl J Med* 1998;339:1642.
152. Bostick PJ, Hoon DS, Cote RJ. Detection of carcinoembryonic antigen messenger RNA in lymph nodes from patients with colorectal cancer [Letter]. *N Engl J Med* 1998;339:1643–1644.
153. Bilchik AJ, Saha S, Wiese D, et al. Molecular staging of early colon cancer on the basis of sentinel node analysis: a multicenter phase II trial. *J Clin Oncol* 2001;19:1128–1136.
154. Fedier A, Fink D. Mutations in DNA mismatch repair genes: implications for DNA damage signaling and drug sensitivity [review]. *Int J Oncol* 2004;24:1039–1047.
155. Ribic CM, Sargent DJ, Moore MJ, et al. Tumor microsatellite-instability status as a predictor of benefit from fluorouracil-based adjuvant chemotherapy for colon cancer. *N Engl J Med* 2003;349:247–257.
156. Bras-Goncalves RA, Rosty C, Laurent-Puig P, et al. Sensitivity to CPT-11 of xenografted human colorectal cancers as a function of microsatellite instability and *p53* status. *Br J Cancer* 2000;82:913–923.
157. Kornmann M, Link KH, Galuba I, et al. Association of time to recurrence with thymidylate synthase and dihydropyrimidine dehydrogenase mRNA expression in stage II and III colorectal cancer. *J Gastrointest Surg* 2002;6:331–337.
158. Kornmann M, Link KH, Lenz HJ, et al. Thymidylate synthase is a predictor for response and resistance in hepatic artery infusion chemotherapy. *Cancer Lett* 1997;118:29–35.
159. Van Triest B, Pinedo HM, Giaccone G, et al. Downstream molecular determinants of response to 5-fluorouracil and antifolate thymidylate synthase inhibitors. *Ann Oncol* 2000;11:385–391.
160. Issaeva N, Bozko P, Enge M, et al. Small molecule RITA binds to *p53*, blocks *p53-HDM-2* interaction and activates *p53* function in tumors. *Nat Med* 2004;10:1321–1328.
161. Arber N, Neugut AI, Weinstein IB, et al. Molecular genetics of small bowel cancer. *Cancer Epidemiol Biomarkers Prev* 1997;6:745–748.
162. Hutchins RR, Bani Hani A, Kojodjojo P, et al. Adenocarcinoma of the small bowel. *ANZ J Surg* 2001;71:428–437.
163. Sellner F. Investigations on the significance of the adenoma-carcinoma sequence in the small bowel. *Cancer* 1990;66:702–715.
164. Planck M, Ericson K, Piotrowska Z, et al. Microsatellite instability and expression of *MLH1* and *MSH2* in carcinomas of the small intestine. *Cancer* 2003;97: 1551–1557.
165. Blaker H, von Herbay A, Penzel R, et al. Genetics of adenocarcinomas of the small intestine: frequent deletions at chromosome 18q and mutations of the *SMAD4* gene. *Oncogene* 2002;21:158–164.
166. Wheeler JM, Warren BF, Mortensen NJ, et al. An insight into the genetic pathway of adenocarcinoma of the small intestine. *Gut* 2002;50:218–223.
167. Arai M, Shimizu S, Imai Y, et al. Mutations of the Ki-*ras*, *p53* and *APC* genes in adenocarcinomas of the human small intestine. *Int J Cancer* 1997;70:390–395.
168. Rashid A, Hamilton SR. Genetic alterations in sporadic and Crohn's-associated adenocarcinomas of the small intestine. *Gastroenterology* 1997;113:127–135.
169. McCarthy DM, Hruban RJ, Argani P, et al. Role of the *DPC4* tumor suppressor gene in adenocarcinoma of the ampulla of Vater: analysis of 140 cases. *Mod Pathol* 2003;16:272–278.
170. Moore PS, Orlandini S, Zamboni G, et al. Pancreatic tumours: molecular pathways implicated in ductal cancer are involved in ampullary but not in exocrine nonductal or endocrine tumorigenesis. *Br J Cancer* 2001;84:253–262.
171. Imai Y, Tsurutani N, Oda H, et al. Genetic instability and mutation of the TGF-beta- receptor-II gene in ampullary carcinomas. *Int J Cancer* 1998;76:407–411.
172. Rodriguez-Bigas MA, Vasen HF, Lynch HT, et al. Characteristics of small bowel carcinoma in hereditary nonpolyposis colorectal carcinoma. International Collaborative Group on HNPCC. *Cancer* 1998;83:240–244.
173. Lauren T. The two histologic main types of gastric carcinoma. *Acta Pathol Microbiol Scand* 1965;64:34.
174. Jinawath N, Furukawa Y, Hasegawa S, et al. Comparison of gene-expression profiles between diffuse- and intestinal-type gastric cancers using a genome-wide cDNA microarray. *Oncogene* 2004;23:6830–6844.
175. Sarbia M, Becker KF, Hofler H. Pathology of upper gastrointestinal malignancies. *Semin Oncol* 2004;31:465–475.
176. Musulen E, Moreno V, Reyes G, et al. Standardized approach for microsatellite instability detection in gastric carcinomas. *Hum Pathol* 2004;35:335–342.
177. Dos Santos NR, Seruca R, Constancia M, et al. Microsatellite instability at multiple loci in gastric carcinoma: clinicopathologic implications and prognosis. *Gastroenterology* 1996;110:38–44.
178. Strickler JG, Zheng J, Shu Q, et al. *p53* mutations and microsatellite instability in sporadic gastric cancer: when guardians fail. *Cancer Res* 1994;54:4750–4755.
179. Hamamoto T, Yokozaki H, Semba S, et al. Altered microsatellites in incomplete-type intestinal metaplasia adjacent to primary gastric cancers. *J Clin Pathol* 1997;50:841–846.
180. El-Rifai W, Powell SM. Molecular biology of gastric cancer. *Semin Radiat Oncol* 2002;12:128–140.
181. Lee HS, Choi SI, Lee HK, et al. Distinct clinical features and outcomes of gastric cancers with microsatellite instability. *Mod Pathol* 2002;15:632–640.
182. Fenoglio-Preiser CM, Wang J, Stemmermann GN, et al. TP53 and gastric carcinoma: a review. *Hum Mutat* 2003;21:258–270.
183. Yao XX, Yin L, Sun ZC. The expression of *hTERT* mRNA and cellular immunity in gastric cancer and precancerosis. *World J Gastroenterol* 2002;8:586–590.
184. Graziano F, Humar B, Guilford P. The role of the E-cadherin gene (*CDH1*) in diffuse gastric cancer susceptibility: from the laboratory to clinical practice. *Ann Oncol* 2003;14:1705–1713.
185. Berx G, Becker KF, Hofler H, et al. Mutations of the human E-cadherin (*CDH1*) gene. *Hum Mutat* 1998;12:226–237.
186. Tamura G, Yin J, Wang S, et al. E-Cadherin gene promoter hypermethylation in primary human gastric carcinomas. *J Natl Cancer Inst* 2000;92:569–573.
187. Sakata K, Tamura G, Endoh Y, et al. Hypermethylation of the *hMLH1* gene promoter in solitary and multiple gastric cancers with microsatellite instability. *Br J Cancer* 2002;86:564–567.
188. Guilford P, Hopkins J, Harraway J, et al. E-cadherin germline mutations in familial gastric cancer. *Nature* 1998;392:402–405.
189. Guilford PJ, Hopkins JB, Grady WM, et al. E-cadherin germline mutations define an inherited cancer syndrome dominated by diffuse gastric cancer. *Hum Mutat* 1999;14:249–255.
190. Gamboa-Dominguez A, Dominguez-Fonseca C, Chavarri-Guerra Y, et al. E-cadherin expression in sporadic gastric cancer from Mexico: exon 8 and 9 deletions are infrequent events associated with poor survival. *Hum Pathol* 2005;36:29–35.
191. Santini V, Kantarjian HM, Issa JP. Changes in DNA methylation in neoplasia: pathophysiology and therapeutic implications. *Ann Intern Med* 2001;134:573–586.
192. Goffin J, Eisenhauer E. DNA methyltransferase inhibitors-state of the art. *Ann Oncol* 2002;13:1699–1716.
193. Wen S, Felley CP, Bouzourene H, et al. Inflammatory gene profiles in gastric mucosa during *Helicobacter pylori* infection in humans. *J Immunol* 2004;172:2595–2606.
194. Meireles SI, Cristo EB, Carvalho AF, et al. Molecular classifiers for gastric cancer and nonmalignant diseases of the gastric mucosa. *Cancer Res* 2004;64:1255–1265.
195. Carlini M, Carboni F, Petric M, et al. Sentinel node in gastric cancer surgery. *J Exp Clin Cancer Res* 2002;21:469–473.
196. Ajisaka H, Miwa K. Micrometastases in sentinel nodes of gastric cancer. *Br J Cancer* 2003;89:676–680.
197. Yamada E, Miyaishi S, Nakazato H, et al. The surgical treatment of cancer of the stomach. *Int Surg* 1980;65:387–399.
198. Boku T, Nakane Y, Minoura T, et al. Prognostic significance of serosal invasion and free intraperitoneal cancer cells in gastric cancer. *Br J Surg* 1990;77:436–439.
199. Bando E, Yonemura Y, Takeshita Y, et al. Intraoperative lavage for cytological examination in 1,297 patients with gastric carcinoma. *Am J Surg* 1999;178:256–262.
200. Ueno H, Yoshida K, Hirai T, et al. Quantitative detection of carcinoembryonic antigen messenger RNA in the peritoneal cavity of gastric cancer patients by real-time quantitative reverse transcription polymerase chain reaction. *Anticancer Res* 2003;23:1701–1708.
201. To EM, Chan WY, Chow C, et al. Gastric cancer cell detection in peritoneal washing: cytology versus RT-PCR for CEA transcripts. *Diagn Mol Pathol* 2003;12:88–95.
202. Ishii T, Fujiwara Y, Ohnaka S, et al. Rapid genetic diagnosis with the transcription-reverse transcription concerted reaction system for cancer micrometastasis. *Ann Surg Oncol* 2004;11:778–785.
203. Mori T, Fujiwara Y, Sugita Y, et al. Application of molecular diagnosis for detection of peritoneal micrometastasis and evaluation of preoperative chemotherapy in advanced gastric carcinoma. *Ann Surg Oncol* 2004;11:14–20.
204. Tay ST, Leong SH, Yu K, et al. A combined comparative genomic hybridization and expression microarray analysis of gastric cancer reveals novel molecular subtypes. *Cancer Res* 2003;63:3309–3316.
205. Hasegawa S, Furukawa Y, Li M, et al. Genome-wide analysis of gene expression in intestinal-type gastric cancers using a complementary DNA microarray representing 23,040 genes. *Cancer Res* 2002;62:7012–7017.
206. Norsett KG, Laegreid A, Midelfart H, et al. Gene expression based classification of gastric carcinoma. *Cancer Lett* 2004;210:227–237.
207. Park JS, Young Yoon S, Kim JM, et al. Identification of novel genes associated with the response to 5-FU treatment in gastric cancer cell lines using a cDNA microarray. *Cancer Lett* 2004;214:19–33.

208. Yoshida K, Tanabe K, Ueno H, et al. Future prospects of personalized chemotherapy in gastric cancer patients: results of a prospective randomized pilot study. *Gastric Cancer* 2003;1:S82–S89.
209. Siewert JR, Stein HJ. Classification of adenocarcinoma of the oesophagogastric junction. *Br J Surg* 1998;85:1457–1459.
210. Spechler SJ, Goyal RK. The columnar-lined esophagus, intestinal metaplasia, and Norman Barrett. *Gastroenterology* 1996;110:614–621.
211. Lin J, Beer DG. Molecular biology of upper gastrointestinal malignancies. *Semin Oncol* 2004;31:476–486.
212. Jenkins GJ, Doak SH, Parry JM, et al. Genetic pathways involved in the progression of Barrett's metaplasia to adenocarcinoma. *Br J Surg* 2002;89:824–837.
213. Wijnhoven BP, Tilanus HW, Dinjens WN. Molecular biology of Barrett's adenocarcinoma. *Ann Surg* 2001;233:322–337.
214. Langan JE, Cole CG, Huckle EJ, et al. Novel microsatellite markers and single nucleotide polymorphisms refine the tylosis with oesophageal cancer (TOC) minimal region on 17q25 to 42.5 kb: sequencing does not identify the causative gene. *Hum Genet* 2004;114:534–540.
215. Xu Y, Selaru FM, Yin J, et al. Artificial neural networks and gene filtering distinguish between global gene expression profiles of Barrett's esophagus and esophageal cancer. *Cancer Res* 2002;62:3493–3497.
216. Kihara C, Tsunoda T, Tanaka T, et al. Prediction of sensitivity of esophageal tumors to adjuvant chemotherapy by cDNA microarray analysis of gene-expression profiles. *Cancer Res* 2001;61:6474–6479.
217. Kato H, Tachimori Y, Watanabe H, et al. Lymph node metastasis in thoracic esophageal carcinoma. *J Surg Oncol* 1991;48:106–111.
218. Nishimaki T, Suzuki T, Suzuki S, et al. Outcomes of extended radical esophagectomy for thoracic esophageal cancer. *J Am Coll Surg* 1998;186:306–312.
219. Law S, Wong J. Two-field dissection is enough for esophageal cancer. *Dis Esophagus* 2001;14:98–103.
220. Shiozaki H, Yano M, Tsujinaka T, et al. Lymph node metastasis along the recurrent nerve chain is an indication for cervical lymph node dissection in thoracic esophageal cancer. *Dis Esophagus* 2001;14:191–196.
221. Yoshioka S, Fujiwara Y, Sugita Y, et al. Real-time rapid reverse transcriptase-polymerase chain reaction for intraoperative diagnosis of lymph node micrometastasis: clinical application for cervical lymph node dissection in esophageal cancers. *Surgery* 2002; 132:34–40.
222. Milne AN, Carvalho R, van Rees BP, et al. Do collision tumors of the gastroesophageal junction exist? A molecular analysis. *Am J Surg Pathol* 2004;28:1492–1498.
223. Goldstein NS, Vincini FA, Hunter S, et al. Molecular clonality relationships in initial carcinomas, ipsilateral breast failures, and distant metastases in patients treated with breast-conserving therapy. *Am J Clin Pathol* 2005;124:1–9.
224. Fredriksson I, Liljegren G, Arnesson LG, et al. Local recurrence in the breast after conservative surgery: a study of prognosis and prognostic factors in 391 women. *Eur J Cancer* 2002;38:1860–1870.
225. Hilgers W, Rosty C, Hahn SA. Molecular pathogenesis of pancreatic cancer. *Hematol Oncol Clin North Am* 2002;16:17–35.
226. Iacobuzio-Donahue CA, Hruban RH. Gene expression in neoplasms of the pancreas: applications to diagnostic pathology. *Adv Anat Pathol* 2003;10:125–134.
227. Cowgill SM, Muscarella P. The genetics of pancreatic cancer. *Am J Surg* 2003;186:279–286.
228. Thayer SP, di Magliano MP, Heiser PW, et al. Hedgehog is an early and late mediator of pancreatic cancer tumorigenesis. *Nature* 2003;425:851–856.
229. Hruban RH, Yeo CJ, Kern SE. Pancreatic cancer. In: Vogelstein B, Kinzler KW, eds. *The Genetic Basis of Human Cancer*, 2nd ed. New York: McGraw-Hill; 2002:659–673.
230. Almoguera C, Shibata D, Forrester K, et al. Most human carcinomas of the exocrine pancreas contain mutant c-K-*ras* genes. *Cell* 1988;53:549–554.
231. Hruban RH, van Mansfeld AD, Offerhaus GJ, et al. K-*ras* oncogene activation in adenocarcinoma of the human pancreas: a study of 82 carcinomas using a combination of mutant-enriched polymerase chain reaction analysis and allele-specific oligonucleotide hybridization. *Am J Pathol* 1993;143:545–554.
232. Yanagisawa A, Ohtake K, Ohashi K, et al. Frequent c-Ki-*ras* oncogene activation in mucous cell hyperplasias of pancreas suffering from chronic inflammation. *Cancer Res* 1993;53:953–956.
233. Tada M, Ohashi M, Shiratori Y, et al. Analysis of K-*ras* gene mutation in hyperplastic duct cells of the pancreas without pancreatic disease. *Gastroenterology* 1996;110:227–231.
234. DiGiuseppe JA, Hruban RH, Offerhaus GA, et al. Detection of K-*ras* mutations in mucinous pancreatic duct hyperplasia from a patient with a family history of pancreatic carcinoma. *Am J Pathol* 1994;144:889–895.
235. Tada M, Omata M, Ohto M. *Ras* gene mutations in intraductal papillary neoplasms of the pancreas: analysis in five cases. *Cancer* 1991;67:634–637.
236. Goggins M, Offerhaus GJA, Hilgers W, et al. Pancreatic adenocarcinomas with DNA replication errors (RER+) are associated with wild-type K-*ras* and characteristic histopathology. *Am J Pathol* 1998;152:1501–1507.
237. Wilentz RE, Goggins M, Redston M, et al. Genetic, immunohistochemical, and clinical features of medullary carcinoma of the pancreas: a newly described and characterized entity. *Am J Pathol* 2000;156:1641–1651.
238. Buchler P, Conejo-Garcia JR, Lehmann G, et al. Real-time quantitative PCR of telomerase mRNA is useful for the differentiation of benign and malignant pancreatic disorders. *Pancreas* 2001;22:331–340.
239. Balcom JH 4th, Keck T, Warshaw AL, et al. Telomerase activity in periampullary tumors correlates with aggressive malignancy. *Ann Surg* 2001;234:344–351.
240. Pearson AS, Chiao P, Zhang L, et al. The detection of telomerase activity in patients with adenocarcinoma of the pancreas by fine needle aspiration. *Int J Oncol* 2000;17:381–385.
241. Sato N, Fukushima N, Maitra A, et al. Gene expression profiling identifies genes associated with invasive intraductal papillary mucinous neoplasms of the pancreas. *Am J Pathol* 2004;164:903–914.
242. Hansel DE, Ashfaq R, Rahman A, et al. A subset of pancreatic adenocarcinomas demonstrates coamplification of topoisomerase IIalpha and *HER2/neu*: use of immunolabeling and multicolor FISH for potential patient screening and treatment. *Am J Clin Pathol* 2005;123:28–35.
243. Uehara H, Nakaizumi A, Tatsuta M, et al. Diagnosis of pancreatic cancer by detecting telomerase activity in pancreatic juice: comparison with K-*ras* mutations. *Am J Gastroenterol* 1999;94:2513–2518.
244. Mizumoto K, Tanaka M. Genetic diagnosis of pancreatic cancer. *J Hepatobiliary Pancreat Surg* 2002;9:39–44.
245. Murakami Y, Yokoyama T, Hiyama E, et al. Successful pre-operative diagnosis of malignant intraductal papillary mucinous tumor of the pancreas by detecting telomerase activity. *Int J Gastrointest Cancer* 2002;31:117–121.
246. Murakami Y, Yokoyama T, Yokoyama Y, et al. Adenosquamous carcinoma of the pancreas: preoperative diagnosis and molecular alterations. *J Gastroenterol* 2003;38:1171–1175.
247. Caldas C, Hahn SA, Hruban RH, et al. Detection of K-*ras* mutations in the stool of patients with pancreatic adenocarcinoma and pancreatic ductal hyperplasia. *Cancer Res* 1994;54:3568–3573.
248. Tada M, Omata M, Kawai S, et al. Detection of *ras* gene mutations in pancreatic juice and peripheral blood of patients with pancreatic adenocarcinoma. *Cancer Res* 1993;53:2472–2474.
249. Niedergethmann M, Rexin M, Hildenbrand R, et al. Prognostic implications of routine, immunohistochemical, and molecular staging in resectable pancreatic adenocarcinoma. *Am J Surg Pathol* 2002;26:1578–1587.
250. Ando N, Nakaio A, Nomoto S, et al. Detection of mutant K-*ras* in dissected paraaortic lymph nodes of patients with pancreatic adenocarcinoma. *Pancreas* 1997;15:374–378.
251. Demeure MJ, Doffek KM, Komorowski RA, et al. Molecular metastases in stage I pancreatic cancer: improved survival with adjuvant chemoradiation. *Surgery* 1998;124:663–669.
252. Demeure MJ, Doffek KM, Komorowski RA, et al. Adenocarcinoma of the pancreas: detection of occult metastases in regional lymph nodes by a polymerase chain reaction-based assay. *Cancer* 1998;83:1328–1334.
253. Tamagawa E, Ueda M, Sugano K, et al. Pancreatic lymph nodal and plexus micrometastases detected by enriched polymerase chain reaction and nonradioisotopic single-strand conformation polymorphism analysis: a new predictive factor for recurrent pancreatic carcinoma. *Clin Cancer Res* 1997;3:2143–2149.
254. van den Berg W, Tascilar M, Offerhaus GJ, et al. Pancreatic mucinous cystic neoplasms with sarcomatous stroma: molecular evidence for monoclonal origin with subsequent divergence of the epithelial and sarcomatous components. *Mod Pathol* 2000;13:86–91.
255. Oberg K. Carcinoid tumors: molecular genetics, tumor biology, and update of diagnosis and treatment. *Curr Opin Oncol* 2002;14:38–45.
256. Leotlela PD, Jauch A, Holtgreve-Grez H, et al. Genetics of neuroendocrine and carcinoid tumours. *Endocr Relat Cancer* 2003;10:437–450.
257. Lohmann DR, Fesseler B, Putz B, et al. Infrequent mutations of the *p53* gene in pulmonary carcinoid tumors. *Cancer Res* 1993;53:5797–5801.
258. Lohmann Dr, Funk A, Niedermeyer HP, et al. Identification of *p53* gene mutations in gastrointestinal and pancreatic carcinoids by nonradioisotopic SSCA. *Virchows Arch B Cell Pathol Incl Mol Pathol* 1993;64:293–296.
259. Younes N, Fulton N, Tanaka R, et al. The presence of K-12 *ras* mutations in duodenal adenocarcinomas and the absence of *ras* mutations in other small bowel adenocarcinomas and carcinoid tumors. *Cancer* 1997;79:1804–1808.
260. Paraskevakou H, Saetta A, Skandalis K, et al. Morphological-histochemical study of intestinal carcinoids and K-*ras* mutation analysis in appendiceal carcinoids. *Pathol Oncol Res* 1999;5:205–210.
261. Stancu M, Wu TT, Wallace C, et al. Genetic alterations in goblet cell carcinoids of the vermiform appendix and comparison with gastrointestinal carcinoid tumors. *Mod Pathol* 2003;16:1189–1198.
262. Li CC, Xu B, Hirokawa M, et al. Alterations of E-cadherin, alpha-catenin and beta-catenin expression in neuroendocrine tumors of the gastrointestinal tract. *Virchows Arch* 2002;440:145–154.
263. Chan A O-O, Kim SG, Bedeir A, et al. CpG island methylation in carcinoid and pancreatic endocrine tumors. *Oncogene* 2003;22:924–934.
264. Marx SJ. Multiple endocrine neoplasia type 1. In: Vogelstein B, Kinzler KW, ed. *The Genetic Basis of Human Cancer*, 2nd ed. New York, McGraw-Hill; 2002:475–499.
265. Jensen RT. Carcinoid and pancreatic endocrine tumors: recent advances in molecular pathogenesis, localization, and treatment. *Curr Opin Oncol* 2000;12:368–377.
266. Debelenko LV, Emmert-Buck MR, Zhuang Z, et al. The multiple endocrine neoplasia type I gene locus is involved in the pathogenesis of type II gastric carcinoids. *Gastroenterology* 1997;113:773–781.
267. Gortz B, Roth J, Krahenmann A, et al. Mutations and allelic deletions of the *MEN1* gene are associated with a subset of sporadic endocrine pancreatic and neuroendocrine tumors and not restricted to foregut neoplasms. *Am J Pathol* 1999;154:429–436.
268. Zhuang Z, Vortmeyer AO, Pack S, et al. Somatic mutations of the *MEN1* tumor suppressor gene in sporadic gastrinomas and insulinomas. *Cancer Res* 1997;57:4682–4686.
269. Wang EH, Ebrahimi SA, Wu AY, et al. Mutation of the *MENIN* gene in sporadic pancreatic endocrine tumors. *Cancer Res* 1998;58:4417–4420.
270. Klein A, Clemens J, Cameron J. Periampullary neoplasms in von Recklinghausen's disease. *Surgery* 1989;106:815–819.
271. Swinburn BA, Yeong ML, Lane MR, et al. Neurofibromatosis associated with somatostatinoma: a report of two patients. *Clin Endocrinol (Oxf)* 1988;28:353–359.
272. Lubensky IA, Pack S, Ault D, et al. Multiple neuroendocrine tumors of the pancreas in von Hippel-Lindau disease patients: histopathological and molecular genetic analysis. *Am J Pathol* 1998;153:223–231.
273. Maioli M, Ciccarese M, Pacifico A, et al. Familial insulinoma: description of two cases. *Acta Diabetol* 1992;29:38–40.
274. Eschbach JW, Rinaldo JA. Metastatic carcinoid: a familial occurrence. *Ann Intern Med* 1962;57:647.
275. Wale RJ, William JA, Veeley AH. Familial occurrence in carcinoid tumors. *Aust NZ J Surg* 1983;53:325.
276. Yeatman TJ, Sharp JV, Kimura AK. Can susceptibility to carcinoid tumors be inherited? *Cancer* 1989;63:390–393.
277. Goebel SU, Heppner C, Burns AL, et al. Genotype/phenotype correlation of multiple endocrine neoplasia type 1 gene mutations in sporadic gastrinomas. *J Clin Endocrinol Metab* 2000;85:116–123.
278. Maitra A, Hansel DE, Argani P, et al. Global expression analysis of well-differentiated pancreatic endocrine neoplasms using oligonucleotide microarrays. *Clin Cancer Res* 2003;9:5988–5995.
279. Fukui H, Takada M, Chiba T, et al. Concurrent occurrence of gastric adenocarcinoma and duodenal neuroendocrine cell carcinoma: a composite tumour or collision tumours? *Gut* 2001;48:853–856.

280. Furlan D, Cerutti R, Genasetti A, et al. Microallelotyping defines the monoclonal or the polyclonal origin of mixed and collision endocrine-exocrine tumors of the gut. *Lab Invest* 2003;83:963–971.
281. Rosenthal DS, Eyre HJ. Hodgkin's disease and non-Hodgkin's lymphomas. In: Murphy GP, Lawrence W Jr, Lenhard RE Jr, eds. *Clinical Oncology*, 2nd ed. Atlanta: *American Cancer Society;* 1995:451–469.
282. Ono H, Kondo H, Saito D, et al. Rapid diagnosis of gastric malignant lymphoma from biopsy specimens: detection of immunoglobulin heavy chain rearrangement by polymerase chain reaction. *Jpn J Cancer Res* 1993;84:813–817.
283. Wundisch T, Neubauer A, Stolte M, et al. B-cell monoclonality is associated with lymphoid follicles in gastritis. *Am J Surg Pathol* 2003;27:882–887.
284. O'Sullivan MJ, Ritter JH, Humhrey PA, et al. Lymphoid lesions of the gastrointestinal tract: a histologic, immunophenotypic, and genotypic analysis of 49 cases. *Am J Clin Pathol* 1998;110:471–477.
285. Wundisch T, Thiede C, Alpen B, et al. Are lymphocytic monoclonality and immunoglobulin heavy chain (IgH) rearrangement premalignant conditions in chronic gastritis? *Microsc Res Tech* 2001;53:414–418.
286. Elenitoba-Johnson KS, Bohling SD, Mitchell RS, et al. PCR analysis of the immunoglobulin heavy chain gene in polyclonal processes can yield pseudoclonal bands as an artifact of low B cell number. *J Mol Diagn* 2000;2:92–96.
287. Taylor JM, Spagnolo DV, Kay PH. B-cell target DNA quantity is a critical factor in the interpretation of B-cell clonality by PCR. *Pathology* 1997;29:309–312.
288. Collins RD. Is clonality equivalent to malignancy: specifically, is immunoglobulin gene rearrangement diagnostic of malignant lymphoma? *Hum Pathol* 1997;28:757–759.
289. Kroft SH. Monoclones, monotypes, and neoplasia pitfalls in lymphoma diagnosis. *Am J Clin Pathol* 2004;121:457–459.
290. Takano Y, Kato Y, Sato Y, et al. Clonal Ig-gene rearrangement in some cases of gastric RLH detected by PCR method. *Pathol Res Pract* 1992;188:973–980.
291. Calvert RJ, Evans PA, Dixon MF. The significance of B-cell clonality in gastric lymphoid infiltrates. *J Pathol* 1996;180:26–32.
292. Algara P, Martinez P, Piris MA. The detection of B-cell monoclonal populations by polymerase chain reaction: accuracy of approach and application in gastric endoscopic biopsy specimens. *Hum Pathol* 1993;24:1184–1188.
293. Iijima T, Inadome Y, Noguchi M. Clonal proliferation of B lymphocytes in the germinal centers of human reactive lymph nodes: possibility of overdiagnosis of B cell clonal proliferation. *Diagn Mol Pathol* 2000;9:132–136.
294. Lee SC, Berg KD, Racke FK, et al. Pseudo-spikes are common in histologically benign lymphoid tissues. *J Mol Diagn* 2000;2:145–152.
295. Chen B, Colleoni GW, Salazar PA, et al. Molecular analysis of gastric washings in the diagnosis and monitoring of gastric lymphomas. *Hum Pathol* 2004;35:582–586.
296. Aiello A, Giardini R, Tondini C, et al. PCR-based clonality analysis: a reliable method for the diagnosis and follow-up monitoring of conservatively treated gastric B-cell MALT lymphomas? *Histopathology* 1999;34:326–330.
297. El-Zimaity HM, El-Zaatari FA, Dore MP, et al. The differential diagnosis of early gastric mucosa-associated lymphoma: polymerase chain reaction and paraffin section immunophenotyping. *Mod Pathol* 1999;12:885–893.
298. Thiede C, Wundish T, Alpern B, et al. Long-term persistence of monoclonal B cells after cure of *Helicobacter pylori* infection and complete histologic remission in gastric mucosa-associated lymphoid tissue B-cell lymphoma. *J Clin Oncol* 2001;19:1600–1609.
299. Isaacson PG. Gastrointestinal lymphomas of T- and B-cell types. *Mod Pathol* 1999;12:151–158.
300. Daum S, Weiss D, Hummel M, et al. Frequency of clonal intraepithelial T lymphocyte proliferations in enteropathy-type intestinal T cell lymphoma, coeliac disease, and refractory sprue. *Gut* 2001;49:804–812.
301. Farstad IN, Lundin KE. Gastrointestinal intraepithelial lymphocytes and T cell lymphomas. *Gut* 2003;52:163–164.
302. Verkarre V, Asnafi V, Lecomte T, et al. Refractory coeliac sprue is a diffuse gastrointestinal disease. *Gut* 2003;52:205–211.
303. Heinrich MC, Rubin BP, Longley BJ, et al. Biology and genetic aspects of gastrointestinal stromal tumors: KIT activation and cytogenetic alterations. *Hum Pathol* 2002;33:484–495.
304. Miettinen M, El-Rifai W, Sobin LH, et al. Evaluation of malignancy and prognosis of gastrointestinal stromal tumors: a review. *Hum Pathol* 2002;33:478–483.
305. Fletcher CD, Berman JJ, Corless C, et al. Diagnosis of gastrointestinal stromal tumors: a consensus approach. *Hum Pathol* 2002;33:459–465.
306. Hirota S, Isozaki K, Moriyama Y, et al. Gain-of-function mutations of *c-kit* in human gastrointestinal stromal tumors. *Science* 1998;279:577–580.
307. Beghini A, Tibiletti MG, Roversi G, et al. Germline mutation in the juxtamembrane domain of the *kit* gene in a family with gastrointestinal stromal tumors and urticaria pigmentosa. *Cancer* 2001;92:657–662.
308. Hirota S, Okazaki T, Kitamura Y, et al. Cause of familial and multiple gastrointestinal autonomic nerve tumors with hyperplasia of interstitial cells of Cajal is germline mutation of the *c-kit* gene. *Am J Surg Pathol* 2000;24:326–327.
309. Hirota S, Nishida T, Isozaki K, et al. Familial gastrointestinal stromal tumors associated with dysphagia and novel type germline mutation of KIT gene. *Gastroenterology* 2002;122:1493–1499.
310. Isozaki K, Terris B, Belghiti J, et al. Germline-activating mutation in the kinase domain of KIT gene in familial gastrointestinal stromal tumors. *Am J Pathol* 2000;157:1581–1585.
311. Maeyama H, Hidaka E, Ota H, et al. Familial gastrointestinal stromal tumor with hyperpigmentation: association with a germline mutation of the *c-kit* gene. *Gastroenterology* 2001;120:210–215.
312. Nishida T, Hirota S, Taniguchi M, et al. Familial gastrointestinal stromal tumours with germline mutation of the KIT gene. *Nat Genet* 1998;19:323–324.
313. Hirota S, Ohashi A, Nishida T, et al. Gain-of-function mutations of platelet-derived growth factor receptor alpha gene in gastrointestinal stromal tumors. *Gastroenterology* 2003;125:660–667.
314. Heinrich MC, Corless CL, Duensing A, et al. PDGFRA activating mutations in gastrointestinal stromal tumors. *Science* 2003;299:708–710.
315. Medeiros F, Corless CL, Duensing A, et al. KIT-negative gastrointestinal stromal tumors: proof of concept and therapeutic implications. *Am J Surg Pathol* 2004;28:889–894.
316. Sakurai S, Hasegawa T, Sakuma Y, et al. Myxoid epithelioid gastrointestinal stromal tumor (GIST) with mast cell infiltrations: a subtype of GIST with mutations of platelet-derived growth factor receptor alpha gene. *Hum Pathol* 2004;35:1223–1230.
317. Lasota J, Dansonka-Mieszkowska A, Stachura T, et al. Gastrointestinal stromal tumors with internal tandem duplications in 3′ end of KIT juxtamembrane domain occur predominantly in stomach and generally seem to have a favorable course. *Mod Pathol* 2003;16:1257–1264.
318. Corless CL, McGreevey L, Haley A, et al. KIT mutations are common in incidental gastrointestinal stromal tumors one centimeter or less in size. *Am J Pathol* 2002;160:1567–1572.
319. Corless CL, McGreevey L, Town A, et al. KIT gene deletions at the intron 10-exon 11 boundary in GI stromal tumors. *J Mol Diagn* 2004;6:366–370.
320. Rubin BP, Singer S, Tsao C, et al. KIT activation is a ubiquitous feature of gastrointestinal stromal tumors. *Cancer Res* 2001;61:8118–8121.
321. Wasag B, Debiec-Rychter M, Pauwels P, et al. Differential expression of KIT/PDGFRA mutant isoforms in epithelioid and mixed variants of gastrointestinal stromal tumors depends predominantly on the tumor site. *Mod Pathol* 2004;17:889–894.
322. Lasota J, Dansonka-Mieszkowska A, Sobin LH, et al. A great majority of GISTs with *PDGFRA* mutations represent gastric tumors of low or no malignant potential. *Lab Invest* 2004;84:874–883.
323. Wardelmann E, Neidt I, Bierhoff E, et al. *c-kit* mutations in gastrointestinal stromal tumors occur preferentially in the spindle rather than in the epithelioid cell variant. *Mod Pathol* 2002;15:125–136.
324. Miettinen M, Sobin LH, Lasota J. Gastrointestinal stromal tumors of the stomach: a clinicopathologic, immunohistochemical, and molecular genetic study of 1765 cases with long-term follow-up. *Am J Surg Pathol* 2005;29:52–68.
325. Antonescu CR, Sommer G, Sarran L, et al. Association of KIT exon 9 mutations with nongastric primary site and aggressive behavior: KIT mutation analysis and clinical correlates of 120 gastrointestinal stromal tumors. *Clin Cancer Res* 2003;9:3329–3337.
326. Miettinen M, Kopczynski J, Makhlouf HR, et al. Gastrointestinal stromal tumors, intramural leiomyomas, and leiomyosarcomas in the duodenum: a clinicopathologic, immunohistochemical, and molecular genetic study of 167 cases. *Am J Surg Pathol* 2003;27:625–641.
327. Sabah M. Cummins R, Leader M, et al. Expression of human telomerase reverse transcriptase in gastrointestinal stromal tumors occurs preferentially in malignant neoplasms. *Hum Pathol* 2004;35:1231–1235.
328. Gunther T, Schneider-Stock R, Hackel C, et al. Telomerase activity and expression of *hTRT* and *hTR* in gastrointestinal stromal tumors in comparison with extragastrointestinal sarcomas. *Clin Cancer Res* 2000;6:1811–1818.
329. Sakurai S, Fukayama M, Kaizaki Y, et al. Telomerase activity in gastrointestinal stromal tumors. *Cancer* 1998;83:2060–2066.
330. Buchdunger E, Cioffi CL, Law N, et al. Abl protein-tyrosine kinase inhibitor STI571 inhibits in vitro signal transduction mediated by *c-kit* and platelet-derived growth factor receptors. *J Pharmacol Exp Ther* 2000;295:139–145.
331. Joensuu H, Roberts PJ, Sarlomo-Rikala M, et al. Effect of the tyrosine kinase inhibitor STI571 in a patient with a metastatic gastrointestinal stromal tumor. *N Engl J Med* 2001;344:1052–1056.
332. Demetri GD, von Mehren M, Blanke CD, et al. Efficacy and safety of imatinib mesylate in advanced gastrointestinal stromal tumors. *N Engl J Med* 2002;347:472–480.
333. von Oosterom A, Judson I, Verweij J, et al. Safety and efficacy of imatinib (STI571) in metastatic gastrointestinal stromal tumours: a phase I study. *Lancet* 2001;358:1421–1423.
334. Singer S, Rubin BP, Lux ML, et al. Prognostic value of KIT mutation type, mitotic activity, and histologic subtype in gastrointestinal stromal tumors. *J Clin Oncol* 2002;20:3898–3905.
335. Tuveson DA, Willis NA, Jacks T, et al. STI571 inactivation of the gastrointestinal stromal tumor c-KIT oncoprotein: biological and clinical implications. *Oncogene* 2001;20:5054–5058.
336. Ma Y, Zeng S, Metcalfe DD, et al. The c-KIT mutation causing human mastocytosis is resistant to STI571 and other KIT kinase inhibitors; kinases with enzymatic site mutations show different inhibitor sensitivity profiles than wild-type kinases and those with regulatory-type mutations. *Blood* 2002;99:1741–1744.
337. Heinrich MC, Corless CL, Demetri GD, et al. Kinase mutations and imatinib response in patients with metastatic gastrointestinal stromal tumor. *J Clin Oncol* 2003;21:4342–4349.
338. Glabbeke M, Van Oosterom AT. Use of c-KIT/PDGFRA mutational analysis to predict the clinical response to imatinib in patients with advanced gastrointestinal stromal tumours entered on phase I and II studies of the EORTC Soft Tissue and Bone Sarcoma Group. *Eur J Cancer* 2004;40:689–695.
339. Demetri GD, Titton RL, Ryan DP, et al. Case records of the Massachusetts General Hospital: weekly clinicopathological exercises—Case 32-2004. A 68-year-old man with a large retroperitoneal mass. *N Engl J Med* 2004;351:1779–1787.
340. Chan GS, Yuen ST, Chan KW. Synovial sarcoma presenting as a polypoid jejunal mass. *Histopathology* 2004;44:191–193.
341. Billings SD, Meisner LF, Cummings OW, et al. Synovial sarcoma of the upper digestive tract: a report of two cases with demonstration of the X;18 translocation by fluorescence in situ hybridization. *Mod Pathol* 2000;13:68–76.
342. Habu S, Okamoto E, Toyosaka A, et al. Synovial sarcoma of the esophagus: report of a case. *Surg Today* 1998;28:401–404.
343. Yamamoto H, Watanabe K, Nagata M, et al. Inflammatory myofibroblastic tumor (IMT) of the pancreas. *J Hepatobiliary Pancreat Surg* 2002;9:116–119.
344. Venkataraman S, Semelka RC, Braga L, et al. Inflammatory myofibroblastic tumor of the hepatobiliary system: report of MR imaging appearance in four patients. *Radiology* 2003;227:758–763.
345. SantaCruz KS, McKinley ET, Powell RD Jr, et al. Inflammatory myofibroblastic tumor of the gastroesophageal junction in childhood. *Pediatr Pathol Mol Med* 2002;21:49–56.
346. Difiore JW, Goldblum JR. Inflammatory myofibroblastic tumor of the small intestine. *J Am Coll Surg* 2002;194:502–506.
347. Kim KA, Park CM, Lee JH, et al. Inflammatory myofibroblastic tumor of the stomach with peritoneal dissemination in a young adult: imaging findings. *Abdom Imaging* 2004;29:9–11.
348. Kie JH, Lee MK, Kim CJ, et al. Primary Ewing's sarcoma of the duodenum: a case report. *Int J Surg Pathol* 2003;11:331–337.

349. Boehm R, Till H, Landes J, et al. Ileoileal intussusception caused by a Ewing sarcoma tumour: an unusual case report. *Eur J Pediatr Surg* 2003;13:272–275.

350. Sarangarajan R, Hill DA, Humphrey PA, et al. Primitive neuroectodermal tumors of the biliary and gastrointestinal tracts: clinicopathologic and molecular diagnostic study of two cases. *Pediatr Dev Pathol* 2001;4:185–191.

351. Drut R, Drut M, Muller C, et al. Rectal primitive neuroectodermal tumor. *Pediatr Pathol Mol Med* 2003;22:391–398.

352. Perek S, Perek A, Sarman K, et al. Primitive neuroectodermal tumor of the pancreas: a case report of an extremely rare tumor. *Pancreatology* 2003;3:352–356.

353. O'Sullivan MJ, Perlman EJ, Furman J. Visceral primitive peripheral neuroectodermal tumors: a clinicopathologic and molecular study. *Hum Pathol* 2001;32:1109–1115.

354. Movahedi-Lankarani S, Hruban RH, Westra WH, et al. Primitive neuroectodermal tumors of the pancreas: a report of seven cases of a rare neoplasm. *Am J Surg Pathol* 2002;26:1040–1047.

355. Bismar TA, Basturk O, Gerald WL, et al. Desmoplastic small cell tumor in the pancreas. *Am J Surg Pathol* 2004;28:808–812.

356. Murray JC, Minifee PK, Trautwein LM, et al. Intraabdominal desmoplastic small round cell tumor presenting as a gastric mural mass with hepatic metastases. *J Pediatr Hematol Oncol* 1996;18:289–292.

357. Yaziji H, Ranaldi R, Verdolini R, et al. Primary alveolar soft part sarcoma of the stomach: a case report and review. *Pathol Res Pract* 2000;196:519–525.

358. Covinsky M, Gong S, Rajaram V, et al. *EWS-ATF1* fusion transcripts in gastrointestinal tumors previously diagnosed as malignant melanoma. *Hum Pathol* 2005;36:74–81.

359. Elmore LW, Harris CC. Hepatocellular carcinoma. In: Vogelstein B, Kinzler KW, eds. *The Genetic Basis of Human Cancer.* 2nd ed. New York: McGraw Hill; 2002:741–750.

360. Nagai H, Terada Y, Tajiri T, et al. Characterization of liver-cirrhosis nodules by analysis of gene-expression profiles and patterns of allelic loss. *J Hum Genet* 2004;49: 246–255.

361. Feitelson MA. *c-myc* overexpression in hepatocarcinogenesis. *Hum Pathol* 2004; 35:1299–1302.

362. Jia L, Wang XW, Harris CC. Hepatitis B virus X protein inhibits nucleotide excision repair. *Int J Cancer* 1999;80:875–879.

363. Wang XW, Forrester K, Yeh H, et al. Hepatitis B virus X protein inhibits *p53* sequence-specific DNA binding, transcriptional activity, and association with transcription factor ERCC3. *Proc Natl Acad Sci USA* 1994;91:2230–2234.

364. Wang XW, Gibson MK, Vermeulen W, et al. Abrogation of *p53*-induced apoptosis by the hepatitis B virus X gene. *Cancer Res* 1995;55:6012–6016.

365. Donato F, Tagger A, Chiesa R, et al. Hepatitis B and C virus infection, alcohol drinking, and hepatocellular carcinoma: a case-control study in Italy. Brescia HCC Study. *Hepatology* 1997;26:579–584.

366. Corrao G, Arico S. Independent and combined action of hepatitis C virus infection and alcohol consumption on the risk of symptomatic liver cirrhosis. *Hepatology* 1998;27:914–919.

367. Ostapowicz G, Watson KJ, Locarnini SA, et al. Role of alcohol in the progression of liver disease caused by hepatitis C virus infection. *Hepatology* 1998;27:1730–1735.

368. Bressac B, Kew M, Wands J, et al. Selective G to T mutations of *p53* gene in hepatocellular carcinoma from southern Africa. *Nature* 1991;350:429–431.

369. Hsu IC, Metcalf RA, Sun T, et al. Mutational hotspot in the *p53* gene in human hepatocellular carcinomas. *Nature* 1991;350:427–428.

370. Tsuda H, Hirohashi S, Shimosato Y, et al. Clonal origin of atypical adenomatous hyperplasia of the liver and clonal identity with hepatocellular carcinoma. *Gastroenterology* 1988;95:1664–1666.

371. Yasui H, Hino O, Ohtake K, et al. Clonal growth of hepatitis B virus-integrated hepatocytes in cirrhotic liver nodules. *Cancer Res* 1992;52:6810–6814.

372. Ponchel F, Puisieux A, Tabone E, et al. Hepatocarcinoma-specific mutant *p53*-249ser induces mitotic activity but has no effect on transforming growth factor beta 1-mediated apoptosis. *Cancer Res* 1994;54:2064–2068.

373. Sakamoto M, Hirohashi S, Tsuda H, et al. Multicentric independent development of hepatocellular carcinoma revealed by analysis of hepatitis B virus integration pattern. *Am J Surg Pathol* 1989;13:1064–1067.

374. Oda T, Tsuda H, Sakamoto M, et al. Different mutations of the *p53* gene in nodule-in-nodule hepatocellular carcinoma as a evidence for multistage progression. *Cancer Lett* 1994;83:197–200.

375. Oda T, Tsuda H, Scarpa A, et al. Mutation pattern of the *p53* gene as a diagnostic marker for multiple hepatocellular carcinoma. *Cancer Res* 1992;52:3674–3678.

376. Chen YJ, Yeh SH, Chen JT, et al. Chromosomal changes and clonality relationship between primary and recurrent hepatocellular carcinoma. *Gastroenterology* 2000;119:431–440.

377. Altimari A, Gruppioni E, Fiorentino M, et al. Genomic allelotyping for distinction of recurrent and de novo hepatocellular carcinoma after orthotopic liver transplantation. *Diagn Mol Pathol* 2005;14:34–38.

378. Flemming P, Tillmann HL, Barg-Hock H, et al. Donor origin of de novo hepatocellular carcinoma in hepatic allografts. *Transplantation* 2003;76:1625–1627.

379. Jeng KS, Sheen IS, Wang YC, et al. Is the vascular endothelial growth factor messenger RNA expression in resectable hepatocellular carcinoma of prognostic value after resection? *World J Gastroenterol* 2004;10:676–681.

380. Ikeguchi M, Ueda T, Sakatani T, et al. Expression of survivin messenger RNA correlates with poor prognosis in patients with hepatocellular carcinoma. *Diagn Mol Pathol* 2002;11:33–40.

381. Park NH, Chung YH, Youn KH, et al. Close correlation of *p53* mutation to microvascular invasion in hepatocellular carcinoma. *J Clin Gastroenterol* 2001;33:397–401.

382. Nagai H, Terada Y, Tajiri T, et al. Characterization of liver-cirrhosis nodules by analysis of gene-expression profiles and patterns of allelic loss. *J Hum Genet* 2004;49: 246–255.

383. Cheung ST, Chen X, Guan XY, et al. Identify metastasis-associated genes in hepatocellular carcinoma through clonality delineation for multinodular tumor. *Cancer Res* 2002;62:4711–4721.

384. Ye QH, Qin LX, Forgues M, et al. Predicting hepatitis B virus-positive metastatic hepatocellular carcinomas using gene expression profiling and supervised machine learning. *Nat Med* 2003;9:416–423.

385. Iizuka N, Oka M, Yamada-Okabe H, et al. Oligonucleotide microarray for prediction of early intrahepatic recurrence of hepatocellular carcinoma after curative resection. *Lancet* 2003;361:923–929.

386. Lee JS, Chu, IS, Heo J, et al. Classification and prediction of survival in hepatocellular carcinoma by gene expression profiling. *Hepatology* 2004;40:667–676.

387. Locker J. A new way to look at liver cancer. *Hepatology* 2004;40:521–523.

388. Ito Y, Matsuura N, Sakon M, et al. Both cell proliferation and apoptosis significantly predict shortened disease-free survival in hepatocellular carcinoma. *Br J Cancer* 1999;81:747–751.

389. Hoshida Y, Moriyama M, Otsuka M, et al. Identification of genes associated with sensitivity to 5-fluorouracil and cisplatin in hepatoma cells. *J Gastroenterol* 2002;37:92–95.

390. Moriyama M, Hoshida Y, Otsuka M, et al. Relevance network between chemosensitivity and transcriptome in human hepatoma cells. *Mol Cancer Ther* 2003;2: 199–205.

391. Iavarone M, Lampertico P, Ronchi G, et al. A prospective study of blood alpha-fetoprotein messenger RNA as a predictor of hepatocellular carcinoma in patients with cirrhosis. *J Viral Hepat* 2003;10:423–426.

392. Jeng KS, Sheen IS, Tsai YC. Does the presence of circulating hepatocellular carcinoma cells indicate a risk of recurrence after resection? *Am J Gastroenterol* 2004;99:1503–1509.

393. Ijichi M, Takayama T, Matsumura M, et al. Alpha-fetoprotein mRNA in the circulation as a predictor of postsurgical recurrence of hepatocellular carcinoma: a prospective study. *Hepatology* 2002;35:853–860.

394. Okuda N, Nakao A, Takeda S, et al. Clinical significance of alpha-fetoprotein mRNA during perioperative period in HCC. *Hepatogastroenterology* 1999;46:381–386.

395. Liu Y, Zhang BH, Qian GX, et al. Expression of AFP mRNA in blood of patients with recurrent hepatocellular carcinoma. *Hepatobiliary Pancreat Dis Int* 2003;2:274–277.

396. Jeng KS, Sheen IS, Wang YC, et al. Prognostic significance of preoperative circulating vascular endothelial growth factor messenger RNA expression in resectable hepatocellular carcinoma: a prospective study. *World J Gastroenterol* 2004;10:643–648.

397. Si MW, Thorson JA, Lauwers GY, et al. Hepatocellular lymphoepithelioma-like carcinoma associated with Epstein Barr virus: a hitherto unrecognized entity. *Diagn Mol Pathol* 2004;13:183–189.

398. Shirabe K, Matsumata T, Maeda T, et al. A long-term surviving patient with hepatocellular carcinoma including lymphocytes infiltration: a clinicopathological study. *Hepatogastroenterology* 1995;42:996–1001.

399. Wada Y, Nakashima O, Kutami R, et al. Clinicopathological study on hepatocellular carcinoma with lymphocytic infiltration. *Hepatology* 1998;27:407–414.

400. Chen PC, Pan CC, Hsu WH, et al. Epstein-Barr virus-associated lymphoepithelioma-like carcinoma of the esophagus. *Hum Pathol* 2003;34:407–411.

401. Lee HS, Chang MS, Yang HK, et al. Epstein-Barr virus-positive gastric carcinoma has a distinct protein expression profile in comparison with Epstein-Barr virus-negative carcinoma. *Clin Cancer Res* 2004;10:1698–1705.

402. Emile JF, Adam R, Sebagh M, et al. Hepatocellular carcinoma with lymphoid stroma: a tumour with good prognosis after liver transplantation. *Histopathology* 2000;37:523–529.

403. Falk H, Herbert J, Crowley S, et al. Epidemiology of hepatic angiosarcoma in the United States: 1964–1974. *Environ Health Perspect* 1981;41:107–113.

404. Hollstein M, Marion MJ, Lehman T, et al. *p53* mutations at A:T base pairs in angiosarcomas of vinyl chloride-exposed factory workers. *Carcinogenesis* 1994;15:1–3.

405. Przygodzki RM, Finkelstein SD, Keohavong P, et al. Sporadic and Thorotrast-induced angiosarcomas of the liver manifest frequent and multiple point mutations in K-*ras*-2. *Lab Invest* 1997;76:153–159.

406. Marion MJ, Froment O, Trepo C. Activation of Ki-*ras* gene by point mutation in human liver angiosarcoma associated with vinyl chloride exposure. *Mol Carcinog* 1991;4:450–454.

407. Soini Y, Welsh JA, Ishak K, et al. *p53* mutations in primary hepatic angiosarcomas not associated with vinyl chloride exposure. *Carcinogenesis* 1995;16:2879–2881.

408. Zietz C, Rossle M, Haas C, et al. MDM-2 oncoprotein overexpression, *p53* gene mutation, and VEGF up-regulation in angiosarcomas. *Am J Pathol* 1998;153: 1425–1433.

409. Vogt S, Schneider-Stock R, Klauck S, et al. Detection of hepatitis C virus RNA in formalin-fixed, paraffin-embedded thin-needle liver biopsy specimens. *Am J Clin Pathol* 2003;120:536–543.

410. de Lamballerie X, Charrel RN, Attoui H, et al. Classification of hepatitis C virus variants in six major types based on analysis of the envelope 1 and nonstructural 5B genome regions and complete polyprotein sequences. *J Gen Virol* 1997;78:45–51.

411. Qian X, Guerrero RB, Plummer TB, et al. Detection of hepatitis C virus RNA in formalin-fixed paraffin-embedded sections with digoxigenin-labeled cRNA probes. *Diagn Mol Pathol* 2004;13:9–14.

412. Svoboda-Newman SM, Greenson JK, Singleton TP, et al. Detection of hepatitis C by RT-PCR in formalin-fixed paraffin-embedded tissue from liver transplant patients. *Diagn Mol Pathol* 1997;6:123–129.

413. Biagini P, Benkoel L, Dodero F, et al. Hepatitis C virus RNA detection by in situ RT-PCR in formalin-fixed paraffin-embedded liver tissue: comparison with serum and tissue results. *Cell Mol Biol* 2001;47:OL167–OL171.

414. Soguero C, Campo E, Ribalta T, et al. Assessment of genotype and molecular evolution of hepatitis C virus in formalin-fixed paraffin-embedded liver tissue from patients with chronic hepatitis C virus infection. *Lab Invest* 2000;80: 851–856.

415. Ikura Y, Ohsawa M, Hai E, et al. Hepatitis C virus genotype testing in paraffin wax embedded liver biopsies for specimen identification. *J Clin Pathol* 2003;56:960–962.

Reproductive Organs

16

CERVIX

Squamous Cell Carcinoma

Cervical cancer remains the most common malignancy and the most common cause of cancer death in women in sub-Sahara Africa, Central America, South Central Asia, and Melanesia, although cervical cancer does not currently rank in the top 10 malignancies in terms of incidence or number of fatalities for women who live in the United States (1).

Genetics

Human papillomavirus (HPV) is the major etiologic factor for cervical cancer and is associated with virtually all cervical squamous cell carcinomas (SCC) (2,3). Over 100 different HPV serotypes have been identified, of which approximately 40 infect the female genital tract. Low-risk types are responsible for genital warts, but high-risk HPV types are associated with invasive carcinoma. Eleven HPV types are consistently classified as high risk, specifically 16, 18, 31, 33, 35, 39, 45, 51, 52, 56, and 58, but recent epidemiologic studies suggest that seven additional types are high risk, specifically 26, 53, 59, 66, 68, 73, and 82 (3–5). Infection with some high-risk HPV types is associated with a greater than 70-fold increased relative risk for cervical SCC or adenocarcinoma (5,6).

Host immune response factors contribute to the probability of persistent HPV infection and progression to cervical neoplasia. A cluster of genes in the HLA region of chromosome 6 is associated with an inherited susceptibility to the transforming properties of high-risk HPV types (7). Impairment of immune function, whether resulting from immunosuppressive therapy associated with organ transplantation (8) or HIV infection (9), has also been shown to be associated with a 5- to 10-fold increased relative risk

of cervical intraepithelial neoplasia (CIN) and invasive carcinoma.

Two viral genes play an important role in cervical carcinogenesis mediated by high-risk HPV types, specifically *E6* and *E7*. The E6 protein binds to the tumor suppressor protein p53, an interaction that leads to rapid degradation of p53 via the ubiquitin pathway. Similarly, interaction of the E7 protein with the RB1 tumor suppressor protein leads to rapid degradation of RB1 via the ubiquitin pathway. The loss of function of p53 and RB1 not only interferes with apoptosis, but also increases unscheduled cellular proliferation, both of which contribute to oncogenesis. Although early observations suggested that polymorphisms in p53 (specifically, polymorphisms at amino acid 72) are associated with altered E6-mediated degradation and an increased susceptibility to tumorigenesis (10), subsequent studies have shown conflicting results (11–13). The role of p53 polymorphisms in the development of invasive cervical carcinoma remains unsettled, and therefore sequence analysis of *TP53* codon 72 currently has no established role in patient management.

Technical Issues in Molecular Testing for Cervical Cancer Screening

There is no doubt that evaluation of exfoliated cervical cells by conventional cytopathology is an effective method for identifying patients with an increased risk of developing cervical carcinoma (based on compiled reports, the sensitivity of conventional cytology for detecting high-grade CIN and SCC ranges between 50% and 95%, with a specificity of at most 90% [reviewed in 14–16]). Given the strong etiologic association between high-risk HPV types and high-grade CIN and carcinoma, a number of molecular genetic approaches focused on detection of high-risk HPV types have been assessed to see if they can provide even more reliable results from exfoliated cervical cells (17).

Telomerase Activity

Both the E6 and E7 oncoproteins of HPV have been shown to activate telomerase (18–21), but the results from assays that measure telomerase activity have not been encouraging. Measured by the telomeric repeat amplification protocol (TRAP) (Chapter 5), the level of telomerase activity does not correlate with the presence of infection by high-risk HPV types in any of the diagnostic categories defined by conventional cytopathology (18,22). Furthermore, the TRAP assay has a sensitivity of only 30% for detecting biopsy-confirmed cases of CIN II to III (18).

Loss of Heterozygosity Analysis

A number of studies have shown that loss of heterozygosity (LOH) in multiple chromosomal regions accumulates in parallel with the progression of CIN to invasive carcinoma to lymphatic metastasis (23–26). However, the relevant loci, which are thought to encode putative tumor suppressor genes, have yet to be completely characterized. In addition, the sensitivity and specificity of LOH analysis in the evaluation of cervical cytology specimens have not been formally evaluated.

Polymerase Chain Reaction

As discussed in more detail in Chapter 22, most polymerase chain reaction (PCR) protocols for HPV testing make use of consensus primers targeted to the viral L1 gene that are, theoretically, capable of amplifying all HPV types that affect the anogenital region. Following amplification, the HPV type can be determined by either DNA sequence analysis (27,28) or membrane hybridization with type-specific probes. However, both approaches are labor intensive and difficult to automate, which makes them poorly suited for screening a large volume of patient specimens. Solution hybridization methods are more suited for high-throughput analysis.

Solution Hybridization

The Hybrid Capture 2 test (HC2, Digene, Gaithersburg, MD) uses pools of synthetic RNA probes to detect 5 low-risk HPV types (types 6, 11, 42, 43, and 44) and 13 high-risk HPV types (types 16, 18, 31, 33, 35, 39, 45, 51, 52, 56, 58, 59, and 68). As shown in Figure 16.1, the method involves three steps. First, DNA is extracted from the cytology specimen (which must be collected in one of a small number of approved transport media) and hybridized in solution to one of the RNA probe cocktails; second, antibodies are used to capture the RNA:DNA hybrids; and third, the bound RNA:DNA hybrids are detected by chemiluminescence, producing an assay readout of relative light units (RLUx). Because the assay is very easy to perform, can be completed within several hours, is not hindered by cross-contamination, and can potentially be automated, the solution hybridization approach is ideally suited for clinical use in high-volume settings.

The Food and Drug Administration (FDA)-approved cutoff value for a positive test (1 pg HPV DNA-polymer, which corresponds to about 5,000 copies of the HPV genome) was specifically selected to provide high sensitivity for identifying CIN II to III and cervical carcinoma (29). Consequently, even though the RLUx measurement provided by the HC2 test is only semi-quantitative, and despite that fact that the test result is not standardized based on the cellularity of the sample, the solution hybridization approach has a very low false negative rate. However, it is worth noting that the HC2 test high-risk probe set does not detect HPV types 26, 53, 66, 73, and 82, which have recently been shown to be most appropriately classified as high-risk types (3).

The HC2 low-risk and high-risk probe sets have limited, but measurable, cross-reactivity (28,30,31), although the clinical significance of this cross-reactivity depends on the patient population (discussed in more detail later). In parallel analysis, there is only fair concordance between HC2 testing using the low-risk probe set and reverse hybridization line probe analysis (LiPA; Chapter 22) and only moderate concordance between HC2 testing using the high-risk probe set and LiPA. This lack of concordance likely reflects the fact that many HPV types detected by LiPA are not specifically targeted by the HC2 assay (28). However, the high concordance between participating laboratories (kappa value, 0.84) in a study of interlaboratory reproducibility demonstrates that the HC2 test is very reliable (32).

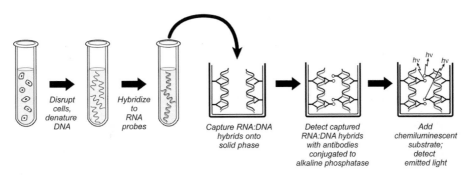

Figure 16.1   Schematic diagram of the Hybrid Capture 2 methodology. After the cells in the liquid-based cytology specimen are lysed, the synthetic RNA probe mixture is added. The RNA:DNA hybrids are captured by antibodies that are coated on the wells of a microtiter plate, and the bound RNA:DNA hybrids are then labeled with reporter antibodies that have been conjugated to alkaline phosphatase (multiple conjugated antibodies bind to each RNA:DNA hybrid, producing significant signal amplification). The alkaline phosphatase enzymes cleave the chemiluminescent substrate, and the emitted light is measured to produce the assay readout of relative light units.

In situ Hybridization

In situ hybridization (ISH) makes it possible to link the presence or absence of HPV infection with the cytomorphology of individual cells. High-thoughput fluorescence in situ hybiridization (FISH) targeting HPV *E6* and *E7* mRNA has been described (33), but chromogeneic in situ hybridization (CISH) is a more widely used used approach (Fig. 16.2). The commercially available INFORM HPV liquid-based kit (Ventana Medical Systems, Inc., Tucson, AZ) employs a probe cocktail that recognizes 13 high-risk HPV types (specifically, types 16, 18, 31, 33, 35, 39, 45, 51, 52, 56, 58, 68, and 70) to yield a chromogenic product that can be visualized by routine light microscopy. In practice, the method has three simple steps; slides prepared from cytology samples or biopsy specimens are treated with an endopeptidase to expose the nuclear DNA, the probe cocktail is hybridized to the treated specimen, and the bound probe is detected through a series of labeled antibodies that are used to generate the chromogenic product.

Several factors can make the CISH result difficult to interpret, including improper specimen handling and the presence of contaminating bacteria and yeast (34). Direct comparison of CISH and solution hybridization by parallel analysis of liquid-based cervical and vaginal cytology specimens with atypical squamous cells of undetermined significance (ASCUS) has shown that that solution hybridization has a higher sensitivity for detecting HPV DNA in women under 40 years of age, and that, of samples that test positive for high-risk HPV DNA, only 20% are positive by both CISH and solution hybridization methods (34). It is difficult to evaluate the significance of these results, however, because the CISH analysis used in the comparison was often not performed within 21 days of sample collection as recommended by the CISH kit manufacturer.

Diagnostic Issues in Molecular Testing for Cervical Cancer Screening

Although DNA-based testing for high-risk HPV types has a higher sensitivity for identifying CIN II, CIN III, or cervical carcinoma in virtually every published study (reviewed in 35), the epidemiology of HPV infection in women constrains the utility of testing in routine clinical practice. Among sexually active women less than 30 years old, the prevalence of high-risk HPV infection is quite high; it is about 35% in the United States, over 40% in some Northern European populations, and over 80% in some South American populations (36–41). However, most HPV infections in women less than 30 years old are transient and clinically insignificant, including those by high-risk HPV types; in this age group, only about 10% of women remain infected after 5 years, and the incidence of cervical cancer is

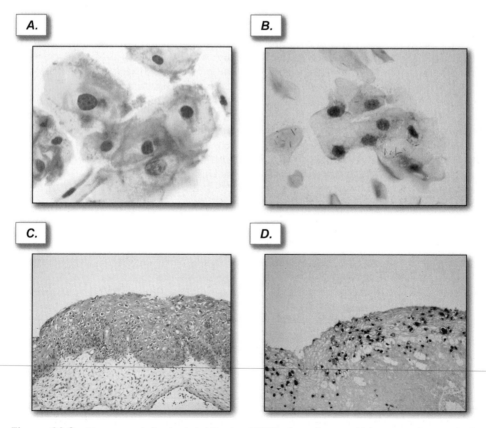

Figure 16.2   Chromogenic in situ hybridization (CISH) of cytology and biopsy specimens. **A**, A conventional PAP smear from a woman less than 30 years old shows ASCUS. **B**, Strong staining by CISH demonstrates the presence of high-risk human papillomavirus (HPV) infection. **C**, A cervical biopsy showing koilocytosis. **D**, Strong staining by CISH demonstrates the presence of high-risk HPV infection. (See color insert.)

very low (2). Molecular testing for high-risk HPV types therefore has a low positive predictive value for CINII, CINIII, and cervical carcinoma in women less than 30 years old, despite the high technical sensitivity and specificity of the various approaches for detecting the HPV virus (36,42–45). In contrast, the prevalence of high-risk HPV infection is less than 10% in women over 40 years old, but this group of women has a greater than 50% chance of developing CIN II, CIN III, or invasive carcinoma (2). Molecular testing for high-risk HPV types among women more than 40 years old therefore has a much higher positive predictive value for CIN II, CIN III, and carcinoma.

Consensus guidelines therefore recommend HPV testing as the preferred strategy for management of women with ASCUS (43,46,47), but recommend that testing for high-risk HPV types should not used to screen women who are under age 30 for cervical cancer. This approach avoids classification of large numbers of women as being at increased risk for CIN II, CIN III, or invasive cervical carcinoma, even though their HPV infection is not clinically significant, thereby limiting unnecessarily intensive follow-up, as well as patient anxiety (2).

Different practice guidelines have been developed for women who are over 30 years old. Because of the decreased prevalence of high-risk HPV infections in women in this age-group, but increased incidence of high-grade dysplasia and invasive carcinoma, a National Institutes of Health-National Cancer Institute workshop recently recommended that HPV DNA testing may be added to routine cervical cytology for women at least age 30 (2).

Analysis of women who are immunosuppressed, whether from HIV infection, post-transplant immunosuppressive drug therapy, or some other cause, has shown that high-risk HPV infections are quite common in this patient population (48). Because the incidence of high-grade cervical dysplasia is higher in HIV-infected women, and because the natural history of disease progression may be different in immunosuppressed women, HPV testing as an adjunct to cervical cytology in this population has little established benefit (49,50).

Diagnostic Issues in Molecular Testing for Clinical Follow-up

High-grade cervical dysplasia recurs in 5% to 15% of women following treatment (51,52). Since high-risk HPV testing has been shown to have a higher predictive value for post-treatment recurrence of CIN II to III than conventional cytopathology, several groups have proposed that high-risk HPV testing should be incorporated into post-treatment screening regimens (53,54). However, formal guidelines have not been developed for this clinical setting.

Cost-effectiveness of Genetic High-risk HPV Testing

Several computer models suggest that DNA-based testing of cervical cytology specimens with ASCUS for high-risk HPV types is a more effective and less costly approach than other triage strategies, including immediate colposcopy or repeat cervical cytology (55,56). However, the data are currently insufficient to determine whether or not the incorporation of reflex HPV testing in cervical cancer screening programs actually does reduce costs or if it is more acceptable to women (35,57). Approximately half of invasive cervical carcinomas in the United States occur in women who do not undergo regular screening (58,59), prompting some health care professionals to question whether more significant decreases in cervical cancer morbidity and mortality could be achieved through an increased emphasis on screening by the conventional Pap test rather than by shifting resources to higher-cost DNA-based testing methods (60). This same concern has also been raised with respect to the implementation of DNA-based testing methods in developing countries (61).

Adenocarcinoma

Genetics

Infection by high-risk HPV types plays an important role in the tumorigenesis of cervical adenocarcinomas, including those of endometrioid, mucinous, or mixed endometrioid and mucinous morphology (62,63). By either PCR-based methods or ISH, high-risk HPV types are identified in 67% to 91% of in situ and invasive adenocarcinomas (62–65).

Role of Molecular Genetic Testing in Diagnosis of Cervical Adenocarcinoma

For some adenocarcinomas that have an endometrioid morphology, it can be difficult to determine whether the tumor is of endometrial origin with extension into the endocervix, or is of endocervical origin with extension into the endometrium. The distinction is important, because the surgical management of primary endocervical carcinoma and primary endometrial carcinoma is different.

Testing for HPV DNA can be quite useful in this setting, because high-risk HPV types are present in the majority of endocervical adenocarcinomas, as noted above. An alternative approach for distinguishing endocervical from endometrial adenocarcinoma is based on immunohistochemical analysis of p16 (as noted previously, the E7 protein from high-risk HPV types binds and inactivates RB1; as a consequence of RB1 inactivation, p16 is overexpressed). About 95% of endocervical adenocarcinomas are immunopositive for p16 expression, whereas virtually 100% of endometrial adenocarcinomas are immunonegative (62). Combined with immunohistochemical analysis of estrogen receptor and progesterone receptor, HPV DNA testing or p16 immunohistochemical analysis therefore provides a reliable approach to determine the origin of endometrioid adenocarcinomas in curettage specimens. As an aside, it is worth mentioning that immunohistochemical analysis of p16 expression in this setting provides an example of the evolution of molecular testing in clinical practice, in which an increased understanding of the genetic basis of tumor development is used to design tests for surrogate markers that do not rely on DNA-based methods.

Minimal Deviation Adenocarcinoma

Minimal deviation adenocarcinoma (MDA), also known as adenoma malignum, is a well-differentiated variety of

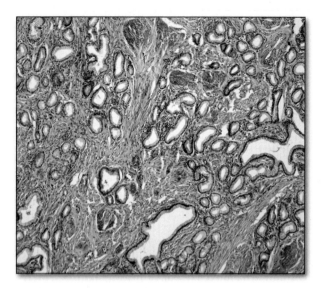

Figure 16.3   Minimal deviation adenocarcinoma (MDA) of the cervix. This tumor type has an increased incidence in women with Putz-Jegher syndrome. A significant percentage of sporadic MDA also harbor mutations in *STK11*. (See text for details.)

mucinous adenocarcinoma (Fig. 16.3) that accounts for far less than 1% of all invasive cervical carcinomas (66). MDA is quite rare in the general population, but has an increased incidence in women who have Putz-Jegher syndrome (67) (another uncommon gynecologic malignancy that is rare in the general population but more frequent in women with Putz-Jegher syndrome is ovarian sex cord tumor with annular tubules [67,68]).

Genetics

Putz-Jegher syndrome is an autosomal dominant disease caused by mutations in the *STK11* tumor suppressor gene at 19p13.3 that encodes a serine threonine kinase (69,70). *STK11* mutations are present in most families affected by the syndrome, although alterations at 19q13.4 are apparently responsible for disease in a subset of kindreds (71).

The spectrum of *STK11* germline mutations includes nonsense mutations, missense mutations, deletions, and inversions, all of which disrupt the protein's kinase domain. Tumorigenesis in patients with Putz-Jegher syndrome is often accompanied by LOH of 19p13.3, consistent with a model in which biallelic inactivation *STK11* occurs through either somatic mutation or LOH of the unaffected allele (72).

Technical Issues in Molecular Genetic Analysis of MDA

LOH of 19p13.3 can be detected in 38% to 100% of sporadic MDA (73,74) and somatic mutations in 0 to 55% of sporadic MDA (73,75). Studies of the mutational profile of sporadic MDA have involved only a small number of cases; thus, the lack of precision in the estimates of the prevalence of the different types of aberrations is not surprising.

Diagnostic Issues in Molecular Genetic Analysis of MDA

Only 5% of conventional endocervical mucinous adenocarcinomas harbors *STK11* mutations (75), and *STK11* mutations are not present in nonmucinous endocervical adenocarcinomas, including endometrioid adenocarcinomas, clear cell adenocarcinomas, and squamous cell carcinomas (75). More importantly, *STK11* mutations are absent in benign endocervical glands, including those with gastric metaplasia (75). If the lack of *STK11* mutations is confirmed in a larger number of benign endocervical glandular proliferations, genetic analysis of *STK11* may prove to be useful in the differential diagnosis of MDA. However, the low prevalence of mutations in sporadic cases of MDA, coupled with the fact that sensitive mutational analysis requires sequencing of most of the coding sequence of the gene, will likely limit the utility of molecular testing in routine practive.

It is noteworthy that MDAs that harbor *STK11* mutations have been shown to have a significantly poorer prognosis than tumors without mutations (75). This result suggests that even if mutational analysis does not have a role in diagnosis, testing may have a role in providing prognostic information and identifying those patients who may benefit from more aggressive therapy.

Putative Collision Tumors

Rare cervical tumors show well-demarcated areas of adenocarcinoma and SCC, and occasionally the question arises as to whether the histologic findings indicate the presence of a single malignancy with divergent differentiation or two independent cervical or lower uterine segment malignancies. Because the distinction can have a significant impact on clinical stage and therapy, molecular testing has been used to define the relationship between the two regions in these tumors. In one small study, LOH analysis using a panel of nine microsatellite markers demonstrated that the different histologic patterns had different clonal origins (76), a result that indicates the clinical utility of testing in problematic cases.

ENDOMETRIUM

Adenocarinoma

Overall, endometrial adenocarcinoma is the most common tumor of the female genital tract in industrialized nations, although the tumor has a lower incidence in developing countries. Clinicopathologically, there are two general types of endometrial cancer (77), and different pathways of oncogenesis appear to underlie the two clinicopathologic types. Type I adenocarcinomas (including endometrioid, mucinous, and secretory adenocarcinomas) are estrogen dependent, low-grade tumors often associated with atypical endometrial hyperplasia. Type I tumors account for 80% to 85% of cases of endometrial adenocarcinoma. Type II adenocarcinomas (serous adenocarcinoma and clear cell adenocarcinoma) are high-grade tumors that are less estrogen dependent. Type I tumors typically arise in a background of atrophic endometrium, and account for 10% to 15% of endometrial adenocarcinomas.

Genetics

Type I endometrial adenocarcinoma

Type I endometrial adenocarcinomas (EA) develop through the accumulation of mutations in at least four different genes (reviewed in reference 78). About 20% to 30% of type I EA show microsatellite instability (MSI) as a result of either mutations or epigenetic modifications of the genes encoding the proteins involved in DNA mismatch repair (79). As a consequence of the MSI, insertions or deletions are common in short tandem repeats (STRs), including mononucleotide repeats that are located within the coding sequence of genes that have an important role in control of signal transduction, apoptosis, and mismatch repair itself (Chapter 2, see also the discussion of hereditary non-polyposis colon cancer [HNPCC] in Chapter 15). The fact that type I EA is the second most common malignancy in patients with HNPCC emphasizes the central role of MSI in the development of this group of endometrial tumors.

From 37% to 61% of type I EA harbor somatic mutations in the tumor suppressor gene *PTEN* located at 10q23, and LOH of 10q23 can be identified in about 40% of cases (women with Cowden syndrome, caused by inherited mutations in *PTEN*, also have an increased risk of type I EA). Mutations in K-*ras* are present in 10% to 30% of cases of type I tumors, and mutations in *CTNNB1* (which encodes β-catenin) are present in 14% to 44%. Figure 16.4 shows one model for the genetic events involved in the development of type I EA.

Type II Endometrial Adenocarcinoma

Type II tumors are characterized by *TP53* mutations and are usually nondiploid (80–82). The presence of MSI and

PTEN mutations in a subset of conventional type II EA, as well as in some mixed adenocarcinomas (such as mixed clear cell and endometrioid adenocarcinomas), suggests that there is some overlap between the two oncogenic pathways, or that some type II EA may develop from conventional type I tumors via accrual of *TP53* or additional mutations (78,83).

Technical and Diagnostic Issues in Molecular Analysis of EA

Molecular genetic analysis of the loci involved in the oncogenesis of types I and II EA is not a sensitive or specific approach for diagnosis of endometrial neoplasms. Test specificity is limited by the fact that genetic aberrations characteristic of type I EA are also present in premalignant proliferations. For example, up to 36% of histologically normal premenopausal endometria contiain glands that do not express *PTEN* because of mutations or deletions (84), and MSI can be detected over 5 years before the onset of adenocarcinoma (85). Test sensitivity is limited by the fact that only a subset of endometrial adenocarcinomas, whether type I or II, harbor mutations at the relevant loci.

Although mutational analysis is not a sensitive or specific method for diagnosis of endometrial adenocarcinoma, characterization of the underlying oncogenic pathways has provided the opportunity to develop a histomorphologic classification for endometrial precancers (termed endometrial intraepithelial neoplasia [EIN]) that correlates more closely with the underlying genetic abnormalities than the conventional classification scheme (86–88). Because the diagnostic criteria for EIN are different from those for conventional atypical endometrial hyperplasia, it is not surprising that about 20% of glandular lesions are classified differently by the EIN scheme versus traditional criteria (89,90), but clinical outcome data suggest that classification by the EIN

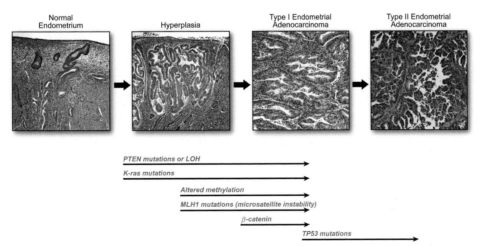

Figure 16.4 Simplified model for the stepwise development of type I endometrial adenocarcinoma. As discussed in the text, a subset of type II endometrial adenocarcinomas have a similar pattern of mutations, which demonstrates that there is some overlap between the oncogenic pathways that give rise to type I and type II tumors, or that some type II adenocarcinomas develop from conventional type I tumors. As an aside, it is noteworthy that the same pattern of mutations involved in development of complex atypical hyperplasia is also involved in the development of the abnormal glandular proliferations in atypical polypoid adenomyoma.

approach is more tightly correlated with the development of endometrial cancer (86–88).

Molecular Analysis of EA to Provide Prognostic Information

It remains unsettled whether or not mutational analysis of the genes involved in the development of EA can provide prognostic information. For example, there are conflicting data regarding whether the presence of K-*ras* mutations correlates with clinical outcome in patients with type I EA (91,92). Similarly, the prognostic significance of MSI in sporadic EA is uncertain; although most tumors with MSI tend to have a high histologic grade (4,93), they are more frequently type I EA and tend to be diagnosed at an earlier stage (94).

Markers other than those directly involved in tumorigenesis have also been evaluated to see if they can provide independent prognostic information. For example, in one small study, telomerase activity as measured by the TRAP assay was shown to be a statistically significant independent predictor of disease progression in patients with endometroid adenocarcinoma (95). However, at present, there is no established role for prognostic molecular testing in the pathologic evaluation of endometrial adenocarcinomas.

Microarray Analysis

Given limited diagnostic and prognostic information that can be obtained by mutational analysis of individual genes, a number of investigators have evaluated the utility of gene expression profiling using microarrays. Although such studies are in their infancy, the early results are noteworthy in that tumor classification based on the pattern of gene expression appears to be highly correlated with classification as type I or type II EA based on routine histomorphologic examination (96,97). However, occasional tumors have a gene expression profile that is inconsistent with their histomorphologic appearance. If the gene expression profile can be shown to more accurately predict patient outcome for those tumors that have disparate molecular and histologic features, microarray analysis may offer the opportunity to identify patients at higher risk who may benefit from more intensive therapy.

Endometrial Stromal Tumors

Endometrial stromal tumors are mesenchymal neoplasms of the uterine corpus that have a range of biologic behavior (98,99). In the current WHO classification scheme (100), endometrial stromal nodule is a benign, well-circumscribed tumor with pushing margins that consists of uniform cells resembling those of normal proliferative-stage endometrial stroma. Endometrial stromal sarcoma (ESS), though histologically similar to endometrial stromal nodule, exhibits myometrial infiltration or lymphovascular invasion. A subset of endometrial stromal tumors exhibit variant morphologic patterns, including smooth muscle differentiation, ovarian sex cord–like/epithelioid patterns, endometrioid glandular structures, or a prominent fibromyxoid component (99,101–105).

It appears that the behavior of ESS is almost entirely a function of stage at diagnosis (98,99,106); thus classification of ESS is currently not based primarily on mitotic rate (100). Tumors that show significant cytologic atypia, have frequent and atypical mitotic figures, and lack a plexiform vasculative are classified as undifferentiated endometrial sarcomas (99).

Genetics of Endometrial Stromal Tumors

The translocation t(7;17)(p15;q21) is a recurring aberration in endometrial stromal tumors (107). The rearrangement produces a fusion gene in which the *JAZF1* gene on chromosome 7 is fused with the *JJAZ1* gene on chromosome 17 (107). In all endometrial stromal tumors thus far characterized, the translocation results in *JAZF1-JJAZ1* fusion transcripts with the same structure (107–109). Another group of endometrial stromal tumors carry rearrangements that involve the 6p11–21 region (110), but the loci involved in the aberrations that cluster in this region have not yet been characterized.

As shown in Figure 16.5, t(7;17)(p15;q21) results in the production of a chimeric protein in which an N-terminal zinc finger domain of JAZF1 is linked to a zinc finger domain and a possible nuclear localization signal in the C-terminal region of JJAZ1 (107). However, the mechanism by which the chimeric protein promotes tumorigenesis remains unknown.

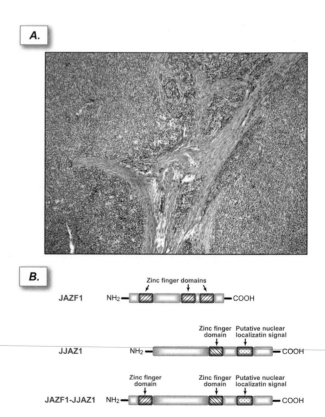

Figure 16.5 The *JAZF1-JJAZ1* fusion is characteristic of endometrial stromal tumors. **A**, An endometrial stromal sarcoma with classic histology. **B**, Schematic diagram of the JZAF1-JJAZ1 chimeric protein that results from the t(7;17)(p15;q21) translocation.

Technical Issues in Molecular Genetic Analysis of Endometrial Stromal Tumors

Conventional cytogenetic analysis demonstrates the t(7;17)(p15;q21) rearrangement in about 43% of cases of endometrial stromal tumors (107–109,111–113). Because published reports that characterize novel translocations are often biased by selective inclusion of positive cases, whether cytogenetic evaluation has this level of sensitivity in prospective use in routine clinical practice is unknown. Although other recurring cytogenetic aberrations have been described, as noted previously, they have not yet been sufficiently characterized to be of diagnostic utility.

FISH-based analysis has been used to demonstrate the t(7;17) translocation in metaphase chromosome spreads and interphase nuclei in a small number of clinical cases and endometrial stromal tumor cell lines (107). Reverse transcriptase polymerase chain reaction (RT-PCR) has been used to detect JAZF1-JJAZ1 fusion transcripts in fresh or FFPE tissue by both non-nested and nested approaches (107–109). Because only a small number of cases have thus far been evaluated, and because the prevalence of the t(7;17) varies between the different categories of endometrial stromal tumors (as discussed later), it has yet to be determined whether or not there are significant differences in the sensitivity and specificity of RT-PCR analysis depending on the tissue substrate or assay design.

Diagnostic Issues in Molecular Genetic Analysis of Endometrial Stromal Tumors

The specificity of the t(7;17) for endometrial stromal tumors is virtually 100%, although only a small number of normal endometrial samples and cellular leiomyomas have been evaluated for rearrangements involving JAZF1-JJAZ1 (107,108). JAZF1-JJAZ1 fusion transcripts have been detected in 100% of endometrial stromal nodules (ESN) thus far evaluated, regardless of whether fresh or FFPE tissue was the substrate for testing (107,108). Of note, the fusion transcript has also been demonstrated in one mixed smooth muscle variant of ESN (108). About 90% of ESS harbor the fusion (virtually all of which have had classic histology), including tumors that arise at extrauterine sites (108). Of the small number of ESS tested to date, none of the morphologic variants (including the epithelioid/sex cord–like variant, mixed smooth muscle variant, and fibromyxoid variants) have tested positive (107,108). Only a very small number of undifferentiated endometrial sarcomas have been evaluated, of which 50% have contained JAZF1-JJAZ1 fusion transcripts (107).

Given the presence of JAZF1-JJAZ fusions in a high proportion of cases of ESN, ESS, and undifferentiated endometrial sarcoma, it is obvious that molecular testing for the rearrangement cannot be used to distinguish between the different groups of endometrial stromal tumor. Furthermore, the low prevalence of the JAZF1-JJAZ1 fusion in ESS with variant morphologic patterns and undifferentiated endometrial sarcoma suggests that molecular testing is of limited utility in the evaluation of these neoplasms, which is unfortunate because tumors in these categories are often the most diagnostically challenging.

The presence of JAZF1-JJAZ1 gene fusions in a subset of ESS and undifferentiated ESS suggests that some of these malignancies develop from ESN (107). It is unknown whether cases of undifferentiated endometrial sarcoma that lack JAZF1-JJAZ1 fusions represent tumors with alternative rearrangements of JAZF1, or JJAZ1, or instead develop through an entirely different oncogenic pathway. In any event, no correlations between the presence of JAZF1-JJAZ1 fusions and patient outcome have so far been described for ESS or undifferentiated endometrial stromal sarcoma, and so molecular analysis of these two tumor types has no role from a prognostic or therapeutic perspective.

Benign Endometrial Polyps

Genetics

Conventional cytogenetic analysis of a large number of benign endometrial polyps has shown that rearrangements involving 12q14-15 and 6p21 are recurring karyotypic abnormalities. As discussed in more detail in Chapter 11 (in the section on lipomas), the 12q14-15 region encodes the high mobility group (HMG) protein HMGA2 (previously known as HMGIC) and the 6p21 region contains the gene encoding the HMG protein HMGA1 (previously known as HMGIY). The HMG proteins are small, acidic, nonhistone chromatin-associated proteins that contain DNA binding domains and an acidic C-terminal domain, and that facilitate formation of transcriptional complexes through protein–DNA and protein–protein interactions. As in other neoplasms (Table 11.7), rearrangements involving HMGA1 or HMGA2 are thought to promote polyp formation through deregulation of the level of expression of the HMG proteins (114,115), consistent with the observation that some endometrial polyps harbor double minute chromosomes containing an amplified and apparently nonarranged HMGA2 gene (116), and that the break point in some tumors with HMGA1 rearrangements is extragenic (117). The fact that the rearrangements involving 12q14-15 and 6p21 are present only in the stroma of endometrial polyps indicates that the epithelial component is not neoplastic (118).

Role of Molecular Genetic Analysis in Diagnosis of Endometrial Polyps

The diagnosis of benign endometrial polyps is straightforward based on routine microscopic examination, and thus there is little need for molecular analysis. The fact that rearrangements of the HMGA2 and HMGA1 loci are characteristic of a variety of other benign and malignant neoplasms is irrelevant, because none of those other neoplasms enter into the differential diagnosis of benign endometrial polyps.

Hydatidiform Moles

Accurate diagnosis of hydatidiform moles is important because of the increased risk of persistent or metastatic gestational trophoblastic disease that follows molar pregnancy (119). Because it is difficult to reliably distinguish early complete and partial molar pregnancies from nonmolar pregnancies based on histologic features alone (120–124), testing based on the genetic features of moles has been used to improve the accuracy of diagnosis. As shown in Table 16.1, hydatidiform moles are characterized by the presence of an abnormal complement of paternal chromosomes

TABLE 16.1

FEATURES OF HYDATIFORM MOLES AND NONMOLAR GESTATIONS

Type	Origins	Karyotype	Findings by Flow Cytometry	Findings by STR DNA Typing
Complete mole	Fertilization of an empty ovum by a single sperm with subsequent duplication (homozygous complete mole); fertilization of an empty ovum by two sperm (heterozygous complete mole)[a]	46,XX (about 85%) 46,XY (about 15%)	Diploid	A single fetal allele that is different from the maternal alleles at the same locus (homozygous complete mole); at least one locus has two non maternal alleles (heterozygous complete mole)
Partial mole	Fertilization of a normal ovum by two sperm (diandric triploidy)[b]	69,XXY (about 70%) 69,XXX (about 27%) 69,XYY (about 3%)	Triploid	At least two loci have three alleles
Nonmolar hydropic gestation	Nonspecific finding	46,XX or 46,XY	Diploid	Normal mendelian inheritance pattern

See reference 129 for complete criteria.
[a]The findings in the extremely rare examples of complete moles that are triploid or aneuploid (130) or biparental (131–133), or that result from confined placental mosaicism (134), are omitted from the table.
[b]The findings in the extremely rare examples of partial moles that are diploid, tetraploid, haploid, or aneuploid (135,136) are also omitted from the table.

(125–128). Complete moles are usually diploid and completely androgenic; most arise through fertilization of an empty ovum by a single haploid sperm with subsequent duplication (homozygous complete mole), while a minority arise from fertilization of an empty ovum by two different sperm (heterozygous complete mole). Biparental complete moles have also been described; these gestations occur repetitively in individual patients in a familial pattern, and the genetic locus responsible for the disease has recently been mapped (131–133). The vast majority of partial moles have a triploid karyotype and arise when a normal ovum is fertilized by two different haploid sperm.

Conventional cytogenetics and flow cytometry have traditionally been used to evaluate the ploidy of putative molar gestations (130). However, both techniques have limitations. Demonstration of diploidy is not specific for a complete mole, because nonmolar products of conception that show hydropic change are usually diploid. Similarly, demonstration of triploidy is consistent with but not necessarily specific for a partial mole, because triploid gestations that have an extra haploid set of chromosomes of maternal origin also occur (digynic triploid gestations do not show histologic features of molar pregnancies, show much longer in utero survival of the triploid fetus, and have a different prognosis than conventional partial molar gestations with diandric triploidy [137–139]).

DNA-based testing can provide greater sensitivity and specificity for diagnosis of molar gestations. Analysis can be performed by a variety of methods, including approaches that target restriction fragment length polymorphisms (RFLPs), sex chromosome markers, variable number of tandem repeats (VNTRs), or histocompatibility loci; interphase FISH; promoter methylation analysis; and short tandem repeat (STR) typing (129,140–151). PCR-based analysis of a panel of STRs is of particular utility because it is very sensitive, virtually always informative, does not require knowledge of paternal alleles, and is technically very straightforward. The use of commercial kits designed for monoplex or multiplex PCR amplification of the *CODIS* loci used for identity testing in forensic settings (Chapter 23) has greatly simplified STR typing and made the method accessible to most molecular genetic laboratories. In practical terms, hydropic villi that suggest a diagnosis of a molar pregnancy (Fig. 16.6) can be easily microdissected from FFPE tissue and their STR profile compared with that of maternal tissue from either the same specimen (i.e., fragments of endometrium) or peripheral blood. Criteria that have been developed to distinguish hydatidiform moles from nonmolar hydrophic gestations (Table 16.1) by STR-based testing indicate that molar pregnancies are underdiagnosed by routine histomorphology and flow cytometry (129), a result that suggests STR-based testing of hydropic gestations may have a role in routine clinical practice.

DNA-based testing is also useful for differentiating complete hydatidiform mole with coexistent fetus (CMCF) from partial mole. Although it is extremely difficult to separate CMCF from partial mole based on morphologic features alone, the distinction has clinical importance because CMCF is associated with an even higher risk of persistent trophoblastic disease than complete mole alone (152). Cytogenetic analysis and flow cytometry have both been used to distinguish between CMCF and partial mole (153–155), but STR analysis appears to be the optimal approach. STR-based analysis not only demonstrates the presence of CMCF, but also provides information on the zygosity of the molar component (134,156,157), a significant advantage given that a heterozygous complete mole in CMCF may confer a higher risk for persistent trophoblastic disease than a homozygous complete mole (152).

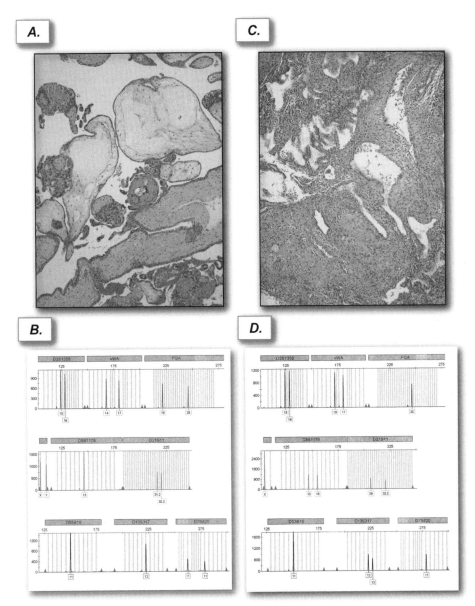

Figure 16.6   Use of STR analysis to evaluate products of conception suspicious for a molar pregnancy. **A**, The histologic features of the villi make it difficult to distinguish between an early molar pregnancy and hydropic change in a nonmolar pregnancy. **B**, DNA typing using a subset of the *CODIS* loci (Table 23.3) on villi microdissected from the tissue block shows a diploid gestation. Parallel analysis on maternal tissue (endometrium microdissected from the tissue block (**C**) shows the maternal genotype (**D**) and demonstrates that the products of conception contain a maternal allele at each locus. Taken together, the findings exclude a complete or partial molar gestation. (See color insert.)

MYOMETRIUM

Leiomyoma

Genetics

Although the cytogenetic abnormalities in leiomyomas are quite heterogeneous, the majority involve rearrangements of the 12q14-15 region that contains the *HMGA2* gene or the 6p21 region that contains the *HMGA1* gene, the same loci involved in the rearrangements characteristic of benign endometrial polyps, as discussed previously. The finding

that the break point in many of the rearrangements lies 3′ or 5′ to the coding region of the HMG genes, and that only a minority of leiomyomas harbor *HMG* fusion transcripts, suggests that deregulation of the level of expression of the HMG proteins is sufficient for tumorigenesis (116,158,159).

Technical Issues in Molecular Genetic Analysis of Leiomyomas

Routine cytogenetic evaluation demonstrates a karyotypic abnormality in about 40% of leiomyomas. Of leiomyomas

TABLE 16.2

RECOMBINATION PARTNERS IN UTERINE LEIOMYOMAS WITH 12q14-15 REARRANGEMENTS

Fusion	Features	Location of Partner Translocation	Reference
HMGA2-HEI10	Homo sapiens enhancer of invasion; unknown function	14q11	160
HMGA2-COX6C	Cytochrome C oxidase subunit VIC	8q22-23	161
HMGA2-RAD51B	Recombinational repair	14q23-24	162
HMGA2-ALDH2	Mitochondrial aldehyde dehydrogenase	12q24.1	163
HMGA2-LPP	Contains LIM domains; regulation of transcription?	3q27-28	164
HMGA2-RTVLH	Retrovirus-like human sequences; unknown function	21q21?	165
HMGA2-LHFP	Unknown	13q12	166

harboring rearrangements of 12q14-15, the partner region is 14q23-24 (the location of *RAD51B*) in about two thirds of cases (158).

Given the wide variety of rearrangements that involve the *HMG* loci (Table 16.2), probe-split FISH methodology is an extremely useful testing approach. The method has been used to demonstrate involvement of *HMGA2* and *HMGA1* in cases with reciprocal translocations, as well as complex rearrangements (118,158). FISH has been primarily performed on metaphase chromosomes in the studies reported to date (118,162,163), but interphase FISH on FFPE tissue is certain to have at least as much utility.

PCR-based methods, including 3'-race and RT-PCR, have also been used to analyze the chromosomal break points and fusion genes characteristic of leiomyomas (158,167). However, the heterogeneity of the rearrangements found in leiomyomas makes PCR a suboptimal approach for comprehensive genetic evaluation of the tumors.

Although both *HMGA2* and *HMGA1* are expressed during development, *HMGA2* is not expressed in normal adult tissues and *HMGA1* is expressed at only low levels (115,168,169), and so RT-PCR based analysis of *HMGA2* or *HMGA1* transcription has been used as an indirect method to detect the presence of rearrangements involving the loci. In fact, *HMGA2* or *HMGA1* expression can be demonstrated in up to 73% of leiomyomas by RT-PCR, and the level of expression is correlated with the presence underlying 12q14-15 or 6p21 rearrangements (167,170). However, the presence of so many different rearrangements involving the *HMG* loci produces significant heterogeneity in the structure of *HMG* transcripts, which makes comprehensive RT-PCR testing impossible. It is worth noting that there is a good correlation between the level of HMGAZ protein expression measured by immunohistochemistry and the level of *HMGAZ* mRNA, but that HMGA1 protein and mRNA levels do not correlate (171). Nonetheless, immunohistochemistry provides a straightforward, though indirect, approach for detecting increased HMG expression due to aberrations of the *HMG* loci (167,170,171).

Diagnostic Issues in Molecular Genetic Analysis of Leiomyomas

As noted above, rearrangements involving 12q14-15 and 6p21 are characteristic of a wide variety of tumors in many anatomic locations. Although most of these other neoplasms do not enter into the diagnosis of uterine leiomyomas, it is important to note that rearrangements of *HMGA2* have been identified in rare examples of myometrial leiomyosarcoma (167). The role of molecular analysis of the *HMG* loci in the diagnosis of problematic myometrial smooth muscle neoplasms has not been evaluated.

Leiomyosarcoma

Leiomyosarcoma accounts for about 1% of uterine malignancies and is the most common pure uterine sarcoma (172). Leiomyosarcomas have a highly variable and complex pattern of cytogenetic aberrations, and no specific abnormalities have emerged that have diagnostic utility (173,174). Of note, rearrangements involving the *HMG* loci are not a feature of leiomyosarcoma, a finding that is consistent with the clinicopathologic fact that leiomyomas are not precursor lesions of leiomyosarcoma. DNA ploidy status as determined by flow cytometry has been reported to have prognostic significance (175), but thus far there are no reports of molecular methods that have a role in diagnostic or prognostic testing.

OVARY

Although ovarian tumors account for only about 30% of malignancies of the female genital tract, in the United

States more women die from ovarian cancer than all other gynecologic cancers combined, and ovarian cancer is the fourth most common cause of cancer deaths in women overall (1). Several clinical syndromes have been associated with an increased risk of ovarian neoplasms, including *BRCA1* syndrome, *BRCA2* syndrome, and HNPCC. Although these syndromes together account for the vast majority of familial ovarian tumors (176), overall the genetic syndromes account for only a minority of ovarian epithelial tumors.

Initial attempts to understand the genetic pathways underlying the tumorigenesis of ovarian neoplasms were hampered by the fact that tumors of different histologic types were frequently lumped together. However, it has become clear within the last decade that even different tumor types within the same general category have different oncogenic pathways (reviewed in 177). Many of the conflicting results in the literature can be traced to studies that do not rigorously separate tumors into specific histologic categories.

Surface Epithelial-Stromal Tumors

Genetics

Molecular analysis has shown that different patterns of genetic aberrations underlie the development of serous, mucinous, endometroid, and clear cell tumors and that there are even differences between benign, borderline, and malignant tumors of the same histologic type (reviewed in 178).

Serous Tumors

Several different genetic mutations underlie the development of serous tumors (179). The vast majority of benign serous cystadenomas are polyclonal, and only 0 to 20% harbor mutations in either K-*ras* or *BRAF*, findings that support the hypothesis that serous cystadenomas develop as hyperplastic expansions of epithelial inclusions (180,181).

Serous borderline tumors (serous cystadenomas of low malignant potential) harbor mutations in either K-*ras* or

BRAF in 27% to 50% of cases, mutations that appear to be mutually exclusive in most tumors (180,182–184). Less than 10% of serous borderline tumors harbor mutations in *TP53* (185).

Well-differentiated (low-grade) serous carcinomas typically contain mutations in K-*ras* or *BRAF* (182,184), and less than 10% harbor mutations in *TP53* (185). In addition, genetic analysis has shown that there is a clonal relationship among the benign, borderline, and fully malignant regions of individual serous tumors (186). These findings support a model (Fig. 16.7) in which the majority of well-differentiated serous carcinomas arise through a stepwise progression from benign serous cystadenoma to serous borderline tumor to invasive well-differentiated serous carcinoma (184,187).

In contrast, high-grade serous carcinomas rarely arise within preexisting borderline or low-grade serous tumors (188). Mutations of K-*ras* or *BRAF* are present in only about 0 to 12% of high-grade serous carcinomas, but even the smallest high-grade serous carcinomas usually harbor *TP53* mutations (179,182,184,185,187,189–191).

Endometroid Tumors

In general, the genetic abnormalities that underlie the development of endometrioid adenocarcinoma of the ovary parallel those involved in the development of endometrioid adenocarcinoma of the endometrium. Somatic mutations in *CTNNB1* are present in 38% to 50% of ovarian endometrioid adenocarcinomas (192,193), *PTEN* in about 15% to 20% (192,194), and K-*ras* in 4% to 36% (183); in addition, 8% to 38% of tumors show evidence of MSI (192,195).

Molecular analysis has also confirmed that endometrioid adenocarcinoma of the ovary often arises via malignant transformation of endometriosis. Evaluation of cases of endometriosis and synchronous endometrioid adenocarcinoma (or synchronous mixed endometrioid and mucinous or clear cell carcinoma) by either *TP53* mutational analysis or LOH analysis has shown that, within individual patients, the two lesions often harbor

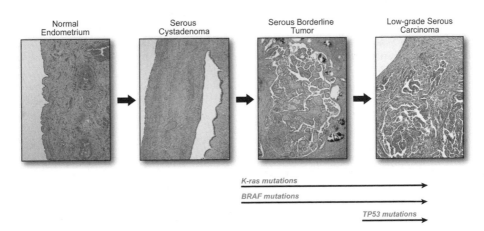

Figure 16.7 Model for the stepwise development of ovarian serous tumors. Well differentiated (low-grade) serous carcinomas can arise via progression from benign serous cystadermas. However, high-grade serous carcinomas have a distinct profile of mutations, which indicates they arise through a distinct oncogenic pathway. (See text for details.)

a pattern of genetic aberrations consistent with a common lineage (196). The relationship between endometriosis and endometrioid carcinoma is further supported by a mouse model in which inactivation of either K-*ras* or *PTEN* is sufficient for development of endometriosis, but mutations in both genes are required for the development of invasive adenocarcinoma (197).

Mucinous Tumors

Mutations in codon 12 or 13 of K-*ras* are a recurrent feature of mucinous ovarian tumors. The observation that the frequency of K-*ras* mutations increases from 14% to 56% in mucinous cystadenomas, to 29% to 73% in mucinous borderline tumors, to 40% to 85% in mucinous carcinomas has been used to support a model in which invasive mucinous carcinomas develop through a stepwise process, from benign to borderline to frankly malignant (198–201). The finding of identical K-*ras* mutations in the benign, borderline, and fully malignant regions of individual mucinous tumors further supports the benign to borderline to adenocarcinoma sequence (198,200).

Clear Cell Tumors

The genetic aberrations that underlie the tumorigenesis of ovarian clear cell carcinoma are incompletely characterized. From 6% to 21% of cases show MSI, but only about 6% of cases contain *PTEN* mutations and none harbor *CTNNB1* mutations (192,202). However, the significance of these results is uncertain because a relatively small number of cases has been evaluated, and because mixed epithelial malignancies that have a clear cell component show a different pattern of genetic abnormalities (192).

Molecular Genetic Analysis for Diagnosis, Prognosis, and Therapy

Despite the description of many key events involved in the oncogenesis of epithelial tumors of the ovary, molecular analysis of individual loci has not been shown to provide any independent diagnostic, prognostic, or therapeutic information. However, a remarkable finding to emerge from microarray analysis is that serous carcinomas can be grouped into two categories defined by the gene expression profiles of ovarian carcinomas that arise in patients with germline mutations in *BRCA1* or *BRCA2* (203), an observation that suggests there are fundamental pathways involved in ovarian epithelial carcinogenesis that have yet to be recognized.

Although the approach does not, at the present time, provide any diagnostic information, gene expression analysis apparently does have some potential for predicting patient response to therapy. In one study, the pattern of gene expression in post-therapy tumor specimens was shown to correlate with clinical outcome (204). Similarly, an animal model system has been used to show that the response of ovarian carcinoma xenografts to paclitaxel therapy correlates with the pattern of expression of a panel of 23 genes (205). Given that epigenetic mechanisms have an important role in the oncogenesis of epithelial neoplasms, as well as in their response to chemotherapy (reviewed in 206,207), it is not surprising that microarray-based genomewide analysis of epigenetic

modifications has been used to stratify patients into statistically significant, clinically relevant prognostic and therapeutic groups (208,209).

SYNCHRONOUS, METACHRONOUS, AND METASTATIC TUMORS

A number of histopathologic and clinical criteria have traditionally been used to distinguish independent synchronous primary tumors from tumor metastasis (210), but classification using these criteria is often ambiguous. DNA-based analysis in this setting is predicated on the assumption that, according to the clonal model of carcinogenesis, all tumors arise from a single cell (211,212). Although the genetic instability that is a hallmark of most malignancies usually produces intratumoral heterogeneity, metastatic or recurrent tumors typically have a genetic profile that is similar enough to the primary neoplasm to establish their relatedness (213–216).

Synchronous Ovarian and Endometrial Neoplasms

Traditional histologic criteria alone can be used to classify most cases of simultaneous ovarian and endometrial involvement (217), and ancillary techniques such as ploidy analysis and immunohistochemistry are often helpful in those cases with inconclusive histomorphologic features. DNA-based testing has also been used as an aid for classification (218); multiple markers must be evaluated to achieve a definitive result, so testing usually involves mutational analysis, X-chromosome inactivation analysis, LOH analysis, or MSI analysis (219–222). In one study in which clinical stage was corrected based on the molecular results, the corrected stage was strongly correlated with clinical outcome (219).

Synchronous Ovarian and Endocervical Neoplasms

DNA-based testing has been used to evaluate synchronous ovarian and endocervical adenocarcinomas that have similar histologic features. In this setting, analysis is focused on detection of HPV DNA because, as discussed previously, high-risk HPV types can be detected in almost 80% of endocervical adenocarcinomas. In one study, DNA-based HPV testing (together with immunohistochemical analysis of estrogen receptor status, progesterone receptor status, and p16 expression) was used to document 10 cases in which ovarian tumors initially classified as synchronous primary neoplasms were shown to actually represent metastatic endocervical adenocarcinoma (223). Detection of HPV DNA in several ovarian tumors provided definitive evidence that the paired endocervical tumors originally interpreted as adenocarcinoma in situ were, in fact, invasive. In addition, detection of HPV DNA in presumed primary ovarian tumors in two patients led to the discovery of occult primary cervical adenocarcinomas.

SUBMICROSCOPIC DISEASE

In practice, most molecular analysis of blood, lymph nodes, or body fluids for detection of submicroscopic disease is performed using RT-PCR assays designed to detect mRNA transcripts that are assumed to be tumor specific. Although the clinical significance of malignant cells detected by only molecular genetic techniques remains to be clarified, two issues confound the utility of analysis from a purely technical perspective, namely the lack of specificity of the marker genes and the lack of morphologic correlation.

Lack of Specificity

As a result of illegitimate transcription, mRNA from marker genes presumed to be specifically expressed by malignant epithelial cells, including cytokeratin-19 (CK-19) and CK-20, are actually present in up to 77% to 100% of peripheral blood samples obtained from patients with no history of malignancy (discussed in detail in the section on molecular staging of colorectal cancer in Chapter 15). Although quantitative RT-PCR can theoretically be used to establish the minimum level of expression that correlates with the presence of viable tumor cells, it can be difficult to distinguish between physiologic expression of a marker gene by a very small number of viable tumor cells versus very low expression resulting from illegitimate transcription by nonmalignant cells.

Lack of Morphologic Correlation

It is impossible to directly evaluate the morphologic features of the cells that are responsible for a positive PCR result because the tissue sample is destroyed during nucleic acid extraction. The lack of specificity of many markers used for RT-PCR analysis, together with the fact that nucleic acids in cellular debris that has drained to lymph nodes can produce a positive PCR result (as demonstrated by the experimental observation that marker genes can be detected in draining or systemic lymph nodes by PCR for up to 4 days following injection of purified cell-free DNA [224]), emphasizes that the lack of direct morphologic correlation is not a mute point.

Peripheral Blood and Lymph Nodes

Sex Cord Stromal Tumors
RT-PCR for CK-20 has been used to detect submicroscopic disease in peripheral blood and lymph nodes in patients with granulosa cell tumors. In one small study the analysis had both high sensitivity and specificity, but the significance of the findings is unknown because no attempt was made to determine if the results correlated with clinical outcome (225).

Germ Cell Tumors
RT-PCR for a variety of transcripts, including those encoding epidermal growth factor receptor (EGFR), germ cell alkaline phosphatese (GCAP), beta human chorionic gonadotropin (β-hCG), and alpha fetoprotein (AFP), has been used to detect tumor cells in either the peripheral blood or progenitor cell harvests from patients with germ cell tumors (226–229). In many of these studies, the molecular results have been shown to correlate with clinical outcome. For example, detection of GCAP transcripts is

associated with a statistically significant reduction in overall survival, and disease-free survival and has a higher predictive value than other known prognostic variables (228). Similarly, detection of β-hCG transcripts is associated with a statistically significant decrease in survival (229).

Epithelial Ovarian Malignancies
Not all molecular testing for submicroscopic disease is based on RT-PCR. One category of tumors for which an alternative approach has been employed is surface epithelial tumors of the ovary. Analysis based on *MLH1* CpG island methylation of plasma DNA has shown that acquisition of an aberrant pattern of epigenetic modification at the time of relapse is associated with a statistically significant decrease in overall survival (230). This testing paradigm is noteworthy not only because it provides information that correlates with clinical outcome, but also because it identifies patients who may be more likely to respond to novel therapies directed against epigenetic alterations.

Cervical Carcinoma
RT-PCR for transcripts encoding CK-19 (231) or SCC antigen (232), as well as PCR for the HPV *E6* gene (233), has been used to detect circulating tumor cells in the peripheral blood of women with cervical cancer. However, the clinical utility of the analysis has yet to be demonstrated because none of the studies have shown that the results correlate with outcome.

Endometrial Adenocarcinoma
RT-PCR for transcripts encoding CK-20 or beta-casein–like protein (BCLP) have been used to detected disseminated tumor cells in the peripheral blood of women with endometrial or cervical malignancies (234,235). However, the presence of mRNA encoding either protein shows no statistically significant correlation with either disease recurrence or overall survival, and so the utility of the analysis in routine clinical practice has yet to be established.

Peritoneal Fluid

A number of studies have evaluated whether molecular approaches can be used to more accurately detect the presence of malignant cells in peritoneal effusions in patients who have gynecologic malignancies. In one report in which nested RT-PCR for transcripts encoding human mammagoblin (hMAM, a glycoprotein expressed by both benign and malignant epithelium from the ovary, uterus, and cervix) was used to test peritoneal effusions in patients with a variety of gynecologic malignancies, there was little correlation between the RT-PCR results and routine cytologic evaluation, and the RT-PCR was positive in 9% of patients without a history of malignant disease (236). Whether the molecular results or routine cytopathologic findings correlated more closely with clinical outcome was not evaluated.

Other studies have analyzed multiple loci to overcome the intrinsic lack of specificity associated with testing focused on single tumor markers. In one report that evaluated patients with ovarian cancer, LOH and MSI analysis of a panel of six microsatellites detected matched novel alleles indicative of the presence of malignant cells in 42% of peritoneal fluid specimens classified as negative by routine cytopathologic examination, including 33% of specimens from patients with stage IA disease (237). However, it is difficult to interpret the significance of the findings because, again, whether the molecular or routine cytopathologic results correlated more closely with clinical outcome was not evaluated. In another report, in which testing involved LOH analysis of four microsatellites combined with mutational analysis of *TP53* and K-*ras*, all peritoneal fluid specimens that harbored a DNA alteration also present in the primary tumor were positive by conventional cytopathologic evaluation (238), and so the technically demanding molecular approach seemed to provide no advantage. In addition, the testing had a sensitivity of just 67% compared with cytopathologic evaluation because only a subset of primary tumors harbored a mutation involving at least one of the marker loci.

A novel approach for analysis of peritoneal fluid specimens from patients with ovarian cancer involves characterization of the pattern of epigenetic changes by methylation-specific PCR of a 15-gene panel (239). Hierarchical cluster analysis of the methylation profile of the 15 genes identifies patient groups that have statistically significant differences in survival. In addition, the patient groupings are also a statistically significant prognostic factor independent of age, International Federation of Gynecology and Obstetrics (FIGO) stage, or tumor grade. Assuming these results can be reproduced in other laboratories, the findings suggest that analysis of epigenetic changes in peritoneal fluid specimens can provide independent, clinically relevant information.

TESTICULAR GERM CELL TUMORS

Testicular germ cell tumors (TGCTs) account for about 98% of all testicular neoplasms. Three different groups of TGCT have been identified by epidemiologic, clinical, and histologic criteria (240). TGCTs that arise in infants and neonates are predominantly teratomas or yoke sac tumors. Tumors that arise in postpubertal males are by far the most common group and include seminomas and nonseminomatous TGCT (Fig. 16.8). The third group of TGCT is spermatocytic seminoma, which predominately occurs in men over 40 years old. Each of the three categories of TGCT has distinct genetic characteristics, but the molecular aberrations in TCGTs that arise in adolescents and young adults are the most well characterized because this group of tumors is the most common.

Aberrations of c-*kit*

Genetics

Mutations in c-*kit* (which encodes a tyrosine kinase receptor; see Fig. 15.6) are present in a subset of testicular seminomas and mixed seminomatous and nonseminomatous germ cell tumors, but are absent in nonseminomatous germ cell tumors (241–244). The most common mutations occur in codon 816 of exon 17, although mutations have been described in other codons of exon 17, and in other exons

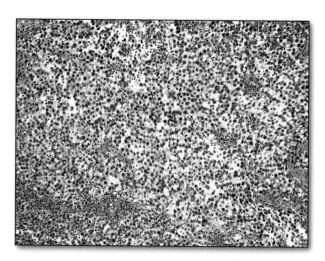

Figure 16.8 Seminoma arising in a postpubertal male. As discussed in the text, c-*kit* mutations and gains of 12p are characteristic features of this group of testicular germ cell tumors.

(241–244). The mutations in exon 17 result in membrane receptors with constitutively activated kinase activity, which is thought to have a key role in tumorigenesis (242,243,245). Consistent with the conventional view that ovarian dysgerminomas are the female counterpart of testicular seminomas, a codon 816 mutation has also been described in an ovarian mixed dysgerminoma and yoke sac tumor (243). Exon 17 c-*kit* mutations have been demonstrated in primary mediastinal seminomas (246), establishing the presence of a similar pattern of genetic alterations in germ cell tumors independent of their anatomic location.

Mutations of c-*kit* are present in 89% to 100% of bilateral TGCT (virtually always in codon 816), but in only a subset of unilateral tumors (discussed more fully later) (244). Because germline c-*kit* mutations are absent in both tumor groups, activating c-*kit* mutations apparently occur early during embryonic development (244).

Technical Issues in Molecular Genetic Analysis of c-*kit*

The sensitivity of testing for c-*kit* mutations in testicular seminomas and mixed seminomatous and nonseminomatous germ cell tumors depends on the approach. When PCR-based analysis is limited to codon 816 of exon 17, mutations are detected in only 1.3% to 5% of cases (243,244); when analysis includes exons 9,11,13, and 17, mutations are detected in about 12% of cases (241). However, the fact that seminomas are frequently aneuploid complicates PCR-based analysis because more abundant wild-type alleles can mask the presence of mutant alleles (247). It is therefore not surprising that the use of denaturing high pressure liquid chromatography (HPLC) to help identify mutant alleles within the PCR product results in an appreciable increase in test sensitivity; with this approach, 26% of cases of seminomas can be shown to harbor mutations in c-*kit* exon 17 (242). Regardless of the method, the reported results are all based on analysis of primarily FFPE tissue, emphasizing that testing can be easily performed in routine practice.

Immunohistochemistry

Immunohistochemical analysis of kit (CD117) typically shows strong membranous expression in the vast majoring of seminomas and dysgerminomas (242,243,248–250). In mixed germ cell tumors, strong membranous staining is limited to the seminomatous component, although focal cytoplasmic staining has been described in nonseminomatous regions (248–250). Thus far, there is no clear correlation between the pattern of underlying c-kit mutations and the pattern of immunohistochemical staining.

Diagnostic, Prognostic, and Therapeutic Issues in Molecular Analysis of c-kit

Mutations in c-kit are characteristic of a number of other neoplasms, including gastrointestinal stromal tumor (GIST), extragastrointestinal GIST, mastocytosis and mast cell leukemia, and rare cases of acute myelogenous leukemia. However, these tumors rarely, if ever, enter into the differential diagnosis of TGCT, and so the fact that they also harbor mutations in c-kit is of no diagnostic relevance. (As an aside, it is interesting to note that the exact same mutations have been reported in exon 11 of seminoma and GIST, and in exon 17 of seminoma and mastocytosis [241]). There are apparently no differences in the clinicopathologic features of TGCT with and without c-kit mutations. Similarly, there is no difference in the outcome of patients with TGCT that do or do not harbor c-kit mutations (241).

Even if genetic testing is not required for diagnosis, mutational analysis may have a role in directing drug therapy. As discussed in more detail in Chapter 15, the activity of tyrosine kinase inhibitors depends on the underlying mutation. Imatinib mesylate (Gleevec) inhibits kit receptors with mutations in the domains encoded by exon 11, but has less of an effect on receptors with mutations encoded by exon 9 or exon 17 (251–253), a pattern of activity that is also seen in seminomas (242). In contrast, indolinone derivatives inhibit kit receptors with mutations in the TK2 domain encoded by exon 17 (254). Therefore, mutational analysis of c-kit may have in role in identifying patients likely to benefit from chemotherapy with tyrosine kinase inhibitors and in selecting the appropriate inhibitor.

Finally, mutational analysis may have a role in identifying those patients at high risk for bilateral disease. As noted above, the observation that the vast majority of patients with bilateral TGCT harbor c-kit codon 816 mutations suggests that mutational analysis that demonstrates a codon 816 mutation should influence the patient's follow-up care (244).

Gain of 12p

Genetics

Virtually all invasive TGCT in the postpubertal age-group harbor gain of 12p, usually in the form of isochrome i(12p) (255,256). The i(12p) is uniparental, so the mechanism of formation involves p-arm doubling with q-arm loss, rather than nonsister exchange (257). Germ cells tumors arising in other sites such as the mediastinum also harbor gain of 12p (255,256). Attempts to identify the genes on 12p responsible for oncogenesis have thus far been unsuccessful (258,259).

Technical Issues in Molecular Genetic Analysis of 12p

Conventional cytogenetic analysis demonstrates an i(12p) in about 50% to 70% of TGCTs (247), although most of the i(12p)-negative cases show other 12p aberrations (260). A number of studies have shown that FISH, using either metaphase chromosome spreads or interphase nuclei, detects 12p abnormalities in 93% to 100% of cases (261,262). FISH-based testing is very straightforward because chromosome 12 centromeric probes are commercially available. Other methods have also been used to demonstrate 12p gain, including comparative genomic hybridization and microarray analysis (263–265), but these other techniques are too cumbersome for routine clinical use.

Diagnostic Issues in Molecular Genetic Analysis of 12p

Because 12p gains are a feature of virtually all TGCTs in the postpubertal age-group regardless of histologic type, and are not associated with response to therapy or survival (255), there is little role for molecular analysis in the routine pathologic evaluation of the tumors. However, testing for 12p amplification can play a role in the diagnosis of germ cell tumors that occur in usual anatomic sites, that present as metastatic disease, or that have the histologic appearance of somatic-type neoplasms. For example, interphase FISH with commercially available probes has been used to demonstrate 12p amplification in cases of metastatic TGCT or primary mediastinal GCT in which the diagnoses based on histopathologic evaluation included adenocarcinoma, sarcoma, and neuroendocrine carcinoma (266). Because 12p amplifications were absent in all tested somatic-type neoplasms, the FISH approach apparently has very high specificity in this clinical setting.

Sex Cord–Stromal Tumors

As discussed in more detail in Chapter 11, mutations in GNAS1 (one of the subunits of the heterotrimeric G proteins) are responsible for McCune-Albright syndrome and are present in a number of neoplasms (Table 11.11). Because sex cord–stromal tumors have been described in association with McCune-Albright syndrome, the role of mutations in GNAS1 and other heterotrimeric G proteins in the development of sporadic tumors has been evaluated.

Genetics

The prevalence of mutations in gip(2), the gene encoding $G\alpha i_2$, another subunit of heterotrimeric G proteins, is uncertain. Although an early study identified mutations in the gene in 30% of ovarian sex cord–stromal tumors (including granulosa tumors and one thecoma) (267), subsequent studies have failed to identify mutations in granulosa cell tumors, Leydig cell tumors, thecomas, androblastomas, or gonadoblastomas (268,269).

Similarly, the prevalence of mutations in the *GNAS1* in sex cord–stromal tumors is uncertain. One study demonstrated the R201C mutation in *GNAS1* in 67% of ovarian and testicular Leydig cell tumors but in no other histologic type of sex cord–stromal tumor (269). However, subsequent reports have failed to identify *GNAS1* mutations in granulosa cell tumors of juvenile or adult type, as well as Leydig cell tumors of ovarian or testicular origin (270,271).

Technical and Diagnostic Issues in Molecular Analysis of Sex Cord–Stromal Tumors

Based on these results, there is no established role for mutational analysis of *gip(2)* or *GNAS1* in the diagnosis of sex cord–stromal tumors. In addition, given that there are no reported differences in the clinicopathologic features of tumors with and without mutations in either of the two genes, there is no established role for mutational analysis as a component of prognostic testing.

VULVA

Squamous Cell Carcinoma

The most common malignant neoplasm of the vulva is SCC. The specific etiology of the majority of cases is unknown, although established risk factors include cigarette smoking (272), lichen sclerosis et atrophicus (273), and chronic granulomatous disease of the vulva (274). HPV infection is associated with only a subset of cases.

HPV Infection

The percentage of SCCs of the vulva that harbor HPV DNA depends on the methodology used in the analysis. By PCR, using either consensus or type specific primers, HPV DNA can be detected in 12% to 89% of cases, and, overall, the most commonly identified types are the high-risk types 16, 18, and 33 (275–277). Although low-risk type 6 or 11 is present in virtually 100% of cases of verrucous carcinoma (278), the presence of HPV infection does not correlate with any other histologic type of vulvar SCC (275–277).

Molecular analysis for HPV DNA has little clinical utility for several reasons. First, and of perhaps most importance, DNA testing is not needed to identify women at high risk for SCC because vulvar lesions can be directly visualized. Second, the presence of HPV infection is not correlated with the presence of lymphovascular invasion, clinical stage, or recurrence and so provides no independent clinical information (275–277).

Cytogenetic Abnormalities

A number of recurring karyotypic abnormalities have been identified in vulvar SCC, including gains of 3q and 11q21 and losses of 3p, 8p, 22q, 10q, and Xp (272,279). Although increasing karyotypic complexity is mirrored by higher tumor grade, ploidy does not correlate with any clinicopathologic features of disease (275).

Other Aberrations

Mutations in *TP53* and *PTEN* (275,280,281) are present in some cases of vulvar SCC. As is true for cervical carcinoma, different *TP53* alleles have been hypothesized to have a role in disease progression, although the data are inconclusive (98). Even though genetic analysis of these loci has provided some insight in to the pathogenesis of vulvar SCC, evaluation of these loci has no established role in diagnostic, prognostic, or therapeutic testing in routine clinical practice.

Sarcomas

A number of sarcomas that are more characteristic of other anatomic sites have been reported as primary tumors of the vulva, including dermatofibrosarcoma protuberans (283) and Ewings sarcoma/peripheral neuroectodermal tumor (284). The issues involved in molecular analysis of these tumor types are discussed in the chapters devoted to the skin (Chapter 18) and soft tissue and bone (Chapter 11).

PROSTATE

Other than malignancies of the skin, adocarcinoma of the prostate is the malignancy with the highest incidence in men in developed countries (1). Geographic, racial, and environmental factors influence the incidence of the tumor, although analysis of these factors is often complicated by superimposed changes in incidence as a result of screening programs (reviewed in 285–288). Although primary neuroendocrine tumors, urothelial carcinomas, ductal adenocarcinomas, and mesenchymal neoplasms account for 2% to 3% of prostatic malignancies, acinar adenocarcinomas are by far the most common tumor.

Genetics

There is strong evidence for a familial predisposition to adenocarcinoma of the prostate. At least seven susceptibility regions have been identified (Table 16.3), and all are associated with an autosomal dominant pattern of inheritance except for *HPCX* (reviewed in 285). Thus far, three specific candidate genes have been identified: *RNASEL* in the *HPC1* region, *HPC2/ELAC2* in the *HPC2* region, and *MSR1* at 8p22-23, but contradictory reports continue to emerge regarding their linkage to hereditary or sporadic disease, and their oncogenic mechanisms remain unknown.

A comprehensive model for the development and progression of sporadic prostate cancer has yet to be developed. A number of chromosomal aberrations are characteristic of sporadic tumors, and a number of individual genes have been implicated in tumor development and progression (reviewed in 285,288). For some genes, such as the tumor suppressor gene *PTEN* and the gene encoding the zinc finger transcription factor KLF-6, mutations and haploinsufficiency are associated with tumor development. For other genes, such as the caretaker gene *GSTP1*, hypermethylation is associated with tumor development. For still other genes, such as those encoding the oxidative enzyme AMACR, the

TABLE 16.3
LOCI LINKED TO A FAMILIAL PREDISPOSITION TO ADENOCARCINOMA OF THE PROSTATE

Locus	Position	Candidate Gene
HPC1	1q24-25	RNASEL
PCAP	1q42.2-43	—
CAPB	1p36	—
HPCX	Xq27-28	—
HPC20	20q13	—
HPC2	17p	HPC2/ELAC2
Not named	8p22-23	MSR1

transmembrane protease hepsin, the cyclin dependent kinase inhibitor p27, and the cell adhesion molecule E-cadherin, the molecular mechanisms responsible for the altered expression associated with tumor progression have yet to be characterized.

Technical and Diagnostic Issues in Molecular Analysis of Prostate Cancer

The College of American Pathologists (CAP) recently concluded that, at the present time, molecular analysis of the various oncogenes and tumor suppressor genes implicated in the development and progression of prostate cancer is not of diagnostic or prognostic value (289).

Even though analysis of individual markers may not have utility, several studies suggest that the overall profile of gene expression may provide clinically relevant information. Microarray analysis has been used to identify gene expression patterns that correlate with prognosis (290,291), and has also been applied to identify novel drug targets (292). Similarly, global patterns of histone modifications have been shown to predict risk of disease recurrence (293). Although these results suggest that simultaneous evaluation of a number of markers may be clinically useful, the approach is largely experimental and does not (yet) have a role in the routine analysis of patient specimens.

Staging

Molecular genetic methods have been evaluated to see if they can provide more accurate preoperative staging information in patients who have biopsy-proven adenocarcinoma. As discussed more fully above (in the section on submicroscopic disease), analyses of this type are all constrained by the lack of specificity of the tumor markers and by the fact that it is usually impossible to evaluate the histopathologic features of the cells that are responsible for a positive molecular result. The specificity limitations of markers commonly used in the setting of prostate cancer are highlighted by the results of RT-PCR–based analysis of prostate specific antigen (PSA) and prostate specific membrane antigen (PSMA). mRNA encoding PSA can be detected in the peripheral blood of roughly 10% to 60% of

men not known to have prostate cancer (294,295), and mRNA encoding PSMA can be detected in 11% of patients with benign prostatic hypertrophy (296).

Peripheral Blood

There is no unequivocal evidence that RT-PCR analysis of peripheral blood provides independent preoperative staging information in men with biopsy-proven prostate cancer. By qualitative or quantitative methods, there are no significant correlations between the level of mRNA encoding PSA and the clinical stage of disease (297–299), and RT-PCR is not as accurate as widely used clinical staging methods (such as Partin Tables) for predicting clinical stage before surgery (300). Even RT-PCR testing for PSA, PSMA, and human kallikrein 2, of lymph nodes and peripheral blood, does not yield improved preoperative staging information versus conventional approaches (301).

Lymph Nodes

Although the results of RT-PCR analysis of PSA transcripts in lymph nodes are correlated with standard pathologic risk factors (including Gleason score, the presence of Gleason patterns 4 or 5, and the presence of lymph node metastases as determined by routine histopathologic examination), it has not been established that the molecular testing provides any independent information (298).

Bone Marrow

The significance of detection of mRNA encoding PSA in bone marrow similarly remains uncertain. When an immunomagnetic method is used to enrich epithelial cells, mRNA encoding PSA can be detected in the bone marrow of 54% of men before radical prostatectomy, 33% of men within 4 months of prostatectomy, and 29% of men more than 5 years after prostatectomy, only a subset of whom develop evidence of recurrent disease (302). The results do not correlate with clinical outcome, so there seems to be little role for testing.

Screening

As noted above, hypermethylation of GSTP1 is associated with the development of prostate cancer. Methylation-specific PCR focused on regulatory sequences of GSTP1 in urine-sediment DNA has therefore been evaluated as an alternative approach for prostate cancer screening, but altered *GSTP1* methylation can be detected in only 27% of patients known to have cancer (303). The relative insensitivity of the testing partially reflects the observation that *GSTP1* methylation changes are present in only about 80% of prostatic adenocarcinomas (303), which emphasizes the fact that only a subset of prostatic adenocarcinomas harbor mutations, epigenetic alterations, or LOH at the markers thus far evaluated. Consequently, regardless of the methodology, screening approaches that focus on individual genetic changes are likely to be of limited sensitivity.

Specimen Identity Issues

Occasionally, residual adenocarcinoma is not identified in a radical prostatectomy specimen, even after the entire gland is submitted for microscopic examination (304,305). Although the phenomenon is well documented and has specifically been referred to as the "vanishing cancer phenomenon" (305), the absence of residual tumor in a radical prostatectomy specimen raises questions about the provenance of the initial biopsy. DNA identity testing (Chapter 23) has been used in this setting to establish whether the initial biopsy and subsequent radical prostatectomy specimens originate from the same patient. In one series, identity testing showed that misidentification of the biopsy specimen was responsible for the vanishing cancer phenomenon in 2.4% of cases (304), a result that raises a number of practical and legal issues regarding the appropriate workup for radical prostatectomy specimens that lack residual tumor.

REFERENCES

1. American Cancer Society. *Statistics for 2005.* http://www.cancer.org/docroot/STT/STT_0.asp.
2. Wright TC Jr, Schiffman M. Adding a test for human papillomavirus DNA to cervical-cancer screening. *N Engl J Med* 2003;348:489–490.
3. Munoz N, Bosch X, de Sanjose S, et al. Screening for genital human papillomavirus: results from an international validation study on human papillomavirus sampling techniques. *Diagn Mol Pathol* 1999;8:26–31.
4. Jacobs MV, de Roda Husman AM, van den Brule AJ, et al. Group-specific differentiation between high- and low-risk human papillomavirus genotypes by general primer-mediated PCR and two cocktails of oligonucleotide probes. *J Clin Microbiol* 1995;33:901–905.
5. Herrero LJ, Lugo-Vicente H. Human papillomavirus and cancer. *Cancer Surv* 1999;33:75–98.
6. International Agency for Research on Cancer, eds. *IARC Monographs on the Evaluation of the Carcinogenic Risks to Humans.* Vol 64. Lyon: IARC Press Publishers; 1995.
7. Gostout BS, Poland GA, Calhoun ES, et al. TAP1, TAP2, and HLA-DR2 alleles are predictors of cervical cancer risk. *Gynecol Oncol* 2003;88:326–332.
8. Birkeland SA, Storm HH, Lamm LU, et al. Cancer risk after renal transplantation in the Nordic countries, 1964–1986. *Int J Cancer* 1995;60:183–189.
9. Frisch M, Biggar RJ, Goedert JJ. Human papillomavirus-associated cancers in patients with human immunodeficiency virus infection and acquired immunodeficiency syndrome. *J Natl Cancer Inst* 2000;92:1500–1510.
10. Storey A, Thomas M, Kalita A, et al. Role of a p53 polymorphism in the development of human papillomavirus-associated cancer. *Nature* 1998;393:229–234.
11. Yamashita T, Yaginuma Y, Saitoh Y, et al. Codon 72 polymorphism of p53 as a risk factor for patients with human papillomavirus-associated squamous intraepithelial lesions and invasive cancer of the uterine cervix. *Carcinogenesis* 1999;20:1733–1736.
12. Yang YC, Chang CL, Chen ML. Effect of p53 polymorphism on the susceptibility of cervical cancer. *Gynecol Obstet Invest* 2001;51:197–201.
13. Koushik A, Platt RW, Franco EL. p53 codon 72 polymorphism and cervical neoplasia: a meta-analysis review. *Cancer Epidemiol Biomarkers Prev* 2004;13:11–22.
14. DeMay RM. The pap smear. In: DeMay RM, ed. *The Art & Science of Cytopathology: Exfoliative Cytology.* Chicago: ASCP Press; 1996:61–205.
15. Koss LG. The Papanicolaou test for cervical cancer detection: a triumph and a tragedy. *JAMA* 1989;261:737–743.
16. van der Graaf Y, Vooijs GP, Gaillaard HL, et al. Screening errors in cervical cytologic screening. *Acta Cytol* 1987;31:434–438.
17. Iftner T, Villa LL. Human papillomavirus technologies. *J Natl Cancer Inst Monogr* 2003;31:80–88.
18. Jarboe EA, Thompson LC, Heinz D, et al. Telomerase and human papillomavirus as diagnostic adjuncts for cervical dysplasia and carcinoma. *Hum Pathol* 2004;35:396–402.
19. Stoppler H, Hartmann DP, Sherman L, et al. The human papillomavirus type 16 E6 and E7 oncoproteins dissociate cellular telomerase activity from the maintenance of telomere length. *J Biol Chem* 1997;272:13332–13337.
20. Klingelhutz AJ, Foster SA, McDougall JK. Telomerase activation by the E6 gene product of human papillomavirus type 16. *Nature* 1996;380:79–82.
21. Anderson S, Shera K, Ihle J, et al. Telomerase activation in cervical cancer. *Am J Pathol* 1997;151:25–31.
22. Jarboe EA, Liaw KL, Thompson LC, et al. Analysis of telomerase as a diagnostic biomarker of cervical dysplasia and carcinoma. *Oncogene* 2002;21:664–673.
23. Larson AA, Liao SY, Stanbridge EJ, et al. Genetic alterations accumulate during cervical tumorigenesis and indicate a common origin for multifocal lesions. *Cancer Res* 1997;57:4171–4176.
24. Kersemaekers AM, Van de Vijver MJ, Kenter GG, et al. Genetic alterations during the progression of squamous cell carcinomas of the uterine cervix. *Genes Chromosomes Cancer* 1999;26:346–354.
25. Lu X, Nikaido T, Toki T, et al. Loss of heterozygosity among tumor suppressor genes in invasive and in situ carcinoma of the uterine cervix. *Int J Gynecol Cancer* 2000;10:452–458.
26. Chatterjee A, Pulido HA, Koul S, et al. Mapping the sites of putative tumor suppressor genes at 6p25 and 6p21.3 in cervical carcinoma: occurrence of allelic deletions in precancerous lesions. *Cancer Res* 2001;61:2119–2123.
27. Feoli-Fonseca JC, Oligny LL, Filion M, et al. A two-tier polymerase chain reaction direct sequencing method for detecting and typing human papillomaviruses in pathological specimens. *Diagn Mol Pathol* 1998;7:317–323.
28. Vernon SD, Unger ER, Williams D. Comparison of human papillomavirus detection and typing by cycle sequencing, line blotting, and hybrid capture. *J Clin Microbiol* 2000;38:651–655.
29. Lorincz AT. Hybrid Capture method for detection of human papillomavirus DNA in clinical specimens: a tool for clinical management of equivocal Pap smears and for population screening. *J Obstet Gynaecol Res* 1996;22:629–636.
30. Peyton CL, Schiffman M, Lorincz AT, et al. Comparison of PCR- and hybrid capture-based human papillomavirus detection systems using multiple cervical specimen collection strategies. *J Clin Microbiol* 1998;36:3248–3254.
31. Castle PE, Schiffman M, Burk RD, et al. Restricted cross-reactivity of hybrid capture 2 with nononcogenic human papillomavirus types. *Cancer Epidemiol Biomarkers Prev* 2002;11:1394–1399.
32. Castle PE, Wheeler CM, Solomon D, et al. Interlaboratory reliability of Hybrid Capture 2. *Am J Clin Pathol* 2004;122:238–245.
33. Narimatsu R, Patterson BK. High-throughput cervical cancer screening using intracellular human papillomavirus E6 and E7 mRNA quantification by flow cytometry. *Am J Clin Pathol* 2005;123:716–723.
34. Schiller CL, Nickolov AG, Kaul KL, et al. High-risk human papillomavirus detection: a split-sample comparison of hybrid capture and chromogenic in situ hybridization. *Am J Clin Pathol* 2004;121:537–545.
35. Wright TC Jr, Schiffman M, Solomon D, et al. Interim guidance for the use of human papillomavirus DNA testing as an adjunct to cervical cytology for screening. *Obstet Gynecol* 2004;103:304–309.
36. Wachtel MS, Boon ME, Korporaal H, et al. Human papillomavirus testing as a cytology gold standard: comparing Surinam with the Netherlands. *Mod Pathol* 2005;18:349–353.
37. Kulasingam SL, Hughes JP, Kiviat NB, et al. Evaluation of human papillomavirus testing in primary screening for cervical abnormalities: comparison of sensitivity, specificity, and frequency of referral. *JAMA* 2002;288:1749–1757.
38. Sherman ME, Lorincz AT, Scott DR, et al. Baseline cytology, human papillomavirus testing, and risk for cervical neoplasia: a 10-year cohort analysis. *J Natl Cancer Inst* 2003;95:46–52.
39. Peyton CL, Gravitt PE, Hunt WC, et al. Determinants of genital human papillomavirus detection in a US population. *J Infect Dis* 2001;183:1554–1564.
40. Giuliano AR, Papenfuss M, Abrahamsen M, et al. Human papillomavirus infection at the United States-Mexico border: implications for cervical cancer prevention and control. *Cancer Epidemiol Biomarkers Prev* 2001;10:1129–1136.
41. Schiffman M, Kjaer SK. Natural history of anogenital human papillomavirus infection and neoplasia. *J Natl Cancer Inst Monogr* 2003;31:14–19.
42. Kendall BS, Bush AC, Olsen CH, et al. Reflex high-risk human papillomavirus testing for women with atypical squamous cells of undetermined significance in cytologic smears: effects since implementation in a large clinical practice. *Am J Clin Pathol* 2005;123:524–528.
43. Guo M, Hu L, Baliga M, et al. The predictive value of p16(INK4a) and hybrid capture 2 human papillomavirus testing for high-grade cervical intraepithelial neoplasia. *Am J Clin Pathol* 2004;122:894–901.
44. Clavel C, Masure M, Bory JP, et al. Human papillomavirus testing in primary screening for the detection of high-grade cervical lesions: a study of 7932 women. *Br J Cancer* 2001;84:1616–1623.
45. Clavel C, Masure M, Bory JP, et al. Hybrid Capture II-based human papillomavirus detection, a sensitive test to detect in routine high-grade cervical lesions: a preliminary study on 1518 women. *Br J Cancer* 1999;80:1306–1311.
46. Solomon D, Schiffman M, Tarone R. Comparison of three management strategies for patients with atypical squamous cells of undetermined significance: baseline results from a randomized trial. *J Natl Cancer Inst* 2001;93:293–299.
47. Wright TC Jr, Cox JT, Massad LS, et al. 2001 Consensus Guidelines for the management of women with cervical cytological abnormalities. *JAMA* 2002;287:2120–2129.
48. Wright TC, Sun XW. Anogenital papillomavirus infection and neoplasia in immunodeficient women. *Obstet Gynecol Clin North Am* 1996;23:861–893.
49. Ellerbrock TV, Chiasson MA, Bush TJ, et al. Incidence of cervical squamous intraepithelial lesions in HIV-infected women. *JAMA* 2000;283:1031–1037.
50. Saslow D, Runowicz CD, Solomon D, et al. American Cancer Society guideline for the early detection of cervical neoplasia and cancer. *CA Cancer J Clin* 2002;52:342–362.
51. Mitchell MF, Tortolero-Luna G, Cook E, et al. A randomized clinical trial of cryotherapy, laser vaporization, and loop electrosurgical excision for treatment of squamous intraepithelial lesions of the cervix. *Obstet Gynecol* 1998;92:737–744.

52. Alvarez RD, Helm CW, Edwards RP, et al. Prospective randomized trial of LLETZ versus laser ablation in patients with cervical intraepithelial neoplasia. *Gynecol Oncol* 1994;52:175–179.
53. Nobbenhuis MA, Meijer CJ, van den Brule AJ, et al. Addition of high-risk HPV testing improves the current guidelines on follow-up after treatment for cervical intraepithelial neoplasia. *Br J Cancer* 2001;84:796–801.
54. Paraskevaidis E, KoliopoulosG, Alamanos Y, et al. Human papillomavirus testing and the outcome of treatment for cervical intraepithelial neoplasia. *Obstet Gynecol* 2001;98:833–836.
55. Kim JJ, Wright TC, Goldie SJ. Cost-effectiveness of alternative triage strategies for atypical squamous cells of undetermined significance. *JAMA* 2002;287:2382–2390.
56. Mandelblatt JS, Lawrence WF, Womack SM, et al. Benefits and costs of using HPV testing to screen for cervical cancer. *JAMA* 2002;287:2372–2381.
57. Hartmann KE, Nanda K, Hall S, et al. Technologic advances for evaluation of cervical cytology: is newer better? *Obstet Gynecol Surv* 2001;56:765–774.
58. Kinney W, Sung HY, Kearney KA, et al. Missed opportunities for cervical cancer screening of HMO members developing invasive cervical cancer (ICC). *Gynecol Oncol* 1998;71:428–430.
59. Cervical cancer. *NIH Consens Statement* 1996;14:1–38.
60. Sawaya GF, Grimes DA. New technologies in cervical cytology screening: a word of caution. *Obstet Gynecol* 1999;94:307–310.
61. Suba EJ, Raab SS, Viet/American Cervical Cancer Prevention Project. Papanicolaou screening in developing countries: an idea whose time has come. *Am J Clin Pathol* 2004;121:315–320.
62. Ansari-Lari MA, Staebler A, Zaino RJ, et al. Distinction of endocervical and endometrial adenocarcinomas: immunohistochemical *p16* expression correlated with human papillomavirus (HPV) DNA detection. *Am J Surg Pathol* 2004;28:160–167.
63. Staebler A, Sherman ME, Zaino RJ, et al. Hormone receptor immunohistochemistry and human papillomavirus in situ hybridization are useful for distinguishing endocervical and endometrial adenocarcinomas. *Am J Surg Pathol* 2002;26:998–1006.
64. Duggan MA, McGregor SE, Benoit JL, et al. The human papillomavirus status of invasive cervical adenocarcinoma: a clinicopathological and outcome analysis. *Hum Pathol* 1995;26:319–325.
65. Pirog EC, Kleter B, Olgac S, et al. Prevalence of human papillomavirus DNA in different histological subtypes of cervical adenocarcinoma. *Am J Pathol* 2000;157:1055–1062.
66. Wright TC Jr, Ferenczy A, Kurman RJ. Carcinoma and other tumors of the cervix. In: Kurman RJ, ed. *Blaustein's Pathology of the Female Genital Tract*, 5th ed. New York: Springer-Verlag; 2002:325–381.
67. Srivatsa PJ, Keeney GL, Podratz KC. Disseminated cervical adenoma malignum and bilateral ovarian sex cord tumors with annular tubules associated with Peutz-Jeghers syndrome. *Gynecol Oncol* 1994;53:256–264.
68. Young RH, Welch WR, Dickersin GR, et al. Ovarian sex cord tumor with annular tubules: review of 74 cases including 27 with Peutz-Jeghers syndrome and four with adenoma malignum of the cervix. *Cancer* 1982;50:1384–1402.
69. Hemminki A, Markie D, Tomlinson IP, et al. A serine/threonine kinase gene defective in Peutz-Jeghers syndrome. *Nature* 1998;391:184–187.
70. Jenne DE, Reimann H, Nezu J, et al. Peutz-Jeghers syndrome is caused by mutations in a novel serine threonine kinase. *Nat Genet* 1998;18:38–43.
71. Buchet-Poyau K, Mehenni H, Radhakrishna U, et al. Search for the second Peutz-Jeghers syndrome locus: exclusion of the *STK13, PRKCG, KLK10*, and *PSCD2* genes on chromosome 19 and the *STK11IP* gene on chromosome 2. *Cytogenet Genome Res* 2002;97:171–178.
72. Miyaki M, Iijima T, Hosono K, et al. Somatic mutations of *LKB1* and beta-catenin genes in gastrointestinal polyps from patients with Peutz-Jeghers syndrome. *Cancer Res* 2000;60:6311–6313.
73. Connolly DC, Katabuchi H, Cliby WA, et al. Somatic mutations in the *STK11/LKB1* gene are uncommon in rare gynecological tumor types associated with Peutz-Jegher's syndrome. *Am J Pathol* 2000;156:339–345.
74. Lee JY, Dong SM, Kim HS, et al. A distinct region of chromosome 19p13.3 associated with the sporadic form of adenoma malignum of the uterine cervix. *Cancer Res* 1998;58:1140–1143.
75. Kuragaki C, Enomoto T, Ueno Y, et al. Mutations in the *STK11* gene characterize minimal deviation adenocarcinoma of the uterine cervix. *Lab Invest* 2003;83:35–45.
76. Kersemaekers AM, van de Vijver MJ, Fleuren GJ, et al. Comparison of the genetic alterations in two epithelial collision tumors of the uterine cervix: A report of two cases. *Int J Gynecol Pathol* 2000;19:225–230.
77. Bokhman JV. Two pathogenetic types of endometrial carcinoma. *Gynecol Oncol* 1983;15:10–17.
78. Matias-Guiu X, Catasus L, Bussaglia E, et al. Molecular pathology of endometrial hyperplasia and carcinoma. *Hum Pathol* 2001;32:569–577.
79. Esteller M, Catasus L, Matias-Guiu X, et al. *hMLH1* promoter hypermethylation is an early event in human endometrial tumorigenesis. *Am J Pathol* 1999;155:1767–1772.
80. Lukes AS, Kohler MF, Pieper CF, et al. Multivariable analysis of DNA ploidy, *p53*, and *HER-2/neu* as prognostic factors in endometrial cancer. *Cancer* 1994;73:2380–2385.
81. Sherman ME, Bur ME, Kurman RJ. *p53* in endometrial cancer and its putative precursors: evidence for diverse pathways of tumorigenesis. *Hum Pathol* 1995;26:1268–1274.
82. Berchuck A, Boyd J. Molecular basis of endometrial cancer. *Cancer* 1995;76:2034–2040.
83. An HJ, Logani S, Isacson C, et al. Molecular characterization of uterine clear cell carcinoma. *Mod Pathol* 2004;17:530–537.
84. Mutter GL, Ince TA, Baak JP, et al. Molecular identification of latent precancers in histologically normal endometrium. *Cancer Res* 2001;61:4311–4314.
85. Faquin WC, Fitzgerald JT, Lin MC, et al. Sporadic microsatellite instability is specific to neoplastic and preneoplastic endometrial tissues. *Am J Clin Pathol* 2000;113:576–582.
86. Mutter GL. Histopathology of genetically defined endometrial precancers. *Int J Gynecol Pathol* 2000;19:301–309.
87. Mutter GL. Endometrial intraepithelial neoplasia (EIN): will it bring order to chaos? The Endometrial Collaborative Group. *Gynecol Oncol* 2000;76:287–290.
88. Mutter GL. Diagnosis of premalignant endometrial disease. *J Clin Pathol* 2002;55:326–331.
89. www.endometrium.org.
90. Ronnett BM, Kurman RJ. Precursor lesions of endometrial carcinoma. In: Kurman RJ, ed. *Blaustein's Pathology of the Female Genital Tract*, 5th ed. New York: Springer Verlag; 2002:467–500.
91. Ito K, Watanabe K, Nasim S, et al. K-*ras* point mutations in endometrial carcinoma: effect on outcome is dependent on age of patient. *Gynecol Oncol* 1996;63:238–246.
92. Caduff RF, Johnston CM, Frank T. Mutations of the Ki-*ras* oncogene in carcinoma of the endometrium. *Am J Pathol* 1995;146:182–188.
93. Kobayashi K, Sagae S, Kudo R, et al. Microsatellite instability in endometrial carcinomas: frequent replication errors in tumors of early onset and/or of poorly differentiated type. *Genes Chromosomes Cancer* 1995;14:128–132.
94. Basil JB, Goodfellow PJ, Rader JS, et al. Clinical significance of microsatellite instability in endometrial carcinoma. *Cancer* 2000;89:1758–1764.
95. Bonatz G, Frahm SO, Klapper W, et al. High telomerase activity is associated with cell cycle deregulation and rapid progression in endometrioid adenocarcinoma of the uterus. *Hum Pathol* 2001;32:605–614.
96. Risinger JI, Maxwell GL, Chandramouli GV, et al. Microarray analysis reveals distinct gene expression profiles among different histologic types of endometrial cancer. *Cancer Res* 2003;63:6–11.
97. Smid-Koopman E, Blok LJ, Helmerhorst TJ, et al. Gene expression profiling in human endometrial cancer tissue samples: utility and diagnostic value. *Gynecol Oncol* 2004;93:292–300.
98. Chang KL, Crabtree GS, Lim-Tan SK, et al. Primary uterine endometrial stromal neoplasms: a clinicopathologic study of 117 cases. *Am J Surg Pathol* 1990;14:415–438.
99. Silverberg SG, Kurman RG, eds. *Atlas of Tumor Pathology: Tumors of the Uterine Corpus and Gestational Trophoblastic Disease*. Vol 3. Washington, DC: Armed Forces Institute of Pathology, Publishers; 1992.
100. Hendrickson MR, Tavassooli FA, Kempson RL, et al. Mesenchymal tumors and related lesions. In: *Pathology and Genetics of Tumours of the Breast and Female Genital Organs*. Lyon: IARC Press; 2003:233–244.
101. Clement PB. The pathology of uterine smooth muscle tumors and mixed endometrial stromal-smooth muscle tumors: a selective review with emphasis on recent advances. *Int J Gynecol Pathol* 2000;19:39–55.
102. Oliva E, Clement PB, Young RH. Endometrial stromal tumors: an update on a group of tumors with a protean phenotype. *Adv Anat Pathol* 2000;7:257–281.
103. Yilmaz A, Rush DS, Soslow RA. Endometrial stromal sarcomas with unusual histologic features: a report of 24 primary and metastatic tumors emphasizing fibroblastic and smooth muscle differentiation. *Am J Surg Pathol* 2002;26:1142–1150.
104. Oliva E, Young RH, Clement PB, et al. Myxoid and fibrous endometrial stromal tumors of the uterus: a report of 10 cases. *Int J Gynecol Pathol* 1999;18:310–319.
105. Clement PB, Scully RE. Endometrial stromal sarcomas of the uterus with extensive endometrioid glandular differentiation: a report of three cases that caused problems in differential diagnosis. *Int J Gynecol Pathol* 1992;11:163–173.
106. Evans HL. Endometrial stromal sarcoma and poorly differentiated endometrial sarcoma. *Cancer* 1982;50:2170–2182.
107. Koontz JI, Soreng AL, Nucci M, et al. Frequent fusion of the *JAZF1* and *JJAZ1* genes in endometrial stromal tumors. *Proc Natl Acad Sci USA* 2001;98:6348–6353.
108. Huang HY, Ladanyi M, Soslow RA. Molecular detection of *JAZF1-JJAZ1* gene fusion in endometrial stromal neoplasms with classic and variant histology: evidence for genetic heterogeneity. *Am J Surg Pathol* 2004;28:224–232.
109. Micci F, Walter CU, Teixeira MR. Cytogenetic and molecular genetic analyses of endometrial stromal sarcoma: nonrandom involvement of chromosome arms 6p and 7p and confirmation of *JAZF1/JJAZ1* gene fusion in t(7;17). *Cancer Genet Cytogenet* 2003;144:119–124.
110. Gunawan B, Schulten HJ, Fuzesi L. Identification of a *BAC* clone overlapping the t(6p12.3) breakpoint in the cell line ESS-1 derived from an endometrial stromal sarcoma. *Cancer Genet Cytogenet* 2003;147:84–86.
111. Amant F, Moerman P, Cadron I, et al. Endometrial stromal sarcoma with a sole t(X;17) chromosome change: report of a case and review of the literature. *Gynecol Oncol* 2003;88:459–462.
112. Dal Cin P, Aly MS, De Wever I, et al. Endometrial stromal sarcoma t(7;17)(p15-21; q12-21) is a nonrandom chromosome change. *Cancer Genet Cytogenet* 1992;63:43–46.
113. Hennig Y, Caselitz J, Bartnitzke S, et al. A third case of a low-grade endometrial stromal sarcoma with a t(7;17)(p14 approximately 21;q11.2 approximately 21). *Cancer Genet Cytogenet* 1997;98:84–86.
114. Sandberg AA. Updates on the cytogenetics and molecular genetics of bone and soft tissue tumors: lipoma. *Cancer Genet Cytogenet* 2004;150:93–115.
115. Hess J. Chromosomal translocations in benign tumors: the HMGI proteins. *Am J Clin Pathol* 1998;109:251–261.
116. Dal Cin P, Wanschura S, Kasmierczak B, et al. Amplification and expression of the *HMGIC* gene in a benign endometrial polyp. *Genes Chromosomes Cancer* 1998;22:95–99.
117. Kazmierczak B, Dal Cin P, Wanschura S, et al. *HMGIY* is the target of 6p21.3 rearrangements in various benign mesenchymal tumors. *Genes Chromosomes Cancer* 1998;23:279–285.
118. Tallini G, Vanni R, Manfioletti G, et al. *HMGI-C* and *HMGI(Y)* immunoreactivity correlates with cytogenetic abnormalities in lipomas, pulmonary chondroid hamartomas, endometrial polyps, and uterine leiomyomas and is compatible with rearrangement of the *HMGI-C* and *HMGI(Y)* genes. *Lab Invest* 2000;80:359–369.
119. Shih I-M, Mazur MT, Kurman RJ. Gestational trophoblastic diseases and related lesions. Kurman RJ, ed. *Blaustein's Pathology of the Female Genital Tract*, 5th ed. New York: Springer Verlag; 2002:1193–1247.
120. Sumithran E, Cheah PL, Susil BJ, et al. Problems in the histological assessment of hydatidiform moles: a study on consensus diagnosis and ploidy status by fluorescent in situ hybridisation. *Pathology* 1996;28:311–315.
121. Howat A, Beck S, Fox H, et al. Can histopathologists reliably diagnose molar pregnancy? *J Clin Pathol* 1993;46:599–602.
122. Javey H, Borazjani G. Discrepancies in the histological diagnosis of hydatidiform mole. *Br J Obstet Gynaecol* 1979;86:480–483.
123. Messerli M, Parmley T, Woodruff J, et al. Inter- and intra-pathologist variability in the diagnosis of gestational trophoblastic neoplasia. *Obstet Gynecol* 1987;69:622–626.
124. Fukunaga M, Katabuchi H, Nagasaka T, et al. Interobserver and Intraobserver variability in the diagnosis of hydatidiform mole. *Am J Surg Pathol* 2005;29:942–947.
125. Trabetti E, Galavotti R, Zanini L, et al. The parental origin of hydatidiform moles and blighted ova: molecular probing with hypervariable DNA polymorphisms. *Mol Cell Probes* 1993;7:325–329.

126. Jacobs PA, Wilson CM, Sprenkle JA, et al. Mechanism of origin of complete hydatidiform moles. *Nature* 1980;286:714–716.
127. Kajii T, Ohama K. Androgenetic origin of hydatidiform mole. *Nature* 1977;268:633–634.
128. Lindor NM, Ney JA, Gaffey TA, et al. A genetic review of complete and partial hydatidiform moles and nonmolar triploidy. *Mayo Clin Proc* 1992;67:791–799.
129. Bell KA, Van Deerlin V, Addya K, et al. Molecular genetic testing from paraffin-embedded tissue distinguishes nonmolar hydropic abortion from hydatidiform mole. *Mol Diagn* 1999;4:11–19.
130. Fukunaga M. Flow cytometric and clinicopathologic study of complete hydatidiform moles with special reference to the significance of cytometric aneuploidy. *Gynecol Oncol* 2001;81:67–70.
131. Helwani MN, Seoud M, Zahed L, et al. A familial case of recurrent hydatidiform molar pregnancies with biparental genomic contribution. *Hum Genet* 1999;105:112–115.
132. Fisher RA, Khatoon R, Paradinas EJ, et al. Repetitive complete hydatidiform mole can be biparental in origin and either male or female. *Hum Reprod* 2000;15:594–598.
133. Hodges MD, Rees HC, Seckl MJ, et al. Genetic refinement and physical mapping of a biparental complete hydatidiform mole locus on chromosome 19q13.4. *J Med Genet* 2003;40:e95.
134. Makrydimas G, Sebire NJ, Thornton SE, et al. Complete hydatidiform mole and normal live birth: a novel case of confined placental mosaicism: case report. *Hum Reprod* 2002;17:2459–263.
135. Jacobs PA, Hunt PA, Matsuura JS, et al. Complete and partial hydatidiform mole in Hawaii: cytogenetics, morphology and epidemiology. *Br J Obstet Gynaecol* 1982;89:258–266.
136. Lage JM, Weinberg DS, Yavner DL, et al. The biology of tetraploid hydatidiform moles: histopathology, cytogenetics, and flow cytometry. *Hum Pathol* 1989;20:419–425.
137. Dietzsch E, Ramsay M, Christianson AL, et al. Maternal origin of extra haploid set of chromosomes in third trimester triploid fetuses. *Am J Med Genet* 1995;58:360–364.
138. McFadden DE, Pantzar JT. Placental pathology of triploidy. *Hum Pathol* 1996;27:1018–1020.
139. Redline RW, Hassold T, Zaragoza MV. Prevalence of the partial molar phenotype in triploidy of maternal and paternal origin. *Hum Pathol* 1998;29:505–511.
140. Keep D, Zaragoza MV, Hassold T, et al. Very early complete hydatidiform mole. *Hum Pathol* 1996;27:708–713.
141. Fisher RA, Newlands ES. Gestational trophoblastic disease: Molecular and genetic studies. *J Reprod Med* 1998;43:87–97.
142. Bateman AC, Hemmatpour SK, Theaker JM, et al. Genetic analysis of hydatidiform moles in paraffin wax embedded tissue using rapid, sequence specific PCR-based HLA class II typing. *J Clin Pathol* 1997;50:288–293.
143. Fisher RA, Newlands ES. Rapid diagnosis and classification of hydatidiform moles with polymerase chain reaction. *Am J Obstet Gynecol* 1993;168:563–569.
144. Fujita N, Tamura S, Shimizu N, et al. Genetic origin analysis of hydatidiform mole and non-molar abortion using the polymerase chain reaction method. *Acta Obstet Gynecol Scand* 1994;73:719–725.
145. Fukuyama R, Takata M, Kudoh J, et al. DNA diagnosis of hydatidiform mole using the polymerase chain reaction. *Hum Genet* 1991;87:216–218.
146. Lane SA, Taylor GR, Ozols B, et al. Diagnosis of complete molar pregnancy by microsatellites in archival material. *J Clin Pathol* 1993;46:346–348.
147. Cho S, Kim SJ. Genetic study of hydatidiform moles by restriction fragment length polymorphisms (RFLPs) analysis. *J Korean Med Sci* 1993;8:446–452.
148. Abeln EC, Cornelisse CJ, Dreef EJ, et al. Molecular identification of a partial hydatidiform mole. *Diagn Mol Pathol* 1997;6:58–63.
149. Lai CY, Chan KY, Khoo US, et al. Analysis of gestational trophoblastic disease by genotyping and chromosome in situ hybridization. *Mod Pathol* 2004;17:40–48.
150. Yver M, Carles D, Bloch B, et al. Determination of DNA ploidy by fluorescence in situ hybridization (FISH) in hydatidiform moles: evaluation of FISH on isolated nuclei. *Hum Pathol* 2004;35:752–758.
151. Xue WC, Chan KY, Feng HC, et al. Promoter hypermethylation of multiple genes in hydatidiform mole and choriocarcinoma. *J Mol Diagn* 2004;6:326–334.
152. Kashimura Y, Tanaka M, Harada N, et al. Twin pregnancy consisting of 46, XY heterozygous complete mole coexisting with a live fetus. *Placenta* 2001;22:323–327.
153. Hirose M, Kimura T, Mitsuno N, et al. DNA flow cytometric quantification and DNA polymorphism analysis in the case of a complete mole with a coexisting fetus. *J Assist Reprod Genet* 1999;16:263–267.
154. Malhotra N, Deka D, Takkar D, et al. Hydatiform mole with coexisting live fetus in dichorionic twin gestation. *Eur J Obstet Gynecol Reprod Biol* 2001;94:301–303.
155. Ruiz-Casares E, Henriques-Gil N, Orera M, et al. Molecular analysis of a gestation consisting of a complete hydatidiform mole and normal dizygotic twin. *J Reprod Med* 2001;46:1041–1045.
156. Wax JR, Pinette MG, Chard R, et al. Prenatal diagnosis by DNA polymorphism analysis of complete mole with coexisting twin. *Am J Obstet Gynecol* 2003;188:1105–1106.
157. Ishii J, Iitsuka Y, Takano H, et al. Genetic differentiation of complete hydatidiform moles coexisting with normal fetuses by short tandem repeat-derived deoxyribonucleic acid polymorphism analysis. *Am J Obstet Gynecol* 1998;179:628–634.
158. Quade BJ, Weremowicz S, Neskey DM, et al. Fusion transcripts involving *HMGA2* are not a common molecular mechanism in uterine leiomyomata with rearrangements in 12q15. *Cancer Res* 2003;63:1351–1358.
159. Bussaglia E, del Rio E, Matias-Guiu X, et al. *PTEN* mutations in endometrial carcinomas: a molecular and clinicopathologic analysis of 38 cases. *Hum Pathol* 2000;31:312–317.
160. Mine N, Kurose K, Konishi H, et al. Fusion of a sequence from *HEI10* (14q11) to the *HMGIC* gene at 12q15 in a uterine leiomyoma. *Jpn J Cancer Res* 2001;92:135–139.
161. Kurose K, Mine N, Doi D, et al. Novel gene fusion of *COX6C* at 8q22–23 to *HMGIC* at 12q15 in a uterine leiomyoma. *Genes Chromosomes Cancer* 2000;27:303–307.
162. Schoenmakers EF, Huysmans C, Van de Ven WJ. Allelic knockout of novel splice variants of human recombination repair gene *RAD51B* in t(12;14) uterine leiomyomas. *Cancer Res* 1999;59:19–23.
163. Kazmierczak B, Hennig Y, Wanschura S, et al. Description of a novel fusion transcript between *HMGI-C*, a gene encoding for a member of the high mobility group proteins, and the mitochondrial aldehyde dehydrogenase gene. *Cancer Res* 1995;55:6038–6039.
164. Petit M, Mols R, Schoenmakers E, et al. LPP, the preferred fusion partner gene of *HMGIC* in lipomas, is a novel member of the LIM protein gene family. *Genomics* 1996;36:118–129.
165. Kazmierczak B, Pohnke Y, Bullerdiek J. Fusion transcripts between the *HMGIC* gene and RTVL-H-related sequences in mesenchymal tumors without cytogenetic aberrations. *Genomics* 1996;38:223–226.
166. Petit M, Schoenmakers E, Huysmans C, et al. *LHFP*, a novel translocation partner gene of *HMGIC* in a lipoma, is a member of a new family of *LHFP*-like genes. *Genomics* 1999;57:438–441.
167. Hisaoka M, Sheng WQ, Tanaka A, et al. *HMGIC* alterations in smooth muscle tumors of soft tissues and other sites. *Cancer Genet Cytogenet* 2002;138:50–55.
168. Reeves R. Molecular biology of HMGA proteins: hubs of nuclear function. *Gene* 2001;277:63–81.
169. Rogalla P, Drechsler K, Frey G, et al. *HMGI-C* expression patterns in human tissues. Implications for the genesis of frequent mesenchymal tumors. *Am J Pathol* 1996;149: 775–779.
170. Gross KL, Neskey DM, Manchanda N, et al. *HMGA2* expression in uterine leiomyomata and myometrium: quantitative analysis and tissue culture studies. *Genes Chromosomes Cancer* 2003;38:68–79.
171. Klotzbucher M, Wasserfall A, Fuhrmann U, et al. Misexpression of wild-type and truncated isoforms of the high-mobility group I proteins *HMGI-C* and *HMGI(Y)* in uterine leiomyomas. *Am J Pathol* 1999;155:1535–1542.
172. Harlow BL, Weiss NS, Lofton S. The epidemiology of sarcomas of the uterus. *J Natl Cancer Inst* 1986;76:399–402.
173. Quade BJ. Pathology, cytogenetics and molecular biology of uterine leiomyomas and other smooth muscle lesions. *Curr Opin Obstet Gynecol* 1995;7:35–42.
174. Han K, Lee W, Harris CP, et al. Comparison of chromosome aberrations in leiomyoma and leiomyosarcoma using FISH on archival tissues. *Cancer Genet Cytogenet* 1994;74: 19–24.
175. Jeffers MD, Oakes SJ, Richmond JA, et al. Proliferation, ploidy and prognosis in uterine smooth muscle tumours. *Histopathology* 1996;29:217–223.
176. Gayther SA, Russell P, Harrington P, et al. The contribution of germline *BRCA1* and *BRCA2* mutations to familial ovarian cancer: no evidence for other ovarian cancer-susceptibility genes. *Am J Hum Genet* 1999;65:1021–1029.
177. Tabassoli F, Devilee P, eds. *Pathology and Genetics of Tumours of the Breast and Female Genital Organs*. Lyon: IARC Press Publishers; 2003.
178. Bell DA. Origins and molecular pathology of ovarian cancer. *Mod Pathol* 2005;18: 19–32.
179. Singer G, Kurman RJ, Chang HW, et al. Diverse tumorigenic pathways in ovarian serous carcinoma. *Am J Pathol* 2002;160:1223–1228.
180. Cuatrecasas M, Erill N, Musulen E, et al. *K-ras* mutations in nonmucinous ovarian epithelial tumors: a molecular analysis and clinicopathologic study of 144 patients. *Cancer* 1998;82:1088–1095.
181. Cheng EJ, Kurman RJ, Wang M, et al. Molecular genetic analysis of ovarian serous cystadenomas. *Lab Invest* 2004;84:778–784.
182. Sieben NL, Macropoulos P, Roemen GM, et al. In ovarian neoplasms, *BRAF*, but not *KRAS*, mutations are restricted to low-grade serous tumours. *J Pathol* 2004;202: 336–340.
183. Mok SC, Bell DA, Knapp RC, et al. Mutation of K-*ras* protooncogene in human ovarian epithelial tumors of borderline malignancy. *Cancer Res* 1993;53:1489–1492.
184. Singer G, Oldt R III, Cohen Y, et al. Mutations in *BRAF* and *KRAS* characterize the development of low-grade ovarian serous carcinoma. *J Natl Cancer Inst* 2003;95:484–486.
185. Singer G, Stohr R, Cope L, et al. Patterns of *p53* mutations separate ovarian serous borderline tumors and low- and high-grade carcinomas and provide support for a new model of ovarian carcinogenesis: a mutational analysis with immunohistochemical correlation. *Am J Surg Pathol* 2005;29:218–224.
186. Wolf NG, Abdul-Karim FW, Schork NJ, et al. Origins of heterogeneous ovarian carcinomas: a molecular cytogenetic analysis of histologically benign, low malignant potential, and fully malignant components. *Am J Pathol* 1996;149:511–520.
187. Singer G, Shih I, Truskinovsky A, et al. Mutational analysis of K-*ras* segregates ovarian serous carcinomas into two types: invasive MPSC (low-grade tumor) and conventional serous carcinoma (high-grade tumor). *Int J Gynecol Pathol* 2003;22:37–41.
188. Bell DA, Scully RE. Early de novo ovarian carcinoma: a study of fourteen cases. *Cancer* 1994;73:1859–1864.
189. Berchuck A, Kohler MF, Marks JR, et al. The *p53* tumor suppressor gene frequently is altered in gynecologic cancers. *Am J Obstet Gynecol* 1994;170:246–252.
190. Wen WH, Reles A, Runnebaum IB, et al. *p53* mutations and expression in ovarian cancers: correlation with overall survival. *Int J Gynecol Pathol* 1999;18:29–41.
191. Pothuri B, Leitao M, Barakat R, et al. Genetic analysis of ovarian carcinoma histogenesis. *Gynecol Oncol* 2001;80:277.
192. Catasus L, Bussaglia E, Rodrigues I, et al. Molecular genetic alterations in endometrioid carcinomas of the ovary: similar frequency of beta-catenin abnormalities but lower rate of microsatellite instability and *PTEN* alterations than in uterine endometrioid carcinomas. *Hum Pathol* 2004;35:1360–1368.
193. Moreno-Bueno G, Gamallo C, Perez-Gallego L, et al. beta-Catenin expression pattern, beta-catenin gene mutations, and microsatellite instability in endometrioid ovarian carcinomas and synchronous endometrial carcinomas. *Diagn Mol Pathol* 2001;10:116–122.
194. Obata K, Morland SJ, Watson RH, et al. Frequent *PTEN/MMAC* mutations in endometrioid but not serous or mucinous epithelial ovarian tumors. *Cancer Res* 1998;58:2095–2097.
195. Liu J, Albarracin CT, Chang KH, et al. Microsatellite instability and expression of hMLH1 and hMSH2 proteins in ovarian endometrioid cancer. *Mod Pathol* 2004;17:75–80.
196. Jiang X, Morland SJ, Hitchcock A, et al. Allelotyping of endometriosis with adjacent ovarian carcinoma reveals evidence of a common lineage. *Cancer Res* 1998;58: 1707–1712.
197. Dinulescu DM, Ince TA, Quade BJ, et al. Role of K-*ras* and *PTEN* in the development of mouse models of endometriosis and endometrioid ovarian cancer. *Nat Med* 2005;11:63–70.
198. Garrett AP, Lee KR, Colitti CR, et al. K-*ras* mutation may be an early event in mucinous ovarian tumorigenesis. *Int J Gynecol Pathol* 2001;20:244–251.
199. Mandai M, Konishi I, Kuroda H, et al. Heterogeneous distribution of K-*ras*-mutated epithelia in mucinous ovarian tumors with special reference to histopathology. *Hum Pathol* 1998;29:34–40.

200. Cuatrecasas M, Villanueva A, Matias-Guiu X, et al. *K-ras* mutations in mucinous ovarian tumors: a clinicopathologic and molecular study of 95 cases. *Cancer* 1997;79:1581–1586.
201. Lee KR, Scully RE. Mucinous tumors of the ovary: a clinicopathologic study of 196 borderline tumors (of intestinal type) and carcinomas, including an evaluation of 11 cases with 'pseudomyxoma peritonei'. *Am J Surg Pathol* 2000;24:1447–1464.
202. Cai KQ, Albarracin C, Rosen D, et al. Microsatellite instability and alteration of the expression of *hMLH1* and *hMSH2* in ovarian clear cell carcinoma. *Hum Pathol* 2004;35:552–559.
203. Jazaeri AA, Yee CJ, Sotiriou C, et al. Gene expression profiles of *BRCA1*-linked, *BRCA2*-linked, and sporadic ovarian cancers. *J Natl Cancer Inst* 2002;94:990–1000.
204. Warrenfeltz S, Pavlik S, Datta S, et al. Gene expression profiling of epithelial ovarian tumours correlated with malignant potential. *Mol Cancer* 2004;3:27.
205. Bani MR, Nicoletti MI, Alkharouf NW, et al. Gene expression correlating with response to paclitaxel in ovarian carcinoma xenografts. *Mol Cancer Ther* 2004;3:111–1121.
206. Balch C, Huang TH, Brown R, et al. The epigenetics of ovarian cancer drug resistance and resensitization. *Am J Obstet Gynecol* 2004;191:1552–1572.
207. Brown R, Hirst GL, Gallagher WM, et al. *hMLH1* expression and cellular responses of ovarian tumour cells to treatment with cytotoxic anticancer agents. *Oncogene* 1997;15:45–52.
208. Strathdee G, Appleton K, Illand M, et al. Primary ovarian carcinomas display multiple methylator phenotypes involving known tumor suppressor genes. *Am J Pathol* 2001;158:1121–1127.
209. Wei SH, Chen CM, Strathdee G, et al. Methylation microarray analysis of late-stage ovarian carcinomas distinguishes progression-free survival in patients and identifies candidate epigenetic markers. *Clin Cancer Res* 2002;8:2246–2252.
210. Warren S, Gates O. Multiple primary tumors: a survey of the literature and a statistical study. *Am J Cancer* 1932;16:1348–1414.
211. Nowell PC. The clonal evolution of tumor cell populations. *Science* 1976;194:23–28.
212. Fialkow PJ. Clonal origin of human tumors. *Biochim Biophys Acta* 1976;458:283–321.
213. Rolston R, Sasatomi E, Hunt J, et al. Distinguishing de novo second cancer formation from tumor recurrence: mutational fingerprinting by microdissection genotyping. *J Mol Diagn* 2001;3:129–132.
214. Goldstein NS, Vicini FA, Hunter S, et al. Molecular clonality determination of ipsilateral recurrence of invasive breast carcinomas after breast-conserving therapy: comparison with clinical and biologic factors. *Am J Clin Pathol* 2005;123:679–689.
215. Heinmoller E, Dietmaier W, Zirngibl H, et al. Molecular analysis of microdissected tumors and preneoplastic intraductal lesions in pancreatic carcinoma. *Am J Pathol* 2000;157:83–92.
216. Hameed O, Pfeifer JD, et al. Classifying "recurrent" breast cancer: lost heterozygosity found. *J Clin Pathol* 2005;123:641–643.
217. Ulbright TM, Roth LM. Metastatic and independent cancers of the endometrium and ovary: a clinicopathologic study of 34 cases. *Hum Pathol* 1985;16:28–34.
218. Tang M, Pires Y, Schultz M, et al. Microsatellite analysis of synchronous and metachronous tumors: a tool for double primary tumor and metastasis assessment. *Diagn Mol Pathol* 2003;12:151–159.
219. Ricci R, Komminoth P, Bannwart F, et al. *PTEN* as a molecular marker to distinguish metastatic from primary synchronous endometrioid carcinomas of the ovary and uterus. *Diagn Mol Pathol* 2003;12:71–78.
220. Emmert-Buck MR, Chuaqui R, Zhuang Z, et al. Molecular analysis of synchronous uterine and ovarian endometrioid tumors. *Int J Gynecol Pathol* 1997;16:143–148.
221. Fujii H, Matsumoto T, Yoshida M, et al. Genetics of synchronous uterine and ovarian endometrioid carcinoma: combined analyses of loss of heterozygosity, *PTEN* mutation, and microsatellite instability. *Hum Pathol* 2002;33:421–428.
222. Fujita M, Enomoto T, Wada H, et al. Application of clonal analysis: differential diagnosis for synchronous primary ovarian and endometrial cancers and metastatic cancer. *Am J Clin Pathol* 1996;105:350–359.
223. Elishaev E, Gilks CB, Miller D, et al. Synchronous and metachronous endocervical and ovarian neoplasms: evidence supporting interpretation of the ovarian neoplasms as metastatic endocervical adenocarcinomas simulating primary ovarian surface epithelial neoplasms. *Am J Surg Pathol* 2005;29:281–294.
224. Yamamoto N, Kato Y, Yanagisawa A, et al. Predictive value of genetic diagnosis for cancer micrometastasis: histologic and experimental appraisal. *Cancer* 1997;80:1393–1398.
225. Altaras MM, Klein A, Zemer R, et al. Detection of tumor circulating cells by cytokeratin 20 in the blood of patients with endometrial carcinoma. *Gynecol Oncol* 2000;78:352–355.
226. Hildebrandt MO, Blaser F, Beyer J, et al. Detection of tumor cells in peripheral blood samples from patients with germ cell tumors using immunocytochemical and reverse transcriptase-polymerase chain reaction techniques. *Bone Marrow Transplant* 1998;22:771–775.
227. Wong IH, Chan AT, Johnson PJ. Molecular analysis of circulating tumor cells in peripheral blood from patients with germ cell tumor: a quantitative approach. *Int J Mol Med* 2000;6:491–494.
228. Hildebrandt M, Rick O, Salama A, et al. Detection of germ-cell tumor cells in peripheral blood progenitor cell harvests: impact on clinical outcome. *Clin Cancer Res* 2000;6:4641–4646.
229. Hara I, Yamada Y, Miyake H, et al. Detection of beta-human chorionic gonadotropin expressing cells by nested reverse transcriptase-polymerase chain reaction in the peripheral blood stem cells of patients with advanced germ cell tumor. *J Urol* 2002;167: 1487–1491.
230. Gifford G, Paul J, Vasey PA, et al. The acquisition of *hMLH1* methylation in plasma DNA after chemotherapy predicts poor survival for ovarian cancer patients. *Clin Cancer Res* 2004;10:4420–4426.
231. Yuan CC, Wang PH, Ng HT, et al. Detecting cytokeratin 19 mRNA in the peripheral blood cells of cervical cancer patients and its clinical-pathological correlation. *Gynecol Oncol* 2002;85:148–153.
232. Stenman J, Lintula S, Hotakainen K, et al. Detection of squamous-cell carcinoma antigen-expressing tumour cells in blood by reverse transcriptase-polymerase chain reaction in cancer of the uterine cervix. *Int J Cancer* 1997;74:75–80.
233. Pao CC, Hor JJ, Yang FP, et al. Detection of human papillomavirus mRNA and cervical cancer cells in peripheral blood of cervical cancer patients with metastasis. *J Clin Oncol* 1997;15:1008–1012.
234. Klein A, Fishman A, Zemer R, et al. Detection of tumor circulating cells by cytokeratin-20 in the blood of patients with granulosa cell tumors. *Gynecol Oncol* 2002;86:330–336.
235. Baba T, Koizumi M, Suzuki T, et al. Specific detection of circulating tumor cells by reverse transcriptase-polymerase chain reaction of a beta-casein-like protein, preferentially expressed in malignant neoplasms. *Anticancer Res* 2001;21:2547–2551.
236. Grunewald K, Haun M, Fiegl M, et al. Mammaglobin expression in gynecologic malignancies and malignant effusions detected by nested reverse transcriptase-polymerase chain reaction. *Lab Invest* 2002;82:1147–1153.
237. Hickey KP, Boyle KP, Jepps HM, et al. Molecular detection of tumour DNA in serum and peritoneal fluid from ovarian cancer patients. *Br J Cancer* 1999;80:1803–1808.
238. Parrella P, Zangen R, Sidransky D, et al. Molecular analysis of peritoneal fluid in ovarian cancer patients. *Mod Pathol* 2003;16:636–640.
239. Muller HM, Millinger S, Fiegl H, et al. Analysis of methylated genes in peritoneal fluids of ovarian cancer patients: a new prognostic tool. *Clin Chem* 2004;50:2171–2173.
240. Reuter VE. Origins and molecular biology of testicular germ cell tumors. *Mod Pathol* 2005;18:S51–S60.
241. Sakuma Y, Sakurai S, Oguni S, et al. Alterations of the c-*kit* gene in testicular germ cell tumors. *Cancer Sci* 2003;94:486–491.
242. Kemmer K, Corless C, Fletcher J, et al. KIT mutations are common in testicular seminomas. *Am J Pathol* 2004;164:305–313.
243. Tian Q, Frierson HF Jr, Krystal GW, et al. Activating c-*kit* gene mutations in human germ cell tumors. *Am J Pathol* 1999;154:1643–1647.
244. Looijenga L, de Leeuw H, van Oorschot M, et al. Stem cell factor receptor (c-KIT) codon 816 mutations predict development of bilateral testicular germ-cell tumors. *Cancer Res* 2003;63:7674–7678.
245. Dibb NJ, Dilworth SM, Mol CD. Switching on kinases: oncogenic activation of *BRAF* and the *PDGFR* family. *Nat Rev Cancer* 2004;4:718–727.
246. Przygodzki RM, Hubbs AE, Zhao FQ, et al. Primary mediastinal seminomas: evidence of single and multiple KIT mutations. *Lab Invest* 2002;82:1369–1375.
247. Chaganti RS, Houldsworth J. Genetics and biology of adult human male germ cell tumors. *Cancer Res* 2000;60:1475–1482.
248. Strohmeyer T, Reese D, Press M. Expression of the c-*kit* proto-oncogene and its ligand stem cell factor (SCF) in normal and malignant human testicular tissue. *J Urol* 1995;153:511–515.
249. Bokemeyer C, Kuczyk MA, Dunn T, et al. Expression of stem-cell factor and its receptor c-*kit* protein in normal testicular tissue and malignant germ-cell tumours. *J Cancer Res Clin Oncol* 1996;122:301–306.
250. Izquierdo MA, Van der Valk P, Van Ark-Otte J, et al. Differential expression of the c-*kit* proto-oncogene in germ cell tumours. *J Pathol* 1995;177:253–258.
251. Frost MJ, Ferrao PT, Hughes TP, et al. Juxtamembrane mutant V560G*kit* is more sensitive to imatinib (STI571) compared with wild-type c-*kit* whereas the kinase domain mutant D816Vkit is resistant. *Mol Cancer Ther* 2002;1:1115–1124.
252. Ma Y, Zeng S, Metcalfe DD, et al. The c-KIT mutation causing human mastocytosis is resistant to STI571 and other KIT kinase inhibitors; kinases with enzymatic site mutations show different inhibitor sensitivity profiles than wild-type kinases and those with regulatory-type mutations. *Blood* 2002;99:1741–1744.
253. Heinrich MC, Blanke CD, Druker BJ, et al. Inhibition of KIT tyrosine kinase activity: a novel molecular approach to the treatment of KIT-positive malignancies. *J Clin Oncol* 2002;20:1692–1703.
254. Liao AT, Chien M, Shenoy N, et al. Inhibition of constitutively active forms of mutant kit by multitargeted indolinone tyrosine kinase inhibitors. *Blood* 2002;100:585–593.
255. Bosl GJ, Ilson DH, Rodriguez E, et al. Clinical relevance of the i(12p) marker chromosome in germ cell tumors. *J Natl Cancer Inst* 1994;86:349–355.
256. Rodriguez E, Mathew S, Mukherjee AB, et al. Analysis of chromosome 12 aneuploidy in interphase cells from human male germ cell tumors by fluorescence in situ hybridization. *Genes Chromosomes Cancer* 1992;5:21–29.
257. Mukherjee AB, Murty W, Rodriguez E, et al. Detection and analysis of origin of i(12p), a diagnostic marker of human male germ cell tumors, by fluorescence in situ hybridization. *Genes Chromosomes Cancer* 1991;3:300–307.
258. Looijenga LH, Zafarana G, Grygalewicz B, et al. Role of gain of 12p in germ cell tumour development. *APMIS* 2003;111:161–173.
259. Henegariu O, Heerema NA, Thurston V, et al. Characterization of gains, losses, and regional amplification in testicular germ cell tumor cell lines by comparative genomic hybridization. *Cancer Genet Cytogenet* 2004;148:14–20.
260. Geurts van Kessel A, Suijkerbuijk RF, Sinke RJ, et al. Molecular cytogenetics of human germ cell tumours: i(12p) and related chromosomal anomalies. *Eur Urol* 1993;23:23–29.
261. Pienkowska-Grela B, Grygalewicz B, Bregula U. Overrepresentation of the short arm of chromosome 12 in seminoma and nonseminoma groups of testicular germ cell tumors. *Cancer Genet Cytogenet* 2002;134:102–108.
262. Smolarek TA, Blough RI, Foster RS, et al. Identification of multiple chromosome 12 abnormalities in human testicular germ cell tumors by two-color fluorescence in situ hybridization (FISH). *Genes Chromosomes Cancer* 1995;14:252–258.
263. Zafarana G, Grygalewicz B, Gillis AJ, et al. 12p-amplicon structure analysis in testicular germ cell tumors of adolescents and adults by array CGH. *Oncogene* 2003;22:7695–7701.
264. Rodriguez S, Jafer O, Goker H, et al. Expression profile of genes from 12p in testicular germ cell tumors of adolescents and adults associated with i(12p) and amplification at 12p11.2-p12.1. *Oncogene* 2003;22:1880–1891.
265. Kraggerud SM, Skotheim RI, Szymanska J, et al. Genome profiles of familial/bilateral and sporadic testicular germ cell tumors. *Genes Chromosomes Cancer* 2002;34:168–174.
266. Kernek KM, Brunelli M, Ulbright TM, et al. Fluorescence in situ hybridization analysis of chromosome 12p in paraffin-embedded tissue is useful for establishing germ cell origin of metastatic tumors. *Mod Pathol* 2004;17:1309–1313.
267. Lyons J, Landis CA, Harsh G, et al. Two G protein oncogenes in human endocrine tumors. *Science* 1990;249:655–659.
268. Shen Y, Mamers P, Jobling T, et al. Absence of the previously reported G protein oncogene (*gip2*) in ovarian granulosa cell tumors. *J Clin Endocrinol Metab* 1996;81:4159–4161.
269. Fragoso MC, Latronico AC, Carvalho FM, et al. Activating mutation of the stimulatory G protein (gsp) as a putative cause of ovarian and testicular human stromal Leydig cell tumors. *J Clin Endocrinol Metab* 1998;83:2074–2078.

270. Hannon TS, King DW, Brinkman AD, et al. Premature thelarche and granulosa cell tumors: a search for FSH receptor and Gs-alpha activating mutations. *J Pediatr Endocrinol Metab* 2002;15:891–895.

271. Vieira TC, Cerutti JM, Dias da Silva MR, et al. Absence of activating mutations in the hot spots of the LH receptor and Gs-alpha genes in Leydig cell tumors. *J Endocrinol Invest* 2002;25:598–602.

272. Teixeira MR, Kristensen GB, Abeler VM, et al. Karyotypic findings in tumors of the vulva and vagina. *Cancer Genet Cytogenet* 1999;111:87–91.

273. Carlson JA, Ambros R, Malfetano J, et al. Vulvar lichen sclerosus and squamous cell carcinoma: a cohort, case control, and investigational study with historical perspective; implications for chronic inflammation and sclerosis in the development of neoplasia. *Hum Pathol* 1998;29:932–948.

274. Sengupta BS. Vulval cancer following or co-existing with chronic granulomatous diseases of vulva: An analysis of its natural history, clinical manifestation and treatment. *Trop Doct* 1981;11:110–114.

275. Lerma E, Matias-Guiu X, Lee SJ, et al. Squamous cell carcinoma of the vulva: study of ploidy, HPV, *p53*, and pRb. *Int J Gynecol Pathol* 1999;18:191–197.

276. Junge J, Poulsen H, Horn T, et al. Prognosis of vulvar dysplasia and carcinoma in situ with special reference to histology and types of human papillomavirus (HPV). *APMIS* 1997;105:963–971.

277. Iwasawa A, Nieminen P, Lehtinen M, et al. Human papillomavirus in squamous cell carcinoma of the vulva by polymerase chain reaction. *Obstet Gynecol* 1997;89:81–84.

278. Kondi-Paphitis A, Deligeorgi-Politi H, Liapis A, et al. Human papilloma virus in verrucus carcinoma of the vulva: an immunopathological study of three cases. *Eur J Gynaecol Oncol* 1998;19:319–320.

279. Worsham MJ, Van Dyke DL, Grenman SE, et al. Consistent chromosome abnormalities in squamous cell carcinoma of the vulva. *Genes Chromosomes Cancer* 1991;3:420–432.

280. Milde-Langosch K, Albrecht K, Joram S, et al. Presence and persistence of HPV infection and *p53* mutation in cancer of the cervix uteri and the vulva. *Int J Cancer* 1995;63:639–645.

281. Holway AH, Rieger-Christ KM, Miner WR, et al. Somatic mutation of *PTEN* in vulvar cancer. *Clin Cancer Res* 2000;6:3228–3235.

282. Brooks LA, Tidy JA, Gusterson B, et al. Preferential retention of codon 72 arginine *p53* in squamous cell carcinomas of the vulva occurs in cancers positive and negative for human papillomavirus. *Cancer Res* 2000;60:6875–6877.

283. Gokden N, Dehner LP, Zhu X, et al. Dermatofibrosarcoma protuberans of the vulva and groin: detection of COL1A1-PDGFB fusion transcripts by RT-PCR. *J Cutan Pathol* 2003;30:190–195.

284. Vang R, Taubenberger JK, Mannion CM, et al. Primary vulvar and vaginal extraosseous Ewing's sarcoma/peripheral neuroectodermal tumor: diagnostic confirmation with CD99 immunostaining and reverse transcriptase-polymerase chain reaction. *Int J Gynecol Pathol* 2000;19:103–109.

285. Rubin MA, De Marzo AM. Molecular genetics of human prostate cancer. *Mod Pathol* 2004;17:380–388.

286. Edwards SM, Eeles RA. Unravelling the genetics of prostate cancer. *Am J Med Genet C Semin Med Genet* 2004;129:65–73.

287. Porkka KP, Visakorpi T. Molecular mechanisms of prostate cancer. *Eur Urol* 2004;45:683–691.

288. Eble JN, Sauter G, Epstein J, et al. Tumours of the prostate. In: Eble JN, ed. *Pathology and Genetics of the Urinary System and Male Genital Organs.* Lyon: IARC Press; 2004:159–215.

289. Bostwick DG, Grignon DJ, Hammond ME, et al. Prognostic factors in prostate cancer. College of American Pathologists Consensus Statement 1999. *Arch Pathol Lab Med* 2000;124:995–1000.

290. Dhanasekaran SM, Barrette TR, Ghosh D, et al. Delineation of prognostic biomarkers in prostate cancer. *Nature* 2001;412:822–826.

291. Singh D, Febbo PG, Ross K, et al. Gene expression correlates of clinical prostate cancer behavior. *Cancer Cell* 2002;1:203–209.

292. Welsh JB, Sapinoso LM, Su AI, et al. Analysis of gene expression identifies candidate markers and pharmacological targets in prostate cancer. *Cancer Res* 2001;61:5974–5978.

293. Seligson DB, Horvath S, Shi T, et al. Global histone modification patterns predict risk of prostate cancer recurrence. *Nature* 2005;435:1262–1266.

294. Chu DC, Chuang CK, Liou YF, et al. The use of real-time quantitative PCR to detect circulating prostate-specific membrane antigen mRNA in patients with prostate carcinoma. *Ann N Y Acad Sci* 2004;1022:157–162.

295. Gao CL, Rawal SK, Sun L, et al. Diagnostic potential of prostate-specific antigen expressing epithelial cells in blood of prostate cancer patients. *Clin Cancer Res* 2003;9:2545–2550.

296. Schmidt B, Anastasiadis AG, Seifert HH, et al. Detection of circulating prostate cells during radical prostatectomy by standardized PSMA RT-PCR: association with positive lymph nodes and high malignant grade. *Anticancer Res* 2003;23:3991–3999.

297. Kurek R, Ylikoski A, Renneberg H, et al. Quantitative PSA RT-PCR for preoperative staging of prostate cancer. *Prostate* 2003;56:263–269.

298. Martinez-Pineiro L, Rios E, Martinez-Gomariz M, et al. Molecular staging of prostatic cancer with RT-PCR assay for prostate-specific antigen in peripheral blood and lymph nodes: comparison with standard histological staging and immunohistochemical assessment of occult regional lymph node metastases. *Eur Urol* 2003;43:342–350.

299. Straub B, Muller M, Krause H, et al. Quantitative real-time RT-PCR for detection of circulating prostate-specific antigen mRNA using sequence-specific oligonucleotide hybridization probes in prostate cancer patients. *Oncology* 2003;65:12–17.

300. Varkarakis J, Deliveliotis C, Sideris D, et al. Preoperative nested reverse transcription-polymerase chain reaction for prostate specific membrane antigen predicts non-organ confined disease in radical prostatectomy specimens. *Urol Res* 2003;31:183–187.

301. Kurek R, Nunez G, Tselis N, et al. Prognostic value of combined "triple"-reverse transcription-PCR analysis for prostate-specific antigen, human kallikrein 2, and prostate-specific membrane antigen mRNA in peripheral blood and lymph nodes of prostate cancer patients. *Clin Cancer Res* 2004;10:5808–5814.

302. Ellis WJ, Pfitzenmaier J, Colli J, et al. Detection and isolation of prostate cancer cells from peripheral blood and bone marrow. *Urology* 2003;61:277–281.

303. Cairns P, Esetller M, Herman JG, et al. Molecular detection of prostate cancer in urine by GSTP1 hypermethylation. *Clin Cancer Res* 2001;7:2727–2730.

304. Cao D, Hafez M, Berg K, et al. Little or no residual prostate cancer at radical prostatectomy: vanishing cancer or switched specimen? A microsatellite analysis of specimen identity. *Am J Surg Pathol* 2005;29:467–473.

305. Goldstein NS, Begin LR, Grody WW, et al. Minimal or no cancer in radical prostatectomy specimens: report of 13 cases of the "vanishing cancer phenomenon". *J Surg Pathol* 1995;19:1002–1009.

Urinary Tract

KIDNEY NEOPLASMS

Renal Cell Carcinoma

Renal cell carcinoma (RCC) affects about 150,000 people worldwide each year, and accounts for about 85% of all renal neoplasms and 2% of all human malignancies. Although RCC occurs in people of all ages, its overall incidence is significantly increased in those between the ages of 50 and 70 years. Most RCC are sporadic, but epidemiologic associations with environmental carcinogens and lifestyle factors (e.g., smoking and obesity) have been demonstrated (1). Although RCCs have traditionally been classified based on morphology, a tumor's underlying pattern of genetic aberrations has recently become an important criterion for diagnosis because it has become clear that recurring genetic aberrations separate tumors with similar microscopic appearance into groups with different clinicopathologic features.

About 1% to 4% of cases of RCC occur as a component of an inherited predisposition syndrome (Table 17.1). A familial predisposition should be suspected whenever an individual patient has multifocal renal tumors, a history of a previous renal tumor, or close relatives who have also been diagnosed with RCC. Even though there are no widely accepted screening guidelines for familial RCC syndromes, it is important to follow up on any suspicion of a hereditary predisposition because the presence of an RCC syndrome has significant implications for both the patient (individuals with hereditary RCC are candidates for nephron-sparing procedures and require close clinical follow-up because they are at risk for recurrent renal tumors throughout their lifetime) and the patient's family. A formal medical genetics consultation is usually used to identify those patients who should undergo mutational analysis (2). However, mutational analysis is performed in only a small number of specialty laboratories (3) because the prevalence of hereditary cases is so low and mutational

analysis is cumbersome, as discussed in more detail later. In any event, genetic analysis of tumor tissue cannot be used to identify syndromic cases because the genes that are responsible for hereditary RCC are also mutated in many sporadic RCC.

Clear Cell Renal Cell Carcinoma

Clear cell RCC accounts for approximately 70% of renal cell carcinomas in adults. A multicentric or bilateral pattern of presentation occurs in less than 5% of tumors overall, but is common in hereditary cancer syndromes.

Genetics

VHL Mutations. Inactivating mutations of the von Hippel-Lindau (*VHL*) tumor suppressor gene at 3p25 are the hallmark of clear cell RCC (4,5). The *VHL* alterations include missense mutations resulting from single base pair (bp) substitutions, in-frame deletions, frame shift mutations (usually caused by the insertion or deletion of a single bp, although insertions or deletions up to 16 bp long have been described), and intronic mutations (which cause the loss of splice acceptor or donor sequences) (5–8), and the mutations are scattered throughout most of the length of all three exons of the gene (Fig. 17.1) without clearly defined mutational hot spots. Loss of heterozygosity (LOH) is also present in up to 98% to 100% of sporadic clear cell RCC with *VHL* mutations (7,8) which supports the hypothesis that biallelic inactivation of the *VHL* gene plays a critical role in the development of the tumor (9) consistent with the markedly increased frequency of clear cell RCC in patients with von Hippel-Lindau syndrome. Similarly, biallelic somatic inactivation of *VHL* is present in sporadic hemangioblastomas, consistent with the fact that the tumor also has a markedly increased frequency in von Hippel-Lindau syndrome (10). About 20% of clear cell RCC do not harbor mutations in the *VHL* gene, but

TABLE 17.1

WELL-CHARACTERIZED HEREDITARY RENAL CELL CARCINOMA PREDISPOSITION SYNDROMES

Syndrome	Frequency of Renal Cell Carcinoma (%)	Gene	Chromosomal Location	Renal Manifestations	Common Associated Manifestations
von Hippel-Lindau	28–45	VHL	3p25	Multiple, bilateral clear cell RCC	Retinal and CNS hemangioblastomas; pheochromocytoma
Hereditary papillary renal carcinoma	20	MET	7q31	Multiple, bilateral type1 papillary RCC	None
Tuberous sclerosis	1–2	TSCI (hamartin) TSC2 (tuberin)	9q34 16p13	Clear cell RCC; multiple, bilateral angiomyolipomas	CNS tubers; cutaneous angiofibromas; lymphangioleiomyomatosis
Hereditary leiomyomatosis and renal carcinoma	Unknown	FH (fumarate hydratase)	1q42–43	Solitary, aggressive collecting duct carcinoma; type 2 papillary RCC	Uterine and cutaneous leiomyomas; leiomyosarcomas
Birt-Hogg-Dubé syndrome	10–15	BHD (folliculin)	17p11.2	Multiple, bilateral oncocytic RCC; clear cell RCC; oncocytoma	Cutaneous fibrofolliculomas; pulmonary cysts; spontaneous pneumothorax
Hyperparathyroidism—jaw tumor	Rare	HRPT2 (parafibromin)	1q25–32	Papillary RCC; mixed epithelioid and stromal neoplasms	Parathyroid carcinoma; ossifying fibromas of the mandible and maxilla
Lynch type 2	2–9	MSH2 MLH1	2p16 3p31	Transitional cell carcinoma of renal pelvis	Carcinoma of the colon, endometrium, ovaries, stomach
Constitutional chromosome 3 translocations	Rare	Various[a]	Various[a]	Multiple, bilateral clear cell RCC	Unknown

[a]See Table 17.2.

nonetheless show decreased VHL protein expression, which suggests that aberrant methylation of a CpG island in the 5′ region of the *VHL* gene may also participate in gene inactivation (11).

The VHL protein has a number of functions, one of which is the regulation of genes controlled by cellular oxygen tension (12–14). Under normoxic conditions, VHL mediates the attachment of a polyubiquitin chain to hypoxia-inducible factor (HIF), which marks HIF for destruction and abolishes HIF-induced expression of a number of proteins, including platelet-derived growth factor (which is angiogenic), transforming growth factor α (which is mitogenic), erythropoietin, and vascular endothelial growth factor (VEGF) (2,10,15,16). A nonfunctional VHL protein therefore results in an altered pattern of gene expression, including increased production of VEGF, which provides an explanation for the therapeutic effect of a neutralizing anti-VEGF antibody in patients with metastatic clear cell RCC (17).

Constitutional Chromosome 3 Translocations. While von Hippel-Lindau disease is the familial syndrome in which the genetic abnormality responsible for clear cell RCC is most well characterized, individuals from families with constitutional chromosome 3 rearrangements also have an increased risk for developing multiple bilateral clear cell RCC (4). The identity of the disrupted genes (Table 17.2) suggests that a number of different pathways are involved in oncogenesis in these families. For example, the t(3;8)(p14;q24) translocation generates a *FHIT-TRC8* fusion gene (18) which may promote tumorigenesis via altered interactions with wild-type VHL protein (25), whereas the t(2;3)(q35;q21) translocation and associated small interstitial deletion appear to result in structural alterations of three separate genes (20,21). In addition, in some families, the constitutional translocation is associated with 3p loss and mutations in *VHL* itself (26).

Nonetheless, the genetic characterization of these syndromes is incomplete. For example, it is unknown whether

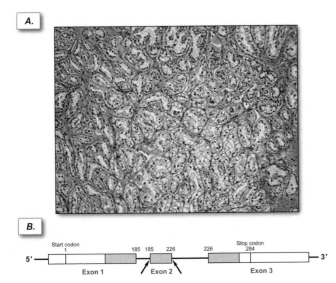

Figure 17.1 Mutations of *VHL* are characteristic of clear cell RCC that occur sporadically or in association with the von Hippel-Lindau syndrome. **A,** A low-grade clear cell RCC that has the typical nested to alveolar pattern and thin-walled vascular septa. **B,** Schematic diagram of the *VHL* gene showing the regions of the gene that harbor mutations (*shaded areas*) in sporadic RCC; over 35 unique mutations have been described in exon 1, over 35 in exon 2, and over 25 in exon 3 (references 6–8). In addition, several unique splice acceptor and splice donor mutations have been described, for example, in introns 1 and 2 (*arrows*).

the precise location of the chromosomal break point in different families with the same rearrangement has any prognostic implications and whether the rearrangements characteristic of the familial chromosome 3 syndromes are responsible for cases of sporadic clear cell RCC that lack mutations in *VHL*. Molecular analysis for constitutional chromosome 3 rearrangements is therefore not yet a part of the routine analysis of RCC.

Tuberous Sclerosis. The incidence of clear cell RCC is also increased in patients with tuberous sclerosis (27). However, biallelic inactivation of either the *TSC1* or *TSC2* locus is not a frequent event in sporadic clear cell RCC (28).

Birt-Hogg-Dubé Syndrome. Individuals with Birt-Hogg-Dubé (BHD) syndrome have an increased risk of RCC (29). The syndrome is due to germline mutations in the *BHD* gene at 17p11.2, which encodes folliculin, a protein of unknown function (30). Somatic mutations in *BHD* are present in 3% to 5% of cases of sporadic RCC, including both clear cell and papillary types (31,32), an observation that is consistent with the fact that renal neoplasms of several different histologic types are a characteristic feature of the BHD syndrome (29).

Other Mutations. Allelotype and deletion mapping studies suggest that still other loci may also be involved in the development of clear cell RCC. Approximately 15% to 30% of sporadic clear cell RCC have losses of chromosomes 5q, 6q, 9q, 10q, 13q, and 17p (33–36), but a direct role for tumor-suppressor genes located at these chromosomal regions in the development of clear cell RCC remains to be demonstrated.

Technical Issues in Molecular Genetic Analysis of Clear Cell RCC

Mutations of *VHL* in clear cell RCC occur in both intronic and exonic sequences; thus, mutational analysis of the gene is not a trivial undertaking. To simplify testing, the various regions of the *VHL* gene are usually first screened for mutations by indirect DNA sequencing methods such as single-strand conformational polymorphism (SSCP) analysis or heteroduplex analysis, with follow-up direct DNA sequence analysis of only the positive regions. When fresh tissue or cell lines are evaluated, comprehensive analysis demonstrates *VHL* mutations in 36% to 57% of sporadic clear cell RCC (6–8). In one study that used formalin-fixed, paraffin-embedded (FFPE) tissue from sporadic clear cell RCC as the substrate for testing, mutations were detected in virtually 100% of cases, but this is probably not a reliable estimate of sensitivity of analysis of FFPE tissue because the study involved only three cases (37).

Because sequence analysis is so cumbersome and LOH at 3p25 is present in such a high percentage of clear cell RCC that harbor biallelic inactivation of *VHL*, demonstration of LOH at 3p25 is often used as an alternative approach to detect aberrations of *VHL*. However, conven-

TABLE 17.2

CONSTITUTIONAL CHROMOSOME 3 REARRANGEMENTS ASSOCIATED WITH HEREDITARY RENAL CLEAR CELL CARCINOMA

Rearrangement	Involved Genes	References
t(3;8)(p14;q24)	*FHIT-TRC8* fusion	18
t(3;6)(p13;q25.1)	Unknown	19
t(2;3)(q35;q21)	*DIRC2* disruption	20
	DIRC3-HSPBA1 fusion	21
t(3;6)(q12;q15)	Unknown	22
t(3;4)(p13;p16)	Unknown	22
t(2;3)(q33;q21)	*DIRC1* disruption	23
t(1;3)(q32;q13.3)	*LSAMP* and *NORE1* disruption	24

tional cytogenetic analysis is an insensitive way to detect 3p LOH, because the method identifies alterations of chromosome 3p in less than 15% of cases (38). Interphase dual-color fluorescence in situ hybridization (FISH) has a greater sensitivity and identifies LOH at the *VHL* locus in greater than 95% of clear cell RCC in patients with von Hippel-Lindau disease (39) and in 36% to 69% of sporadic clear cell RCC (38,40,41), including a significant percentage of cases that show no abnormalities by routine cytogenetic analysis (38). Southern blot analysis of genomic DNA has also been used to detect LOH and when optimized can detect 3p LOH in up to 90% of cases (6–8,42–44). LOH can be demonstrated in up to 80% of informative cases by SSCP (8) and in up to 91% of cases by microsatellite analysis (36,41,45). A combination of FISH and PCR-based microsatellite analysis seems to achieve the greatest sensitivity for detecting LOH (6,41,44).

Recently, rapid detection of *VHL* exon deletions by quantitative PCR has been described as a highly sensitive method for identification of patients with von Hippel-Lindau syndrome (46). However, the utility of this approach for analysis of sporadic cases of clear cell RCC has not yet been evaluated.

Diagnostic Issues in Molecular Genetic Analysis of Clear Cell RCC

Biallelic inactivation of the *VHL* gene is specific for clear cell RCC, whether occurring in the context of von Hippel-Lindau syndrome or in sporadic tumors. Conventional cytogenetics, Southern blot, and direct DNA sequence analysis have all shown that *VHL* mutations are not a feature of other renal neoplasms, including papillary RCC, oncocytoma, or tumors classified as chromophilic or chromophobic RCC (1,6–8,37,40,47). However, 3p LOH has been detected in a number of other tumor types, including a subset of renal oncocytomas, mesotheliomas, follicular thyroid carcinomas, and bladder malignancies (6,36,37,48,49).

Admittedly, from a diagnostic perspective, for most cases of conventional clear cell RCC there is little need to perform molecular analysis of the *VHL* gene. However, the specificity of *VHL* mutations for clear cell RCC can be used to confirm that a tumor with an ambiguous morphologic appearance is actually a phenotypic variant of clear cell RCC. For example, conventional cytogenetics, FISH, and microsatellite analysis can be used to show that some epithelial neoplasms with cytologic features of clear cell RCC but a papillary architecture do, in fact, harbor a pattern of genetic abnormalities indicative of clear cell RCC (45,50), an important distinction given the prognostic differences between clear cell RCC and papillary RCC. LOH analysis of polymorphic microsatellite markers coupled with SSCP mutational analysis of the *VHL* gene has been used to distinguish poorly differentiated clear cell RCC with a rhabdoid phenotype from rhabdoid tumor of the kidney and other poorly differentiated malignancies (51). Molecular analysis of the *VHL* locus can be used to distinguish cystic clear cell RCC from other types of cystic renal tumors (52), to differentiate clear cell RCC from renal neoplasms with a clear cell morphology that are associated with *TFE3* gene rearrangements (see later discussion), and to discriminate metastatic clear cell RCC from independent synchronous or metachronous tumors that may also have

a clear cell morphology (53,54). In these settings, molecular analysis can successfully be performed on both FFPE and fresh tissue (45,51), underscoring the utility of genetic testing in routine clinical practice.

Prognostic Issues in Molecular Genetic Analysis of Clear Cell RCC

Even if molecular analysis does not have a role in the diagnosis of most clear cell RCC encountered in routine surgical pathology, genotype-phenotype correlations in patients with von Hippel-Lindau syndrome suggest that mutational analysis of the *VHL* gene in patients with sporadic clear cell RCC can potentially be used to provide prognostic information. For example, different *VHL* mutations are associated with a different spectrum of clinical disease and different defects in HIF regulation (55–57) that may correlate with the response to treatment directed against specific proteins whose expression is regulated by HIF, such as the anti-VEGF therapy discussed previously.

In addition to analysis of the *VHL* locus itself, global gene expression profiling has been shown to provide prognostic information in clear cell RCC. Microarray analysis has shown that the gene expression profile of nonaggressive clear cell RCC (those tumors associated with 100% patient survival after 5 years) is significantly distinct from the profile of aggressive clear cell RCC (tumors associated with 0% patient survival after 5 years) and that the expression pattern of a set of approximately 40 genes more accurately predicts patient survival than traditional TNM staging (58). Gene expression analysis has also been used to define groups of genes associated with significant differences in overall survival, even among patients with metastatic RCC (59). Although gene expression analysis is, at present, not part of the routine pathologic evaluation of clear cell RCC, these results indicate the potential that the methodology has for stratifying patients into clinically meaningful prognostic and therapeutic groups.

Papillary Renal Cell Carcinoma

Papillary RCC accounts for approximately 10% of renal cell carcinomas and can occur sporadically or as a hereditary syndrome (Table 17.1). Morphologically, two types of papillary RCC have been described. In type 1 tumors, small epithelial cells with scant cytoplasm are arranged in a single layer on the tumor papillae. In type 2 tumors, the epithelial cells have a higher cytologic grade and abundant eosinophilic cytoplasm and form a pseudo-stratified layer on the papillary cores (1).

Genetics

Hereditary Papillary RCC. Hereditary papillary renal carcinoma is an autosomal dominant syndrome for which the sole manifestation is multiple bilateral type 1 papillary RCC (2,47). The syndrome is due to missense mutations of the *MET* proto-oncogene at chromosomal region 7q31 (60), which encodes the receptor tyrosine kinase that binds hepatocyte growth factor (61). Missense mutations result in amino acid substitutions in the activation loop or adenosine triphosphate (ATP)-binding pocket of the tyrosine kinase domain of MET (11,60,62,63) (Fig. 17.2) that cause

A.

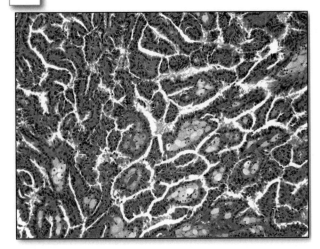

B.

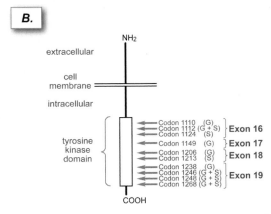

Figure 17.2 Mutations of *MET* are characteristic of papillary RCC. **A,** A typical low-grade papillary RCC showing a single layer of cuboidal cells that covers fibrovascular stalks, with prominent stromal xanthoma cells. **B,** Schematic diagram of the missense mutations of the *MET* proto-oncogene found in papillary RCC. The mutations cluster in the exons encoding the intracellular kinase domain, and there is overlap between the germline (*G*) mutations in hereditary cases and the mutations in sporadic (*S*) cases.

ligand-independent receptor activation (64), although ligand binding is still required for full activation of the mutant receptor proteins (2). Mutations in *MET* can be detected in about 86% of kindreds with hereditary papillary RCC (60,65), but the tumors that develop in this background typically also show trisomy 7 resulting from nonrandom duplication of the chromosome harboring the mutant *MET* gene (66,67).

Sporadic Papillary RCC. Activating missense mutations in *MET* also occur in about 13% of patients with papillary RCC that do not have a family history of renal tumors (62,63,68). However, surprisingly, approximately half of patients with presumed sporadic papillary RCC turn out to harbor germline *MET* mutations, and consequently the prevalence of *MET* mutations in true sporadic papillary RCC is even lower (62,63). Sporadic papillary RCCs that harbor *MET* mutations have a type 1 morphology,

although not all type 1 sporadic papillary RCC harbor *MET* mutations (62,63).

The most common cytogenetic aberrations in sporadic papillary RCC are trisomy or tetrasomy 7, trisomy 17, and (in male patients) loss of chromosome Y (69). In addition, a small subset of cases show trisomy 12, 16, or 20, interstitial LOH at 3p, or allelic loss at 9p13 (which is associated with a worse clinical outcome) (69–72).

Hereditary Leiomyomatosis and Renal Cell Cancer. Hereditary leiomyomatosis and renal cell cancer (HLRCC) is caused by a germline mutation in the *FH* gene encoding the enzyme fumarate hydratase (73) (Table 17.1). The RCCs that are associated with this rare autosomal dominant tumor syndrome have primarily a papillary type 2 histology. However, DNA sequence analysis has demonstrated that mutations of the *FH* gene are not a feature of sporadic papillary RCC of either type 1 or type 2 (74).

Other Mutations. One study reported that 94% of papillary RCC, of both type 1 and type 2 subgroups, harbor the same single bp substitution in intron 17 (IVS17 + 43T > A) of the *c-kit* gene (75). The mutation is apparently not characteristic of either conventional clear cell RCC or chromophobe RCC, is not present in adjacent non-neoplastic renal tissue, and is not associated with any known single-nucleotide polymorphism. Because the point mutation is not near a splice site, its role in the pathogenesis of papillary RCC is uncertain, and it is unknown whether or not the mutation correlates with any other clinicopathologic features of papillary RCC.

Technical Issues in Molecular Genetic Analysis of Papillary RCC

Although all of the mutations in *MET* occur in the tyrosine kinase domain (Fig. 17.2), this functional domain is encoded by four different exons (76). For the sake of efficiency, these four exons are often screened for mutations by indirect methods such as SSCP before direct DNA sequence analysis (60,62,63,77).

The trisomy 7, trisomy 17, and loss of chromosome Y that are characteristic of sporadic papillary RCC can be detected by routine cytogenetic analysis in over 69% of cases (69), although this level of sensitivity is derived from a series of preselected cases and so is likely not a reliable estimate of the sensitivity of cytogenetic analysis in routine clinical practice. When interphase FISH is used to evaluate chromosomal aneuploidy in papillary RCC, trisomy 7 can be detected in 88% to 100% of cases, trisomy 17 in about 70% of cases, loss of Y in about 85% of cases in males, and combined +7, +17, −Y in 56% to 71% of cases (78,79).

Diagnostic Issues in Molecular Analysis of Papillary RCC

A number of primary renal tumors can enter into the differential diagnosis of type 1 papillary RCC, including clear cell RCC, collecting duct carcinoma, carcinomas associated with *TFE3* fusion genes (discussed below), and even mesonephric adenoma. Molecular genetic analysis for +7, +17, −Y (characteristic of type 1 papillary RCC) by either conventional cytogenetics or FISH, combined with demonstration of LOH at 3p (characteristic of clear cell RCC), can be used to distinguish sporadic type 1 papillary RCC with a prominent clear cell morphology from clear cell RCC (45,50). Similarly, analysis for +7, +17, −Y combined with testing for *TFE3* fusion transcripts can be used to distinguish papillary RCC from tumors with rearrangements of *TFE3* (the difficulty of this differential diagnosis based on morphologic features alone is demonstrated by the fact that many carcinomas now known to harbor *TFE3* rearrangements were classified as papillary RCC before the recognition that, based on their genetic features, they comprise a separate group). Whether analysis for +7, +17, −Y can be used to distinguish papillary RCC from mesonephric adenoma is unsettled; in one study, almost 75% of mesonephric adenomas harbored the same pattern of aneuploidy as papillary RCC (80), but more recent reports have not detected changes in chromosome number in mesonephric adenoma that are characteristic of papillary RCC (reviewed in 81).

The prevalence of *MET* mutations in sporadic papillary RCC is so low that mutation analysis has little clinical utility for diagnosis in routine clinical practice. On the other hand, because some studies have suggested that up to half of patients whose tumor harbors *MET* mutations also harbor germline *MET* mutations, as noted previously, it could be argued that there is a role for *MET* mutational analysis in cases of presumed sporadic papillary RCC to detect occult hereditary papillary RCC. However, retrospective analysis of an unselected series of patients performed to specifically address this question showed that the prevalence of germline *MET* mutations in individuals with papillary RCC but without additional evidence for a genetic disposition (such as a positive family history, young age, or bilateral disease) approaches 0% (77).

As noted previously, the clinicopathologic significance of the IVS17 + 43T > A of *c-kit* is uncertain; therefore DNA sequence analysis for the mutation is not routinely performed.

Renal Cell Carcinoma Associated with Xp11.2 Rearrangements

This category of RCC is defined by a group of rearrangements involving the *TFE3* gene at Xp11.2 (Table 17.3). The tumors primarily affect children and young adults (97,101), although they also occasionally occur in older adults (102,106). In general, the carcinomas are composed of clear cells with a papillary growth pattern, although there are some morphologic differences between tumors with different *TFE3* fusion partners (1,85,97,107). Even though Xp11.2-associated carcinomas apparently account for 24% to 41% of renal cell carcinomas in children and young adults (108,109), they are nonetheless rare tumors, and their clinical behavior has yet to be well characterized.

Genetics

As shown in Table 17.3, five different fusion genes have been described in the Xp11.2-associated carcinomas. Most of the rearrangements are balanced translocations, although one of the fusion genes is produced by an inversion. Heterogeneity in the site of the translocation break point in *PRCC-TFE3* fusions (84,85) produces a set of chimeric proteins with slightly different structure (Fig. 17.3). There is similar heterogeneity (82,83,110) in the site of the translocation break points in *ASPL-TFE3* fusions (Fig. 11.12). The significance of the resulting variation in structure of the encoded chimeric proteins remains unknown, but thus far structural differences in *PRCC-TFE3* fusions and *ASPL-TFE3* fusions have not been correlated with any clinical or pathologic features in the resulting tumors (82,85,97). Because only single cases

---

TABLE 17.3

TRANSLOCATION-ASSOCIATED PRIMARY RENAL NEOPLASMS

Neoplasm	Translocation	References
Xp11.1-associated carcinomas		
ASPL-TFE3 carcinoma	t(X;17)(p11.2;q25)	82, 83
PRCC-TFE3 carcinoma	t(X;1)(p11.2;q21)	84, 85
PSF-TFE3 carcinoma	t(X;1)(p11.2;p34)	86
NonO-TFE3 carcinoma	inv(X)(p11.2;q12)	86
CLTC-TFE3 carcionma	t(X;17)(p11.2;q23)	87
Neoplasms with TFEB fusions		
Alpha-TFEB tumors	t(6;11)(p21;q13)	88, 89
Sarcomas		
EWS/PNET	t(11;22)(q24;q12)[a]	90–92
Synovial sarcoma	t(X;18)(p11;q11)[b]	93–95
Clear cell sarcoma	t(12;22)(q13;q12)	96
Alveolar rhabdomyosarcoma	t(1;13)(p36;q14)	97
	t(2;13)(q35;q14)	
Congenital mesoblastic nephroma (cellular and mixed types)	t(2;15)(p13;q25)	98, 99
Desmoplastic small round cell tumor	t(11;22)(p13;q12)[a]	100

[a]See Table 11.1 for more details
[b]See Table 11.2 for more details

Given that all of the chimeric proteins are overexpressed (as discussed later), they are thought to exert their oncogenic effect as constitutively produced transcriptional activators (112,113). However, TFE3 chimeric proteins may cause transcriptional deregulation through other mechanisms. Because PRCC, NonO, and PSF are RNA splicing factors (86,112), it has been suggested that *TFE3* fusions with one of these three partners also contribute to tumorigenesis through disruption of RNA processing (86). The recent demonstration that *PRCC-TFE3* disrupts mitotic checkpoint control (114) suggests yet another mechanism by which *TFE3* fusions are oncogenic.

Finally, it should be noted that the *ASPL-TFE3* fusion characteristic of Xp11.2-associated RCC is also a hallmark of alveolar soft part sarcoma (110,115). However, as discussed in more detail in Chapter 11, the rearrangement that produces the fusion in alveolar soft part sarcoma is nonreciprocal. Thus, the *ASPL-TFE3* fusion gene provides the first example of an oncogenic chimeric gene that can arise from either a balanced or unbalanced translocation.

Technical Issues in Molecular Genetic Analysis of Xp11.2-associated RCC

Even though conventional cytogenetic analysis was used to characterize the various translocations that are the hallmark of RCC with *TFE3* fusion genes, these studies cannot be used to estimate the sensitivity of cytogenetic analysis because they selectively reported positive cases. The sensitivity of cytogenetics in routine evaluation of RCCs is therefore unknown, even for patient populations that consist of children and young adults, although some of the method's limitations are suggested by the fact that the inv(X)(p11.2;q12) responsible for the *NonO-TFE3* fusion is not evident in standard karyotypes (86) and by the fact that the t(X;17)(p11.2;q23) is often correctly identified only after the presence of the *CLTC-TFE3* fusion is first identified by RT-PCR (87).

Northern and Southern blot analysis have been used to demonstrate the rearrangements characteristic of the Xp11.2-associated carcinomas (82–84,86). However, because both methods are cumbersome and can be performed only when frozen tissue is available for analysis, their usefulness is restricted. The negative impact of the requirement for frozen tissue on the utility of the techniques in routine practice is emphasized by the fact that frozen tissue was available in only 0 to 18% of Xp11.2-associated carcinomas in two recent series (85,102).

For Xp11.2-associated RCC in which the underlying karyotypic abnormality is known, RT-PCR can be used to demonstrate the associated *TFE3* fusion transcript in virtually 100% of cases (82–87). However, because of the number of *TFE3* fusion partners and the structural heterogeneity of the resulting chimeric genes, RT-PCR evaluation of cases in which the underlying translocation is unknown requires comprehensive analysis by a panel of primers specific for all the known fusion transcript types. RT-PCR testing has thus far been limited to fresh tissue, but because fresh tissue is available in only a small minority of tumors, as noted previously, the method must be adapted for use with FFPE tissue if RT-PCR testing is to have a meaningful role in routine clinical practice.

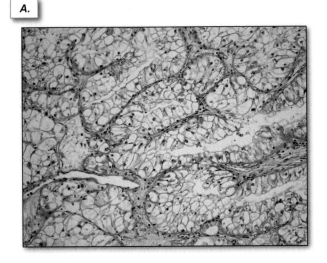

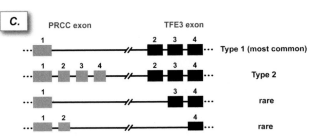

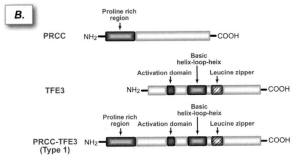

Figure 17.3 Xp11.2-associated renal carcinomas harbor rearrangements of the *TFE3* gene. **A,** A renal carcinoma from a 6-year-old girl that shows several of the features that are characteristic of Xp11.2-associated carcinomas; the tumor is composed of cells with voluminous clear cytoplasm and well-defined cell borders, arranged in a nested growth pattern. **B,** Schematic diagram of PRCC-TFE3 chimeric proteins formed by the t(X;17)(p11.2;q25) translocation that is one of the rearrangements characteristic of Xp11.2-associated renal carcinomas. In the most common chimeric protein, the N-terminal proline rich region of PRCC is linked to the full-length TFE3 protein. **C,** Because the translocation break point can be located within different introns of *PRCC* and *TFE3*, the fusion gene and resulting transcripts (and chimeric proteins) show structural heterogeneity (exons are numbered according to reference 85). (See Fig. 11.12 for a diagram of *ASPL-TPE3* fusions that are present in another subset of Xp11.2-associated renal carcinomas.)

with *PSF-TFE3*, *NonO-TFE3*, or *CLTC-TFE3* fusions have been described, it is unknown whether there is also variability in the precise site of the translocation break point in these fusion genes (86,87).

TFE3 is a member of the MiT subfamily of basic helix-loop-helix leucine-zipper transcription factors, and most *TFE3* fusions retain the full-length *TFE3* coding region (111).

FISH can be used to test for the genetic aberrations in Xp11.2-associated RCC. Using metaphase chromosomes, probe-splitting methodology has been used to demonstrate the t(X;17) translocation associated with the *AFPL-TFE3* fusion gene (82) and the inv(X) associated with the *NonO-TFE3* fusion gene (86). Probe-fusion methodology has been used with metaphase chromosomes to show the presence of the t(X;1) associated with *PSF-TFE3* fusion genes (86). However, given that *TFE3* can recombine with several different genes, the probe-split approach will likely be a more efficient way to identify rearrangements in cases of Xp.11.2-associated carcinomas.

Immunohistochemistry. A polyclonal antibody against the C-terminal region of TFE3 can be used for immuno-histochemical analysis of carcinomas with Xp11.2 rearrangements because this region of TFE3 is retained in all the chimeric proteins. Intense nuclear immunoreactivity is present in 95% of renal neoplasms known to harbor an Xp11.2 fusion gene (102) and in about 88% of renal neoplasms with suggestive morphology (102,107). Because native TFE3 is ubiquitously expressed, immunohistochemical assays must be optimized on known positive and negative cases to adjust the assay sensitivity to minimize false positive results (102).

Diagnostic Issues in Molecular Genetic Analysis of Xp11.2-associated RCC

As noted above, *ASPL-TFE3* fusion genes are also characteristic of alveolar soft part sarcoma. From a practical point of view, this fact usually creates no diagnostic uncertainty because Xp11.2-associated RCC and alveolar soft part sarcoma have different clinical presentations. Formally, even if faced with a case in which the diagnosis was in doubt, it would still be possible to definitively classify the tumor based on whether the Xp11.2 rearrangement was balanced or unbalanced (82,115).

Molecular techniques for detecting *TFE3* fusion transcripts and immunohistochemistry using antibodies against the C-terminal region of the TFE3 protein have both shown that Xp11.2 rearrangements are not a characteristic feature of any other primary renal neoplasm, including conventional clear cell RCC, conventional papillary RCC, chromophobe RCC, oncocytoma, Wilms' tumor, clear cell sarcoma of the kidney, angiomyolipoma, and collecting duct carcinoma (82,107). Testing for *TFE3* rearrangements can therefore be used to distinguish Xp11.2-associated RCC from clear cell or papillary RCC, which can be quite difficult based on morphologic features alone (as noted previously, carcinomas now known to harbor *TFE3* rearrangements were, in fact, usually classified as clear cell or papillary RCC before their recognition as a separate group [4]). The utility of molecular genetic or immunohistochemical analysis in the differential diagnosis of RCC in young patients, as well as adult conventional clear cell RCC and unclassified RCC, is emphasized by two recent clinical series (102,107).

Renal Neoplasms with *TFEB* Fusion Genes

This category of renal neoplasm most often occurs in children or young adults, although cases have also been described in older adults (116,117). Cytologically, the tumor is composed of cells with abundant clear to granular eosinophilic cytoplasm suggestive of clear cell RCC, but mitoses are rare and necrosis is absent. Architecturally, the tumor does not have a well-developed papillary morphology. The neoplasm shows strong immunoreactivity for HMB-45 and MelanA, but shows no expression of cytokeratin or epithelial membrane antigen.

Genetics

The translocation t(6;11)(p21;q13) is responsible for formation of the *alpha-TFEB* fusion gene that is characteristic of the tumor (88,89). *Alpha* is an intronless, nonprotein encoding gene with unknown function. *TFEB* is a member of the MiT subfamily of basic helix-loop-helix leucine-zipper transcription factors, which also includes *TFE3* as noted above. In all the cases thus far characterized, the translocation break point occurs in exon 1 of *TFEB*, upstream of the initiation codon (Fig. 17.4), and consequently the *alpha* promoter drives expression of the fusion gene. Because a stop codon in *alpha* is present 3′ of the translocation break point, the translated fusion protein consists only of native full-length TFEB (88,89). Tumorigenesis is therefore a consequence of disregulated *TFEB* expression rather than altered protein structure.

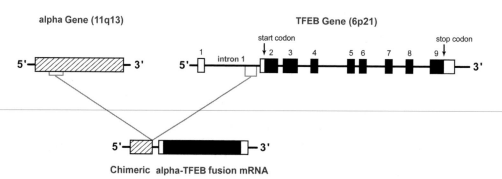

Figure 17.4 Schematic diagram of the t(6;11)(p21;q13) that gives rise to so-called *alpha-TFEB* renal neoplasms. The translocation break points in *alpha* and intron 1 of *TFEB* are clustered; all produce fusion genes that encode the native full-length TFEB protein.

Technical Issues in Molecular Genetic Analysis of Renal Neoplasms with *TFEB* Fusions

Conventional cytogenetic analysis was central to the recognition of this group of renal tumors because it demonstrated the presence of the characteristic t(6;11)(p21;q13) translocation (88,89). However, the sensitivity of cytogenetic analysis for evaluation of renal neoplasms thought to harbor *TFEB* fusions in routine practice, even in patients from the pediatric and young adult age-groups, has not been formally evaluated.

Even though the native *alpha* transcript is approximately 7.5 kb long and intron 1 of *TFEB* is over 43 kb long, the t(6;11) translocation can be detected by either Southern or northern blot hybridization using only a limited number of probes because the position of the chromosomal break point is clustered in specific regions in *alpha* and *TFEB* (88,89). Nonetheless, because both hybridization methods are cumbersome and require fresh tissue for analysis, their utility in routine use is limited.

RT-PCR analysis of t(6;11)-associated renal neoplasms has shown *alpha-TFEB* fusion transcripts in virtually all tumors in which fresh tissue was available for analysis and in the single tumor in which FFPE tissue was tested (88,89,118). Probe-splitting and probe-fusion FISH have also been used to detect *alpha-TFEB* rearrangements in metaphase chromosomes and interphase nuclei (89). However, analysis of a larger number of cases, including tumors not preselected on the basis of the presence of the t(6;11)(p21;q13), and tumors not expected to harbor *TFEB* rearrangements, is necessary to more fully characterize the utility of RT-PCR and FISH in routine clinical practice.

Immunohistochemistry. Strong nuclear expression of TFEB protein can be detected by immunohistochemistry in t(6;11) associated renal tumors, but not in normal tissue or other neoplasms (89,118), consistent with the model that *alpha-TFEB* fusion gene produces disregulated *TFEB* expression. Renal neoplasms with *TFEB* fusions are also immunopositive for HMB-45 and MelanA, two proteins whose expression is normally activated by the transcription factor MITF (119). Because TFEB and MITF have homologous DNA binding domains, bind to a common DNA sequence, and may even form heterodimers (89,97), the fact that t(6;11)-associated tumors express HMB-45 and MelanA is not unexpected.

Diagnostic Issues in Molecular Genetic Analysis of Renal Neoplasms with *TFEB* Fusions

Two reports have emphasized that the morphologic features of renal tumors with the t(6;11) show a great deal of overlap with conventional clear cell RCC (116,117), a fact that emphasizes the usefulness of molecular genetic analysis for *alpha-TFEB* fusions in the differential diagnosis. However, it is also possible, given the unique immunoprofile of t(6;11)-associated neoplasms, that immunohistochemistry may supplant molecular analysis in the diagnostic workup of suspected cases.

Chromophobe RCC

Chromophobe RCC (Fig. 17.5) accounts for approximately 5% of renal cell carcinomas (1). Morphologically, the tumor is composed of cells with abundant cytoplasm and distinct cell borders, but because the cytoplasm often shows very pale staining, it can be difficult to distinguish chromophobe RCC from oncocytoma or clear cell RCC by morphology alone. However, the unique pattern of genetic aberrations in chromophobe RCC demonstrates that the tumor is not related to either of the latter two neoplasms. An uncommon eosinophilic variant characterized by abundant eosinophilic cytoplasm has also been described (120).

Genetics

Chromophobe RCC, including the eosinophilic variant, is characterized by loss of multiple whole chromosomes, most frequently 1, 2, 6, 10, 13, 16, 21, and Y (121,122), but the identity of relevant loci has yet to be determined.

Technical Issues in Molecular Genetic Analysis of Chromophobe RCC

The recurring loss of multiple whole chromosomes characteristic of chromophobe RCC has been detected by a number of molecular techniques, including conventional cytogenetic analysis (122–124), DNA ploidy analysis by flow cytometry and quantitative image analysis (125), comparative genomic hybridization (CGH) (126), and FISH (121,127). Taken together, these studies indicate that only 11% to 33% of chromophobe RCC have a normal chromosomal complement, but the lack of parallel analysis of the same cases by the different methods makes it

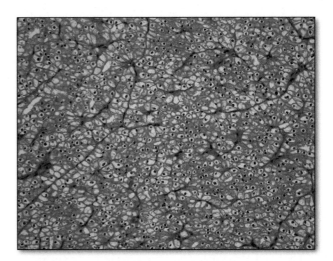

Figure 17.5 Chromophobe RCC is characterized genetically by loss of multiple chromosomes, most frequently 1, 2, 6, 10, 13, 16, 21, and Y. The illustrated tumor shows the morphologic features typical of chromophobe RCC, including cells with granular to clear cytoplasm and very prominent cell borders, oriented along thin vascular septa.

difficult to compare the sensitivity and specificity of the techniques.

Diagnostic Issues in Molecular Genetic Analysis of Chromophobe RCC

The pattern of chromosomal loss in chromophobe RCC is not a feature of any other renal neoplasm and so is a useful adjunct for diagnosis when present. The utility of molecular analysis was emphasized in one study in which interphase FISH for chromosomes 2, 6, 10, and 17 was used to distinguish renal oncocytoma from the chromophobe RCC, two tumors that can show significant morphologic similarity (122).

Congenital Mesoblastic Nephroma

Congenital mesoblastic nephroma (CMN) is a low-grade fibroblastic sarcoma of the infantile kidney that accounts for about 2% of all pediatric renal neoplasms (1,101). Roughly 90% of cases occur within the first year of life, and virtually none occur in children over the age of 3 years. The tumor is usually associated with an excellent prognosis; 95% of cases do not recur, and chemotherapy following complete excision is not required because hematogenous metastasis is very rare. Local recurrences, which occur in about 5% of cases, are thought be due to incomplete primary excision.

Morphologically, CMN is usually divided into three subtypes (1). Classic CMN (25% of cases) has an architectural and cytologic pattern identical to that of infantile fibromatosis, consisting of fascicles of bland fibroblastic/myofibroblastic cells that dissect apart the normal renal parenchyma. Cellular CMN (66% of cases) is cytologically identical to congenital/infantile fibrosarcoma (CIF), but has a pushing border and is composed of cells with a higher mitotic rate that may have a primitive or embryonal morphology with focal necrosis. Mixed CMN (10% of cases) is a neoplasm that has features of both classic and cellular CMN (Fig. 17.6). As discussed later, the classic and cellular subtypes are not simply different morphologic pattern of the same tumor, but instead are genetically distinct neoplasms.

Genetics

The translocation t(12;15)(p13;q25) produces an *ETV6-NTRK3* fusion gene that is the hallmark of CMN (98,99). Although trisomies of chromosomes 8, 11, and 17 are nearly as common as the t(12;15), the translocation is thought to be the initial transforming event, while the polysomy is considered a secondary event that is responsible for tumor progression to a more mitotically active phenotype (101,128).

The *ETV6-NTRK3* fusion gene encodes a protein in which the N-terminal helix-loop-helix dimerization domain of the highly expressed ETV6 transcription factor (also known as TEL) is fused to the tyrosine kinase domain of NTRK3 (also known as TRKC) (Fig. 11.5). The chimeric protein is thought to undergo ligand-independent,

A.

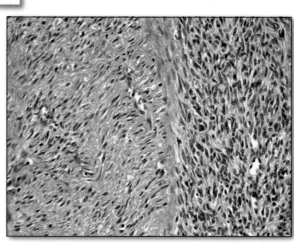

B.

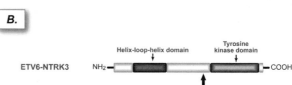

Figure 17.6   The translocation t(12;15)(p13;q25) that produces an *ETV6-NTRK3* fusion is the hallmark of cellular and mixed congenital mesoblastic nephroma. **A,** A mixed CMN from a 2-week-old boy; the region of the tumor with the morphology of cellular type CMN (*right half*) abruptly merges with the region that has the morphology of classic type CMN (*left half*). **B,** Schematic diagram of the ETV6-NTRK3 chimeric protein; the *arrow* indicates the fusion junction. (See Fig. 11.5 for more detail regarding native *ETV6* and *NTRK3*.)

helix-loop-helix–mediated dimerization with subsequent activation of the tyrosine kinase activity of NTRK3, producing a constitutively active protein tyrosine kinase that has potent transforming activity through a number of different cell activation pathways (129,130). In all cases of CMN so far described, the t(12;15) translocation break point occurs within intron 5 of *ETV6* and intron 12 of *NTRK3* (131).

Technical Issues in Molecular Genetic Analysis of CMN

Even though the t(12;15)(p13;q25) translocation is a recurrent finding in CMN, the regions exchanged between chromosomes 12 and 15 are so similar in size and banding characteristics that the translocation can be easily overlooked when evaluated by conventional cytogenetic banding methods. Because the translocation is difficult to identify by conventional cytogenetics, FISH-based testing can be more useful for demonstrating the rearrangement. Interphase FISH performed via a probe-split methodology on FFPE specimens has been used to show rearrangement of the *ETV6* locus consistent with *ETV6-NTRK3* fusions in 50% to 100% of cellular CMN and virtually 100% of mixed CMN, although only a very small number of cases has been evaluated to date (99,132). Interphase FISH on

FFPE tissue sections has been used to demonstrate trisomy 11 and 8 in a subset of cases harboring the *ETV6* region rearrangement (99,132).

When performed on cases of CMN in which fresh tissue is available for analysis, RT-PCR demonstrates an *ETV6-NTRK3* fusion transcript in 89% to 100% of cellular CMN and virtually 100% of mixed CMN, but in 0% of classic CMN (98,99). RT-PCR also has been adapted for use with FFPE tissue. In one study, analysis of FFPE specimens showed *ETV6-NTRK3* transcripts in 92% of cellular CMN, 0% of classic CMN, and 0% of mixed CMN (133); it is noteworthy that the lack of detection of *ETV6-NTRK3* fusions in mixed CMN was not interpreted as a sign of reduced test sensitivity, but rather as an indication that mixed CMN may actually represent a genetically heterogeneous group of neoplasms, an interpretation that emphasizes the difficulty in objectively evaluating test performance when the reference standard for the diagnosis itself is uncertain.

Diagnostic Issues in Molecular Genetic Analysis of CMN

The *ETV6-NTRK3* fusion gene is also the hallmark of CIF (131), as discussed in more detail in Chapter 11. Cellular and mixed types of CMN are therefore considered to be renal forms of CIF (1,101). Classic CMN does not harbor the *ETV6-NTRK3* rearrangement; thus, it is a distinct neoplasm rather than merely an architectureal variant of cellular or mixed CMN.

The *ETV6-NTRK3* fusion gene has not been detected in a variety of other primary renal tumors that enter into the differential diagnosis of CMN, including rhabdoid tumor, clear cell sarcoma of the kidney, and Wilms' tumor (98,133). The utility of molecular genetic analysis for diagnosis of challenging pediatric renal neoplasms is demonstrated by a recent study in which RT-PCR detection of *ETV6-NTRK3* transcripts in routinely processed FFPE tissue was used to distinguish cellular CMN from rhabdoid tumor and clear cell sarcoma of the kidney (133).

However, the *ETV6-NTFK3* rearrangement has been described in tumors of other cellular lineages (Table 11.3), including rare cases of acute myeloid leukemia (134–136) and the distinct variant of invasive ductal carcinoma known as secretory carcinoma (137,138). The *ETV6-NTRK3* fusion in acute leukemia and secretory breast carcinoma is identical at the molecular level to the fusion in CMN, emphasizing that aberrant tyrosine kinase signaling by a chimeric *ETV6-NTRK3* protein is a common oncogenetic mechanism across a number of different cell types (129,130).

Rhabdoid Tumor

Rhabdoid tumor of the kidney (RTK) is a highly aggressive neoplasm of infants and young children. RTK accounts for approximately 2% of pediatric renal neoplasms, is most common during the first 3 years of life, and is extremely uncommon in patients over the age of 3 years (1,101). Although the name RTK reflects the fact that the malignant cells have prominent hyaline intracytoplasmic inclusions that resemble those of rhabdomyoblasts, RTK does not demonstrate muscle differentiation. About 15% of RTK are associated with malignant neoplasms that resemble Ewing sarcoma/peripheral neuroectodermal tumor (EWS/PNET) in the posterior fossa of the central nervous system (CNS) that have clinical and pathologic features of second primaries rather than metastases (1).

Genetics

The characteristic genetic abnormality of RTK is somatic biallelic alteration of the hSNF5 locus (also known as INI1/SMARCB1) at 22q11.2 (139). The types of alteration include homozygous deletion, hemizygous deletion (with inactivation of the remaining allele by nonsense mutations, frame shift mutations, or intragenic deletions), and biallelic mutation without evidence of chromosome 22q11.2 deletion (139,140). hSNF5 encodes a protein that is a member of the ATP-dependent chromatin-remodeling complex (141,142), although the precise mechanism by which loss-of-function mutations promote oncogenesis remains unknown.

For most RTK, the biallelic alterations of *hSNF5* are a somatic event, and no correlation of individual mutations with prognosis has been described (140). In contrast, germline mutations of the gene are responsible for the rhabdoid predisposition syndrome, a hereditary disease characterized by renal or extrarenal malignant rhabdoid tumors and a variety of tumors of the CNS, including central EWS/PNET, medulloblastoma, and choroid plexus carcinoma (143–145).

Technical Issues in Molecular Genetic Analysis of RTK

Interphase FISH and PCR-based microsatellite LOH analysis can be used to demonstrate homozygous deletion of the *hSNF5* locus in approximately 16% to 20% of RTK (139,140,144,145), but use of FFPE tissue may be associated with decreased sensitivity (140). In RTK without homozygous deletion of the *hSNF5* locus, DNA sequence analysis demonstrates nonsense or missense mutations in the retained allele in 60% to 84% of cases (139,140). However, DNA sequence analysis is cumbersome because mutations in *hSNF5* occur over most of the length of the gene, and so it is necessary to evaluate all 9 exons of the gene or the complete transcript.

Routine cytogenetic analysis can be used to detect deletions of 22q, often in association with a translocation (140,146–149), but the method lacks the sensitivity to detect small-scale structural changes and point mutations of *hSNF5* that are so frequently responsible for the gene's inactivation in RTK. Southern blot hybridization has been used to demonstrate aberrations in the *hSNF5*, but because the method requires a large amount of fresh tissue and is unable to detect small-scale mutations, its usefulness in routine practice is limited (139).

Immunohistochemistry. Using an monoclonal antibody against *hSNF5/INI1*, virtually 100% of RTK (as well as extrarenal malignant rhabdoid tumors) lack strong diffuse nuclear staining, as expected based on the underlying genetic abnormality (150). In contrast, positive nuclear staining is present in virtually all pediatric tumors that can show rhabdoid features, including EWS/PNET, Wilms' tumor, DSRCT, clear cell sarcoma, CMN, undifferentiated sarcoma, and rhabdomyosarcoma, although synovial sarcoma and epithelioid sarcoma exhibit variable or focal nuclear staining (150).

Diagnostic Issues in Molecular Genetic Analysis of RTK

Biallelic loss-of-function mutations of *hSNF5* are also characteristic of malignant rhabdoid tumors that arise in the CNS or soft tissue of infants and children, as discussed in more detail in Chapter 11. However, inactivation of *hSNF5* is not a recurring feature of any other renal neoplasm that commonly enters into the differential diagnosis of RTK, including cellular CMN, Wilms' tumor, clear cell sarcoma of the kidney, EWS/PNET, renal medullary carcinoma, and even synovial sarcoma (95,151). A variety of other renal and extrarenal malignancies can show rhabdoid features (Fig. 17.7), including carcinomas and sarcomas (152–156); however these tumors usually occur in adults and careful morphologic examination usually demonstrates that the rhabdoid phenotype is merely a poorly differentiated component of the underlying neoplasm, and so the clinicopathologic features are usually sufficient to exclude RTK without mutational analysis of *hSNF5*.

Nephroblastoma (Wilms' Tumor)

Wilms' tumor is the most common renal malignancy in the pediatric age-group, and 98% of cases occur in children under 10 years old (1). The staging and classification of nephroblastoma is based on the extent of disease and histopathologic features of the tumor, and, with multimodality therapy, over 85% of patients with even advanced-stage disease can be cured (157).

Genetics

Although nephroblastoma was one of the original paradigms of the two-hit model of cancer formation, it is now thought that a number of genetic events contribute to tumorigenesis.

WT1 Gene. The observation that approximately 30% of patients with the WAGR syndrome (*W*ilms' tumor, *a*niridia, *g*enitourinary anomalies, and mental *r*etardation) develop nephroblastoma led to identification of the *WT1* gene at 11p13. The WT1 protein is a zinc finger transcription factor that is not only critical for normal kidney and gonad development (158,159), but also functions as a tumor suppressor (160), and so it is not surprising that germline mutations in WT1 underlie developmental syndromes that have an associated increased risk of Wilms' tumor (Table 17.4). Nonetheless, only about 5% of Wilms' tumors arise in patients with germline *WT1* mutations and only 6% to

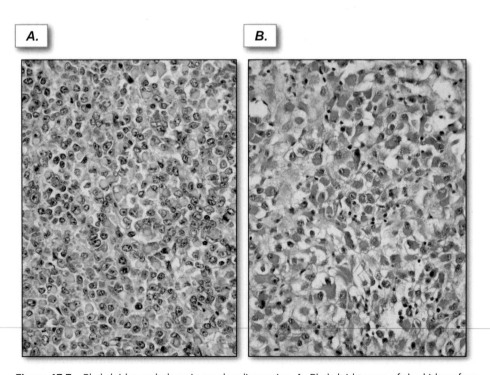

Figure 17.7 Rhabdoid morphology in renal malignancies. **A,** Rhabdoid tumor of the kidney from a 3-day-old girl showing the characteristic vesicular nuclei with prominent nucleoli, prominent globular hyaline intracytoplasmic inclusions, and a sheet-like growth pattern. Rhabdoid tumor of the kidney is characterized by biallelic inactivation of *hSNF5*. **B,** Clear cell RCC with prominent rhabdoid features arising in a 53-year-old man. Tumors with this morphology harbor the same pattern of *VHL* aberrations as conventional clear cell RCC.

TABLE 17.4

CLINICAL SYNDROMES ASSOCIATED WITH WILMS' TUMOR

Syndrome	Gene	Mutation	Locus	Clinical Features	Risk of Wilms' Tumor
WAGR[a]	WT1	Deletion	11p13	Wilms tumor; aniridia; genitourinary anomalies; mental retardation; delayed-onset renal failure	30%
Denys-Drash	WT1	Missense mutations in zinc finger regions of WT1 protein	11p13	Ambiguous genitalia; diffuse mesangial sclerosis	90%
Frasier	WT1	Point mutation in intron 9 donor splice site	11p13	Ambiguous genitalia; streak gonads; focal segmental glomerulosclerosis	Low (case reports)
Beckwith-Wiedemann	WT2	Unknown, but associated with loss of imprinting of several genes	11p15	Organomegaly; omphalocele; hemihypertrophy	5%
Familial predisposition to Wilms' tumor	FWT1 (WT4) FWT2	Unknown Unknown	17q13 19q13	Autosomal dominant inheritance with incomplete penetrance	15%–25% for FWT1; unknown for FWT2

[a]Wilms' tumor, aniridia, genitourinary anomalies, and mental retardation.

18% of tumors are due to sporadic *WT1* mutations (161–164). Even though it is possible that epigenetic changes or post-transcriptional mRNA modifications contribute to tumorigenesis in some cases (165,166), it is clear that many Wilms' tumors arise from genetic alterations at loci other than *WT1*.

WT2 Region. The discovery of *WT2* stemmed from the observation that the 11p15 region is linked with the Beckwith-Widemann syndrome, which is itself associated with a 5% to 10% risk of Wilms' tumor. The 11p15 region is commonly referred to the *WT2* locus, although the region actually contains at least 10 imprinted genes (167,168).

FWT1 and FWT2 Genes. About 1% to 2% of Wilms' tumors arise in individuals from kindreds that show a familial predisposition to Wilms' tumor without linkage to the *WT1* gene at 11p13. At least two different loci are involved, *FWT1* at 17q13 and *FWT2* at 19q13 (169–172). Additional tumor susceptibility genes must also exist because still other kindreds show no linkage to *WT1*, *FWT1*, or *FWT2* (172,173).

Other Markers. Up to 75% of Wilms' tumors with anaplastic histology harbor *TP53* mutations, whereas mutations are uncommon in tumors with favorable histology; thus, it has been suggested that analysis of *TP53* may be of some prognostic utility (174–177). Allelic imbalance/LOH of the deleted in colorectal cancer (*DCC*) gene has also been shown to provide statistically independent prognostic information (178). Surveys of gene expression profiles have even been used to provide information of diagnostic or prognostic utility (179–181). Nonetheless, molecular genetic analysis of Wilms' tumor is currently experimental, and the standard tumor workup does not include evaluation of any specific genes or chromosomal regions.

Other Tumor Types

A number of malignancies that characteristically involve the soft tissue have also been described as primary tumors of the kidney (Table 17.3), including EWS/PNET, desmoplastic small round cell tumor, synovial sarcoma, clear cell sarcoma (malignant melanoma of soft parts), and alveolar rhabdomyosarcoma. The genetic aberrations characteristic of these tumors, as well as the technical and diagnostic issues associated with their evaluation by molecular testing, are the same whether the neoplasms arise in the kidney or soft tissue (see Chapter 11).

GLOMERULAR DISEASE

The genetic bases of the glomerular diseases responsible for various hematuria syndromes, congenital nephrotic syndromes, and hereditary lipidoses have recently been characterized (Table 17.5). The histologic, ultrastructural, genetic, and clinical features of the various glomerular diseases are summarized in several excellent reviews (200–206).

Genetics

Congenital Hematuria Syndromes
Mutations in the *COLIVA5* gene (207,208) are responsible for X-linked Alport syndrome (Fig. 17.8). Approximately 85% of cases of X-linked Alport syndrome are familial; the

TABLE 17.5

GENETIC BASIS OF GLOMERULAR DISEASE

Disease	Inheritance	Gene	Protein	References
Congenital hematuria syndromes				
Autosomal recessive Alport syndrome	Autosomal recessive	COLIVA3[a] COLIVA4	α3 Chain of collagen IV α4 Chain of collagen IV	182, 183
Autosomal dominant Alport syndrome	Autosomal dominant	COLIVA3[b] COLIVA4	α3 Chain of collagen IV α4 Chain of collagen IV	182, 183
X-linked Alport syndrome	X-linked	COLIVA5	α5 Chain of collagen IV	184
Thin basement membrane nephropathy	Autosomal dominant	COLIVA3[b] COLIVA4	α3 Chain of collagen IV α4 Chain of collagen IV	182, 183
Nail-Patella syndrome	Autosomal dominant	LMX1B	Transcription factor	185
Congenital nephrotic syndromes				
Finnish type	Autosomal recessive	NPHS1	Nephrin	186
Familial steroid resistant focal segmental glomerulosclerosis	Autosomal recessive	NPHS2 SRN1 at 1q25–31	Podocin Unknown	187 188
Sporadic steroid resistant focal segmental glomerulosclerosis	—	NPHS2	Podocin	189, 190
Familial focal segmental glomerulosclerosis	Autosomal dominant	ACTN4 TRPC6	α-Actinin-4 Membrane cation channel	191 192
Glomuler disease as a component of a developmental/tumor syndrome				
Frasier syndrome (focal segmental glomerulosclerosis)	—	WT1	Transcription factor	193
Denys-Drash syndrome (diffuse mesangial sclerosis)	—	WT1	Transcription factor	194
Renal lipidoses				
Fabry's disease	X-linked	α-GalA	Enzyme α-galactosidase A	195, 196
Lipoprotein glomerulopathy	Unknown	ApoE	Apolipoprotein E	197
Lecithin cholesterol acyl transferase deficiency (fish-eye disease)	Autosomal recessive	LCAT	Lecithin cholesterol acyltransferase	198
Dense deposit disease	Autosomal recessive	HF1	Complement factor H	199
Other				
IgA nephropathy	Unknown	IGAN-1 at 6q22–23	Unknown	200

[a]Disease is due to biallelic inactivation of either gene.
[b]Disease is due to inactivation of only one allele of either gene.

other 15% of cases are apparently due to de novo germline mutations. Over 360 different mutations in COLIVA5 have been reported so far (209), and although this genetic heterogeneity parallels the clinical heterogeneity of X-linked Alport syndrome, the mechanism by which individual mutations lead to different phenotypes is not entirely clear (210,211).

Mutations in two other type IV collagen genes, specifically COLIVA3 and COLIVA4, are responsible for autosomal recessive Alport syndrome, autosomal dominant Alport syndrome, and thin basement membrane nephropathy (Fig. 17.8), which helps explain the clinical overlap between these diseases (201,203,207,208,212). Although in most cases the genetic aberrations are familial, sporadic mutations in COLIVA3 or COLIVA4 may account for as high

as 30% of cases (201). Dozens of unique mutations in COLIVA3 and COLIVA4 have been described (209), but there are few correlations between specific mutations and either disease severity or the pattern of altered basement membrane structure (201,213), and the pathways through which the different mutations lead to the various patterns of clinical disease remain largely unknown (201–203).

The Nail-Patella syndrome is due to mutations in the LMX1B gene. More than 90 different mutations in the gene have been reported, and although this genetic heterogeneity mirrors the clinical variability of the syndrome, the mechanism by which the mutations cause differences in disease severity is unclear (214). LMX1B encodes a transcription factor that, among other functions, is responsible for regulation of matrix protein production by podocytes

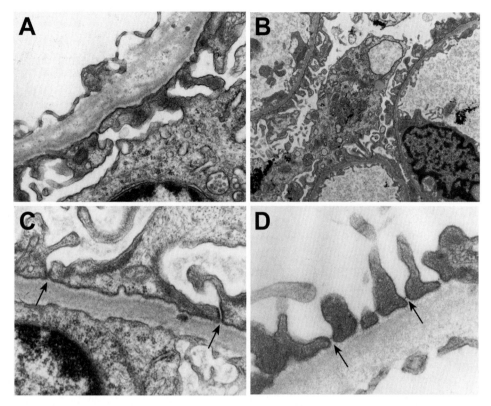

Figure 17.8   Ultrastructure of monogenetic glomerular diseases. Glomerular basement membrane splitting is a characteristic finding in X-linked Alport syndrome and is present in about 92% of cases (**A,** magnification 40,000×). However, about 8% of cases of X-linked Alport syndrome show a diffusely thin glomerular basement membrane that is more typical of autosomal dominant thin basement membrane nephropathy (**B,** magnification 12,000×). In Finnish type nephropathy, the podocyte foot processes are fused and the slit pore (*arrows*) between foot processes is empty (**C,** magnification 172,000×). In a normal kidney, slit diaphragms (*arrows*) bridge adjacent foot processes (**D,** magnification 120,000×). (Electron micrographs courtesy Dr. Helen Liapis, Washington University School of Medicine.)

(185,214). In addition, *LMX1B* is involved in regulation of expression of other podocyte proteins, including NPHS2 (mutated in steroid resistant focal segmental glomerulosclerosis, as discussed later) and CD2AP (deficiency of which causes congenital nephrotic syndrome in a mouse model) (215,216).

Congenital Nephrotic Syndromes

Finnish type focal segmental glomerulosclerosis (FSGS) is due to a wide variety of mutations in the *NPHS1* gene. *NPHS1* encodes the protein nephrin, which is a major component of the slit diaphragm (Fig. 17.8) between prodocyte foot processes (186,204,205). Although two specific *NPHS1* mutations account for 95% of syndromic cases in Finland, over 30 different mutations have been described in cases in other geographic regions (204,205,217).

Recessive (steroid resistant) FSGS is due to mutations in the *NPHS2* gene that encodes the protein podocin. Podocin also localizes to the podocyte and apparently interacts directly with nephrin (187,204,205). Mutations in *NPHS2* are also responsible for disease in 20% to 30% of children who have sporadic steroid resistant nephrotic syndrome (204,205). A number of different *NPHS2*

mutations have been described, some of which correlate with the pattern of clinical disease (204).

A subset of cases of autosomal dominant FSGS are due to mutations in *ACTN4* gene, which encodes the protein α-actinin-4. Mutations in *ACTN4* are thought to alter the mechanical properties of podocytes by changing the affinity of the α-actinin interaction with actin (218). Missense mutations in the *TRPC6* gene are responsible for other cases of autosomal dominant FSGS (192). *TRPC6* encodes a membrane cation channel, and the fact that missense mutations alter calcium signaling suggests that disease in these patients may be amendable to pharmacologic manipulation of the channel (192).

Developmental Syndromes

Donor splice site point mutations in intron 9 of the *WT1* gene are responsible for Frasier syndrome, which is associated with FSGS (193). Missense mutations in the zinc finger regions of WT1 are responsible for Denys-Drash syndrome, which is associated with diffuse mesangial sclerosis (194).

Renal Lipidoses

Fabry's disease, which is associated with the classic ultrastructural finding of myeloid bodies, is due to mutations in the *α-GalA* gene that encodes the enzyme α-galactosidase A. Hundreds of different mutations in *α-GalA* have been linked to Fabry's disease, and although the severity of disease in general parallels the reduction of enzymatic activity, family members with the same mutation often show differences in disease severity. Numerous mutations have also been described in the genes responsible for other hereditary lipidoses, but as is true for Fabry's disease, it is often difficult to predict the ultrastructural pathology or severity of disease based on a specific mutation.

Technical Issues in Molecular Genetic Analysis of Glomerular Disease

For some diseases, in specific patient populations, genetic analysis is technically straightforward. For example, because only two mutations in the *NPHS1* gene account for over 95% of cases of congenital nephrotic syndrome in Finland, disease screening by molecular methods is inexpensive and highly sensitive (204). Similarly, only a limited number of *WT1* mutations are associated with Frasier syndrome and Denys-Drash syndrome; thus, DNA sequence analysis of only a limited region of the *WT1* gene can still provide a highly sensitive testing method.

However, from a purely technical standpoint, molecular testing for mutations in the genes associated with many of the other glomerular diseases is complicated by several factors. First, as noted above, a large number of different mutations has been described in the genes that are responsible for many of the diseases. The mutations are not clustered into well-defined hot-spots, and so analysis is not a trivial undertaking because it involves analysis of virtually the entire target gene. Second, specific mutations are not tightly correlated with disease severity, so analysis must include testing for the full range of mutations, regardless of the patient's clinical symptoms. Third, the pattern of mutations in many of the diseases includes missense and nonsense mutations, splice site mutations, small insertions and deletions, gross insertions and deletions, duplications, and even complex rearrangements. Consequently, it is difficult to detect the entire range of mutations by one testing methodology, and a variety of techniques must be combined to achieve high test sensitivity. For these reasons, mutational analysis is primarily performed by specialty laboratories (219,220).

Diagnostic Issues in Molecular Genetic Analysis of Glomerular Disease

Even though comprehensive mutational analysis of the genes associated with glomerular disease is a daunting task, there are several clinical settings in which testing is indicated. First, as noted above, heterogeneity in the severity of disease, even among family members known to harbor the same mutation, can make it difficult to clinically determine whether a specific individual is a disease carrier. In addition, because sporadic mutations are responsible for a significant percentage of many types of genetic glomerular disease, an absence of familial renal disease can be an unreliable guide to whether an individual harbors a mutation. Since the phenotype of the patient (or the

patient's family) is such an unreliable guide to his or her genotype, molecular testing may be required to definitively establish the presence of a mutation. Second, genetic testing may be required to ensure that a patient's relative under consideration as a renal transplant donor does not carry the mutation. Given that the absence of clinical disease cannot be used to exclude the presence of a mutation, especially for FSGS, genetic analysis can be the only definitive way to ensure that the relative is not a disease carrier. Third, genetic testing can be the only method to establish the diagnosis in those cases in which the morphologic, immunohistochemical, and ultrastructural features of the renal biopsy are ambiguous. In all of these settings, genetic testing should be performed only in consultation with a medical geneticist because of the implications of a positive test result for the patient and the patient's family.

There is little role for genetic analysis to determine an individual patient's prognosis. As has already been noted, the same mutation can cause disease of varying severity, and, as yet, there are no known tests that can predict an individual patient's clinical course even when the precise mutation is known.

BLADDER NEOPLASMS

Invasive Urothelial Carcinoma

Urothelial carcinoma is the seventh most common malignancy worldwide and accounts for 2% to 3% of all malignancies (1,221). The World Health Organization (WHO) International Society of Urologic Pathology (ISUP) consensus classification system (222) has been shown to correlate with both immunophenotypic findings and clinical outcome (223) and is the most widely used classification scheme.

Genetics

Invasive transitional cell carcinomas (TCC) usually harbor multiple genetic abnormalities, ranging from gross structural aberrations of several different chromosomal regions, to single bp substitutions in oncogenes and tumor suppressor genes (224–226). Detailed molecular analysis has shown that the pattern of genetic abnormalities in muscle invasive TCC is consistent with a model in which low-grade, superficial bladder cancers accumulate genetic alterations as they progress to advanced muscle invasive tumors (227).

Role of Molecular Genetic Testing for Diagnosis

In general there is no established value for molecular genetic analysis in the diagnosis of TCC because the presence of mutations shows no clear-cut association with tumor stage or grade (228,229). As examples, although over 40% of invasive TCC harbor mutations in H-*ras*, the presence or type of mutation does not correlate with tumor stage or grade (230–232); the mutational status or expression level of cyclin-dependent kinases does not appear to correlate with tumor grade or stage (225,233–235); and inactivation of the retinoblastoma gene *RB1*, usually a consequence of LOH resulting from 13q deletions with mutation of the remaining allele, is not strongly associated with muscle invasion (224,225,236,237).

Role of Molecular Genetic Testing for Evaluation of Prognosis

Even though molecular analysis does not have a defined role for diagnosis of TCC, some genetic aberrations have been correlated with prognosis. For example, the presence of aneuploid cell populations or mutations in specific genes (including *TP53*, *p21*, and genes encoding proteins of the epidermal growth factor receptor pathway) has been shown to be prognostic determinates in patients with bladder cancer (225), and mutations in *TP53* appear to have prognostic significance independent of tumor stage and grade when *p21* expression is absent (238,239). If clinical trials confirm that mutational status of any (or all) of these loci correlates with treatment outcome, molecular testing may have a role in the pathologic evaluation of TCC independent of any role in diagnosis.

The role of molecular genetic analysis for evaluation of prognosis may eventually extend to analysis of genes involved in the cellular response to chemotherapy. Allelic differences at a number of loci, including those that encode dihydropyrimidine dehydrogenase (DPD, an enzyme involved in the catabolism of 5-fluorouracil) (240), cytochrome P450 enzymes (which have a role in the metabolism of ifosfamide, vinblastine, paclitaxel, and docetaxel) (241,242), and glutathione S-transferase (responsible for conjugating platinum complexes and alkylating agents to glutathione) (243) are known to underlie individual variation in the metabolism of a number of chemotherapeutic agents. However, because TCCs often harbor mutations, epigenetic modifications, or altered patterns of gene expression that affect the cytotoxic effect of chemotherapeutic drugs within the tumor itself (225), the most informative analysis will likely require testing of tumor tissue as well as normal somatic cells (225).

Role of Molecular Genetic Testing for Staging

Molecular genetic techniques have been used to identify occult metastases that are not evident by routine clinical and histopathologic evaluation. For example, RT-PCR has been used to detect expression of uroplakin II (UPII) and cytokeratin-20 (CK-20) in the peripheral blood of patients with urothelial cancer (244). Despite the fact that expression of these markers in peripheral blood may not be 100% specific for the presence of malignant cells, (e.g., CK-20 has been detected in the peripheral blood of up to 100% of patients with no history of malignancy [245–248] as discussed in more detail in Chapter 15), detection of UPII and CK-20 transcripts correlates with disease stage, correlates with recurrence-free survival in patients with superficial stage disease, and is an independent prognostic factor in patients with superficial stage disease (244). If confirmed by other groups, these results suggest that molecular genetic demonstration of submicroscopic disease may provide independent prognostic information, even if it has yet to be established whether testing for submicroscopic metastatic disease should be incorporated into traditional staging schemes.

Role of Molecular Genetic Testing for Screening

Patients who have a history of superficial urothelial carcinoma of the bladder (pT stage pTa, pTis, or pT1) have up to a 40% risk of recurrence or later development of an upper urinary tract tumor (249). Despite its high specificity, routine cytologic examination of urine specimens has limited sensitivity for detecting these subsequent tumors. Consequently, there has been much interest in alternative molecular approaches to detect urothelial carcinoma in urine specimens.

Fluorescence in Situ Hybridization

One approach consists of a multitarget, multicolor FISH assay that employs four probes, including a probe for the pericentromeric region of chromosome 3, the pericentromeric region of chromosome 7, the pericentromeric of chromosome 17, and chromosome region 9p21 (250,251). Using slightly different criteria for interpreting the test result as positive based on the number of cells that show polysomy (a gain of two or more different chromosomes based on the chromosome 3, 17, and 17 probes), gain of a single chromosome, or homozygous loss of the 9p21 region, the FISH assay has been shown for patients with biopsy-proven urothelial carcinoma to have an overall sensitivity of 81% to 87% and a specificity of 92% to 97%, a level of performance that is superior to that of conventional cytology (250,251). More precisely, the sensitivity of FISH and cytology are 100% and 78%, respectively, for patients with pTis tumors; 95% and 60% for patients with pT1-pT4 tumors, respectively, and 97% and 71%, respectively, for patients with grade 3 tumors, all differences that are statistically significant (251). In addition, there is also a trend for increased FISH sensitivity in detection of pTa and grade 2 tumors (251). Consequently, a kit based on the four probes (UroVysion, Vysis/Abbott, Downer's Grove, IL) has been approved by the Food and Drug Administration (FDA) for monitoring urothelial carcinoma patients for tumor recurrence.

A number of follow-up studies have confirmed that the sensitivity of the UroVysion FISH assay exceeds that of conventional cytology, with a specificity that is at least equivalent to that of conventional cytology (252–255). Follow-up studies have also shown that the multitarget FISH approach has a sensitivity and specificity that is superior to that of immunoassays for tumor-associated proteins in voided urine specimens, hemoglobin dipstick tests for hematuria, and assays for telomerase activity (255,256). However, it is important to recognize that reports evaluating the performance of the UroVysion FISH test often use different criteria for scoring the FISH signal pattern (252,253,256), and so it is unclear whether these studies would have obtained similar results using the criteria for test interpretation suggested by the manufacturer of the UroVysion kit.

Polymerase Chain Reaction

PCR-based microsatellite analysis of DNA extracted from urine sediment has a sensitivity of 77% for detecting urothelial carcinoma, and the pattern of microsatellite alterations correlates with both the grade and stage of the tumor (257). When free DNA in urine is the substrate for analysis, testing has a sensitivity of 50%, which increases to 64% when coupled with microsatellite analysis of paired peripheral blood samples (258). However, because analysis was not performed on control urine samples in the studies that report these measures of test performance, the specificity of microsatellite-based testing is unknown. In addition, the upper limit of sensitivity of testing is constrained by the fact that only 72% to 87% of invasive TCC harbor LOH, length alterations, or allelic gain at marker microsatellite loci (257,258).

Telomerase

Regulation of telomere length is altered in urothelial carcinomas (261); therefore, telomerase metabolism assays have been evaluated as screening approaches (the TRAP assay for telomerase expression, as well as the RT-PCR assay for hTERT mRNA expression, are discussed in detail in Chapter 5). The TRAP assay has a sensitivity that ranges from 7% to 85% in voided urine specimens and up to 86% in bladder wash specimens and a specificity that ranges from 78% to 100%, indices of test performance that are comparable to those of urine cytology (260,261). The hTERT assay has a sensitivity of 57% to 92% when urine samples are evaluated, and from 76% to 94% when bladder washings are evaluated with an overall specificity that ranges from 92% to 98% (260,262,263). In some settings, particularly for the detection of low-grade transitional cell carcinoma, the higher sensitivity of the hTERT assay compared with routine urine cytology is statistically significant (260,262). Some reports have demonstrated that the combined use of telomerase analysis and urine cytology has a higher sensitivity than either test alone (261).

Noninvasive Urothelial Neoplasms

Noninvasive low-grade papillary bladder neoplasms (pTa, grade 1–2) are considered to be genetically stable. These tumors may have a few cytogenetic changes and mutations, but gene amplifications, TP53 mutations, and DNA aneuploidy are rare (225,227,264–266). In contrast, high-grade noninvasive urothelial neoplasms (stage pTa, grade 3 or carcinoma in-situ) are genetically unstable and show high levels of gene amplifications, TP53 mutations, and aneuploidy (265–269). However, molecular testing to distinguish grade 1–2 versus grade 3 pTa noninvasive tumors, or to distinguish stage pTa versus pT1 tumors, does not have the sensitivity or specificity to be of use in routine clinical practice (268–273).

Other Tumor Types

A wide variety of nonepithelial malignancies have also been described as primary tumors of the bladder, including malignant round cell tumors such as EWS/PNET (274,275) and neuroblastoma (276,277) and spindle cell tumors such as inflammatory myofibroblastic tumor (278–280) and extragastrointestinal stromal tumor (281). The genetic aberrations characteristic of these tumor types, as well as

the technical and diagnostic issues associated with their evaluation by molecular testing, are the same whether the neoplasms arise in the bladder or at more conventional sites (Chapters 11 and 12).

REFERENCES

1. Eble JN, Sauter G, Epstein JI, et al, eds. *Pathology and Genetics of Tumours of the Urinary System and Male Genital Organs: World Health Organization Classification of Tumours.* Lyon: IARC Press; 2004.
2. Pavlovich CP, Schmidt LS. Searching for the hereditary causes of renal-cell carcinoma. *Nat Rev Cancer* 2004;4:381–393.
3. http://www.genetests.org/
4. Bodmer D, van den Hurk W, van Groningen JJ, et al. Understanding familial and non-familial renal cell cancer. *Hum Mol Genet* 2002;11:2489–2498.
5. Latif F, Tory K, Gnarra J, et al. Identification of the von Hippel-Lindau disease tumor suppressor gene. *Science* 1993;260:1317–1320.
6. Foster K, Prowse A, van den Berg A, et al. Somatic mutations of the von Hippel-Lindau disease tumour suppressor gene in non-familial clear cell renal carcinoma. *Hum Mol Genet* 1994;3:2169–2173.
7. Shuin T, Kondo K, Torigoe S, et al. Frequent somatic mutations and loss of heterozygosity of the von Hippel-Lindau tumor suppressor gene in primary human renal cell carcinomas. *Cancer Res* 1994;54:2852–2855.
8. Gnarra JR, Tory K, Weng Y, et al. Mutations of the *VHL* tumour suppressor gene in renal carcinoma. *Nat Genet* 1994;7:85–90.
9. Knudson AG. Hereditary cancer, oncogenes, and antioncogenes. *Cancer Res* 1985;45:1437–1443.
10. George DJ, Kaelin WG Jr, et al. The von Hippel-Lindau protein, vascular endothelial growth factor, and kidney cancer. *N Engl J Med* 2003;349:419–421.
11. Herman JG, Latif F, Weng Y, et al. Silencing of the *VHL* tumor-suppressor gene by DNA methylation in renal carcinoma. *Proc Natl Acad Sci USA* 1994;91:9700–9704.
12. Kim W, Kaelin WG Jr. The von Hippel-Lindau tumor suppressor protein: new insights into oxygen sensing and cancer. *Curr Opin Genet Dev* 2003;13:55–60.
13. Pugh CW, Ratcliffe PJ. The von Hippel-Lindau tumor suppressor, hypoxia-inducible factor-1 (HIF-1) degradation, and cancer pathogenesis. *Semin Cancer Biol* 2003;13:83–89.
14. Maxwell PH, Wiesener MS, Chang GW, et al. The tumour suppressor protein *VHL* targets hypoxia-inducible factors for oxygen-dependent proteolysis. *Nature* 1999;399:271–275.
15. Siemeister G, Weindel K, Mohrs K, et al. Reversion of deregulated expression of vascular endothelial growth factor in human renal carcinoma cells by von Hippel-Lindau tumor suppressor protein. *Cancer Res* 1996;56:2299–2301.
16. Knebelmann B, Ananth S, Cohen HT, et al. Transforming growth factor *alpha* is a target for the von Hippel-Lindau tumor suppressor. *Cancer Res* 1998;58:226–231.
17. Yang JC, Haworth L, Sherry RM, et al. A randomized trial of bevacizumab, an antivascular endothelial growth factor antibody, for metastatic renal cancer. *N Engl J Med* 2003;349:427–434.
18. Gemmill RM, West JD, Boldog F, et al. The hereditary renal cell carcinoma 3;8 translocation fuses FHIT to a patched-related gene, TRC8. *Proc Natl Acad Sci USA* 1998;95:9572–9877.
19. Kovacs G, Brusa P, de Riese W. Tissue-specific expression of a constitutional 3;6 translocation: development of multiple bilateral renal-cell carcinomas. *Int J Cancer* 1989;43:422–427.
20. Bodmer D, Eleveld M, Kater-Baats E, et al. Disruption of a novel MFS transporter gene, DIRC2, by a familial renal cell carcinoma-associated t(2;3)(q35;q21). *Hum Mol Genet* 2002;11:641–649.
21. Bodmer D, Schepens M, Eleveld MJ, et al. Disruption of a novel gene, DIRC3, and expression of DIRC3-HSPBAP1 fusion transcripts in a case of familial renal cell cancer and t(2;3)(q35;q21). *Genes Chromosomes Cancer* 2003;38:107–116.
22. Geurts van Kessel A, Wijnhoven H, Bodmer D, et al. Renal cell cancer: chromosome 3 translocations as risk factors. *J Natl Cancer Inst* 1999;91:1159–1160.
23. Druck T, Podolski J, Byrski T, et al. The DIRC1 gene at chromosome 2q33 spans a familial RCC-associated t(2;3)(q33;q21) chromosome translocation. *J Hum Genet* 2001;46:583–589.
24. Chen J, Lui WO, Vos MD, et al. The t(1;3) breakpoint-spanning genes LSAMP and NORE1 are involved in clear cell renal cell carcinomas. *Cancer Cell* 2003;4:405–413.
25. Gemmill RM, Bemis LT, Lee JP, et al. The TRC8 hereditary kidney cancer gene suppresses growth and functions with *VHL* in a common pathway. *Oncogene* 2002;21:3507–3516.
26. Schmidt L, Li F, Brown RS, et al. Mechanism of tumorigenesis of renal carcinomas associated with the constitutional chromosome 3;8 translocation. *Cancer J Sci Am* 1995;1:191.
27. Lendvay TS, Marshall FF. The tuberous sclerosis complex and its highly variable manifestations. *J Urol* 2003;169:1635–1642.
28. Parry L, Maynard JH, Patel A, et al. Analysis of the TSC1 and TSC2 genes in sporadic renal cell carcinomas. *Br J Cancer* 2001;85:1226–1230.
29. Schmidt LS, Warren MB, Nickerson ML, et al. Birt-Hogg-Dube syndrome, a genodermatosis associated with spontaneous pneumothorax and kidney neoplasia, maps to chromosome 17p11.2. *Am J Hum Genet* 2001;69:876–882.
30. Nickerson ML, Warren MB, Toro JR, et al. Mutations in a novel gene lead to kidney tumors, lung wall defects, and benign tumors of the hair follicle in patients with the Birt-Hogg-Dube syndrome. *Cancer Cell* 2002;2:157–164.
31. Khoo SK, Kahnoski K, Sugimura J, et al. Inactivation of BHD in sporadic renal tumors. *Cancer Res* 2003;63:4583–4587.
32. da Silva NF, Gentle D, Hesson LB, et al. Analysis of the Birt-Hogg-Dube (BHD) tumour suppressor gene in sporadic renal cell carcinoma and colorectal cancer. *J Med Genet* 2003;40:820–824.
33. Fukunaga K, Wada T, Matsumoto H, et al. Renal cell carcinoma: allelic loss at chromosome 9 using the fluorescent multiplex-polymerase chain reaction technique. *Hum Pathol* 2002;33:910–914.

34. Morita R, Ishikawa J, Tsutsumi M, et al. Allelotype of renal cell carcinoma. *Cancer Res* 1991;51:820–823.

35. Brooks JD, Bova GS, Marshall FF, et al. Tumor suppressor gene allelic loss in human renal cancers. *J Urol* 1993;150:1278–1283.

36. Foster K, Crossey PA, Cairns P, et al. Molecular genetic investigation of sporadic renal cell carcinoma: analysis of allele loss on chromosomes 3p, 5q, 11p, 17 and 22. *Br J Cancer* 1994;69:230–234.

37. Zhuang Z, Gnarra JR, Dudley CF, et al. Detection of von Hippel-Lindau disease gene mutations in paraffin-embedded sporadic renal cell carcinoma specimens. *Mod Pathol* 1996;9:838–842.

38. Decker HH, Klauck SM, Lawrence JB, et al. Cytogenetic and fluorescence in situ hybridization studies on sporadic and hereditary tumors associated with von Hippel-Lindau syndrome (VHL). *Cancer Genet Cytogenet* 1994;77:1–13.

39. Pack SD, Zbar B, Pak E, et al. Constitutional von Hippel-Lindau (VHL) gene deletions detected in VHL families by fluorescence in situ hybridization. *Cancer Res* 1999;59:5560–5564.

40. Moch H, Schraml P, Bubendorf L, et al. Intratumoral heterogeneity of von Hippel-Lindau gene deletions in renal cell carcinoma detected by fluorescence in situ hybridization. *Cancer Res* 1998;58:2304–2309.

41. Heinze F, Kovacs G. Identifying *BAC* clones for diagnosis of conventional renal cell carcinoma by FISH. *Histopathology* 2002;41:308–312.

42. van der Hout AH, van der Vlies P, Wijmenga C, et al. The region of common allelic losses in sporadic renal cell carcinoma is bordered by the loci *D3S2* and *THRB*. *Genomics* 1991;11:537–542.

43. van der Hout AH, van den Berg E, van der Vlies P, et al. Loss of heterozygosity at the short arm of chromosome 3 in renal-cell cancer correlates with the cytological tumour type. *Int J Cancer* 1993;53:353–357.

44. Stolle C, Glenn G, Zbar B, et al. Improved detection of germline mutations in the von Hippel-Lindau disease tumor suppressor gene. *Hum Mutat* 1998;12:417–423.

45. Salama ME, Worsham MJ, DePeralta-Venturina M. Malignant papillary renal tumors with extensive clear cell change: a molecular analysis by microsatellite analysis and fluorescence in situ hybridization. *Arch Pathol Lab Med* 2003;127:1176–1181.

46. Hoebeeck J, van der Luijt R, Poppe B, et al. Rapid detection of VHL exon deletions using real-time quantitative PCR. *Lab Invest* 2005;85:24–33.

47. Choyke PL, Glenn GM, Walther MM, et al. Hereditary renal cancers. *Radiology* 2003;226:33–46.

48. Meloni AM, White RD, Sandberg AA. -Y,-1 as recurrent anomaly in oncocytoma. *Cancer Genet Cytogenet* 1992;61:108–109.

49. Brauch H, Tory K, Linehan WM, et al. Molecular analysis of the short arm of chromosome 3 in five renal oncocytomas. *J Urol* 1990;143:622–624.

50. Fuzesi L, Gunawan B, Bergmann F, et al. Papillary renal cell carcinoma with clear cell cytomorphology and chromosomal loss of 3p. *Histopathology* 1999;35:157–161.

51. Shannon B, Stan Wisniewski Z, Bentel J, et al. Adult rhabdoid renal cell carcinoma. *Arch Pathol Lab Med* 2002;126:1506–1510.

52. Truong LD, Choi YJ, Shen SS, et al. Renal cystic neoplasms and renal neoplasms associated with cystic renal diseases: pathogenetic and molecular links. *Adv Anat Pathol* 2003;10:135–159.

53. Wick MR, Ritter JH, Humphrey PA, et al. Clear cell neoplasms of the endocrine system and thymus. *Semin Diagn Pathol* 1997;14:183–202.

54. Ritter JH, Mills SE, Gaffey MJ, et al. Clear cell tumors of the alimentary tract and abdominal cavity. *Semin Diagn Pathol* 1997;14:213–219.

55. Zbar B, Kishida T, Chen F, et al. Germline mutations in the Von Hippel-Lindau disease (VHL) gene in families from North America, Europe, and Japan. *Hum Mutat* 1996;8:348–357.

56. Friedrich CA. Genotype-phenotype correlation in von Hippel-Lindau syndrome. *Hum Mol Genet* 2001;10:763–767.

57. Clifford SC, Cockman ME, Smallwood AC, et al. Contrasting effects on HIF-1α regulation by disease-causing pVHL mutations correlate with patterns of tumourigenesis in von Hippel-Lindau disease. *Hum Mol Genet* 2001;10:1029–1038.

58. Takahashi M, Rhodes DR, Furge KA, et al. Gene expression profiling of clear cell renal cell carcinoma: gene identification and prognostic classification. *Proc Natl Acad Sci USA* 2001;98:9754–9759.

59. Vasselli JR, Shih JH, Iyengar SR, et al. Predicting survival in patients with metastatic kidney cancer by gene-expression profiling in the primary tumor. *Proc Natl Acad Sci USA* 2003;100:6958–6963.

60. Schmidt L, Duh FM, Chen F, et al. Germline and somatic mutations in the tyrosine kinase domain of the *MET* proto-oncogene in papillary renal carcinomas. *Nat Genet* 1997;16:68–73.

61. Bottaro DP, Rubin JS, Faletto DL, et al. Identification of the hepatocyte growth factor receptor as the c-*met* proto-oncogene product. *Science* 1991;251:802–804.

62. Schmidt L, Junker K, Nakaigawa N, et al. Novel mutations of the *MET* proto-oncogene in papillary renal carcinomas. *Oncogene* 1999;18:2343–2350.

63. Lubensky IA, Schmidt L, Zhuang Z, et al. Hereditary and sporadic papillary renal carcinomas with c-*met* mutations share a distinct morphological phenotype. *Am J Pathol* 1999;155:517–526.

64. Jeffers M, Schmidt L, Nakaigawa N, et al. Activating mutations for the *MET* tyrosine kinase receptor in human cancer. *Proc Natl Acad Sci USA* 1997;94:11445–11450.

65. Schmidt L, Junker K, Weirich G, et al. Two North American families with hereditary papillary renal carcinoma and identical novel mutations in the *MET* proto-oncogene. *Cancer Res* 1998;58:1719–1722.

66. Zhuang Z, Park WS, Pack S, et al. Trisomy 7-harbouring non-random duplication of the mutant *MET* allele in hereditary papillary renal carcinomas. *Nat Genet* 1998;20:66–69.

67. Fischer J, Palmedo G, von Knobloch R, et al. Duplication and overexpression of the mutant allele of the *MET* proto-oncogene in multiple hereditary papillary renal cell tumours. *Oncogene* 1998;17:733–739.

68. Takaki Y, Furihata M, Yoshikawa C, et al. Sporadic bilateral papillary renal carcinoma exhibiting c-*met* mutation in the left kidney tumor. *J Urol* 2000;163:1241–1242.

69. Kovacs G, Fuzesi L, Emanual A, et al. Cytogenetics of papillary renal cell tumors. *Genes Chromosomes Cancer* 1991;3:249–255.

70. Velickovic M, Delahunt B, Storkel S, et al. VHL and *FHIT* locus loss of heterozygosity is common in all renal cancer morphotypes but differs in pattern and prognostic significance. *Cancer Res* 2001;61:4815–4819.

71. Morrissey C, Martinez A, Zatyka M, et al. Epigenetic inactivation of the *RASSF1A* 3p21.3 tumor suppressor gene in both clear cell and papillary renal cell carcinoma. *Cancer Res* 2001;61:7277–7281.

72. Schraml P, Muller D, Bednar R, et al. Allelic loss at the *D9S171* locus on chromosome 9p13 is associated with progression of papillary renal cell carcinoma. *J Pathol* 2000;190:457–461.

73. Tomlinson IP, Alam NA, Rowan AJ, et al. Germline mutations in FH predispose to dominantly inherited uterine fibroids, skin leiomyomata and papillary renal cell cancer. *Nat Genet* 2002;30:406–410.

74. Kiuru M, Lehtonen R, Arola J, et al. Few FH mutations in sporadic counterparts of tumor types observed in hereditary leiomyomatosis and renal cell cancer families. *Cancer Res* 2002;62:4554–4557.

75. Lin ZH, Han EM, Lee ES, et al. A distinct expression pattern and point mutation of c-*kit* in papillary renal cell carcinomas. *Mod Pathol* 2004;17:611–616.

76. Duh FM, Scherer SW, Tsui LC, et al. Gene structure of the human *MET* proto-oncogene. *Oncogene* 1997;15:1583–1586.

77. Lindor NM, Dechet CB, Greene MH, et al. Papillary renal cell carcinoma: analysis of germline mutations in the *MET* proto-oncogene in a clinic-based population. *Genet Test* 2001;5:101–106.

78. Kattar MM, Grignon DJ, Wallis T, et al. Clinicopathologic and interphase cytogenetic analysis of papillary (chromophilic) renal cell carcinoma. *Mod Pathol* 1997;10:1143–1150.

79. Brunelli M, Eble JN, Zhang S, et al. Gains of chromosomes 7, 17, 12, 16, and 20 and loss of Y occur early in the evolution of papillary renal cell neoplasia: a fluorescence in situ hybridization study. *Mod Pathol* 2003;16:1053–1059.

80. Brown JA, Anderl KL, Borell TJ, et al. Simultaneous chromosome 7 and 17 gain and sex chromosome loss provide evidence that renal metanephric adenoma is related to papillary renal cell carcinoma. *J Urol* 1997;158:370–374.

81. Brunneli M, Eble JN, Zhang S, et al. Metanephric adenoma lacks the gains of chromosomes 7 and 17 and loss of Y that are typical of papillary renal cell carcinoma and papillary adenoma. *Mod Pathol* 2003;16:1060–1063.

82. Argani P, Antonescu CR, Illei PB, et al. Primary renal neoplasms with the *ASPL-TFE3* gene fusion of alveolar soft part sarcoma: a distinctive tumor entity previously included among renal cell carcinomas of children and adolescents. *Am J Pathol* 2001;159:179–192.

83. Heimann P, El Housni H, Ogur G, et al. Fusion of a novel gene, *RCC17*, to the *TFE3* gene in t(X;17)(p11.2;q25.3)-bearing papillary renal cell carcinomas. *Cancer Res* 2001;61:4130–4135.

84. Weterman MA, Wilbrink M, Geurts van Kessel A. Fusion of the transcription factor *TFE3* gene to a novel gene, *PRCC*, in t(X;1)(p11;q21)-positive papillary renal cell carcinomas. *Proc Natl Acad Sci USA* 1996;93:15294–15298.

85. Argani P, Antonescu CR, Couturier J, et al. *PRCC-TFE3* renal carcinomas: morphologic, immunohistochemical, ultrastructural, and molecular analysis of an entity associated with the t(X;1)(p11.2;q21). *Am J Surg Pathol* 2002;26:1553–1566.

86. Clark J, Lu YJ, Sidhar SK, et al. Fusion of splicing factor genes *PSF* and *NonO* (*p54nrb*) to the *TFE3* gene in papillary renal cell carcinoma. *Oncogene* 1997;15:2233–2239.

87. Argani P, Lui MY, Couturier J, et al. A novel *CLTC-TFE3* gene fusion in pediatric renal adenocarcinoma with t(X;17)(p11.2;q23). *Oncogene* 2003;22:5374–5378.

88. Kuiper RP, Schepens M, Thijssen J, et al. Upregulation of the transcription factor TFEB in t(6;11)(p21;q13)-positive renal cell carcinomas due to promoter substitution. *Hum Mol Genet* 2003;12:1661–1669.

89. Davis IJ, His BL, Arroyo JD, et al. Cloning of an α-TFEB fusion in renal tumors harboring the t(6;11)(p21;q13) chromosome translocation. *Proc Natl Acad Sci USA* 2003;100:6051–6056.

90. Quezado M, Benjamin DR, Tsokos M. *EWS/FLI-1* fusion transcripts in three peripheral primitive neuroectodermal tumors of the kidney. *Hum Pathol* 1997;28:767–771.

91. Marley EF, Liapis H, Humphrey PA, et al. Primitive neuroectodermal tumor of the kidney: another enigma: a pathologic, immunohistochemical, and molecular diagnostic study. *Am J Surg Pathol* 1997;21:354–359.

92. Parham DM, Roloson GJ, Feely M, et al. Primary malignant neuroepithelial tumors of the kidney: a clinicopathologic analysis of 146 adult and pediatric cases from the National Wilms' Tumor Study Group Pathology Center. *Am J Surg Pathol* 2001;25:133–146.

93. Kim DH, Sohn JH, Lee MC, et al. Primary synovial sarcoma of the kidney. *Am J Surg Pathol* 2000;24:1097–1104.

94. Argani P, Faria PA, Epstein JL, et al. Primary renal synovial sarcoma: molecular and morphologic delineation of an entity previously included among embryonal sarcomas of the kidney. *Am J Surg Pathol* 2000;24:1087–1096.

95. Jun SY, Choi J, Kang GH, et al. Synovial sarcoma of the kidney with rhabdoid features: report of three cases. *Am J Surg Pathol* 2004;28:634–637.

96. Rubin BP, Fletcher JA, Renshaw AA. Clear cell sarcoma of soft parts: report of a case primary in the kidney with cytogenetic confirmation. *Am J Surg Pathol* 1999;23:589–594.

97. Argani P, Ladanyi M. Distinctive neoplasms characterised by specific chromosomal translocations comprise a significant proportion of paediatric renal cell carcinomas. *Pathology* 2003;35:492–498.

98. Knezevich SR, Garnett MJ, Pysher TJ, et al. *ETV6-NTRK3* gene fusions and trisomy 11 establish a histogenetic link between mesoblastic nephroma and congenital fibrosarcoma. *Cancer Res* 1998;58:5046–5048.

99. Rubin BP, Chen CJ, Morgan TW, et al. Congenital mesoblastic nephroma t(12;15) is associated with *ETV6-NTRK3* gene fusion: cytogenetic and molecular relationship to congenital (infantile) fibrosarcoma. *Am J Pathol* 1998;153:1451–1458.

100. Su MC, Jeng YM, Chu YC, et al. Desmoplastic small round cell tumor of the kidney. *Am J Surg Pathol* 2004;28:1379–1383.

101. Argani P, Ladanyi M. Recent advances in pediatric renal neoplasia. *Adv Anat Pathol* 2003;10:243–260.

102. Argani P, Lal P, Hutchinson B, et al. Aberrant nuclear immunoreactivity for TFE3 in neoplasms with *TFE3* gene fusions: a sensitive and specific immunohistochemical assay. *Am J Surg Pathol* 2003;27:750–761.

103. Dijkhuizen T, van den Berg E, Storkel S, et al. Distinct features for chromophilic renal cell cancer with Xp11.2 breakpoints. *Cancer Genet Cytogenet* 1998;104:74–76.
104. Meloni AM, Dobbs RM, Pontes JE, et al. Translocation (X;1) in papillary renal cell carcinoma: a new cytogenetic subtype. *Cancer Genet Cytogenet* 1993;65:1–6.
105. Zattara-Cannoni H, Daniel L, Roll P, et al. Molecular cytogenetics of t(X;1)(p11.2;q21) with complex rearrangements in a renal cell carcinoma. *Cancer Genet Cytogenet* 2000;123:61–64.
106. Perot C, Boccon-Gibod L, Bouvier R, et al. Five new cases of juvenile renal cell carcinoma with translocations involving Xp11.2: a cytogenetic and morphologic study. *Cancer Genet Cytogenet* 2003;143:93–99.
107. Bruder E, Passera O, Harms D, et al. Morphologic and molecular characterization of renal cell carcinoma in children and young adults. *Am J Surg Pathol* 2004;28:1117–1132.
108. Chian-Garcia CA, Torres-Cabala CA, Eyler R, et al. Renal cell carcinoma in children and young adults: a clinicopathologic and immunohistochemical study of 14 cases. *Mod Pathol* 2003;16:145A.
109. Renshaw AA, Granter SR, Fletcher JA, et al. Renal cell carcinomas in children and young adults: increased incidence of papillary architecture and unique subtypes. *Am J Surg Pathol* 1999;23:795–802.
110. Ladanyi M, Lui MY, Antonescu CR, et al. The der(17)t(X;17)(p11;q25) of human alveolar soft part sarcoma fuses the *TFE3* transcription factor gene to *ASPL*, a novel gene at 17q25. *Oncogene* 2001;20:48–57.
111. Takebayashi K, Chida K, Tsukamoto I, et al. The recessive phenotype displayed by a dominant negative microphthalmia-associated transcription factor mutant is a result of impaired nucleation potential. *Mol Cell Biol* 1996;16:1203–1211.
112. Skalsky YM, Ajuh PM, Parker C, et al. *PRCC*, the commonest *TFE3* fusion partner in papillary renal carcinoma is associated with pre-mRNA splicing factors. *Oncogene* 2001;20:178–187.
113. Weterman MAJ, van Groningen JJ, Jansen A, et al. Nuclear localization and transactivating capacities of the papillary renal cell carcinoma-associated TFE3 and PRCC (fusion) proteins. *Oncogene* 2000;19:69–74.
114. Weterman MA, van Groningen JJ, Tertoolen L, et al. Impairment of *MAD2B-PRCC* interaction in mitotic checkpoint defective t(X;1)-positive renal cell carcinomas. *Proc Natl Acad Sci USA* 2001;98:13808–13813.
115. Sandberg AA, Bridge JA. Updates on the cytogenetics and molecular genetics of bone and soft tissue tumors: alveolar soft part sarcoma. *Cancer Genet Cytogenet* 2002;136:1–9.
116. Dijkhuizen T, van den Berg E, Storkel S, et al. Two cases of renal cell carcinoma, clear cell type, revealing a t(6;11)(p21;q13). *Cancer Genet Cytogenet* 1996;91:141.
117. Argani P, Hawkins A, Griffin CA, et al. A distinctive pediatric renal neoplasm characterized by epithelioid morphology, basement membrane production, focal *HMB45* immunoreactivity, and t(6;11)(p21.1;q12) chromosome translocation. *Am J Pathol* 2001;158:2089–2096.
118. Argani P, Lae M, Hutchinson B, et al. Renal carcinomas with the t(6;11)(p21;q12): clinicopathologic features and demonstration of the specific *alpha-TFEB* gene fusion by immunohistochemistry, RT-PCR, and DNA PCR. *Am J Surg Pathol* 2005;29:230–240.
119. Du J, Miller AJ, Widlund HR, et al. MLANA/MART1 and SILV/PMEL17/GP100 are transcriptionally regulated by MITF in melanocytes and melanoma. *Am J Pathol* 2003; 163:333–343.
120. Thoenes W, Storkel S, Rumpelt HJ, et al. Chromophobe cell renal carcinoma and its variants: a report on 32 cases. *J Pathol* 1988;155:277–287.
121. Brunelli M, Eble JN, Zhang S, et al. Eosinophilic and classic chromophobe renal cell carcinomas have similar frequent losses of multiple chromosomes from among chromosomes 1, 2, 6, 10, and 17, and this pattern of genetic abnormality is not present in renal oncocytoma. *Mod Pathol* 2005;18:161–169.
122. Kovacs A, Kovacs G. Low chromosome number in chromophobe renal cell carcinomas. *Genes Chromosomes Cancer* 1992;4:267–368.
123. Gunawan B, Bergmann F, Braun S, et al. Polyploidization and losses of chromosomes 1, 2, 6, 10, 13, and 17 in three cases of chromophobe renal cell carcinomas. *Cancer Genet Cytogenet* 1999;110:57–61.
124. Iqbal MA, Akhtar M, Ali MA. Cytogenetic findings in renal cell carcinoma. *Hum Pathol* 1996;27:949–954.
125. Akhtar M, Chantziantoniou N. Flow cytometric and quantitative image cell analysis of DNA ploidy in renal chromophobe cell carcinoma. *Hum Pathol* 1998;29:1181–1188.
126. Speicher MR,Schoell B, du Manoir S, et al. Specific loss of chromosomes 1, 2, 6, 10, 13, 17, and 21 in chromophobe renal cell carcinomas revealed by comparative genomic hybridization. *Am J Pathol* 1994;145:356–364.
127. Iqbal MA, Akhtar M, Ulmer C, et al. FISH analysis in chromophobe renal-cell carcinoma. *Diagn Cytopathol* 2000;22:3–6.
128. Schofield DE, Yunis EJ, Fletcher JA. Chromosome aberrations in mesoblastic nephroma. *Am J Pathol* 1993;143:714–724.
129. Lannon CL, Martin MJ, Tognon CE, et al. A highly conserved NTRK3 C-terminal sequence in the ETV6-NTRK3 oncoprotein binds the phosphotyrosine binding domain of insulin receptor substrate-1: an essential interaction for transformation. *J Biol Chem* 2004;279:6225–6234.
130. Ladanyi M. Aberrant ALK tyrosine kinase signaling: different cellular lineages, common oncogenic mechanisms. *Am J Pathol* 2000;157:341–345.
131. Knezevich SR, McFadden DE, Tao W, et al. A novel *ETV6-NTRK3* gene fusion in congenital fibrosarcoma. *Nat Genet* 1998;18:184–187.
132. Adem C, Gisselsson D, Dal Cin PD, et al. *ETV6* rearrangements in patients with infantile fibrosarcomas and congenital mesoblastic nephromas by fluorescence in situ hybridization. *Mod Pathol* 2001;14:1246–1251.
133. Argani P, Fritsch M, Kadkol S, et al Detection of the *ETV6-NTRK3* chimeric RNA of infantile fibrosarcoma/cellular congenital mesoblastic nephroma in paraffin-embedded tissue: application to challenging pediatric renal stromal tumors. *Mod Pathol* 2000; 13:29–36.
134. Eguchi M, Eguchi-Ishimae M, Tojo A, et al. Fusion of *ETV6* to neurotrophin-3 receptor TRKC in acute myeloid leukemia with t(12;15)(p13;q25). *Blood* 1999;93:1355–1563.
135. Alessandri AJ, Knezevich SR, Mathers JA, et al. Absence of t(12;15) associated *ETV6-NTRK3* fusion transcripts in pediatric acute leukemias. *Med Pediatr Oncol* 2001; 37:415–416.
136. Eguchi M, Eguchi-Ishimai M. Absence of t(12;15) associated *ETV6-NTRK3* fusion transcripts in pediatric acute leukemias [Letter]. *Med Pediatr Oncol* 2001;37:417.
137. Tognon C, Knezevich SR, Huntsman D, et al. Expression of the *ETV6-NTRK3* gene fusion as a primary event in human secretory breast carcinoma. *Cancer Cell* 2002;2:367–376.
138. Diallo R, Schaefer KL, Bankfalvi A, et al. Secretory carcinoma of the breast: a distinct variant of invasive ductal carcinoma assessed by comparative genomic hybridization and immunohistochemistry. *Hum Pathol* 2003;34:1299–1305.
139. Versteege I, Sevenet N, Lange J, et al. Truncating mutations of *hSNF5/INI1* in aggressive paediatric cancer. *Nature* 1998;394:203–206.
140. Biegel JA, Tan L, Zhang F, et al. Alterations of the *hSNF5/INI1* gene in central nervous system atypical teratoid/rhabdoid tumors and renal and extrarenal rhabdoid tumors. *Clin Cancer Res* 2002;8:3461–3467.
141. Kalpana GV, Marmon S, Wang W, et al. Binding and stimulation of HIV-1 integrase by a human homolog of yeast transcription factor *SNF5*. *Science* 1994;266:2002–2006.
142. Muchardt C, Sardet C, Bourachot B, et al. A human protein with homology to *Saccharomyces cerevisiae SNF5* interacts with the potential helicase hbrm. *Nucleic Acids Res* 1995;23:1127–1132.
143. Lee HY, Yoon CS, Sevenet N, et al. Rhabdoid tumor of the kidney is a component of the rhabdoid predisposition syndrome. *Pediatr Dev Pathol* 2002:395–399.
144. Kusafuka T, MIao J, Yoneda A, et al. Novel germ-line deletion of *SNF5/INI1/SMARCB1* gene in neonate presenting with congenital malignant rhabdoid tumor of kidney and brain primitive neuroectodermal tumor. *Genes Chromosomes Cancer* 2004;40:133–139.
145. Sevenet N, Sheridan E, Amram D, et al. Constitutional mutations of the *hSNF5/INI1* gene predispose to a variety of cancers. *Am J Hum Genet* 1999;65:1342–1348.
146. Shashi V, Lovell MA, von Kap-herr C, et al. Malignant rhabdoid tumor of the kidney: involvement of chromosome 22. *Genes Chromosomes Cancer* 1994;10:49–54.
147. Biegel JA, Allen CS, Kawasaki K, et al. Narrowing the critical region for a rhabdoid tumor locus in 22q11. *Genes Chromosomes Cancer* 1996;16:94–105.
148. Rosty C, Peter M, Zucman J, et al. Cytogenetic and molecular analysis of a t(1;22)(p36;q11.2) in a rhabdoid tumor with a putative homozygous deletion of chromosome 22. *Genes Chromosomes Cancer* 1998;21:82–89.
149. Rousseau-Merck MF, Versteege I, Legrand I, et al. *hSNF5/INI1* inactivation is mainly associated with homozygous deletions and mitotic recombinations in rhabdoid tumors. *Cancer Res* 1999;59:3152–3156.
150. Hoot AC, Russo P, Judkins AR, et al. Immunohistochemical analysis of *hSNF5/INI1* distinguishes renal and extra-renal malignant rhabdoid tumors from other pediatric soft tissue tumors. *Am J Surg Pathol* 2004;28:1485–1491.
151. Weeks DA, Beckwith JB, Mierau GW, et al. Renal neoplasms mimicking rhabdoid tumor of kidney: a report from the National Wilms' Tumor Study Pathology Center. *Am J Surg Pathol* 19911;5:1042–1054.
152. Gokden N, Nappi O, Swanson P, et al. Renal cell carcinoma with rhabdoid features. *Am J Surg Pathol* 2000;24:1329–1338.
153. Shannon BA, Cohen RJ. Rhabdoid differentiation of chromophobe renal cell carcinoma. *Pathology* 2003;35:228–230.
154. Wick MR, Ritter JH, Dehner LP. Malignant rhabdoid tumors: a clinicopathologic review and conceptual discussion. *Semin Diagn Pathol* 1995;12:233–248.
155. Guillou L, Wadden C, Coindre JM, et al. "Proximal-type" epithelioid sarcoma, a distinctive aggressive neoplasm showing rhabdoid features: clinicopathologic, immunohistochemical, and ultrastructural study of a series. *Am J Surg Pathol* 1997;21:130–146.
156. Parham DM, Weeks DA, Beckwith JB. The clinicopathologic spectrum of putative extrarenal rhabdoid tumors: an analysis of 42 cases studied with immunohistochemistry or electron microscopy. *Am J Surg Pathol* 1994;18:1010–1029.
157. Green DM, Coppes MJ, Breslow NE, et al. Wilms tumor. In: Pizzo PA, ed. *Principles and Practice of Pediatric Oncology*. Philadelphia: Lippincott-Raven; 1997:733–759.
158. Dome JS, Coppes MJ. Recent advances in Wilms tumor genetics. *Curr Opin Pediatr* 2002;14:5–11.
159. Coppes MJ, Huff V, Pelletier J. Denys-Drash syndrome: relating a clinical disorder to genetic alterations in the tumor suppressor gene *WT1*. *J Pediatr* 1993;123:673–678.
160. Huff V. Wilms tumor genetics. *Am J Med Genet* 1998;79:260–267.
161. Lee SB, Haber DA. Wilms tumor and the *WT1* gene. *Exp Cell Res* 2001;264:74–99.
162. Diller L, Ghahremani M, Morgan J, et al. Constitutional *WT1* mutations in Wilms' tumor patients. *J Clin Oncol* 1998;16:3634–3640.
163. Varanasi R, Bardeesy N, Petruzzi MJ, et al. Fine structure analysis of the *WT1* gene in sporadic Wilms tumors. *Proc Natl Acad Sci USA* 1994;91:3554–3558.
164. Gessler M. Konig A, Arden K, et al. Infrequent mutation of the *WT1* gene in 77 Wilms' tumors. *Hum Mutat* 1994;3:212–222.
165. Baudry D, Hamelin M, Cabanis MO, et al. *WT1* splicing alterations in Wilms' tumors. *Clin Cancer Res* 2000;6:3957–3965.
166. Mares J, Kriz V, Weinhausel A, et al. Methylation changes in promoter and enhancer regions of the *WT1* gene in Wilms' tumours. *Cancer Lett* 2001;166:165–171.
167. Maher ER, Reik W. Beckwith-Wiedemann syndrome: imprinting in clusters revisited. *J Clin Invest* 2000;105:247–252.
168. Steenman M, Westerveid A, Mannens M. Genetics of Beckwith-Wiedemann syndrome-associated tumors: common genetic pathways. *Genes Chromosomes Cancer* 2000;28: 1–13.
169. Rahman N, Arbour L, Tonin P, et al. Evidence for a familial Wilms' tumour gene (*FWT1*) on chromosome 17q12-q21. *Nat Genet* 1996;13:461–463.
170. Rahman N, Abidi F, Ford D, et al. Confirmation of *FWT1* as a Wilms' tumour susceptibility gene and phenotypic characteristics of Wilms' tumour attributable to *FWT1*. *Hum Genet* 1998;103:547–556.
171. McDonald JM, Douglass EC, Fisher R, et al. Linkage of familial Wilms' tumor predisposition to chromosome 19 and a two-locus model for the etiology of familial tumors. *Cancer Res* 1998;58:1387–1390.
172. Ruteshouser EC, Huff V. Familial Wilms tumor. *Am J Med Genet* 2004;129C:29–34.
173. Rapley EA, Barfoot R, Bonaiti-Pellie C, et al. Evidence for susceptibility genes to familial Wilms tumour in addition to *WT1*, *FWT1* and *FWT2*. *Br J Cancer* 2000;83:177–183.
174. Beniers AJ, Efferth T, Fuzesi L, et al. *p53* expression in Wilms' tumor: a possible role as prognostic factor. *Int J Oncol* 2001;18:133–139.
175. Bardeesy N, Falkoff D, Petruzzi MJ, et al. Anaplastic Wilms' tumour, a subtype displaying poor prognosis, harbours *p53* gene mutations. *Nat Genet* 1994;7:91–97.
176. Malkin D, Sexsmith E, Yeger H, et al. Mutations of the *p53* tumor suppressor gene occur infrequently in Wilms' tumor. *Cancer Res* 1994;54:2077–2079.

177. Bardeesy N, Beckwith JB, Pelletier J. Clonal expansion and attenuated apoptosis in Wilms' tumors are associated with *p53* gene mutations. *Cancer Res* 1995;55:215–219.
178. Ramburan A, Chetty R, Hadley GP, et al. Microsatellite analysis of the *DCC* gene in nephroblastomas: pathologic correlations and prognostic implications. *Mod Pathol* 2004;17:89–95.
179. Lu YJ, Williamson D, Wang R, et al. Expression profiling targeting chromosomes for tumor classification and prediction of clinical behavior. *Genes Chromosomes Cancer* 2003;38:207–214.
180. Williams RD, Hing SN, Greer BT, et al. Prognostic classification of relapsing favorable histology Wilms tumor using cDNA microarray expression profiling and support vector machines. *Genes Chromosomes Cancer* 2004;41:65–79.
181. Takahashi M, Yang XJ, Lavery TT, et al. Gene expression profiling of favorable histology Wilms tumors and its correlation with clinical features. *Cancer Res* 2002;62:6598–6605.
182. Badenas C, Praga M, Tazon B, et al. Mutations in the *COL4A4* and *COL4A3* genes cause familial benign hematuria. *J Am Soc Nephrol* 2002;13:1248–1254.
183. Buzza M, Wilson D, Savige J. Segregation of hematuria in thin basement membrane disease with haplotypes at the loci for Alport syndrome. *Kidney Int* 2001;59:1670–1676.
184. Barker DF, Hostikka SL, Zhou J, et al. Identification of mutations in the *COL4A5* collagen gene in Alport syndrome. *Science* 1990;248:1224–1227.
185. Dreyer SD, Zhou G, Baldini A, et al. Mutations in *LMX1B* cause abnormal skeletal patterning and renal dysplasia in nail patella syndrome. *Nat Genet* 1998;19:47–50.
186. Kestila M, Lenkerri U, Mannikko M, et al. Positionally cloned gene for a novel glomerular protein—nephrin—is mutated in congenital nephrotic syndrome. *Mol Cell* 1998; 1:575–582.
187. Boute N, Gribouval O, Roselli S, et al. *NPHS2*, encoding the glomerular protein podocin, is mutated in autosomal recessive steroid-resistant nephrotic syndrome. *Nat Genet* 2000;24:349–354.
188. Fuchshuber A, Jean G, Gribouval O, et al. Mapping a gene (*SRN1*) to chromosome 1q25-q31 in idiopathic nephrotic syndrome confirms a distinct entity of autosomal recessive nephrosis. *Hum Mol Genet* 1995;4:2155–2158.
189. Caridi G, Bertelli R, Carrea A, et al. Prevalence, genetics, and clinical features of patients carrying podocin mutations in steroid-resistant nonfamilial focal segmental glomerulosclerosis. *J Am Soc Nephrol* 2001;12:2742–2746.
190. Karle SM, Uetz B, Ronner V, et al. Novel mutations in *NPHS2* detected in both familial and sporadic steroid-resistant nephrotic syndrome. *J Am Soc Nephrol* 2002;13:388–393.
191. Kaplan JM, Kim SH, North KN, et al. Mutations in *ACTN4*, encoding alpha-actinin-4, cause familial focal segmental glomerulosclerosis. *Nat Genet* 2000;24:251–256.
192. Winn MP, Conlon PJ, Lynn KL, et al. A mutation in the TRPC6 cation channel causes familial focal segmental glomerulosclerosis. *Science* 2005;308:1801–1804.
193. Barbaux S, Niaudet P, Gubler MC, et al. Donor splice-site mutations in *WT1* are responsible for Frasier syndrome. *Nat Genet* 1997;17:467–470.
194. Pelletier J, Bruening W, Kashtan C, et al. Germline mutations in the Wilms' tumor suppressor gene are associated with abnormal urogenital development in Denys-Drash syndrome. *Cell* 1991;67:437–447.
195. Pastores GM, Lien YH. Biochemical and molecular genetic basis of Fabry disease. *J Am Soc Nephrol* 2002;13:S130–S133.
196. Grunfeld JP, Chauveau D, Levy M. Anderson-Fabry disease: its place among other genetic causes of renal disease. *J Am Soc Nephrol* 2002;13:S126–S129.
197. Liberopoulos E, Siamopoulos K, Elisaf M. Apolipoprotein E and renal disease. *Am J Kidney Dis* 2004;43:223–233.
198. Kuivenhoven JA, Pritchard H, Hill J, et al. The molecular pathology of lecithin:cholesterol acyltransferase (LCAT) deficiency syndromes. *J Lipid Res* 1997;38:191–205.
199. Dragon-Durey MA, Fremeaux-Bacchi V, Loirat C, et al. Heterozygous and homozygous factor h deficiencies associated with hemolytic uremic syndrome or membranoproliferative glomerulonephritis: report and genetic analysis of 16 cases. *J Am Soc Nephrol* 2004;15:787–795.
200. Scolari F. Inherited forms of IgA nephropathy. *J Nephrol* 2003;16:317–320.
201. Savige J, Rana K, Tonna S, et al. Thin basement membrane nephropathy. *Kidney Int* 2003;64:1169–1178.
202. Liapis H, Gokden N, Hmiel P, et al. Histopathology, ultrastructure, and clinical phenotypes in thin glomerular basement membrane disease variants. *Hum Pathol* 2002; 33:836–845.
203. Kashtan CE. Familial hematuria due to type IV collagen mutations: Alport syndrome and thin basement membrane nephropathy. *Curr Opin Pediatr* 2004; 16:177–181.
204. Pollak MR. The genetic basis of FSGS and steroid-resistant nephrosis. *Semin Nephrol* 2003;23:141–146.
205. Jalanko H, Patrakka J, Tryggvason K, et al. Genetic kidney diseases disclose the pathogenesis of proteinuria. *Ann Med* 2001;33:526–533.
206. Liapis H, Foster K, Theodoropoulou E, et al. Phenotype/genotype correlations in the ultrastrucdture of monogenetic glomerular diseases. *Ultrastruct Pathol* 2004;28: 181–197.
207. Hudson BG, Tryggvason K, Sundaramoorthy M, et al. Alport's syndrome, Goodpasture's syndrome, and type IV collagen. *N Engl J Med* 2003;348:2543–2556.
208. Mazzucco G, Barsotti P, Muda AO, et al. Ultrastructural and immunohistochemical findings in Alport's syndrome: a study of 108 patients from 97 Italian families with particular emphasis on *COL4A5* gene mutation correlations. *J Am Soc Nephrol* 1998; 9:1023–1031.
209. http://archive.uwcm.ac.uk/uwcm/mg/hgmd0.html
210. Kashtan CE. Alport syndromes: phenotypic heterogeneity of progressive hereditary nephritis. *Pediatr Nephrol* 2000;14:502–512.
211. Jais JP, Knebelmann B, Giatras I, et al. X-linked Alport syndrome: natural history in 195 families and genotype-phenotype correlations in males. *J Am Soc Nephrol* 2000; 11:649–657.
212. Steele DJ, Michaels PJ. Case records of the Massachusetts General Hospital: weekly clinicopathological exercises. Case 40-2004: a 42-year-old woman with long-standing hematuria. *N Engl J Med* 2004;351:2851–2859.
213. Buzza M, Dagher H, Wang YY, et al. Mutations in the *COL4A4* gene in thin basement membrane disease. *Kidney Int* 2003;63:447–453.
214. Bongers EM, Gubler MC, Knoers NV. Nail-patella syndrome: overview on clinical and molecular findings. *Pediatr Nephrol* 2002;17:703–712.
215. Miner JH, Morello R, Andrews KL, et al. Transcriptional induction of slit diaphragm genes by Lmx1b is required in podocyte differentiation. *J Clin Invest* 2002;109:1065–1072.
216. Shih NY, Li J, Karpitskii V, et al. Congenital nephrotic syndrome in mice lacking CD2-associated protein. *Science* 1999;286:312–315.
217. Patrakka J, Kestila M, Wartiovaara J, et al. Congenital nephrotic syndrome (NPHS1): features resulting from different mutations in Finnish patients. *Kidney Int* 2000; 58:972–980.
218. Wachsstock DH, Schwartz WH, Pollard TD. Affinity of *alpha*-actinin for actin determines the structure and mechanical properties of actin filament gels. *Biophys J* 1993; 65:205–214.
219. http://www.cc.utah.edu/~cla6202/ASHP.htm#GT
220. http://www.moldiag.com/en/cgi/fmsearch.cgi
221. Parkin DM, Whelan SL, Ferlay J, et al. eds. *Cancer Incidence in Five Continents*. IARC Scientific Publications No. 155. Lyon: IARC Press; 2003.
222. Epstein JI, Amin MB, Reuter VR, et al. The World Health Organization/International Society of Urological Pathology consensus classification of urothelial (transitional cell) neoplasms of the urinary bladder. Bladder Consensus Conference Committee. *Am J Surg Pathol* 1998;22:1435–1448.
223. Yin H, Leong AS. Histologic grading of noninvasive papillary urothelial tumors: validation of the 1998 WHO/ISUP system by immunophenotyping and follow-up. *Am J Clin Pathol* 2004;121:679–687.
224. Al-Sukhun S, Hussain M. Molecular biology of transitional cell carcinoma. *Crit Rev Oncol Hematol* 2003;47:181–193.
225. Ragjavan D. Molecular targeting and pharmacogenomics in the management of advanced bladder cancer. *Cancer* 2003;97:2083–2089.
226. Munro NP, Knowles MA. Fibroblast growth factors and their receptors in transitional cell carcinoma. *J Urol* 2003;169:675–682.
227. Diaz-Cano SJ, Blanes A, Rubio J, et al. Molecular evolution and intratumor heterogeneity by topographic compartments in muscle-invasive transitional cell carcinoma of the urinary bladder. *Lab Invest* 2000;80:279–289.
228. Richter J, Beffa L, Wagner U, et al. Patterns of chromosomal imbalances in advanced urinary bladder cancer detected by comparative genomic hybridization. *Am J Pathol* 1998;153:1615–1621.
229. Simon R, Burger H, Brinkschmidt C, et al. Patterns of chromosomal aberrations in urinary bladder tumours and adjacent urothelium. *J Pathol* 2002;198:115–120.
230. Cattan N, Saison-Behmoaras T, Mari B, et al. Screening of human bladder carcinomas for the presence of Ha-*ras* codon 12 mutation. *Oncol Rep* 2000;7:497–500.
231. Fitzgerald JM, Ramchurren N, Rieger K, et al. Identification of H-*ras* mutations in urine sediments complements cytology in the detection of bladder tumors. *J Natl Cancer Inst* 1995;87:129–133.
232. Knowles MA, Williamson M. Mutation of H-*ras* is infrequent in bladder cancer: confirmation by single-strand conformation polymorphism analysis, designed restriction fragment length polymorphisms, and direct sequencing. *Cancer Res* 1993;53:133–139.
233. Liukkonen T, Lipponen P, Raitanen M, et al. Evaluation of *p21WAF1/CIP1* and cyclin D1 expression in the progression of superficial bladder cancer. Finbladder Group. *Urol Res* 2000;28:285–292.
234. Suwa Y, Takano Y, Iki M, et al. Cyclin D1 protein overexpression is related to tumor differentiation, but not to tumor progression or proliferative activity, in transitional cell carcinoma of the bladder. *J Urol* 1998;160:897–900.
235. Wagner U, Suess K, Luginbuhl T, et al. Cyclin D1 overexpression lacks prognostic significance in superficial urinary bladder cancer. *J Pathol* 1999;188:44–50.
236. Cordon-Cardo C, Reuter VE. Alterations of tumor suppressor genes in bladder cancer. *Semin Diagn Pathol* 1997;14:123–132.
237. Korkolopoulou P, Christodoulou P, Konstantinidou AE, et al. Cell cycle regulators in bladder cancer: a multivariate survival study with emphasis on *p27Kip1*. *Hum Pathol* 2000;31:751–760.
238. Esrig D, Elmajian D, Groshen S, et al. Accumulation of nuclear *p53* and tumor progression in bladder cancer. *N Engl J Med* 1994;331:1259–1264.
239. Stein JP, Ginsberg DA, Grossfield GD, et al. Effect of *p21WAF1/CIP1* expression on tumor progression in bladder cancer. *J Natl Cancer Inst* 1998;90:1072–1079.
240. Harris BE, Song R, Soong S, et al. Relationship between dihydropyrimidine dehydrogenase activity and plasma 5-fluorouracil levels with evidence for circadian variation of enzyme activity and plasma drug levels in cancer patients receiving 5-fluorouracil by protracted continuous infusion. *Cancer Res* 1990;50:197–201.
241. Harris JW, Rahman A, Kim BR, et al. metabolism of taxol by human hepatic microsomes and liver slices: participation of cytochrome P450 3A4 and an unknown P450 enzyme. *Cancer Res* 1994;54:4026–4035.
242. Royer I, Monsarrat B, Sonnier M, et al. metabolism of docetaxel by human cytochromes P450: interactions with paclitaxel and other antineoplastic drugs. *Cancer Res* 1996;56:58–65.
243. Waxman DJ. Glutathione S-transferases: role in alkylating agent resistance and possible target for modulation chemotherapy—a review. *Cancer Res* 1990;50:6449–6454.
244. Okegawa T, Kinjo M, Nutahara K, et al. Value of reverse transcription polymerase chain assay in peripheral blood of patients with urothelial cancer. *J Urol* 2004;171: 1461–1466.
245. Denis MG, Lipart C, Leborgne J, et al. Detection of disseminated tumor cells in peripheral blood of colorectal cancer patients. *Int J Cancer* 1997;74:540–544.
246. Jung R, Petersen K, Kruger W, et al. Detection of micrometastasis by cytokeratin 20 RT-PCR is limited due to stable background transcription in granulocytes. *Br J Cancer* 1999;81:870–873.
247. Bustin SA, Gyselman VG, Siddiqi S, et al. Cytokeratin 20 is not a tissue-specific marker for the detection of malignant epithelial cells in the blood of colorectal cancer patients. *Int J Surg Investig* 2000;2:49–57.
248. Vlems FA, Diepstra JH, Cornelissen IM, et al. Investigations for a multi-marker RT-PCR to improve sensitivity of disseminated tumor cell detection. *Anticancer Res* 2003; 23:179–186.
249. Rabbani F, Perrotti M, Russo P, et al. Upper-tract tumors after an initial diagnosis of bladder cancer: argument for long-term surveillance. *J Clin Oncol* 2001;19:94–100.
250. Sokolova IA, Halling KC, Jenkins RB, et al. The development of a multitarget, multicolor fluorescence in situ hybridization assay for the detection of urothelial carcinoma in urine. *J Mol Diagn* 2000;2:116–123.

251. Halling KC, King W, Sokolova IA, et al. A comparison of cytology and fluorescence in situ hybridization for the detection of urothelial carcinoma. *J Urol* 2000;164:1768–1775.

252. Veeramachaneni R, Nordberg ML, Shi R, et al. Evaluation of fluorescence in situ hybridization as an ancillary tool to urine cytology in diagnosing urothelial carcinoma. *Diagn Cytopathol* 2003;28:301–307.

253. Skacel M, Fahmy M, Brainard JA, et al. Multitarget fluorescence in situ hybridization assay detects transitional cell carcinoma in the majority of patients with bladder cancer and atypical or negative urine cytology. *J Urol* 2003;169:2101–2105.

254. Bubendorf L, Grilli B, Sauter G, et al. Multiprobe FISH for enhanced detection of bladder cancer in voided urine specimens and bladder washings. *Am J Clin Pathol* 2001;116:79–86.

255. Sarosdy MF, Schellhammer P, Bokinsky G, et al. Clinical evaluation of a multi-target fluorescent in situ hybridization assay for detection of bladder cancer. *J Urol* 2002;168:1950–1954.

256. Halling KC, King W, Sokolova IA, et al. A comparison of BTA stat, hemoglobin dipstick, telomerase and Vysis UroVysion assays for the detection of urothelial carcinoma in urine. *J Urol* 2002;167:2001–2006.

257. Berger AP, ParsonW, Stenzl A, et al. Microsatellite alterations in human bladder cancer: detection of tumor cells in urine sediment and tumor tissue. *Eur Urol* 2002;41:532–539.

258. Utting M, Werner W, Dahse R, et al. Microsatellite analysis of free tumor DNA in urine, serum, and plasma of patients: a minimally invasive method for the detection of bladder cancer. *Clin Cancer Res* 2002;8:35–40.

259. Suzuki T, Suzuki Y, Fujioka T. Expression of the catalytic subunit associated with telomerase gene in human urinary bladder cancer. *J Urol* 1999;162:2217–2220.

260. Bialkowska-Hobrzanska H, Bowles L, Bukala B, et al. Comparison of human telomerase reverse transcriptase messenger RNA and telomerase activity as urine markers for diagnosis of bladder carcinoma. *Mol Diagn* 2000;5:267–277.

261. Eissa S, Labib RA, Mourad MS, et al. Comparison of telomerase activity and matrix metalloproteinase-9 in voided urine and bladder wash samples as a useful diagnostic tool for bladder cancer. *Eur Urol* 2003;44:687–694.

262. Melissourgos N, Kastrinakis NG, Davilas I, et al. Detection of human telomerase reverse transcriptase mRNA in urine of patients with bladder cancer: evaluation of an emerging tumor marker. *Urology* 2003;62:362–367.

263. Isurugi K, Suzuki Y, Tanji S, et al. Detection of the presence of catalytic subunit mRNA associated with telomerase gene in exfoliated urothelial cells from patients with bladder cancer. *J Urol* 2002;168:1574–1577.

264. Cordon-Cardo C, Dalbagni G, Saez GT, et al. p53 mutations in human bladder cancer: genotypic versus phenotypic patterns. *Int J Cancer* 1994;56:347–353.

265. Sauter G, Gasser TC, Moch H, et al. DNA aberrations in urinary bladder cancer detected by flow cytometry and FISH. *Urol Res* 1997;25:S37–S43.

266. Zhang FF, Arber DA, Wilson TG, et al. Toward the validation of aneusomy detection by fluorescence in situ hybridization in bladder cancer: comparative analysis with cytology, cytogenetics, and clinical features predicts recurrence and defines clinical testing limitations. *Clin Cancer Res* 1997;3:2317–2328.

267. Fujimoto K, Yamada Y, Okajima E, et al. Frequent association of p53 gene mutation in invasive bladder cancer. *Cancer Res* 1992;52:1393–1398.

268. Simon R, Burger H, Brinkschmidt C, et al. Chromosomal aberrations associated with invasion in papillary superficial bladder cancer. *J Pathol* 1998;185:345–351.

269. Richter J, Jiang F, Gorog JP, et al. Marked genetic differences between stage pTa and stage pT1 papillary bladder cancer detected by comparative genomic hybridization. *Cancer Res* 1997;57:2860–2864.

270. Sauter G, Mihatsch MJ. Pussycats and baby tigers: non-invasive (pTa) and minimally invasive (pT1) bladder carcinomas are not the same! *J Pathol* 1998;185:339–341.

271. Knowles MA. What we could do now: molecular pathology of bladder cancer. *Mol Pathol* 2001;54:215–221.

272. Stein JP, Grossfeld GD, Ginsberg DA, et al. Prognostic markers in bladder cancer: a contemporary review of the literature. *J Urol* 1998;160:645–659.

273. Williams SG, Buscarini M, Stein JP. Molecular markers for diagnosis, staging, and prognosis of bladder cancer. *Oncology* 2001;15:1461–776.

274. Colecchia M, Dagrada GP, Poliani, et al. Immunophenotypic and genotypic analysis of a case of primary peripheral primitive neuroectodermal tumour (pPNET) of the urinary bladder [Letter]. *Histopathology* 2002;40:103–113.

275. Kruger S, Schmidt H, Kausch I, et al. Primitive neuroectodermal tumor (PNET) of the urinary bladder. *Pathol Res Pract* 2003;199:751–754.

276. Entz-Werle N, Marcellin L, Becmeur F, et al. The urinary bladder: an extremely rare location of pediatric neuroblastoma. *J Pediatr Surg* 2003;38:E10–E12.

277. Saez C, Marquez C, Quiroga E, et al. Neuroblastoma of the urinary bladder in an infant clinically detected by hematuria. *Med Pediatr Oncol* 2000;35:488–492.

278. Freeman A, Geddes N, Munson P, et al. Anaplastic lymphoma kinase (ALK 1) staining and molecular analysis in inflammatory myofibroblastic tumours of the bladder: a preliminary clinicopathological study of nine cases and review of the literature. *Mod Pathol* 2004;17:765–771.

279. Debiec-Rychter M, Marynen P, Hagemeijer A, et al. ALK-ATIC fusion in urinary bladder inflammatory myofibroblastic tumor. *Genes Chromosomes Cancer* 2003;38:187–190.

280. Tsuzuki T, Magi-Galluzzi C, Epstein JI, et al. ALK-1 expression in inflammatory myofibroblastic tumor of the urinary bladder. *Am J Surg Pathol* 2004;28:1609–1614.

281. Lasota J, Carlson JA, Miettinen M. Spindle cell tumor of urinary bladder serosa with phenotypic and genotypic features of gastrointestinal stromal tumor. *Arch Pathol Lab Med* 2000;124:894–897.

Skin

MELANOMA

Melanoma is responsible for less than 4% of all skin cancers worldwide, but accounts for the greatest number of skin cancer–related deaths. Both constitutional and behavioral factors are associated with an increased risk of the disease. Constitutional risk factors, which are fixed, include a sun-sensitive phenotype (freckling, fair skin), number of nevi (acquired or atypical), and a hereditary predisposition syndrome (familial atypical mole and melanoma syndrome, xeroderma pigmentosa) (1,2). Behavioral risk factors, which are potentially modifiable, include exposures to doses of ultraviolet light that lead to sunburns. Worldwide, there is an increasing incidence of melanoma; while surveillance efforts have been successful in detecting thin melanomas that are potentially more curable, there has not been a significant change in the incidence of thick melanomas or the overall mortality rate.

Genetics of Cutaneous Melanoma

Hereditary Melanoma

As shown in Figure 18.1, germline mutations account for at most 12% of melanomas. Mutations in two genes, cyclin-dependent kinase inhibitor 2A (CDKN2A) and cyclin-dependent kinase 4 (CDK4), have been associated with a high risk of disease in the familial atypical mole and melanoma (FAMM) syndrome. Mutations in the melanocortin-1 receptor, DNA repair proteins, vitamin D receptor, glutathione S-transferase, cytochrome P450 CYP2D6, and epidermal growth factor are associated with a smaller increased risk of disease (1,2).

The CDKN2A gene contains four exons and encodes two different tumor suppressor proteins, p16 and p14^{ARF} (Fig. 18.2). Wild-type p16 sequesters CDK4 kinase, which prevents CDK4 binding to cyclin D, and thereby prevents phosphorylation of RB1; wild-type p14^{ARF} interacts with the

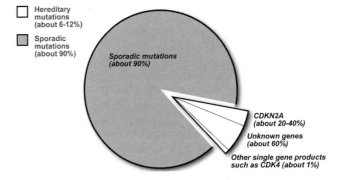

Figure 18.1 Germline mutations account for only a small subset of melanomas.

protein MDM2, which limits MDM2-controlled destruction of p53 (3,4). Thus, CDKN2A mutations contribute to hereditary melanoma through disregulation of major pathways of cell cycle control. Mutations in CDKN2A associated with hereditary melanoma include single base substitutions and deletions that alter the function of p16 alone, p14^{ARF} alone, or both (4–6). CDKN2A mutations have also been detected in a subset of sporadic melanomas (7–9).

Since mutated p16 exerts its oncogenic affect through an altered interaction with the CDK4 protein, it is not surprising that mutations in the CDK4 gene have also been associated with hereditary melanoma, as well as sporadic melanoma (10–12). Linkage analysis of melanoma-prone kindreds has recently shown that another melanoma susceptibility locus is present on chromosome 1p22 (13), but the identity of the relevant gene(s) has not yet been determined.

It is interesting to note that even though mutations in CDKN2A and CDK4 ultimately exert their effect through p53 and RB1, an increased incidence of melanoma is not a significant feature of patients who have germline mutations in TP53 or RB1 (4).

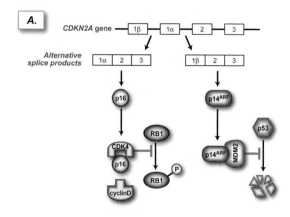

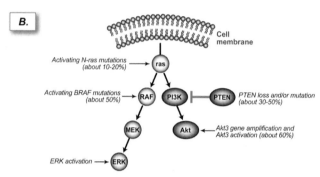

Figure 18.2 Schematic diagram of oncogenic pathways in cutaneous melanoma. **A,** Common pathways in hereditary melanoma. The *CDKN2A* gene encodes both the p16 and p14[ARF] proteins, which are produced through alternative splicing of *CDKN2A* transcripts. Wild-type p16 sequesters CDK4 kinase, which blocks cyclin D binding, and so prevents phosphorylation of RB1. Wild-type p14[ARF] interacts with MDM2, limiting the degradation of p53. Mutations in *CDKN2A* therefore disrupt two major pathways of cell cycle control. **B,** Common pathways in sporadic melanoma. Mutation or activation of different components of the canonical *ras* pathway produce aberrant activation of *ERK* or *Akt3*, which is thought to promote the development of melanoma by stimulation of cell proliferation and inhibition of apoptosis.

Sporadic Melanoma

As shown in Figure 18.2, a second pathway of melanoma oncogenesis also exists, the ras/RAF/MEK/ERK pathway. Overall, about 10% to 20% of sporadic melanomas harbor mutations in the *ras* gene family (14,15) and about 50% harbor mutations in *BRAF* (16,17). A small subset of cases shows constitutive *ERK* activation even though somatic *ERK* mutations are not present; because *ERK* activation is ultimately triggered by the interaction of extracellular ligands with cell surface receptors, constitutive activation of *ERK* is thought to represent the acquisition of autocrine growth factor loops by malignant melanocytes (18,19).

As is also shown in Figure 18.2, ras proteins activate the PI3K cascade as well as the BRAF cascade, and consequently it is not surprising that aberrations of the PI3K cascade have also been detected in sporadic melanoma. For example, loss of heterozygosity (LOH) of *PTEN* is present in 30% to 50% of melanomas (20,21) and about 10% of melanomas harbor *PTEN* mutations (22,23); however, it is interesting that patients with Cowden disease (which is

due to inherited *PTEN* mutations) do not display a significantly increased incidence of melanoma. More than 60% of melanomas show constitutive activation of *AKT3*, which in a subset of cases is due to amplification of the *AKT3* gene (24,25).

Mutations at a number of other loci have also been described in sporadic melanoma, many of which correlate with patient survival (1,26). Analysis of some classes of mutations is limited by the fact that they can be detected only by advanced genetic techniques such as spectral karyotyping or microarray analysis (27,28).

Genetics of Other Subtypes of Melanoma

Several subtypes of melanoma have underlying genetic pathways that are different from those characteristic of cutaneous melanoma.

Ocular and Mucosal Melanoma

Uveal melanoma has phenotypic associations with FAMM syndrome and oculodermal melanocytosis; linkages with other hereditary syndromes are less well established (29). The most common genetic aberrations include abnormalities of chromosome 3 (monosomy 3 in about 40% of cases, although partial deletions of 3p or 3q also occur), abnormalities of chromosome 8 (including polysomy 8, isochromosome 8q, and amplification of 8q23-24 [which contains the *C-myc* locus]), and abnormalities of chromosome 6 (isochromosome 6p) (29–35). The fact that *ERK* is constitutively activated in virtually all uveal melanomas demonstrates that the ras/BRAF/MET/ERK pathway is involved in oncogenesis, but *ras* and *BRAF* mutations are exceedingly rare (29).

Acral Melanoma

Comparative genomic hybridization (CGH) has shown that high-level amplification of specific chromosomal regions is often present in acral melanomas, most frequently 11q13, 22q11-13, and 5p15 (36). Since the pattern of chromosomal gains is distinct from that found in superficial spreading melanoma, it has been suggested that acral melanoma is a distinct clinicopathologic entity that has a pathogenesis different from that of conventional cutaneous melanoma (36).

Technical and Diagnostic Issues in Molecular Genetic Analysis of Melanoma

DNA Content

Changes in DNA content that can be detected by flow cytometry are a characteristic feature of melanoma. However, because roughly 50% of melanomas have a diploid DNA content (37), analysis of DNA content is not a reliable marker of malignancy. Similarly, LOH analysis shows such substantial overlap in the pattern of microsatellite loss between benign and malignant melanocyte proliferations that the methodology has no diagnostic utility (38).

Several reports suggest that more focused chromosomal analysis by CGH may be useful in some specific settings. For example, a subset of Spitz nevi harbor gain of chromosomal 11p in the absence of other chromosomal abnormalities (discussed in more detail later), and detection of 11p gain by either metaphase CGH or high-resolution array-based CGH may prove useful for distinguishing Spitz nevi from melanoma (39,40). Similarly, CGH analysis of atypical nodular proliferations arising in congenital nevi in children demonstrates a pattern of aberrations that exclusively involves entire chromosomes (41). Even if additional studies confirm the reliability of CGH in clinical use, the practical advantages of CGH (the approach can be applied to formalin-fixed, paraffin-embedded [FFPE] tissue and so can be used without sacrificing potentially diagnostic tissue, and can be used in cases for which the need for genetic analysis is only apparent after histopathologic evaluation) are still limited by the cumbersome methodology (Chapter 6).

Sequence Analysis

Only about 50% of melanomas harbor *BRAF* mutations, but as high as 80% of benign nevi also harbor *BRAF* mutations, including the V599E mutation that is characteristic of melanoma (17,42), and, furthermore, there is no evidence that benign nevi with *BRAF* mutations progress to malignancy. Consequently, mutational analysis of *BRAF* provides neither the diagnostic sensitivity nor specificity to be useful in the analysis of challenging cases. The same limitations constrain the diagnostic utility of sequence analysis of other loci that are involved in the oncogenesis of melanoma, and therefore histologic examination by a trained dermatopathologist remains the gold standard for diagnosis (1,4).

Gene Activation or Expression Analysis

Although the clinical role of activation analysis in the diagnosis of problematic pigmented lesions has not been evaluated, it is likely that such testing would have limited sensitivity because *ERK* and *AKT3* are only abnormally activated in a subset of melanomas. Similarly, analysis of the level of expression of individual genes does not appear to have diagnostic utility (reviewed in references 1 and 43). For example, even though in situ hybridization (ISH) studies have shown focal or complete loss of melastatin expression in over 50% of invasive cutaneous melanomas, over 20% of benign nevi also show a gradient of reduced expression with increased dermal depth (44).

Microarray Analysis

Microarray analysis has been used to identify genomewide patterns of gene expression that correlate with normal skin, benign nevi, primary melanoma, and metastatic melanoma (45,46). However, microarray analysis is still experimental, and its role in diagnosis of challenging cases has yet to be established.

Prognostic and Therapeutic Issues in Molecular Genetic Analysis of Melanoma

From a prognostic standpoint, there are no clinical differences between melanomas that do or do not harbor specific mutations in the oncogenic pathways described previously. Similarly, although associations with prognosis have been

described for a number of individual loci, none have been shown to have a level of reliability that is required for clinical use (1,43).

Even if mutational analysis of individual genes has no role from a diagnostic or prognostic standpoint, the analysis may still have a role in defining patient groups that are likely to respond to novel therapies. For example, the kinase inhibitor BAY 43-9006 is currently undergoing phase I and phase II clinical evaluation because it has been shown to inhibit the growth of melanoma cell lines harboring the *BRAF* V599E mutation (4,47,48). Likewise, methylation analysis may be useful for identifying patients who would benefit from treatment with drugs that interfere with DNA methyltransferase (2) because decreased *CDKN2A* expression in some tumors (especially ocular melanomas) has been shown to be due to transcriptional repression as a consequence of aberrant CpG island methylation (49). Microarray gene expression analysis also has been used to stratify patients into groups that correlate with outcome, often results that more accurately predict outcome than clinicopathologic findings or cytogenetic changes (29).

Genetic Testing in Hereditary Melanoma

The issue of a familial syndrome often arises when a patient has multiple dysplastic nevi or a personal history of melanoma, but since the penetrance of many mutations associated with familial melanoma is quite low and is influenced by environmental factors, it is often difficult to determine whether the kindred is affected by hereditary melanoma (1). Several laboratories now offer mutational analysis of *CDKN2A*, but because differences in penetrance make it difficult to predict the onset and severity of disease in an individual carrier, because it can be difficult to determine whether a sequence variation is a mutation or merely a polymorphism, and because such a small subset of familial melanoma is due to *CDKN2A* sequence variants, testing should only be performed in the context of formal medical genetic counseling (50,51).

Staging

Most molecular staging assays use reverse transcriptase polymerase chain reaction (RT-PCR) to detect transcripts of marker genes whose expression is presumed to be limited to malignant melanocytes and are designed to detect submicroscopic disease (i.e., disease that is not evident by routine light microscopy) in lymph nodes or peripheral blood. Although the clinical significance of malignant cells that can be detected only by molecular genetic methods remains to be clarified from a clinical perspective (27,43,52,53), several issues confound the utility of analysis from a purely technical perspective, including the lack of specificity of marker genes and the lack of morphologic correlation.

Lack of Specificity

The lack of specificity of many of the marker genes is best illustrated in the setting of evaluation of sentinel lymph nodes (SLNs). Using a variety of pigment cell–specific targets for RT-PCR analysis, including tyrosinase, tyrosinase-related proteins types 1 and 2, MART-1, and pmel-17, marker transcripts are detected in 50% to 60% (or more) of patients, although only 20% to 30% of patients with invasive melanoma will experience a disease recurrence (27,43,52). Various explanations have been offered to account for this high false positive rate, all of which are based on the extreme sensitivity of the RT-PCR assays (which are routinely capable of detecting one melanoma cell in 10^6 to 10^7 background cells). The explanations include detection of normal marker expression by rare Schwann cells, nodal nevus cell inclusions (Fig. 18.3), or malignant melanocytes incapable of tumor progression (52); detection of abnormal marker expression by lymphocytes or endothelial cells because of illegitimate transcription (52); and detection of nucleic acids within cellular debris that has drained to lymph nodes in the absence of viable tumor cells (54). Quantitative RT-PCR can theoretically be used to establish a minimum level of expression that correlates with the presence of viable malignant cells (55), but in practice it may still be difficult to distinguish between expression of a marker gene by a very small number of viable tumor cells versus amplification of mRNA from illegitimate transcription by nonmalignant cells, nucleic acid debris, or nodal nevi.

Lack of Morphologic Correlation

The specificity of immunohistochemical evaluation of SLNs is optimized by the fact that the architecture and cytologic features of the immunopositive cells can be used as a guide to their diagnostic significance. However, it is impossible to directly evaluate the morphologic features of the cells that are responsible for a positive RT-PCR result because the tissue sample is destroyed during nucleic acid extraction. The significance of this limitation is underscored by the fact that nodal nevi in SLNs occur more frequently in patients with melanoma-associated cutaneous nevi (56). Although benign nodal nevi can be distinguished from metastases by routine light microscopy, it is difficult to discern the difference based on the pattern of marker expression by RT-PCR.

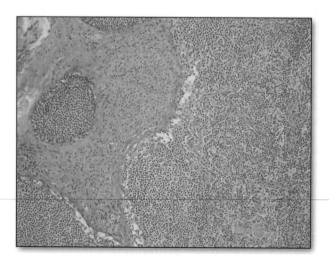

Figure 18.3 A nodal nevus in a sentinel lymph node (SLN) from a patient with cutaneous melanoma. Although nodal nevi can be distinguished from metastatic melanoma by routine light microscopy, they are a likely source of false positive results when SLN are evaluated by RT-PCR.

Testing for Submicroscopic Disease in SLNs

Several initial studies suggested that RT-PCR–based analysis of SLNs identified a patient population that has a significantly decreased disease-free survival and overall survival versus patients whose lymph nodes are negative by RT-PCR (57,58). However, interpretation of the significance of these initial studies (and many that have followed) is complicated by the fact that histopathologic evaluation of the lymph nodes did not include immunohistochemical analysis of multiple tissue levels, and by the fact that the period of follow-up was relatively short. These limitations are emphasized by a recent report that found that submicroscopic disease detected by RT-PCR for tyrosinase (mRNA) identified patients at a higher risk for recurrence than histopathologic evaluation (in which evaluation of the SLN included immunohistochemical staining for both S100 and HMB45) after a median follow-up of 42 months, but that after a median follow-up of 67 months for the same group of patients, the RT-PCR result did not show a statistically significant correlation with recurrence (59). Several clinical trials that have been designed to specifically address the role of RT-PCR analysis of SLNs will hopefully clarify the clinical relevance of assays for submicroscopic disease (53,60).

Many authors have made the point that although the extreme technical sensitivity of RT-PCR analysis of SLNs may limit the predictive value of a positive result, the predictive value of a negative result is actually quite high (27,43,52). Most studies that have evaluated SLNs, regardless of the marker mRNA used in testing, have shown that patients with a negative RT-PCR result have a statistically significant lower overall recurrence rate and higher survival rate than patients who test positive.

Testing for Submicroscopic Disease in Peripheral Blood

Some reports have demonstrated that detection of transcripts presumed to be produced by circulating malignant melanocytes correlates with advanced clinical stage (reviewed in reference 11). However, because malignant cells are apparently shed only intermittently into the circulation (61,62), assay results may depend on the sampling protocol. Furthermore, different PCR approaches (e.g., nested PCR or PCR for a number of different markers) yield results that may not be directly comparable between different studies (63,64). Consequently, it remains to be definitively established that testing for submicroscopic disease in peripheral blood provides independent and reliable prognostic or staging information.

DYSPLASTIC NEVI

Genetics

The pattern of genetic abnormalities that is characteristic of dysplastic nevi is quite complex and includes allelic loss, microsatellite instability (MSI), and mutations in a wide variety of tumor suppressor genes, oncogenes, and growth factors (65). Because a subset of the abnormalities that are present in dysplastic nevi is also present in cutaneous melanomas, at least some dysplastic nevi are thought to represent melanocytic lesions at an intermediate stage in the multistep process of melanoma tumorigenesis. From a diagnostic perspective, the significant overlap between the genetic changes in dysplastic nevi and melanoma means that molecular analysis of displastic nevi lacks the specificity needed for clinical utility.

SPITZ NEVI

Genetics

The complex cytogenetic abnormalities typical of melanoma are not a feature of Spitz nevi (66,67). Although Spitz nevi generally are not aneuploid, about 25% of cases show gain of 11p, frequently due to isochromosome 11p (39,40). In addition, about 80% of Spitz nevi with isochromosome 11p harbor a mutated H-*ras* allele on the additional chromosome (68). In contrast to normal melanocytes and melanoma, mutations in *BRAF* are rarely present in Spitz nevi (17).

Technical and Diagnostic Issues in Molecular Genetic Analysis of Spitz Nevi

The utility of mutational analysis of *ras* gene family members and *BRAF* for distinguishing Spitz nevi from melanoma has recently been demonstrated (69).

A recent report has also emphasized the utility of CGH using high-resolution arrays for distinguishing Spitz nevi from melanoma (39). Although the fact that only a subset of Spitz nevi harbors gain of 11p limits the sensitivity of the approach when confined to analysis of chromosome 11, the overall pattern of changes in Spitz nevi (no significant changes in copy number except for gain of 11p) is so different from that of melanomas (complicated changes in copy number involving many chromosomal regions as well as entire chromosomes) that genomewide CGH can differentiate the two lesions even in the absence of gain of 11p.

BASAL CELL CARCINOMA

Basal cell carcinoma (BCC) is the most common cancer in the United States and has a yearly incidence of over 1,000,000 cases (70). The tumor occurs most commonly in fair-skinned individuals, usually on sun-exposed surfaces.

Genetics

Heritable Syndromes. As shown in Table 18.1, BCC occurs as part of several heritable syndromes. The basal cell nevus syndrome is due to mutations in the *PTCH1* gene, which encodes a transmembrane protein that is a component of the sonic hedgehog (SHH) signal transduction pathway. In wild-type cells (Fig. 18.4), PTCH1 inhibits

TABLE 18.1

HEREDITARY CANCER SYNDROMES WITH CUTANEOUS MANIFESTATIONS

Clinical Features	Syndromes	Inheritance	Genes	Cutaneous Tumors
Cutaneous malignancies with occasional visceral tumors	Familial atypical mole and melanoma syndrome	AD (though polygenic)	CDKN2A, CDK4, other	Melanoma
	Nevoid basal cell carcinoma syndrome (Gorlin's syndrome)	AD	PTCH1	Multiple BCC
	Xeroderma pigmentosum	AR	Various XP genes (Chapter 2)	SCC, BCC, melanoma
Benign skin tumors with extracutaneous malignancies	Cowden syndrome	AD	PTEN	Facial trichilemmomas, acral keratosis
	Muir-Torre syndrome	AD	MSH2, MLH1	Sebaceous tumors
	Gardner's syndrome	AD	APC (Figure 15.2)	Epidermoid cysts
	Multiple endocrine neoplasia 1	AD	MEN1	Facial angiofibromas
	Tuberous sclerosis	AD	TSC1, TSC2	Angiofibromas
	Neurofibromatosis type 1	AD	NF1	Neurofibromas
	Neurofibromatosis type 2	AD	NF2	Schwannomas
	Birt-Hogg-Dubé syndrome	AD	BHD	Fibrofolliculomas, trichodiscomas, acrochordons
	Familial cylindromatosis	AD	CYLD1	Cylindromas
	Multiple cutaneous and uterine leiomyomatosis	AD	MCUL1	Leiomyomas
Non-neoplastic skin lesions with visceral tumors	Carney complex	AD	PRKARIα; others at 2p16	Lentiginosis, myxomas
	Multiple endocrine neoplasia 2A	AD	RET	Cutaneous lichen amyloidosis
	Peutz-Jeghers syndrome	AD	STK11/LKB1	Mucocutaneous macular hyperpigmentation
Cutaneous malignancies associated with abnormalities of the basement membrane zone	Recessive dystrophic epidermolysis bullosa	AR	COL7A1	SCC

AD, autosomal dominant; AR, autosomal recessive; BCC, basal cell carcinoma; SCC, squamous cell carcinoma.

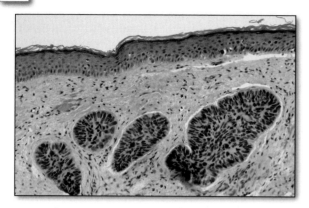

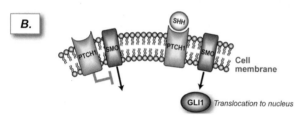

Figure 18.4 Oncogenic pathways in basal cell carcinoma (BCC). **A**, A basal cell carcinoma arising in sun-damaged skin. **B**, Schematic diagram of the sonic hedgehog signal transduction pathway. Wild-type PTCH1 inhibits SMO signaling in the absence of SHH (and so blocks GLI1 translocation to the nucleus and subsequent transcriptional activation of target genes). Hereditary mutations in *PTCH1* are responsible for the basal cell nevus syndrome. Somatic mutations in *PTCH1*, *SMO*, and *SHH* have been detected in sporadic BCC; the somatic mutations in *PTCH1* are consistent with UV-induced damage, underscoring the relationship between BCC and sun exposure.

signaling by the transmembrane protein SMO in the absence of SHH, and so GLI1 translocation to the nucleus (and subsequent transcription of its target genes) does not occur (71, 72). Because the SHH transduction pathway in normal epidermal cells not only promotes proliferation, but also inhibits cell cycle exit and terminal differentiation, inactivating mutations of *PTCH1* promote oncogenesis by abrogating the inhibition provided by the wild-type *PTCH1*.

Sporadic BCC

Almost half of sporadic BCCs harbor *PTCH1* mutations, as do many BCCs that arise in the context of xeroderma pigmentosum. In both settings, the pattern of *PTCH1* mutations is consistent with ultraviolet (UV)-induced damage (73,74), underscoring the link between BCC and sun exposure. As could be anticipated based on Figure 18.4, a subset of sporadic and xeroderma pigmentosum–associated BCCs harbor activating mutations in the *SMO* gene (75). Mutations in the *SHH* gene have also been detected in sporadic BCC. UV-induced mutations at other loci may have a role in the development of BCC, including *TP53* (73,76).

Technical and Diagnostic Issues in Molecular Genetic Analysis of BCC

Because the diagnosis of BCC is straightforward based on routine light microscopy, there is no role for molecular testing in the diagnosis of BCC. Although rare BCCs metastasize, there is no association between the pattern of mutations and the propensity for metastasis and so there is no role for testing for prognostic purposes. Even though a more complete understanding of the genetic pathway underlying the development of BCC suggests several novel targets for drug therapy (77), treatment is currently based on excision, or, for superficial BCC, topical application of imiquimod (Aldara), and so there is also no role for testing to guide therapy.

SQUAMOUS CELL CARCINOMA

Squamous cell carcinoma (SCC) of the skin is the second most common tumor in the United States, with an annual incidence of approximately 250,000 cases (70). However, SCC is biologically more aggressive than BCC and metastasizes in up to 12% of cases.

Genetics

SCC typically arises from precursor lesions in a sequence that includes actinic keratosis, in situ SCC, invasive SCC, and metastatic SCC, and this morphologic progression is thought to reflect a sequential accumulation of genetic changes (72,73,76). Genes that have an important role in oncogenesis in immunocompetent individuals include *TP53*, *ras* (as well as other genes in the ras activation pathway), and *CDKN2A*; however, the range of mutations at each locus is extremely variable, every tumor does not harbor mutations in the same set of genes, and different tumors accumulate mutations in a different sequence (71–73,76). UV-induced mutagenesis is the primary environmental factor responsible for tumorigenesis (73), as emphasized by the observation that most mutations in *TP53* in cutaneous SCC are C→T or CC→TT transitions characteristic of UV radiation–mediated damage (Chapter 2). SCC also frequently harbors structural chromosomal abnormalities, specifically LOH at 3p, 9p, 9q, 13q, 17p, and 17q.

As shown in Table 18.1, some hereditary syndromes are associated with an increased incidence of cutaneous SCC. It is interesting to note that for some of the diseases, the responsible genes do not encode proteins that are directly involved in the multistep process of tumorigenesis, but instead encode proteins that indirectly promote tumorigenesis through an effect on genome integrity or even chronic wounding injury (78).

In immunocompetent patients, human papilloma virus (HPV) is associated with cutaneous SCC in only a few specific settings, specifically anogenital SCC (79) and rare cases of digital SCC (80). As discussed in more detail in the context of cervical carcinoma (Chapter 16), the oncogenic effect of high-risk HPV types in anogenital infections is due to the virally encoded E7 and E6 proteins, which functionally inactivate cellular RB1 and p53, respectively.

Technical and Diagnostic Issues in Molecular Genetic Analysis of SCC

The oncobiology of cutaneous SCC imposes fundamental limitations on the diagnostic sensitivity and specificity of genetic analysis in the evaluation of the tumor, regardless of the testing approach. Test sensitivity is limited by the fact that only a subset of SCCs harbors the same mutations in the same set of genes. Test specificity is limited by the fact that genetic changes that are present in invasive SCC also occur in premalignant lesions (73,76), as illustrated by the data for *TP53* mutations: only about 90% of invasive SCCs harbor *TP53* mutations (81), but over 70% of actinic keratoses contain *TP53* mutations (82), and *TP53* mutations are also present in about 60% of the histologically normal cells adjacent to invasive SCC (83). The limitations on test sensitivity and specificity are largely a moot point, however, because the diagnosis of cutaneous SCC is usually straightforward by routine histopathologic evaluation.

Although therapeutic decisions for patients who have SCC are not currently based on the results of genetic testing, several novel drugs are under development that could potentially target the various proteins involved in the oncogenesis of SCC (77). If the activity of these new drugs is shown to be dependent on the presence of specific mutations, molecular testing may have a role in directing therapy by identifying the chemotherapeutic regimen most likely to benefit individual patients.

DERMATOFIBROSARCOMA PROTUBERANS

Dermatofibrosarcoma protuberans (DFSP) is a nodular or plaquelike fibrohistiocytic tumor of low-grade or intermediate malignant potential. The tumor usually diffusely infiltrates the dermis and subcutaneous tissues, and although it has a propensity for local recurrence, distant metastasis is rare. Although a well-described phenomenon, fibrosarcomatous change in DFSP is actually quite rare (84).

Genetics

Two cytogenetic changes are characteristic of DFSP, the t(17;22)(q22;q13) reciprocal translocation, and supernumerary ring chromosomes derived from the translocation (85,86). Both aberrations produce a fusion gene in which the collagen type Iα1 gene (*COLIA1*) on chromosome 17 is fused with the platelet-derived growth factor B-chain gene (*PDGFB*) on chromosome 22 (87). DFSP is, in fact, the first example of a tumor in which the same gene fusion produces a linear derivative chromosome or as a supernumerary ring chromosome. Chromosomal break points have been identified in about 20 different introns of *COLIA1* (Fig. 18.5), and consequently there is tremendous structural heterogeneity in *COLIA1-PDGFB* fusion genes even though the break point is almost always in intron 1 of *PDGFB* (88). A variety of other recurrent structural and numerical abnormalities have been described in DFSP in addition to the t(17;22) rearrangement, including trisomy 8 (present in about one third of cases) and trisomy 5 (present less frequently) (89,90).

The *COLIA1-PDGFB* rearrangement replaces the strong, negative regulatory sequences that are normally upstream of the *PDGFB* gene with the promoter of the *COLIA1* gene (91,92). It is thought that the ensuing unregulated production of *PDGFB* results in autocrine stimulation of the PDGF receptor, which promotes tumorigenesis (87,89,93).

Because the PDGF receptor is a tyrosine kinase that shows a high degree of specific inhibition by imatinib mesylate (Gleevec), the hypothesized autocrine loop that results from unregulated production of PDGFB provides a rationale for treatment of DFSP with the drug. Laboratory data have shown that cell lines expressing the COLIA1-PDGFB chimeric protein are inhibited by imatinib mesylate, and, of more importance, recent clinical reports demonstrate that a subset of patients with metastatic DFSP show at least a partial response to treatment with the drug (94,95).

Technical Issues in Molecular Genetic Analysis of DFSP

Because the *COLIA1-PDGFB* rearrangement involves a limited region upstream of exon 2 of the *PDGFB* gene, Southern blot analysis can be used to demonstrate the presence of *PDGFB* rearrangements indicative of the translocation (87). However, given the heterogeneity in the location of the translocation break points in *COLIA1*, Southern blot analysis of the *COLIA1* gene is impractical.

FISH-based analysis has been successfully employed to demonstrate the *COLIA1-PDGFB* rearrangement in metaphase chromosomes by spectral karyotyping or via the use of probes that are specific for the *PDGFB* and *COLIA1* loci (87,96–99). FISH-based analysis of interphase nuclei should make a wider range of cases amenable to testing.

RT-PCR is a reliable and sensitive method for detecting *COLIA1-PDGFB* fusion transcripts. However, the considerable heterogeneity in the location of the *COLIA1* break point necessitates the use of multiple primers that span virtually the entire *COLIA1* gene, which is easily accomplished in a multiplex format (87,88). When fresh tissue is used as the substrate for testing, *COLIA1-PDGFB* fusion transcripts can be detected in about 97% of cases of DFSP (as well as in giant cell fibroblastoma and Bednar tumor, as discussed later). RT-PCR has been adapted for use with FFPE tissue (100), although only about 85% of DFSP can be shown to harbor *COLIA1-PDGFB* fusion transcripts when testing is performed on fixed specimens (100,101), a statistically significant reduction in sensitivity. Because the many regions of sequence similarity between the various *COLIA1* exons can give rise to spurious PCR products, it is advisable to confirm the product's identity by DNA sequence analysis to exclude false positive results (89).

Specificity of the *COLIA1-PDGFB* Gene Fusion

As expected, the *COLIA1-PDGFB* fusion gene is a characteristic feature of the pigmented variant of DFSP known as Bednar tumor (89,100) as well as the granular cell variant of DFSP (102). Also as expected, the fusion gene is present in fibrosarcomatous areas that evolve out of cases of typical DFSP (103).

The *COLIA1-PDGFB* fusion gene is also characteristic of giant cell fibroblastoma (GCF). This observation, together with the similar clinical, pathologic, and histologic features of DFSP and GCF, indicates that the two tumors are merely adult and pediatric presentations of a single tumor entity (85,87–89,101,104,105). At the molecular level, the pattern of *COLIA1-PDGFB* fusion genes in GCF and DFSP is indistinguishable.

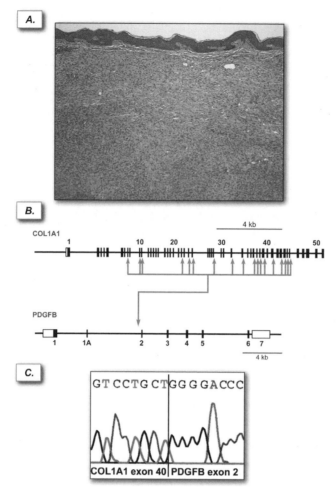

Figure 18.5 *The COLIA1-PDGFB* gene fusion is characteristic of dermatofibrosarcoma protuberans (DFSP). **A,** DFSP arising in the skin of the groin; the photomicrograph illustrates the tumor's storiform pattern and growth immediately beneath a thinned epidermis. **B,** The translocation break point that produces the *COLIA1-PDGFB* fusion can occur in a wide region of the *COLIA1* gene, but almost always occurs in intron 1 of *PDGFB*. **C,** Multiplex RT-PCR analysis of the groin neoplasm shows an in-frame fusion between *COL1A1* exon 40 and *PDGFB* exon 2, consistent with the diagnosis of DFSP (See color insert.)

COLIA1-PDGFB fusion transcripts with structural features typical of those occurring in DFSP also have been demonstrated in superficial adult fibrosarcomas that lack the histologic features of conventional DFSP (106). Based on this finding, it has been suggested that superficial adult fibrosarcomas represent a higher grade and more advanced stage of DFSP with fibrosarcomatous transformation (106), but this hypothesis awaits confirmation by analysis of additional cases.

COLIA1-PDGFB gene fusions have not been detected in a number of other tumors with a histologic similarity to DFSP, including conventional fibrosarcoma, congenital/infantile fibrosarcoma, dermatofibroma, and malignant fibrocyticytoma (100).

Prognostic Significance of Transcript Type

There appears to be no correlation between the location of the translocation break point within *COLIA1* and patient age, tumor site, histologic pattern, or prognosis. Molecular analysis has not revealed any features that predict fibrosarcomatous or metastatic evolution.

KAPOSI'S SARCOMA

Kaposi's sarcoma (KS) is a low-grade vascular neoplasm (Figure 18.6) that is the most common neoplasm in patients with acquired immunodeficiency syndrome (AIDS). Four clinical forms of KS have been described: an indolent sarcoma that usually involves the lower extremities of elderly men of Mediterranean or eastern European origin, a form that occurs in association with long-term immunosuppressive therapy (usually in transplant recipients), an endemic form in younger adults and children in central Africa, and a human immunodeficiency virus (HIV)-associated form (107). Histologically, KS has traditionally been divided into three histologic stages—patch, plaque, and nodular—which form a morphologic continuum.

Genetics

KS-associated herpesvirus(KSHV), also known as human herpesvirus-8 (HHV-8), has been identified as the causative agent of KS (108). The virus has a primary tropism for endothelial cells and B-lymphocytes, although it can infect other cell types with much lower efficiency (109). The genome of KSHV has been sequenced, and, as with other members of the gamma herpesvirus subfamily, the virus encodes proteins that can produce latent infection (109).

Technical Issues in Molecular Genetic Analysis of KS

PCR-based testing of FFPE tissue detects HHV-8 sequences in 88% to 100% of cases of KS, regardless of the clinical form or histologic stage of disease (110–113). RT-PCR of FFPE tissue, in which transcripts encoding the latency-associated nuclear antigen (LANA) are the target mRNA, detects HHV-8 in virtually 100% of cases of KS (114). In situ RT-PCR of FFPE tissue also has been described, again with a sensitivity of virtually 100% (115). However, RT-PCR approaches suffer from a lack of specificity because of their high intrinsic sensitivity, in that the methods are capable of detecting intralesional blood mononuclear cells that are infected with HHV-8 even when the neoplastic cell population itself is not infected (114,116).

Immunohistochemistry

Monoclonal antibodies to LANA-1 strongly stain the nuclei of the spindle cells lining the vascular channels of KS. Immunostaining has a sensitivity of 92% to 100%, with a specificity that is virtually 100% because immunoreactivity is not seen in other vascular lesions (including angiosarcoma or kaposiform hemangioendothelioma) or spindle cell lesions (including dermatofibrosarcoma protuberans, pirogenetic granuloma, or spindle melanoma) (117–119). In parallel analysis, immunohistochemistry shows higher specificity than RT-PCR for *LANA* transcripts (114), an example of how knowledge of the molecular mechanisms underlying tumorigenesis can lead to assays that are both more specific and less cumbersome than nucleic acid–based tests.

Diagnostic Issues in Molecular Genetic Analysis of KS

Even though HHV-8 was initially identified based on its epidemiologic association with KS, it has subsequently been shown to be associated with effusion lymphomas (107,120,121) and to be present in at least a subset of cases of multicentric Castleman's disease (121,122), primary pulmonary hypertension (123), and inflammatory myofibroblastic tumor (124). The virus has even been detected in reactive mesothelium (125). Because these diseases rarely enter into the differential diagnosis of KS, PCR-based methods are useful for confirming the diagnosis of KS, especially at an early stage of disease evolution or in patients with an unusual clinical presentation (115,126).

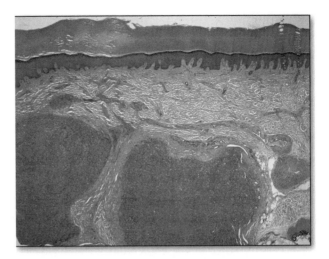

Figure 18.6 Kaposi's sarcoma (nodular stage). Human herpesvirus-8 (HHV-8), the causative agent of Kaposi's sarcoma, can be detected in virtually 100% of cases regardless of the clinical form or histologic stage of disease.

However, it is important to note that molecular analysis of vascular lesions for HHV-8 lacks 100% diagnostic specificity because some endothelial neoplasms other than KS have been reported to harbor HHV-8, including angiosarcoma (up to 29% of cases in one series, by PCR and Southern blot analysis) (127,128), pyogenic granuloma (by PCR and Southern blot analysis) (129), retiform hemangioendothelioma (130), angiolymphoid hyperplasia with eosinophilia (131), and hemangioma (127). As discussed previously, it is possible that the extreme sensitivity of PCR is responsible for false positive test results in some lesions other than KS, although the fact that the unexpected presence of HHV-8 was confirmed by two independent methods in some reports suggests that endothelial neoplasms other than KS may, in fact, harbor the virus. In any event, the cumulative data indicate that only exceedingly rare vascular lesions other than KS harbor HHV-8 (111–114,119); thus a positive molecular result must be interpreted in the context of all the clinicopathologic, serologic, and immunohistochemical features of the case to ensure that the problematic lesion is not just a misdiagnosed KS.

LYMPHOMA

The World Health Organization–European Organization for the Research and Treatment of Cancer (WHO-EORTC) classification of cutaneous lymphomas is based on the combined clinical, histopathologic, immunophenotypic, and molecular features of the various categories of cutaneous T-cell lymphomas, natural killer (NK)-cell lymphomas, and cutaneous B-cell lymphomas (132).

Currently, the molecular features of lymphoid infiltrates are usually evaluated by PCR rather than Southern hybridization because PCR-based analysis can be performed on small samples of fresh or FFPE tissue and can be completed within only a few hours.

Cutaneous T-cell Lymphomas

Cutaneous T-cell lymphomas (CTCL) comprise a group of lymphoproliferative diseases that are composed of cells with a dominant T-cell clonality and an abnormal immunophenotype that occur in characteristic clinico-pathologic settings. Analysis of T-cell clonality is based on detection of clonal T-cell receptor (*TCR*) gene rearrangements. PCR-based testing is most frequently performed using primers for the TCR γ-chain locus (*TCRγ*), although assays based on analysis of the β-chain or δ-chain of the TCR also have been described (133). Several different methods can be used to separate and visualize the PCR products following amplification, including simple poly-acrylimide gel electrophoresis, single-strand conformational polymorphism (SSCP) analysis, denaturing gradient gel electrophoresis (DGGE), temperature gradient gel electrophoresis (TGGE), and heteroduplex analysis. Although most assays are performed on nucleic acids extracted from tissue specimens (Fig. 18.7), in situ approaches have also been developed (134).

Technical Issues in Molecular Genetic Analysis of CTCL

PCR-based testing for T-cell clonality is subject to several technical limitations regardless of which TCR locus is evaluated. First, sensitivity is critically dependent on primer design. Optimized primers for *TCRγ* can detect at least 90% of rearrangements, but because the *TCRβ* and *TCRδ* genes have a larger number of V and J regions, multiple primer sets are required to achieve a similar test sensitivity when these loci are the target of analysis (Chapter 13). Second, there are no standard criteria to determine whether or not a dominant PCR product represents a monoclonal population, and so there is variability in the interpretation of the product profile, even when evaluated by quantitative methods. Third, because of dilutional effects, analysis based on a very low quantity of input DNA is more likely to yield pseudo-clonal bands and is also more likely to miss true clonal populations. The wide variety of primers used in PCR testing, as well as the number of different methods to separate and visualize the amplification products, no doubt contributes to the wide range of test performance reported by different groups (134–136).

Diagnostic Issues in Molecular Genetic Analysis of CTCL

The presence of a monoclonal T-cell population based on PCR testing is not synonymous with the presence of a malignant T-cell population (133,136,137). For example, clonal *TCR* rearrangements are present in up to 25% of patients with lichen planus (133,138,139) and in up to 49% of cases of lichen sclerosis et atrophicus (140). For diseases in which the inflammatory infiltrate lies within the spectrum of premalignant T-cell dyscrasias, such as pityriasis lichenoides chronica and pityriasis lichenoides et varioliformis acuta, T-cell clonality analysis does not identify the patients in whom disease will transform into cutaneous

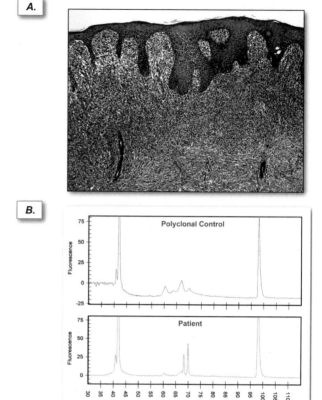

Figure 18.7   T-cell clonality analysis. **A,** Biopsy of the edge of an ulcerated lesion from a 60-year-old man who presented with multiple skin plaques and patches. The biopsy shows a cellular infiltrate with epidermotropism; immunohistochemistry showed that the majority of the lymphocytes are T-cells. **B,** T-cell clonality analysis using PCR for *TCRγ* rearrangements shows a polyclonal pattern in a normal control (*upper panel*, the large peaks at 42 and 98 seconds are calibration standards). However, PCR for *TCRγ* rearrangements performed on the patient's skin biopsy shows two dominant peaks (*lower panel*), consistent with a clonal T-cell population in which the malignant clone has undergone rearrangement of both *TCRγ* genes. Together with the clinical, morphologic, and immunohistochemical findings, the results are indicative of cutaneous T-cell lymphoma.

lymphoma (141,142). Consequently, virtually all investigators who have evaluated the role of molecular clonality tests for diagnosis of cutaneous T-cell infiltrates emphasize that the results should be interpreted only in the context of the clinical setting and histologic and immunophenotypic features of the infiltrate (133,135–137,143).

Microarray Analysis

In experimental settings, microarray analysis has been shown to provide information that can supplement routine histopathology, immunohistochemistry, and PCR-based T-cell clonality assays for classification of cutaneous T-cell infiltrates. For example, cDNA microarrays have been used to identify consistent differences in the pattern of expression of six genes that can be used to identify early-stage mycosis fungoides with 97% accuracy (144). Microarrays also have been used to provide prognostic information. For example, analysis of cDNA from patients with leukemic-phase CTCL has identified a set of ten genes whose expression profile can be used to predict 6-month survival regardless of tumor burden at diagnosis (145), a finding that suggests analysis may be useful for identifying those patients who may benefit from more aggressive treatment. Finally, microarray analysis also has been used to predict response to therapy. For example, different profiles of gene expression have been identified in CTCL cell lines that are susceptible or resistant to treatment with interferon-α (146), which indicates the potential of the approach to not only optimize treatment regimens for individual patients, but also identify novel therapeutic targets.

Cutaneous B-cell Lymphomas

Clonality Assays

PCR-based testing for B-cell clonality is usually performed using consensus primers to the V and J regions of the *IgH* locus. Regardless of whether immunoglobulin heavy- or light-chain genes are used as the target in the amplification, testing is subject to the same technical limitations discussed above for PCR-based T-cell clonality assays (147). And because the presence of a monoclonal population is again not synonymous with the presence of a malignant population, the molecular B-cell clonality results must be integrated with the clinical, histopathologic, and immunophenotypic features of the infiltrate.

Assays for Recurring Translocations

Some types of cutaneous B-cell lymphoma contain recurring translocations, although the identity and prevalence of the translocations are often quite different between morphologically similar primary cutaneous B-cell lymphomas and primary nodal B-cell lymphomas (132). The technical and diagnostic issues associated with testing for the translocations in cutaneous B-cell lymphomas by cytogenetic analysis, metaphase FISH, interphase FISH, and RT-PCR are the same as with testing for translocations characteristic of primary nodal B-cell lymphomas (Chapter 13).

Microarray Analysis

Gene expression profiles have been used to distinguish different types of cutaneous B-cell lymphomas, as well as to distinguish cutaneous B-cell lymphomas from their nodal counterparts (148,149). As with microarray analysis of cutaneous T-cell lymphomas, microarray approaches are still largely experimental, but in addition to their diagnostic applications, they also have potential utility for predicting prognosis or response to therapy.

REFERENCES

1. Carlson JA, Slominski A, Linette GP, et al. Biomarkers in melanoma: predisposition, screening and diagnosis. *Expert Rev Mol Diagn* 2003;3:163–184.
2. Hull C, Larson A, Leachman S. Pharmacogenetic candidate genes for melanoma. *Pharmacogenomics* 2003;4:753–765.
3. Hayward NK. Genetics of melanoma predisposition. *Oncogene* 2003;22:3053–3062.
4. Chudnovsky Y, Khavari PA, Adams AE. Melanoma genetics and the development of rational therapeutics. *J Clin Invest* 2005;115:813–824.
5. Piepkorn M. Melanoma genetics: an update with focus on the *CDKN2A(p16)/ARF* tumor suppressors. *J Am Acad Dermatol* 2000;42:705–726.
6. Harland M, Mistry S, Bishop DT, et al. A deep intronic mutation in CDKN2A is associated with disease in a subset of melanoma pedigrees. *Hum Mol Genet* 2001; 10:2679–2686.
7. Flores JF, Walker GJ, Glendening JM, et al. Loss of the p16INK4a and p15INK4b genes, as well as neighboring 9p21 markers, in sporadic melanoma. *Cancer Res* 1996; 56:5023–5032.
8. Cachia AR, Indsto JO, McLaren KM, et al. CDKN2A mutation and deletion status in thin and thick primary melanoma. *Clin Cancer Res* 2000;6:3511–3515.
9. Kumar R, Smeds J, Lundh Rozell B, et al. Loss of heterozygosity at chromosome 9p21 (INK4-p14ARF locus): homozygous deletions and mutations in the p16 and p14ARF genes in sporadic primary melanomas. *Melanoma Res* 1999;9:138–147.
10. Zuo L, Weger J, Yang Q, et al. Germline mutations in the p16INK4a binding domain of CDK4 in familial melanoma. *Nat Genet* 1996;12:97–99.
11. Soufir N, Avril MF, Chompret A, et al. Prevalence of p16 and CDK4 germline mutations in 48 melanoma-prone families in France. The French Familial Melanoma Study Group. *Hum Mol Genet* 1998;7:209–216.
12. Tsao H, Benoit E, Sober AJ, et al. Novel mutations in the p16/CDKN2A binding region of the cyclin-dependent kinase-4 gene. *Cancer Res* 1998;58:109–113.
13. Gillanders E, Juo SH, Holland EA, et al. Localization of a novel melanoma susceptibility locus to 1p22. *Am J Hum Genet* 2003;73:301–313.
14. Demunter A, Stas M, Degreef H, et al. Analysis of N- and K-ras mutations in the distinctive tumor progression phases of melanoma. *J Invest Dermatol* 2001;117:1483–1489.
15. Gorden A, Osman I, Gai W, et al. Analysis of BRAF and N-ras mutations in metastatic melanoma tissues. *Cancer Res* 2003;63:3955–3957.
16. Davies H, Bignell GR, Cox C, et al. Mutations of the BRAF gene in human cancer. *Nature* 2002;417:949–954.
17. Yazdi AS, Palmedo G, Flaig MJ, et al. Mutations of the BRAF gene in benign and malignant melanocytic lesions. *J Invest Dermatol* 2003;121:1160–1162.
18. Satyamoorthy K, Li G, Gerrero MR, et al. Constitutive mitogen-activated protein kinase activation in melanoma is mediated by both BRAF mutations and autocrine growth factor stimulation. *Cancer Res* 2003;63:756–759.
19. Smalley KS. A pivotal role for ERK in the oncogenic behaviour of malignant melanoma? *Int J Cancer* 2003;104:527–532.
20. Herbst RA, Weiss J, Ehnis A, et al. Loss of heterozygosity for 10q22-10qter in malignant melanoma progression. *Cancer Res* 1994;54:3111–3114.
21. Healy E, Rehman I, Angus B, et al. Loss of heterozygosity in sporadic primary cutaneous melanoma. *Genes Chromosomes Cancer* 1995;12:152–156.
22. Guldberg P, thor Straten P, Birck A, et al. Disruption of the MMAC1/PTEN gene by deletion or mutation is a frequent event in malignant melanoma. *Cancer Res* 1997;57: 3660–3663.
23. Teng DH, Hu R, Lin H, et al. MMAC1/PTEN mutations in primary tumor specimens and tumor cell lines. *Cancer Res* 1997;57:5221–5225.
24. Dhawan P, Singh AB, Ellis DL, et al. Constitutive activation of Akt/protein kinase B in melanoma leads to up-regulation of nuclear factor-kappaB and tumor progression. *Cancer Res* 2002;62:7335–7342.
25. Stahl JM, Sharma A, Cheung M, et al. Deregulated Akt3 activity promotes development of malignant melanoma. *Cancer Res* 2004;64:7002–7010.
26. Garraway LA, Widlund HR, Rubin MA, et al. Integrative genomic analyses identify MITF as a lineage survival oncogene amplified in malignant melanoma. *Nature* 2005; 436:117–122.
27. McMasters KM. Molecular staging of melanoma: sensitivity, specificity, and the search for clinical significance. *Ann Surg Oncol* 2003;10:336–337.
28. Sargent LM, Nelson MA, Lowry DT, et al. Detection of three novel translocations and specific common chromosomal break sites in malignant melanoma by spectral karyotyping. *Genes Chromosomes Cancer* 2001;32:18–25.
29. Singh AD, Damato B, Howard P, et al. Uveal melanoma: genetic aspects. *Ophthalmol Clin North Am* 2005;18:85–97.
30. Horsman DE, Sroka H, Rootman J, et al. Monosomy 3 and isochromosome 8q in a uveal melanoma. *Cancer Genet Cytogenet* 1990;45:249–253.
31. Sisley K, Cottam DW, Rennie IG, et al. Non-random abnormalities of chromosomes 3, 6, and 8 associated with posterior uveal melanoma. *Genes Chromosomes Cancer* 1992; 5:197–200.
32. Prescher G, Bornfeld N, Becher R. Nonrandom chromosomal abnormalities in primary uveal melanoma. *J Natl Cancer Inst* 1990;82:1765–1769.
33. Singh AD, Boghosian-Sell L, Wary KK. Cytogenetic findings in primary uveal melanoma. *Cancer Genet Cytogenet* 1994;72:109–115.
34. Tschentscher F, Prescher G, Horsman DE, et al. Partial deletions of the long and short arm of chromosome 3 point to two tumor suppressor genes in uveal melanoma. *Cancer Res* 2001;61:3439–3442.
35. Parrella P, Fazio VM, Gallo AP, et al. Fine mapping of chromosome 3 in uveal melanoma: identification of a minimal region of deletion on chromosomal arm 3p25.1–p25.2. *Cancer Res* 2003;63:8507–8510.
36. Bastian BC, Kashani-Sabet M, Hamm H, et al. Gene amplifications characterize acral melanoma and permit the detection of occult tumor cells in the surrounding skin. *Cancer Res* 2000;60:1968–1973.
37. Martin G, Halwani F, Shibata H, et al. Value of DNA ploidy and S-phase fraction as prognostic factors in stage III cutaneous melanoma. *Can J Surg* 2000;43:29–34.
38. Maitra A, Gazdar AF, Moore TO, et al. Loss of heterozygosity analysis of cutaneous melanoma and benign melanocytic nevi: laser capture microdissection demonstrates clonal genetic changes in acquired nevocellular nevi. *Hum Pathol* 2002;33:191–197.
39. Harvell JD, Kohler S, Zhu S, et al. High-resolution array-based comparative genomic hybridization for distinguishing paraffin-embedded Spitz nevi and melanomas. *Diagn Mol Pathol* 2004;13:22–25.
40. Bastian BC. Molecular genetics of melanocytic neoplasia: practical applications for diagnosis. *Pathology* 2004;36:458–461.
41. Bastian BC, Xiong J, Frieden IJ, et al. Genetic changes in neoplasms arising in congenital melanocytic nevi: differences between nodular proliferations and melanomas. *Am J Pathol* 2002;161:1163–1169.
42. Pollock PM, Harper UL, Hansen KS, et al. High frequency of BRAF mutations in nevi. *Nat Genet* 2003;33:19–20.

43. Carlson JA, Slominski A, Linette GP, et al. Biomarkers in melanoma: staging, prognosis and detection of early metastases. *Expert Rev Mol Diagn* 2003;3:303–330.

44. Deeds J, Cronin F, Duncan LM. Patterns of melastatin mRNA expression in melanocytic tumors. *Hum Pathol* 2000;31:1346–1356.

45. Haqq C, Nosrati M, Sudilovsky D, et al. The gene expression signatures of melanoma progression. *Proc Natl Acad Sci USA* 2005;102:6092–6097.

46. Hoek K, Rimm DL, Williams KR, et al. Expression profiling reveals novel pathways in the transformation of melanocytes to melanomas. *Cancer Res* 2004;64:5270–5282.

47. Tuveson DA, Weber BL, Herlyn M. BRAF as a potential therapeutic target in melanoma and other malignancies. *Cancer Cell* 2003;4:95–98.

48. Bollag G, Freeman S, Lyons JF, et al. Raf pathway inhibitors in oncology. *Curr Opin Investig Drugs* 2003;4:1436–1441.

49. Van der Velden PA, Metzelaar-Blok JA, Berman W, et al. Promoter hypermethylation: a common cause of reduced p16(INK4a) expression in uveal melanoma. *Cancer Res* 2001;61:5303–5306.

50. Hansen CB, Wadge LM, Lowstuter K, et al. Promoter hypermethylation: a common cause of reduced p16(INK4a) expression in uveal melanoma. *Cancer Res* 2001;61:5303–5306.

51. Tsao H, Niendorf K. Genetic testing in hereditary melanoma. *J Am Acad Dermatol* 2004;51:803–808.

52. Davids V, Kidson SH, Hanekom GS. Melanoma patient staging: histopathological versus molecular evaluation of the sentinel node. *Melanoma Res* 2003;13:313–324.

53. Roberts AA, Cochran AJ. Pathologic analysis of sentinel lymph nodes in melanoma patients: current and future trends. *J Surg Oncol* 2004;85:152–161.

54. Yamamoto N, Kato Y, Yanagisawa A, et al. Predictive value of genetic diagnosis for cancer micrometastasis: histologic and experimental appraisal. *Cancer* 1997;80:1393–1398.

55. Abrahamsen HN, Nexo E, Steiniche T, et al. Quantification of melanoma mRNA markers in sentinel nodes: pre-clinical evaluation of a single-step real-time reverse transcriptase-polymerase chain reaction assay. *J Mol Diagn* 2004;6:253–259.

56. Holt JB, Sanguesza OP, Levine EA, et al. Nodal melanocytic nevi in sentinel lymph nodes: correlation with melanoma-associated cutaneous nevi. *Am J Clin Pathol* 2004;121:58–63.

57. Shivers SC, Wang X, Li W, et al. Molecular staging of malignant melanoma: correlation with clinical outcome. *JAMA* 1998;280:1410–1415.

58. Blaheta HJ, Ellwanger U, Schittek B, et al. Examination of regional lymph nodes by sentinel node biopsy and molecular analysis provides new staging facilities in primary cutaneous melanoma. *J Invest Dermatol* 2000;114:637–642.

59. Kammula US, Ghossein R, Bhattacharya S, et al. Serial follow-up and the prognostic significance of reverse transcriptase-polymerase chain reaction–staged sentinel lymph nodes from melanoma patients. *J Clin Oncol* 2004;22:3989–3996.

60. Reintgen D, Pendas S, Jakub J, et al. National trials involving lymphatic mapping for melanoma. The Multicenter Selective Lymphadenectomy Trial, the Sunbelt Melanoma Trial and the Florida Melanoma Trial. *Semin Oncol* 2004;31:363–373.

61. Reinhold U, Ludtke-Handjery HC, Schnautz S, et al. The analysis of tyrosinase-specific mRNA in blood samples of melanoma patients by RT-PCR is not a useful test for metastatic tumor progression. *J Invest Dermatol* 1997;108:166–169.

62. Curry BJ, Myers K, Hersey P. Utility of tests for circulating melanoma cells in identifying patients who develop recurrent melanoma. *Recent Results Cancer Res* 2001;158:211–230.

63. Schrader AJ, Probst-Kepper M, Grosse J, et al. Molecular and prognostic classification of advanced melanoma: a multi-marker microcontamination assay of peripheral blood stem cells. *Melanoma Res* 2000;10:355–362.

64. Max N, Wolf K, Thiel E, et al. Quantitative nested real-time RT-PCR specific for tyrosinase transcripts to quantitative minimal residual disease. *Clin Chim Acta* 2002;317:39–46.

65. Hussein MR, Wood GS. Molecular aspects of melanocytic dysplastic nevi. *J Mol Diagn* 2002;4:71–80.

66. Bastian BC, Wesselmann U, Pinkel D, et al. Molecular cytogenetic analysis of Spitz nevi shows clear differences to melanoma. *J Invest Dermatol* 1999;113:1065–1069.

67. Bastian BC, Olshen A, LeBoit PE, et al. Classifying melanocytic tumors based on DNA copy number changes. *Am J Pathol* 2003;163:1765–1770.

68. Bastian BC, LeBoit PE, Pinkel D. Mutations and copy number increase of HRAS in Spitz nevi with distinctive histopathological features. *Am J Pathol* 2000;157:967–972.

69. van Dijk MCRF, Bensen MR, Ruiter DJ. Analysis of mutations in B-RAF, N-RAS, and H-RAS genes in the differential diagnosis of Spitz nevus and Spitzoid melanoma. *AM J Surg Pathol* 2005;29:1145–1151.

70. Christenson LJ, Borrowman TA, Vachon CM, et al. Incidence of basal cell and squamous cell carcinomas in a population younger than 40 years. *JAMA* 2005;294:681–90

71. Ridky TW, Khavari PA. Pathways sufficient to induce epidermal carcinogenesis. *Cell Cycle* 2004;3:621–624.

72. Tsai KY, Tsao H. The genetics of skin cancer. *Am J Med Genet C Semin Med Genet* 2004;131C:82–92.

73. Hussein MR. Ultraviolet radiation and skin cancer: molecular mechanisms. *J Cutan Pathol* 2005;32:191–205.

74. Kim MY, Park HJ, Baek SC. Mutations of the p53 and PTCH gene in basal cell carcinomas: UV mutation signature and strand bias. *J Dermatol Sci* 2002;29:1–9.

75. Couve-Privat S, Bouadjar B, Avril MF, et al. Significantly high levels of ultraviolet-specific mutations in the smoothened gene in basal cell carcinomas from DNA repair-deficient xeroderma pigmentosum patients. *Cancer Res* 2002;62:7186–7189.

76. Backvall H, Asplund A, Gustafsson A, et al. Genetic tumor archeology: microdissection and genetic heterogeneity in squamous and basal cell carcinoma. *Mutat Res* 2005; 571:65–79.

77. Green CL, Khavari PA. Targets for molecular therapy of skin cancer. *Semin Cancer Biol* 2004;14:63–69.

78. Ortiz-Urda S, Garcia J, Green C, et al. Type VII collagen is required for Ras-driven human epidermal tumorigenesis. *Science* 2005;307:1773–1776.

79. Frisch M. On the etiology of anal squamous carcinoma. *Dan Med Bull* 2002; 49:194–209.

80. Alam M, Caldwell JB, Eliezri YD. Human papillomavirus-associated digital squamous cell carcinoma: literature review and report of 21 new cases. *J Am Acad Dermatol* 2003;48:385–393.

81. Leffell DJ. The scientific basis of skin cancer. *J Am Acad Dermatol* 2000;42:18–22.

82. Campbell C, Quinn AG, Ro YS, et al. p53 mutations are common and early events that precede tumor invasion in squamous cell neoplasia of the skin. *J Invest Dermatol* 1993;100:746–748.

83. Backvall H, Stromberg S, Gustafsson A, et al. Mutation spectra of epidermal p53 clones adjacent to basal cell carcinoma and squamous cell carcinoma. *Exp Dermatol* 2004;13:643–650.

84. Mentzel T, Beham A, Katenkamp D, et al. Fibrosarcomatous ("high-grade") dermatofibrosarcoma protuberans: clinicopathologic and immunohistochemical study of a series of 41 cases with emphasis on prognostic significance. *Am J Surg Pathol* 1998;22:576–587.

85. Pedeutour F, Simon MP, Minoletti F, et al. Ring 22 chromosomes in dermatofibrosarcoma protuberans are low-level amplifiers of chromosome 17 and 22 sequences. *Cancer Res* 1995;55:2400–2403.

86. Pedeutour F, Simon MP, Minoletti F, et al. Translocation t(17;22)(q22;q13), in dermatofibrosarcoma protuberans: a new tumor-associated chromosome rearrangement. *Cytogenet Cell Genet* 1996;72:171–174.

87. Simon MP, Pedeutour F, Sirvent N, et al. Deregulation of the platelet-derived growth factor B-chain gene via fusion with collagen gene COL1A1 in dermatofibrosarcoma protuberans and giant-cell fibroblastoma. *Nat Genet* 1997;15:95–98.

88. O'Brien KP, Seroussi E, Dal Cin P, et al. Various regions within the alpha-helical domain of the COL1A1 gene are fused to the second exon of the PDGFB gene in dermatofibrosarcomas and giant-cell fibroblastomas. *Genes Chromosomes Cancer* 1998;23:187–193.

89. Sirvent N, Maire G, Pedeutour F. Genetics of dermatofibrosarcoma protuberans family of tumors: from ring chromosomes to tyrosine kinase inhibitor treatment. *Genes Chromosomes Cancer* 2003;37:1–19.

90. Sandberg AA, Bridge JA. Updates on the cytogenetics and molecular genetics of bone and soft tissue tumors: dermatofibrosarcoma protuberans and giant cell fibroblastoma. *Cancer Genet Cytogenet* 2003;140:1–12.

91. Dirks RP, Jansen HJ, Onnekink C, et al. DNase-I-hypersensitive sites located far upstream of the human c-sis/PDGF-B gene comap with transcriptional enhancers and a silencer and are preceded by (part of) a new transcription unit. *Eur J Biochem* 1993;216:487–495.

92. Rao CD, Pech M, Robbins KC, et al. The 5' untranslated sequence of the c-sis/platelet-derived growth factor 2 transcript is a potent translational inhibitor. *Mol Cell Biol* 1988;8:284–292.

93. Greco A, Fusetti L, Villa R, et al. Transforming activity of the chimeric sequence formed by the fusion of collagen gene COL1A1 and the platelet derived growth factor b-chain gene in dermatofibrosarcoma protuberans. *Oncogene* 1998;17:1313–1319.

94. Maki RG, Awan RA, Dixon RH, et al. Differential sensitivity to imatinib of 2 patients with metastatic sarcoma arising from dermatofibrosarcoma protuberans. *Int J Cancer* 2002;100:623–626.

95. Rubin BP, Schuetze SM, Eary JF, et al. Molecular targeting of platelet-derived growth factor B by imatinib mesylate in a patient with metastatic dermatofibrosarcoma protuberans. *J Clin Oncol* 2002;20:3586–3591.

96. Vanni R, Faa G, Dettori T, et al. A case of dermatofibrosarcoma protuberans of the vulva with a COL1A1/PDGFB fusion identical to a case of giant cell fibroblastoma. *Virchows Arch* 2000;437:95–100.

97. Gisselsson D, Hoglund M, O'Brien KP, et al. A case of dermatofibrosarcoma protuberans with a ring chromosome 5 and a rearranged chromosome 22 containing amplified COL1A1 and PDGFB sequences. *Cancer Lett* 1998;133:129–134.

98. Sonobe H, Furihata M, Iwata J, et al. Dermatofibrosarcoma protuberans harboring t(9;22)(q32;q12.2). *Cancer Genet Cytogenet* 1999;110:14–18.

99. Navarro M, Simon MP, Migeon C, et al. COL1A1-PDGFB fusion in a ring chromosome 4 found in a dermatofibrosarcoma protuberans. *Genes Chromosomes Cancer* 1998;23:263–266.

100. Wang J, Hisaoka M, Shimajiri S, et al. Detection of COL1A1-PDGFB fusion transcripts in dermatofibrosarcoma protuberans by reverse transcription-polymerase chain reaction using archival formalin-fixed, paraffin-embedded tissues. *Diagn Mol Pathol* 1999;8:113–119.

101. Gokden N, Dehner LP, Zhu X, et al. Dermatofibrosarcoma protuberans of the vulva and groin: detection of COL1A1-PDGFB fusion transcripts by RT-PCR. *J Cutan Pathol* 2003;30:190–195.

102. Maire G, Pedeutour F, Coindre JM. COL1A1-PDGFB gene fusion demonstrates a common histogenetic origin for dermatofibrosarcoma protuberans and its granular cell variant. *Am J Surg Pathol* 2002;26:932–937.

103. Wang J, Morimitsu Y, Okamoto S, et al. COL1A1-PDGFB fusion transcripts in fibrosarcomatous areas of six dermatofibrosarcomas protuberans. *J Mol Diagn* 2000;2:47–52.

104. Dal Cin P, Sciot R, de Wever I, et al. Cytogenetic and immunohistochemical evidence that giant cell fibroblastoma is related to dermatofibrosarcoma protuberans. *Genes Chromosomes Cancer* 1996;15:73–75.

105. Maire G, Martin L, Michalak-Provost S, et al. Fusion of COL1A1 exon 29 with PDGFB exon 2 in a der(22)t(17;22) in a pediatric giant cell fibroblastoma with a pigmented Bednar tumor component: evidence for age-related chromosomal pattern in dermatofibrosarcoma protuberans and related tumors. *Cancer Genet Cytogenet* 2002;134:156–161.

106. Sheng WQ, Hashimoto H, Okamoto S, et al. Expression of COL1A1-PDGFB fusion transcripts in superficial adult fibrosarcoma suggests a close relationship to dermatofibrosarcoma protuberans. *J Pathol* 2001;194:88–94.

107. Hengge UR, Ruzicka T, Tyring SK, et al. Update on Kaposi's sarcoma and other HHV8 associated diseases. I. Epidemiology, environmental predispositions, clinical manifestations, and therapy. *Lancet Infect Dis* 2002;2:281–292.

108. Chang Y, Cesarman E, Pessin MS, et al. Identification of herpesvirus-like DNA sequences in AIDS-associated Kaposi's sarcoma. *Science* 1994;266:1865–1869.

109. Verma SC, Robertson ES. Molecular biology and pathogenesis of Kaposi sarcoma-associated herpesvirus. *FEMS Microbiol Lett* 2003;222:155–163.

110. Moore PS, Chang Y. Detection of herpesvirus-like DNA sequences in Kaposi's sarcoma in patients with and without HIV infection. *N Engl J Med* 1995;332:1181–1185.

111. Kazakov DV, Prinz BM, Michaelis S, et al. Study of HHV-8 DNA sequences in archival biopsies from lesional skin of Kaposi's sarcoma, various mesenchymal tumors and related reactive conditions. *J Cutan Pathol* 2002;29:279–281.

112. Jin YT, Tsai ST, Yan JJ, et al. Detection of Kaposi's sarcoma-associated herpesvirus-like DNA sequence in vascular lesions: a reliable diagnostic marker for Kaposi's sarcoma. *Am J Clin Pathol* 1996;105:360–363.

113. Dictor M, Rambech E, Way D, et al. Human herpesvirus 8 (Kaposi's sarcoma-associated herpesvirus) DNA in Kaposi's sarcoma lesions, AIDS Kaposi's sarcoma cell lines,

endothelial Kaposi's sarcoma simulators, and the skin of immunosuppressed patients. *Am J Pathol* 1996;148:2009–2016.

114. Hammock L, Reisenauer A, Wang W, et al. Latency-associated nuclear antigen expression and human herpesvirus-8 polymerase chain reaction in the evaluation of Kaposi sarcoma and other vascular tumors in HIV-positive patients. *Mod Pathol* 2005;18: 463–468.

115. Nuovo M, Nuovo G. Utility of HHV8 RNA detection for differentiating Kaposi's sarcoma from its mimics. *J Cutan Pathol* 2001;28:248–255.

116. Kazakov DV, Schmid M, Adams V, et al. HHV-8 DNA sequences in the peripheral blood and skin lesions of an HIV-negative patient with multiple eruptive dermatofibromas: implications for the detection of HHV-8 as a diagnostic marker for Kaposi's sarcoma. *Dermatology* 2003;206:217–221.

117. Patel RM, Goldblum JR, Hsi ED. Immunohistochemical detection of human herpes virus-8 latent nuclear antigen-1 is useful in the diagnosis of Kaposi sarcoma. *Mod Pathol* 2004;17:456–460.

118. Robin YM, Guillou L, Michels JJ, et al. Human herpesvirus 8 immunostaining: a sensitive and specific method for diagnosing Kaposi sarcoma in paraffin-embedded sections. *Am J Clin Pathol* 2004;121:330–334.

119. Cheuk W, Wong KO, Wong CS, et al. Immunostaining for human herpesvirus 8 latent nuclear antigen-1 helps distinguish Kaposi sarcoma from its mimickers. *Am J Clin Pathol* 2004;121:335–342.

120. Cesarman E, Chang Y, Moore PS, et al. Kaposi's sarcoma-associated herpesvirus-like DNA sequences in AIDS-related body-cavity-based lymphomas. *N Engl J Med* 1995; 332:1186–1191.

121. Dupin N, Fisher C, Kellam P, et al. Distribution of human herpesvirus-8 latently infected cells in Kaposi's sarcoma, multicentric Castleman's disease, and primary effusion lymphoma. *Proc Natl Acad Sci USA* 1999;96:4546–4551.

122. Du MQ, Liu H, Diss TC, et al. Kaposi sarcoma-associated herpesvirus infects monotypic (IgM lambda) but polyclonal naive B cells in Castleman disease and associated lymphoproliferative disorders. *Blood* 2001;97:2130–2136.

123. Cool CD, Rai PR, Yeager ME, et al. Expression of human herpesvirus 8 in primary pulmonary hypertension. *N Engl J Med* 2003;349:1113–1122.

124. Gomez-Roman JJ, Ocejo-Vinyals G, Sanchez-Velasco P, et al. Presence of human herpesvirus-8 DNA sequences and overexpression of human IL-6 and cyclin D1 in inflammatory myofibroblastic tumor (inflammatory pseudotumor). *Lab Invest* 2000;80: 1121–1126.

125. Bryant-Greenwood P, Sorbara L, Filie AC, et al. Infection of mesothelial cells with human herpes virus 8 in human immunodeficiency virus-infected patients with Kaposi's sarcoma, Castleman's disease, and recurrent pleural effusions. *Mod Pathol* 2003;16:145–153.

126. Insabato L, Di Vizio D, Terracciano LM, et al. Primary Kaposi sarcoma of the bowel in a HIV-negative patient. *J Surg Oncol* 2001;76:197–200.

127. McDonagh DP, Liu J, Gaffey MJ, et al. Detection of Kaposi's sarcoma-associated herpesvirus-like DNA sequence in angiosarcoma. *Am J Pathol* 1996;149:1363–1368.

128. Gyulai R, Kemeny L, Kiss M, et al. Herpesvirus-like DNA sequence in angiosarcoma in a patient without HIV infection. *N Engl J Med* 1996;334:540–541.

129. Hisaoka M, Hashimoto H, Iwamasa T. Diagnostic implication of Kaposi's sarcoma-associated herpesvirus with special reference to the distinction between spindle cell hemangioendothelioma and Kaposi's sarcoma. *Arch Pathol Lab Med* 1998;122:72–76.

130. Schommer M, Herbst RA, Brodersen JP, et al. Retiform hemangioendothelioma: another tumor associated with human herpesvirus type 8? *J Am Acad Dermatol* 2000; 42:290–292.

131. Gyulai R, Kemeny L, Kiss M, et al. HHV8 DNA in angiolymphoid hyperplasia of the skin. *Lancet* 1996;347:1837.

132. Willemze R, Jaffe ES, Burg G, et al. WHO-EORTC classification for cutaneous lymphomas. *Blood* 2005;105:3768–3785.

133. Holm N, Flaig MJ, Yazdi AS, et al. The value of molecular analysis by PCR in the diagnosis of cutaneous lymphocytic infiltrates. *J Cutan Pathol* 2002;29:447–452.

134. Magro CM, Nuovo GJ, Crowson AN. The utility of the in situ detection of T-cell receptor beta rearrangements in cutaneous T-cell-dominant infiltrates. *Diagn Mol Pathol* 2003;12:133–141.

135. Guitart J, Kaul K. A new polymerase chain reaction-based method for the detection of T-cell clonality in patients with possible cutaneous T-cell lymphoma. *Arch Dermatol* 1999;135:158–162.

136. LeBoit PE. Cutaneous lymphocytic infiltrates: let's get real. *Am J Dermatopathol* 2005; 27:182–184.

137. Bergman R. How useful are T-cell receptor gene rearrangement studies as an adjunct to the histopathologic diagnosis of mycosis fungoides? *Am J Dermatopathol* 1999; 21:498–502.

138. Saunder CA, Kind P, Flaig M, et al. Genotypic analysis in cutaneous lymphoproliferative disease: a reliable test? *J Cutan Pathol* 1998;25:511.

139. Schiller PI, Flaig MJ, Puchta U, et al. Detection of clonal T cells in lichen planus. *Arch Dermatol Res* 2000;292:568–569.

140. Lukowsky A, Muche JM, Serry W, et al. Detection of expanded T cell clones in skin biopsy samples of patients with lichen sclerosus et atrophicus by T cell receptor-gamma polymerase chain reaction assays. *J Invest Dermatol* 2000;115:254–259.

141. Magro C, Crowson AN, Kovatich A, et al. Pityriasis lichenoides: a clonal T-cell lymphoproliferative disorder. *Hum Pathol* 2002;33:788–795.

142. Dereure O, Levi E, Kadin ME. T-Cell clonality in pityriasis lichenoides et varioliformis acuta: a heteroduplex analysis of 20 cases. *Arch Dermatol* 2000;136:1483–1486.

143. Bakels V, van Oostveen J, van der Putte S, et al. Immunophenotyping and gene rearrangement analysis provide additional criteria to differentiate between cutaneous T-cell lymphomas and pseudo-T-cell lymphomas. *Am J Pathol* 1997;150:1941–1949.

144. Tracey L, Villuendas R, Dotor AM, et al. Mycosis fungoides shows concurrent deregulation of multiple genes involved in the TNF signaling pathway: an expression profile study. *Blood* 2003;102:1042–1050.

145. Kari L, Loboda A, Nebozhyn M, et al. Classification and prediction of survival in patients with the leukemic phase of cutaneous T cell lymphoma. *J Exp Med* 2003;197:1477–1488.

146. Tracey L, Villuendas R, Ortiz P, et al. Identification of genes involved in resistance to interferon-alpha in cutaneous T-cell lymphoma. *Am J Pathol* 2002;161:1825–1837.

147. Kerl H, Kodama K, Cerroni L. Diagnostic principles and new developments in primary cutaneous B-cell lymphomas. *J Dermatol Sci* 2004;34:167–175.

148. Staudt LM. Molecular diagnosis of the hematologic cancers. *N Engl J Med* 2003; 348:1777–1785.

149. Vermeer M, Dijkman R, Hoefnagel JJ, et al. Identification of gene expression profiles that segregate patients with distinct primary cutaneous large B cell lymphoma. *J Invest Dermatol* 2003;121:158.

Lung and Mediastinum

19

NON–SMALL CELL LUNG CANCER AND SMALL CELL LUNG CANCER

Lung cancer is the most common malignancy worldwide and is also the leading cause of cancer-related death worldwide (1). Cigarette smoking is responsible for about 85% of the attributable risk of lung cancer; radiation exposure and environmental carcinogens such asbestos and arsenic are associated with smaller attributable risks (2–5). The biochemistry of mutagenesis caused by cigarette smoking is reasonably well described, even if the identity of the individual loci that are the targets of mutation is uncertain (6–8). The mechanism of carcinogenesis for other risk factors, such as arsenic exposure, is not well characterized (9,10). Similarly, even though epidemiologic studies have shown that there is approximately a 2-fold increase in lung cancer in the first-degree relatives of patients with lung cancer (3), neither the

major susceptibility genes (11), the modifier genes (which may enhance the carcinogenic potential of tobacco smoke and other occupational or environmental lung carcinogens) (12,13), nor the so-called addiction genes (which may predispose individuals to cigarette smoking) have been identified (14,15).

At the genetic level, both non–small cell lung carcinoma (NSCLC) and small cell lung carcinoma (SCLC) are thought to develop through a multistep process (Fig. 19.1) in which an initial mutation in a single cell provides its progeny with a selective growth advantage, a single cell from within this expanded clone acquires a second mutation that provides a further growth advantage, and so on, until a fully malignant carcinoma emerges. However, as could be anticipated based on the markedly different pathologic features of NSCLC and SCLC, the pattern of molecular changes in the two categories of lung carcinoma are significantly different. As Table 19.1

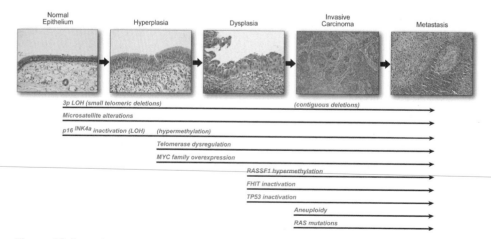

Figure 19.1 Multistep model of non–small cell lung carcinoma (NSCLC) oncogenesis. The model emphasizes that NSCLC arises via an accumulation of somatically acquired genetic alternations, although there is some heterogeneity in the sequence of genetic changes and the individual loci involved. (Modified from reference 16).

TABLE 19.1

EXAMPLES OF COMMON GENETIC ALTERATIONS IN LUNG CANCER

Genetic Alteration	SCLC[a]	NSCLC[b]
Frequent allelic loss	3p, 4p, 4q, 5q, 8p, 10q, 13q, 17p, 22q	3p, 6q, 8p, 9p, 13q, 17p, 19q
ras mutations	Rare	15–20%
BCL2 expression	75%–95%	10–35%
myc family overexpression	15%–30%	5–10%
RB1 inactivation	~90%	15–30%
TP53 inactivation	80%–90%	~50%
p16^{INK4a} inactivation	0–10%	30–70%
FHIT inactivation	~75%	50–75%
RARβ promoter hypermethylation	70%	40%
RASSF1 promoter methylation	>90%	~40%
Genetic instability	High	Low-intermediate
Telomerase activity	100%	80–90%

Adapted from references 2, 16, 19.
[a]Small cell lung carcinoma.
[b]Non–small cell lung carcinoma.

shows, the pattern of aberrations includes gross structural changes (with loss or gain of segments of multiple different chromosomes), numerical chromosome changes, gene amplifications, point mutations, and epigenetic gene silencing. The mutated loci include proto-oncogenes that contribute to growth stimulation by autocrine and paracrine pathways, tumor suppressor genes, genes involved in the regulation of apoptosis, and genes encoding proteins that govern cellular interaction with the extracellular matrix (reviewed in 2,16–19).

Figure 19.1 emphasizes that, for NSCLC, the sequential accumulation of genetic and epigenetic changes that culminates in the development of invasive carcinoma is accompanied by a progression of morphologic changes in the epithelium. Although a multistep accumulation of somatically acquired genetic alterations underlies development of SCLC, a similar of morphologic changes in the epithelium is not characteristic of SCLC.

Technical and Diagnostic Issues in Molecular Genetic Analysis of Lung Cancer

Even though both NSCLC and SCLC are thought to develop through a stepwise accumulation of genetic abnormalities, Figure 19.1 and Table 19.1 emphasize that every tumor does not harbor the same mutations in the same set of genes, and that different tumors acquire mutations in a different sequence (2,16–19). Consequently, the oncobiology of lung carcinomas imposes fundamental limitations on the technical and diagnostic sensitivity and specificity of genetic analysis, regardless of the testing approach. Test sensitivity is limited by the fact that only a subset of lung carcinomas, whether NSCLC or SCLC, harbors a mutation at each of the relevant loci. Similarly, specificity is limited by the fact that virtually every genetic change present in invasive carcinomas is also present in a subset of premalignant lesions (20).

In situ Hybridization

TP53 mutations are present in a high percentage of NSCLC and SCLC, and demonstration of loss of heterozygosity (LOH) of chromosome 3p by fluorescence in situ hybridization (FISH) is a useful way to establish the presence of *TP53* alterations because LOH of 3p is highly correlated with biallelic inactivation of the gene. FISH analysis of metaphase chromosome spreads is a suboptimal approach because it is constrained not only by the availability of fresh tissue, but also by the fact that metaphase chromosomes can be obtained from only 40% to 60% of cases of NSCLC for which fresh tissue is available, and as few as 20% of cases of SCLC for which fresh tissue is available (21). Analysis of interphase nuclei overcomes these limitations.

A dual-color FISH assay has been described that makes it possible to detect imbalances between the long and short arms of chromosome 3 in interphase nuclei of about 80% of primary lung carcinomas, and that can even be used to detect malignant cells with chromosomal imbalance within a background of normal cells in pleural effusions (22,23). However, the sensitivity of the approach is limited by the fact that at most 90% of SCLC and 65% of NSCLC harbor loss of 3p; test specificity is limited by the fact that imbalance is present in many premalignant lesions because 3p loss is an early event in tumor development. FISH approaches that simultaneously target multiple loci on different chromosomes achieve a higher level of sensitivity and specificity, and some multitarget multicolor FISH assays have been shown to perform at least as well as cytology in the setting of lung cancer screening (24,25), as discussed in more detail later.

Polymerase Chain Reaction–based Analysis of Gene Expression

In an attempt to overcome the intrinsic limitations on test sensitivity and specificity imposed by the fact that only a subset of lung carcinomas harbor a mutation at any marker locus, quantitative empirical indexes have been developed that incorporate the level of expression of several different genes (26,27). For example, an index value calculated from the level of expression of *C-myc*, *E2F*, and *p21* as measured by modified quantitative reverse transcriptase polymerase chain reaction (RT-PCR) analysis has been shown to have 100% sensitivity for correctly classifying fine-needle aspiration (FNA) biopsies, while paired conventional cytomorphologic evaluation has a sensitivity of only 75% (26). Although there is little need to determine index values for cases in which the cytologic and morphologic findings are diagnostic, this result suggests that quantitative RT-PCR can be used to augment the findings in biopsies that are non-diagnostic by routine light microscopy. However, the index value's specificity of 93% indicates that analysis of a small panel of genes cannot entirely overcome the fact that altered gene expression profiles are present in premalignant lesions.

Telomere Metabolism

Whether measured by the traditional or telomeric repeat amplification protocol (TRAP assay; Chapter 5), or by semi-quantitative modifications of the method, telomerase activity is detected in 79% to 91% of NSCLC and in virtually 100% of SCLC (28–30). Furthermore, there is a statistically significant correlation between the level of telomerase activity and tumor type; the highest activity is present in SCLC, and among NSCLC, the lowest activity is present in adenocarcinomas (28). Similarly, in analysis limited primarily to NSCLC, in situ hybridization (ISH) for human telomerase RNA component (hTERC) and mRNA encoding human telomerase reverse transcriptase (*hTERT*) has shown a sensitivity of 100 and 94%, respectively for the diagnosis of carcinoma (28).

However, the specificity of assays for telomerase activity or telomerase component enzymes is not well characterized, because most studies have failed to evaluate preneoplastic epithelial lesions as well as carcinomas. This is not a moot point because dysregulated telomere metabolism is known to be one component of the multistage pathogenesis of lung carcinoma, and is present in precursor lesions as well as carcinomas (31).

From a prognostic standpoint, telomerase activity has been shown to be significantly higher in poorly differentiated tumors and to have a significant association with overall survival (28,32,33). However, the prognostic information provided by analysis of telomerase metabolism does not appear to be independent of stage and grade by multivariant analysis, which limits the utility of the testing in routine practice.

Altered DNA Methylation

Changes in the level of methylation of the promoter region of specific genes, as well as the global pattern of DNA methylation, are characteristic features of lung cancer (reviewed in references 16,18). Altered promoter methylation, usually measured by methylation-specific PCR (Chapter 5), has been shown to correlate with the diagnosis and prognosis for a number of different genes, including those encoding cell cycle regulators (such as $p16^{INK4a}$), nuclear receptors (such as $RAR\beta$), her tumor suppressors (such as *FHIT*), and cell surface adhesions (such as *CDH13* and *ECAD*) (reviewed in 16–18). Changes in the global pattern of DNA methylation are often measured using a monoclonal antibody that recognizes 5-methylcytosine (34). Although global changes correlate with tumor size and clinical stage, hyperplastic and dysplastic lesions also show altered levels of immunostaining.

Microarray Expression Analysis

Given the problems of sensitivity and specificity associated with diagnostic or prognostic analysis of single loci, a number of studies have evaluated the utility of microarray analysis of gene expression in the pathologic evaluation of lung NSCLC and SCLC. These studies have shown that gene expression profiles can discriminate SCLC from pulmonary carcinoid tumors, squamous cell carcinomas, and adenocarcinomas and can even be used to classify pulmonary adenocarcinomas into subgroups with statistically significant differences in prognosis (35–38). Gene expression profiles can also be used to distinguish primary lung adenocarcinomas from metastatic adenocarcinomas and can even indicate the likely anatomic origin of the metastatic tumors (36).

Most of the genes that can be used to define the different diagnostic or prognostic groups encode proteins that are neuroendocrine markers, growth factor receptors, regulators of cell growth and proliferation, or involved in the control of apoptosis. Although there is little overlap in the identity of the genes between studies reported by different groups, a recent cross-study comparison showed that the level of agreement is more than would be expected by chance (39), one of the first demonstrations that there is an underlying small set of genes whose expression profile can be reproducibly identified as having a statistically significant correlation with tumor groupings or patient outcome. Even if oligonucleotide arrays are a useful basic science tool, it remains to be shown that they are the optimum platform for evaluating profiles of gene expression in clinical practice. It is likely that intrinsic limitations on the precision of measurement using oligonucleotide arrays will limit their routine laboratory use, and that quantitative RT-PRC may provide a less cumbersome and more reliable method for assessment of expression levels once the relevant genes are identified (40).

In most studies, gene expression analysis is performed on tissue samples obtained from the definitive surgical excision of the neoplasm. However, gene expression analysis may be applicable to an even broader group of patient specimens. For example, gene expression profiling using oligonucleotide microarrays has been successfully performed on needle biopsy and brushing specimens in which excess tissue was available beyond that needed for pathologic diagnosis (41). In this study, enough excess tissue was present in 88% of patients to perform the microarray analysis, and the expression profile derived from the biopsy and brushing specimens had an accuracy of 86% for predicting the histologic tumor type and 87% of predicting patient outcome. These results suggest that microarray analysis of biopsy specimens can be used to identify patients who may benefit from neoadjuvant therapy before primary excision of their tumor, or to guide selection of the most appropriate therapy regimen for those patients with unresectable tumors.

Role of Molecular Genetic Testing for Screening

By current methods of diagnosis and treatment, 85% of patients with lung cancer will succumb to their disease; most patients who will become long-term survivors have NSCLC detected at an early clinical stage (42). Although patients with preinvasive or micro-invasive tumors have a survival rate of greater than 90%, they constitute less than 1% of newly diagnosed cases (42). Some studies have shown that molecular genetic analysis can detect genetic or epigenetic alterations from months to years before a definitive diagnosis of carcinoma (42–45), and so it has been suggested that screening by molecular genetic techniques may have a role in the routine monitoring of patients who are at high risk of lung cancer. In fact, at least one prospective clinical trial is testing this hypothesis (46).

However, the risk status for development of a fully malignant carcinoma is complex, even in high-risk patients (47). Furthermore, the clinical approach to a patient for whom testing indicates an extremely high likelihood of the presence of a fully malignant carcinoma, but for whom a neoplasm cannot be detected by imaging studies, has yet to be defined. Whether screening involves evaluation of sputum or specimens obtained by bronchoscopy, the molecular genetic approaches used in the analysis are all limited by the fact that every tumor does not harbor the same mutations in the same set of genes, and by the fact that different tumors acquire mutations in a different sequence, as discussed in detail previously (48–51).

Sputum Samples

One approach to molecular analysis of sputum involves the detection of point mutations in the genes that frequently harbor mutations in lung carcinomas. It is difficult to compare studies of this type because the results are often not stratified by tumor type (even though there is marked variation in the percentage of NSCLC versus SCLC tested), different loci are evaluated (or different regions of the same loci), and the mutational analysis is performed by different approaches (including SSCP, DGGE, or restriction fragment length polymorphism [RFLP] analysis, with or without laser capture microdissection to enrich the population of cells for those that show cytologic atypia). Given the technical variation among studies, it is not surprising that the reported sensitivity for detecting *TP53* mutations in the sputum of patients with known lung cancer ranges from 8% to 56% (43,52–54) and ranges from 10% to 45% for detecting mutations in K-*ras* (53–55). Furthermore, because most studies have limited analysis to samples from patients known to have cancer, the specificity of testing is unknown, although one report suggests that mutational analysis of *TP53* has a specificity of 98% (52). Since many studies do not perform parallel cytologic analysis, it is also difficult to compare mutational analysis with routine cytologic evaluation which, for the sake of comparison, is generally

reported to have a sensitivity of 60% when three satisfactory sputum samples are evaluated (56,57).

Alternatively, RT-PCR testing has been used to demonstrate mRNA from genes not normally expressed by non-neoplastic lung tissue. For example, RT-PCR designed to simultaneously detect transcripts from melanoma antigen gene (*MAGE*) subtypes A1-A6 has a sensitivity of 54% in random sputum samples and over 70% in induced sputum samples in patients known to have lung cancer and a specificity of about 98% (58). In paired analysis, the level of performance of the RT-PCR assay is superior to conventional cytology or telomerase activity measured by the TRAP assay.

Another approach has focused on detection of epigenetic changes associated with lung carcinoma, specifically changes in DNA methylation. Even though most studies use the methylation-specific PCR technique, it is again difficult to compare published reports because of differences in the marker loci evaluated, and because the results from patients with NSCLC and SCLC are often not reported separately (45). In any event, analysis limited to one marker has limited utility; for example, detection of an aberrant $p16^{INK4a}$ promoter region methylation pattern has a sensitivity of only 35% (53). In contrast, analysis of multiple markers significantly increases test sensitivity; combined evaluation of the promoter regions of *p16* and *MGMT* has a reported sensitivity of virtually 100% (47). This latter result provides the rationale for clinical trials seeking to validate the hypothesis that detection of methylation markers in exfoliated cells in sputum cells can be used to assess the relative risk that a patient has early lung cancer (45,46).

Similarly, parallel testing by a number of different techniques (including mutational analysis and methylation analysis) of several different loci (including *TP53*, K-*ras*, and $p16^{INK4a}$) has also been shown to provide better overall sensitivity and specificity (53,54), although some parallel testing approaches are so cumbersome that they are poorly suited for use in routine clinical practice. Multitarget, multicolor interphase FISH analysis using a panel of four different probes (to 7p12 including *EGFR*, 8q24 including *myc*, 5p15.2, and 6p11-q11) that is commercially available (LAVysion, Vysis, Downer's Grove, IL) combined with cytologic evaluation has likewise been shown to provide a higher test sensitivity for detection of carcinoma than either method alone (59).

Samples Obtained by Bronchoscopy

The same types of mutation analysis that have been performed on sputum samples have also been applied to bronchoalveolar lavage (BAL) specimens. And, as with studies evaluating sputum samples, it is difficult to compare published reports analyzing BAL specimens because the results are often not stratified by tumor type, different loci are evaluated, and the analysis is performed by different techniques (42,60). Nonetheless, mutational analysis of *TP53* has a reported sensitivity ranging from 8% to 22% for NSCLC (53,61), with a specificity of 88% in the one study in which patients without lung carcinoma were evaluated (53). Mutational analysis of K-*ras* has a reported sensitivity of 9% to 31% for NSCLC but 0% for SCLC (53,61,62), and therefore a specificity of virtually 100% for NSCLC (54,62).

Several other molecular approaches have also been used to evaluate BAL fluid. Methylation-specific PCR analysis of the $p16^{INK4a}$ promoter region has a sensitivity of 22% to 24% for identifying patients with SCLC or NSCLC (54,61), with a specificity of 88% in a study that also involved testing of samples from patients with benign lung disease (54). Microsatellite instability (MSI) analysis has an overall sensitivity ranging from 6% to 40% for SCLC or NSCLC, although test performance depends on whether analysis is restricted to the cell-free lavage supernatants or the cell pellet itself (61,63). Telomerase activity as measured by the TRAP assay has a sensitivity of 70% and a specificity of 92% for the diagnosis of NSCLC, a level of performance that is superior to routine cytologic examination, although combined TRAP and cytologic evaluation apparently provides the highest level of test performance (64). Even testing based on detection of mitochondrial DNA mutations has been performed, although the protocol is so time and labor intensive that the method is not feasible in routine practice (65).

And, not surprisingly, a number of studies have shown that higher test sensitivity and specificity can be achieved when different approaches are used in parallel. However, combined analysis can be so involved that it has virtually no applicability to routine testing of patient specimens; for example, the testing protocol in one study involved mutational analysis of TP53 (by direct sequencing and a plaque hybridization assay), mutational analysis of K-ras (by a ligation assay and a mutant-enriched PCR technique), methylation status of the p16 promoter (by methylation-specific PCR), and MSI (using a panel of 15 markers) (61). A less complicated approach to combined analysis is provided by multitarget multicolor interphase FISH using a panel of four different probes (to 7p12 including EGFR, 8q24 including myc, 5p15.2, and the centromeric region of chromosome 1 or chromosome 6), a technique that has a sensitivity of up to 82% and 73% and a specificity of up to 82% and 87% for detection of carcinoma in bronchial washing and brushing specimens, respectively (24,25). The assay is very straightforward technically because the probe mixture is available commercially (LAVysion, Vysis, Downer's Grove, IL), and in some settings, improved sensitivity and specificity can be obtained when the FISH results are combined with the findings from routine cytologic evaluation (24).

Role of Molecular Genetic Analysis in Staging

Some studies have evaluated whether molecular analysis of lymph nodes or peripheral blood can provide more accurate staging information for patients who have lung carcinoma. In practice, most assays use RT-PCR to detect the messenger ribonucleic acid (mRNA) transcripts of marker genes whose expression is presumed to be limited to the malignant epithelial cells. Although the clinical significance of malignant cells that can be detected only by molecular testing (often referred to as submicroscopic disease) remains to be clarified from a clinical perspective, two issues confound the utility of analysis from a purely technical perspective—the lack of specificity of the marker genes and the lack of morphologic correlation.

Lack of Specificity

Transcripts encoding proteins presumed to be specifically expressed by malignant epithelial cells of NSCLC or SCLC, such as cytokeratin 19 (CK-19), CK-20, and HuD, can be detected by RT-PCR in lymph nodes, peripheral blood samples, or bone marrow specimens in patients with no history of malignancy (66–69). For example, transcripts encoding CK-19 can be detected in the peripheral blood of up to 61% of samples from healthy donors (69), CK-20 in the peripheral blood and lymph nodes of up to 100% of patients with no history of malignancy (66,70–72), and HuD in up to 100% of normal individuals (67). Explanations for these high false positive rates include the fact that some genes are expressed at low levels by the endothelial cells and fibroblasts within lymph nodes (either physiologically or as a result of illegitimate transcription) and the fact that the RT-PCR method is so sensitive that it can detect nucleic acids within cellular debris that has drained to lymph nodes even in the absence of viable tumor cells (73).

Lack of Morphologic Correlation

The specificity of immunohistochemical evaluation of lymph nodes and bone marrow is optimized by the fact that the architectural and cytologic features of immunopositive cells can be used as guide to their diagnostic significance. However, it is impossible to directly evaluate the morphologic features of the cells that are responsible for a positive PCR result because the tissue sample is destroyed during nucleic acid extraction. Because the lack of specificity of many of the markers used for RT-PCR analysis of lymph nodes can lead to false positive results, as could the presence of benign mesothelial inclusions (74), the fact that the PCR-based results cannot be confirmed by direct morphologic correlation is not a trivial point.

Lymph Nodes

To avoid the nonspecificity issues associated with RT-PCR–based detection of marker gene expression, PCR has been used to focus on identification of marker gene mutations known to be present in the patient's primary tumor. In one study, this approach demonstrated TP53 or K-ras mutations in the DNA from regional lymph nodes in 78% of patients who had stage I disease based on routine histologic evaluation and confirmed the presence of lymph node metastases in 100% of patients who had stage II or stage III disease based on conventional histopathologic evaluation (75). However, the clinical significance of these findings is uncertain for several reasons (76). First, the presence of submicroscopic disease detected by PCR was not associated with a statistically significant difference in overall survival or disease-specific survival in patients with stage I disease. Second, the histologic evaluation of the lymph nodes was based on hematoxylin and eosin (H&E)-stained sections only, without supplementary immunohistochemical stains for epithelial markers. Given that immunohistochemical stains demonstrate metastatic disease in 15% to 25% of lymph nodes in NSCLC patients whose nodes are negative based on examination of H&E-stained sections alone (77–79), it is not clear that the molecular testing provides information that could not be obtained more simply and more inexpensively by routine immunohistochemical analysis.

Molecular analysis has also been used to study nodes obtained from staging procedures prior to definitive therapy. Although mediastinoscopy (with routine histopathologic evaluation of the sampled lymph nodes) has an 89% sensitivity and almost 100% specificity for detection of metastases in patients with NSCLS, it is an invasive procedure. Endoscopic ultrasound-guided FNA (EUS-FNA) provides a less invasive approach for sampling lymph nodes that can be used to significantly increase the sensitivity and specificity of imaging techniques such as computer tomography and positron emission tomography (80–82). The utility of molecular genetic analysis as an approach to increase the sensitivity of the pathologic evaluation of the lymph node biopsies obtained from EUS-FNA has been evaluated in one study, but the results are not encouraging. RT-PCR for transcripts encoding hTERT failed to detect metastases in 37% of lymph nodes that were positive by routine histopathologic examination and had a false positive rate of 28% based on the histologic findings in the subsequent surgical resection specimens (83).

Peripheral Blood

Molecular methods have also been used to detect submicroscopic disease in peripheral blood. The different approaches have included RT-PCR detection of marker gene transcripts (66,69), analysis of microsatellite alterations, including instability and LOH (84), and evaluation of epigenetic changes by methylation-specific PCR (33). As expected, the published reports emphasize that the significance of a positive result is critically dependent on both the individual markers and test methodology (66,69). However, from a broader perspective, the role of molecular analysis of peripheral blood remains undefined because prospective studies have yet to demonstrate that the presence of submicroscopic metastases detected by genetic testing has any implications for patient therapy or outcome.

Role of Molecular Genetic Analysis in Choice of Therapy

Apart from any diagnostic or prognostic applications, molecular testing may have a role in identifying which patients are most likely to benefit from a specific chemotherapeutic regimen.

EGFR Inhibitors

By way of background, signaling through the EGFR is normally triggered by the binding of any of several growth factors (including epidermal growth factor [EGF] and TGF-α). Growth factor binding induces receptor dimerization, and the subsequent autophosphorylation and transphosphorylation mediated by the receptor's tyrosine kinase domain lead to activation of downstream proliferative and cell survival signals. Multiple different mechanisms of dysregulated EGFR activation and subsequent intracellular signaling have been described (Fig. 19.2), including deletions and missense mutations in the extracellular domain of the receptor (common in glioblastomas), deletions of the regulatory

intracellular domains (also characteristic of glioblastomas), and small deletions or missense mutations of the kinase domain (present in a subset of lung cancers).

Despite the fact that the drug gefitinib (Iressa) targets the EGFR tyrosine kinase domain (86), and that increased EGFR expression is present in from 40% to 80% of NSCLC (87), neither the level of receptor expression nor its phosphorylation state correlates with tumor responsive to the drug. Furthermore, clinical studies shown that gefitinib overall has only minimal effect on patients with advanced NSCLC, with or without concomitant traditional chemotherapy (88–91). However, DNA sequence analysis of EGFR in the small subset of patients who did respond to gefitinib therapy shows that 93% of patients harbor EGFR mutations affecting the receptor's kinase domain (92,93), including missense mutations and small deletions (Fig. 19.2), that functionally render the receptor more sensitive to gefitinib inhibition (92,94). The pattern of mutations that make the EGFR more sensitive to gefitinib inhibition is more common in adenocarcinomas than other types of NSCLC, more frequent in women, and more frequent in patients from Japan than the United States, which precisely mirrors the clinical characteristics of patients who show a clinical response to the drug, although the ethnic and environmental factors that are responsible for this skewed pattern of mutations are as yet unknown (88,89,93). It is interesting to note that the terminal respiratory unit (TRU) type of pulmonary adenocarcinoma (Fig. 19.3) shows an extremely high overlap with the clinical and pathologic features of those patients who respond to gefitinib therapy (95).

A recent clinical trial has demonstrated a survival benefit in patients with NSCLC treated with erlotinib (Tarceva), another drug that inhibits the tyrosine kinase activity of EGFR (96). However, the molecular and clinical predictors of treatment outcome are different for erlotinib than for gefitinib (97); the presence of an EGFR mutation may increase responsiveness to erlotinib, but is not indicative of improved survival.

Finally, it should be noted that the demonstration that only a subset of EGFR mutations correlate with clinical response to gefitinib has important implications for the design of clinical trials. The fact that the subgroup of patients with a durable clinical responses to gefitinib was identified only after clinical trials had failed to demonstrate a clinically significant overall response rate, or any correlation with the level of EGFR expression or activation, indicates that the traditional criteria for patient selection and data analysis in clinical trials of novel chemotherapeutic drugs may be inadequate (98,99). Trials that incorporate molecular genetic analysis to select patients whose mutations correlate with the presumed mechanism of drug activity will not only be more likely to identify a therapeutic benefit associated with a new drug (especially if the probable responders make up only a small percentage of the patient population) but will also limit the potential toxicity and treatment, delay associated with the clinical trial for patients who are unlikely to benefit from the drug.

Drugs that Interfere with DNA Methylation

A number of drugs that interfere with the enzymatic pathways involved in DNA methylation and demethylation are

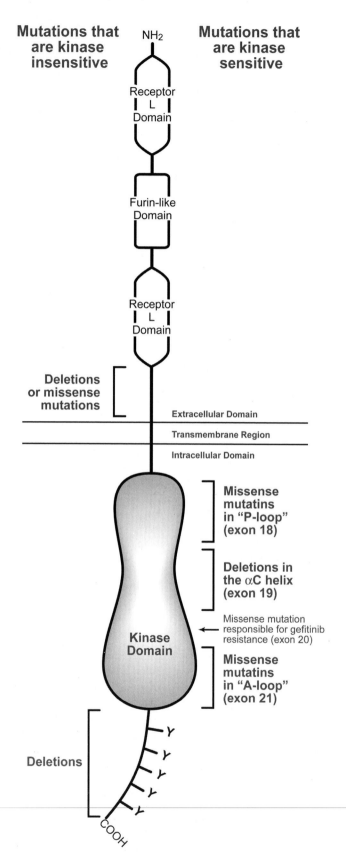

Mutations that are kinase insensitive

NH₂

Receptor L Domain

Furin-like Domain

Receptor L Domain

Deletions or missense mutations

Extracellular Domain

Transmembrane Region

Intracellular Domain

Kinase Domain

Deletions

COOH

Mutations that are kinase sensitive

Missense mutatins in "P-loop" (exon 18)

Deletions in the αC helix (exon 19)

Missense mutation responsible for gefitinib resistance (exon 20)

Missense mutatins in "A-loop" (exon 21)

Figure 19.2 Schematic diagram of the epidermal growth factor receptor (EGFR) showing the relative positions of the two receptor ligand (*L*) domains, the furin-like domain, the tyrosine kinase domain, and the carboxy-terminal regulatory domain (which harbors several tyrosine residues whose phosphorylation is responsible for receptor activation). The left side of the diagram indicates the position of mutations common in glioblastomas that are insensitive to kinase inhibitors but are more likely to respond to the neutralizing antibody cetuximab (Erbitux). The right side indicates the location of the deletions and mutations in the kinase domain that render NSCLC sensitive to kinase inhibitors such as gefitinib. The position of a missense mutation in exon 20 that leads to gefitinib-resistance in NSCLC that harbor P-loop, A-loop or αC helix mutations is also shown (85).

methylation, although the use of DAC in vivo is complicated by the fact that pharmacologically active dosages are usually accompanied by systemic toxicity (100). Zebularine and (−)-epigallocatechin-3-gallate both inhibit cytosine DNA methyltransferase, but in contrast to DAC can be taken chronically without systemic toxicity (101,102). Selenium is a demethylating agent that apparently also acts via inhibition of cytosine DNA methyltransferase (103). Sodium phenylbutyrate is a histone deactylase inhibitor that may have synergistic effects with DAC (104), as expected based on the links between histone deacetylation and DNA methylation (Chapter 1). The availability of these drugs suggests that even if DNA methylation analysis has no role in the diagnosis of lung cancer, testing may still have a role for identifying patients with known lung cancer who may benefit from chemotherapy with these compounds, or for identifying patients at high risk for developing lung cancer who may benefit from chemoprevention using these drugs. At least one clinical trial is already evaluating the efficacy of long-term selenium supplementation for decreasing the incidence of second primary tumors in patients who have undergone curative surgery for stage I NSCLC (45).

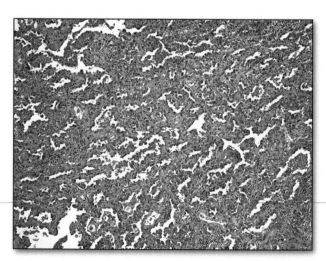

Figure 19.3 The terminal respiratory unit (TRU) type of pulmonary adenocarcinoma is highly correlated with response to kinase inhibitor therapy. TRU morphology is characterized by differentiation to type II pneumocytes, Clara cells, and/or bronchiolar epithelium (see reference 97).

currently available or undergoing clinical trials for treatment of lung carcinoma. The drug 5-aza-2′-deoxycytidine (DAC) is a demethylating agent that has been shown to lead to the reexpression of genes silenced by promoter

NEUROENDOCRINE TUMORS

Neuroendocrine tumors account for 20% to 25% of all lung neoplasms and include carcinoid tumor (low-grade neuroendocrine carcinoma), atypical carcinoid tumor (intermediate-grade neuroendocrine carcinoma), and SCLC and large cell neuroendocrine carcinoma (high-grade neuroendocrine carcinoma) (Fig. 19.4). Carcinoid and atypical carcinoid tumors together account for 1% to 2% of all primary lung neoplasms; SCLC and large cell neuroendocrine carcinoma (LCNEC) together account for about 20% to 25% (105).

Genetics

Low-grade and Intermediate Grade Neuroendocrine Carcinoma

Pulmonary carcinoid and atypical carcinoid tumors harbor some, but not all, of the genetic changes that are characteristic of other foregut neuroendocrine tumors (those arising in the esophagus, stomach, pancreas, and duodenum proximal to the ampulla of Vater). Deletions and mutations of the *MEN1* gene and LOH of 11q are relatively common in pulmonary carcinoid and atypical carcinoid tumors, whereas mutations of *TP53*, mutations of K-*ras*, and LOH of 18q and 18p are rare (reviewed in 106,107).

Despite the many genetic similarities between pulmonary carcinoid and atypical carcinoid, the two tumors show several recurring genetic differences (Table 19.2). By microsatellite analysis, LOH of 11q13 (which harbors the *MEN1* gene) is present in a greater percentage of atypical carcinoids than typical carcinoids (108–110). Microsatellite analysis has also shown different patterns of LOH between typical and atypical carcinoid tumors for several tumor suppressor genes, including *FHIT*, *RB1*, and *TP53* (111,112), and has demonstrated a higher rate of X chromosome deletions in atypical than typical carcinoids (113). Comparative genomic hybridization has shown differences in the prevalence of 10q and 13q losses between typical and atypical carcinoid tumors (109), and it is interesting to note that comparative genomic hybridization has also demonstrated that thymic neuroendocrine tumors harbor a pattern of cytogenetic aberrations that is completely different from that of foregut carcinoid tumors, a finding that is consistent with the different clinicopathologic features of thymic neuroendocrine tumors (114).

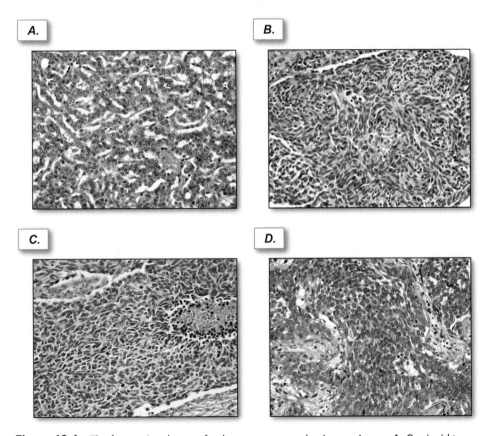

Figure 19.4   The four major classes of pulmonary neuroendocrine carcinoma. **A,** Carcinoid tumor (low-grade neuroendocrine carcinoma). **B,** Atypical carcinoid (intermediate-grade neuroendocrine carcinoma; note the mitotic figures and necrosis). **C,** SCLC. **D,** Large-cell neuroendocrine carcinoma (LCNEC). Both SCLC and LCNEC are high-grade neuroendocrine carcinomas. As discussed in the text, carcinoid tumor, atypical carcinoid tumor, and SCLC have a different profile of genetic aberrations (see also Tables 19.1 and 19.2), but there are few significant genetic differences between the SCLC and LCNEC types of high-grade neuroendocrine carcinoma.

TABLE 19.2

EXAMPLES OF COMMON GENETIC ALTERATIONS IN PULMONARY NEUROENDOCRINE TUMOURS[a]

Genetic Alteration	Carcinoid Tumor (low-grade neuroendocrine carcinoma)	Atypical Carcinoid (intermediate-grade neuroendocrine carcinoma)
MEN1 mutation	Common	Common
LOH of 11q13	0–70%	50%–100%
Regions of frequent LOH	11q13	11q13, 10q, 13q, X
RAS mutations	Rare	Rare
RB1 inactivation	Rare	50%
TP53 inactivation	Rare	50%
FHIT inactivation	Rare	40%

[a]See Table 19.1 for common genetic alterations in SCLC.
[b]Compiled from references 106, 107, 109–113.

High-grade Neuroendocrine Carcinoma

As discussed above, the pattern of mutations and epigenetic changes that underlies the development of high-grade neuroendocrine carcinoma differs from that of adenocarcinoma and squamous cell carcinoma (SCC). Although the recent World Health Organization (WHO) classification separates high-grade neuroendocrine carcinoma into the SCLS and large cell neuroendocrine carcinoma (LCNEC) categories (105), the significant histopathologic overlap and clinical behavior of SCLC and LCNEC has led to the suggestion that the two categories should be reclassified as a single high-grade neuroendocrine tumor group (115,116). The proposed reclassification is supported by several types of genetic analysis, including LOH analysis, mutational analysis of TP53, and gene expression profiling, all of which show that SCLC and LCNEC have a different profile of aberrations than carcinoid and atypical carcinoid tumors, but tend not to show a significantly different pattern of molecular changes from each other (111,112).

Diagnostic and Prognostic Features of Molecular Genetic Analysis of Neuroendocrine Tumors

The morphology and immunoprofile of low-grade, intermediate-grade, and high-grade neuroendocrine carcinoma are well defined (117). However, there is no established role for molecular genetic analysis in diagnosis. Given the heterogeneity in the prevalence of genetic aberrations as determined by LOH analysis of microsatellite loci, comparative genomic hybridization, and mutational analysis of specific genes (108–111), the accumulated data indicate that testing by any of these techniques lacks the sensitivity and specificity to be of clinical utility in routine practice.

Even if there is no role for genetic testing for diagnosis of neuroendocrine tumors, several studies have suggested that molecular analysis may play a role in providing prognostic information. For example, microsatellite analysis has shown that LOH at 5q21 is associated with a poor survival in patients with carcinoid tumors (107–112), and that allelic losses of the X chromosome are associated with a worse clinical outcome in patients with atypical carcinoid tumors (113). Gene expression profiling of high-grade neuroendocrine carcinoma has been used to detect a pattern of gene expression that correlates with improved survival; specifically, expression of a panel of 740 genes identifies a group of patients with an 83% 5-year survival (118), a remarkable finding because the 5-year survival of unselected patients is only 12% or lower. Of note, the gene expression analysis could not distinguish SCLC from LCNEC, and there were no significant differences in survival between patients with SCLC and LCNEC.

COMBINED VERSUS COLLISION TUMORS

Some lung carcinomas have a mixed small cell and non–small cell morphology, and molecular analysis has been used to define the relationship between the two regions in these tumors. Mutational analysis of specific genes (specifically, TP53 or K-ras) and LOH analysis of microsatellite loci at a number of chromosomal locations (including 3p, 5p, 9p, 13q, 17p, and 18q) has demonstrated a clonal relationship in tumors that show a mixture of SCLC and SCC morphologies (119,120). However, the relationship between tumors that show mixed SCLC and adenocarcinoma histology remains to be established. In the small number of cases that have thus far been evaluated, the pattern of TP53 mutations and chromosome 3p LOH is ambiguous and does not definitely establish whether the malignancies are collision tumors that develop from separate clones or combined neoplasms in which the two components result from clonal diversion that occurs at an early stage of tumor growth (119).

PRIMARY VERSUS METASTATIC TUMORS

The presence of a solitary lung nodule in a patient known to have an extrathoracic carcinoma presents a difficult diagnostic challenge (121). In some settings, for example, in patients with a history of head and neck SCC (HNSSC), lung metastases and primary lung SCC have such a high degree of morphologic similarity that they often cannot be distinguished based on histopathologic evaluation (117). However, the difference has important prognostic and therapeutic implications because metastatic disease is rarely curable, but an independent primary lung tumor is usually treated with curative intent.

Molecular clonality determination using LOH analysis of microsatellite loci on chromosomes 3p and 9p has been shown to be useful in this situation. In cases in which standard clinical and histopathologic parameters could not unambiguously establish whether a solitary SSC in the lung represented a primary lung tumor or metastatic HNSCC, the pattern of LOH could definitely establish whether the tumor represented a metastasis or an independent lung tumor in 91% of cases (122). The finding that the majority of solitary lung nodules in patients who have a history of HNSCC represent metastatic disease is consistent with the clinical fact that this group of patients has a very poor survival rate (123). Although clonality analysis involving multiple microsatellite loci is admittedly cumbersome, it clearly has clinical utility because the testing is informative in such a high percentage of cases and because the results significantly influence patient care.

PULMONARY CHONDROID HAMARTOMA

Pulmonary chondroid hamartoma is a benign tumor that consists of varying combinations of cartilage, connective tissue, smooth muscle, fat, and lung epithelium. Despite its name, the presence of recurring clonal genetic aberrations indicates that the lesion is a benign neoplasm.

Genetics

Conventional cytogenetic analysis of a large number of pulmonary chondroid hamartomas (PCH) has demonstrated recurring clonal karyotypic abnormalities involving 12q14-15 or 6p21. In tumors with aberrations involving 12q14-15, the gene encoding the high mobility group (HMG) protein HMGA2 (previously known HMGIC) is consistently rearranged (124–126). In tumors with rearrangements of 6p21, the gene encoding the HMG protein HMGA1 (previously known as HMGIY) is consistently rearranged (124–127). HMG proteins are small, acidic, nonhistone, chromatin-associated proteins that do not exhibit transcriptional activity themselves, but facilitate formation of transcriptional complexes through protein–DNA and protein–protein interactions. Both HMGA2 and HMGA1 contain three DNA binding domains (which bind to the minor groove of adenine and thymine-rich [AT-rich] DNA sequences and are therefore referred to as AT hooks) and an acidic C-terminal domain, and both have important roles during growth and development (128). The fact that the rearrangements involving *HMGA2* or *HMGA1* are

present in the stromal but not the epithelial component of PCH indicates that the epithelial component of PCH is not neoplastic, but is merely entrapped.

The wide variety of karyotypic alterations in PCH indicates that a number of different loci can partner with the *HMGA2* and *HMGA1* loci to promote tumorigenesis. By analogy with the involvement of the same two genes in the development of a wide variety of other benign mesenchymal tumors (Table 11.7), it is thought that the loci involved in HMG rearrangements in PCH have no specific role in tumor development beyond merely separating the DNA-binding domains of the HMG proteins from their acidic C-terminal domains (129), or beyond simple deregulation of the level of expression of the *HMG* genes themselves (128,130,131). The demonstration that some PCHs harbor HMG rearrangements with chromosomal break points that lie 3' or 5' to the coding region of the genes (124,125,127,132) supports the hypothesis that deregulation of HMG expression alone is sufficient to promote tumor development.

Some of the rearrangements in PCH have been characterized at a DNA sequence level. The relatively common translocation t(3;12)(q27-28;q14-15) results in the formation of an *HMGA2-LPP* fusion gene in which exons 1 to 3 of *HMGA2* are fused to exons 9 to 11 of *LPP*, forming a chimeric protein in which the three AT-hook of *HMGA2* are fused to two LIM domains of *LPP* (Fig. 19.5). LIM

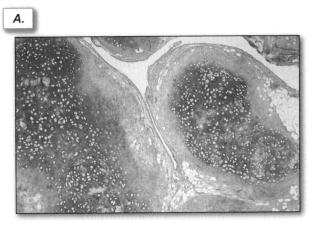

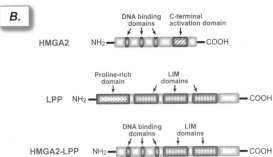

Figure 19.5 *HMG* fusions are characteristic of pulmonary chondroid hamartoma (PCH). **A,** A PCH with prominent islands of cartilage, an outer rim of mesenchyme that includes fat, and invaginated cleftlike spaces lined by respiratory type epithelium. **B,** Schematic diagram of the HMGA2-LPP chimeric protein that results from the t(3;12)(q27-28;q14-15) that is relatively common in PCH. The most common structure of the HMGAZ-LPP fusion protein that results from from the t(3; 12) is illustrated.

domains are cysteine rich, zinc-binding protein sequences present in transcription regulatory proteins, some of which have a role in cell signaling and development (124). It is interesting to note that the exact same fusion gene also has been described in lipomas (133).

The t(12;14)(q15;q23-24) translocation produces a fusion between *HMGA2* and *RAD51B*. *RAD51B* encodes a protein kinase essential for DNA repair by homologous recombination (Chapter 2), and it is again interesting to note that the *HMGA2-RAD51L* fusion is a recurring feature of uterine leiomyomas (134).

Technical Issues in Molecular Genetic Analysis of PCH

Routine cytogenetic evaluation of PCH shows a rearrangement involving 12q14-15 or 6p21 in about 60% of cases (125,126); series that report a much higher prevalence of translocations have focused on preselected groups of cases (124,127). Approximately 85% of PCH with an abnormal karyotype have rearrangements involving 12q14-15, while about 15% have rearrangements involving 6p21 (125,126). Given the marked heterogeneity in the karyotypic abnormalities that are associated with PCH, the genomewide screen provided by conventional cytogenetic analysis makes the method ideally suited for the evaluation of PCH.

FISH was an essential component of the experimental approach used to identify many of the 12q14-15 and 6p21 rearrangements in PCH (124–126,132,134). The probe-split FISH technique has been used to demonstrate rearrangements involving *HMGA2* or *HMGA1* in 70% to 76% of cases, and combined cytogenetic analysis and FISH can identify rearrangements of the *HMGA2* or *HMGA1* loci in up to 80% of cases (125,126). FISH is especially helpful in confirming the involvement of the *HMG* loci in cases with complex rearrangements (135). In the studies reported to date, FISH has been performed on metaphase chromosomes, so the utility of interphase FISH for the demonstration of rearrangements involving *HMGA2* and *HMGA1* loci has yet to be formally evaluated. Nonetheless, because of the heterogeneity of the chromosomal rearrangements that involve the 12q14-15 and 6p21 regions, probe-split FISH will almost certainly be a more sensitive approach than probe-fusion FISH.

PCR-based methods, including RT-PCR, 3′-RACE, and 5′-RACE, have been used to characterize the break points and fusion genes found in PCH (124,125,132,133). Given the variety of structural rearrangements that involve *HMGA2* and *HMGA1* in PCH, RT-PCR is not ideally suited for routine evaluation of the tumors. Sensitive testing would require a number of primer sets to detect all the known fusion genes, and even then would not detect transcripts from fusion genes that have yet to be characterized (136).

Immunohistochemistry

Both *HMGA2* and *HMGA1* are expressed during development and in a wide variety of human malignancies, but *HMGA2* is not expressed in normal adult tissues, and *HMGA1* is expressed at only very low levels (126,128,137). Aberrant expression of *HMGA2* or *HMGA1* detected

immunohistochemically in PCH therefore correlates with chromosomal aberrations at 12q14-15 or 6p21 (126). Immunoreactivity for *HMGA2* and *HMGA1* is present in about 20% of PCH without rearrangements involving 12q14-15 or 6p21 (126), which suggests that immunohistochemistry may be more sensitive than molecular methods for demonstrating deregulated gene expression at these two loci.

Diagnostic Issues in Molecular Genetic Analysis of PCH

As noted previously, rearrangements involving *HMGA2* and *HMGA1* are also involved in the development of a wide variety of other benign mesenchymal tumors, and some other benign mesenchymal neoplasms harbor the exact same gene fusions that are present in PCH. Rare malignant soft tissue tumors have also been shown to harbor rearrangements involving the 12q14-15 region (138). However, from a diagnostic point of view, the fact that rearrangements of *HMGA2* and *HMGA1* are also characteristic of a number of benign and malignant mesenchymal tumors other than PCH is of little relevance, because most of these other neoplasms do not enter into the differential diagnosis of PCH.

TUMORS OF SALIVARY GLAND TYPE

Pleomorphic Adenoma

Pleomorphic adenoma (PA) (also known as benign mixed tumor) is the most common benign tumor of the major and minor salivary glands, and cases have been described in the lung (117,139). PA of the lung (Fig. 19.6) occurs within or adjacent to a bronchus and can present as either a polypoid endobronchial lesion or a peripheral tumor without apparent involvement of an airway (140).

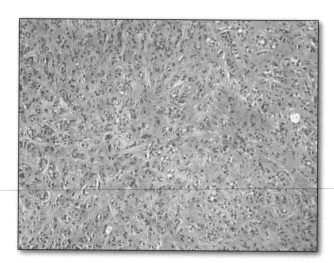

Figure 19.6 Pleomorphic adenoma (PA) arising in the trachea of a 64-year-old woman. Rearrangements involving the *HMGA2* locus at 12q14-15 are frequently present in PA, as rearrangements of the *PLAG1* locus at 8q12. (See Chapter 21.)

The genetics of PA, as well as the technical and diagnostic issues involved in the evaluation of the tumor by molecular techniques, are discussed in detail in Chapter 21. However, it is worth noting here that one of the genetic aberrations characteristic of PA is rearrangement of the *HMGA2* locus at 12q14-15, which is also rearranged in PCH, as discussed previously.

Mucoepidermoid Carcinoma

Mucoepidermoid carcinoma (MEC) is the most common malignant salivary gland tumor, but accounts for only 0.1% to 0.2% of primary lung carcinomas (117). Primary pulmonary MEC usually arises in the main or lobar bronchi, but cases in the peripheral lung that arise in segmental bronchi have been described.

The genetics of the t(11;19)(q21;p13) translocation that is the hallmark of MEC are described in more detail in Chapter 21, as are the technical and diagnostic issues involved in the molecular genetic analysis of MEC. The original molecular characterization of the t(11;19) translocation included several cases that arose within the lung (141,142), formally establishing that MECs of the lung harbor the same molecular abnormalities as tumors that arise in the salivary glands of the head and neck.

PLEURAL EFFUSIONS

Epithelial Malignancies

Demonstration of malignant cells in a pleural effusion has a profound effect on prognosis, and can lead to either withholding or intensification of therapy depending on the clinical setting. Even though conventional cytologic evaluation of pleural effusions for detection of malignant cells has a specificity that approaches 100%, cytology has a sensitivity of only 50% to 95% (143,144). Consequently, a number of different genetic methods have been studied as potential tests for evaluation of pleural effusions, but regardless of the molecular approach, testing for epithelial malignancies has three general limitations. First, molecular analysis that focuses on a single genetic locus has an intrinsically limited sensitivity, as discussed in detail previously. Second, transcripts of marker genes presumed to be specifically expressed by malignant cells often can be detected in benign effusions because the genes are transcribed at a low level by inflammatory cells and mesothelial cells. Third, because the tissue substrate is destroyed when nucleic acids are extracted (as is required for other than in situ approaches), it is not possible to evaluate the morphologic features of the cells that are responsible for a positive test result.

PCR-based Methods

Markers whose expression is restricted to primary lung carcinomas (e.g., surfactant protein A) have a specificity of virtually 100% for detecting malignant epithelial cells from primary lung carcinomas, but have no utility in testing for a wider range of carcinomas (145). Markers present in a wider range of carcinomas (e.g., mucin gene transcripts or variant CD44 transcripts produced by alternative splicing) are therefore often more useful targets, especially in quantitative RT-PCR testing formats (146–150), and can be used to discriminate between malignant and benign pleural fluids with a sensitivity of up to 96% and a specificity of up to 92% (146,151). Some quantitative methods are based on modified competitive formats that are cumbersome and costly (151), and so are not ideally suited for routine clinical use. RT-PCR analysis that employs the dye SYBR green (Chapter 5) provides a more straightforward method for quantitative analysis. Using *GA733-2* as the marker (*GA733-2* encodes the epithelial glycoprotein recognized by the monoclonal antibody BerEP4), expression thresholds have been identified that yield a sensitivity of 96% and specificity of 98% for correct diagnosis of metastatic effusions from BerEP4-positive primary tumors (152). This result demonstrates that quantitative RT-PCR in this setting is a useful method for distinguishing marker expression due to the presence of a very small number of tumor cells from background transcription by benign cells.

Telomerase-based Methods

When used to evaluate effusions (of pleural as well as pericardial or peritoneal origin) for the presence of malignant epithelial cells, TRAP analysis of cell extracts has a sensitivity of 76% and a specificity of 74% to 94% (153,154). The assay provides little, if any, increase in sensitivity or specificity compared with routine cytology, and thus it is difficult to justify the added time and expense of the analysis, or to recommend the assay as a suitable replacement for cytology for routine diagnostic purposes (155). In contrast, the utility of testing by in situ TRAP is much higher; because the in situ approach makes it possible to determine the morphology of the TRAP-positive cells, and to distinguish malignant cells from proliferative mesothelial cells and lymphocytes, the method has a sensitivity to 95% and a specificity of virtually 100% (156).

Lymphomas

In situ RT-PCR has been used in the context of lymphoproliferative disorders to overcome the lack of morphologic correlation that is traditionally associated with genetic analysis of effusion specimens. In one study, the technique was applied to sections of FFPE tissue from patients with primary effusion lymphoma, a distinct subtype of large B-cell lymphoma defined by the presence of human herpesvirus-8 (HHV-8) in the tumor (157,158). The T0.7 mRNA of HHV-8 that is expressed in latent infections was the target in the analysis, and although the number of cases analyzed was admittedly quite small, testing was positive in 100% of cases (159). The significance of a testing approach that permits direct genotype-phenotype correlation is emphasized by the recent demonstration that benign mesothelial cells can also be infected by HHV-8 in immunodeficient patients (160).

Sarcomas

RT-PCR has also been applied to malignant effusions to document the presence of fusion transcripts characteristic of specific tumor types. For example, the finding of a *PAX3-FKHR* fusion transcript characteristic of alveolar rhabdomyosarcoma (Chapter 11) was used to establish the diagnosis in a child who presented with a pleural effusion that contained malignant small round cells with scattered large atypical cells, but who had no prior history of rhabdomyosarcoma (161).

MIDLINE CARCINOMA WITH NUT REARRANGEMENT

NUT-rearranged carcinoma (NRC) is an extremely aggressive carcinoma that occurs in children, adolescents, and young adults (162–164). All of the cases of NRC reported to date involve midline structures, including the mediastinum, thymus, lung, trachea, nasopharynx, and sinus and orbit. A single case arising below the diaphragm (involving the bladder) has also been described (164). Morphologically, the tumor consists of discohesive undifferentiated cells that have scant cytoplasm, prominent nucleoli, and show varying degrees of squamous differentiation, but no evidence of glandular differentiation. The cell type that gives rise to the tumor is unknown, and the tumor is invariably unresponsive to even combined chemoradiotherapy.

Genetics

The hallmark of NRC is rearrangement of the *NUT* gene at 15q13 (164). The majority of cases harbor the translocation t(15;19)(q13;p13.1), which produces a *BRD4-NUT* fusion gene in which the 5′ region of *BRD4* is fused to the 3′ region of *NUT* (Fig. 19.7). In all cases in which the sequence of *BRD4-NUT* fusion transcripts has been determined, the translocation produces a fusion gene in which *BRD4* exon 10 is fused to *NUT* exon 2 (165). It is notable that two alternative BRD4 isoforms are normally produced as a result of alternative splicing, and so the translocation break point results in fusion transcripts from the longer isoform, while the shorter isoform remains unaltered (162), although the physiologic significance of this finding is unknown. In about 25% of NRC that harbor rearrangements of *NUT*, *BRD4* is not involved; the identity of the partner gene(s) in these variant cases is not yet known (164).

In the BRD4-NUT chimeric protein, the N-terminal region of BRD4 that contains several different functional domains is linked to almost the entire length of the native NUT protein. BRD4 has an important role in regulation of cellular proliferation and is widely expressed in adult tissue (165–167). NUT harbors a putative nuclear localization signal, although the protein's function is unknown and its expression in the adult is limited to the testes (165). Therefore even though the translocation results in

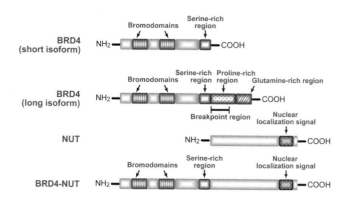

Figure 19.7   *BRD4-NUT* fusions are characteristic of midline carcinomas with *NUT* rearrangements. The schematic diagram shows the location of the proline-rich region and glutamine-rich region that are present in the long isoform of BRD4, but are not present in the short isoform. Because the break point region in *BDR4* in t(15;19)(q13;p13.1) rearrangements that produce BRD4-NUT chimeric proteins is within the region of the gene encoding the proline-rich region, only the long isoform of BDR4 is altered by the translocation. (Modified from references 162 and 165).

constitutive production of a chimeric protein that combines different functional domains within a single molecule, the details of the mechanism by which the chimeric protein induces tumorigeneis are not yet known.

Technical Issues in Molecular Genetic Analysis of NRC

The translocation t(15;19) was originally identified by routine cytologic evaluation, although the limits of conventional chromosome banding techniques can create some ambiguity as to the precise break point within the 15q12 and 19p13 regions (168). The fact that a karyotype has been successfully produced in most of the cases reported to date (162,168–171) most likely reflects a reporting bias.

Metaphase FISH has been used to document the presence of rearrangements in the 15q12-13 and 19p13.1-13.3 regions (162) and has been shown to be especially useful for identifying rearrangements in these regions in cases that harbor complex translocations (168). Interphase FISH by probe-split methodology has been developed for use with FFPE tissue (162,163). The utility of the interphase FISH approach is suggested by the findings of one large study of FFPE tissue from cases of poorly differentiated carcinomas arising in young patients; in this case series, 8% of tumors were shown to harbor *BRD4-NUT* fusions, and an additional 3% of cases were shown to harbor rearrangements of *NUT* without involvement of *BRD4* (164).

RT-PCR has been used to demonstrate the presence of *BRD4-NUT* fusion transcripts in cases of NRC (165). However, thus far the assay has been applied only to NRC cell lines known to harbor the t(15;19)(q13;p13.1) translocation, so the performance characteristics of an RT-PCR–based approach for detecting fusion transcripts in either fresh or FFPE tissue is unknown. In any event, because about 25% of NRC with *NUT* rearrangements harbor variant translocations, RT-PCR based on detection of

BRD4-NET fusions will have a sensitivity that is lower than probe-split FISH analysis of *NUT*.

Immunohistochemistry

The fact that NUT is normally expressed only in testes suggests that immunohistochemistry using antibodies against NUT protein could potentially be used to identify NRC (165). However, immunohistochemical detection of overexpressed chimeric NUT proteins has yet to be described.

Diagnostic Issues in Molecular Genetic Analysis of NRC

NRC does not have a specific morphologic pattern and can arise at a variety of anatomic sites, and so the tumor is currently defined on the basis of rearrangements involving *NUT* (164). In the absence of molecular testing for definitive diagnosis, NRC has been classified as neuroblastoma, primary lung carcinoma, lymphoma, nonseminomatous germ cell tumor, teratocarcinoma, thymic carcinoma, poorly differentiated SCC, or undifferentiated carcinoma (163,164,168). Although NRC is not common, the fact that the neoplasm accounts for approximately 11% of tumors in some patient populations (164) indicates the clinical significance of molecular testing for correct diagnosis.

Role of Molecular Genetic Analysis for Prognostic Testing in NRC

NRCs that harbor *BRD4-NUT* fusions are rapidly progressive malignancies, and most patients succumb to their disease within about 6 months (163,164,168). In the small number of cases thus far described, *NUT*-variant NRC has been associated with a less aggressive course, with patients surviving as long as 1 to 3 years (164). Analysis of the type of *NUT* rearrangement can therefore provide prognostic information, even though patients with NRC are not stratified into different therapeutic groups based on the results of molecular testing.

CYSTIC FIBROSIS

Cystic fibrosis (CF) is a chronic progressive disease with an autosomal recessive inheritance. The disease is due to mutations in the *CFTR* gene at 7q31.2 that encodes the cAMP-dependent Cl^- channel also referred to as the cystic fibrosis transmembrane conductance regulator (CFTR). In the absence of normal CFTR protein, epithelial membranes become relatively impermeable to Cl^-, which together with secondary effects on transmembrane movement of Na^+ and water results in the production of abnormal viscid mucus. The thick inspissated mucus is the common underlying link for the clinical features of CF, including chronic infective bronchopulmonary disease, pancreatic insufficiency with intestinal obstruction, biliary sclerosis, and chronic sinusitis (reviewed in 172).

Genetics

The incidence of CF varies among racial and ethnic groups. Among Caucasions of northern or central European ancestry, the incidence is 1 in 2,500, an incidence that makes CF the most common lethal autosomal recessive disorder in this population. In contrast, the incidence of CF is only 1 in 10,500 among Native Americans, 1 in 11,500 among Hispanics, 1 in 14,000 among blacks, and only 1 in 25,500 among Asians. Over 1,300 different CFTR mutations have been described in patients with CF (173), including nonsense, missense, frame shift, deletion, insertion, and splice site mutations. Even though ΔF508 accounts for approximately 70% of mutations in Caucasian populations, taken together the 70 most common mutations still account for only about 90% of CF cases. Variability in the clinical spectrum of disease associated with specific CFTR mutations indicates that modifier loci exist, only a few of which have been characterized (174–176).

Role of Molecular Analysis in CF

Screening

Whereas a role for genetic testing is well established in some settings (e.g., for adults with a family history of CF or for partners of patients with CF), a role for general screening (e.g., of all couples seeking preconception or prenatal care or for all newborns) remains a matter of debate (177,178). In the context of neonatal screening, it has been convincingly established that screening programs substantially decrease the age of diagnosis and consequently have a significant impact on disease sequella (179), although the large number of mutations makes it difficult to design a program that approaches 100% sensitivity (177). In any event, because screening can be performed on any somatic tissue (usually peripheral blood), it usually does not fall under the purview of diagnostic surgical pathology.

Choice of Therapy

The availability of a number of drug therapies that have activity only for specific classes of mutant CFTR proteins (180–182) has identified a potential role for mutational analysis of the *CFTR* gene. For example, the drug 4-phenylbutyrate increases expression of the ΔF508 CFTR protein in the cell membrane through nonspecific stimulation of gene transcription and modulation of the interactions with chaperone proteins that are involved in CFTR folding. Various phosphatase inhibitors can correct defective function of CFTR proteins that contain G551D or ΔF508 mutations (181,183). The aminoglycoside gentamicin can be used to enhance production of full-length CFTR protein molecules from *CFTR* genes that harbor nonsense mutations by promoting amino acid misincorporation during translation (184,185); although nonsense mutations account for only 2% to 5% of CF cases worldwide, they are present in almost 60% of Ashkenazi Jewish patients with CF. However, as with mutational analysis in the context of screening for CF, molecular testing performed to optimize treatment can be performed on any somatic tissue and so is not likely to be performed in the context of diagnostic surgical pathology.

PRIMARY PULMONARY HYPERTENSION

Primary (or idiopathic) pulmonary hypertension (PPH) occurs in familial and sporadic forms that cannot be distinguished from one another by the histopathologic findings in lung tissue (186) (Fig. 19.8). The endothelial cells in the plexiform lesions of patients with PPH are monoclonal, show microsatellite instability (MSI), and possess an abnormal pattern of expression of genes controlling cellular growth and apoptosis, a constellation of findings that suggests the endothelial cells may be neoplastic (187–189). In contrast, the endothelial cells in the plexiform lesions of patients with secondary pulmonary hypertension are polyclonal.

Genetics

Familial PPH

About 50% of cases of inherited PPH are due to mutations in the *BMPR2* gene (190,191), which encodes the bone morphogenetic protein receptor type-2 involved in pulmonary arterial smooth muscle cell mitosis (192). Exonic mutations are responsible for most cases, although it is likely that more extensive sequence analysis will demonstrate intronic or promoter mutations in a significant subset of the remaining cases (186). Carriers of *BMPR2* mutations not only have lifetime risk of 15% to 20% for developing PPH (186), but also have an increased risk for developing PPH after exposure to

a number of different appetite suppressants, including fenfluramine, dexfenfluramine, and amfepramone (193,194). Of note, mutations in *BMPR2* have also been detected in about 6% of a mixed cohort of children and adults with pulmonary arterial hypertension resulting from congenital cardiac anomalies (195).

A subset of patients with hereditary hemorrhagic telangiectasia and coexistant inherited PPH harbors mutations in activin-like kinase type-1 (*ALK1*) (186,196). *ALK1* is a member of the TGFβ superfamily (as is *BMPR2*) and is thought to be involved in vascular differentiation and proliferation (197). Some individual patients with inherited *ALK1* mutations have disease that is clinically and histologically identical to PPH caused by *BMPR2* mutations (196).

Sporadic PPH

Based on current data, only about 10% of patients with sporadic PPH have a somatic mutation in *BMPR2* (191,198). In contrast, 50% to 62% of patients with sporadic PPH show pulmonary infection with HHV-8 based on PCR analysis of DNA extracted from plexiform lesions using primers that target the *ORF72* region of the HHV-8 viral genome, or immunohistochemical detection of the HHV-8 latency-associated nuclear antigen 1 (LANA-1) (198,199). Pulmonary hypertension thus joins the growing list of diseases associated with HHV-8 infection, which includes all clinical types of Kaposi's sarcoma (Chapter 18), primary effusion lymphoma, and multicentric Castleman's disease (200,201).

Technical and Diagnostic Issues and Molecular Testing of PPH

Thus far, it appears that mutations in *BMPR2* and *ALK1* do not cluster in specific regions of the gene in either familial or sporadic PPH, and so mutational analysis requires screening of the entire coding sequence of the genes (186,196). This finding, together with the fact that the diagnosis of PPH is established based on the clinical and histologic features of the disease, indicates that molecular analysis of *BMPR2* and *ALK1* has little utility in routine clinical practice. Although it could be argued that there is a role for mutational analysis in presumed sporadic cases of PPH to exclude occult hereditary disease, testing in this setting would involve germline rather than lesional tissue (and given the implications of a positive result for the patient and the patient's family, testing in this setting should ideally be performed in conjunction with a formal medical genetics consultation). Similarly, because the presence of *BMPR2* or *ALK1* mutations has not been associated with clinical outcome or response to therapy, there is also no role for molecular analysis in the context of prognostic testing.

As far as PCR-based testing for HHV-8 is concerned, amplification of *ORF72* from the DNA of plexiform lesions has a specificity of 93% for PPH versus secondary pulmonary hypertension and a specificity of 100% for PPH versus unrelated lung disease (198). In addition, a positive PCR result shows virtually 100% correlation with

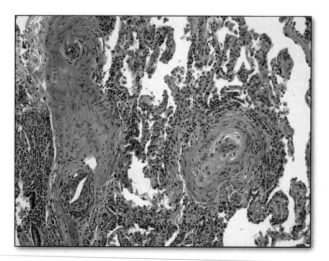

Figure 19.8 Photomicrograph of vascular lesions within the lung of a woman who underwent lung transplantation for primary pulmonary hypertension (PPH). Note the intimal proliferation as well as the medial hypertrophy. Hereditary cases of PPH are due to mutations in BMPR2 (a protein involved in pulmonary arterial smooth muscle cell mitosis). Hereditary cases of PPH associated with hereditary hemorrhagic telangiectasia are due to mutations in ALK1 (a protein involved in vascular differentiation and proliferation). In contrast, most cases of sporadic PPH are associated with human herpesvirus-8 infection. (See text for details).

immunohistochemical detection of the LANA-1 protein (198,199). Given the ease of immunohistochemical detection, the latter result suggests that immunostains may well supplant molecular testing for detection of the virus, even though PCR can easily be performed on FFPE tissue (198).

From a diagnostic perspective, the role of HHV-8 testing has not yet been established. Even though HHV-8 is also responsible for Kaposi's sarcoma and several lymphoproliferative disorders, as noted previously, these neoplasms have a different clinicopathologic setting from PPH and rarely enter into the differential diagnosis. Similarly, because no differences in survival or response to therapy have been demonstrated for PPH associated with HHV-8 infection, and because it is unknown whether the presence of HHV-8 is associated with a higher likelihood of disease recurrence after lung transplantation, there appears to be no role for testing from a prognostic or therapeutic prospective. Furthermore, because approximately 20% of patients who show HHV-8 infection by PCR also harbor *BMPR2* mutations (198), the presence of the virus cannot be used to exclude hereditary causes of PPH.

PULMONARY LYMPHANGIOLEIOMYOMATOSIS

Lymphangioleiomyomatosis (LAM) is an interstitial lung disease characterized by a proliferation of smooth muscle cells that results in cystic parenchymal destruction and chronic, progressive respiratory failure (202) (Fig. 19.9). Pulmonary LAM occurs as a hereditary disease in association with tuberous sclerosis complex (TSC) or sporadically in patients without the signs and symptoms of TSC. For patients who develop end-stage pulmonary LAM, lung transplantation is the only effective therapy.

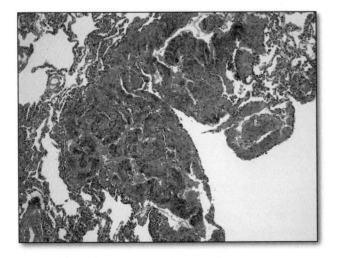

Figure 19.9 Photomicrograph of the lung from a woman who underwent lung transplantation for pulmonary lymphangioleiomyomatosis (LAM). Note the bundles of immature-appearing smooth muscle cells within the interstitium, associated with cystic spaces. Hereditary cases of pulmonary LAM occur in association with tuberous sclerosis complex caused by mutations in *TSC1* or *TSC2*. Sporadic cases are caused by somatic mutations in *TSC1* or *TSC2*. (See text for details.)

Genetics

TSC is a tumor suppressor gene syndrome characterized by seizures, mental retardation, angiofibromas, and renal angiomyolipomas. The disease is caused by mutations in the *TSC1* gene at 9q34 or the *TSC2* gene at 16p13 (203,204). *TSC1* encodes hamartin, a protein that has a role in cytoskeletal rearrangements, and *TSC2* encodes the protein tuberin, which interacts with hamartin and also appears to have a role in cell cycle control (205,206). Traditionally, LAM was thought to occur in only about 4% of women with TSC, but it has recently been demonstrated that one third of patients with TSC have radiographic evidence of pulmonary cysts consistent with LAM (207).

The sporadic form of pulmonary LAM is quite rare, and only about 500 to 1,000 women in the United States are known to have the disease (202). Most patients with sporadic LAM harbor somatic mutations in *TSC2*, but rare cases of sporadic LAM resulting from somatic mutations in *TSC1* have also been described (208,209).

Recurrent pulmonary LAM following lung transplantation has been described (210–213). Several studies have definitively established that the cells producing the recurrent lesions are of recipient origin (210,214), which suggests that either migration or metastatic spread of smooth muscle cells is responsible for the recurrent lesions. This result is consistent with the observation that LAM cells can be identified in the body fluids and blood of patients with TSC-related LAM (215), and is also consistent with the finding that the pulmonary lesions and renal angiomyolipomas of patients with sporadic LAM harbor the same somatic mutation (208,209).

Technical Issues in Molecular Genetic Analysis of LAM

The aberrations in *TSC1* and *TSC2* responsible for pulmonary LAM include nonsense mutations, missense mutations, splice site mutations, insertions, and deletions and are scattered throughout virtually the entire coding region of both genes. Consequently, mutational analysis is not only time consuming, but yields different estimates for the prevalence of alterations in patients with pulmonary LAM, depending on the method employed. In patients with TSC-related LAM, the detection rate of germline *TSC1* or *TSC2* mutations varies from 37% to 83%; not surprisingly, the highest detection rate is achieved by comprehensive analysis using a variety of mutational screening methods (209,216). Similarly, estimates of the prevalence of *TSC1* or *TSC2* mutations in patients with sporadic LAM range from 14% to 71%, depending on the method used to screen for mutations (208,209).

Diagnostic Issues in Molecular Genetic Analysis of LAM

The clinicopathologic and morphologic features of pulmonary LAM are pathognomonic, and therefore molecular analysis is not required for diagnosis. Even though mutations in exon 40 or 41 of *TSC2* in patients with TCS are apparently associated with a higher incidence of pulmonary LAM (216), it has not been demonstrated that screening to identify patients at greater risk can be used to direct early intervention that achieves a better clinical outcome. Because specific mutations have not been correlated with outcome for pulmonary LAM, and detection of LAM cells in blood or body fluids is also not correlated with either the presence of pulmonary LAM or the severity of disease (216), there is little role for mutational analysis from either a prognostic or therapeutic perspective.

Nonetheless, it has recently been emphasized that variability in the clinical manifestations of TSC can produce pulmonary LAM with a presentation that mimics sporadic disease, even though germline mutations are present in one of the TSC genes (217). This report suggests that the role of germline testing in patients with presumed sporadic LAM should be reappraised because a positive result would have a profound impact on the patient's family.

SARCOMAS

A number of spindle cell malignancies that most commonly occur in the soft tissue have been described as primary tumors of the lung and mediastinum, including inflammatory myofibroblastic tumor (218–221) and synovial sarcoma (222–224). Similarly, a number of malignant round cell tumors that more typically involve the soft tissue have also been described as primary malignancies of the lung and thorax, including alveolar rhabdomyosarcoma (161,225), Ewing sarcoma/peripheral neuroectodermal tumor (226), and desmoplastic small round cell tumor (227). The issues involved in the molecular analysis of these tumors are discussed in detail in Chapter 11.

LYMPHOMAS

At least 95% of pulmonary lymphomas are B-cell non-Hodgkin lymphomas, tumors that can represent either a primary lung malignancy or secondary involvement from a known lymphoma at another site. About 75% to 80% of primary lymphomas are low-grade neoplasms, mostly mucosa-associated lymphoid tissue (MALT) lymphomas. The other 20% to 25% of primary B-cell tumors are high-grade malignant lymphomas (228–230).

As discussed in more detail in Chapter 13, molecular analysis of B-cell lymphomas has traditionally been performed by Southern hybridization using probes for immunoglobulin heavy-chain genes. However, the clinical utility of Southern hybridization in routine practice is limited by the requirement for a relatively large sample of unfixed tissue. Consequently, most molecular analysis is based on PCR using consensus primers to the V and J regions of the IgH locus, although several factors limit PCR testing on a purely technical level. First, sensitivity depends on primer design. Individual primer pairs can only detect about 95% of V and J regions, so multiple primer sets are required to achieve optimum test sensitivity (the fact that there are no standardized primer sets, and that different investigators use different primer sets, often complicates comparison of results reported in different studies). Second, there are no standard criteria to determine whether or not a dominant

PCR product represents a monoclonal population. Third, because of dilution effects, analysis based on a very low quantity of DNA is not only more likely to miss a clonal population (231,232), but also more likely to yield pseudo-clonal bands (233–235).

Similarly, the diagnostic specificity of PCR analysis is limited even when a monoclonal B-cell proliferation is detected, because the presence of a monoclonal B-cell population is not synonymous with B-cell lymphoma (236,237). Monoclonal or oligoclonal B-cell infiltrates have been documented in autoimmune diseases, including Sjögren's syndrome (238,239), in the inflammatory response associated with carcinoma (240,241), and in benign lymphoid tissue (241,242). Even physiologic antigen-specific responses have been shown to generate small clonal B-cell populations (231,232).

Analysis of Biopsy or Excision Specimens

The utility of PCR-based analysis for evaluation of low-grade B-cell MALT lymphomas is highlighted by several reports in which diagnosis based solely on the morphologic features of the lymphoid infiltrate was complicated by the presence of additional pathology. Even though diffuse infiltrates of small to intermediate size lymphocytes with irregular contours and pale cytoplasm were present in these cases, with associated lymphoepithelial lesions, the regions suggestive of MALT lymphoma merged with reactive lymphoid follicles or areas of caseating necrosis associated with mycobacterial (243) or fungal infection (244). The demonstration of a dominant band by IgH PCR testing provided the confirmatory evidence needed to establish the diagnosis of MALT lymphoma. As an aside, PCR-based testing has also been used to establish the diagnosis of MALT lymphoma at unusual sites within the mediastinum, including the thymus (245).

Analysis of BAL Fluid

Because the clonality of bronchoalveolar lymphocytes reflects the clonality of the associated pulmonary infiltrate (246) (Fig. 19.10), PCR testing of BAL fluid can sometimes be used to eliminate the need for open lung biopsy. In one prospective study of over 100 consecutive patients in which there was a clinical suspension of primary or secondary pulmonary non-Hodgkin lymphoma (B-NHL), B-cell clonality analysis of BAL fluid performed by IgH PCR showed a sensitivity of 83% and specificity of 86% for diagnosis of primary pulmonary B-NHL and a sensitivity of 75% and specificity of 83% for diagnosis of secondary pulmonary involvement by B-cell lymphoproliferative disorders (247). However, careful analysis demonstrated that the profile of the dominant PCR product bands fell into "strong" and "weak" groups and that a "strong" B-cell clonal population had 97% specificity for pulmonary B-NHL, while a "weak" clonal population was present in 38% of patients with autoimmune disease involving the lung, including Sjögren's syndrome, pulmonary vasculitis, and dermatopolymyositis. Although the low specificity of "weak" clonal bands makes the utility of the analysis uncertain in

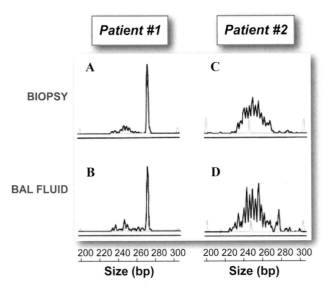

Figure 19.10 Example of *IgH* PCR-based clonality analysis of bronchoalveolar lavage (BAL) fluid. For Patient 1, electrophoresis of the PCR product shows a single dominant peak of the same size in both the biopsy specimen (*A*), and BAL fluid (*B*), indicative of a clonal B-cell population. When a dominant peak of this type is present in a tissue biopsy that is diagnostic of lymphoma, it is assumed to represent the malignant B-cell population. For Patient 2, electrophoresis of the PCR product shows a gaussian distribution of fragment sizes in both the biopsy specimen (*C*), and BAL fluid (*D*), indicative of a polyclonal B-cell population. (Modified from Zompi S, Couderc LJ, Cadranel J, et al. Clonality analysis of alveolar B lymphocytes contributes to the diagnostic strategy in clinical suspicion of pulmonary lymphoma. *Blood* 2004; 103: 3208–3215. Copyright American Society of Hematology, used with permission

patients with autoimmune or chronic infectious diseases, the results suggest that detection of a "strong" B-cell clonal population in BAL fluid can be used to identify patients likely to have primary B-NHL (and who therefore should have a biopsy for formal diagnosis) and to identify the presence of secondary pulmonary involvement in patients known to have B-NHL at another site (for whom a pulmonary biopsy can be avoided).

REFERENCES

1. Ferlay J, Bray F, Pisani P, et al, eds. *GLOBOCAN 2002: Cancer Incidence, Mortality and Prevalence Worldwide.* Lyon, France: IARC Press; 2004. Available at: http://www.dep.iarc.fr
2. Mitsuuchi Y, Testa JR. Cytogenetics and molecular genetics of lung cancer. *Am J Med Genet* 2002;115:183–188.
3. Ahsan H, Thomas DC. Lung cancer etiology: independent and joint effects of genetics, tobacco, and arsenic. *JAMA* 2004;292:3026–3029.
4. Chen CL, Hsu LI, Chiou HY, et al. Ingested arsenic, cigarette smoking, and lung cancer risk: a follow-up study in arseniasis-endemic areas in Taiwan. *JAMA* 2004;292: 2984–2990.
5. Jonsson S, Thorsteinsdottir U, Gudbjartsson DF, et al. Familial risk of lung carcinoma in the Icelandic population. *JAMA* 2004;292:2977–2983.
6. Hecht SS. Tobacco smoke carcinogens and lung cancer. *J Natl Cancer Inst* 1999; 91:1194–1210.
7. Pryor WA. Cigarette smoke radicals and the role of free radicals in chemical carcinogenicity. *Environ Health Perspect* 1997;105:875–882.
8. Pfeifer GP, Denissenko MF, Olivier M, et al. Tobacco smoke carcinogens, DNA damage and p53 mutations in smoking-associated cancers. *Oncogene* 2002;21:7435–7451.
9. Yang C, Frenkel K. Arsenic-mediated cellular signal transduction, transcription factor activation, and aberrant gene expression: implications in carcinogenesis. *J Environ Pathol Toxicol Oncol* 2002;21:331–342.
10. Tchounwou PB, Patlolla AK, Centeno JA. Carcinogenic and systemic health effects associated with arsenic exposure:a critical review. *Toxicol Pathol* 2003;31:575–588.
11. Bailey-Wilson JE, Amos CI, Pinney SM, et al. A major lung cancer susceptibility locus maps to chromosome 6q23-25. *Am J Hum Genet* 2004;75:460–474.
12. Divine KK, Gilliland FD, Crowell RE, et al. The XRCC1 399 glutamine allele is a risk factor for adenocarcinoma of the lung. *Mutat Res* 2001;461:273–278.
13. Weu Q, Cheng L, Hong WK, et al. Reduced DNA repair capacity in lung cancer patients. *Cancer Res* 1996;56:4103–4107.
14. Carter B, Long T, Cinciripini P. A meta-analytic review of the *CYP2A6* genotype and smoking behavior. *Nicotine Tob Res* 2004;6:221–227.
15. Feng Y, Niu T, Xing H, et al. A common haplotype of the nicotine acetylcholine receptor alpha 4 subunit gene is associated with vulnerability to nicotine addiction in men. *Am J Hum Genet* 2004;75:112–121.
16. Wistuba II, Gazdar AF. Characteristic genetic alterations in lung cancer. *Methods Mol Med* 2003;74:3–28.
17. Fong KM, Sekido Y, Gazdar AF, et al. Lung cancer. 9: Molecular biology of lung cancer: clinical implications. *Thorax* 2003;58:892–900.
18. Sekido Y, Fong KM, Minna JD. Molecular genetics of lung cancer. *Annu Rev Med* 2003;54:73–87.
19. Wistuba II, Gazdar AF, Minna JD. Molecular genetics of small cell lung carcinoma. *Semin Oncol* 2001;28:3–13.
20. Woenckhaus M, Grepmeier U, Wild P, et al. Multitarget FISH and LOH analyses at chromosome 3p in non-small cell lung cancer and adjacent bronchial epithelium. *Am J Clin Pathol* 2005;123:752–761.
21. Testa JR, Liu Z, Feder M, et al. Advances in the analysis of chromosome alterations in human lung carcinomas. *Cancer Genet Cytogenet* 1997;95:20–32.
22. Truong K, Gerbault-Seureau M, Guilly MN, et al. Quantitative fluorescence in situ hybridization in lung cancer as a diagnostic marker. *J Mol Diagn* 1999;1:33–37.
23. Truong K, Boenders J, Maciorowski Z, et al. Signal amplification of FISH for automated detection using image cytometry. *Anal Cell Pathol* 1997;13:137–146.
24. Bubendorf L, Muller P, Joos L, et al. Multitarget FISH analysis in the diagnosis of lung cancer. *Am J Clin Pathol* 2005;123:516–523.
25. Sokolova IA, Bubendorf L, O'Hare A, et al. A fluorescence in situ hybridization-based assay for improved detection of lung cancer cells in bronchial washing specimens. *Cancer* 2002;96:306–315.
26. Warner KA, Crawford EL, Zaher A, et al. The c-myc x E2F-1/p21 interactive gene expression index augments cytomorphologic diagnosis of lung cancer in fine-needle aspirate specimens. *J Mol Diagn* 2003;5:176–183.
27. DeMuth JP, Jackson CM, Weaver DA, et al. The gene expression index c-myc x E2F-1/p21 is highly predictive of malignant phenotype in human bronchial epithelial cells. *Am J Respir Cell Mol Biol* 1998;19:18–24.
28. Kumaki F, Kawai T, Hiroi S, et al. Telomerase activity and expression of human telomerase RNA component and human telomerase reverse transcriptase in lung carcinomas. *Hum Pathol* 2001;32:188–195.
29. Shay JW. Telomerase in human development and cancer. *J Cell Physiol* 1997;173: 266–270.
30. Meeker AK, Coffey DS. Telomerase: a promising marker of biological immortality of germ, stem, and cancer cells: a review. *Biochemistry (Mosc)* 1997;62:1323–1331.
31. Yashima K, Litzky LA, Kaiser L, et al. Telomerase expression in respiratory epithelium during the multistage pathogenesis of lung carcinomas. *Cancer Res* 1997;57:2373–2377.
32. Albanell J, Lonardo F, Rusch V, et al. High telomerase activity in primary lung cancers: association with increased cell proliferation rates and advanced pathologic stage. *J Natl Cancer Inst* 1997;89:1609–1615.
33. Esteller M, Sanchez-Cespedes M, Rosell R, et al. Detection of aberrant promoter hypermethylation of tumor suppressor genes in serum DNA from non-small cell lung cancer patients. *Cancer Res* 1999;59:67–70.
34. Piyathilake CJ, Frost AR, Bell WC, et al. Altered global methylation of DNA: an epigenetic difference in susceptibility for lung cancer is associated with its progression. *Hum Pathol* 2001;32:856–862.
35. Wigle DA, Jurisica I, Radulovich N, et al. Molecular profiling of non-small cell lung cancer and correlation with disease-free survival. *Cancer Res* 2002;62:3005–3008.
36. Bhattacharjee A, Richards WG, Staunton J, et al. Classification of human lung carcinomas by mRNA expression profiling reveals distinct adenocarcinoma subclasses. *Proc Natl Acad Sci USA* 2001;98:13790–13795.
37. Garber ME, Troyanskaya OG, Schluens K, et al. Diversity of gene expression in adenocarcinoma of the lung. *Proc Natl Acad Sci USA* 2001;98:13784–13789.
38. Beer DG, Kardia SL, Huang CC, et al. Gene-expression profiles predict survival of patients with lung adenocarcinoma. *Nat Med* 2002;8:816–824.
39. Parmigiani G, Garrett-Mayer ES, Anbazhagan R, et al. A cross-study comparison of gene expression studies for the molecular classification of lung cancer. *Clin Cancer Res* 2004;10:2922–2927.
40. O'Sullivan M, Budhraja V, Sadovsky Y, et al. Tumor heterogeneity affects the precision of microarray analysis. *Diagn Mol Pathol* 2005;14:65–71.
41. Borczuk AC, Shah L, Pearson GD, et al. Molecular signatures in biopsy specimens of lung cancer. *Am J Respir Crit Care Med* 2004;170:167–174.
42. Gazdar AF, Minna JD. Molecular detection of early lung cancer. *J Natl Cancer Inst* 1999;91:299–301.
43. Chen JT, Ho WL, Cheng YW, et al. Detection of p53 mutations in sputum smears precedes diagnosis of non-small cell lung carcinoma. *Anticancer Res* 2000;20: 2687–2690.
44. Mao L, Hruban RH, Boyle JO, et al. Detection of oncogene mutations in sputum precedes diagnosis of lung cancer. *Cancer Res* 1994;54:1634–1637.
45. Belinsky SA. Gene-promoter hypermethylation as a biomarker in lung cancer. *Nat Rev Cancer* 2004;4:707–717.
46. Prindiville SA, Byers T, Hirsch FR, et al. Sputum cytological atypia as a predictor of incident lung cancer in a cohort of heavy smokers with airflow obstruction. *Cancer Epidemiol Biomarkers Prev* 2003;12:987–993.
47. Palmisano WA, Divine KK, Saccomanno G, et al. Predicting lung cancer by detecting aberrant promoter methylation in sputum. *Cancer Res* 2000;60:5954–5958.
48. Wistuba II, Lam S, Behrens C, et al. Molecular damage in the bronchial epithelium of current and former smokers. *J Natl Cancer Inst* 1997;89:1366–1373.
49. Nelson MA, Wymer J, Clements N Jr. Detection of K-ras gene mutations in non-neoplastic lung tissue and lung cancers. *Cancer Lett* 1996;103:115–121.
50. Yakubovskaya MS, Spiegelman V, Luo FC, et al. High frequency of K-ras mutations in normal appearing lung tissues and sputum of patients with lung cancer. *Int J Cancer* 1995;63:810–814.

51. Franklin WA, Gazdar AF, Haney J, et al. Widely dispersed *p53* mutation in respiratory epithelium: a novel mechanism for field carcinogenesis. *J Clin Invest* 1997;100:2133–2137.
52. Wang B, Li L, Yao L, et al. Detection of *p53* gene mutations in sputum samples and their implications in the early diagnosis of lung cancer in suspicious patients. *Chin Med J* 2001;114:694–697.
53. Kersting M, Friedl C, Kraus A, et al. Differential frequencies of *p16(INK4a)* promoter hypermethylation, *p53* mutation, and K-*ras* mutation in exfoliative material mark the development of lung cancer in symptomatic chronic smokers. *J Clin Oncol* 2000;18: 3221–3229.
54. Keohavong P, Gao WM, Zheng KC, et al. Detection of K-*ras* and *p53* mutations in sputum samples of lung cancer patients using laser capture microdissection microscope and mutation analysis. *Anal Biochem* 2004;324:92–99.
55. Zhang L, Gao WM, Gealy R, et al. Comparison of K-*ras* gene mutations in tumour and sputum DNA of patients with lung cancer. *Biomarkers* 2003;8:156–161.
56. Bocking A, Biesterfeld S, Chatelain R, et al. Diagnosis of bronchial carcinoma on sections of paraffin-embedded sputum: sensitivity and specificity of an alternative to routine cytology. *Acta Cytol* 1992;36:37–47.
57. Popp W, Rauscher H, Ritschka L, et al. Diagnostic sensitivity of different techniques in the diagnosis of lung tumors with the flexible fiberoptic bronchoscope: comparison of brush biopsy, imprint cytology of forceps biopsy, and histology of forceps biopsy. *Cancer* 1991;67:72–75.
58. Jheon S, Hyun DS, Lee SC, et al. Lung cancer detection by a RT-nested PCR using MAGE A1: 6 common primers. *Lung Cancer* 2004;43:29–37.
59. Varella-Garcia M, Kittelson J, Schulte AP, et al. Multi-target interphase fluorescence in situ hybridization assay increases sensitivity of sputum cytology as a predictor of lung cancer. *Cancer Detect Prev* 2004;28:244–251.
60. Hu YC, Sidransky D, Ahrendt SA. Molecular detection approaches for smoking associated tumors. *Oncogene* 2002;21:7289–7297.
61. Ahrendt SA, Chow JT, Xu LH, et al. Molecular detection of tumor cells in bronchoalveolar lavage fluid from patients with early stage lung cancer. *J Natl Cancer Inst* 1999;91:332–339.
62. Mills NE, Fishman CL, Scholes J, et al. Detection of K-*ras* oncogene mutations in bronchoalveolar lavage fluid for lung cancer diagnosis. *J Natl Cancer Inst* 1995;87: 1056–1060.
63. Carstensen T, Schmidt B, Engel E, et al. Detection of cell-free DNA in bronchial lavage fluid supernatants of patients with lung cancer. *Ann NY Acad Sci* 2004;1022: 202–210.
64. Xinarianos G, Scott FM, Liloglou T, et al. Evaluation of telomerase activity in bronchial lavage as a potential diagnostic marker for malignant lung disease. *Lung Cancer* 2000;28:37–42.
65. Fliss MS, Usadel H, Caballero OL, et al. Facile detection of mitochondrial DNA mutations in tumors and bodily fluids. *Science* 2000;287:2017–2019.
66. Jung R, Petersen K, Kruger W, et al. Detection of micrometastasis by cytokeratin 20 RT-PCR is limited due to stable background transcription in granulocytes. *Br J Cancer* 1999;81:870–873.
67. Tora M, Barbera VM, Real FX. Detection of *HuD* transcripts by means of reverse transcriptase and polymerase chain reaction: implications for the detection of minimal residual disease in patients with small cell lung cancer. *Cancer Lett* 2000;161:157–164.
68. Costa J. Caution neophiles! *Lab Invest* 1997;77:211–212.
69. Dingemans AM, Brakenhoff RH, Postmus PE, et al. Detection of cytokeratin-19 transcripts by reverse transcriptase-polymerase chain reaction in lung cancer cell lines and blood of lung cancer patients. *Lab Invest* 1997;77:213–220.
70. Bustin SAV, Siddiqi S, Ahmed S, et al. Quantification of cytokeratin 20, carcinoembryonic antigen and guanylyl cyclase C mRNA levels in lymph nodes may not predict treatment failure in colorectal cancer patients. *Int J Cancer* 2004;108:412–417.
71. Soeth E, Vogel I, Roder C, et al. Comparative analysis of bone marrow and venous blood isolates from gastrointestinal cancer patients for the detection of disseminated tumor cells using reverse transcription PCR. *Cancer Res* 1997;57:3106–3110.
72. Bustin SA, Gyselman VG, Siddiqi S, et al. Cytokeratin 20 is not a tissue-specific marker for the detection of malignant epithelial cells in the blood of colorectal cancer patients. *Int J Surg Investig* 2000;2:49–57.
73. Yamamoto N, Kato Y, Yanagisawa A, et al. Predictive value of genetic diagnosis for cancer micrometastasis: histologic and experimental appraisal. *Cancer* 1997;80:1393–1398.
74. Argani P, Rosai J. Hyperplastic mesothelial cells in lymph nodes: report of six cases of a benign process that can stimulate metastatic involvement by mesothelioma or carcinoma. *Hum Pathol* 1998;29:339–346.
75. Ahrendt SA, Yang SC, Roig CM, et al. Molecular assessment of lymph nodes in patients with resected stage I non-small cell lung cancer: preliminary results of a prospective study. *J Thorac Cardiovasc Surg* 2002;123:466–473.
76. D'Amico TA. Molecular biologic substaging of non-small cell lung cancer. *J Thorac Cardiovasc Surg* 2002;123:409–410.
77. Goldstein NS, Mani A, Chmielewski G, et al. Immunohistochemically detected micrometastases in peribronchial and mediastinal lymph nodes from patients with T1, N0, M0 pulmonary adenocarcinomas. *Am J Surg Pathol* 2000;24:274–279.
78. Passlick B, Izbicki JR, Kubuschok B, et al. Immunohistochemical assessment of individual tumor cells in lymph nodes of patients with non-small-cell lung cancer. *J Clin Oncol* 1994;12:1827–1832.
79. Dobashi K, Sugio K, Osaki T, et al. Micrometastatic *P53*-positive cells in the lymph nodes of non-small-cell lung cancer: prognostic significance. *J Thorac Cardiovasc Surg* 1997;114:339–346.
80. Valk PE, Pounds TR, Hopkins DM, et al. Staging non-small cell lung cancer by whole-body positron emission tomographic imaging. *Ann Thorac Surg* 1995;60: 1573–1581.
81. Dales RE, Stark RM, Raman S. Computed tomography to stage lung cancer: approaching a controversy using meta-analysis. *Am Rev Respir Dis* 1990;141:1096–1101.
82. Wallace MB, Silvestri GA, Sahai AV, et al. Endoscopic ultrasound-guided fine needle aspiration for staging patients with carcinoma of the lung. *Ann Thorac Surg* 2001;72:1861–1867.
83. Wallace MB, Block M, Hoffman BJ, et al. Detection of telomerase expression in mediastinal lymph nodes of patients with lung cancer. *Am J Respir Crit Care Med* 2003; 167:1670–1675.
84. Chen XQ, Stroun M, Magnenat JL, et al. Microsatellite alterations in plasma DNA of small cell lung cancer patients. *Nat Med* 1996;2:1033–1035.
85. Kobayashi S, Boggon TJ, Dayaram T, et al. EGFR mutation and resistance of non-small-cell lung cancer to gefitinib. *N Engl J Med* 2005;352:786–792.
86. Wakeling AE, Guy SP, Woodburn JR, et al. ZD1839 (Iressa): an orally active inhibitor of epidermal growth factor signaling with potential for cancer therapy. *Cancer Res* 2002;62:5749–5754.
87. Arteaga CL. *ErbB*-targeted therapeutic approaches in human cancer. *Exp Cell Res* 2003;284:122–130.
88. Kris MG, Natale RB, Herbst RS, et al. Efficacy of gefitinib, an inhibitor of the epidermal growth factor receptor tyrosine kinase, in symptomatic patients with non-small cell lung cancer: a randomized trial. *JAMA* 2003;290:2149–2158.
89. Fukuoka M, Yano S, Giaccone G, et al. Multi-institutional randomized phase II trial of gefitinib for previously treated patients with advanced non-small-cell lung cancer. *J Clin Oncol* 2003;21:2237–2246.
90. Giaccone G, Herbst RS, Manegold C, et al. Gefitinib in combination with gemcitabine and cisplatin in advanced non-small-cell lung cancer: a phase III trial: INTACT 1. *J Clin Oncol* 2004;22:777–784.
91. Herbst RS, Giaccone G, Schiller JH, et al. Gefitinib in combination with paclitaxel and carboplatin in advanced non-small-cell lung cancer: a phase III trial: INTACT 2. *J Clin Oncol* 2004;22:785–794.
92. Lynch TJ, Bell DW, Sordella R, et al. Activating mutations in the epidermal growth factor receptor underlying responsiveness of non-small-cell lung cancer to gefitinib. *N Engl J Med* 2004;350:2129–2139.
93. Paez JG, Janne PA, Lee JC, et al. *EGFR* mutations in lung cancer: correlation with clinical response to gefitinib therapy. *Science* 2004;304:1497–1500.
94. Sordella R, Bell DW, Haber DA, et al. Gefitinib-sensitizing *EGFR* mutations in lung cancer activate anti-apoptotic pathways. *Science* 2004;305:1163–1167.
95. Yatabe Y, Kosaka T, Takahashi T, et al. *EGFR* mutation is specific for terminal respiratory unit type adenocarcinoma. *Am J Surg Pathol* 2005;29:633–639.
96. Shepherd FA, Rodrigues-Pereira J, Ciuleanu T, et al. Erlotinib in previously trated non-small-cell lung cancer. *N Engl J Med* 2005;353:123–132.
97. Tsao MS, Sakurada K, Cutz JC, et al. Erlotinib in lung cancer: molecular and clinical predictors of outcome. *N Engl J Med* 2005;353:133–144.
98. Minna JD, Gazdar AF, Sprang SR, et al. Cancer: a bull's eye for targeted lung cancer therapy. *Science* 2004;304:1458–1461.
99. Arteaga CL. Selecting the right patient for tumor therapy. *Nat Med* 2004;10: 577–578.
100. Jones PA, Baylin SB. The fundamental role of epigenetic events in cancer. *Nat Rev* Genet 2002;3:415–428.
101. Cheng JC, Matsen CB, Gonzales FA, et al. Inhibition of DNA methylation and reactivation of silenced genes by zebularine. *J Natl Cancer Inst* 2003;95:399–409.
102. Fang MZ, Wang Y, Ai N, et al. Tea polyphenol (−)-epigallocatechin-3-gallate inhibits DNA methyltransferase and reactivates methylation-silenced genes in cancer cell lines. *Cancer Res* 2003;63:7563–7570.
103. Fiala ES, Staretz ME, Pandya GA, et al. Inhibition of DNA cytosine methyltransferase by chemopreventive selenium compounds, determined by an improved assay for DNA cytosine methyltransferase and DNA cytosine methylation. *Carcinogenesis* 1998;19:597–604.
104. Cameron EE, Bachman KE, Myohanen S, et al. Synergy of demethylation and histone deacetylase inhibition in the re-expression of genes silenced in cancer. *Nat Genet* 1999;21:103–107.
105. Travis WD, Colby TV, Corrin B, et al, eds. *World Health Organization International Histological Classification of Tumours: Histological Typing of Lung and Pleural Tumours.* Berlin: Springer; 1999.
106. Oberg K. Carcinoid tumors: molecular genetics, tumor biology, and update of diagnosis and treatment. *Curr Opin Oncol* 2002;14:38–45.
107. Leotlela PD, Jauch A, Holtgreve-Grez H, et al. Genetics of neuroendocrine and carcinoid tumours. *Endocr Relat Cancer* 2003;10:437–450.
108. Debelenko LV, Brambilla E, Agarwal S, et al. Identification of *MEN1* gene mutations in sporadic carcinoid tumors of the lung. *Hum Mol Genet* 1997;6:2285–2290.
109. Walch AK, Zitzelsberger HF, Aubele MM, et al. Typical and atypical carcinoid tumors of the lung are characterized by 11q deletions as detected by comparative genomic hybridization. *Am J Pathol* 1998;153:1089–1098.
110. Petzmann S, Ullmann R, Klemen H, et al. Loss of heterozygosity on chromosome arm 11q in lung carcinoids. *Hum Pathol* 2001;32:333–338.
111. Kobayashi Y, Tokuchi Y, Hashimoto T, et al. Molecular markers for reinforcement of histological subclassification of neuroendocrine lung tumors. *Cancer Sci* 2004;95:334–341.
112. Onuki N, Wistuba II, Travis WD, et al. Genetic changes in the spectrum of neuroendocrine lung tumors. *Cancer* 1999;85:600–607.
113. D'Adda T, Bottarelli L, Azzoni C, et al. Malignancy-associated X chromosome allelic losses in foregut endocrine neoplasms: further evidence from lung tumors. *Mod Pathol* 2005;18:795–805.
114. Pan CC, Jong YJ, Chen YJ. Comparative genomic hybridization analysis of thymic neuroendocrine tumors. *Mod Pathol* 2005;18:358–364.
115. Cerilli LA, Ritter JH, Mills SE, et al. Neuroendocrine neoplasms of the lung. *Am J Clin Pathol* 2001;116:65–96.
116. Marchevsky AM, Gal AA, Shah S, et al. Morphometry confirms the presence of considerable nuclear size overlap between "small cells" and "large cells" in high-grade pulmonary neuroendocrine neoplasms. *Am J Clin Pathol* 2001;116:466–472.
117. Colby T, Koss M, Travis W, eds. *Atlas of Tumor Pathology: Tumors of the Lower Respiratory Tract.* Washington, DC: Armed Forces Institute of Pathology; 1995:517–546.
118. Jones MH, Virtanen C, Honjoh D, et al. Two prognostically significant subtypes of high-grade lung neuroendocrine tumours independent of small-cell and large-cell neuroendocrine carcinomas identified by gene expression profiles. *Lancet* 2004;363: 775–781.
119. Murase T, Takino H, Shimizu S, et al. Clonality analysis of different histological components in combined small cell and non-small cell carcinoma of the lung. *Hum Pathol* 2003;34:1178–1184.
120. Huang J, Behrens C, Wistuba II, et al. Clonality of combined tumors. *Arch Pathol Lab Med* 2002;126:437–441.

121. Askin FB. Something old? Something new? Second primary or pulmonary metastasis in the patient with known extrathoracic carcinoma. *Am J Clin Pathol* 1993;100:4–5.

122. Leong PP, Rezai B, Koch WM, et al. Distinguishing second primary tumors from lung metastases in patients with head and neck squamous cell carcinoma. *J Natl Cancer Inst* 1998;90:972–977.

123. Schwartz LH, Ozsahin M, Zhang GN, et al. Synchronous and metachronous head and neck carcinomas. *Cancer* 1994;74:1933–1938.

124. Schoenmakers EF, Wanschura S, Mols R, et al. Recurrent rearrangements in the high mobility group protein gene, *HMGI-C*, in benign mesenchymal tumours. *Nat Genet* 1995;10:436–444.

125. Kazmierczak B, Rosigkeit J, Wanschura S, et al. *HMGI-C* rearrangements as the molecular basis for the majority of pulmonary chondroid hamartomas: a survey of 30 tumors. *Oncogene* 1996;12:515–521.

126. Tallini G, Vanni R, Manfioletti G, et al. *HMGI-C* and *HMGI(Y)* immunoreactivity correlates with cytogenetic abnormalities in lipomas, pulmonary chondroid hamartomas, endometrial polyps, and uterine leiomyomas and is compatible with rearrangement of the *HMGI-C* and *HMGI(Y)* genes. *Lab Invest* 2000;80:359–369.

127. Kazmierczak B, Wanschura S, Rommel B, et al. Ten pulmonary chondroid hamartomas with chromosome 6p21 breakpoints within the HMG-I(Y) gene or its immediate surroundings. *J Natl Cancer Inst* 1996;88:1234–1236.

128. Hess JL. Chromosomal translocations in benign tumors: the HMGI proteins. *Am J Clin Pathol* 1998;109:251–261.

129. Geurts JM, Schoenmakers EF, Roijer E, et al. Expression of reciprocal hybrid transcripts of *HMGIC* and *FHIT* in a pleomorphic adenoma of the parotid gland. *Cancer Res* 1997;57:13–17.

130. Sandberg AA. Updates on the cytogenetics and molecular genetics of bone and soft tissue tumors: lipoma. *Cancer Genet Cytogenet* 2004;150:93–115.

131. Merscher S, Marondel I, Pedeutour F, et al. Identification of new translocation breakpoints at 12q13 in lipomas. *Genomics* 1997;46:70–77.

132. Xiao S, Lux ML, Reeves R, et al. *HMGI(Y)* activation by chromosome 6p21 rearrangements in multilineage mesenchymal cells from pulmonary hamartoma. *Am J Pathol* 1997;150:901–910.

133. Rogalla P, Lemke I, Kazmierczak B, et al. An identical *HMGIC-LPP* fusion transcript is consistently expressed in pulmonary chondroid hamartomas with t(3;12)(q27–28;q14–15). *Genes Chromosomes Cancer* 2000;29:363–366.

134. Blank C, Schoenmakers EF, Rogalla P, et al. Intragenic breakpoint within *RAD51L1* in a t(6;14)(p21.3;q24) of a pulmonary chondroid hamartoma. *Cytogenet Cell Genet* 2001; 95:17–19.

135. Gregori-Romero MA, Lopez-Gines C, Cerda-Nicolas M, et al. Recombinations of chromosomal bands 10q24, 12q14-q15, and 14q24 in two cases of pulmonary chondroid hamartoma studied by fluorescence in situ hybridization. *Cancer Genet Cytogenet* 2003; 142:153–157.

136. Rogalla P, Lemke I, Bullerdiek J. Absence of *HMGIC-LHFP* fusion in pulmonary chondroid hamartomas with aberrations involving chromosomal regions 12q13 through 15 and 13q12 through q14. *Cancer Genet Cytogenet* 2002;133:90–93.

137. Rogalla P, Drechsler K, Frey G, et al. *HMGI-C* expression patterns in human tissues: implications for the genesis of frequent mesenchymal tumors. *Am J Pathol* 1996;149:775–779.

138. Hisaoka M, Sheng WQ, Tanaka A, et al. *HMGIC* alterations in smooth muscle tumors of soft tissues and other sites. *Cancer Genet Cytogenet* 2002;138:50–55.

139. Tanigaki T, Shoyama Y, Iwasaki M, et al. Pleomorphic adenoma in the lung. *Monaldi Arch Chest Dis* 2002;57:30–32.

140. Sakamoto H, Uda H, Tanaka T, et al. Pleomorphic adenoma in the periphery of the lung: report of a case and review of the literature. *Arch Pathol Lab Med* 1991;115:393–396.

141. Tonon G, Modi S, Wu L, et al. t(11;19)(q21;p13) translocation in mucoepidermoid carcinoma creates a novel fusion product that disrupts a Notch signaling pathway. *Nat Genet* 2003;33:208–223.

142. Enlund F, Behboudi A, Andren Y, et al. Altered Notch signaling resulting from expression of a *WAMTP1-MAML2* gene fusion in mucoepidermoid carcinomas and benign Warthin's tumors. *Exp Cell Res* 2004;292:21–28.

143. Motherby H, Nadjari B, Friegel P, et al. Diagnostic accuracy of effusion cytology. *Diagn Cytopathol* 1999;20:350–357.

144. Sahn SA. Malignancy metastatic to the pleura. *Clin Chest Med* 1998;19:351–361.

145. Saitoh H, Shimura S, Fushimi T, et al. Detection of surfactant protein-A gene transcript in the cells from pleural effusion for the diagnosis of lung adenocarcinoma. *Am J Med* 1997;103:400–404.

146. Okamoto I, Morisaki T, Sasaki J, et al. Molecular detection of cancer cells by competitive reverse transcription-polymerase chain reaction analysis of specific CD44 variant RNAs. *J Natl Cancer Inst* 1998;90:307–315.

147. Yan PS, Ho SB, Itzkowitz SH, et al. Expression of native and deglycosylated colon cancer mucin antigens in normal and malignant epithelial tissues. *Lab Invest* 1990; 63:698–706.

148. O'Connell JT, Shao ZM, Drori E, et al. Altered mucin expression is a field change that accompanies mucinous (colloid) breast carcinoma histogenesis. *Hum Pathol* 1998;29: 1517–1523.

149. Balague C, Gambus G, Carrato C, et al. Altered expression of *MUC2*, *MUC4*, and *MUC5* mucin genes in pancreas tissues and cancer cell lines. *Gastroenterology* 1994;106:1054–1061.

150. Ho SB, Shekels LL, Toribara NW, et al. Mucin gene expression in normal, preneoplastic, and neoplastic human gastric epithelium. *Cancer Res* 1995;55:2681–2690.

151. Yu CJ, Shew JY, Liaw YS, et al. Application of mucin quantitative competitive reverse transcription polymerase chain reaction in assisting the diagnosis of malignant pleural effusion. *Am J Respir Crit Care Med* 2001;164:1312–1318.

152. Nagel H, Werner C, Hemmerlein B, et al. Real-time reverse transcription-polymerase chain reaction assay for GA733-2 mRNA in the detection of metastatic carcinoma cells in serous effusions. *Am J Clin Pathol* 2003;120:888–901.

153. Yang CT, Lee MH, Lan RS, et al. Telomerase activity in pleural effusions: diagnostic significance. *J Clin Oncol* 1998;16:567–573.

154. Braunschweig R, Yan P, Guilleret I, et al. Detection of malignant effusions: comparison of a telomerase assay and cytologic examination. *Diagn Cytopathol* 2001;24:174–180.

155. Braunschweig R, Guilleret I, Delacretaz F, et al. Pitfalls in TRAP assay in routine detection of malignancy in effusions. *Diagn Cytopathol* 2001;25:225–230.

156. Zendehrokh N, Dejmek A. Telomere repeat amplification protocol (TRAP) in situ reveals telomerase activity in three cell types in effusions: malignant cells, proliferative mesothelial cells, and lymphocytes. *Mod Pathol* 2005;18:189–196.

157. Jaffe ES, Harris NL, Stein H, et al, eds. *World Health Organization Classification of Tumours: Pathology and Genetics of Tumour of Haematopoietic and Lymphoid Tissues.* Lyon, France: IARC Press; 2001.

158. Gaildano G, Carbone A. Primary effusion lymphoma: a liquid phase lymphoma of fluid-filled body cavities. *Adv Cancer Res* 2001;80:115–146.

159. Wakely PE Jr, Menezes G, Nuovo GJ. Primary effusion lymphoma: cytopathologic diagnosis using in situ molecular genetic analysis for human herpesvirus 8. *Mod Pathol* 2002;15:944–950.

160. Bryant-Greenwood P, Sorbara L, Filie AC, et al. Infection of mesothelial cells with human herpes virus 8 in human immunodeficiency virus-infected patients with Kaposi's sarcoma, Castleman's disease, and recurrent pleural effusions. *Mod Pathol* 2003;16: 145–153.

161. Theunissen P, Cremers M, van der Meer S, et al. Cytologic diagnosis of rhabdomyosarcoma in a child with a pleural effusion: a case report. *Acta Cytol* 2004; 48:249–253.

162. French CA, Miyoshi I, Aster JC, et al. *BRD4* bromodomain gene rearrangement in aggressive carcinoma with translocation t(15;19). *Am J Pathol* 2001;159:1987–1992.

163. Rahbar R, Vargas SO, Miyamoto CR, et al. The role of chromosomal translocation (15;19) in the carcinoma of the upper aerodigestive tract in children. *Otolaryngol Head Neck Surg* 2003;129:698–704.

164. French CA, Kutok JL, Faquin WC, et al. Midline carcinoma of children and young adults with *NUT* rearrangement. *J Clin Oncol* 2004;22:4135–4139.

165. French CA, Miyoshi I, Kubonishi I, et al. *BRD4-NUT* fusion oncogene: a novel mechanism in aggressive carcinoma. *Cancer Res* 2003;63:304–307.

166. Maruyama T, Farina A, Dey A, et al. A Mammalian bromodomain protein, brd4, interacts with replication factor C and inhibits progression to S phase. *Mol Cell Biol* 2002;22:6509–6520.

167. Houzelstein D, Bullock SL, Lynch DE, et al. Growth and early postimplantation defects in mice deficient for the bromodomain-containing protein Brd4. *Mol Cell Biol* 2002;22: 3794–3802.

168. Toretsky JA, Jenson J, Sun CC, et al. Translocation (11;15;19): a highly specific chromosome rearrangement associated with poorly differentiated thymic carcinoma in young patients. *Am J Clin Oncol* 2003;26:300–306.

169. Kubonishi I, Takehara N, Iwata J, et al. Novel t(15;19)(q15;p13) chromosome abnormality in a thymic carcinoma. *Cancer Res* 1991;51:3327–3328.

170. Kees UR, Mulcahy MT, Willoughby ML. Intrathoracic carcinoma in an 11-year-old girl showing a translocation t(15;19). *Am J Pediatr Hematol Oncol* 1991;13:459–464.

171. Lee AC, Kwong YI, Fu KH, et al. Disseminated mediastinal carcinoma with chromosomal translocation (15;19): a distinctive clinicopathologic syndrome. *Cancer* 1993;72: 2273–2276.

172. Rowe SM, Miller S, Sorscher EJ. Cystic fibrosis. *N Engl J Med* 2005;352:1992–2001.

173. http://www.genet.sickkids.on.ca/cftr/.

174. Hadd AG, Laosinchai-Wolf W, Novak CR, et al. Microsphere bead arrays and sequence validation of 5/7/9T genotypes for multiplex screening of cystic fibrosis polymorphisms.*J Mol Diagn* 2004;6:348–355.

175. Sontag MK, Accurso FJ. Gene modifiers in pediatrics: application to cystic fibrosis. *Adv Pediatr* 2004;51:5–36.

176. Sangiuolo F, D'Apice MR, Gambardella S, et al. Toward the pharmacogenomics of cystic fibrosis:an update. *Pharmacogenomics* 2004;5:861–878.

177. Balinsky W, Zhu CW. Pediatric cystic fibrosis: evaluating costs and genetic testing. *J Pediatr Health Care* 2004;18:30–34.

178. National Institute of Health. Genetic testing for cystic fibrosis. National Institutes of Health Consensus Development Conference Statement on genetic testing for cystic fibrosis. *Arch Intern Med* 1999;159:1529–1539.

179. Farrell PM, Kosorok MR, Rock MJ, et al. Early diagnosis of cystic fibrosis through neonatal screening prevents severe malnutrition and improves long-term growth. Wisconsin Cystic Fibrosis Neonatal Screening Study Group. *Pediatrics* 2001;107:1–13.

180. Powell K, Zeitlin PL. Therapeutic approaches to repair defects in deltaF508 CFTR folding and cellular targeting. *Adv Drug Deliv Rev* 2002;54:1395–1408.

181. Roomans G. Pharmacological treatment of the ion transport defect in cystic fibrosis. *Expert Opin Investig Drugs* 2001;10:1–19.

182. Lukacs GL, Durie PR. Pharmacologic approaches to correcting the basic defect in cystic fibrosis. *N Engl J Med* 2003;349:1401–1404.

183. Yang H, Shelat AA, Guy RK, et al. Nanomolar affinity small molecule correctors of defective Delta F508-CFTR chloride channel gating. *J Biol Chem* 2003;278: 35079–35085.

184. Wilschanski M, Yahav Y, Yaacov Y, et al. Gentamicin-induced correction of CFTR function in patients with cystic fibrosis and *CFTR* stop mutations. *N Engl J Med* 2003; 349:1433–1441.

185. Howard MT, Shirts BH, Petros LM, et al. Sequence specificity of aminoglycoside-induced stop condon readthrough: potential implications for treatment of Duchenne muscular dystrophy. *Ann Neurol* 2000;48:164–169.

186. Newman JH, Trembath RC, Morse JA, et al. Genetic basis of pulmonary arterial hypertension: current understanding and future directions. *J Am Coll Cardiol* 2004;43: 33S–39S.

187. Lee SD, Shroyer KR, Markham NE, et al. Monoclonal endothelial cell proliferation is present in primary but not secondary pulmonary hypertension. *J Clin Invest* 1998;101:927–934.

188. Voelkel NF, Cool C, Lee SD, et al. Primary pulmonary hypertension between inflammation and cancer. *Chest* 1998;114:225S–230S.

189. Yeager ME, Halley GR, Golpon HA, et al. Microsatellite instability of endothelial cell growth and apoptosis genes within plexiform lesions in primary pulmonary hypertension. *Circ Res* 2001;88:E2–E11.

190. Deng Z, Morse JH, Slager SL, et al. Familial primary pulmonary hypertension (gene *PPH1*) is caused by mutations in the bone morphogenetic protein receptor-II gene. *Am J Hum Genet* 2000;67:737–744.

191. Tuder RM, Cool CD, Yeager M. The pathobiology of pulmonary hypertension: endothelium. *Clin Chest Med* 2001;22:405–418:

192. Takeda M, Otsuka F, Nakamura K, et al. Characterization of the bone morphogenetic protein (BMP) system in human pulmonary arterial smooth muscle cells isolated from a sporadic case of primary pulmonary hypertension: roles of BMP type IB receptor (activin receptor-like kinase-6) in the mitotic action. *Endocrinology* 2004;145:4344–4354.

193. Abramowicz MJ, Van Haecke P, Demedts M, et al. Primary pulmonary hypertension after amfepramone (diethylpropion) with *BMPR2* mutation. *Eur Respir J* 2003;22:560–562.

194. Humbert M, Deng Z, Simonneau G, et al. *BMPR2* germline mutations in pulmonary hypertension associated with fenfluramine derivatives. *Eur Respir J* 2002;20:518–523.

195. Roberts KE, McElroy JJ, Wong WP, et al. *BMPR2* mutations in pulmonary arterial hypertension with congenital heart disease. *Eur Respir J* 2004;24:371–374.

196. Trembath RC, Thomson JR, Machado RD, et al. Clinical and molecular genetic features of pulmonary hypertension in patients with hereditary hemorrhagic telangiectasia. *N Engl J Med* 2001;345:325–334.

197. Schulick AH, Taylor AJ, Zuo W, et al. Overexpression of transforming growth factor beta1 in arterial endothelium causes hyperplasia, apoptosis, and cartilaginous metaplasia. *Proc Natl Acad Sci USA* 1998;95:6983–6988.

198. Cool CD, Rai R, Yeager ME, et al. Expression of human herpesvirus 8 in primary pulmonary hypertension. *N Engl J Med* 2003;349:1113–1122.

199. Bull TM, Cool CD, Serls AE, et al. Primary pulmonary hypertension, Castleman's disease and human herpesvirus-8. *Eur Respir J* 2003;22:403–407.

200. Cesarman E. Kaposi's sarcoma-associated herpesvirus:the high cost of viral survival. *N Engl J Med* 2003;349:1107–1109.

201. Weiss RA, Whitby D, Talbot S, et al. Human herpesvirus type 8 and Kaposi's sarcoma. *J Natl Cancer Inst Monogr* 1998;23:51–54.

202. Pacheco-Rodriguez G, Kristof A, Stevens L, et al. Giles F. Filley Lecture. Genetics and gene expression in lymphangioleiomyomatosis. *Chest* 2002;121:56S-60S.

203. van Slegtenhorst M, de Hoogty R, Hermans C, et al. Identification of the tuberous sclerosis gene *TSC1* on chromosome 9q34. *Science* 1997;277:805–808.

204. European Chromosome 16 Tuberous Sclerosis Consortium. Identification and characterization of the tuberous sclerosis gene on chromosome 16. The European Chromosome 16 Tuberous Sclerosis Consortium. *Cell* 1993;75:1305–1315.

205. Lamb RF, Roy C, Diefenbach TJ, et al. The TSC1 tumour suppressor hamartin regulates cell adhesion through ERM proteins and the GTPase Rho. *Nat Cell Biol* 2000;2:281–287.

206. Aicher LD, Campbell JS, Yeung RS. Tuberin phosphorylation regulates its interaction with hamartin: two proteins involved in tuberous sclerosis. *J Biol Chem* 2001;276:21017–21021.

207. Moss J, Avila NA, Barnes PM, et al. Prevalence and clinical characteristics of lymphangioleiomyomatosis (LAM) in patients with tuberous sclerosis complex. *Am J Respir Crit Care Med* 2001;164:669–671.

208. Carsillo T, Astrinidis A, Henski E. Mutations in the tuberous sclerosis complex gene *TSC2* are a cause of sporadic pulmonary lymphangioleiomyomatosis. *Proc Natl Acad Sci USA* 2000;97:6085–6090.

209. Sato T, Seyama K, Fujii H, et al. Mutation analysis of the *TSC1* and *TSC2* genes in Japanese patients with pulmonary lymphangioleiomyomatosis. *J Hum Genet* 2002;47:20–28.

210. Karbowniczek M, Astrinidis A, Balsara B, et al. Recurrent lymphangiomyomatosis after transplantation: genetic analyses reveal a metastatic mechanism. *Am J Respir Crit Care Med* 2003;167:976–982.

211. O'Brien JD, Lium JH, Parosa JF, et al. Lymphangiomyomatosis recurrence in the allograft after single-lung transplantation. *Am J Respir Crit Care Med* 1995;151:2033–2036.

212. Nine JS, Yousem SA, Paradis IL, et al. Lymphangioleiomyomatosis: recurrence after lung transplantation. *J Heart Lung Transplant* 1994;13:714–719.

213. Bittmann I, Dose TB, Muller C, et al. Lymphangioleiomyomatosis: recurrence after single lung transplantation. *Hum Pathol* 1997;28:1420–1423.

214. Bittmann I, Rolf B, Amann G, et al. Recurrence of lymphangioleiomyomatosis after single lung transplantation: new insights into pathogenesis. *Hum Pathol* 2003;34:95–98.

215. Crooks DM, Pacheco-Rodriguez G, DeCastro RM, et al. Molecular and genetic analysis of disseminated neoplastic cells in lymphangioleiomyomatosis. *Proc Natl Acad Sci USA* 2004;101:17462–17467.

216. Dabora S, Jozwiak S, Franz D, et al. Mutational analysis in a cohort of 224 tuberous sclerosis patients indicates increased severity of *TSC2*, compared with TSC1, disease in multiple organs. *Am J Hum Genet* 2001;68:64–80.

217. Sato T, Seyama K, Kumasaka T, et al. A patient with *TSC1* germline mutation whose clinical phenotype was limited to lymphangioleiomyomatosis. *J Intern Med* 2004;256:166–173.

218. Lawrence B, Perez-Atayde A, Hibbard MK, et al. *TPM3-ALK* and *TPM4-ALK* oncogenes in inflammatory myofibroblastic tumors. *Am J Pathol* 2000;157:377–384.

219. Cook JR, Dehner LP, Collins MH, et al. Anaplastic lymphoma kinase (ALK) expression in the inflammatory myofibroblastic tumor: a comparative immunohistochemical study. *Am J Surg Pathol* 2001;25:1364–1371.

220. Sakurai H, Hasegawa T, Watanabe S, et al. Inflammatory myofibroblastic tumor of the lung. *Eur J Cardiothorac Surg* 2004;25:155–159.

221. Zennaro H, Laurent F, Vergier B, et al. Inflammatory myofibroblastic tumor of the lung (inflammatory pseudotumor): uncommon cause of solitary pulmonary nodule. *Eur Radiol* 1999;9:1205–1207.

222. Hisaoka M, Hashimoto H, Iwamasa T, et al. Primary synovial sarcoma of the lung: report of two cases confirmed by molecular detection of *SYT-SSX* fusion gene transcripts. *Histopathology* 1999;34:205–210.

223. Okamoto S, Hisaoka M, Daa T, et al. Primary pulmonary synovial sarcoma: a clinicopathologic, immunohistochemical, and molecular study of 11 cases. *Hum Pathol* 2004;35:850–856.

224. Suster S, Moran CA. Primary synovial sarcomas of the mediastinum: a clinicopathologic, immunohistochemical, and ultrastructural study of 15 cases. *Am J Surg Pathol* 2005;29:569–578.

225. Saha S, Rogers AG, Earle GF, et al. Primary pulmonary rhabdomyosarcoma: a long-term survivor. *J Ky Med Assoc* 2002;100:496–498.

226. O'Sullivan MJ, Perlman EJ, Furman J, et al. Visceral primitive peripheral neuroectodermal tumors: a clinicopathologic and molecular study. *Hum Pathol* 2001;321109–1115.

227. Syed S, Haque AK, Hawkins HK, et al. Desmoplastic small round cell tumor of the lung. *Arch Pathol Lab Med* 2002;126:1226–1228.

228. Li G, Hansmann ML, Zwingers T, et al. Primary lymphomas of the lung: morphological, immunohistochemical and clinical features. *Histopathology* 1990;16:519–531.

229. Maejima S, Kitano K, Ichikawa S, et al. T-cell non-Hodgkin's lymphoma of the lung. *Intern Med* 1993;32:403–447.

230. Fiche M, Caprons F, Berger F, et al. Primary pulmonary non-Hodgkin's lymphomas. *Histopathology* 1995;26:529–537.

231. Wundisch T, Neubauer A, Stolte M, et al. B-cell monoclonality is associated with lymphoid follicles in gastritis. *Am J Surg Pathol* 2003;27:882–887.

232. O'Sullivan MJ, Ritter JH, Humphrey PA, et al. Lymphoid lesions of the gastrointestinal tract: a histologic, immunophenotypic, and genotypic analysis of 49 cases. *Am J Clin Pathol* 1998;110:471–477.

233. Iijima T, Inadome Y, Noguchi M. Clonal proliferation of B lymphocytes in the germinal centers of human reactive lymph nodes: possibility of overdiagnosis of B cell clonal proliferation. *Diagn Mol Pathol* 2000;9:132–136.

234. Elenitoba-Johnson KS, Bohling SD,Mitchell RS, et al. PCR analysis of the immunoglobulin heavy chain gene in polyclonal processes can yield pseudoclonal bands as an artifact of low B cell number. *J Mol Diagn* 2000;2:92–96.

235. Taylor JM, Spagnolo DV, Kay PH. B-cell target DNA quantity is a critical factor in the interpretation of B-cell clonality by PCR. *Pathology* 1997;29:309–312.

236. Collins RD. Is clonality equivalent to malignancy: specifically, is immunoglobulin gene rearrangement diagnostic of malignant lymphoma? *Hum Pathol* 1997;28:757–759.

237. Kroft SH. Monoclones, monotypes, and neoplasia pitfalls in lymphoma diagnosis. *Am J Clin Pathol* 2004;121:457–459.

238. Gellrich S, Rutz S, Borkowski A, et al. Analysis of *V(H)-D-J(H)* gene transcripts in B cells infiltrating the salivary glands and lymph node tissues of patients with Sjogren's syndrome. *Arthritis Rheum* 1999;42:240–247.

239. De Vita S, Bolocchi M, Sorrentino D, et al. Characterization of prelymphomatous stages of B cell lymphoproliferation in Sjogren's syndrome. *Arthritis Rheum* 1997;40:318–331.

240. Calvert RJ, Evans PA, Dixon MF. The significance of B-cell clonality in gastric lymphoid infiltrates. *J Pathol* 1996;180:26–32.

241. Algara P, Martinez P, Piris MA. The detection of B-cell monoclonal populations by polymerase chain reaction: accuracy of approach and application in gastric endoscopic biopsy specimens. *Hum Pathol* 1993;24:1184–1188.

242. Lee SC, Berg KD, Racke FK, et al. Pseudo-spikes are common in histologically benign lymphoid tissues. *J Mol Diagn* 2000;2:145–152.

243. Inadome Y, Ikezawa T, Oyasu R, et al. Malignant lymphoma of bronchus-associated lymphoid tissue (BALT) coexistent with pulmonary tuberculosis. *Pathol Int* 2001;51:807–811.

244. Mhawech P, Krishnan B, Shahab I. Primary pulmonary mucosa-associated lymphoid tissue lymphoma with associated fungal ball in a patient with human immunodeficiency virus infection. *Arch Pathol Lab Med* 2000;124:1506–1509.

245. McCluggage WG, McManus K, Qureshi R, et al. Low-grade B-cell lymphoma of mucosa-associated lymphoid tissue (MALT) of thymus. *Hum Pathol* 2000;31:255–259.

246. Philippe B, Delfau-Larue MH, Epardeau B, et al. B-cell pulmonary lymphoma: gene rearrangement analysis of bronchoalveolar lymphocytes by polymerase chain reaction. *Chest* 1999;115:1242–1247.

247. Zompi S, Couderc LJ, Cadranel J, et al. Clonality analysis of alveolar B lymphocytes contributes to the diagnostic strategy in clinical suspicion of pulmonary lymphoma. *Blood* 2004;103:3208–3215.

INVASIVE CARCINOMA

Except for nonmelanoma skin cancer, invasive breast carcinoma is the most common malignancy among women. In developed countries, a woman's lifetime risk of developing invasive breast carcinoma is over 13% (1), although in less developed countries the lifetime risk is lower. As shown in Figure 20.1, only a minority of breast cancer cases in women occur in families with evidence of an inherited susceptibility to breast cancer. For the vast majority of cases, tumor development is the result of the interaction of hormone and reproductive factors, diet and diet-related factors, environmental influences, lifestyle factors, and susceptibility genes (2–5).

Genetics of Familial Breast Cancer Syndromes

A number of inherited syndromes (Table 20.1) are associated with an increased incidence of breast cancer and other malignancies.

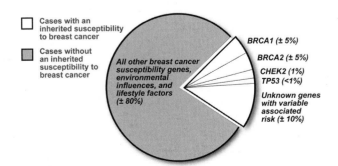

Figure 20.1 Genetics of breast cancer. Note that only about 20% of cases occur in families with evidence of an inherited predisposition to breast cancer, and that even within this group, only about half are associated with mutations in well-characterized susceptibility genes.

BRCA1 Syndrome

Infiltrating breast carcinomas that arise in women who harbor *BRCA1* mutations have an earlier onset, often before age 40, and tend occur without a prior in situ component (2,6). *BRCA1* mutations are present in 20% to 30% of high-risk breast cancer families overall (the exact percentage differs by country and racial background), but *BRCA1* mutations are extremely rare in sporadic cases of invasive breast cancer (2,3,7). Over 1,500 different mutations have been characterized, including frame shift mutations, splice site mutations, and single base pair (bp) substitutions that cause missense and nonsense mutations, all evenly scattered throughout the gene (3). The lack of BRCA1 protein expression in a majority of high-grade invasive breast cancers indicates that the gene may also be inactivated by gross chromosomal rearrangements or promoter hypermethylation (8–12). In practice, mutational analysis is complicated by the fact that assays for BRCA1 function have yet to be developed, and so it is impossible to classify up to 20% of all single bp substitutions as benign polymorphisms versus disease-associated mutations (3,13). In addition, given the wide variety of aberrations, mutational analysis has up to a 20% to 30% false negative rate, regardless of whether the protein truncation assay, multiplex heteroduplex analysis, single-strand conformational polymorphism (SSCP) analysis, or direct sequencing based on polymerase chain reaction (PCR) amplification of specific regions of the gene is used for testing.

The *BRCA1* gene encodes a protein that is 1,863 amino acids long. The protein cannot be assigned to any known protein family, although several functional domains in BRCA1 are found in other proteins (Fig. 20.2). BRCA1 protein expression and phosphorylation are linked to the cell cycle, and although characterization of the full range of BRCA1 functions is ongoing, BRCA1 is known to have a role in transcriptional regulation, the cellular response to DNA damage, and development (reviewed in reference 3).

TABLE 20.1

INHERITED SYNDROMES WITH AN INCREASED SUSCEPTIBILITY TO BREAST CANCER

Syndrome	Gene	Sites of Associated Malignancies	Inheritance
BRCA1 syndrome	BRCA1	Ovary, colon, liver, endometrium, cervix, fallopian tube, peritoneum	Autosomal dominant
BRCA2 syndrome	BRCA2	Ovary, fallopian tube, prostate, pancreas, gallbladder, stomach, skin (melanoma)	Autosomal dominant
Unnamed	CHEK2	Breast	Not established
Li-Fraumeni syndrome	TP53	Soft tissue, brain, adrenal	Autosomal dominant
Cowden syndrome	PTEN	Skin, thyroid, cerebellum, colon	Autosomal dominant
Hereditary non-polyposis colorectal cancer (including Lynch II and Muir-Torre syndromes)	MLH1 MSH2 MSH6 MLH3 PMS2	Colon, endometrium, small intestine, ovary, ureter/renal pelvis, hepatobiliary tract, brain, skin	Autosomal dominant
Peutz-Jeghers syndrome	STK11	Small intestine, ovary, cervix, testis, pancreas	Autosomal dominant
Ataxia telangiectasia	ATM	Breast	Autosomal recessive

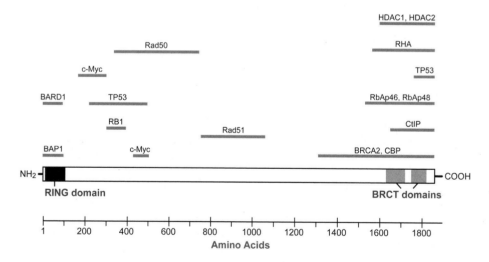

Figure 20.2 Schematic diagram of the BRCA1 protein, including its functional domains. The wide range of BRCA1 functions is suggested by the activities of the numerous other proteins that interact with BRCA1; BAP1 is a deubiquitinating enzyme, CtIP is a transcriptional repressor, RbAp46 and RbAp48 are RB1 binding proteins, RHA is an RNA helicase, HDAC1 and HDAC2 are histone deacetylases, CBP is a transcriptional coactivator that is also a histone acetyltransferase, Rad50 and RAD51 are involved in DNA repair, and BARD1 is involved in regulation of the cell cycle (modified from reference 14).

BRCA2 Syndrome

BRCA2 mutations are present in about 10% to 20% of high-risk breast cancer families, although the prevalence is higher in certain racial groups (2,3). *BRCA2* mutations are also associated with about a 100-fold increase in relative risk for breast cancer in males. Almost 1,900 distinct mutations, and polymorphisms in the gene have been detected (13). About 80% of mutations are nonsense mutations, or

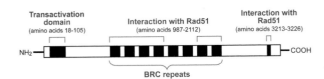

Figure 20.3 Schematic diagram of the functional domains of the BRCA2 protein. Each consensus BRC repeat is 26 amino acids long, but only some of the repeats appear to interact with RAD51 (15,16).

small insertions or deletions that change the reading frame, which result in the production of a truncated protein. However, for about 20% of sequence changes that are due to single bp substitutions, it is unclear whether the alteration represents a benign polymorphism or a disease-causing mutation. As with *BRCA1*, mutational analysis is hampered by the fact that the sequence changes span the entire coding region of the gene without well-defined mutational hot spots. Mutations in *BRCA2* are extremely rare in cases of sporadic breast cancer.

The *BRCA2* gene encodes a protein that is 3,418 amino acids long. Mutations in the *BRCA2* gene have helped identify functional domains in the protein (Fig. 20.3), but none of the domains shows homology to structural motifs that have been previously defined in other proteins. BRCA2 expression is regulated by the cell cycle, and although functional characterization is still incomplete, the protein appears to have a role in development, gene transcription, and the cellular response to DNA damage (2–5).

Li-Fraumeni Syndrome

Germline mutations in *TP53* account for only about 1% of familial breast cancer, even among high-risk families (17,18). About 75% of the mutations are missense or nonsense mutations resulting from single bp substitutions (19,20). Although mutations are scattered throughout the gene, they are more frequent in exons 5 to 8, which encode the protein's DNA binding domain, and codons 245, 248, 273 appear to be relative hot spots (21). Somatic mutations in *TP53* are present in 20% to 50% of sporadic breast cancers (22). Most *TP53* missense mutations lead to accumulation of a stable but inactive protein in tumor cells (9,23), but some mutations do not yield a stable protein, and wild-type protein may accumulate a response to cellular stress or DNA damage. Consequently, in most studies of *TP53* status, DNA sequence analysis shows a stronger correlation with the clinical features of disease than immunohistochemical analysis (24–27).

Cowden Syndrome (Multiple Hamartoma Syndrome)

Germline mutations in *PTEN* are responsible for Cowden syndrome (28,29) and for the allelic Bannayan-Riley-Ruvalcaba syndrome (characterized by lipomatosis, hemangiomatosis, macrocephaly, and a speckled penis) (30–32). Using strict diagnostic criteria, 70% to 80% of individuals with Cowden syndrome harbor germline *PTEN* mutations, and women in this group have a lifetime risk of

invasive breast cancer as high as 50% (30). However, it is difficult to estimate the lifetime risk of breast cancer precisely because some germline sequence differences in *PTEN* represent polymorphisms rather than disease-associated mutations (33), and because the *PTEN* mutation frequency and breast cancer risk drops when diagnostic criteria for Cowden syndrome are relaxed (reviewed in 2). *PTEN* mutations are very rare in sporadic breast cancers and tumors that arise in breast cancer families without manifestations of Cowden syndrome (33,34). Recent data demonstrating that loss of PTEN activity predicts resistance to trastuzmab therapy suggest that evaluation of the level of PTEN expression may have a role in identifying patients likely to be unresponsive to standard therapy even in the absence of coding mutations (35).

Ataxia Telangiectasia

As discussed in detail in Chapter 2, mutations in the *ATM* gene are responsible for ataxia telangiectasia. Over 300 different mutations have been characterized, including truncating mutations resulting from nonsense or frame shift mutations and mutations that effect mRNA splicing (36–38). Individuals who are homozygous or compound heterozygous for mutations in *ATM* have an elevated risk for breast cancer, but the contribution of heterozygous mutations to familial or sporadic breast cancer is apparently minimal (3,4,39).

Hereditary Nonpolyposis Colorectal Cancer

As also discussed in more detail in Chapter 2, mutations in a number of different mismatch repair genes cause the microsatellite instability (MSI) that underlies heredity nonpolyposis colorectal cancer (HNPCC). Women who have the Muir-Torre syndrome (a variant of HNPCC) have an increased risk of breast cancer (40). However, sporadic mutations in mismatch repair genes have only a negligible contribution to breast cancer oncogenesis (41).

CHEK2 associated

The *CHEK2* gene (also known as *cds1* and *RAD53*) encodes a G2 checkpoint kinase that is activated in response to DNA damage. The low-penetrance, kinase-deficient allele 1100delC has recently been shown to confer about a 2-fold increased risk for invasive breast cancer in women and about a 10-fold increased risk of invasive breast carcinoma in men (42,43). However, the frequency of the 1100delC allele varies considerably between different ethnic populations (42–44) and may have an overall frequency as low as 0.3% in some North American populations (44). Other polymorphisms of the *CHEK2* gene are not associated with an increased risk of breast cancer (45,46).

Others

Specific alleles of a number of other genes have been associated with breast cancer susceptibility, including genes encoding proteins involved in recombination and DNA repair such as *RAD51* (47), oncogenes such as H-*ras* (48,49), and genes encoding various enzymes involved in the metabolism of carcinogens, estrogen biosynthesis, and estrogen metabolism (reviewed in 4,50). For most of these genes, the DNA sequence differences that correlate with an increased risk of breast cancer have been identified, although the biochemical basis of the increased risk is generally not well characterized.

Genetics of Sporadic Infiltrating Breast Cancer

Mutational analysis, comparative genomic hybridization (51,52), loss of heterozygosity (LOH) testing (53,54), and gene expression profiling (55) have all shown that the development of invasive breast carcinoma is a multistep process (2,3), as is true for epithelial malignancies of many anatomic sites. Sporadic invasive breast carcinomas harbor a number of mutations (Table 20.2) that result in activation of oncogenes and inactivation of tumor suppressor genes, and alterations in the expression of growth factors and receptors, intercellular signaling molecules, cell surface adhesion molecules, and extracellular proteases (reviewed in 3,4,56–58).

In general, oncogene activation usually occurs through amplification, historically demonstrated by Southern blot hybridization, FISH, comparative genomic hybridization

(CGH), or gene expression analysis by quantitative PCR or immunohistochemistry. Inactivation of tumor suppressor genes usually occurs via biallelic mutation, through deletions, point mutations, or often a combination of both; demonstration of LOH by cytogenetic analysis, CGH, or microsatellite analysis is usually interpreted as evidence of biallelic inactivation even in the absence of formal mutational analysis of the retained allele. Altered promoter methylation is thought to account for those cases that show decreased expression of a specific tumor suppressor despite the lack of any evidence of a mutation.

Technical Issues in Molecular Genetic Analysis of Infiltrating Breast Carcinoma

Cytogenetic Analysis

Conventional cytogenetic analysis is not a part of the routine laboratory evaluation of invasive breast carcinoma for two principle reasons. First, in unselected series, a karyotype can be derived from only about 11% of cases (59). Second, even though the karyotype of infiltrating breast carcinomas correlates with the clinicopathologic features of disease, recurring cytogenetic abnormalities that have diagnostic or prognostic utility are not a feature of invasive breast carcinoma, except for the rare secretory

TABLE 20.2
ALTERATIONS IN SPORADIC BREAST CANCER

Protein	Modification	Frequency(%)
Growth factor receptors		
EGFR	Overexpression	3
HER-2/neu	Overexpression	20–40
FGFR1	Overexpression	10
FGFR2	Overexpression	12
IGFR2	Inactivation	5–10
Growth factors		
FGF1/FGF4	Overexpression	20–30
TGFα	Overexpression	Unknown
Intracellular signaling molecules		
H-ras	Mutation	5–10
c-src	Overexpression	50–70
Cell cycle regulators		
TP53	Mutation/inactivation	20–60
RB1	Inactivation	20
Cyclin D1	Overexpression	35–45
Adhesion molecules and proteases		
E-cadherin	Reduced/absent	60–70
P-cadherin	Reduced/absent	30
Cathepsin D	Overexpression	20–24
Matrix metalloproteinases	Increased expression	20–80
Other proteins		
bcl-2	Overexpression	30–45
c-myc	Amplification	5–20
RB1CC1	Inactivation	20

variant discussed below (60). Comparative genomic hybridization has been shown to be a robust and reproducible method for detection of DNA copy number alterations that is well suited to analysis of breast tumors, even for cases in which only nanogram quantities of DNA from formalin-fixed, parafin-embedded (FFPE) tissue are available (61). The method has been used to correlate patterns of chromosomal gain and loss with outcome in specific subgroups of breast cancer patients (62), but the technique is so cumbersome that it is not well suited for use in routine practice.

DNA Ploidy and S Fraction Analysis

Evaluation of the tumor's mitotic rate is part of routine histologic grading of infiltrating carcinoma (63) because it correlates with prognosis (64,65). However, it is not clear that DNA ploidy and S fraction measurements provide independent prognostic information (66–68). Consequently, neither the College of American Pathologists (CAP) nor the American Society of Clinical Oncologists (ASCO) include DNA ploidy and S fraction measurements as prognostic factors (69,70).

Mutational Analysis of Individual Genes

Mutational analysis of sporadic cases of infiltrating breast carcinoma is not a routine component of the pathologic evaluation for several reasons. First, for most loci that show somatic mutations in sporadic cases of infiltrating breast carcinoma, it is uncertain whether or not the presence of a mutation is associated with prognosis or response to therapy (reviewed in 2–4,56,57). Second, alterations of many markers that have been shown to be strongly associated with prognosis and response to therapy can be detected by immunohistochemical staining (e.g., estrogen receptor, progesterone receptor), eliminating the need for molecular genetic analysis, with the noteworthy exception of HER2/neu as discussed below. However, mutational analysis is indicated for those cases in which a hereditary breast cancer syndrome is suspected (71); since testing in this setting is performed to identify germline mutations, it is best performed on somatic tissue (such as peripheral blood) rather than tumor tissue. Given the significant psychologic and medical implications of a positive test result, for the patient as well as the patient's family, mutational analysis of BRCA1, BRCA2, TP53, and so on should be performed only after the patient has been appropriately counseled by a medical geneticist (71–74).

HER2/neu Analysis

In patients with infiltrating breast carcinoma, overexpression of the HER2/neu oncoprotein is an independent marker of poor clinical outcome (75–79), response to various chemotherapeutic regimens (56,80,81), and therapeutic benefit from treatment with the anti-HER2/neu antibody trastuzumab (82–85). Even though trastuzumab is approved for treatment of patients in a number of different clinical settings (56), it is important to accurately identify patients whose tumors overexpress HER2/neu, because the drug is associated with significant cardiotoxicity (86).

Overexpression of the protein is primarily due to amplification of the HER2/neu gene on chromosome 17q12, and so a number of molecular genetic methods can be used for HER2/neu analysis (87). Southern blot analysis is cumbersome and requires a large amount of fresh tissue, which makes the technique impractical for routine use in a clinical laboratory, as does the fact that the method is not ideally suited to quantitative analysis (because tumor specimens used for testing contain a variable mixture of malignant cells, benign breast tissue, and inflammatory cells). The same factors limit the clinical utility of northern blot analysis of HER2/neu mRNA expression and immunoblot analysis (also known as western blot analysis) of HER2/neu protein (56,88). In contrast, interphase FISH is ideally suited for routine use because the approach can be used with FFPE tissue, permits analysis that is limited to just the population of malignant cells, and is quantitative.

Fluorescence in situ Hybridization (FISH)

Interphase FISH has been validated for use as a screening test for selection of patients for trastuzumab therapy because a positive result identifies those patients who have a greater benefit from chemotherapy with the drug (89). Two interphase FISH assays are approved by the Food and Drug Administration (FDA) for evaluation of HER2/neu gene amplification (90). The PathVysion HER2 Probe kit employs two probes in a dual-color approach, one probe for the chromosome 17 centromere and one probe for the HER2/neu gene; the level of HER2/neu gene amplification is quantified as the ratio of HER2/neu gene copies per chromosome 17 copy, and a ratio of 2.0 or greater is defined as a positive test result. The Inform HER2/neu test employs a probe for the HER2/neu gene alone; amplification is scored on the basis of the absolute HER2/neu gene copy number per tumor cell nucleus, and a copy number per tumor nucleus greater than 4.0 is defined as a positive test result.

It is important to note that the two assays do not yield equivalent results for all patients. For example, testing performed via the PathVysion method that showed chromosome 17 polysomy without gene amplification would be scored as negative, whereas testing via the Inform method would be scored as positive. This difference is not a moot point because patients scored as negative by the PathVysion method would not be eligible for trastuzumab therapy despite the fact that they have an increased HER2/neu gene copy number. Even though 25% to 30% of tumors show chromosome 17 polysomy (91,92), the clinical difference between the two methods may have been overestimated because a parallel comparison of the two methods produces discrepant results in only 4% of cases (93). Paired analysis has shown that there is a strong correlation between the level of HER2/neu amplification measured by FISH in fine-needle aspirates of breast tumors and the corresponding excised tumor specimens (94).

Interphase FISH does have some disadvantages, including a high cost and an intrinsic time-intensive test interpretation (56,92). Consequently, interphase FISH testing is usually incorporated into an algorithm in which immunohistochemical analysis is the primary screening method, as discussed below.

Immunohistochemistry

Immunohistochemical analysis of HER2/neu expression has recently been recommended by an international panel as the screening method of choice, provided that strict quality control and quality assurance measures are maintained (95,96). Two commercially available kits, HercepTest and Pathway, have been approved by the FDA for immunohistochemical analysis of HER2/neu expression. Both kits have been approved for determining the eligibility of patients for therapy with trastuzumab. When membrane staining is scored according to the system approved by the FDA (97), immunohistochemistry produces an interpretable result in over 90% of cases. Numerous studies have shown that the concordance rate between positive (3+) membrane immunostaining and HER2/neu amplification by FISH is in the range of 80% to 100%, that the concordance rate between negative (0 or 1+) immunostaining and a lack of HER2/neu amplification by FISH is over 90%, but that the concordance rate between indeterminate or intermediate (2+) immunostaining and HER2/neu amplification by FISH is only 10% to 35% (91–93,98–103), although the correlation between HER2/neu gene amplification by FISH and protein overexpression by immunohistochemistry depends somewhat on whether the PathVysion or Inform assay is used in the analysis (104,105). It is interesting to note that the poor correlation between indeterminate (2+) immunostaining and FISH may help explain the finding from phase III clinical trials that, as a group, patients whose tumors have an indeterminate (2+) score do not show a benefit from trastuzumab therapy (89).

Given the low concordance rate between FISH and immunohistochemistry for those infiltrating carcinomas with indeterminate (2+) membrane staining, a widely used test algorithm (Fig. 20.4) involves screening of all cases by immunohistochemistry, with secondary testing by FISH for those cases with an indeterminate (2+) membrane staining (56,92,106). Given the high level of agreement among pathologists in scoring the immunohistochemical result on the 0 to 3+ scale (92), this algorithm should help to minimize disconcordance in HER2/neu testing between reference and community-based laboratories (95, 107).

PCR-based Analysis

Several studies have compared HER2/neu protein expression by immunohistochemistry, HER2/neu amplification by FISH (using the PathVysion kit), and quantitative PCR using the LightCycler system (Roche Diagnostics, Indianapolis, IN). These studies have shown that there is an 83% to 98% concordance between FISH and quantitative PCR and that FISH and quantitative PCR show 100% concordance for tumors scored as negative (0 or 1+) by immunohistochemistry, 63% to 96% concordance for tumors scored as intermediate (2+), and 100% concordance for tumors scored as positive (3+) (108,109). Because HER2/neu transcripts can be amplified from 94% of cases when FFPE tissue is the substrate for testing, quantitative PCR analysis can be easily performed on routinely processed tissue specimens, although optimum test performance is only achieved using microdissected tumor specimens, regardless of whether fresh or FFPE

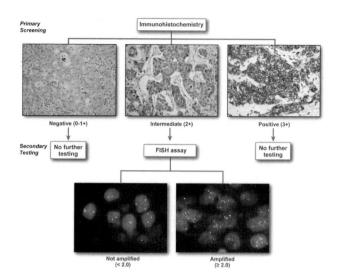

Figure 20.4 Testing algorithm for tissue-based HER2/neu analysis in breast cancer. All cases are primarily screened for HER2/neu overexpression by immunohistochemistry. Secondary testing by FISH analysis is only performed on cases with an intermediate (2+) level of immunohistochemical staining. In this illustration, primary screening was performed by HercepTest immunohistochemical staining; 0 indicates no membrane staining, 1+ indicates partial membrane staining in more than 10% of cells without circumferential staining, 2+ indicates thin circumferential membrane staining in more than 10% of cells, and 3+ indicates thick circumferential membrane staining in more than 10% of cells. Secondary screening was performed by the PathVysion FISH assay, where HER2 amplification is indicated by a ratio of HER2 (red signals) to chromosome 17 (green signals) that is 2.0 or greater. (See color insert.)

tissue is analyzed (108,109). Measurement of the level of HER2/neu gene amplification by a competitive PCR approach produces results that show an excellent correlation with the results of the quantitative PCR method (110).

Chromogenic in situ Hybridization Analysis

Chromogenic in situ hybridization (CISH) has been used as an alternative methodology for detection of HER2/neu amplification and shows excellent concordance with the results of FISH-based testing (111–113). However, the CISH result is simpler to score because the slides can be evaluated by routine light microscopy, a technical feature of the approach that also makes it very easy to correlate the genotype and phenotype of individual cells.

Diagnostic and Prognostic Issues in Molecular Genetic Analysis of Infiltrating Breast Carcinoma

Molecular genetic analysis of individual genes shows neither the sensitivity nor the specificity to distinguish invasive ductal from invasive lobular carcinoma or to distinguish invasive carcinoma from in situ disease. Even though specific markers cannot reliably distinguish most subtypes of infiltrating carcinoma (with the exception of secretory carcinoma, as discussed later), the fact that mutations in BRCA1 have been associated with medullary carcinoma (114–117) suggests that it is nonetheless prudent in cases of this subtype of invasive ductal carcinoma to include a comment in the pathology report suggesting clinical follow-up to exclude BRCA1 syndrome.

Even though genetic analysis of individual genes has little role in the diagnosis of individual tumors, molecular evaluation of individual loci does play an important role in stratifying patients into appropriate treatment groups. Analysis of *HER2/neu* is the best example of the use of molecular testing to direct therapy, as discussed in detail previously. Analysis of *TP53* may have a similar role because specific mutations of the gene are associated with clinical outcome, response to specific chemotherapy regimens, and response to radiation therapy (118–124). Parallel analysis of multiple markers rather than individual loci may provide the most reliable prognostic and therapeutic information (57,58,92,125).

Microarray-based Gene Expression Analysis of Invasive Tumors

Using current guidelines for defining prognostic and treatment groups of patients with infiltrating carcinoma, up to 85% of patients without axillary node metastasis are candidates for adjuvant systemic therapy, although as many as 70% to 80% of these patients do not develop distant metastases and therefore probably do not need adjuvant therapy (126,127). Several studies suggest that gene expression analysis is potentially capable of providing a molecular classification that more accurately predicts prognosis and the need for therapy. Using a microarray for almost 25,000 human genes, a so-called prognosis profile of 70 genes has been developed that is an independent factor in predicting disease outcome in young patients with stage I or II breast cancer (128,129). The prognosis profile is a strong independent predictor of disease outcome, both in terms of an increased risk for distant metastasis and a lower overall survival for both node-negative and node-positive patients. Similarly, patterns of gene expression in breast carcinoma specimens have been identified that can predict lymph node metastases, relapse, and survival (130,131). Although there is admittedly some question as to whether the size of the included breast tumors and differing adjuvant therapy protocols introduced bias into these studies (132), the results suggest that gene expression analysis can identify patients who have such a low risk of recurrence that adjuvant therapy can be safely omitted. In fact, a prospective randomized clinical trial has been designed to determine whether the 70 gene expression profile can, in fact, be used to direct therapy; patients will be randomized into treatment groups based on the risk of recurrence as assessed by either conventional histopathologic criteria or by the 70 gene expression profile (133), which marks the first time that the role of microarray analysis in directing clinical therapy will be evaluated by a prospective clinical trial.

Other microarray analyses have attempted to identify gene expression profiles that can be used to predict patient subgroups that have an optimal response to a particular therapy. The functional status of hormone receptor pathways has been evaluated as a guide for endocrine therapy (134,135), and limited sets of genes have been identified that stratify patients at the time of diagnosis into subgroups

with statistically different probabilities of response to endocrine therapy (136,137). For example, transcriptional profiling has been used to predict a complete pathologic response to neoadjuvant multiagent chemotherapy (including paclitaxel and 5-fluorouracil (5-FU), doxorubicin, and cyclophosphamide) with 81% accuracy (138) and to define patterns of gene expression that correlate with the response of infiltrating breast cancer to docetaxel (139,140).

A number of technical innovations may extend the range of specimens that is available for microarray analysis and increase the accuracy of the results. First, expression analysis of mRNA from very small samples of fresh tissue has been shown to be both feasible and practical (141,142). Consequently, it is now possible to microdissect viable tumor cells from background inflammatory cells, stromal cells, and normal epithelium, providing the opportunity for even more precise analysis of gene expression changes that correlate with prognosis and response to therapy. In addition, methods for evaluating very small tissue samples will make it possible to avoid biases that crept into earlier microarray studies that were limited to relatively large tumors because of the volume of tissue required for testing (132). Second, there are reports of methods that produce highly reproducible gene expression profiles from even small amounts of RNA isolated from formalin-fixed tissues (143). Although the reliability of expression profiles obtained from FFPE tissue remains uncertain (Chapter 9), the ability to analyze FFPE tissue would markedly expand the number of cases amenable to analysis, both clinically and experimentally. Third, once clinically relevant gene clusters are identified, it may be possible to perform multigene reverse transcriptase PCR (RT-PCR) and so eliminate the need for costly and cumbersome microarray analysis. Multigene RT-PCR holds great promise for tailoring therapy to individual patients, as shown by one recent study in which RT-PCR performed on a panel of 21 genes from FFPE tissue was used to categorize node-negative patients into groups with a low, intermediate, or high risk of recurrence (144). The so-called recurrence score derived from the RT-PCR provided statistically significant prognostic information independent of patient age and tumor size and was also a statistically significant predictor of overall survival.

IN SITU CARCINOMA AND OTHER NONINVASIVE PROLIFERATIVE LESIONS

Even though the relationship between in situ proliferations and invasive carcinoma is quite complex, a variety of data support a model in which there is a precursor relationship between at least a subset of in situ neoplasms and invasive lobular and ductal carcinoma (131,145–147). In situ lesions, especially in situ lesions adjacent to invasive carcinoma, often harbor aberrations characteristic of invasive carcinoma, including mutations in the genes encoding E cadherin, HER2/neu, cyclin D1, and TP53 (3, 148,149). LOH has also been demonstrated in a variety of noninvasive proliferative lesions, including lobular carcinoma in situ (150,151) and ductal carcinoma in situ (148, 152–155).

However, the biologic significance of LOH data from neoplasms of the breast must be interpreted with caution, because normal breast parenchyma (156,157), non-neoplastic breast tissue adjacent to carcinoma (158), and even the stromal component of in situ carcinoma (52) can all show LOH.

Microarray analysis of gene expression also supports a precursor relationship between at least a subset of in situ neoplasms and invasive lobular and ductal carcinoma (54,131), even though the significance of all of the differences between benign breast tissue, in situ neoplasms, and invasive carcinoma remains to be more thoroughly evaluated (159).

SECRETORY BREAST CARCINOMA

Secretory breast carcinoma (SBC) is a rare variant of infiltrating ductal carcinoma. The tumor was originally described in children and adolescents (160), but additional reports have made it clear that the neoplasm has an equal incidence in adults (161). Histologically, secretory carcinoma has three morphologic patterns, including a microcystic (honeycomb) pattern that can simulate thyroid follicles, a compact solid pattern, and a tubular pattern, which are present in varying combinations in individual tumors.

Genetics

The translocation t(12;15)(p13;q25) that produces an *ETV6-NTRK3* fusion gene is the hallmark of secretary breast carcinoma (162,163). The *ETV6-NTRK3* fusion (Fig. 20.5) encodes a protein in which the N-terminal helix-loop-helix dimerization domain of the highly expressed ET V6 transcription factor (also known as TEL) is fused to the tyrosine kinase domain of NTRK3 (also known as TRKC). The chimeric protein is thought to undergo ligand-independent, helix-loop-helix–mediated dimerization with subsequent activation of the tyrosine kinase activity of NTRK3, producing a constitutively active protein tyrosine kinase that has transforming activity through a number of different cell activation pathways (164,165).

The t(12;15) translocation break point in all cases of SBC evaluated to date occurs within intron 5 of *ETV6* and intron 12 of *NTRK3* (162,166). Interestingly, the fusion transcripts in SBC do not contain *NTRK3* exon 16 which encodes a 42 bp insert within the protein tyrosine kinase domain of NTRK3. When present, the 14 amino acids encoded by the insert decrease the activity of the NTRK3 protein kinase, but the significance of the alternative pattern of mRNA processing in the pathogenesis of SBC remains unknown (167,168).

Technical Issues in Molecular Genetic Analysis of SBC

Cytogenetic analysis has been used to identify the t(12;15)(p13;q25) translocation in SBC (162). However, because the regions that are exchanged between chromosomes 12 and 15 are so similar in size and banding characteristics, the translocation can be easily overlooked when evaluated by conventional banding methods (169–171).

In routine practice, RT-PCR or FISH is most often used to identify the *NTV6-NTRK3* fusion. Even when FFPE tissue is used as a substrate for testing, RT-PCR demonstrates *ETV6-NTRK3* fusion transcripts in 92% of cases (162). Dual-color FISH, using either the probe splitting or probe fusion approach, demonstrates the characteristic rearrangement in from 75% to 100% of cases (162,163).

Diagnostic Issues in Molecular Genetic Analysis of SBC

The *ETV6-NTRK3* fusion characteristic of SBC is not a recurrent feature of any other type of breast neoplasm (162,163). When evaluated by RT-PCR or FISH, only 0% to 2% of conventional infiltrating ductal carcinomas harbor the *ETV6-NTRK3* rearrangement, and the fusion has not been detected in infiltrating lobular carcinoma, mucinous carcinoma, signet ring carcinoma, papillary carcinoma, or medullary carcinoma (163). CGH analysis and immunohistochemistry also indicate that SBC is a malignancy distinct from conventional infiltrating ductal carcinoma (172).

Although the t(12;15) is the hallmark of SBC, the same aberration is also characteristic of several other neoplasms, including congenital/infantile fibrosarcoma (169–171), cellular and mixed type congenital mesoblastic nephroma (169, 171, 173, 174), and rare cases of acute myeloid leukemia (175,176). The presence of *ETV6-NTRK3* fusions in all of these tumors, which emphasizes that aberrant tyrosine kinase signaling by a chimeric ETV6-NTRK3 fusion protein is a common oncogenic mechanism across a number of different cell types (162,165).

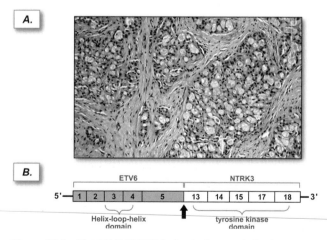

Figure 20.5 The *ETV6-NTRK3* fusion is characteristic of secretory breast carcinoma (SBC). **A,** Photomicrograph of SBC from an 8-year-old girl with a breast mass. **B,** Schematic diagram of the fusion transcript encoding the chimeric ETV6-NTRK3 protein. Note that exons 1 to 5 of *ETV6* are fused in frame with exons 13 to 16 and 17 to 18 of *NTRK3*. The functional domains of ETV6 and NTRK3 encoded by the transcript are indicated; the *arrow* shows the position of the fusion junction.

FIBROADENOMA

Occasional fibroadenomas have been described that harbor rearrangements involving the *HMGA2* gene (177, 178), an aberration that has been described in a wide variety of other benign mesenchymal tumor types (Chapter 11 and Table 11.7). Testing for rearrangements in *HMGA2* has little utility in the evaluation of fibroadenomas, however, because such a small percentage of cases harbor the abnormality (179) and the rearrangement also has been described in phyllodes tumor (180).

SALIVARY GLAND-LIKE NEOPLASMS

Tumors that morphologically resemble pleomorphic adenoma (benign mixed tumor) of the salivary glands occur, albeit rarely, as primary breast tumors (2). Whether or not they share the same pattern of recurring translocations that is characteristic of pleomorphic adenomas of the major and minor salivary glands (Chapter 21) is unknown. Very rare cases of primary mucoepidermoid carcinoma of the breast have also been described (2), but again it is unknown whether they share the same translocation that is the hallmark of mucoepidermoid carcinoma of the salivary glands (Chapter 21).

SARCOMAS

Sarcomas that classically occur in the soft tissue or skin also occur, though rarely, as primary tumors of the breast. For example, cases of Ewing sarcoma/peripheral neuroectodermal tumor (181), alveolar rhabdomyosarcoma (182,183), alveolar soft part sarcoma (184), dermatofibrosarcoma protuberans (185), and inflammatory myofibroblastic tumor (186) have all been described that originated in the breast. The molecular genetic features of these tumors have been shown to be the same whether they occur in the breast or at more conventional sites (Chapter 11).

MOLECULAR GENETIC ANALYSIS OF SENTINEL LYMPH NODES

Sentinel lymph node biopsy has been developed as a method to identify the subset of patients who harbor clinically occult lymph node metastases, thereby sparing the remainder of patients the morbidity of unnecessary regional lymphadenectomy. However, the role of sentinel node (SN) biopsy as a component of standard of care therapy continues to be evaluated, as does the optimum method for pathologic evaluation of the excised nodes (187–191). Although the use of multiple hematoxylin and eosing (H&E)-stained sections, supplemented with immunohistochemical stains for epithelial markers, is the most widely used approach for evaluating SN from patients with breast cancer, PCR has been evaluated as a method for assessment of SN. However, several aspects of PCR-based analysis introduce uncertainty into the interpretation of the test result.

Lack of Specificity

Tumor Markers

A wide variety of markers presumed to be specific for epithelial cells have been evaluated, including cytokeratin-19 (CK-19), CK-20, carcinoembryonic antigen (CEA) prolactin-inducible protein, mucin-1 (MUC-1) epithelial glycoprotein-2, mammaglobin, mammaglobin B, and others. However, RT-PCR amplification detects messenger ribonucleic acid (mRNA) from these genes in a significant percentage (up to 100% in some studies) of control lymph nodes obtained from patients with no history of malignancy, a lack of specificity that is evident in virtually every study in which control lymph nodes have been evaluated (reviewed in 187,192,193). There are several explanations for this high false positive rate. Some genes (e.g., *CK-19*) are expressed at low levels by normal components of lymph nodes, including endothelial cells and fibroblasts (194). A low level of mRNA expression from other genes may arise as the result of illegitimate transcription (195,196). And, benign epithelium can even be displaced into axillary lymph nodes by biopsy procedures (197,198).

A number of approaches can be used to increase RT-PCR–based test specificity, including amplification of a panel of mRNA markers and amplification of a marker sequence known to harbor a mutation in the primary tumor (199). Quantitative RT-PCR can also be used to increase the specificity of a positive result and increase the correlation between the results of molecular testing and routine histopathologic analysis or immunohistochemical staining (200,201). However, even using quantitative RT-PCR, it can still be difficult to distinguish whether a low level of mRNA originates from benign lymph node components or a very small number of malignant cells.

Detection of Cellular Debris

RT-PCR is so sensitive that the method can detect nucleic acids that have drained to lymph nodes in the absence of viable tumor cells. In fact, in one well-controlled model system, target sequences could be amplified from draining or systemic lymph nodes by PCR up to 4 days after injection of cell-free purified DNA (202). Because SNs are by definition the first nodes in the lymphatic drainage from the primary tumor, it is likely that they can contain cellular debris that can yield a positive PCR result even in the absence of metastatic disease.

Lack of Morphologic Correlation

Correct interpretation of immunopositive cells in SNs requires correlation of the cells' immunoreactivity with their cytologic features (187,188). However, the SN tissue used for RT-PCR analysis is destroyed by mRNA extraction and direct morphologic confirmation of the result is therefore impossible. This is not a moot point because, as noted previously, several different scenarios can produce false positive RT-PCR results.

Clinical Significance of a Positive Test Result

The extreme technical sensitivity of RT-PCR makes it possible to routinely detect 1 malignant cell within 10^6 benign cells (Chapters 5 and 8), and so molecular analysis makes it possible to detect micrometastatic disease that consists of individual cells. Although the majority of large studies with long-term follow-up suggest that there is a distinct survival disadvantage for metastases as small as 0.2 mm (187,188,191), the clinical significance of metastases that consist of only individual cells remains uncertain. Although one small study has suggested that SN metastases detected only by RT-PCR analysis do not predict a poor clinical outcome (192), the data from a number of ongoing large prospective, randomized, clinical trials are required to definitively establish whether or not occult metastases detected only by RT-PCR predict further node involvement, prognosis, or the need for adjuvant systemic treatment (187,191).

DETECTION OF SUBMICROSCOPIC DISEASE

Molecular genetic analysis, again primarily via RT-PCR methodology, has been used to correlate clinical outcome with the presence of submicroscopic disease (generally defined as metastatic disease that can be detected by RT-PCR, but not by routine light microscopy or immunohistochemical stains) in peripheral blood, bone marrow, or leukapheresis products. Molecular evidence of bone marrow involvement is a statistically significant predictor of disease recurrence (203,204), but because detection of metastatic disease by immunohistochemistry also provides statistically significant prognostic information (205,206), it will remain unknown whether or not genetic analysis provides any independent information until a set of the same cases is evaluated by parallel molecular and immunohistochemical testing. The relationship between the presence of submicroscopic peripheral blood involvement and patient outcome is less certain (207–212), although detection of circulating tumor cells by immunohistochemical-based methods is clearly an independent predictor of outcome in some settings (213). However, as with analysis of SN, technical features of RT-PCR methodology introduce uncertainties into the interpretation of the test result.

Lack of Marker Specificity

The specificity of the mRNA markers used in RT-PCR assays to detect submicroscopic metastases is often quite low. Transcripts encoding CEA, CK-19, and MUC-1 have been detected in the peripheral blood of up to 45% of healthy donors; likewise, transcripts encoding CEA, CK-19, HER2/neu (also known as erb-B2), and MUC-1 (among others) have been detected in the bone marrow of up to 70% of healthy individuals (193,200,214–220). Some of the nonspecificity is due to intrinsic biologic phenomena such as illegitimate transcription, but purely technical factors also affect the assay, including the type of blood preservative and the time interval between sample collection and processing (221,222). The use of modified test approaches, such as amplification of multiple markers, competitive RT-PCR, and quantitative RT-PCR, has been shown to limit the number of false positive test results (217,218,220). However, as with RT-PCR evaluation of SN, it can still be difficult to distinguish whether a low level of mRNA originates from benign blood components or a very small number of malignant cells.

Variability in Marker Expression by Malignant Cells

RT-PCR analysis of infiltrating breast carcinoma tumor specimens and cell lines has demonstrated that variability in the level of expression of a number of marker mRNAs (including those encoding CK-19, mammaglobin, HER2/neu, epithelial glycoprotein-2 [EG-2], and MUC-5B) can be a source of false negative test results (200,216–218). This finding suggests that optimal test performance can be achieved only if the marker mRNAs expressed by the patient's primary tumor are identified before RT-PCR testing of blood or bone marrow for submicroscopic disease.

Variability in Sampling Protocol

Just as biopsy procedures have been shown to displace benign breast epithelial cells into lymph nodes (197,198), surgical manipulation at the time of biopsy or excision can produce a shower of circulating tumor cells (223). Consequently, it is possible that the timing of blood or bone marrow sampling following a biopsy or excision may have a significant impact on test results.

Clinical Significance of a Positive Test Result

The significance of occult blood or bone marrow disease identified only by RT-PCR remains unclear. Most studies that have demonstrated a correlation between submicroscopic disease and patient outcome have been either small or retrospective and have not used the results of molecular analysis to stratify patients into different treatment groups. Until large prospective randomized clinical studies with long-term follow-up are completed, the role of molecular genetic testing for detection of submicroscopic disease will remain uncertain.

ANALYSIS OF SYNCHRONOUS AND METACHRONOUS TUMORS

Bilateral breast carcinoma occurs in 1% to 15% of patients with breast cancer, and 2% to 15% of women with unilateral carcinoma develop recurrent disease after primary therapy. Consequently, synchronous or metachronous breast carcinomas in these settings raise the question as to whether the two tumors represent recurrence or metastasis of one primary malignancy or two independent primary malignancies. The difference is clinically important for staging, prognosis and therapy because metastatic disease is rarely curable, but a second primary tumor is usually treated with curative intent. Because the pattern of microsatellite allelic imbalance has been shown to be the same between primary tumors and subsequent recurrences

(224,225), microsatellite analysis can be used to objectively establish the clonality relationship between tumors in this clinical setting (the technical aspects of clonality determination by microsatellite analysis are discussed in detail in Chapters 5 and 23).

Approximately 6% of patients whose primary infiltrating carcinoma is treated with breast-conserving therapy will develop a second invasive carcinoma in the same breast, referred to as an ipsilateral breast failure (226). Traditionally, clinical and pathologic criteria have been used to determine whether the ipsilateral breast failure represents a second primary tumor or metastasis, although the tumor classifications produced by this approach are not highly correlated with clinical outcome (226). In contrast, the classifications provided by clonality analysis show much better correlation with patient outcome (224,227), and so it is not surprising that the results of molecular analysis differ in 38% to 43% of cases from the classification provided by traditional clinical and pathologic criteria (224,227). Although clonality analysis is somewhat cumbersome because it involves analysis of at least 20 microsatellite markers, it is informative in about 80% of cases and so provides the opportunity to significantly affect the care of women with ipsilateral breast failures (224,227).

Molecular genetic analysis of microsatellite loci has also been used to establish the clonality relationship between bilateral invasive carcinomas (228–230). Although in this setting traditional clinical and pathologic criteria can distinguish unrelated primary tumors from metastases with high accuracy, molecular clonality analysis can still be of use in cases for which traditional criteria are indeterminate (228–230).

Finally, molecular clonality analysis using microsatellite loci has also been used to demonstrate that reappearance of ipsilateral ductal carcinoma in situ (DCIS) most often represents recurrence of the initial tumor (usually with genetic progression) rather than a second tumor, even when the recurrence occurs as long as 15 years after the initial disease (231). Although this finding has limited diagnostic relevance, it has implications for the surgical approach to excision of DCIS (232,233).

REFERENCES

1. http://www.cancer.org/docroot/STT/stt_0.asp.
2. Tavassoli FA, Devilee P, eds. *Pathology and Genetics of Tumours of the Breast and Female Genital Organs: World Health Organization Classification of Tumours.* Lyon: IARC Press; 2003.
3. Couch FJ, Weber BL. Breast cancer. In: Vogelstein B, Kinzler KW, ed. *The Genetic Basis of Human Cancer*, 2d ed. New York: McGraw-Hill; 2002:549–581.
4. Lymberis SC, Parhar PK, Katsoulakis E, et al. Pharmacogenomics and breast cancer. *Pharmacogenomics* 2004;5:31–55.
5. Wooster R, Weber BL. Breast and ovarian cancer. *N Engl J Med* 2003;348:2339–2347.
6. Miki Y, Swensen J, Shattuck-Eidens D, et al. A strong candidate for the breast and ovarian cancer susceptibility gene BRCA1. *Science* 1994;266:66–71.
7. Merajver SD, Pham TM, Caduff RF, et al. Somatic mutations in the BRCA1 gene in sporadic ovarian tumours. *Nat Genet* 1995;9:439–443.
8. Cornelis RS, Devilee P, van Vliet M, et al. Allele loss patterns on chromosome 17q in 109 breast carcinomas indicate at least two distinct target regions. *Oncogene* 1993;8:781–785.
9. Hanssen AM, Fryns JP. Cowden syndrome. *J Med Genet* 1995;32:117–119.
10. Catteau A, Harris WH, Xu CF, et al. Methylation of the BRCA1 promoter region in sporadic breast and ovarian cancer: correlation with disease characteristics. *Oncogene* 1999;18:1957–1965.
11. Russell PA, Pharoah PD, De Foy K, et al. Frequent loss of BRCA1 mRNA and protein expression in sporadic ovarian cancers. *Int J Cancer* 2000;87:317–321.
12. Wilson CA, Ramos L, Villasenor MR, et al. Localization of human BRCA1 and its loss in high-grade, non-inherited breast carcinomas. *Nat Genet* 1999;21:236–240.
13. http://research.nhgri.nih.gov/bic/.
14. Lee JS, Chung JH. Diverse functions of BRCA1 in the DNA damage response. *Exp Rev Mol Med* 2001;1–9. http://www.expertreviews.org/01003131h.htm
15. Chen CF, Chen PL, Zhong Q, et al. Expression of BRC repeats in breast cancer cells disrupts the BRCA2-RAD51 complex and leads to radiation hypersensitivity and loss of G(2)/M checkpoint control. *J Biol Chem* 1999;274:32931–32935.
16. Bignell G, Micklem G, Stratton MR, et al. The BRC repeats are conserved in mammalian BRCA2 proteins. *Hum Mol Genet* 1997;6:53–58.
17. Sidransky D, Tokino T, Helzlsouer K, et al. Inherited p53 gene mutations in breast cancer. *Cancer Res* 1992;52:2984–2986.
18. Borresen AL, Andersen TI, Garber J, et al. Screening for germ line TP53 mutations in breast cancer patients. *Cancer Res* 1992;52:3234–3236.
19. Malkin D, Li FP, Strong LC, et al. Germ line p53 mutations in a familial syndrome of breast cancer, sarcomas, and other neoplasms. *Science* 1990;250:1233–1238.
20. Srivastava S, Zou ZQ, Pirollo K, et al. Germ-line transmission of a mutated p53 gene in a cancer-prone family with Li-Fraumeni syndrome. *Nature* 1990;348:747–749.
21. Kleihues P, Schauble B, zur Hausen A, et al. Tumors associated with p53 germline mutations: a synopsis of 91 families. *Am J Pathol* 1997;150:1–13.
22. de Jong MM, Nolte IM, te Meerman GJ, et al. Genes other than BRCA1 and BRCA2 involved in breast cancer susceptibility. *J Med Genet* 2002;39:225–242.
23. Pharoah PD, Day NE, Caldas C. Somatic mutations in the p53 gene and prognosis in breast cancer: a meta-analysis. *Br J Cancer* 1999;80:1968–1973.
24. Fitzgibbons PL, Page DL, Weaver D, et al. Prognostic factors in breast cancer. College of American Pathologists Consensus Statement 1999. *Arch Pathol Lab Med* 2000;124:966–978.
25. Soussi T, Beroud C. Assessing TP53 status in human tumours to evaluate clinical outcome. *Nat Rev Cancer* 2001;1:233–240.
26. Rosen PP, Lesser ML, Arroyo CD, et al. p53 in node-negative breast carcinoma: an immunohistochemical study of epidemiologic risk factors, histologic features, and prognosis. *J Clin Oncol* 1995;13:821–830.
27. Reed W, Hannisdal E, Boehler PJ, et al. The prognostic value of p53 and c-erb B-2 immunostaining is overrated for patients with lymph node negative breast carcinoma: a multivariate analysis of prognostic factors in 613 patients with a follow-up of 14–30 years. *Cancer* 2000;88:804–813.
28. Liaw D, Marsh DJ, Li J, et al. Germline mutations of the PTEN gene in Cowden disease, an inherited breast and thyroid cancer syndrome. *Nat Genet* 1997;16:64–67.
29. Nelen MR, Padberg GW, Peeters EA, et al. Localization of the gene for Cowden disease to chromosome 10q22–23. *Nat Genet* 1996;13:114–116.
30. Marsh DJ, Coulon V, Lunetta KL, et al. Mutation spectrum and genotype-phenotype analyses in Cowden disease and Bannayan-Zonana syndrome, two hamartoma syndromes with germline PTEN mutation. *Hum Mol Genet* 1998;7:507–515.
31. Marsh DJ, Dahia PL, Zheng Z, et al. Germline mutations in PTEN are present in Bannayan-Zonana syndrome. *Nat Genet* 1997;16:333–334.
32. Marsh DJ, Kum JB, Lunetta KL, et al. PTEN mutation spectrum and genotype-phenotype correlations in Bannayan-Riley-Ruvalcaba syndrome suggest a single entity with Cowden syndrome. *Hum Mol Genet* 1999;8:1461–1472.
33. Zhou XP, Hampel H, Roggenbuck J, et al. A 39-bp deletion polymorphism in PTEN in African American individuals: implications for molecular diagnostic testing. *J Mol Diagn* 2002;4:114–117.
34. Carroll BT, Couch FJ, Rebbeck TR, et al. Polymorphisms in PTEN in breast cancer families. *J Med Genet* 1999;36:94–96.
35. Pandolfi PP. Breast cancer: loss of PTEN predicts resistance to treatment. *N Engl J Med* 2004;351:2337–2338.
36. Gilad S, Chessa L, Khosravi R, et al. Genotype-phenotype relationships in ataxia-telangiectasia and variants. *Am J Hum Genet* 1998;62:551–561.
37. Sandoval N, Platzer M, Rosenthal A, et al. Characterization of ATM gene mutations in 66 ataxia telangiectasia families. *Hum Mol Genet* 1999;8:69–79.
38. Teraoka SN, Telatar M, Becker-Catania S, et al. Splicing defects in the ataxia-telangiectasia gene, ATM: underlying mutations and consequences. *Am J Hum Genet* 1999;64:1617–1631.
39. Fitzgerald MG, Bean JM, Hegde SR, et al. Heterozygous ATM mutations do not contribute to early onset of breast cancer. *Nat Genet* 1997;15:307–310.
40. Anderson DE. An inherited form of large bowel cancer: Muir's syndrome. *Cancer* 1980;45:1103–1107.
41. Anbazhagan R, Fujii H, Gabrielson E. Microsatellite instability is uncommon in breast cancer. *Clin Cancer Res* 1999;5:839–844.
42. Meijers-Heijboer H, van den Ouweland A, Klijn J, et al. Low-penetrance susceptibility to breast cancer due to CHEK2 1100delC in noncarriers of BRCA1 or BRCA2 mutations. *Nat Genet* 2002;31:55–59.
43. Vahteristo P, Bartkova J, Eerola H, et al. A CHEK2 genetic variant contributing to a substantial fraction of familial breast cancer. *Am J Hum Genet* 2002;71:432–438.
44. Offit K, Pierce H, Kirchhoff T, et al. Frequency of CHEK2 1100delC in New York breast cancer cases and controls. *BMC Med Genet* 2003;4:1.
45. Schutte M, Seal S, Barfoot R, et al. Variants in CHEK2 other than 1100delC do not make a major contribution to breast cancer susceptibility. *Am J Hum Genet* 2003;72:1023–1028.
46. Kuschel B, Auranen A, Gregory CS, et al. Common polymorphisms in checkpoint kinase 2 are not associated with breast cancer risk. *Cancer Epidemiol Biomarkers Prev* 2003;12:809–812.
47. Kato M, Yano K, Matsuo F, et al. Identification of Rad51 alteration in patients with bilateral breast cancer. *J Hum Genet* 2000;45:133–137.
48. Krontiris TG, DiMartino NA, Colb M, et al. Unique allelic restriction fragments of the human Ha-ras locus in leukocyte and tumour DNAs of cancer patients. *Nature* 1985;313:369–374.
49. Krontiris TG, Devlin B, Karp DD, et al. An association between the risk of cancer and mutations in the HRAS1 minisatellite locus. *N Engl J Med* 1993;329:517–523.
50. Dunning AM, Healey CS, Pharoah PD, et al. A systematic review of genetic polymorphisms and breast cancer risk. *Cancer Epidemiol Biomarkers Prev* 1999;8:843–854.
51. Gunther K, Merkelbach-Bruse S, Amo-Takyi BK, et al. Differences in genetic alterations between primary lobular and ductal breast cancers detected by comparative genomic hybridization. *J Pathol* 2001;193:40–47.

52. Roylance R, Gorman P, Harris W, et al. Comparative genomic hybridization of breast tumors stratified by histological grade reveals new insights into the biological progression of breast cancer. *Cancer Res* 1999;59:1433–1436.
53. Moinfar F, Man YG, Arnould L, et al. Concurrent and independent genetic alterations in the stromal and epithelial cells of mammary carcinoma: implications for tumorigenesis. *Cancer Res* 2000;60:2562–2566.
54. Kurose K, Hoshaw-Woodard S, Adeyinka A, et al. Genetic model of multi-step breast carcinogenesis involving the epithelium and stroma: clues to tumour-microenvironment interactions. *Hum Mol Genet* 2001;10:1907–1913.
55. Ma XJ, Salunga R, Tuggle JT, et al. Gene expression profiles of human breast cancer progression. *Proc Natl Acad Sci USA* 2003;100:5974–5979.
56. Ross JS, Linette GP, Stec J, et al. Breast cancer biomarkers and molecular medicine. *Expert Rev Mol Diagn* 2003;3:573–585.
57. Ross JS, Linette GP, Stec J, et al. Breast cancer biomarkers and molecular medicine. II. *Expert Rev Mol Diagn* 2004;4:169–188.
58. Hodgson SV, Morrison PJ, Irving M. Breast cancer genetics: unsolved questions and open perspectives in an expanding clinical practice. *Am J Med Genet* 2004;129:56–64.
59. Gebhart E, Bruderlein S, Augustus M, et al. Cytogenetic studies on human breast carcinomas. *Breast Cancer Res Treat* 1986;8:125–138.
60. Adeyinka A, Mertens F, Idvall I, et al. Cytogenetic findings in invasive breast carcinomas with prognostically favourable histology: a less complex karyotypic pattern? *Int J Cancer* 1998;79:361–364.
61. DeVries S, Nyante S, Korkola J, et al. Array-based comparative genomic hybridization from formalin-fixed, paraffin-embedded breast tumors. *J Mol Diagn* 2005;7:65–71.
62. Isola JJ, Kallioniemi OP, Chu LW, et al. Genetic aberrations detected by comparative genomic hybridization predict outcome in node-negative breast cancer. *Am J Pathol* 1995;147:905–911.
63. Frierson HF Jr, Wolber RA, Berean KW, et al. Interobserver reproducibility of the Nottingham modification of the Bloom and Richardson histologic grading scheme for infiltrating ductal carcinoma. *Am J Clin Pathol* 1995;103:195–198.
64. Fisher ER, Redmond C, Fisher B, et al. Pathologic findings from the National Surgical Adjuvant Breast and Bowel Projects (NSABP): prognostic discriminants for 8-year survival for node-negative invasive breast cancer patients. *Cancer* 1990;65:2121–2128.
65. Garne JP, Aspegren K, Linell F, et al. Primary prognostic factors in invasive breast cancer with special reference to ductal carcinoma and histologic malignancy grade. *Cancer* 1994;73:1438–1448.
66. Frierson HF Jr. Ploidy analysis and S-phase fraction determination by flow cytometry of invasive adenocarcinomas of the breast. *Am J Surg Pathol* 1991;15:358–367.
67. Auer G, Eriksson E, Azavedo E, et al. Prognostic significance of nuclear DNA content in mammary adenocarcinomas in humans. *Cancer Res* 1984;44:394–396.
68. Keyhani-Rofagha S, O'Toole RV, Farrar WB, et al. Is DNA ploidy an independent prognostic indicator in infiltrative node-negative breast adenocarcinoma? *Cancer* 1990; 65:1577–1582.
69. Bast RC Jr., Ravdin P, Hayes DF, et al. 2000 update of recommendations for the use of tumor markers in breast and colorectal cancer: clinical practice guidelines of the American Society of Clinical Oncology. *J Clin Oncol* 2001;19:1865–1878.
70. Hammond ME, Fitzgibbons PL, Compton CC, et al. College of American Pathologists Conference XXXV: solid tumor prognostic factors-which, how and so what? Summary document and recommendations for implementation. Cancer Committee and Conference Participants. *Arch Pathol Lab Med* 2000;124:958–965.
71. Sifri R, Gangadharappa S, Acheson LS. Identifying and testing for hereditary susceptibility to common cancers. *CA Cancer J Clin* 2004;54:309–326.
72. Petty EM, Killeen AA. *BRCA1* mutation testing: controversies and challenges. *Clin Chem* 1997;43:6–8.
73. Botkin JR, Smith KR, Croyle RT, et al. Genetic testing for a *BRCA1* mutation: prophylactic surgery and screening behavior in women 2 years post testing. *Am J Med Genet* 2003;118A:201–209.
74. Burke W, Daly M, Garber J, et al. Recommendations for follow-up care of individuals with an inherited predisposition to cancer. II. *BRCA1* and *BRCA2*. Cancer Genetics Studies Consortium. *JAMA* 1997;277:997–1003.
75. Tandon AK, Clark GM, Chamness GC, et al. *HER-2/neu* oncogene protein and prognosis in breast cancer. *J Clin Oncol* 1989;7:1120–1128.
76. Paik S, Hazan R, Fisher ER, et al. Pathologic findings from the National Surgical Adjuvant Breast and Bowel Project: prognostic significance of erbB-2 protein overexpression in primary breast cancer. *J Clin Oncol* 1990;8:103–112.
77. Press MF, Bernstein L, Thomas PA, et al. *HER-2/neu* gene amplification characterized by fluorescence in situ hybridization: poor prognosis in node-negative breast carcinomas. *J Clin Oncol* 1997;15:2894–2904.
78. Sjogren S, Inganas M, Lindgren A, et al. Prognostic and predictive value of *c-erbB-2* overexpression in primary breast cancer, alone and in combination with other prognostic markers. *J Clin Oncol* 1998;16:462–469.
79. Slamon DJ, Clark GM, Wong SG, et al. Human breast cancer: correlation of relapse and survival with amplification of the *HER-2/neu* oncogene. *Science* 1987;235: 177–182.
80. Muss HB, Thor AD, Berry DA, et al. *c-erbB-2* expression and response to adjuvant therapy in women with node-positive early breast cancer. *N Engl J Med* 1994;330: 1260–1266.
81. Paik S, Bryant J, Park C, et al. *erbB-2* and response to doxorubicin in patients with axillary lymph node-positive, hormone receptor-negative breast cancer. *J Natl Cancer Inst* 1998;90:1361–1370.
82. Baselga J, Tripathy D, Mendelsohn J, et al. Phase II study of weekly intravenous trastuzumab (Herceptin) in patients with *HER2/neu*-overexpressing metastatic breast cancer. *Semin Oncol* 1999;26:78–83.
83. Cobleigh MA, Vogel CL, Tripathy D, et al. Multinational study of the efficacy and safety of humanized anti-HER2 monoclonal antibody in women who have *HER2*-overexpressing metastatic breast cancer that has progressed after chemotherapy for metastatic disease. *J Clin Oncol* 1999;17:2639–2648.
84. Vogel CL, Cobleigh MA, Tripathy D, et al. Efficacy and safety of trastuzumab as a single agent in first-line treatment of *HER2*-overexpressing metastatic breast cancer. *J Clin Oncol* 2002;20:719–726.
85. Slamon DJ, Leyland-Jones B, Shak S, et al. Use of chemotherapy plus a monoclonal antibody against *HER2* for metastatic breast cancer that overexpresses *HER2*. *N Engl J Med* 2001;344:783–792.
86. Sparano JA. Cardiac toxicity of trastuzumab (Herceptin): implications for the design of adjuvant trials. *Semin Oncol* 2001;28:20–27.
87. Slamon DJ, Godolphin W, Jones LA, et al. Studies of the *HER-2/neu* proto-oncogene in human breast and ovarian cancer. *Science* 1989;244:707–712.
88. Pauletti G, Godolphin W, Press MF, et al. Detection and quantitation of *HER-2/neu* gene amplification in human breast cancer archival material using fluorescence in situ hybridization. *Oncogene* 1996;13:63–72.
89. Department of Health and Human Services, Food and Drug Administration, Center for Drug Evaluation and Research. Oncology Drugs Advisory Committee, 58th Meeting, September 2, 1998. P.M. session: Biologics license application (BLA) 98–0369: Herceptin (trastuzumab), Genentech, Inc. [meeting minutes]. Available at http://www.fda.gov/cder/biologics/review/trasgen092598r1p1.pdf and http://www.fda.gov/cder/biologics/review/trasgen092598rlp2.pdf; see also http://www.fda.gov/ohrms/dockets/ac/01/briefing/3815b1_08_HER2%20FISH.htm.
90. Hicks DG, Tubbs RR. Assessment of the *HER2* status in breast cancer by fluorescence in situ hybridization: a technical review with interpretive guidelines. *Hum Pathol* 2005;36:250–261.
91. Pauletti G, Dandekar S, Rong HM, et al. Assessment of methods for tissue-based detection of the *HER-2/neu* alteration in human breast cancer: a direct comparison of fluorescence in situ hybridization and immunohistochemistry. *J Clin Oncol* 2000;18:3651–3664.
92. Yaziji H, Goldstein LC, Barry TS, et al. *HER-2* testing in breast cancer using parallel tissue-based methods. *JAMA* 2004;291:1972–1977.
93. Lal P, Salazar PA, Hudis CA, et al. *HER-2* testing in breast cancer using immunohistochemical analysis and fluorescence in situ hybridization: a single-institution experience of 2,279 cases and comparison of dual-color and single-color scoring. *Am J Clin Pathol* 2004;121:631–636.
94. Beatty BG, Bryant R, Wang W, et al. *HER-2/neu* detection in fine-needle aspirates of breast cancer: fluorescence in situ hybridization and immunocytochemical analysis. *Am J Clin Pathol* 2004;122:246–255.
95. Paik S, Bryant J, Tan-Chiu E, et al. Real-world performance of *HER2* testing: National Surgical Adjuvant Breast and Bowel Project experience. *J Natl Cancer Inst* 2002; 94:852–854.
96. Bilous M, Dowsett M, Hanna W, et al. Current perspectives on *HER2* testing: a review of national testing guidelines. *Mod Pathol* 2003;16:173–182.
97. Jacobs TW, Gown AM, Yaziji H, et al. Specificity of HercepTest in determining *HER-2/neu* status of breast cancers using the United States Food and Drug Administration-approved scoring system. *J Clin Oncol* 1999;17:1983–1987.
98. Hammock L, Lewis M, Phillips C, et al. Strong HER-2/neu protein overexpression by immunohistochemistry often does not predict oncogene amplification by fluorescence in situ hybridization. *Hum Pathol* 2003;34:1043–1047.
99. Jimenez RE, Wallis T, Tabasczka P, et al. Determination of *Her-2/Neu* status in breast carcinoma: comparative analysis of immunohistochemistry and fluorescent in situ hybridization. *Mod Pathol* 2000;13:37–45.
100. Lebeau A, Deimling D, Kaltz C, et al. *Her-2/neu* analysis in archival tissue samples of human breast cancer: comparison of immunohistochemistry and fluorescence in situ hybridization. *J Clin Oncol* 2001;19:354–363.
101. Tubbs RR, Pettay JD, Roche PC, et al. Discrepancies in clinical laboratory testing of eligibility for trastuzumab therapy: apparent immunohistochemical false-positives do not get the message. *J Clin Oncol* 2001;19:2714–2721.
102. Perez EA, Roche PC, Jenkins RB, et al. *HER2* testing in patients with breast cancer: poor correlation between weak positivity by immunohistochemistry and gene amplification by fluorescence in situ hybridization. *Mayo Clin Proc* 2002;77:148–154.
103. Ridolfi RL, Jamehdor MR, Arber JM. *HER-2/neu* testing in breast carcinoma: a combined immunohistochemical and fluorescence in situ hybridization approach. *Mod Pathol* 2000;13:866–873.
104. Varshney D, Zhou YY, Geller SA, et al. Determination of *HER-2* status and chromosome 17 polysomy in breast carcinomas comparing HercepTest and PathVysion FISH assay. *Am J Clin Pathol* 2004;121:70–77.
105. Lal P, Salazar PA, Ladanyi M, et al. Impact of polysomy 17 on *HER-2/neu* immunohistochemistry in breast carcinomas without *HER-2/neu* gene amplification. *J Mol Diagn* 2003;5:155–159.
106. Yaziji H, Gown AM. Accuracy and precision in *HER2/neu* testing in breast cancer: are we there yet? *Hum Pathol* 2004;35:143–146.
107. Roche PC, Suman VJ, Jenkins RB, et al. Concordance between local and central laboratory *HER2* testing in the breast intergroup trial N9831. *J Natl Cancer Inst* 2002; 94:855–857.
108. Merkelbach-Bruse S, Wardelmann E, Behrens P, et al. Current diagnostic methods of *HER-2/neu* detection in breast cancer with special regard to real-time PCR. *Am J Surg Pathol* 2003;27:1565–1570.
109. Gjerdrum LM, Sorensen BS, Kjeldsen E, et al. Real-time quantitative PCR of microdissected paraffin-embedded breast carcinoma: an alternative method for *HER-2/neu* analysis. *J Mol Diagn* 2004;6:42–51.
110. Millson A, Suli A, Hartung L, et al. Comparison of two quantitative polymerase chain reaction methods for detecting *HER2/neu* amplification. *J Mol Diagn* 2003;5:184–190.
111. Tanner M, Gancberg D, Di Leo A, et al. Chromogenic in situ hybridization: a practical alternative for fluorescence in situ hybridization to detect *HER-2/neu* oncogene amplification in archival breast cancer samples. *Am J Pathol* 2000;157:1467–1472.
112. Zhao J, Wu R, Au A, et al. Determination of *HER2* gene amplification by chromogenic in situ hybridization (CISH) in archival breast carcinoma. *Mod Pathol* 2002;15: 657–665.
113. Bhargava R, Lal P, Chen B. Chromogenic in situ hybridization for the detection of *HER-2/neu* gene amplification in breast cancer with an emphasis on tumors with borderline and low-level amplification: does it measure up to fluoroscence in situ hybridization? *Am J Clin Pathol* 2005;123:237–243.
114. Stratton MR. Pathology of familial breast cancer: differences between breast cancers in carriers of *BRCA1* or *BRCA2* mutations and sporadic cases. Breast Cancer Linkage Consortium. *Lancet* 1997;349:1505–1510.

115. Marchal C,Weber B, de Lafontan B, et al. Nine breast angiosarcomas after conservative treatment for breast carcinoma: a survey from French comprehensive Cancer Centers. *Int J Radiat Oncol Biol Phys* 1999;44:113–119.
116. Armes JE, Egan AJ, Southey MC, et al. The histologic phenotypes of breast carcinoma occurring before age 40 years in women with and without *BRCA1* or *BRCA2* germline mutations: a population-based study. *Cancer* 1998;83:2335–2345.
117. Eisinger F, Jacquemier J, Charpin C, et al. Mutations at *BRCA1*: the medullary breast carcinoma revisited. *Cancer Res* 1998;58:1588–1592.
118. Berns EM, van Staveren IL, Look MP, et al. Mutations in residues of *TP53* that directly contact DNA predict poor outcome in human primary breast cancer. *Br J Cancer* 1998;77:1130–1136.
119. Borresen AL, Andersen TI, Eyfjord JE, et al. *TP53* mutations and breast cancer prognosis: particularly poor survival rates for cases with mutations in the zinc-binding domains. *Genes Chromosomes Cancer* 1995;14:71–75.
120. Kucera E, Speiser P, Gnant M, et al. Prognostic significance of mutations in the *p53* gene, particularly in the zinc-binding domains, in lymph node- and steroid receptor positive breast cancer patients. Austrian Breast Cancer Study Group. *Eur J Cancer* 1999; 35:398–405.
121. Geisler S, Lonning PE, Aas T, et al. Influence of *TP53* gene alterations and c-*erbB-2* expression on the response to treatment with doxorubicin in locally advanced breast cancer. *Cancer Res* 2001;61:2505–2512.
122. Aas T, Borresen AL, Geisler S, et al. Specific *P53* mutations are associated with de novo resistance to doxorubicin in breast cancer patients. *Nat Med* 1996;2:811–814.
123. Bergh J, Norberg T, Sjogren S, et al. Complete sequencing of the *p53* gene provides prognostic information in breast cancer patients, particularly in relation to adjuvant systemic therapy and radiotherapy. *Nat Med* 1995;1:1029–1034.
124. Berns EM, Foekens JA, Vossen R, et al. Complete sequencing of *TP53* predicts poor response to systemic therapy of advanced breast cancer. *Cancer Res* 2000;60:2155–2162.
125. Coradini D, Daidone MG. Biomolecular prognostic factors in breast cancer. *Curr Opin Obstet Gynecol* 2004;16:49–55.
126. Fiets WE, Nortier JW. A multigene RT-PCR assay used to predict recurrence in early breast cancer: two presentations with contradictory results. *Breast Cancer Res* 2004; 6:185–187.
127. Caldas C, Aparicio SA. The molecular outlook. *Nature* 2002;415:484–485.
128. van't Veer LJ, Dai H, van de Vijver MJ, et al. Gene expression profiling predicts clinical outcome of breast cancer. *Nature* 2002;415:530–536.
129. van de Vijver MJ, He YD, van't Veer LJ, et al. A gene-expression signature as a predictor of survival in breast cancer. *N Engl J Med* 2002;347:1999–2009.
130. Huang E, Cheng SH, Dressman H, et al. Gene expression predictors of breast cancer outcomes. *Lancet* 2003;361:1590–1596.
131. Aubele M, Mattis A, Zitzelsberger H, et al. Extensive ductal carcinoma in situ with small foci of invasive ductal carcinoma: evidence of genetic resemblance by CGH. *Int J Cancer* 2000;85:82–86.
132. Master SR, Mies C. Gene-expression profiles and breast-cancer prognosis. *Adv Anat Pathol* 2003;10:338–346.
133. Hampton T. Breast cancer gene chip study under way: can new technology help predict treatment success? *JAMA* 2004;291:2927–2930.
134. Ellis MJ. Breast cancer gene expression analysis: the case for dynamic profiling. *Adv Exp Med Biol* 2003;532:223–234.
135. Dressman MA, Walz TM, Barnes L, et al. Genes that co-cluster with estrogen receptor alpha in microarray analysis of breast biopsies. *Pharmacogenomics J* 2001;1:135–141.
136. Glinsky GV, Higashiyama T, Glinskii AB, et al. Classification of human breast cancer using gene expression profiling as a component of the survival predictor algorithm. *Clin Cancer Res* 2004;10:2272–2283.
137. Hayashi SI. Prediction of hormone sensitivity by DNA microarray. *Biomed Pharmacother* 2004;58:1–9.
138. Ayers M, Symmans WF, Stec J, et al. Gene expression profiling of fine needle aspirations of breast cancer identifies genes associated with complete pathologic response to Neoadjuvant taxol/FAC chemotherapy. *J Clin Oncol* 2004;22:2284–2293.
139. Chang JC, Wooten EC, Tsimelzon A, et al. Gene expression profiling for the prediction of therapeutic response to docetaxel in patients with breast cancer. *Lancet* 2003;362:362–369.
140. Herbst RS, Khuri FR. Mode of action of docetaxel: a basis for combination with novel anticancer agents. *Cancer Treat Rev* 2003;29:407–415.
141. Glanzer JG, Eberwine JH. Expression profiling of small cellular samples in cancer: less is more. *Br J Cancer* 2004;90:1111–1114.
142. Sotiriou C, Powles TJ, Dowsett M, et al. Gene expression profiles derived from fine needle aspiration correlate with response to systemic chemotherapy in breast cancer. *Breast Cancer Res* 2002;4:R3.
143. Bibikova M, Talantov D, Chudin E, et al. Quantitative gene expression profiling in formalin-fixed, paraffin-embedded tissues using universal bead arrays. *Am J Pathol* 2004;165:1799–1807.
144. Paik S, Shak S, Tang G, et al. A multigene assay to predict recurrence of tamoxifen-treated, node-negative breast cancer. *N Engl J Med* 2004;351:2817–2826.
145. Vos CB, Cleton-Jansen AM, Berx G, et al. E-cadherin inactivation in lobular carcinoma in situ of the breast: an early event in tumorigenesis. *Br J Cancer* 1997;76: 1131–1133.
146. Amari M, Moriya T, Ishida T, et al. Loss of heterozygosity analyses of asynchronous lesions of ductal carcinoma in situ and invasive ductal carcinoma of the human breast. *Jpn J Clin Oncol* 2003;33:556–562.
147. Nyante SJ, Devries S, Chen YY, et al. Array-based comparative genomic hybridization of ductal carcinoma in situ and synchronous invasive lobular cancer. *Hum Pathol* 2004;35:759–763.
148. Allred DC, Mohsin SK, Fuqua SA. Histological and biological evolution of human premalignant breast disease. *Endocr Relat Cancer* 2001;8:47–61.
149. Acs G, Lawton TJ, Rebbeck TR, et al. Differential expression of E-cadherin in lobular and ductal neoplasms of the breast and its biologic and diagnostic implications. *Am J Clin Pathol* 2001;115:85–98.
150. Lakhani SR, Collins N, Sloane JP, et al. Loss of heterozygosity in ductal carcinoma in situ of the breast. *J Pathol* 1995;175:195–201.
151. Nayar R, Zhuang Z, Merino MJ, et al. Loss of heterozygosity on chromosome 11q13 in lobular lesions of the breast using tissue microdissection and polymerase chain reaction. *Hum Pathol* 1997;28:277–282.
152. Fujii H, Szumel R, Marsh C, et al. Genetic progression, histological grade, and allelic loss in ductal carcinoma in situ of the breast. *Cancer Res* 1996;56:5260–5265.
153. Munn KE, Walker RA, Varley JM. Frequent alterations of chromosome 1 in ductal carcinoma in situ of the breast. *Oncogene* 1995;10:1653–1657.
154. Maitra A, Wistuba II, Washington C, et al. High-resolution chromosome 3p allelotyping of breast carcinomas and precursor lesions demonstrates frequent loss of heterozygosity and a discontinuous pattern of allele loss. *Am J Pathol* 2001;159:119–130.
155. O'Connell P, Pekkel V, Fuqua SA, et al. Analysis of loss of heterozygosity in 399 premalignant breast lesions at 15 genetic loci. *J Natl Cancer Inst* 1998;90:697–703.
156. Lakhani SR, Chaggar R, Davies S, et al. Genetic alterations in 'normal' luminal and myoepithelial cells of the breast. *J Pathol* 1999;189:496–503.
157. Larson PS, de las Morenas A, Cupples LA, et al. Genetically abnormal clones in histologically normal breast tissue. *Am J Pathol* 1998;152:1591–1598.
158. Deng G, Lu Y, Zlotnikov G, et al. Loss of heterozygosity in normal tissue adjacent to breast carcinomas. *Science* 1996;274:2057–2059.
159. Luzzi V, Holtschlag V, Watson MA. Expression profiling of ductal carcinoma in situ by laser capture microdissection and high-density oligonucleotide arrays. *Am J Pathol* 2001;158:2005–2010.
160. Page DL, Anderson TJ. Uncommon types of invasive carcinoma. In: *Diagnostic Histopathology of the Breast*. Edinburgh: Churchill Livingstone; 1987;236–239.
161. Oberman HA. Secretory carcinoma of the breast in adults. *Am J Surg Pathol* 1980;4:465–470.
162. Tognon C, Knezevich SR, Huntsman, et al. Expression of the *ETV6-NTRK3* gene fusion as a primary event in human secretory breast carcinoma. *Cancer Cell* 2002;2:367–376.
163. Makretsov N, He M, Hayes M, et al. Fluorescence in situ hybridization study of *ETV6-NTRK3* fusion gene in secretory breast carcinoma. *Genes Chromosomes Cancer* 2004; 40:152–157.
164. Lannon CL, Martin MJ, Tognon CE, et al. A highly conserved *NTRK3* C-terminal sequence in the ETV6-NTRK3 oncoprotein binds the phosphotyrosine binding domain of insulin receptor substrate-1: an essential interaction for transformation. *J Biol Chem* 2004;279:6225–6234.
165. Ladanyi M. Aberrant ALK tyrosine kinase signaling: different cellular lineages, common oncogenic mechanisms. *Am J Pathol* 2000;157:341–345.
166. Grabellus F, Worm K, Willruth A, et al. *ETV6-NTRK3* gene fusion in a secretory carcinoma of the breast of a male-to-female transsexual. *Breast* 2005;14:71–74.
167. Ichaso N, Rodriguez RE, Martin-Zanca D, et al. Genomic characterization of the human *trkC* gene. *Oncogene* 1998;17:1871–1875.
168. Barbacid M. The Trk family of neurotrophin receptors. *J Neurobiol* 1994;25:1386–1403.
169. Rubin BP, Chen CJ, Morgan TW, et al. Congenital mesoblastic nephroma t(12;15) is associated with *ETV6-NTRK3* gene fusion: cytogenetic and molecular relationship to congenital (infantile) fibrosarcoma. *Am J Pathol* 1998;153:1451–1458.
170. Knezevich SR, McFadden DE, Tao W, et al. A novel *ETV6-NTRK3* gene fusion in congenital fibrosarcoma. *Nat Genet* 1998;18:184–187.
171. Adem C, Gisselsson D, Dal Cin PD, et al. *ETV6* rearrangements in patients with infantile fibrosarcomas and congenital mesoblastic nephromas by fluorescence in situ hybridization. *Mod Pathol* 2001;14:1246–1251.
172. Diallo R, Schaefer KL, Bankfalvi A, et al. Secretory carcinoma of the breast: a distinct variant of invasive ductal carcinoma assessed by comparative genomic hybridization and immunohistochemistry. *Hum Pathol* 2003;34:1299–1305.
173. Knezevich SR, Garnett MJ, Pysher TJ, et al. *ETV6-NTRK3* gene fusions and trisomy 11 establish a histogenetic link between mesoblastic nephroma and congenital fibrosarcoma. *Cancer Res* 1998;58:5046–5048.
174. Argani P, Fritsch M, Kadkol S, et al. Detection of the *ETV6-NTRK3* chimeric RNA of infantile fibrosarcoma/cellular congenital mesoblastic nephroma in paraffin-embedded tissue: application to challenging pediatric renal stromal tumors. *Mod Pathol* 2000; 13:29–36.
175. Eguchi M, Eguchi-Ishimae M, Tojo A, et al. Fusion of *ETV6* to neurotrophin-3 receptor TRKC in acute myeloid leukemia with t(12;15)(p13;q25). *Blood* 1999;93:1355–1563.
176. Eguchi M, Eguchi-Ishimai M. Absence of t(12;15) associated *ETV6-NTRK3* fusion transcripts in pediatric acute leukemias [Letter]. *Med Pediatr Oncol* 2001;37:417.
177. Staats B, Bonk U, Wanschura S, et al. A fibroadenoma with a t(4;12) (q27;q15) affecting the *HMGI-C* gene, a member of the high mobility group protein gene family. *Breast Cancer Res Treat* 1996;38:299–303.
178. Schoenmakers EF, Wanschura S, Mols R, et al. Recurrent rearrangements in the high mobility group protein gene, *HMGI-C*, in benign mesenchymal tumours. *Nat Genet* 1995;10:436–444.
179. Calabrese G, Di Virgilio C, Cianchetti E, et al. Chromosome abnormalities in breast fibroadenomas. *Genes Chromosomes Cancer* 1991;3:202–204.
180. Birdsall SH, MacLennan KA, Gusterson BA. t(6;12)(q23;q13) and t(10;16)(q22;p11) in a phyllodes tumor of breast. *Cancer Genet Cytogenet* 1992;60:74–77.
181. Sezer O, Jugovic D, Blohmer JU, et al. CD99 positivity and *EWS-FLI1* gene rearrangement identify a breast tumor in a 60-year-old patient with attributes of the Ewing family of neoplasms. *Diagn Mol Pathol* 1999;8:120–124.
182. Hays DM, Donaldson SS, Shimada H, et al. Primary and metastatic rhabdomyosarcoma in the breast: neoplasms of adolescent females: a report from the Intergroup Rhabdomyosarcoma Study. *Med Pediatr Oncol* 1997;29:181–189.
183. Binokay F, Soyupak SK, Inal M, et al. Primary and metastatic rhabdomyosarcoma in the breast: report of two pediatric cases. *Eur J Radiol* 2003;48:282–284.
184. Luna Vega AR, Vetto JT, Kinne DW. Primary sarcomas of the breast in women under 20 years of age. *N Y State J Med* 1992;92:497–498.
185. Karcnik TJ, Miller JA, Fromowitz F, et al. Dermatofibrosarcoma protuberans of the breast: a rare malignant tumor simulating benign disease. *Breast J* 1999;5:262–263.
186. Zardawi IM, Clark D, Williamsz G. Inflammatory myofibroblastic tumor of the breast: a case report. *Acta Cytol* 2003;47:1077–1081.
187. Cserni G, Amendoeira I, Apostolikas N, et al. Pathological work-up of sentinel lymph nodes in breast cancer: review of current data to be considered for the formulation of guidelines. *Eur J Cancer* 2003;39:1654–1667.

188. Pfeifer JD. Sentinel lymph node biopsy. *Am J Clin Pathol* 1999;112:599–602.
189. Jakub JW, Cox CE, Pippas AW, et al. Controversial topics in breast lymphatic mapping. *Semin Oncol* 2004;31:324–332.
190. Fielding LP. Prognostic factor development: an important caution from a small study. *Cancer* 1997;80:1363–1365.
191. Quan ML, Cody HS 3rd. Missed micrometastatic disease in breast cancer. *Semin Oncol* 2004;31:311–317.
192. Sakaguchi M, Virmani A, Dudak MW, et al. Clinical relevance of reverse transcriptase-polymerase chain reaction for the detection of axillary lymph node metastasis in breast cancer. *Ann Surg Oncol* 2003;10:117–125.
193. Bostick PJ, Chatterjee S, Chi DD, et al. Limitations of specific reverse-transcriptase polymerase chain reaction markers in the detection of metastases in the lymph nodes and blood of breast cancer patients. *J Clin Oncol* 1998;16:2632–2640.
194. Traweek ST, Liu J, Battifora H. Keratin gene expression in non-epithelial tissues: detection with polymerase chain reaction. *Am J Pathol* 1993;142:1111–1118.
195. Burchill SA, Bradbury MF, Pittman K, et al. Detection of epithelial cancer cells in peripheral blood by reverse transcriptase-polymerase chain reaction. *Br J Cancer* 1995;71:278–281.
196. Bader BL, Magin TM, Hatzfeld M, et al. Amino acid sequence and gene organization of cytokeratin no. 19, an exceptional tail-less intermediate filament protein. *EMBO J* 1986;5:1865–1875.
197. Youngson BJ, Cranor M, Rosen PP. Epithelial displacement in surgical breast specimens following needling procedures. *Am J Surg Pathol* 1994;18:896–903.
198. Diaz NM, Cox CE, Ebert M, et al. Benign mechanical transport of breast epithelial cells to sentinel lymph nodes. *Am J Surg Pathol* 2004;28:1641–1645.
199. Ouellette RJ, Richard D, Maicas E. RT-PCR for mammaglobin genes, *MGB1* and *MGB2*, identifies breast cancer micrometastases in sentinel lymph nodes. *Am J Clin Pathol* 2004;121:637–643.
200. Schroder CP, Ruiters MH, de Jong S, et al. Detection of micrometastatic breast cancer by means of real time quantitative RT-PCR and immunostaining in perioperative blood samples and sentinel nodes. *Int J Cancer* 2003;106:611–618.
201. Inokuchi M, Ninomiya I, Tsugawa K, et al. Quantitative evaluation of metastases in axillary lymph nodes of breast cancer. *Br J Cancer* 2003;89:1750–1756.
202. Yamamoto N, Kato Y, Yanagisawa A, et al. Predictive value of genetic diagnosis for cancer micrometastasis: histologic and experimental appraisal. *Cancer* 1997;80: 1393–1398.
203. Jung YS, Lee KJ, Kim HJ, et al. Clinical significance of bone marrow micrometastasis detected by nested RT-PCR for keratin-19 in breast cancer patients. *Jpn J Clin Oncol* 2003;33:167–172.
204. Nogi H, Takeyama H, Uchida K, et al. Detection of *MUC1* and keratin 19 mRNAs in the bone marrow by quantitative RT-PCR predicts the risk of distant metastasis in breast cancer patients. *Breast Cancer* 2003;10:74–81.
205. Landys K, Persson S, Kovarik J, et al. Prognostic value of bone marrow biopsy in operable breast cancer patients at the time of initial diagnosis: results of a 20-year median follow-up. *Breast Cancer Res Treat* 1998;49:27–33.
206. Diel IJ, Kaufmann M, Costa SD, et al. Micrometastatic breast cancer cells in bone marrow at primary surgery: prognostic value in comparison with nodal status. *J Natl Cancer Inst* 1996;88:1652–1658.
207. Bossolasco P, Ricci C, Farina G, et al. Detection of micrometastatic cells in breast cancer by RT-PCR for the mammaglobin gene. *Cancer Detect Prev* 2002;26:60–63.
208. Cooper BW, Moss TJ, Ross AA, et al. Occult tumor contamination of hematopoietic stem-cell products does not affect clinical outcome of autologous transplantation in patients with metastatic breast cancer. *J Clin Oncol* 1998;16:3509–3517.
209. Vannucchi AM, Bosi A, Glinz S, et al. Evaluation of breast tumour cell contamination in the bone marrow and leukapheresis collections by RT-PCR for cytokeratin-19 mRNA. *Br J Haematol* 1998;103:610–617.
210. Brockstein BE, Ross AA, Moss TJ, et al. Tumor cell contamination of bone marrow harvest products: clinical consequences in a cohort of advanced-stage breast cancer patients undergoing high-dose chemotherapy. *J Hematother* 1996;5:617–624.
211. Pedrazzoli P, Battaglia M, Da Prada GA, et al. Role of tumor cells contaminating the graft in breast cancer recurrence after high-dose chemotherapy. *Bone Marrow Transplant* 1997;20:167–169.
212. Schulze R, Schulze M, Wischnik A, et al. Tumor cell contamination of peripheral blood stem cell transplants and bone marrow in high-risk breast cancer patients. *Bone Marrow Transplant* 1997;19:1223–1228.
213. Cristofanilli M, Budd GT, Ellis MJ, et al. Circulating tumor cells, disease progression, and survival in metastatic breast cancer. *N Engl J Med* 2004;351:781–791.
214. Dent GA, Civalier CJ, Brecher ME, et al. *MUC1* expression in hematopoietic tissues. *Am J Clin Pathol* 1999;111:741–747.
215. Wulf GG, Jurgens B, Liersch T, et al. Reverse transcriptase/polymerase chain reaction analysis of parathyroid hormone-related protein for the detection of tumor cell dissemination in the peripheral blood and bone marrow of patients with breast cancer. *J Cancer Res Clin Oncol* 1997;123:514–521.
216. de Graaf H, Maelandsmo GM, Ruud P, et al. Ectopic expression of target genes may represent an inherent limitation of RT-PCR assays used for micrometastasis detection: studies on the epithelial glycoprotein gene *EGP-2*. *Int J Cancer* 1997;72:191–196.
217. Leone F, Perissinotto E, Viale A, et al. Detection of breast cancer cell contamination in leukapheresis product by real-time quantitative polymerase chain reaction. *Bone Marrow Transplant* 2001;27:517–523.
218. Berois N, Varangot M, Sonora C, et al. Detection of bone marrow-disseminated breast cancer cells using an RT-PCR assay of *MUC5B* mRNA. *Int J Cancer* 2003;103:550–555.
219. Zippelius A, Kufer P, Honold G, et al. Limitations of reverse-transcriptase polymerase chain reaction analyses for detection of micrometastatic epithelial cancer cells in bone marrow. *J Clin Oncol* 1997;15:2701–2708.
220. Trummer A, Kadar J, Arseniev L, et al. Competitive cytokeratin 19 RT-PCR for quantification of breast cancer cells in blood cell suspensions. *J Hematother Stem Cell Res* 2000;9:275–284.
221. Becker S, Becker-Pergola G, Fehm T, et al. Time is an important factor when processing samples for the detection of disseminated tumor cells in blood/bone marrow by reverse transcription-PCR. *Clin Chem* 2004;50:785–786.
222. Traystman MD, Cochran GT, Hake SJ, et al. Comparison of molecular cytokeratin 19 reverse transcriptase polymerase chain reaction (CK19 RT-PCR) and immunocytochemical detection of micrometastatic breast cancer cells in hematopoietic harvests. *J Hematother* 1997;6:551–561.
223. Diaz NM, Mayes JR, Vrcel V, et al. Breast epithelial cells in dermal angiolymphatic spaces: a manifestation of benign mechanical transport. *Hum Pathol* 2005;36:310–313.
224. Schlechter BL, Yang Q, Larson PS, et al. Quantitative DNA fingerprinting may distinguish new primary breast cancer from disease recurrence. *J Clin Oncol* 2004;22: 1830–1838.
225. Regitnig P, Moser R, Thalhammer M, et al. Microsatellite analysis of breast carcinoma and corresponding local recurrences. *J Pathol* 2002;198:190–197.
226. Goldstein NS, Kestin L, Vicini F, et al. Factors associated with ipsilateral breast failure and distant metastases in patients with invasive breast carcinoma treated with breast-conserving therapy: a clinicopathologic study of 607 neoplasms from 583 patients. *Am J Clin Pathol* 2003;120:500–527.
227. Goldstein NS, Vicini FA, Hunter S, et al. Molecular assay clonality determination of ipsilateral recurrence of invasive breast carcinomas after breast-conserving therapy: comparison with clinical and biologic factors. *Am J Clin Pathol*. 2005;123:679–689.
228. Kung FY, Tse GM, Lo KW, et al. Metachronous bilateral mammary metaplastic and infiltrating duct carcinomas: a molecular study for clonality. *Hum Pathol* 2002;33: 677–679.
229. Tse GM, Kung FY, Chan AB, et al. Clonal analysis of bilateral mammary carcinomas by clinical evaluation and partial allelotyping. *Am J Clin Pathol* 2003;120:168–174.
230. Regitnig P, Ploner F, Maderbacher M, et al. Bilateral carcinomas of the breast with local recurrence: analysis of genetic relationship of the tumors. *Mod Pathol* 2004;17:597–602.
231. Lininger RA, Fujii H, Man YG, et al. Comparison of loss heterozygosity in primary and recurrent ductal carcinoma in situ of the breast. *Mod Pathol* 1998;11:1151–1159.
232. Johnson JE, Page DL, Winfield AC, et al. Recurrent mammary carcinoma after local excision: a segmental problem. *Cancer* 1995;75:1612–1618.
233. Ohtake T, Abe R, Kimijima I, et al. Intraductal extension of primary invasive breast carcinoma treated by breast-conservative surgery: computer graphic three-dimensional reconstruction of the mammary duct-lobular systems. *Cancer* 1995;76:32–45.

Head and Neck

SQUAMOUS CELL CARCINOMA

Established risk factors for squamous cell carcinoma (SCC) include cigarette smoking, use of smokeless tobacco, excess alcohol consumption, and, especially in Asia, the habit of chewing betel quid. A diet high in fruits and fresh vegetables, as well as high in antioxidants, appears to be protective.

Genetics

A multistep model of tumorigenesis of head and neck SCC has been proposed (Fig. 21.1) in which the progression from dysplasia to invasive carcinoma to metastasis is due to the accumulation of genetic mutations (1–3). There are two key features of the model, first, that tumor initiation and progression are associated with overlapping genetic events, and second, that it is not necessarily the order of genetic events but rather the accumulation of mutations that leads to progression. Although the range of genetic alterations in SCC (reviewed in references 4–9) includes mutations in tumor suppressor genes (such as TP53, RB1, and p16), mutations in oncogenes (such as CCND1 and EGFR), loss of heterozygosity (LOH) at multiple loci (including 3p, 4p, 5q, 8p, 10p, 18q, and 21q), and recurring gross chromosomal changes (including deletions of 1p, 4, 5q, 6q, 9p, 11, 13q, 18q, 21q, and gains of 3q, 8q, 11q, 16p, 17q, 19, 20q, 22q), no single alteration is present in every invasive SCC (Table 21.1).

Molecular Genetic Testing in Diagnosis and Prognosis of SCC

Even though the overall pattern of genetic changes correlates with progression from premalignant to malignant disease, alterations at individual loci are present in premalignant lesions as well as invasive carcinoma, and no single alteration appears to be present in all invasive SCC. Molecular analysis limited to a single locus has neither the sensitivity nor specificity to be of clinical utility (5,10).

The data concerning TP53 illustrate this point. Even though the prevalence of TP53 mutations varies by anatomic site within the head and neck, and even though there is a distinct mutational spectrum at specific sites, the same pattern of mutations can be seen in precursor lesions as well as invasive carcinoma (5,10,11). Conversely, TP53 aberrations can be detected in only about 50% to 80% of cases of SCC by polymerase chain reaction (PCR) or LOH testing (5,11,12). The presence or type of mutation does not strongly correlate with outcome for patients with invasive SCC, and thus there is also little role for evaluation of TP53 status from a prognostic standpoint (5,10,11). Finally, detection of TP53 mutations often does not even show a high correlation with the presence of abnormal p53 expression measured by immunohistochemistry (reviewed in reference 5).

Since individual markers usually fail to provide definitive diagnostic or prognostic information, many studies have evaluated whether analysis of the pattern of genetic alterations at groups of loci is more useful. LOH analysis performed using a panel of microsatellites has shown that distinctive profiles of allelic loss correlate with less aggressive (verrucous, papillary, and conventional well-differentiated) versus more aggressive (basaloid, sarcomatoid, and conventional high-grade) SCC categories, tumor stage, nodal status, and clinical outcome (6,8). Prognostic implications in the pattern of mitochondrial DNA mutations have also been evaluated (13). However, because different studies have employed different marker loci and different tumor groupings, it is difficult to directly compare the results of individual series or interpret the significance of contradictory results.

Gene expression profiling has been used to investigate whether changes in patterns of gene expression provide more relevant information than mutational analysis (14). Although microarray analysis of head and neck SCC

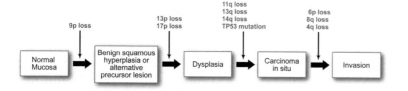

Figure 21.1 Model of the genetic progression that leads to squamous cell carcinoma (SCC) of the head and neck (compiled from references 1 and 2). The sequence of alterations is not as well defined as for colorectal adenocarcinoma (Figure 15.1); nonetheless, the data indicate that overlapping genetic events occur during initiation and progression and that it is not the order of genetic events but rather the accumulation of mutations that leads to progression. That fact that many of the regions of recurring chromosomal loss harbor proto-oncogenes (*CCND1*, which encodes cyclin D1 is at 11q) or tumor suppressor genes (*p16/CDKN2* is at 9p, *RB1* is at 13q) suggests that these specific genes are the sites of mutation, but the data regarding many individual loci are not yet conclusive.

TABLE 21.1

RECURRING GENETIC ABERRATIONS IN SQUAMOUS CELL CARCINOMA OF THE HEAD AND NECK

Gene or Chromosomal Region	Type of Alteration	Approximate Frequency (%)
ras family	Mutation	5–35
p21	Overexpression	30–90
p16/CDKN2	Mutation	50–66
	Hypermethylation	20
EGFR	Overexpression	40–90
Her2/neu	Overexpression	40
TP53	Mutation	50–80
CCND1	Amplification	30–50
EMS1	Amplification (coamplified with *CCND1*)	30–50
RB1	Loss of heterozygosity	15–60
	Loss of expression	10–75
3p, 4p, 5q, 8p, 10p, 18q, and 21q	Loss of heterozygosity	20–50

Compiled from references 4 to 9.

is still largely experimental, several reports suggest that gene expression profiling may have clinical utility for assigning patients into prognostic or high-risk groups that may benefit from more aggressive treatment (15). Studies that have focused on SCC arising in the hypopharynx have shown that the pattern of expression of a cluster of less than 120 genes correlates with the likelihood of metastasis at the time of surgery (16,17) and within 3 years after surgery (15). Similarly, transcriptional patterns that stratify patients into subgroups that have clinically different outcomes in terms of disease-specific and overall survival (18) or recurrence-free survival (18,19) have also been identified, even when patients are not grouped together on the basis of the anatomic site of the primary tumor.

Microarray analysis has also been used to identify changes in gene expression that are characteristic of head and neck SCC cell lines that are cisplatin-resistant (20), although it has not been shown that the same changes correlate with the development of cisplatin resistance in vivo or that patterns of gene expression in the primary tumor can be used to predict which patients are likely to become

resistant to cisplatin chemotherapy. Nonetheless, the basic science observations suggest that microarray analysis holds great potential for identifying patients likely to benefit from alternative chemotherapeutic regimens.

Evaluation of Surgical Margins

Given that complete surgical excision of the primary tumor is the most important prognostic factor for SCC of the head and neck, molecular genetic analysis of the margins of excision has been used in attempts to increase the accuracy of traditional histopathologic evaluation. In one study, molecular testing directed at detecting *TP53* mutations known to be present in the primary tumor identified at least one positive margin in 52% of patients with tumors deemed to be completely excised based on conventional histopathologic evaluation (21). Furthermore, the presence of positive margins by PCR-based analysis showed a statistically significant correlation with patient outcome; in 38% of patients with positive margins by molecular testing SCC recurred locally within the median follow-up time of 17 months, whereas none of the patients with negative margins experienced recurrence (21). Similarly, a quantitative methylation-specific PCR method (MS-PCR) has been used to detect promoter hypermethylation of *p16* and the O6-methylguanine-DNA-methyltransferase (*MGMT*) gene in 50% of patients undergoing excision of head and neck SCC whose tumors were not present at the excision margin based on frozen section evaluation (22). A significant advantage of the quantitative MS-PCR method is that the analysis can be performed in less than 5 hours, a time frame short enough that the assay results are available intraoperatively.

Despite these promising reports, the utility of molecular analysis of surgical margins remains unclear for several reasons. First, presence of the target genetic alteration may not be specific for invasive carcinoma, but may instead be a change that is also present in premalignant surface epithelial cells (23–25). Second, the prevalence of mutations at specific loci in invasive SCC is rather low. In the studies noted above, only 43% of the study cases harbored *TP53* mutations and only 46% showed hypermethylation of the *p16* and *MGMT* promoters (21,22). The fact that genetic aberrations at the target loci are present in less than half of patients significantly limits the utility of the approach in routine practice. Third, whether or not histopathologic evaluation of additional hematoxylin and eosin (H&E)-stained sections of the margin or immunohistochemical stains for epithelial markers would provide the same or even more precise clinical information has not been evaluated (26,27). However, a hint of the information that could be provided by simple histopathologic evaluation of additional levels is provided by the observation that almost one quarter of patients found to have positive excision margins by molecular analysis were found to have positive margins on review of additional frozen sections or deeper levels of the routinely processed tissue (21).

Evaluation of Lymph Nodes

Molecular genetic analysis has also been used to detect micrometastatic disease in lymph nodes from patients undergoing excision for head and neck SCC. In one study, PCR-based analysis designed to detect *TP53* mutations known to be present in the patient's primary tumor identified occult metastases in 21% of lymph nodes that were negative by routine histopathologic evaluation, but the molecular findings did not result in an altered overall clinical disease stage (overall TNM stage) in any of the patients with primary disease (21). This result suggests that the clinical utility of the extra molecular analysis may be limited (26).

In the context of molecular evaluation of sentinel lymph nodes (SN), a rapid quantitative reverse transcriptase PCR (RT-PCR) approach has been described that can be completed in just 2 hours. Applied to mRNA encoding SCC antigen (also known as leupin, a serine proteinase inhibitor), the assay has such a short turnaround time that it has been used to document metastatic disease intraoperatively, which makes it possible to incorporate the results into the decision as to whether or not the primary surgical excision should include a neck dissection (28,29). The high specificity of the approach is demonstrated by the finding that for all patients who had SN metastases detected via the intraoperative quantitative RT-PCR, at least one positive SN was identified by subsequent histopathologic examination.

However, the role of molecular genetic analysis of lymph nodes in the evaluation of patients with head and neck SSC remains unsettled for several reasons. First, as described in more detail in Chapters 15 and 20 regarding molecular testing of SN from colorectal and breast cancer patients, respectively, many markers are not 100% specific for the presence of malignant cells (30–33). Explanations for false positive results include the fact that the marker gene may be expressed at low levels by normal components of lymph nodes such as endothelial cells or fibroblasts or that the mRNA may arise as a result of illegitimate transcription. Molecular analysis designed to demonstrate metastatic disease by detecting a mutation known to be present in the patient's primary tumor obviously provides a much higher degree of specificity (21). Second, the extremely high technical sensitivity of PCR makes it possible to amplify target loci from nucleic acids within cellular debris that has drained to lymph nodes even in the absence of viable tumor cells (34). Although quantitative RT-PCR can be used to establish a minimal level of gene expression to increase the specificity of a positive result, it can still be difficult to distinguish among a very low level of gene expression resulting from physiologic transcription by a very small number of tumor cells, illegitimate transcription by nonmalignant cells, or amplification of mRNA from cell debris (35). Third, because the lymph node sample is destroyed during nucleic acid extraction, the PCR result cannot be correlated with the microscopic findings in the tissue itself. Given that ectopic salivary gland tissue is present in many lymph nodes of the head and neck, and that the ectopic glands would produce a positive PCR result for the epithelial markers that have been studied (28), the inability to confirm the results of molecular analysis by histopathologic evaluation is not a moot point. Fourth, it has not been established that molecular analysis provides information that would not be evident from a more thorough evaluation of the lymph nodes by examination of additional routine sections or sections immunostained for epithelial markers.

Analysis of Serum

Molecular genetic methods have also been use to detect metastatic disease in peripheral blood and serum of patients with SCC, although the way in which the test results should be incorporated into standardized staging schemes remains unclear. For example, microsatellite instability (MSI) or LOH analysis based on PCR amplification of a panel of 10 microsatellite loci has shown that detection of the same profile of alterations in a patient's serum as in the primary tumor identifies those individuals most likely to develop metastases, with the highest statistical significance among patients with recurrent disease (36). However, because the prevalence of MSI or LOH is only 45% in SCC of the head and neck, the predictive value of a negative test result is rather limited. Nonetheless, studies of this type suggest that molecular analysis of peripheral blood may eventually be used to identify patient subgroups at high risk for distant metastases that may benefit from more intensive or alternative therapy (36).

Role of Molecular Genetic Testing in Screening

A wide variety of molecular approaches have been used to evaluate whether or not molecular markers can be used to detect malignant cells in saliva. The approaches include analysis of microsatellite alterations (including either MSI or LOH) (37), mutational analysis of genes encoded by mitochondrial DNA (38), and analysis of abnormal promoter methylation (39).

However, the utility of molecular analysis in this setting is limited by the same technical issues that affect molecular analysis in the evaluation of surgical margins. Because only a subset of invasive SCC harbors aberrations at the marker loci, the sensitivity of analysis ranges from only 31% for analysis of mitochondrial DNA mutations (38) to 79% for the evaluation of MSI or LOH (37). Similarly, the prevalence of the genetic alterations in premalignant epithelial cells is unknown, and thus the specificity of the target aberrations is unknown. Finally, from a purely practical perspective, the advantage of molecular analysis versus a thorough clinical examination (which is not an invasive procedure) has yet to be demonstrated.

Testing for Human Papilloma Virus

Among SCC of the head and neck, the prevalence of human papilloma virus (HPV) infection is highest in tumors arising in the tonsils. About half of tonsillar SCC harbor the virus, and 90% to 100% of the infections are due to the high-risk type 16 (40,41). Patients with HPV-associated tonsillar cancer have a lower risk of relapse within 3 years after diagnosis, a better overall survival, and a better disease-specific survival, prognostic features that are independent of TNM stage, nodal status, age, and gender (40,41). However, despite these prognostic differences, it is not yet established whether or not the results of HPV testing can be used to stratify patients into treatment groups that influence clinical outcome.

The association of HPV infection with SCC at other sites in the oral cavity and oropharynx is less certain. Some reports suggest that HPV infection is associated with a survival benefit for oropharyngeal SCC (42–44), some have found no significant association with tumor behavior (45), and some have shown that HPV-associated tumors are more aggressive (46). These conflicting results may be due to technical issues related to the sensitivity and specificity of the different methods used to detect the virus and may also be an artifact of the relatively small number of cases in each series. However, it is also possible that there are biologic differences in the oncogenesis and tumor biology of SCC arising at different sites in the oral cavity and oropharynx (41). The relationship between HPV infection and SCC at sites outside of the tonsil must be more well defined before HPV testing will have a role in this setting.

LEUKOPLAKIA

Oral leukoplakia, a white patch of mucosa that will not rub off, has a number of causes. Cases resulting from chronic trauma, lichen planus, or lupus erythematosus are benign. Cases associated with smoking, use of smokeless tobacco, or chewing betel quid are precancerous, and up to 18% undergo malignant transformation. For those cases with biopsy-proven dysplasia, the rate of malignant transformation is even higher, ranging from 16% to 33% (47).

Genetics

Of the various molecular markers that have been evaluated by different techniques (including LOH analysis, mutational analysis, and gene expression analysis), DNA ploidy appears to have the most significance because invasive SCC eventually develops in 84% of aneuploid lesions and 60% of tetraploid lesions, but only 3% of diploid lesions. Among patients with aneuploid lesions, the cumulative disease-free survival rate is only 16%, while it is 40% among patients with tetraploid lesions, and 97% among patients with diploid lesions (48). In fact, one study found that the only patients with leukoplakia who died of oral cancer were those with aneuploid lesions and that 72% of patients with aneuploid lesions died of invasive carcinoma within 5 years (49).

Technical Issues in the Evaluation of Aneuploidy in Oral Leukoplakia

The methodology used to measure ploidy in cases of leukoplakia is quite complex. First, the areas of the lesion that show dysplasia are collected by microdissection, and the epithelial fragments are processed to yield isolated nuclei that are suspended in a monolayer and stained. Next, the DNA content of at least 300 nuclei is measured by digital microscopy. Finally, the data from the individual nuclei is used to construct a histogram that is the basis of the actual ploidy determination (48). This involved methodology is obviously poorly suited for routine laboratory use, and so the clinical utility of ploidy analysis may depend on whether or not simplified methodologies can be developed.

NASOPHARYNGEAL CARCINOMA

Nasopharyngeal carcinoma is associated with Epstein-Barr Virus (EBV) infection. Although the tumor is endemic in southeast Asia, and to a lesser extent in northern Africa, EBV is present in almost every primary tumor regardless of the geographic origin of the patient or the degree of tumor differentiation (50–54). These data suggest that while EBV expression is required for tumor initiation, full expression of a malignant phenotype is dependent on a genetic predisposition and environmental factors (55,56). Even though molecular analysis is rarely required to diagnose nasopharyngeal carcinoma, patients with recurrent tumor have a poor prognosis, and consequently there has been much interest in developing methods that can identify patients at high risk for recurrence who might benefit from more aggressive primary therapy and for detecting relapse at an earlier stage which may improve the outcome of salvage therapy (57).

Several groups have shown that the level of EBV DNA in plasma or serum in patients with nasopharyngeal carcinoma correlates with the presence of distant metastases, overall survival, and relapse survival (57–59), and that changes in the plasma or serum EBV DNA levels after completion of therapy also are powerful predictors of overall survival and relapse-free survival (57,60). Because there is sequence variation between different clones of EBV, testing can even be designed to demonstrate that the circulating EBV DNA is from the same clone present in the patient's nasopharyngeal carcinoma (57,61).

Microarray analysis has also been used to examine the pattern of gene expression in nasopharyngeal carcinoma in an attempt to identify novel prognostic markers or therapeutic targets. Comparison of nasopharyngeal carcinoma with normal nasopharyngeal tissue shows changes in the level of expression of genes encoding growth factors and cytokines, as well as proteins involved in control of the cell cycle or regulation of apoptotic pathways (62). Although microarray expression analysis is not currently a component of the pathologic evaluation of nasopharyngeal carcinoma, this study suggests that gene expression profiling may become an important method for stratifying patients into prognostic and therapeutic groups.

Finally, it must be noted that EBV infection is not specific for nasopharyngeal carcinoma but has also been detected in SCC arising in anatomic sites outside of the nasopharynx, most often the oral cavity and tongue. By a variety of molecular techniques, including PCR, Southern blot hybridization, and in situ hybridization, EBV infection has been demonstrated in 15% to 75% of head and neck SCC (63,64). Although a relationship between EBV infection and well-differentiated SCC has been suggested, as has a correlation between EBV infection and clinical outcome (63), demonstration of EBV infection in SCC outside the nasopharynx currently has no established role in diagnostic or prognostic testing. Similarly, even though the virus can be detected in metastatic disease within lymph nodes (63,64), molecular analysis of EBV has no role in assessing clinical stage.

SALIVARY GLANDS

Pleomorphic Adenoma

Depending on the clinical series, pleomorphic adenoma (benign mixed tumor) constitutes 45% to 74% of all salivary gland neoplasms, which makes the tumor the most common benign neoplasm of the major and minor salivary glands and the most common salivary gland tumor overall (65). All pleomorphic adenomas (PAs) contain both epithelial and mesenchymal-like components, but based on immunohistochemical and ultrastructural evidence, PA is apparently of epithelial origin; the mesenchymal areas consist predominately of neoplastic modified myoepithelial cells (65–68).

Genetics

Conventional cytogenetic analysis of a large number of PAs (Fig. 21.2) has demonstrated karyotypic abnormalities in 50% to 80% of cases (69,70). About 40% of tumors harbor rearrangements involving 8q12, about 8% of cases harbor rearrangements of 12q15, and about 25% of cases contain

gross structural abnormalities or translocations at other sites. There appear to be no consistent correlations between the clinical features of PAs and their cytogenetic aberrations, and no definite relationships exist between the different cytogenetic abnormalities and the incidence of recurrence or malignant transformation.

PLAG1 Rearrangements

The *PLAG1* gene is consistently rearranged in tumors with aberrations involving 8q12. So far, three different fusion genes have been described (Table 21.2). In the vast majority of cases, a t(3;8) translocation produces a *CTNNB1-PLAG1* fusion gene in which the partner is β-catenin (71). A small percentage of tumors harbors a t(5;8) translocation that produces an *LIFR-PLAG1* fusion gene in which the partner is the leukemia inhibitory factor receptor (72) or a cryptic rearrangement that produces an *SII-PLAG1* fusion gene in which the partner encodes the transcription elongation factor SII (73). In all three fusion genes, the chromosomal break point is located in the first intron of *PLAG1* (which is about 25 kb long), and so the rearrangements are essentially promoter-swapping events in which the upstream 5′ regulatory elements of *PLAG1* are replaced by the promoter regions of the fusion partner. Alternative processing of the transcripts from all three fusion genes gives rise to a population of mRNAs that lack exon 2 of *PLAG1*, which does not appear to have any functional consequences.

PLAG1 encodes a zinc finger transcription factor that is normally developmentally regulated. Although the *PLAG1* fusion partners all have different cellular functions, they share a high level of expression in normal salivary gland, and consequently the dysregulated expression of PLAG1 that results from the promoter-swapping is thought to be responsible for the development of PA (71–73). In this context, it is interesting to note that PLAG1 overexpression is also present in a majority of PAs that have a normal karyotype (73), although the genetic basis for the activation of *PLAG1* in these cases is unknown.

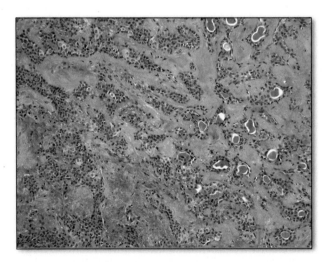

Figure 21.2 Pleomorphic adenoma (PA) of the parotid gland. In this region, the tumor shows ductal structures, small epithelial islands, and areas of myxoid stroma, only a few of the numerous architectural patterns that are characteristic of PA. Rearrangements of *PLAG1* and *HMGA2* are typical of PA (Table 21.2).

TABLE 21.2

REARRANGEMENTS IN PLEOMORPHIC ADENOMA

Fusion Gene	Cytogenetic Aberration	Partner Gene	References
PLAG1 rearrangements			
CTNNB1-PLAG1	t(3;8)(p21;q12)	β-Catenin	71
LIFR-PLAG1	t(5;8)(p13;q12)	Leukemia inhibitory factor receptor	72
SII-PLAG1	Cryptic	Transcription elongation factor SII	73
HMGA2 rearrangements			
HMGA2-FHIT and FHIT-HMGA2[a]	t(3;12)(p14.2;q15)	Fragile histidine triad gene	74
HMGA2-NFIB	ins(9;12)(p23;q12q15)	Nuclear protein involved in transcriptional regulation	75
HMGA2 3′ untranslated region	Complex rearrangement including t(1;12)(p22;q15)	Not applicable[b]	76

[a]Both of the reciprocal fusion transcripts were present in the reported case.
[b]The break point in the 3′ untranslated region of HMGA2 results in the removal of 8 AUUUA motifs thought to function as mRNA-destabilizing motifs.

HMGA2 Rearrangements

In PAs with aberrations involving 12q15, the HMGA2 gene (previously known as HMGIC) is consistently rearranged. HMGA2 encodes one of the high mobility group (HMG) proteins, which are small, acidic, nonhistone chromatin-associated proteins. HMGA2 contains three DNA binding domains and an acidic C-terminal domain and has an important role during growth and development (77). The DNA binding domains bind to the minor groove of adenine and thymine-rich (AT-rich) DNA sequences and are therefore referred to as AT hooks (78), and although HMGA2 does not exhibit transcriptional activity itself, it facilitates formation of transcriptional complexes through protein–DNA and protein–protein interactions.

Three different HMGA2 rearrangements have thus far been described (Table 21.2). The translocation t(3;12) produces a fusion gene in which the partner is the FHIT fragile histidine triad gene at 3p14.2 (74), and cases that harbor the rearrangement ins(9;12)(p23;q12q15) produce a fusion between HMGA2 and the NFIB gene that encodes a member of the human nuclear factor I proteins involved in transcriptional regulation (75). A rearrangement has also been described in which the chromosomal break point is in the 3′ untranslated region of HMGA2, a structural change that leaves the coding region of the gene intact but removes multiple AUUUA motifs that may function as mRNA-destabilizing motifs (76).

The diversity of HMGA2 translocation partners, together with the fact that the break point can occur outside of the coding region of the gene, suggests that the partner genes have no specific role in tumor development beyond simple deregulation of the level of expression of HMGA2 itself (77,79,80) or beyond physical separation of the DNA binding domains from the acidic C-terminal domain of HMGA2 (74,81).

Technical Issues in the Molecular Genetic Analysis of PA

PLAG1 Rearrangements

Given the variety of chromosomal rearrangements associated with PA, conventional cytogenetic evaluation is ideally suited for evaluating PAs, and, as noted above, routine cytogenetic evaluation can be used to demonstrate an abnormal karyotype in 50% to 80% of cases (69,70). However, additional molecular analysis can detect PLAG1 aberrations in 60% of tumors that have a normal karyotype (73).

Although metaphase FISH using a break-apart methodology was an essential component of the experimental approach used to identify several of the 8q12 rearrangements characteristic of PA (71,72), the utility of interphase FISH for detection of PLAG1 rearrangements remains to be formally evaluated. In any event, because a number of different rearrangements involve PLAG1, probe-split FISH will likely be a more sensitive approach in routine use than probe-fusion FISH.

PCR-based methods, including 5′-RACE and RT-PCR, have also been used to detect the fusion genes characteristic of PA (71–73). In tumors known to harbor a translocation characteristic of PA, RT-PCR demonstrates the associated fusion transcript in 100% of cases when fresh tissue is used as the substrate for analysis (71,72). In tumors with a normal karyotype, RT-PCR using a panel of primers demonstrates PLAG1 fusion transcripts in 60% of cases (73), although the number of different loci that can be rearranged in PA makes comprehensive evaluation by RT-PCR cumbersome. The application of RT-PCR for the evaluation of formalin-fixed, paraffin-embedded (FFPE) tissue from cases of PA has not been described.

Northern blot analysis has shown that PLAG1 activation is a consistent feature of PA, whether or not chromosomal aberrations are evident by conventional cytogenetic analysis, as noted above. Specifically, up to 100% of tumors with 8q12 aberrations show overexpression of *PLAG1* transcripts (71–73), and 76% with a normal karyotype also shown *PLAG1* activation (73). However, 18% of malignant salivary gland tumors also show *PLAG1* activation, which limits the utility of northern blot analysis for the diagnosis of salivary gland tumors (73).

Although polyclonal anti-PLAG1 antibody preparations are available (82) and have been used to show increased nuclear staining in other tumor types that harbor *PLAG1* fusions (as discussed below), the utility of immunohistochemical staining for PLAG1 in the diagnosis of PA has not been evaluated.

HMGA2 Rearrangements

As noted above, conventional cytogenetic analysis demonstrates rearrangements involving 12q15 in about 8% of cases (69,70). No studies have formally evaluated the technique prospectively, so the reported prevalence of 12q15 rearrangements in PA may not accurately reflect the sensitivity of cytogenetic analysis for detecting 12q15 rearrangements in routine clinical practice.

Metaphase FISH analysis using a break-apart approach has been used to help identify many of the 12q15 rearrangements in cases of PA (74–76), but the utility of interphase FISH for the demonstration of *HMGA2* rearrangements remains to be formally evaluated. As is the case with the *PLAG1* locus, the variety of *HMGA2* aberrations described in PA suggests that probe-split FISH will likely turn out to be a more sensitive and less cumbersome approach in routine use than probe-fusion FISH.

PCR-based methods, including 3'-RACE and RT-PCR, have been used to characterize the break points in *HMGA2* fusion genes (74–76). In tumors known to harbor structural changes of 12q15, RT-PCR has been used with fresh tissue to demonstrate fusion transcripts in virtually 100% of cases and is especially useful for confirming the presence of fusion genes in cases with a complex karyotype (74,76). The use of RT-PCR for identification of *HMGA2* fusion transcripts in FFPE tissue has not been evaluated.

HMGA2 is not expressed in normal adult tissues (77,83–85), although aberrant expression of HMGA2 is present in many tumor types that harbor chromosomal aberrations of 12q15 (discussed in more detail later). Consequently, even though immunohistochemical analysis of PA has not been reported, it is likely that HMGA2 expression will be present in the subset of PAs that harbor 12q15 rearrangements.

Diagnostic Issues in Molecular Genetic Analysis of PA

PLAG1 Rearrangements

Aberrations of *PLAG1* are not a characteristic finding in normal salivary gland tissue or any other benign salivary gland neoplasm (71,73,75). However, because the same pattern of *PLAG1* rearrangements is present in carcinoma ex pleomorphic adenoma (as discussed later), molecular analysis cannot be used to separate benign from malignant tumors.

It is interesting to note that rearrangements of *PLAG1* are also a characteristic feature of lipoblastoma (86). The *PLAG1* fusion partners in lipoblastoma are, at least in the cases reported to date, different from those described in pleomorphic adenoma (discussed in more detail in Chapter 11). Although the presence of *PLAG1* fusion genes in both lipoblastoma and PA is noteworthy from a tumor biology perspective, it obviously has little impact on molecular testing of salivary gland neoplasms because lipoblastoma is not in the differential diagnosis of PA.

HMGA2 Rearrangements

As is true for rearrangements of 8q12, cytogenetic data show that PA is the only benign salivary gland neoplasm that harbors rearrangements of 12q15. As is also true for the *PLAG1* locus, the same pattern of *HMGA2* rearrangements is present in carcinoma ex pleomorphic adenoma, and so molecular analysis cannot be used to distinguish benign from malignant tumors.

As shown in Table 11.7, one of the remarkable features of rearrangements involving 12q15 is that alterations of the same region are characteristic of a variety of benign (77,87,88) and malignant (89,90) tumors involving a wide variety of anatomic sites. However, the *HMGA2* fusion partners found in PA have not (yet) been documented in any of these other tumor types. From a diagnostic viewpoint, the fact that *HMGA2* is also involved in the development of a number of mesenchymal neoplasms is of limited importance because the tumors listed in Table 11.7 rarely, if ever, enter into the differential diagnosis of PA.

Carcinoma ex Pleomorphic Adenoma

The proportion of PAs that undergoes malignant transformation ranges from 2% to 23% in different series, although the longer a PA has been present, the greater the risk (65,91).

Genetics

Less than two dozen carcinoma ex pleomorphic adenomas (CexPA) have been characterized by routine cytogenetic analysis (reviewed in reference 81). Approximately 53% of cases harbor rearrangements of 8q12, presumably involving the *PLAG1* locus; about 20% harbor aberrations involving 12q15, presumably involving the *HMGA2* locus. Given that rearrangements of *PLAG1* and *HGMA2* are characteristic of PA as discussed above, recurring aberrations involving these loci is not an unanticipated finding. The percentage of cases with rearrangements of either 8q12 or 12q15 suggests that neither locus shows a significantly higher propensity to produce CexPA from PA, although the number of cases that has thus far been evaluated is admittedly quite small.

About 40% of CexPA show evidence of gene amplification manifested as double minute chromosomes (dmin) or homogeneously staining regions (hsr). In the few cases studied in detail by molecular genetic approaches, the amplified region consisted of 12q14-15, including *HMGA2*, *CDK4*, and *MDM2* (81,92). Because dmin and hsr are not recurring features of PA and because amplification of the 12q14-15 region is characteristic of other malignant tumors (including atypical lipomatous tumor/well-differentiated liposarcoma, as discussed in Chapter 11), the cytogenetic findings suggest that amplification and overexpression of genes in the 12q14-15 region contributes to malignant transformation of PA. Other recurrent genetic abnormalities that may also contribute to the development of CexPA include polysomy 7, deletion of the chromosomal region distal to 5q22, and mutations or overexpression of *TP53* (81,93).

Given the small number of cases of CexPA that have been evaluated, the sensitivity and specificity of routine cytogenetic analysis to detect dmin and hsr for the diagnosis of CexPA remains unknown. The role of testing by other molecular genetic techniques to demonstrate 12q14-15 amplifications also remains unknown.

Mucoepidermoid Carcinoma

Mucoepidermoid carcinoma (MEC) is the most common malignant salivary gland tumor. Slightly more than 50% of cases occur in the major salivary glands, about 20% originate in the minor salivary glands of the palate, and approximately 20% arise in the buccal mucosa, lips, retromolar region, or tongue (65). Histologically, as its name implies, MEC contains mucous and epidermoid cells, but in most tumors these cell types are outnumbered by intermediate cells (65).

Genetics

Rearrangements involving 11q21 and 19p13 are the hallmark of MEC, regardless of whether the tumor originates in major salivary glands, minor salivary glands, or bronchial glands (94–97), but there is no correlation between the presence of the rearrangement and tumor grade or stage. The rearrangements produce a fusion gene between *MECT1* (also known as *WAMTP1* and *TORC1*) at 19p13 with the *MAML2* gene at 11q21 (96,97). In all tumors that have been characterized thus far, the translocation break point occurs in intron1 of *MECT1* (which is about 60 kb long) and intron1 of *MAML2* (which is about 250 kb long), producing a gene in which exon 1 of *MECT1* is fused to exons 2 to 5 of *MAML2*. Other recurring rearrangements (involving region 1q32, 5p15, 6q21-25, 7q22, and 15q22) and numerical abnormalities (including gains of chromosomes 2, 3, 5, 7, 18, 20, and X, and loss of chromosome Y) have also been described (98–103), but the identity of the relevant genes is unknown.

The protein encoded by *MECT1* is a potent coactivator of genes regulated by cAMP response elements (also known as CREs) (104,105); specifically, MECT1 interacts with CREB, a protein that directly binds to CREs. The *MAML2* gene product is a transcriptional coactivator in the Notch signaling pathway, a regulatory pathway that influences many critical cellular processes, including proliferation, apoptosis, and differentiation (106–108). In the MECT1-MAML2 chimeric protein, the N-terminal region of MECT1 that binds CREB replaces the N-terminal basic domain of MAML2 (Fig. 21.3). It is therefore likely that the fusion protein causes activation of CREB-responsive genes (109) and ligand-independent activation of Notch target genes (96), thereby promoting tumorigenesis through disruption of two different signaling pathways.

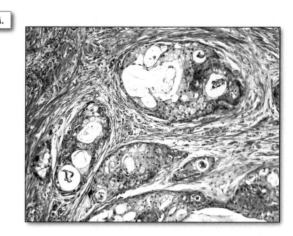

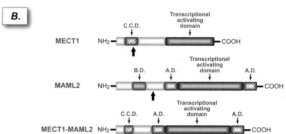

Figure 21.3   The translocation t(11;19)(q21;p13) that produces an *MECT1-MAML2* gene fusion is characteristic of mucoepidermoid carcinoma. **A,** Low-grade MEC arising in minor salivary gland tissue showing a close association of epidermoid cells and mucinous cells in some of the tumor nests. **B,** Schematic diagram of the structure of the MECT1-MAML2 chimeric protein. In the cases thus far described, the breakpoint has always occurred at the same location (*bold arrows*); CCD, coil-coil domain involved in binding to CREB; BD, basic domain involved in binding to the ankyrin repeat domain of Notch receptors; AD, acidic domain. The precise boundaries of the transcriptional activating domains in *MECT1* and *MAML2* have not been mapped.

Technical Issues in Molecular Genetic Analysis of MEC

The rearrangements that give rise to *MECT1-MAML2* gene fusions can occur as a reciprocal translocation t(11;19) (q21;p13), as well as part of more complicated translocations or other chromosomal changes (109,110). Rearrangements involving 11q21 and 19p13 can be detected in 27% to 63% of MEC by conventional cytogenetic analysis of G-banded chromosomes (97,109,110), but spectral karyotyping has also been used to demonstrate the rearrangements (96).

In situ hybridization analysis has also been used to demonstrate the presence of *MECT1-MAML2* gene fusions by a number of approaches, including probe-fusion (97) and probe-split FISH on metaphase chromosomes (97, 98,109), and probe-split chromogenic in situ hybridization (CISH) on interphase nuclei in sections of FFPE tissue (109). In one report in which conventional cytogenetic analysis, probe-split FISH on metaphase chromosomes, and probe-split CISH on interphase nuclei were directly compared, each of the three techniques had a sensitivity of about 50% and a specificity of 100%, although each technique demonstrated rearrangements in a different subsets of cases (109). However, because this latter study evaluated cases based on the availability of fresh tissue, cultured tissue, or cell lines, the performance characteristics of FISH- or CISH-based analysis in routine practice remains to be determined.

RT-PCR has also been used to detect *MECT1-MAML2* rearrangements. When fresh tissue, cultured tissue, or cell lines are used as the substrate for testing, fusion transcripts are detected in 70% to 100% of MEC (96,97,109), and in parallel analysis, RT-PCR has a higher sensitivity than either metaphase FISH or interphase CISH (109). However, the selection of cases for RT-PCR analysis in these studies was based on the availability of fresh tissue, cultured tissue, or cell lines, or the presence of a known *MECT1-MAML2* rearrangement based on prior karyotypic- or in situ hybridization–based analysis, and so the results undoubtedly reflect a selection bias. Until RT-PCR is used to test unselected series of MEC, including cases for which only FFPE tissue is available, the sensitivity and specificity of the approach in routine practice will remain unknown.

Diagnostic Issues in Molecular Genetic Analysis of MEC

MECT1-MAML2 fusions have not been detected in normal salivary glands (97,109), in polymorphous low-grade adenocarcinoma or acinic cell carcinoma (109), or in a group of 20 nonmucoepidermoid carcinomas, the histologic type of which was not otherwise specified (96). However, the translocation t(11;19)(q21;p13) has been described in a subset of Warthin's tumors (97,111,112), with associated expression of *MECT1-MAML2* fusion transcripts (97). The histogenesis of Warthin's tumor and MEC are thought to be distinct (66,113–115), and so the presence of the same genetic aberration in both tumor types may merely be an indication that the t(11;19) translocation, while more common in MEC, is nonetheless not absolutely specific. However, because several reports have documented coexistence of both MEC and Warthin's tumor within the same salivary gland lesion (65,109,116,117), it is possible that the occurrence of the translocation t(11;19)(q21;p13) in Warthin's tumor may actually be due to the presence of an unrecognized MEC.

Warthin's Tumor

Warthin's tumor, also known as papillary cystadenoma lymphomatosum, is the second most common benign tumor of the parotid gland (65). The neoplasm (Fig. 21.4) consists of cystic spaces lined by a bilayered oncocytic epithelium within a supporting stroma that contains abundant lymphocytes (65). Although the vast majority of Warthin's tumors occur in the parotid gland, rare cases arise in the submandibular glands or the oral cavity.

Genetics

As noted above, the translocation t(11;19)(q21;p13) has been described in Warthin's tumor, and based on the single case studied by molecular analysis, the resulting *MECT1-MAML2* fusion gene is identical in Warthin's tumor and mucoepidermoid carcinoma (97). Apparently identical translocations have been described in other Warthin's tumors by a number of groups (111,112,118).

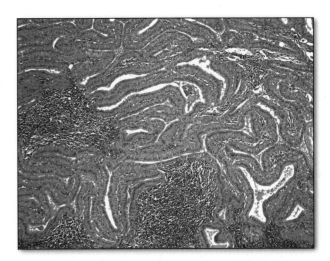

Figure 21.4 Warthin's tumor arising in the parotid gland showing the typical bilayered epithelium and supporting lymphoid stroma. Rare cases of Warthin's tumor have been shown to harbor the same t(11;19)(q21;p13) and *MECT1-MAML2* fusion characteristic of mucoepidermoid carcinoma (Figure 21.3).

Technical and Diagnostic Issues of Molecular Genetic analysis of Warthin's Tumor

Given the apparent rarity of Warthin's tumors that harbor an *MECT1-MAML2* fusion (109), and the fact that Warthin's tumor can coexist with MEC within the same salivary gland lesion (65,109,116,117), molecular analysis of a Warthin's tumor that demonstrates the fusion should raise suspicion that the tumor may harbor an occult MEC. Consequently, it would seem prudent to extensively sample cases of Warthin's tumor in which an *MECT1-MAML2* fusion is identified to ensure that an MEC was not simply overlooked.

Sarcomas

A number of malignant small round cell tumors and spindle cell sarcomas that characteristically arise in soft tissue have also been described as primary tumors of the salivary glands. Examples include Ewing sarcoma/peripheral neuroectodermal tumor (119,120), alveolar rhabdomyosarcoma (121,122), and synovial sarcoma (123). The molecular genetic features of these tumors, as well as the technical and diagnostic issues involved in their analysis by molecular genetic methods, are discussed in detail in Chapter 11.

REFERENCES

1. Califano J, van der Riet P, Westra W, et al. Genetic progression model for head and neck cancer: implications for field cancerization. *Cancer Res* 1996;56:2488–2492.
2. Field JK. The role of oncogenes and tumour-suppressor genes in the aetiology of oral, head and neck squamous cell carcinoma. *J R Soc Med* 1995;88:35–39.
3. Ha PK, Benoit NE, Yochem R, et al. A transcriptional progression model for head and neck cancer. *Clin Cancer Res* 2003;9:3058–3064.
4. Rosin MP, Cheng X, Poh C, et al. Use of allelic loss to predict malignant risk for low-grade oral epithelial dysplasia. *Clin Cancer Res* 2000;6:357–362.
5. Gleich LL, Salamone FN. Molecular genetics of head and neck cancer. *Cancer Control* 2002;9:369–378.
6. Choi HR, Roberts DB, Johnigan RH, et al. Molecular and clinicopathologic comparisons of head and neck squamous carcinoma variants: common and distinctive features of biological significance. *Am J Surg Pathol* 2004;28:1299–1310.

7. Koch W. Sidransky D. Molecular markers of radiation effectiveness in head and neck squamous cell carcinoma. *Semin Radiat Oncol* 2004;14:130–138.
8. Rybicki BA, Savera AT, Gomez JA, et al. Allelic loss and tumor pathology in head and neck squamous cell carcinoma. *Mod Pathol* 2003;16:970–979.
9. Bochmuhl U, Wolf G, Schmidt S, et al. Genomic alterations associated with malignancy in head and neck cancer. *Head Neck* 1998;20:145–151.
10. Kim MM, Califano JA. Molecular pathology of head-and-neck cancer. *Int J Cancer* 2004;112:545–553.
11. Bosch FX, Ritter D, Enders C, et al. Head and neck tumor sites differ in prevalence and spectrum of *p53* alterations but these have limited prognostic value. *Int J Cancer* 2004; 111:530–538.
12. Gleich LL, Li YQ. The loss of heterozygosity in retinoblastoma and *p53* suppressor genes as a prognostic indicator for head and neck cancer. *Laryngoscope* 1996;106: 1378–1381.
13. Poetsch M, Petersmann A, Lignitz E, et al. Relationship between mitochondrial DNA instability, mitochondrial DNA large deletions, and nuclear microsatellite instability in head and neck squamous cell carcinomas. *Diagn Mol Pathol* 2004;13:26–32.
14. Sotiriou C, Lothaire P, Dequanter D, et al. Molecular profiling of head and neck tumors. *Curr Opin Oncol* 2004;16:211–214.
15. Cromer A, Carles A, Millon R, et al. Identification of genes associated with tumorigenesis and metastatic potential of hypopharyngeal cancer by microarray analysis. *Oncogene* 2004;23:2484–2498.
16. Roepman P, Wessels LF, Kettelarij N, et al. An expression profile for diagnosis of lymph node metastases from primary head and neck squamous cell carcinomas. *Nat Genet* 2005;37:182–186.
17. O'Donnell RK, Kupferman M, Wei SJ, et al. Gene expression signature predicts lymphatic metastasis in squamous cell carcinoma of the oral cavity. *Oncogene* 2005;24: 1244–1251.
18. Belbin TJ, Singh B, Barber I, et al. Molecular classification of head and neck squamous cell carcinoma using cDNA microarrays. *Cancer Res* 2002;62:1184–1190.
19. Chung CH, Parker JS, Karaca G, et al. Molecular classification of head and neck squamous cell carcinomas using patterns of gene expression. *Cancer Cell* 2004;5:489–500.
20. Higuchi E, Oridate N, Furuta Y, et al. Differentially expressed genes associated with CIS-diamminedichloroplatinum (II) resistance in head and neck cancer using differential display and CDNA microarray. *Head Neck* 2003;25:187–193.
21. Brennan JA, Mao L, Hruban RH, et al. Molecular assessment of histopathological staging in squamous-cell carcinoma of the head and neck. *N Engl J Med* 1995;332:429–435.
22. Goldenberg D, Harden S, Masayesva BG, et al. Intraoperative molecular margin analysis in head and neck cancer. *Arch Otolaryngol Head Neck Surg* 2004;130:39–44.
23. van Oijen MGCT, Slootweg PJ. Oral field cancerization: carcinogen-induced independent events or micrometastatic deposits? *Cancer Epidemiol Biomarkers Prev* 2000;9: 249–256.
24. Qin GZ, Park JY, Chen SY, et al. A high prevalence of *p53* mutations in pre-malignant oral erythroplakia. *Int J Cancer* 1999;80:345–348.
25. van der Toorn PP, Veltman JA, Bot FJ, et al. Mapping of resection margins of oral cancer for *p53* overexpression and chromosome instability to detect residual (pre)malignant cells. *J Pathol* 2001;193:66–72.
26. Slootweg PJ, Hordijk GJ, Schade Y, et al. Treatment failure and margin status in head and neck cancer: a critical view on the potential value of molecular pathology. *Oral Oncol* 2002;38:500–503.
27. Batsakis JG. Surgical excision margins: a pathologist's perspective. *Adv Anat Pathol* 1999;6:140–148.
28. Hamakawa H, Onishi A, Sumida T, et al. Intraoperative real-time genetic diagnosis for sentinel node navigation surgery. *Int J Oral Maxillofac Surg* 2004;33:670–675.
29. Hamakawa H, Fukizumi M, Bao Y, et al. Genetic diagnosis of micrometastasis based on SCC antigen mRNA in cervical lymph nodes of head and neck cancer. *Clin Exp Metastasis* 1999;17:593–599.
30. Cserni G, Amendoeira I, Apostolikas N, et al. Pathological work-up of sentinel lymph nodes in breast cancer: review of current data to be considered for the formulation of guidelines. *Eur J Cancer* 2003;39:1654–1667.
31. Bostick PJ, Chatterjee S, Chi DD, et al. Limitations of specific reverse-transcriptase polymerase chain reaction markers in the detection of metastases in the lymph nodes and blood of breast cancer patients. *J Clin Oncol* 1998;16:2632–2640.
32. Vlems FA, Diepstra JH, Cornelissen IM, et al. Investigations for a multi-marker RT-PCR to improve sensitivity of disseminated tumor cell detection. *Anticancer Res* 2003; 23:179–186.
33. Zippelius A, Kufer P, Honold G, et al. Limitations of reverse-transcriptase polymerase chain reaction analyses for detection of micrometastatic epithelial cancer cells in bone marrow. *J Clin Oncol* 1997;15:2701–2708.
34. Yamamoto N, Kato Y, Yanagisawa A, et al. Predictive value of genetic diagnosis for cancer micrometastasis: histologic and experimental appraisal. *Cancer* 1997;80: 1393–1398.
35. Sumida T, Hamakawa H, Kayahara H, et al. Clinical usefulness of telomerase assay for the detection of lymph node metastasis in patients with oral malignancy. *Arch Pathol Lab Med* 2000;124:398–400.
36. Nawroz-Danish H, Eisenberger CF, Yoo GH, et al. Microsatellite analysis of serum DNA in patients with head and neck cancer. *Int J Cancer* 2004;111:96–100.
37. Spafford MF, Koch WM, Reed AL, et al. Detection of head and neck squamous cell carcinoma among exfoliated oral mucosal cells by microsatellite analysis. *Clin Cancer Res* 2001;7:607–612.
38. Fliss MS, Usadel H, Caballero OL, et al. Facile detection of mitochondrial DNA mutations in tumors and bodily fluids. *Science* 2000;287:2017–2019.
39. Rosas SL, Koch W, da Costa Carvalho MG, et al. Promoter hypermethylation patterns of p16, O6-methylguanine-DNA-methyltransferase, and death-associated protein kinase in tumors and saliva of head and neck cancer patients. *Cancer Res* 2001;61:939–942.
40. Mellin H, Friesland S, Lewensohn R, et al. Human papillomavirus (HPV) DNA in tonsillar cancer: clinical correlates, risk of relapse, and survival. *Int J Cancer* 2000;89: 300–304.
41. Li W, Thompson CH, O'Brien CJ, et al. Human papillomavirus positivity predicts favourable outcome for squamous carcinoma of the tonsil. *Int J Cancer* 2003;106: 553–558.
42. Gillison ML, Koch WM, Capone RB, et al. Evidence for a causal association between human papillomavirus and a subset of head and neck cancers. *J Natl Cancer Inst* 2000; 92:709–720.
43. Lindel K, Beer KT, Laissue J, et al. Human papillomavirus positive squamous cell carcinoma of the oropharynx: a radiosensitive subgroup of head and neck carcinoma. *Cancer* 2001;92:805–813.
44. Ritchie JM, Smith EM, Summersgill KF, et al. Human papillomavirus infection as a prognostic factor in carcinomas of the oral cavity and oropharynx. *Int J Cancer* 2003; 104:336–344.
45. Brandwein M, Zeitlin J, Nuovo GJ, et al. HPV detection using "hot start" polymerase chain reaction in patients with oral cancer: a clinicopathological study of 64 patients. *Mod Pathol* 1994;7:720–727.
46. Cattani P, Hohaus S, Bellacosa A, et al. Association between cyclin D1 (*CCND1*) gene amplification and human papillomavirus infection in human laryngeal squamous cell carcinoma. *Clin Cancer Res* 1998;4:2585–2589.
47. Greenspan D, Jordan RC. The white lesion that kills: aneuploid dysplastic oral leukoplakia. *N Engl J Med* 2004;350:1382–1384.
48. Sudbo J, Kildal W, Risberg B, et al. DNA content as a prognostic marker in patients with oral leukoplakia. *N Engl J Med* 2001;344:1270–1278.
49. Sudbo J, Lippman SM, Lee JJ, et al. The influence of resection and aneuploidy on mortality in oral leukoplakia. *N Engl J Med* 2004;350:1405–1413.
50. Pathmanathan R, Prasad U, Chandrika G, et al. Undifferentiated, nonkeratinizing, and squamous cell carcinoma of the nasopharynx: variants of Epstein-Barr virus-infected neoplasia. *Am J Pathol* 1995;146:1355–1367.
51. Tsai ST, Jin YT, Su IJ. Expression of *EBER1* in primary and metastatic nasopharyngeal carcinoma tissues using in situ hybridization: a correlation with WHO histologic subtypes. *Cancer* 1996;77:231–236.
52. Chang YS, Tyan YS, Liu ST, et al. Detection of Epstein-Barr virus DNA sequences in nasopharyngeal carcinoma cells by enzymatic DNA amplification. *J Clin Microbiol* 1990;28:2398–2402.
53. Wu TC, Mann RB, Epstein JL, et al. Abundant expression of *EBER1* small nuclear RNA in nasopharyngeal carcinoma: a morphologically distinctive target for detection of Epstein-Barr virus in formalin-fixed paraffin-embedded carcinoma specimens. *Am J Pathol* 1991;138:1461–1469.
54. Chen CL, Wen WN, Chen JY, et al. Detection of Epstein-Barr virus genome in nasopharyngeal carcinoma by in situ DNA hybridization. *Intervirology* 1993;36:91–98.
55. Lu SJ, Day NE, Degos L, et al. Linkage of a nasopharyngeal carcinoma susceptibility locus to the HLA region. *Nature* 1990;346:470–471.
56. Chien YC, Chen JY, Liu MY, et al. Serologic markers of Epstein-Barr virus infection and nasopharyngeal carcinoma in Taiwanese men. *N Engl J Med* 2001;345:1877–1882.
57. Lin JC, Wang WY, Chen KY, et al. Quantification of plasma Epstein-Barr virus DNA in patients with advanced nasopharyngeal carcinoma. *N Engl J Med* 2004;350: 2461–2470.
58. Lo YM, Chan LY, Lo KW, et al. Quantitative analysis of cell-free Epstein-Barr virus DNA in plasma of patients with nasopharyngeal carcinoma. *Cancer Res* 1999;59:1188–1191.
59. Lin JC, Chen KY, Wang WY, et al. Detection of Epstein-Barr virus DNA the peripheral-blood cells of patients with nasopharyngeal carcinoma: relationship to distant metastasis and survival. *J Clin Oncol* 2001;19:2607–2615.
60. Ngan RK, Lau WH, Yip TT, et al. Remarkable application of serum EBV *EBER-1* in monitoring response of nasopharyngeal cancer patients to salvage chemotherapy. *Ann N Y Acad Sci* 2001;945:73–79.
61. Wang WY, Chien YC, Jan JS, et al. Consistent sequence variation of Epstein-Barr virus nuclear antigen 1 in primary tumor and peripheral blood cells of patients with nasopharyngeal carcinoma. *Clin Cancer Res* 2002;8:2586–2590.
62. Xie L, Xu L, He Z, et al. Identification of differentially expressed genes in nasopharyngeal carcinoma by means of the Atlas human cancer cDNA expression array. *J Cancer Res Clin Oncol* 2000;126:400–406.
63. Kobayashi I, Shima K, Saito I, et al. Prevalence of Epstein-Barr virus in oral squamous cell carcinoma. *J Pathol* 1999;189:34–39.
64. Shimakage M, Horii K, Tempaku A, et al. Association of Epstein-Barr virus with oral cancers. *Hum Pathol* 2002;33:608–614.
65. Ellis GL, Auclair PL. *Tumors of the Salivary Glands*. Washington, DC: Armed Forces Institute of Pathology; 1996.
66. Dardick I, Ostrynski VL, Ekem JK, et al. Immunohistochemical and ultrastructural correlates of muscle-actin expression in pleomorphic adenomas and myoepitheliomas based on comparison of formalin and methanol fixation. *Virchows Arch A Pathol Anat Histopathol* 1992;421:95–104.
67. Dardick I, van Nostrand AW. Myoepithelial cells in salivary gland tumors: revisited. *Head Neck Surg* 1985;7:395–408.
68. Dardick I, van Nostrand AW, Phillips MJ. Histogenesis of salivary gland pleomorphic adenoma (mixed tumor) with an evaluation of the role of the myoepithelial cell. *Hum Pathol* 1982;13:62–75.
69. Sandros J, Stenman G, Mark J. Cytogenetic and molecular observations in human and experimental salivary gland tumors. *Cancer Genet Cytogenet* 1990;44:153–167.
70. Bullerdiek J, Wobst G, Meyer-Bolte K, et al. Cytogenetic subtyping of 220 salivary gland pleomorphic adenomas: correlation to occurrence, histological subtype, and in vitro cellular behavior. *Cancer Genet Cytogenet* 1993;65:27–31.
71. Kas K, Voz ML, Roijer E, et al. Promoter swapping between the genes for a novel zinc finger protein and beta-catenin in pleiomorphic adenomas with t(3;8)(p21;q12) translocations. *Nat Genet* 1997;15:170–174.
72. Voz ML, Astrom AK, Kas K, et al. The recurrent translocation t(5;8)(p13;q12) in pleomorphic adenomas results in upregulation of *PLAG1* gene expression under control of the LIFR promoter. *Oncogene* 1998;16:1409–1416.
73. Astrom AK, Voz ML, Kas K, et al. Conserved mechanism of *PLAG1* activation in salivary gland tumors with and without chromosome 8q12 abnormalities: identification of *SII* as a new fusion partner gene. *Cancer Res* 1999;59:918–923.
74. Geurts JM, Schoenmakers EF, Roijer E, et al. Expression of reciprocal hybrid transcripts of *HMGIC* and *FHIT* in a pleomorphic adenoma of the parotid gland. *Cancer Res* 1997;57:13–17.
75. Geurts JM, Schoenmakers EF, Roijer E, et al. Identification of *NFIB* as recurrent translocation partner gene of *HMGIC* in pleomorphic adenomas. *Oncogene* 1998;16:865–872.

76. Geurts JM, Schoenmakers EF, Van de Ven WJ. Molecular characterization of a complex chromosomal rearrangement in a pleomorphic salivary gland adenoma involving the 3'-UTR of *HMGIC*. *Cancer Genet Cytogenet* 1997;95:198–205.

77. Hess J. Chromosomal translocations in benign tumors: the HMGI proteins. *Am J Clin Pathol* 1998;109:251–261.

78. Ashar HR, Fejzo M, Tkachenko A, et al. Disruption of the architectural factor HMGI-C: DNA-binding AT hook motifs fused in lipomas to distinct transcriptional regulatory domains. *Cell* 1995;82:57–65.

79. Sandberg AA. Updates on the cytogenetics and molecular genetics of bone and soft tissue tumors: lipoma. *Cancer Genet Cytogenet* 2004;150:93–115.

80. Merscher S, Marondel I, Pedeutour F, et al. Identification of new translocation breakpoints at 12q13 in lipomas. *Genomics* 1997;46:70–77.

81. Roijer E, Nordkvist A, Strom AK, et al. Translocation, deletion/amplification, and expression of *HMGIC* and *MDM2* in a carcinoma ex pleomorphic adenoma. *Am J Pathol* 2002;160:433–440.

82. Astrom A, D'Amore ES, Sainati L, et al. Evidence of involvement of the *PLAG1* gene in lipoblastomas. *Int J Oncol* 2000;16:1107–1110.

83. Reeves R. Molecular biology of HMGA proteins: hubs of nuclear function. *Gene* 2001; 277:63–81.

84. Tallini G, Vanni R, Manfioletti G, et al. *HMGI-C* and *HMGI(Y)* immunoreactivity correlates with cytogenetic abnormalities in lipomas, pulmonary chondroid hamartomas, endometrial polyps, and uterine leiomyomas and is compatible with rearrangement of the *HMGI-C* and *HMGI(Y)* genes. *Lab Invest* 2000;80:359–369.

85. Rogalla P, Drechsler K, Frey G, et al. *HMGI-C* expression patterns in human tissues: implications for the genesis of frequent mesenchymal tumors. *Am J Pathol* 1996; 149:775–779.

86. Hibbard MK, Kozakewich HP, Dal Cin P, et al. *PLAG1* fusion oncogenes in lipoblastoma. *Cancer Res* 2000;60:4869–4872.

87. Schoenmakers EF, Wanschura S, Mols R, et al. Recurrent rearrangements in the high mobility group protein gene, *HMGI-C*, in benign mesenchymal tumours. *Nat Genet* 1995;10:436–444.

88. Tallini G, Dal Cin P, Rhoden KJ, et al. Expression of *HMGI-C* and *HMGI(Y)* in ordinary lipoma and atypical lipomatous tumors: immunohistochemical reactivity correlates with karyotypic alterations. *Am J Pathol* 1997;151:37–43.

89. Dahlen A, Mertens F, Rydholm A, et al. Fusion, disruption, and expression of *HMGA2* in bone and soft tissue chondromas. *Mod Pathol* 2003;16:1132–1140.

90. Hisaoka M, Sheng WQ, Tanaka A, et al. *HMGIC* alterations in smooth muscle tumors of soft tissues and other sites. *Cancer Genet Cytogenet* 2002;138:50–55.

91. Eneroth CM, Zetterberg A. Malignancy in pleomorphic adenoma: a clinical and microspectrophotometric study. *Acta Otolaryngol* 1974;77:426–432.

92. Rao PH, Murty VV, Louie DC, et al. Nonsyntenic amplification of *MYC* with *CDK4* and *MDM2* in a malignant mixed tumor of salivary gland. *Cancer Genet Cytogenet* 1998; 105:160–163.

93. Nordkvist A, Roijer E, Bang G, et al. Expression and mutation patterns of *p53* in benign and malignant salivary gland tumors. *Int J Oncol* 2000;16:477–483.

94. Johansson M, Mandahl N, Johansson L, et al. Translocation 11;19 in a mucoepidermoid tumor of the lung. *Cancer Genet Cytogenet* 1995;80:85–86.

95. Stenman G, Petursdottir V, Mellgren G, et al. A child with a t(11;19)(q14–21;p12) in a pulmonary mucoepidermoid carcinoma. *Virchows Arch* 1998;433:579–581.

96. Tonon G, Modi S, Wu L, et al. t(11;19)(q21;p13) translocation in mucoepidermoid carcinoma creates a novel fusion product that disrupts a Notch signaling pathway. *Nat Genet* 2003;33:208–213.

97. Enlund F, Behboudi A, Andren Y, et al. Altered Notch signaling resulting from expression of a *WAMTP1-MAML2* gene fusion in mucoepidermoid carcinomas and benign Warthin's tumors. *Exp Cell Res* 2004;292:21–28.

98. Tonon G, Gehlhaus KS, Yonescu R, et al. Multiple reciprocal translocations in salivary gland mucoepidermoid carcinomas. *Cancer Genet Cytogenet* 2004;152:15–22.

99. Sandros J, Mark J, Happonen R, et al. Specificity of 6q- markers and other recurrent deviations in human malignant salivary gland tumors. *Anticancer Res* 1988;8:637–643.

100. Jin Y, Mertens F, Limon J, et al. Characteristic karyotypic features in lacrimal and salivary gland carcinomas. *Br J Cancer* 1994;70:42–47.

101. Martins C, Fonseca I, Roque L, et al. Malignant salivary gland neoplasms: a cytogenetic study of 19 cases. *Eur J Cancer B Oral Oncol* 1996;32B:128–132.

102. El-Naggar AK, Lovell M, Killary A, et al. Trisomy 5 as the sole chromosomal abnormality in a primary mucoepidermoid carcinoma of the minor salivary gland. *Cancer Genet Cytogenet* 1994;76:96–99.

103. El-Naggar AK, Lovell M, Killary A, et al. Genotypic characterization of a primary mucoepidermoid carcinoma of the parotid gland by cytogenetic, fluorescence in situ hybridization, and DNA ploidy analysis. *Cancer Genet Cytogenet* 1996;89:38–43.

104. Conkright MD, Canettieri G, Screaton R, et al. TORCs: transducers of regulated CREB activity. *Mol Cell* 2003;12:413–423.

105. Iourgenko V, Zhang W, Mickanin C, et al. Identification of a family of cAMP response element-binding protein coactivators by genome-scale functional analysis in mammalian cells. *Proc Natl Acad Sci USA* 2003;100:12147–12152.

106. Artavanis-Tsakonas S, Matsuno K, Fortini ME. Notch signaling. *Science* 1995;268:225–232.

107. Wu L, Aster JC, Blacklow SC. MAML1, a human homologue of *Drosophila* mastermind, is a transcriptional co-activator for NOTCH receptors. *Nat Genet* 2000;26:484–489.

108. Mumm JS, Kopan R. Notch signaling: from the outside in. *Dev Biol* 2000;228:151–165.

109. Martins C, Cavaco B, Tonon G, et al. A study of *MECT1-MAML2* in mucoepidermoid carcinoma and Warthin's tumor of salivary glands. *J Mol Diagn* 2004;6:205–210.

110. Miltelman F, Johansson B, Mertens F. Mitelman database of chromosome aberrations in cancer. http://cgap.nci.nih.gov/Chromosomes/Mitelman.

111. Bullerdiek J, Haubrich J, Meyer K, et al. Translocation t(11;19)(q21;p13.1) as the sole chromosome abnormality in a cystadenolymphoma (Warthin's tumor) of the parotid gland. *Cancer Genet Cytogenet* 1988;35:129–132.

112. Mark J, Dahlenfors R, Stenman G, et al. A human adenolymphoma showing the chromosomal aberrations del (7)(p12p14–15) and t(11;19)(q21;p12–13). *Anticancer Res* 1989;9:1565–1566.

113. Seifert G, Brocheriou C, Cardesa A, et al. WHO International Histological Classification of Tumours: tentative histological classification of salivary gland tumours. *Pathol Res Pract* 1990;186:555–581.

114. Warnnock GR. Papillary cystadenoma lymphomatosum (Warthin's tumor). In: Ellis GL, Auclair PL, Gnepp DR, eds. *Surgical Pathology of the Salivary Glands*. Philadelphia: WB Saunders; 1991:187–201.

115. Auclair PL, Ellis GL. Mucoepidermoid carcinoma of the major salivary glands: clinical and histopathologic analysis of 234 cases with evaluation of grading criteria. *Cancer* 1998;82:1217–1224.

116. Seifert G. Mucoepidermoid carcinoma in a salivary duct cyst of the parotid gland: contribution to the development of tumours in salivary gland cysts. *Pathol Res Pract* 1996;192:1211–1217.

117. Williamson JD, Simmons BH, El-Naggar AK, et al. Mucoepidermoid carcinoma involving Warthin tumor: a report of five cases and review of the literature. *Am J Clin Pathol* 2000;114:564–570.

118. Mark J, Dahlenfors R, Stenman G, et al. Chromosomal patterns in Warthin's tumor: a second type of human benign salivary gland neoplasm. *Cancer Genet Cytogenet* 1990;46:35–39.

119. Helsel JC, Mrak RE, Hanna E, et al. Peripheral primitive neuroectodermal tumor of the parotid gland region: report of a case with fine-needle aspiration findings. *Diagn Cytopathol* 2000;22:161–166.

120. Deb RA, Desai SB, Amonkar PP, et al. Primary primitive neuroectodermal tumour of the parotid gland. *Histopathology* 1998;33:375–378.

121. Valencerina Gopez E, Dauterman J, Layfield LJ. Fine-needle aspiration biopsy of alveolar rhabdomyosarcoma of the parotid: a case report and review of the literature. *Diagn Cytopathol* 2001;24:249–252.

122. De M, Banerjee A, Graham I, et al. Alveolar rhabdomyosarcoma of the parotid gland. *J Laryngol Otol* 2001;115:155–157.

124. Grayson W, Nayler SJ, Jena GP. Synovial sarcoma of the parotid gland: a case report with clinicopathological analysis and review of the literature. *S Afr J Surg* 1998;36:32–35.

Infectious Diseases

The histopathologic findings in routinely processed tissue sometimes provide the first evidence that an infectious etiology underlies the patient's disease, in which case microbiologic culture of the specimen is not possible. In this situation, molecular genetic approaches frequently have higher sensitivity than standard special stains and can often provide information not typically available from special stains, such as species-specific identification and drug sensitivity (Table 22.1). Molecular methods are also a useful way to detect organisms that cannot be cultured (e.g., human papilloma virus [HPV]) or that are notorious for their slow growth in culture (e.g., *Mycobacterium tuberculosis*).

Many of the molecular approaches used to detect pathogens in tissue specimens are adaptations of tests originally designed for automated, high-throughput testing in the clinical microbiology laboratory. Consequently, the tests often employ methodologies that are not commonly encountered in molecular genetic analysis of neoplasms.

BACTERIA

Mycobacteria

Molecular testing for mycobacteria in fixed tissue samples is driven by three clinical realities. First, conventional histochemical stains for acid-fast bacteria lack the sensitivity of microbiologic cultures and are time-consuming to evaluate. Second, it is not possible to discriminate many

---

TABLE 22.1

EXAMPLES OF THE UTILITY OF MOLECULAR GENETIC TESTING IN SURGICAL PATHOLOGY

Reasons for testing
Cultures not sent
Treatment started before cultures were sent
Organism not culturable
Culture period is long
Cultures are negative but there is a high clinical suspicion of infection
Evaluate the response to treatment

Uses for testing
Identification and/or speciation of infectious agent
Drug sensitivity testing
Quantitation of viral load
Detection of cultured organism in tissue itself
Demonstration of an etiologic link between disease and pathogen

mycobacterial species by conventional histochemical stains. Third, microbiologic culture of mycobacteria can take as long as 4 to 6 weeks.

Conventional PCR

Polymerase chain reaction (PCR) is one of the most common molecular approaches used to detect mycobacteria in formalin-fixed, paraffin-embedded (FFPE) tissue. In most studies, the PCR target is the highly conserved gene that encodes the 65-kDa heat shock protein (hsp) (1–6), but other target loci include the genes encoding 16S rRNA (7) or the repetitive insertion element IS6110 (8). PCR testing has been successfully applied to FFPE tissue from a wide variety of sites, including the respiratory tract, gastrointestinal tract, genitourinary tract, skin, bone, liver, and lymph nodes (1,2,5,7,8) and has also been applied to cytology specimens (6).

In general, PCR-based methods have a higher sensitivity than histochemical stains, such as the Ziehl-Neelsen (ZN) stain. In paired analysis in which either FFPE tissue or cytology specimens were the substrate for analysis, the ZN stain detected mycobacteria in only 40% to 58% of cases that were culture positive, while PCR detected mycobacteria in 78% to 100% of cases (1,7,9). In another study, the sensitivity of PCR was shown to be virtually 100% for tissue specimens in which corresponding blood or tissue cultures were positive (8). Not surprisingly, the sensitivity of detection is decreased in paucibacillary specimens (4,10,11), the setting in which the PCR is most likely to produce a false negative result when compared with culture.

Even though the gene encoding the 65-kDa hsp is highly conserved, sequence differences make it possible to use a combined approach to determine the mycobacterial species in infected tissue (Fig. 22.1). The protocol is straightforward: PCR is used to amplify the region of the 65-kDa *hsp* gene, which shows the greatest sequence diversity between different mycobacterial species, and then the PCR product is digested by a panel of restriction endonucleases to produce a pattern of fragments that identifies the particular mycobacterial species (3,5). Although this approach can be used to speciate virtually 100% of cases caused by *Mycobacterium tuberculosis* complex infection, it has less utility for classification of nontuberculous mycobacteria (5). For nontuberculous infections, DNA sequence analysis of the PCR product often provides more information than restriction endonuclease digestion (5).

Although the specificity of PCR-based detection of mycobacteria in tissue samples is quite high, several reports suggest that it is less than 100%. Not surprisingly, the specificity is dependent on the method used to confirm the identity of the PCR product. In one study, restriction endonuclease digestion demonstrated that the PCR product was a nonspecific artifact in 14% of cases, even in some cases in which the PCR product was of the correct size (1).

Alternative Exponential Amplification Methodologies

As noted above, a number of approaches originally developed for use in the clinical microbiology laboratory have also been adapted for use with processed tissue specimens.

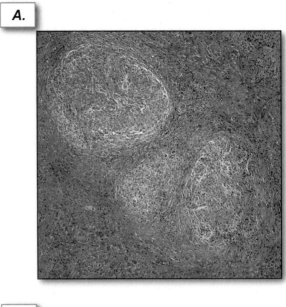

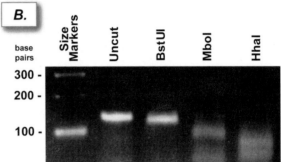

Figure 22.1 Use of PCR coupled with restriction enzyme digestion to identify mycobacterial infection. **A,** Sections of a right neck mass in a 50-year-old man showed granulomatous inflammation, but cultures were not sent at the time of excision. **B,** PCR using primers for the mycobacterial gene encoding the 65-kDA heat shock protein showed a 133-bp product indicative of mycobacterial infection; digestion of the PCR product with *BstU1* yielded a 120-bp fragment, digestion with *Mbo1* yielded bands of about 80 bp and 50 bp, and digestion with *Hha1* yielded bands of about 75 bp and 65 bp. This restriction pattern is indicative of *Mycobacterium fortuitum* according to the established algorithm (reference 8).

One such technique involves isothermal amplification of the IS6110 sequence of mycobacterial species by the method known as strand displacement amplification (12–14). As shown in Figure 22.2, the method has two stages. In the target generation stage, two primers are used to copy the target region; in the exponential amplification stage, a restriction endonuclease is used to nick the DNA copies. Iterative cycles of nicking and displacement produce DNA strands capable of binding the opposite strand primers, producing exponential amplification of the target region, which can be detected in real time through the use of fluorophore-labeled probes. Because the same specialized DNA polymerase is used in both the target generation and exponential amplification stages and because the amplification step does not require DNA melting for primer binding, the reaction can be performed in one tube at one temperature, which not only decreases the time of the test (to about 1 hour), but also decreases the risk of cross-contamination.

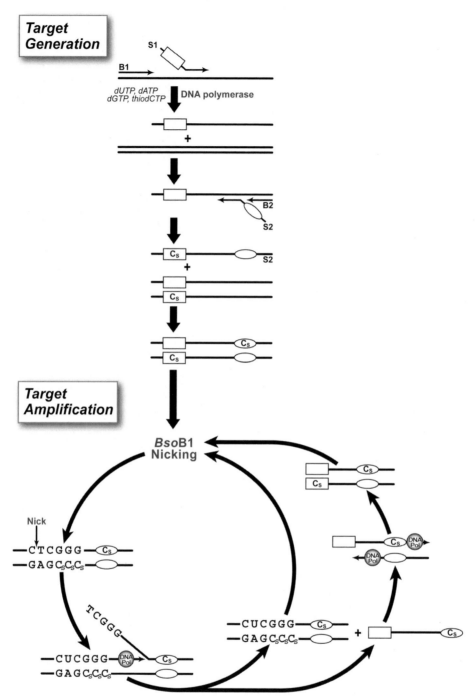

Figure 22.2 Schematic diagram of strand displacement amplification. In the Target Generation stage, a mixture of the DNA template, a specialized DNA polymerase, dATP, dUTP, dGTP, and thiodCTP (dCTP in which one of the phosphate groups is substituted by a thiol group), primers that contain the sequence recognized by the *BsoB1* restriction enzyme (S1 and S2), and bumper primers (B1 and B2) are mixed together in a single tube. Extension of the bumper primers displaces the newly synthesized DNA strands primed by the S1 and S2 primers (Cs indicates strands that contain thiodCTP as a result of DNA synthesis, versus strands that contain unmodified dCTP from the S1 and S2 primers). In the Target Amplification stage, the *BsoB1* enzyme nicks its recognition site (the presence of the thiodCTP makes the site refractory to double-stranded cleavage). The DNA polymerase binds to the nick and synthesizes a new strand, simultaneously displacing the downstream strand. As a result, the double-stranded target is recreated, which serves as a target for iterative rounds of *BsoB1* nicking and DNA polymerization. In addition, the displaced single strand can bind to the opposite strand primer, which generates another copy of the target after extension by DNA polymerase, producing exponential amplification of the target sequence. Note that although the Target Amplification stage is only diagramed for the *BsoB1* site generated by primer S1, identical iterative cycles of nicking and amplification occur from the *BsoB1* site generated by primer S2. A fluorophore-labeled probe also present in the reaction mixture (not diagrammed) is used to quantitate the amplification in real-time. (Modified from reference 12.)

Transcription-mediated amplification is another isothermal amplification method originally designed for use in the clinical microbiology laboratory that has subsequently been applied to processed tissue samples. This technique targets RNA and, as is shown in Figure 22.3, also has two stages (15,16). In the target generation stage, primers that incorporate ribonucleic acid (RNA) polymerase binding sites are used to prime reverse transcription of the RNA target, producing multiple cDNA copies. In the amplification stage, RNA polymerase transcribes the cDNA intermediates, producing RNA molecules that themselves become the targets of reverse transcription. Together, the reverse transcription and RNA polymerization steps produce exponential amplification of the RNA target, which is detected at the

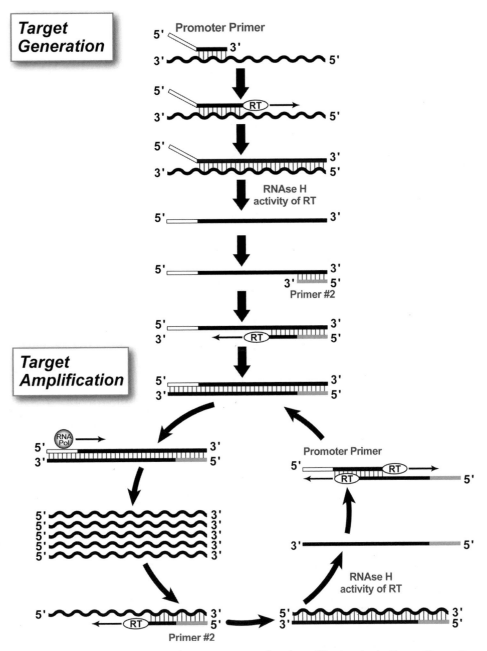

Figure 22.3 Schematic diagram of transcription-mediated amplification. In the Target Generation stage, reverse transcriptase (RT) is used to produce a cDNA copy of the RNA template using a "promoter primer" that includes an RNA polymerase promoter sequence (in this diagram, *solid lines* represent DNA, *wavy lines* represent RNA). The RNAse H activity of RT degrades the RNA strand of the RNA–DNA heteroduplex; the second DNA strand is then produced by RT by extension of primer #2. In the Target Amplification stage, the enzyme T7 RNA polymerase recognizes the RNA polymerase promoter sequence and transcribes multiple RNA copies from the double-stranded DNA. Each of these RNA molecules serves as a template to produce a cDNA copy by extension of primer #2, leading to production of additional double-stranded DNA templates via the same steps as in the Target Generation stage, producing exponential amplification of the target sequence. The reaction product is usually quantitated by use of a chemiluminescent reaction (15,17,18,20).

end of the assay using novel fluorophore-labeled DNA probes (15,17,18,20).

When used prospectively on FFPE tissue with granulomatous inflammation from patients known to have tuberculosis, commercially available strand displacement amplification kits (e.g., BDProbeTec, Becton Dickinson Microbiology Systems, Franklin Lakes, NJ) have a sensitivity of 91% and a specificity of virtually 100% (19). However, the test has a sensitivity of only 40% when applied to archived FFPE tissue of patients known to have tuberculosis, although most false negative results are obtained from specimens that are 3 to 5 years old (19). When used to test archived FFPE pleural biopsy specimens from patients known to have tuberculosis, a commercially available transcription-mediated amplification kit (e.g., AMTDT, Gen-Probe Inc., San Diego, CA) for detecting *M. tuberculosis* has a sensitivity of 53% (20). This level of sensitivity compares favorably with testing via the commercially available LCxMTB kit (Abbott Laboratories Abott Park, IL), an assay based on ligase chain reaction (Chapter 5) that has a sensitivity of 63% and a specificity of 100% (20). However, it is worth noting that these commercially available assays essentially target only organisms of the *M. tuberculosis* complex, which, depending on the patient population, may account for only a subset of disease resulting from mycobacterial infection.

Drug Susceptibility Testing

M. tuberculosis resistance to rifampicin is often associated with isoniazid resistance, and so testing for rifampicin resistance can be used to identify strains of the bacterium likely to be multidrug resistant (21,22). Because rifampicin resistance is known to be due to mutations in the *rpoB* gene (23), mutational analysis can be used to predict drug response. For example, an assay based on single-strand conformational polymorphism analysis (SSCP; Chapter 7) has been used to detect the presence of *rpoB* mutations in lymph node aspirates of 32% of patients diagnosed with tuberculous lymphadenitis (9). Although this result suggests a role for mutational analysis of tissue specimens, its significance is uncertain because the SSCP findings were not correlated with the results of conventional microbiologic resistance testing or with patient response to therapy.

Similarly, direct DNA sequence analysis and heteroduplex analysis (Chapter 7) have been used to detect missense mutations in the *folP1* gene responsible for dapsone resistance in *Mycobacterium leprae*, with 93% correlation between the two methods (24). Even though the assay requires skin biopsies fixed in ethanol, the results are significant since conventional susceptibility testing involves mouse foot pad inoculation because *M. leprae* can not be cultivated on artificial medium (25).

Helicobacter pylori

H. pylori is a gram-negative bacterium associated with a range of disorders including chronic gastritis, peptic ulcer disease, gastric adenocarcinoma, and gastric mucosa-associated lymphoid tissue (MALT) lymphoma. It is interesting to note that the closely related bacterium *C. jejuni* has recently been shown to be associated with immuno-proliferative small intestinal disease (also known as alpha chain disease), a lymphoma that also arises within small intestinal MALT (26).

PCR

Although the genome of *H. pylori* is remarkable for the polymorphism between different clinical isolates, PCR-based methods have nonetheless been developed that permit successful detection of virtually all reported forms of *H. pylori* by PCR from either fresh or FFPE tissue (27–29), including the nonculturable coccoid form of the organism (27). The most common target loci in PCR assays include the *16S rRNA* gene (27), urease gene (29,30), and arbitrarily chosen regions of the *H. pylori* genome (28), although a wide variety of other targets have also been successfully employed (reviewed in 31). In general, PCR-based assays are more sensitive and specific than routine histopathologic examination, culture, and urea breath testing (32).

Recently developed real-time quantitative PCR methods that target the *23S rRNA* gene permit simultaneous detection of *H. pylori* and antibiotic resistant testing (discussed below). For detection of the pathogen, these assays have been shown to have a sensitivity of 96% to 100% and a specificity of 95% to 98% when performed on fresh gastric biopsy specimens, while microbiologic culture and routine histopathologic evaluation have sensitivities of up to 91% and 88%, respectively, in parallel analysis (30,33,34).

Drug Susceptibility Testing

A combination of antimicrobial drugs is used to treat *H. pylori* infection, but a meta-analysis of published studies demonstrate that treatment failure is strongly linked to the presence of macrolide resistance resulting from mutations in the *23S rRNA* gene (35). Real-time quantitative PCR that targets the mutated region of the *23S rRNA* gene shows a 96% to 98% concordance with culture-based sensitivity testing when fresh gastric biopsy specimens are the substrate for analysis (30,33). In cases in which there is a discrepancy between culture-based and PCR-based sensitivity testing, a mixed infection of both susceptible and resistant strains is invariably present (30,33). It is worth noting that the sensitivity of PCR-based testing for macrolide-resistant *H. pylori* strains depends on the biopsy protocol and is optimized if multiple sites in both the antrum and the corpus are sampled at the time of upper endoscopy (36).

A fluorescence in situ hybridization (FISH)-based method has been developed that also makes it possible to perform simultaneous testing for *H. pylori* infection and macrolide-resistance on routinely processed FFPE tissue. The commercially available test, CreaFast *H. pylori* Combi Kit (SeaPro Diagnostics Ltd., Liverpool, UK), employs three oligonucleotide probes designed to detect the most prevalent *23S rRNA* mutations that are responsible for macrolide-resistance (37,38). When applied to sections of FFPE tissue of gastric biopsies, the test has virtually 100% sensitivity for detecting the presence of *H. pylori* infection, and shows 90% to 100% correlation with culture-based sensitivity testing (37–39). The approach also makes it possible to determine the antibiotic sensitivity of the nonculturable coccoid form of the organism (38,39).

Other Bacterial Pathogens

PCR has been used to detect *Bacillus anthracis* organisms in patient specimens associated with bioterrorism (40,41) or accidental environmental release from bioweapons facilities (42). The most sensitive testing involves analysis of multiple loci, including genes from the *B. anthracis* virulence plasmids and may require an increased number of amplification cycles when applied to analysis of FFPE tissue (41). PCR can detect the pathogen's DNA even from biopsy specimens obtained at least 3 days after initiation of antibiotic therapy (41), which enhances the utility of testing because it makes it possible to confirm infection even in patients for whom the initial differential diagnosis did not include anthrax. Taken together, these reports suggest that molecular genetic testing may have an important role in the evaluation of cases of suspected bioterrorism. One study has suggested that immunohistochemical analysis has a much higher sensitivity for the diagnosis of cutaneous anthrax than PCR, but because the details of the PCR protocol were not reported, it is difficult to evaluate the significance of the result (40).

Unanticipated Results

Not unexpectedly, PCR-based testing of tissue samples occasionally produces unanticipated results. For example, some studies (many of which involve a nested approach in order to achieve maximum test sensitivity) have detected mycobacterial DNA in 7% to 14% of cases of sarcoidosis (2,8). Although the results were confirmed by repeat testing and DNA sequence analysis of the PCR products, it nonetheless remains unclear whether the findings are due to incorrect clinical diagnoses, specimen cross-contamination, or an association of sarcoidosis with mycobacterial infection as has been suggested by other sporadic reports (2,43–45). Similarly, PCR for genes present in *Yersinia enterocolitica* and *Y. pseudotuberculosis*, the two *Yersinia* species that cause human gastrointestinal disease, yields a positive result in 31% of resection specimens of patients with known Crohn's disease (46). Although it is easy to dismiss such unanticipated results as false positives due to poor laboratory technique or specimen cross-contamination, it is also possible that the results are an indication of an unrecognized component of the disease process. Nonetheless, it would seem imprudent to base diagnosis or therapy on unexpected findings unless they are verified by independent techniques.

FUNGI

Microbiologic diagnosis of fungal infection can be challenging because many fungal pathogens are difficult to culture (especially if antifungal therapy has been initiated) and grow very slowly. Consequently, even if the need for microbiologic cultures is recognized at the time of surgery, diagnosis may still rely on histologic identification of fungal pathogens in tissue sections. When a paucity of organisms

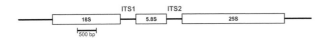

Figure 22.4 Schematic diagram of the fungal gene cluster encoding ribosomal RNAs 18S, 5.8S, and 25S. The location of the two internal transcribed spacer regions ITS1 and ITS2 is shown. Because this gene cluster is highly variable between different fungi, the indicated scale is only approximate.

or an ambiguous morphology complicates histologic diagnosis, ancillary testing using DNA-based methods can be helpful. The two techniques that have the most utility in this setting are PCR and ISH.

PCR

Most PCR assays target sequences within the fungal rRNA genes (Fig. 22.4). PCR can be performed using universal primers that bind to highly conserved sequences in the region, followed by direct or indirect DNA sequence analysis of the PCR product to identify the specific fungal pathogen (47,48). Alternatively, sequence differences in the *18S rRNA* gene can be used to design primers that are specific for individual fungal pathogens (49).

The universal primer PCR approach utilizes primers that bind to regions of sequence homology in the internal transcribed spacer (ITS) regions to amplify ITS1, 5.8S rRNA, and ITS2 sequences. Because the ITS regions vary in both sequence and length between different fungal pathogens, primers that bind to conserved regions in ITS1 and ITS2 can be used to identify specific fungi based on either the size of the PCR product as determined by simple gel electrophoresis or the PCR product's sequence (50–52). PCR analysis with universal primers has been shown to have a sensitivity of 83% and a specificity of virtually 100% for identifying a wide range of pathogenic fungi in specimens collected by scarification from the active edges of from patients with dermatomycoses, including *Trichophyton* spp., *Microsporum gypseum*, and a variety of yeasts including *Candida* spp. (52). Similarly, a modified multiplex PCR designed to identify eight common fungal pathogens, including *Aspergillus flavus*, *A. fumigatus*, *Candida albicans*, *C. krusei*, *C. glabrata*, *C. parapsilosis*, *C. tropicalis*, and *Cryptococcus neoformans* has been shown to have a sensitivity for each of the pathogens comparable to that of PCR performed separately for each of the fungi (51,53,54). In parallel analysis, the multiplex PCR has a sensitivity of 95%, compared with 35% and 60% for microbiologic culture and routine histopathologic evaluation, respectively (51).

Testing for *Sporothrix schenckii*, the fungus responsible for cutaneous sporotrichosis, provides one example of a setting in which PCR using pathogen-specific *18S rRNA* primers has been performed. Testing is necessary because cutaneous sporotrichosis often presents as a nonspecific granulomatous reaction and the paucity of organisms in infected tissue makes it difficult to identify the fungus by routine histopathologic evaluation (55). When fresh tissue is the substrate for analysis, a nested PCR approach for *18S rRNA*, microbiologic culture, and fungal identification by periodic acid–Schiff (PAS) stain have sensitivities of 91%, 67%, and 58%, respectively; PCR and culture both have a specificity of 100% (49). However, the specificity of PCR testing is decreased significantly when colonization by nonpathogenic organisms is present (56), a indication that there are *18S rRNA* sequence similarities between fungi that are often not accounted for during primer design.

Sequence polymorphisms of the mitochondrial large subunit rRNA gene have also been used as a target in PCR tests to identify fungal pathogens in tissue specimens (57,58). This approach has been used to discriminate between *Pneumocystis carinii* and *P. jirovecii* in FFPE lung tissue from immunocompetent children who were victims of sudden infant death syndrome (58), which emphasizes that PCR-based identification of fungal pathogens can be successfully applied to routinely processed tissue.

Quantitative PCR (Q-PCR) methods have also been developed for detection of fungal pathogens in tissue specimens. In general, the sensitivity and specificity of these assays varies based on the C_t chosen as a cutoff for a positive test result (59). However, when optimized, Q-PCR using universal primers for the *18S rRNA* gene has a higher sensitivity for detecting fungal infection than either direct microscopy or microbiologic culture alone, and the identity of the pathogen based on the Q-PCR is 100% concordant with the results of microbiologic culture (47).

In situ Hybridization

Several studies have shown that ISH can be used to determine the genus or species of yeastlike and filamentous fungi in tissue sections for which definitive identification based on routine light microscopy is difficult or impossible. One set of probes allows differentiation of five different yeastlike organisms (specifically *Blastomyces dermatitidis*, *Coccidioides immitis*, *Cyrptococcus neoformans*, *Histoplasma capsulatum*, and *Sporothrix schenckii*) based on sequence differences in their *18S rRNA* and *28S rRNA* genes (60). Although routine histologic evaluation of tissue sections stained with Grocott's methanemine silver (GMS) has a slightly greater sensitivity than ISH overall, ISH makes it possible to accurately identify rare or atypical organisms that cannot be definitely classified solely on morphologic features (60). Similarly, probes for genus-specific sequence differences in the *18S rRNA* and *5S rRNA* genes can be used to distinguish filamentous fungi, including *Aspergillus*, *Zygomycetes*, and *Candida* in sections of routinely processed FFPE tissue with a sensitivity of 95% to 100% (which favorably compares with the sensitivity of histologic examination of either GMS- or PAS-stained sections), although the specificity of ISH is dependent on the genus of the fungus (61,62).

Aspergillus, *Fusarium*, and *Pseudallescheria* can be especially difficult to differentiate in routinely processed tissue sections, even by GMS or PAS stains, because all have a septae branched hyphal morphology. Using a panel of probes against *5S rRNA*, *18S rRNA*, and *28S rRNA* sequences specific for each genus, ISH has a sensitivity of 85% for detecting the presence of fungi in routinely processed tissue versus 100% by morphologic examination of GMS- or PAS-stained sections, when microbiologic culture is the gold standard (63). However, in contrast to morphologic examination of GMS- or PAS-stained sections, ISH has 100% specificity for identification of the genus of the fungal pathogen and can

even be used to document the presence of mixed fungal infections (63).

VIRUSES

Molecular genetic techniques, including PCR-based methods, ISH, and isothermal amplification can be used to detect the presence of viruses in cytology or tissue specimens and identify the cell types that are infected by the virus. Other techniques such as Q-PCR and branch DNA (bDNA) methodology (discussed later) make it possible to quantitate the viral lode, which often has prognostic and therapeutic implications.

Molecular methods offer several advantages over the traditional microbiologic or serologic methods that are used to diagnose viral infection. Viral culture, widely considered the reference standard, often takes days to weeks, and requires stringent specimen transport and storage conditions to preserve viral infectivity. Similarly, direct immunofluorescent antibody staining often requires stringent specimen transport and storage conditions. Serologic tests are often of little utility within the first several weeks of infection and may produce false negatives in patients who are immunocompromized.

Human Papilloma Virus

PCR

Most PCR protocols for HPV testing make use of consensus primers targeted to the viral *L1* gene that are potentially capable of detecting all HPV types that affect the anogenital region. The widely used MY09/11 primer set amplifies a region of the *L1* gene that is about 450 bp long (64), but nondegenerate primer pools that target the *L1* gene can be used to detect an even broader range of HPV types (65,66). Primer sets that amplify shorter regions of the *L1* gene can be used to increase the sensitivity of analysis (67–71), especially when testing FFPE tissue. Following amplification using consensus primers, the HPV type can be determined by either DNA sequence analysis (72,73) or membrane hybridization with type-specific probes (see later discussion). However, both approaches are labor intensive and difficult to automate, which makes them poorly suited for screening a large volume of patient specimens. Solution hybridization methods (discussed later) are more well suited for high-throughput analysis.

Membrane Hybridization

In the reverse hybridization line probe assay (LiPA), PCR is performed using a pool of primers for the *L1* gene, and the PCR product is hybridized to a membrane that is arrayed with oligonucleotide probes specific for individual HPV types (71,74–76) (the phrase reverse hybridization in the assay name reflects the fact that the probe is bound to the membrane rather than the target nucleic acid strand, the reverse of the usual scenario for filter hybridization assays, as discussed in Chapter 6). The bound PCR product is detected via a chromogenic reaction, and its position in the array indicates the HPV type (Fig. 22.5). Comparison of direct DNA sequence analysis and LiPA has shown that PCR followed by direct sequence analysis is more sensitive (73). Initially, there was only moderate concordance between PCR and LiPA for identification of specific HPV types, but more recent versions of the LiPA assay have a higher specificity for a broader range of HPV types.

Solution Hybridization Methods

The Hybrid Capture 2 test (HC2, marketed by Digene Gaithersburg, MD) utilizes two pools of synthetic RNA

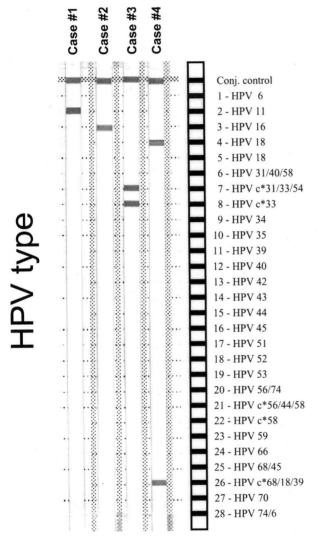

probes to detect five low-risk HPV types (types 6, 11, 42, 43, and 44) or 13 high-risk HPV types (16, 18, 31, 33, 35, 39, 45, 51, 52, 56, 58, 59, and 68). The method involves three steps: DNA is extracted from the specimen and hybridized in solution to either probe cocktail, the DNA-RNA hybrids are captured by antibodies specific for RNA:DNA hybrids, and the bound RNA:DNA hybrids are detected using a chemiluminescent probe (see Fig. 16.1). As discussed in more detail in Chapter 16, the HC2 test has a very high sensitivity and, because the low-risk and high-risk probes have limited cross-reactivity, testing also has high specificity (73,77,78). Because the assay is easy to perform, can be completed within several hours, is not hindered by cross-contamination, and can potentially be automated, the method is ideally suited for clinical use in high-volume settings.

In parallel analysis, there is only fair concordance between HC2 testing using the low-risk probe set and LiPA (kappa value, 0.21) and moderate concordance between HC2 testing using the high-risk probe set and LiPA (kappa value, 0.56), findings that reflect the fact that many of the HPV types detected by LiPA are not specifically targeted by the HC2 assay (73). However, the high concordance between participating laboratories (kappa value, 0.84) in a study of interlaboratory reproducibility demonstrates that the HC2 test is very reliable (79).

In situ Hybridization

Chromogenic in situ hybridization (CISH) is an approach that not only makes it possible to link the presence or absence of HPV infection with the cytomorphology of individual cells, but also makes it possible to determine whether nor not the viral genome is integrated into the host genome (80). As discussed in more detail in Chapter 16, the widely used commercially available INFORM HPV method (Ventana Medical Systems, Inc., Tucson, AZ) utilizes a probe cocktail that recognizes high-risk HPV types 16, 18, 31, 33, 35, 39, 45, 51, 52, 56, 58, 68, and 70 to generate a chromogenic product that can be visualized by routine microscopy (Fig. 16.2). Comparison of HPV CISH and HC2 solution hybridization by parallel analysis of liquid-based cervical/vaginal cytology specimens with atypical squamous cells of undetermined significance (ASCUS) has shown that, of the samples that tested positive for high-risk HPV DNA, only 20% were positive by both the CISH and solution hybridization methods (81). In addition, solution hybridization had a higher sensitivity for women under 40 years of age (81). However, it is difficult to evaluate the significance of these results because the ISH analysis was often not performed within 21 days of sample collection as recommended by the CISH kit manufacturer.

Figure 22.5 A line-probe assay (LiPA) for human papillomavirus (HPV) by the INNO-LiPA HPV genotyping assay (Innogenetics Inc., Alpharetta, GA). The HPV type is indicated by the position at which the PCR product binds to the filter paper strip, using the key to the right. Case 1: HPV type 11 from an anal condyloma. Case 2: HPV type 16 from a cervical biopsy with high-grade squamous dysplasia. Case 3: HPV type 33 from SCC of the base of the tongue (positive hybridization to the c*33 probe [line 8] and the c*31/33/54 probe [line 7] indicates infection with HPV type 33 alone rather than a mixed infection). Case 4: HPV type 18 from SCC of the tonsil (positive hybridization to the 18 probe [line 4] and c*68/18/39 probe [line 26] indicates infection with HPV type 18 alone rather than a mixed infection). (Cases 3 and 4 courtesy Dr. Sushama Patil and Dr. Samir El-Mofty, Washington University School of Medicine, St. Louis, MO.)

Hepatitis C Virus

PCR

As discussed in more detail in Chapter 15, reverse transcriptase PCR (RT-PCR) methods used to detect hepatitis C virus (HCV) in liver biopsy specimens focus on the 5' noncoding region of the virus that is highly conserved between the (at least) 6 genotypes and more than 90 subtypes of HCV that have been described worldwide (82). When applied to liver specimens from patients who show serologic evidence of infection, analysis of fresh tissue has a sensitivity of 86% to 88% and analysis of FFPE tissue has a sensitivity of 69% to 98%, which compare favorably with the sensitivity of testing by routine histology, immunohistochemical staining, and ISH of 72%, 47% to 80%, and 42% to 95%, respectively (83–86). However, maximal RT-PCR test sensitivity can be achieved only via a nested RT-PCR approach (83,86) or when the PCR products are evaluated by Southern blot hybridization (87). When applied to liver specimens from patients who are serum antibody negative, RT-PCR testing detects evidence of HCV infection in about 50% of patients, a level of sensitivity that again compares favorably with the sensitivity of testing by immunohistochemisty or ISH of 69% and 50%, respectively (83,86).

Although in situ RT-PCR has also been used to detect HCV infection in FFPE tissue, several factors mitigate against the use of this assay in routine practice. First, the methodology is technically demanding. Second, the sensitivity of the technique is lower than that of other methodologies; specifically, for analysis of FFPE tissue from patients who are serum antibody positive, in situ RT-PCR has a sensitivity of only 54% to 67% for detecting HCV (88,89) versus the 69% to 98% sensitivity of traditional RT-PCR (83,84,86).

In situ Hybridization

ISH methods used to detect HCV in liver biopsy specimens also focus on the highly conserved 5' noncoding region of the virus. Because the HCV viral genome consists of a single-stranded, positive-sense RNA, ISH methods use either cDNA probes or cRNA probes (also known as riboprobes). Although early reports suggested that ISH had low sensitivity, more recent studies have shown that the approach has a sensitivity that is comparable to that of RT-PCR for analysis of serum antibody positive or negative patients, as noted previously (84).

Membrane Hybridization

A commercially available LiPA assay (INNO-LiPA, Innogenetics Inc., Alpharetta, GA) provides one of the most straightforward approaches for HCV genotype determination. Thus far the assay has been applied only to the analysis of blood, but it has shown a high degree of correlation with other HCV genotyping methods (90,91). Because testing is informative when applied to blood, it is unclear whether the method provides any additional information if applied to tissue specimens.

Branched DNA

The viral load of HCV correlates with prognosis and response to therapy, as does the viral load of hepatitis B virus (HBV). bDNA analysis is a novel proprietary method (Bayer Health Care, Tarrytown, NY) for quantifying viral load and, as shown in Figure 22.6, is essentially a hybridization-based amplification methodology (92). The approach has been shown to be a highly reliable and reproducible method for analysis of not only HCV (93,94) and HBV (95), but also a number of other viral pathogens, including human immunodeficiency virus (HIV) (96,97). The results of bDNA analysis are also highly correlated with traditional Q-PCR or transcription-mediated amplification methods (94–97). bDNA analysis has thus far been applied only to blood samples, but the method's simplicity and high reproducibility suggest that it will likely have utility when modified for use with tissue specimens. A recent cost analysis indicates that the approach is not well suited for use in developing countries (98).

Epstein-Barr Virus

In situ Hybridization

Two different types of nonradioactive ISH have been used to detect EBV infection in a wide range of tumor types. The most common method is a DNA-ISH assay directed against

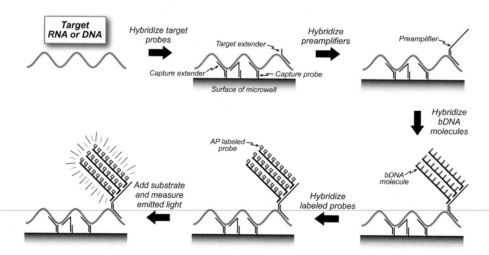

Figure 22.6 Schematic diagram of branched DNA (bDNA) methodology. The assay employs plastic 96-well plates that have "capture" probes attached to the surface of each microwell. The target nucleic acid binds to the well via hybridization to "capture extender" probes, and hybridization of the bDNA molecule is accomplished via "target extender" and "preamplifer" probes. Bound bDNA molecules are detected quantitatively by alkaline phosphatase–conjugated "labeled probes," which generate a chemiluminescent signal when a dioxetane substrate is added to the well.

BamH1W sequences that are repeated 7 to 14 times in the genome of most EBV strains (99,100); the probe used in the assay can be obtained commercially (ENZO Biochemical, Inc., New York, NY). In contrast, RNA-ISH uses a mixture of antisense probes that target small nontranslated virally encoded *EBER1* and *EBER2* transcripts; because *EBER1* and *EBER2* transcripts are present at roughly 10^7 copies per cell in both latent and lytic EBV infections, the RNA-ISH assay is very sensitive (101–103). Although *EBER* antisense probes can be produced by standard techniques (72), the probes are most often obtained from commercial vendors (e.g., Biogenex, San Ramon, CA). DNA-ISH and RNA-ISH can be used to test for EBV in FFPE tissue (Fig. 22.7), and both methodologies make it possible to correlate histopathologic changes of disease with the specific cell types that are infected (87,99,102,103).

PCR

A quantitative PCR methodology has been described that targets five highly conserved segments of the EBV genome (87). When applied to FFPE tissue from a variety of tumor types, Q-PCR testing shows 100% correlation with RNA-ISH analysis when all five EBV genomic markers are analyzed, but the sensitivity of the Q-PCR is significantly lower if it involves analysis of only a subset of the marker loci (87). Notably, the Q-PCR methodology is both more rapid and less labor intensive than RNA-ISH.

Respiratory Viruses

Two of the most common laboratory techniques for detecting respiratory virus are viral culture (which is often limited by an extended growth period and stringent specimen requirements) and immunofluorescent staining (which is often limited by difficulty in test interpretation and stringent specimen requirements). Although PCR assays have been developed for many individual viruses, a multiplex RT-PCR assay for seven common respiratory viruses (specifically, adenovirus, influenza types A and B, respiratory syncytial virus, and parainfluenza types 1, 2, and 3) is one of the most efficient molecular approaches thus far described (104). The multiplex assay not only has a specificity of 100% for each viral pathogen, but also has a sensitivity for each virus that is superior to direct immunofluorescent staining alone or combined immunofluorescent staining and viral culture.

Coronavirus

A nested RT-PCR assay has been described (105) for detection of the coronavirus responsible for severe acute respiratory syndrome (SARS) (106,107). The method can be applied to FFPE tissue from both open lung biopsies and necropsy specimens, a feature of the assay that is important given the virulence of the pathogen (105). The rapidity and simplicity of the approach make it ideally suited for diagnosis given the epidemiology of SARS outbreaks.

RNA-ISH performed using DNA probes or riboprobes to a variety of viral transcripts has also been used to detect the virus that causes SARS (105,108–110), but thus far the methodology has primarily been used to characterize the pathobiology of infection (108,111). Even though the results of RNA-ISH and PCR are highly correlated (105), ISH testing will likely have only a limited role for clinical diagnosis of SARS because PCR analysis is fast and less labor intensive.

Smallpox

Although the last cases of human smallpox disease were reported in 1979, potential use of the virus as an agent of bioterrorism has emphasized the limitations of traditional

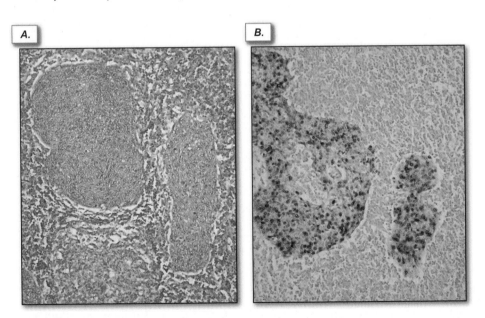

Figure 22.7 Chromogenic in situ hybridization (CISH) for detection of Epstein-Barr virus (EBV). **A,** A lymphoepithelial-like carcinoma involving the thymus, mediastinum, and lung of a 13-year-old girl. **B,** CISH using EBER probes shows positive nuclear staining in over 95% of the epithelial cells, but not the inflammatory cells, a result that confirms the diagnosis of lymphoepithelial-like carcinoma. (See color insert.)

laboratory methods for diagnosis (112,113). Even with a heightened index of suspension, routine histopathologic evaluation cannot reliably distinguish smallpox infection from other virally induced vesicle diseases, including varicella-zoster and disseminated herpes simplex (114,115). Consequently, there has been increased interest in the use of molecular techniques to collect more rapid and accurate laboratory diagnosis.

A DNA-ISH assay has been developed that shows 100% specificity for distinguishing smallpox from varicella-zoster and disseminated herpes simplex, with 100% sensitivity (114). The ISH assay can be applied to routinely processed FFPE tissue and can be completed within 4 hours, technical features that make the assay well suited for rapid and specific identification of smallpox infection. As an aside, control testing using probes for varicella-zoster and herpes simplex has also demonstrated that one third of cases diagnosed as disseminated herpes simplex actually represent varicella-zoster, which further indicates the difficulty of differentiating virally induced vesicle diseases based on histopathologic features alone (114).

A quantitative PCR assay has been developed to distinguish *Variola* from *Orthopox* species infections of human tissues (116). Although the assay has been used successfully with FFPE tissue, it is difficult to determine its sensitivity and specificity because such a small number of cases has been evaluated and because paired analysis by other methodologies has not been performed.

Microarrays

The use of microarray analysis of gene expression profiles for diagnosis of viral infections has also been described. Using customized oligonucleotides, an array has been developed that can detect and distinguish between related serotypes of over 100 different viral pathogens, including picornaviruses, rhinoviruses, orthomyxoviruses, paramyxoviruses, nidoviruses, retroviruses, adenoviruses, papillomaviruses, and herpesviruses (117). Thus far, microarray analysis has been used to evaluate only nasal lavage specimens and has not been used with either fresh or FFPE tissue specimens. However, because it is essentially impossible to screen for such a wide variety of pathogens by routine culture, PCR, or even multiplex PCR, the microarray approach may have a higher sensitivity than traditional methods, especially because it can detect mixed viral infections that likely go unrecognized by traditional molecular methods (117).

Novel Disease Associations

Molecular analysis of diseases traditionally not considered to have a viral etiology has produced some unexpected findings. As examples, ISH analysis has demonstrated latent EBV infection or cytomegalovirus (CMV) infection in synovial tissue in several different types of autoimmune chronic arthritis, including rheumatoid arthritis and psoriatic arthritis (102). PCR has shown the presence of herpes simplex virus (HSV) in 88% of histologically positive temporal artery biopsies from patients with clinically suspected giant cell arthritis and in 53% of biopsies that are histologically negative from patients with clinically suspected giant

cell arthritis (118). RT-PCR has even revealed the presence of human herpesvirus-8 (HHV) DNA sequences in 100% of cases of pulmonary inflammatory myofibroblastic tumor (119). Although such findings are provocative, until they are repeated by other groups or independent methodologies, it is premature to use the molecular tests as the basis for diagnosis.

PROTOZOANS

Worldwide, tens of millions of immunocompetent individuals suffer from diseases caused by protozoans, although in the United States clinical disease caused by this group of organisms is primarily encountered in immunocompromized patients. A variety of molecular techniques has been used to increase the accuracy or timeliness of diagnosis of protozoan infections using tissue specimens, a few examples of which follow.

Toxoplasmosis

Several different PCR-based assays for *Toxoplasma gondii*, the etiologic agent of toxoplasmosis, have been developed. The assays have clinical utility because serologic diagnosis of active infection is unreliable since IgM levels do not correlate with recent infection and since reactivation of disease is not always accompanied by changes in antibody levels (120,121).

Although it is difficult to compare the sensitivity and specificity of different approaches because of a lack of standardization, PCR assays have an overall sensitivity of 50% to 80% for diagnosis of prenatal infection, higher than either traditional cell culture or mouse inoculation (reviewed in 122). In one recent study in which two widely used primer pairs (both of which target the *B1* gene, which is repeated about 35 times in the organism's genome) were compared in parallel testing of blood or fresh tissue from placenta, the primer pairs had markedly different sensitivities. Furthermore, both pairs were associated with the amplification of spurious amplification products in 8% to 31% of cases, and optimal performance was achieved only when the identity of the PCR product was confirmed by either Southern blot analysis or direct DNA sequence analysis (123).

Quantitative-PCR methods have also been used to detect *T. gondii* infection. Using primers designed to amply the *B1* gene, Q-PCR shows 100% correlation with the results of nested PCR when routinely processed FFPE fetal tissue specimens are the substrate for analysis (121). However, up to 100-fold higher sensitivity is achieved when a 529-bp element that is repeated more than 300 times in the genome of the parasite is the target of the Q-PCR assay (120). Selection of an appropriate C_t quantitative threshold, coupled with melting curve analysis to confirm the identity of the PCR product, can be used to maintain 100% assay specificity despite the marked increase in sensitivity. Although the Q-PCR assay has thus far been used primarily to test amniotic fluid specimens, the extreme sensitivity and high specificity of the approach suggests that it is well suited for use with tissue specimens.

Leishmaniasis

About 12 million people worldwide suffer from disease caused by parasites of the genus *Leishmania* (124). The spectrum of disease depends on the species of the parasite, and ranges from a limited number of cutaneous ulcers, to mucocutaneous or systemic involvement as a result of metastasis or dissemination via the blood or lymphatics. The appropriate clinical treatment, either topical or systemic chemotherapy, is therefore dependent on identification of the species responsible for infection. Although routine histopathologic examination of tissue biopsies can be used to detect the parasite in 16% to 74% of cases (125), the organism cannot be speciated based on morphology alone, and so identification has historically relied on enzyme electrophoresis, DNA hybridization, or genomewide survey based on restriction fragment length polymorphism (RFLP) analysis (126,127), all of which are labor-intensive techniques that require a relative large sample for testing.

A number of PCR-based approaches have been used to increase the accuracy and ease of testing. In these assays, a number of different loci have served as targets, including repetitive nuclear DNA sequences and genes encoding rRNA. However, assays that target kinetoplast DNA are some of the most useful. PCR using primers that amplify a 120-bp fragment of kinetoplast DNA can be used to identify the parasite in either fresh or FFPE tissue from cutaneous biopsies with a sensitivity of 92% to 100% and a specificity of 100% (128–130); this PCR approach has a higher sensitivity than all other diagnostic methods that have been evaluated, including serologic testing, microbiologic culture, routine histopathologic evaluation, and immunohistochemical staining (130). A polymorphism specific PCR method has also been developed, which, when applied to the five major species responsible for endemic New World cutaneous leishmaniasis, permits subgenus and species identification of parasites with 100% sensitivity and 100% specificity compared with the results of microbiologic culture (131). The utility of this latter approach in actual clinical practice is suggested by the fact that the reported level of accuracy was achieved by analysis of FFPE biopsy samples.

Intestinal Parasites

Microsporidia are obligate intracellular parasites and are a cause of diarrhea and disseminated infection, especially in patients with immunocompromise resulting from HIV infection (132). At least six different protozoans have been associated with human microsporidiosis, some of which are morphologically indistinguishable. Because different pathogenic microsporidia can have different sensitivities to antimicrobial agents, molecular testing provides an opportunity to establish the diagnosis and direct therapy (133). A nested PCR that targets the gene encoding the small subunit rRNA gene of microsporidia has been described that can be used with fresh tissue specimens for species-specific detection of four different pathogens, including *Encephalitozoon cuniculi*, *E. hellem*, *E. (Septata) intestinalis*, and *Enterocytozoon bieneusi*.

Similarly, PCR targeted to genes encoding 18S rRNA or oocyst wall proteins can be used to document infection with *Cryptosporidium*, a major cause of diarrheal disease worldwide, especially in immunocompromized patients because of either HIV infection or primary immunodeficiency syndromes (134). When applied to fresh liver tissue, PCR has a markedly higher sensitivity than traditional microbiologic analysis by modified ZN staining or immunofluorescence, and DNA sequence analysis of the PCR product makes it possible to determine the *Cryptosporidium* species responsible for infection (134). The clinical relevance of molecular testing is demonstrated by the finding that PCR-based detection of infection, even in asymptomatic patients, correlates with diarrhea and cholangiopathy following transplant-associated immunosuppression (134).

REFERENCES

1. Ghossein RA, Ross DG, Salomon RN, et al. Rapid detection and species identification of mycobacteria in paraffin-embedded tissues by polymerase chain reaction. *Diagn Mol Pathol* 1992;1:185–191.
2. Popper HH, Winter E, Hofler G. DNA of *Mycobacterium tuberculosis* in formalin-fixed, paraffin-embedded tissue in tuberculosis and sarcoidosis detected by polymerase chain reaction. *Am J Clin Pathol* 1994;101:738–741.
3. Cook SM, Bartos RE, Pierson CL, et al. Detection and characterization of atypical mycobacteria by the polymerase chain reaction. *Diagn Mol Pathol* 1994;3:53–58.
4. Perosio PM, Frank TS. Detection and species identification of mycobacteria in paraffin sections of lung biopsy specimens by the polymerase chain reaction. *Am J Clin Pathol* 1993;100:643–647.
5. Schulz S, Cabras AD, Kremer M, et al. Species identification of mycobacteria in paraffin-embedded tissues: frequent detection of nontuberculous mycobacteria. *Mod Pathol* 2005;18:274–282.
6. Shim JJ, Cheong HJ, Kang EY, et al. Nested polymerase chain reaction for detection of *Mycobacterium tuberculosis* in solitary pulmonary nodules. *Chest* 1998;113:20–24.
7. Hardman WJ, Benian GM, Howard T, et al. Rapid detection of mycobacteria in inflammatory necrotizing granulomas from formalin-fixed, paraffin-embedded tissue by PCR in clinically high-risk patients with acid-fast stain and culture-negative tissue biopsies. *Am J Clin Pathol* 1996;106:384–389.
8. Vago L, Barberis M, Gori A, et al. Nested polymerase chain reaction for *Mycobacterium tuberculosis* IS6110 sequence on formalin-fixed paraffin-embedded tissues with granulomatous diseases for rapid diagnosis of tuberculosis. *Am J Clin Pathol* 1998;109:411–415.
9. Gong G, Lee H, Kang GH, et al. Nested PCR for diagnosis of tuberculous lymphadenitis and PCR-SSCP for identification of rifampicin resistance in fine-needle aspirates. *Diagn Cytopathol* 2002;26:228–231.
10. Degitz K, Steidl M, Neubert U, et al. Detection of mycobacterial DNA in paraffin-embedded specimens of lupus vulgaris by polymerase-chain reaction. *Arch Dermatol Res* 1993;285:168–170.
11. Wichitwechkarn J, Karnjan S, Shuntawuttisettee S, et al. Detection of *Mycobacterium leprae* infection by PCR. *J Clin Microbiol* 1995;33:45–49.
12. Little MC, Andrews J, Moore R, et al. Strand displacement amplification and homogeneous real-time detection incorporated in a second-generation DNA probe system, BDProbeTecET. *Clin Chem* 1999;45:777–784.
13. Hellyer TJ, Nadeau JG. Strand displacement amplification: a versatile tool for molecular diagnostics. *Expert Rev Mol Diagn* 2004;4:251–261.
14. Walker GT, Fraiser MS, Schram JL, et al. Strand displacement amplification: an isothermal, in vitro DNA amplification technique. *Nucleic Acids Res* 1992;20:1691–1696.
15. http://www.gen-probe.com/pdfs/pi/IN0013F-01revc.pdf.
16. Hill CS. Molecular diagnostic testing for infectious diseases using TMA WD technology. *Expert Rev Mol Diagn* 2001;1:445–455.
17. Arnold LJ Jr, Hammond PW, Wiese WA, et al. Assay formats involving acridinium-ester-labeled DNA probes. *Clin Chem* 1989;35:1588–1594.
18. Ishiguro T, Saitoh J, Horie R, et al. Intercalation activating fluorescence DNA probe and its application to homogeneous quantification of a target sequence by isothermal sequence amplification in a closed vessel. *Anal Biochem* 2003;314:77–86.
19. Johansen IS, Thomsen VO, Forsgren A, et al. Detection of *Mycobacterium tuberculosis* complex in formalin-fixed, paraffin-embedded tissue specimens with necrotizing granulomatous inflammation by strand displacement amplification. *J Mol Diagn* 2004;6:231–236.
20. Ruiz-Manzano J, Manterola JM, Gamboa F, et al. Detection of *Mycobacterium tuberculosis* in paraffin-embedded pleural biopsy specimens by commercial ribosomal RNA and DNA amplification kits. *Chest* 2000;118:648–655.
21. Heym B, Honore N, Truffot-Pernot C, et al. Implications of multidrug resistance for the future of short-course chemotherapy of tuberculosis: a molecular study. *Lancet* 1994;344:293–298.
22. Watterson SA, Wilson SM, Yates MD, et al. Comparison of three molecular assays for rapid detection of rifampin resistance in *Mycobacterium tuberculosis*. *J Clin Microbiol* 1998;36:1969–1973.
23. Telenti A, Imboden P, Marchesi F, et al. Detection of rifampicin-resistance mutations in *Mycobacterium tuberculosis*. *Lancet* 1993;341:647–650.
24. Williams DL, Pittman TL, Gillis TP, et al. Simultaneous detection of *Mycobacterium leprae* and its susceptibility to dapsone using DNA heteroduplex analysis. *J Clin Microbiol* 2001;39:2083–2088.
25. Shepard CC. A kenetic method for the study of activity of drugs against *Mycobacterium leprae* in mice. *Int J Lepr* 1967;35:429–435.

26. Lecuit M, Abachin E, Martin A, et al. Immunoproliferative small intestinal disease associated with *Campylobacter jejuni*. *N Engl J Med* 2004;350:239–248.
27. Ho S, Hoyle JA, Lewis FA, et al. Direct polymerase chain reaction test for detection of *Helicobacter pylori* in humans and animals. *J Clin Microbiol* 1991;29:2543–2549.
28. Valentine JL, Arthur RR, Mobley HL, et al. Detection of *Helicobacter pylori* by using the polymerase chain reaction. *J Clin Microbiol* 1991;29:689–695.
29. Clayton CL, Kleanthous H, Coates PJ, et al. Sensitive detection of *Helicobacter pylori* by using polymerase chain reaction. *J Clin Microbiol* 1992;30:192–200.
30. Schabereiter-Gurtner C, Hirschl AM, Dragosics B, et al. Novel real-time PCR assay for detection of *Helicobacter pylori* infection and simultaneous clarithromycin susceptibility testing of stool and biopsy specimens. *J Clin Microbiol* 2004;42(9):4512–4518.
31. Ruzsovics A, Molnar B, Tulassay Z. Deoxyribonucleic acid-based diagnostic techniques to detect *Helicobacter pylori* [Review]. *Aliment Pharmacol Ther* 2004;19:1137–1146.
32. Fabre R, Sobhani I, Laurent-Puig P, et al. Polymerase chain reaction assay for the detection of *Helicobacter pylori* in gastric biopsy specimens: comparison with culture, rapid urease test, and histopathological tests. *Gut* 1994;35:905–908.
33. Lascols C, Lamarque D, Costa JM, et al. Fast and accurate quantitative detection of *Helicobacter pylori* and identification of clarithromycin resistance mutations in *H. pylori* isolates from gastric biopsy specimens by real-time PCR. *J Clin Microbiol* 2003;41: 4573–4577.
34. Maeda S, Yoshida H, Matsunaga H, et al. Detection of clarithromycin-resistant *Helicobacter pylori* strains by a preferential homoduplex formation assay. *J Clin Microbiol* 2000;38:210–214.
35. Houben MH, van de Beek D, Hensen EF, et al. A systematic review of *Helicobacter pylori* eradication therapy: the impact of antimicrobial resistance on eradication rates. *Aliment Pharmacol Ther* 1999;13:1047–1055.
36. Masuda H, Hiyama T, Yoshihara M, et al. Necessity of multiple gastric biopsies from different sites for detection of clarithromycin-resistant *Helicobacter pylori* strains. *Scand J Gastroenterol* 2003;38:942–946.
37. Russmann H, Adler K, Haas R, et al. Rapid and accurate determination of genotypic clarithromycin resistance in cultured *Helicobacter pylori* by fluorescent in situ hybridization. *J Clin Microbiol* 2001;39:4142–4144.
38. Trebesius K, Panthel K, Strobel S, et al. Rapid and specific detection of *Helicobacter pylori* macrolide resistance in gastric tissue by fluorescent in situ hybridisation. *Gut* 2000;46:608–614.
39. Juttner S, Vieth M, Miehlke S, et al. Reliable detection of macrolide-resistant *Helicobacter pylori* via fluorescence in situ hybridization in formalin-fixed tissue. *Mod Pathol* 2004;17:684–689.
40. Shieh WJ, Guarner J, Paddock C, et al. The critical role of pathology in the investigation of bioterrorism-related cutaneous anthrax. *Am J Pathol* 2003;163:1901–1910.
41. Levine SM, Perez-Perez G, Olivares A, et al. PCR-based detection of *Bacillus anthracis* in formalin-fixed tissue from a patient receiving ciprofloxacin. *J Clin Microbiol* 2002; 40:4360–4362.
42. Jackson PJ, Hugh-Jones ME, Adair DM, et al. PCR analysis of tissue samples from the 1979 Sverdlovsk anthrax victims: the presence of multiple *Bacillus anthracis* strains in different victims. *Proc Natl Acad Sci USA* 1998;95:1224–1229.
43. Graham DY, Markesich DC, Kalter DC, et al. Mycobacterial aetiology of sarcoidosis. *Lancet* 1992;340:52–53.
44. Richter E, Greinert U, Kirsten D, et al. Assessment of mycobacterial DNA in cells and tissues of mycobacterial and sarcoid lesions. *Am J Respir Crit Care Med* 1996;153: 375–380.
45. Bocart D, Lecossier D, De Lassence A, et al. A search for mycobacterial DNA in granulomatous tissues from patients with sarcoidosis using the polymerase chain reaction. *Am Rev Respir Dis* 1992;145:1142–1148.
46. Lamps LW, Madhusudhan KT, Havens JM, et al. Pathogenic Yersinia DNA is detected in bowel and mesenteric lymph nodes from patients with Crohn's disease. *Am J Surg Pathol* 2003;27:220–227.
47. Imhof A, Schaer C, Schoedon G, et al. Rapid detection of pathogenic fungi from clinical specimens using LightCycler real-time fluorescence PCR. *Eur J Clin Microbiol Infect Dis* 2003;22:558–560.
48. Kobayashi M, Togitani K, Machida H, et al. Molecular polymerase chain reaction diagnosis of pulmonary mucormycosis caused by *Cunninghamella bertholletiae*. *Respirology* 2004;9:397–401.
49. Hu S, Chung WH, Hung SI, et al. Detection of *Sporothrix schenckii* in clinical samples by a nested PCR assay. *J Clin Microbiol* 2003;41:1414–1418.
50. Kirby A, Chapman C, Hassan I, et al. The diagnosis of hepatosplenic candidiasis by DNA analysis of tissue biopsy and serum. *J Clin Pathol* 2004;57:764–765.
51. Hendolin PH, Paulin L, Koukila-Kahkola P, et al. Panfungal PCR and multiplex liquid hybridization for detection of fungi in tissue specimens. *J Clin Microbiol* 2000; 38:4186–4192.
52. Turin L, Riva F, Galbiati G, et al. Fast, simple and highly sensitive double-rounded polymerase chain reaction assay to detect medically relevant fungi in dermatological specimens. *Eur J Clin Invest* 2000;30:511–518.
53. Sandhu GS, Kline BC, Stockman L, et al. Molecular probes for diagnosis of fungal infections. *J Clin Microbiol* 1995;33:2913–2919.
54. Spreadbury C, Holden D, Aufauvre-Brown A, et al. Detection of *Aspergillus fumigatus* by polymerase chain reaction. *J Clin Microbiol* 1993;31:615–621.
55. Belknap BS. Sporotrichosis. *Dermatol Clin* 1989;7:193–202.
56. Bialek R, Feucht A, Aepinus C, et al. Evaluation of two nested PCR assays for detection of *Histoplasma capsulatum* DNA in human tissue. *J Clin Microbiol* 2002;40:1644–1647.
57. Wakefield AE, Pixley FJ, Banerji S, et al. Detection of *Pneumocystis carinii* with DNA amplification. *Lancet* 1990;336:451–453.
58. Chabe M, Vargas SL, Eyzaguirre I, et al. Molecular typing of *Pneumocystis jirovecii* found in formalin-fixed paraffin-embedded lung tissue sections from sudden infant death victims. *Microbiology* 2004;150:1167–1672.
59. Rantakokko-Jalava K, Laaksonen S, Issakainen J, et al. Semiquantitative detection by real-time PCR of *Aspergillus fumigatus* in bronchoalveolar lavage fluids and tissue biopsy specimens from patients with invasive aspergillosis. *J Clin Microbiol* 2003;41: 4304–4311.
60. Hayden RT, Qian X, Roberts GD, et al. In situ hybridization for the identification of yeastlike organisms in tissue section. *Diagn Mol Pathol* 2001;10:15–23.
61. Hayden RT, Qian X, Procop GW, et al. In situ hybridization for the identification of filamentous fungi in tissue section. *Diagn Mol Pathol* 2002;11:119–126.
62. Kobayashi M, Sonobe H, Ikezoe T, et al. In situ detection of *Aspergillus* 18S ribosomal RNA in invasive pulmonary aspergillosis. *Intern Med* 1999;38:563–569.
63. Hayden RT, Isotalo PA, Parrett T, et al. In situ hybridization for the differentiation of *Aspergillus*, *Fusarium*, and *Pseudallescheria* species in tissue section. *Diagn Mol Pathol* 2003; 12:21–26.
64. Manos MM, Ting Y, Wright DK, et al. Use of polymerase chain reaction amplification for detection of genital papillomavirus. *Cancer Cells* 1989;29:20–27.
65. Gravitt PE, Peyton CL, Apple RJ, et al. Genotyping of 27 human papillomavirus types by using L1 consensus PCR products by a single-hybridization, reverse line blot detection method. *J Clin Microbiol* 1998;36:3020–3027.
66. Gravitt PE, Peyton CL, Alessi TQ, et al. Improved amplification of genital human papillomaviruses. *J Clin Microbiol* 2000;38:357–361.
67. de Roda Husman AM, Walboomers JM, van den Brule AJ, et al. The use of general primers GP5 and GP6 elongated at their 3′ ends with adjacent highly conserved sequences improves human papillomavirus detection by PCR. *J Gen Virol* 1995; 76:1057–1062.
68. Jacobs MV, Snijders PJ, van den Brule AJ, et al. A general primer GP5+/GP6(+)-mediated PCR-enzyme immunoassay method for rapid detection of 14 high-risk and 6 low-risk human papillomavirus genotypes in cervical scrapings. *J Clin Microbiol* 1997; 35:791–795.
69. de Roda Husman AM, Walboomers JM, van den Brule AJ, et al. The use of general primers GP5 and GP6 elongated at their 3′ ends with adjacent highly conserved sequences improves human papillomavirus detection by PCR. *J Gen Virol* 1995; 76:1057–1062.
70. Kleter B, van Doorn LJ, ter Schegget J, et al. Novel short-fragment PCR assay for highly sensitive broad-spectrum detection of anogenital human papillomavirus. *Am J Pathol* 1998;153:1731–1739.
71. Kleter B, van Doorn LJ, Schrauwen L, et al. Development and clinical evaluation of a highly sensitive PCR-reverse hybridization line probe assay for detection and identification of anogenital human papillomavirus. *J Clin Microbiol* 1999;37:2508–2517.
72. Feoli-Fonseca JC, Oligny LL, Filion M, et al. A two-tier polymerase chain reaction direct sequencing method for detecting and typing human papillomaviruses in pathological specimens. *Diagn Mol Pathol* 1998;7:317–323.
73. Vernon SD, Unger ER, Williams D. Comparison of human papillomavirus detection and typing by cycle sequencing, line blotting, and hybrid capture. *J Clin Microbiol* 2000;38:651–655.
74. Lu DW, El-Mofty SK, Wang HL. Expression of p16, Rb, and p53 proteins in squamous cell carcinomas of the anorectal region harboring human papillomavirus DNA. *Mod Pathol* 2003;16:692–699.
75. van den Brule AJ, Pol R, Fransen-Daalmeijer N, et al. GP5+/6+ PCR followed by reverse line blot analysis enables rapid and high-throughput identification of human papillomavirus genotypes. *J Clin Microbiol* 2002;40:779–787.
76. Tabrizi SN, Stevens M, Chen S, et al. Evaluation of a modified reverse line blot assay for detection and typing of human papillomavirus. *Am J Clin Pathol* 2005;123:896–899.
77. Peyton CL, Schiffman M, Lorincz AT, et al. Comparison of PCR- and hybrid capture-based human papillomavirus detection systems using multiple cervical specimen collection strategies. *J Clin Microbiol* 1998;36:3248–3254.
78. Castle PE, Schiffman M, Burk RD, et al. Restricted cross-reactivity of hybrid capture 2 with nononcogenic human papillomavirus types. *Cancer Epidemiol Biomarkers Prev* 2002; 11:1394–1399.
79. Castle PE, Wheeler CM, Solomon D, et al. Interlaboratory reliability of Hybrid Capture 2. *Am J Clin Pathol* 2004;122:238–245.
80. Fujii T, Masumoto N, Saito M, et al. Comparison between in situ hybridization and real-time PCR technique as a means of detecting the integrated form of human papillomavirus 16 in cervical neoplasia. *Diagn Mol Pathol* 2005;14:103–108.
81. Schiller CL, Nickolov AG, Kaul KL, et al. High-risk human papillomavirus detection: a split-sample comparison of hybrid capture and chromogenic in situ hybridization. *Am J Clin Pathol* 2004;121:537–545.
82. de Lamballerie X, Charrel RN, Attoui H, et al. Classification of hepatitis C virus variants in six major types based on analysis of the envelope 1 and nonstructural 5B genome regions and complete polyprotein sequences. *J Gen Virol* 1997;78:45–51.
83. Svoboda-Newman SM, Greenson JK, Singleton TP, et al. Detection of hepatitis C by RT-PCR in formalin-fixed paraffin-embedded tissue from liver transplant patients. *Diagn Mol Pathol* 1997;6:123–129.
84. Qian X, Guerrero RB, Plummer TB, et al. Detection of hepatitis C virus RNA in formalin-fixed paraffin-embedded sections with digoxigenin-labeled cRNA probes. *Diagn Mol Pathol* 2004;13:9–14.
85. Lau GK, Davis GL, Wu SP, et al. Hepatic expression of hepatitis C virus RNA in chronic hepatitis C: a study by in situ reverse-transcription polymerase chain reaction. *Hepatology* 1996;23:1318–1323.
86. Vogt S, Schneider-Stock R, Klauck S, et al. Detection of hepatitis C virus RNA in formalin-fixed, paraffin-embedded thin-needle liver biopsy specimens. *Am J Clin Pathol* 2003;120:536–543.
87. Ryan JL, Fan H, Glaser SL, et al. Epstein-Barr virus quantitation by real-time PCR targeting multiple gene segments: a novel approach to screen for the virus in paraffin-embedded tissue and plasma. *J Mol Diagn* 2004;6:378–385.
88. Biagini P, Benkoel L, Dodero F, et al. Hepatitis C virus RNA detection by in situ RT-PCR in formalin-fixed paraffin-embedded liver tissue: comparison with serum and tissue results. *Cell Mol Biol* 2001;47, Online Pub:OL167–171.
89. Lidonnici K, Lane B, Nuovo GJ. Comparison of serologic analysis and in situ localization of PCR-amplified cDNA for the diagnosis of hepatitis C infection. *Diagn Mol Pathol* 1995;4:98–107.
90. Nolte FS, Green AM, Fiebelkorn KR, et al. Clinical evaluation of two methods for genotyping hepatitis C virus based on analysis of the 5′ noncoding region. *J Clin Microbiol* 2003;41:1558–1564.
91. Ansaldi F, Torre F, Bruzzone BM, et al. Evaluation of a new hepatitis C virus sequencing assay as a routine method for genotyping. *J Med Virol* 2001;63:17–21.
92. Urdea MS. Synthesis and characteristics of branched DNA (bDNA) for the direct and quantitative detection of CMB, HBV, HCV, and HIV. *Clin Chem* 1993;39:725–726.

93. Elbeik T, Surtihadi J, Destree M, et al. Multicenter evaluation of the performance characteristics of the bayer VERSANT HCV RNA 3.0 assay (bDNA). *J Clin Microbiol* 2004;42:563–569.

94. Hendricks DA, Friesenhahn M, Tanimoto L, et al. Multicenter evaluation of the VERSANT HCV RNA qualitative assay for detection of hepatitis C virus RNA. *J Clin Microbiol* 2003;41:651–656.

95. Yao JD, Marcel GH, Oon LL, et al. Multicenter evaluation of the VERSANT hepatitis B virus DNA 3.0 assay. *J Clin Microbiol* 2004;42:800–806.

96. Gleaves CA, Welle J, Campbell M, et al. Multicenter evaluation of the Bayer VERSANT HIV-1 RNA 3.0 assay: analytical and clinical performance. *J Clin Virol* 2002;25: 205–216.

97. Katsoulidou A, Papachristou E, Petrodaskalaki M, et al. Comparison of three current viral load assays for the quantitation of human immunodeficiency virus type 1 RNA in plasma. *J Virol Methods* 2004;121:93–99.

98. Elbeik T, Delassandro R, Chen YM, et al. Global cost modeling analysis of HIV-1 and HCV viral load assays. *Expert Rev Pharmacoecon Outcomes Res* 2003;3383–3407.

99. Leenman EE, Panzer-Grumayer RE, Fischer S, et al. Rapid determination of Epstein-Barr virus latent or lytic infection in single human cells using in situ hybridization. *Mod Pathol* 2004;17:1564–1572.

100. Weiss LM, Strickler JG, Warnke RA, et al. Epstein-Barr viral DNA in tissues of Hodgkin's disease. *Am J Pathol* 1987;129:86–91.

101. Modrow S, Falke D, Truyen U. Herpesviren. In: Modrow S, FAlke D, Truyen U, eds. *Molekulare Virologie*, 2nd ed. Heidelberg, Berlin: Spectrum Akademischer Verlag; 2003: 514–613.

102. Mehraein Y, Lennerz C, Ehlhardt S, et al. Latent Epstein-Barr virus (EBV) infection and cytomegalovirus (CMV) infection in synovial tissue of autoimmune chronic arthritis determined by RNA- and DNA-in situ hybridization. *Mod Pathol* 2004;17: 781–789.

103. Chang KL, Chen YY, Shibata D, et al. Description of an in situ hybridization methodology for detection of Epstein-Barr virus RNA in paraffin-embedded tissues, with a survey of normal and neoplastic tissues. *Diagn Mol Pathol* 1992;1:246–255.

104. Syrmis MW, Whiley DM, Thomas M, et al. A sensitive, specific, and cost-effective multiplex reverse transcriptase-PCR assay for the detection of seven common respiratory viruses in respiratory samples. *J Mol Diagn* 2004;6:125–131.

105. Chow KC, Hsiao CH, Lin TY, et al. Detection of severe acute respiratory syndrome-associated coronavirus in pneumocytes of the lung. *Am J Clin Pathol* 2004;121:574–580.

106. Drosten C, Gunther S, Preiser W, et al. Identification of a novel coronavirus in patients with severe acute respiratory syndrome. *N Engl J Med* 2003;348:1967–1976.

107. Ksiazek TG, Erdman D, Goldsmith CS, et al. A novel coronavirus associated with severe acute respiratory syndrome. *N Engl J Med* 2003;348:1953–1966.

108. Shieh WJ, Hsiao CH, Paddock CD, et al. Immunohistochemical, in situ hybridization, and ultrastructural localization of SARS-associated coronavirus in lung of a fatal case of severe acute respiratory syndrome in Taiwan. *Hum Pathol* 2005;36:303–309.

109. Nakajima N, Asahi-Ozaki Y, Nagata N, et al. SARS coronavirus-infected cells in lung detected by new in situ hybridization technique. *Jpn J Infect* Dis 2003;56:139–141.

110. To KF, Tong JH, Chan PK, et al. Tissue and cellular tropism of the coronavirus associated with severe acute respiratory syndrome: an in-situ hybridization study of fatal cases. *J Pathol* 2004;202:157–163.

111. Ding Y, He L, Zhang Q, et al. Organ distribution of severe acute respiratory syndrome (SARS) associated coronavirus (SARS-CoV) in SARS patients: implications for pathogenesis and virus transmission pathways. *J Pathol* 2004;203:622–630.

112. Marennikova SS, Gurvich EB, Yumasheva MA. Laboratory diagnosis of smallpox and similar viral diseases by means of tissue culture methods: differentiation of smallpox virus from varicella, vaccinia, cowpox and herpes viruses. *Acta Virol* 1964;127:135–142.

113. Swanepoel R, Cruickshank JG. Smallpox in Rhodesia and the use of the electron microscope in the diagnosis of this and other diseases. *Cent Afr J Med* 1972;18:68–72.

114. Nuovo GJ, Plaza JA, Magro C, et al. Rapid diagnosis of smallpox infection and differentiation from its mimics. *Diagn Mol Pathol* 2003;12:103–107.

115. Rendtorff RC, Fowinkle EW. Herpes simplex skin lesions simulating smallpox. *JAMA* 1965;192:998–1000.

116. Schoepp RJ, Morin MD, Martinez MJ, et al. Detection and identification of Variola virus in fixed human tissue after prolonged archival storage. *Lab Invest* 2004;84:41–48.

117. Wang D, Coscoy L, Zylberberg M, et al. Microarray-based detection and genotyping of viral pathogens. *Proc Natl Acad Sci USA* 2002;99:15687–15692.

118. Powers JF, Bedri S, Hussein S, et al. High prevalence of herpes simplex virus DNA in temporal arteritis biopsy specimens. *Am J Clin Pathol* 2005;123:261–264.

119. Gomez-Roman JJ, Sanchez-Velasco P, Ocejo-Vinyals G, et al. Human herpesvirus-8 genes are expressed in pulmonary inflammatory myofibroblastic tumor (inflammatory pseudotumor). *Am J Surg Pathol* 2001;25:624–629.

120. Reischl U, Bretagne S, Kruger D, et al. Comparison of two DNA targets for the diagnosis of toxoplasmosis by real-time PCR using fluorescence resonance energy transfer hybridization probes. *BMC Infect Dis* 2003;3:7.

121. Lin MH, Chen TC, Kuo TT, et al. Real-time PCR for quantitative detection of *Toxoplasma gondii*. *J Clin Microbiol* 2000;38:4121–4125.

122. Buchbinder S, Blatz R, Rodloff AC. Comparison of real-time PCR detection methods for B1 and P30 genes of *Toxoplasma gondii*. *Diagn Microbiol Infect Dis* 2003;45:269–271.

123. Chabbert E, Lachaud L, Crobu L, et al. Comparison of two widely used PCR primer systems for detection of toxoplasma in amniotic fluid, blood, and tissues. *J Clin Microbiol* 2004;42:1719–1722.

124. Desjeux P. Leishmaniasis: current situation and new perspectives. *Comp Immunol Microbiol Infect Dis* 2004; 27: 305–318.

125. Kalter DC. Laboratory tests for the diagnosis and evaluation of leishmaniasis. *Dermatol Clin* 1994;12:37–50.

126. Barker CD. DNA diagnosis of human leishmaniasis. *Parasitol* 1987; 3:177–184.

127. Le Blancq SM, Lanham SM, Evans DA. Comparative isoenzyme profiles of old and new world leishmania. In: Peters W, Killick-Kendrick R, eds. *The Leishmaniases in Biology and Medicine*. London: Academic Press; 1987:543–551.

128. Romero GA, Guerra MV, Paes MG, et al. Sensitivity of the polymerase chain reaction for the diagnosis of cutaneous leishmaniasis due to *Leishmania (Viannia) guyanensis*. *Acta Trop* 2001;79:225–229.

129. Safaei A, Motazedian MH, Vasei M. Polymerase chain reaction for diagnosis of cutaneous leishmaniasis in histologically positive, suspicious and negative skin biopsies. *Dermatology* 2002;205:18–24.

130. de Oliveira CI, Oliveira F, Favali CB, et al. Clinical utility of polymerase chain reaction-based detection of *Leishmania* in the diagnosis of American cutaneous leishmaniasis. *Clin Infect Dis* 2003;37:e149–e153.

131. Mimori T, Sasaki J, Nakata M, et al. Rapid identification of *Leishmania* species from formalin-fixed biopsy samples by polymorphism-specific polymerase chain reaction. *Gene* 1998;210:179–186.

132. Schwartz DA, Sobottka I, Leitch GJ, et al. Pathology of microsporidiosis: emerging parasitic infections in patients with acquired immunodeficiency syndrome. *Arch Pathol Lab Med* 1996;120:173–188.

133. Kock NP, Petersen H, Fenner T, et al. Species-specific identification of microsporidia in stool and intestinal biopsy specimens by the polymerase chain reaction. *Eur J Clin Microbiol Infect Dis* 1997;16:369–376.

134. McLauchlin J, Amar CF, Pedraza-Diaz S, et al. Polymerase chain reaction-based diagnosis of infection with *Cryptosporidium* in children with primary immunodeficiencies. *Pediatr Infect Dis J* 2003;22:329–335.

Identity Determination

Scientific methods for identity determination were initially based on variations in protein markers, including ABO blood group antigens, serum proteins, red blood cell enzymes, and human leukocyte antigens (1). The proteins' variations in all these systems are the result of genetic polymorphisms, and thus identity determination in these systems is essentially based on indirect detection of underlying DNA sequence differences. More direct DNA-based approaches for identity determination use hypervariable regions of DNA, specifically minisatellites (also known as variable number of tandem repeat loci, or VNTRs) or microsatellites (also known as short tandem repeat loci, or STRs). The use of VNTRs to produce a DNA fingerprint was first described in 1985 (2), and soon afterward DNA-based identity determination was applied to forensic testing (3–5). Increased knowledge of the structure and sequence of the human genome (6) has greatly multiplied the number of potentially useful loci for identity determination.

Although the advantages of direct DNA-based identification analysis have been most widely publicized in forensics and parentage studies (7,8), testing also has a role in the routine practice of surgical pathology. The clinical settings in which DNA typing has been described include resolution of specimen identity issues, differentiation of synchronous and metachronous tumors from metastases, evaluation of tumors in transplant recipients, evaluation of bone marrow engraftment, and demonstration of natural chimerism. DNA typing has also been used in the diagnosis of hydatidiform moles, as discussed in more detail in Chapter 16.

MATCHING PROBABILITY

As with all approaches to identity determination, direct DNA-based methods are used to ascertain whether two samples share a common source. When the two DNA profiles are different, the result indicates that the samples originated from different people and a common origin is excluded (rare exceptions to this general rule can be caused by natural chimerism (see later discussion), somatic mosacism [9–11], and somatic mutation [12–14], as listed in Table 23.1). When the two DNA profiles are the same, the result indicates that the samples either originated from the same source or originated from two different people who happen to be identical at the evaluated loci by random chance (Table 23.1 also lists rare exceptions to this general rule).

When two specimens have the same profile, excluding from discussion the exceptions in Table 23.1, interpretation of the result is dependent on the probability that the same profile would occur by random chance alone. An estimate of this probability is typically provided in the form of a profile frequency, which is an indication of the number of times the same profile would be seen in a reference population. For many loci there are a large number of alleles, each at low frequency, and population genetics theory is required to accurately estimate profile frequencies based on data collected for each locus of interest from different population groups, often Caucasian, African American, Hispanic, and Asian (8). Allele frequencies from different loci are multiplied together to obtain the frequency of the complete DNA profile, usually expressed as "1 in X" (e.g., 1 in 1 billion), where X denotes the number of people who would need to be sampled, on average, to see the profile once. With this information, the likelihood ratio (LR) can be determined, where the LR is defined as the probability of finding the test sample's profile if the reference sample donor were the true donor compared with the probability of finding the test sample's profile if someone else were the true donor (8). In the simplest case, LR is merely the reciprocal of the profile frequency (e.g., given the profile found in the test sample, it is 1 billion times more likely that it originates from the reference sample donor than from a random person).

The power of discrimination (P_d) of a test depends on the LR of the test result. Because LR ultimately depends on the number of alleles evaluated and the allele frequencies in the population under study, a test that relies on a single

TABLE 23.1 EXCEPTIONS THAT CAN COMPLICATE IDENTITY DETERMINATION BY DNA TYPING	
Exceptions	**Comments**
Different DNA profiles originate from the same individual	
Natural chimerism[a]	Occurs in fraternal twins; usually manifested as different DNA profiles in hematopoietic tissues versus somatic tissues
Iatrogenic chimerism	Occurs after bone marrow or solid organ transplantation; can also occur after a recent blood transfusion
Fetal microchimerism	Occurs after pregnancy as a result of trafficking of fetal cells in the maternal circulation
Somatic mosaicism[b]	Can result from de novo mutations, reversion to normal of inherited mutations, or numerical or structural chromosomal abnormalities
Somatic mutation	Occurs in neoplasms; usually manifested as different DNA profiles in the tumor resulting from mutations at primer binding sites, deletions, duplications, improper segregation of entire chromosomes, point mutations, loss of heterozygosity, microsatellite instability, etc.
The same DNA profile originates from different people	
Monozygous twins	
Closely related family members	
Inbred populations	
Random chance	

[a] Chimerism is the presence in a single individual of two (or more) cell lineages derived from different zygotes.
[b] Mosaicism is the presence in a single individual of genetically distinct cell lineages derived from the same zygote.

locus with a limited number of alleles will have a low LR, whereas a test that involves multiple loci can easily have an LR in the trillions. The allele frequencies for a large number of genetic loci have been cataloged, and it is standard practice when working with unknown cases to report probabilities for different major racial groups because allele frequencies vary among populations (8,15–17). Objective criteria for assessing the significance of an LR in a health care setting have been proposed (18,19).

IDENTITY TESTING METHODS

Some of the first DNA polymorphisms described that were amenable to direct evaluation were VNTRs, which can be detected by restriction fragment length polymorphism (RFLP) analysis. RFLP analysis was therefore one of the initial DNA-based technologies that was widely used for identity testing (20–24). However, identity determination by direct RFLP analysis is cumbersome, labor intensive, and is limited by the large quantity of intact DNA required for testing.

Polymerase chain reaction (PCR)-based approaches for DNA typing greatly expanded the range of testing because PCR-based methods require such small amounts of DNA and can be performed on fresh, fixed, or even partially degraded specimens. PCR-based methods also expanded the range of polymorphisms amenable to testing to include single nucleotide polymorphisms (SNPs) and STRs as well as VNTRs (Table 23.2).

Single Nucleotide Polymorphism Analysis

The first widely used PCR-based approach for analysis of SNRs in the context of identity determination was the reverse dot blot system (25). By reverse dot blot analysis, several polymorphic genetic loci are amplified in a multiplex PCR reaction using biotin-labeled primers, and the PCR product DNA is then hybridized to a membrane strip that contains sequence-specific oligonucleotide (SSO) probes for each of the alleles bound in an array of small circular regions or "dots." The hybridization to the membrane strip is performed under stringent conditions so that each allele in the labeled PCR product hybridizes only with the complementary SSO probe on the membrane. A colorimetric system is used to detect the biotin label of the bound PCR product DNA, and the

TABLE 23.2

METHODS FOR DNA TYPING

Polymorphism	Structural Basis	Likelihood Ratio	Methods of Analysis	Examples of Commercial Reagents
Single nucleotide polymorphism	Single nucleotide change	Hundreds to thousands	Allele-specific PCR Reverse dot blots	No longer marketed
Minisatellites (variable number of tandem repeats or VNTRs)	Tandem repeats of core sequences that range from 14 to about 500 bp long; each locus has from several to several hundred repeats of the core sequence	Millions to billions	Restriction fragment length polymorphism (RFLP) analysis PCR amplification (known as AmpFLPs)	No longer marketed
Microsatellites (short tandem repeats or STRs)	Tandem repeats of core sequences that range from 1 to 13 bp long; each locus has from several to several dozen repeats of the core sequence	Thousands to trillions, depending on the number of loci evaluated	Multiplex PCR of autosomal chromosomes Multiplex PCR of Y chromosome	AmpFLSTR kits (Applied Biosystems); PowerPlex and GenePrint System kits (Promega) Y-PLEX kits (Reliagene Technologies)

pattern of dots on the hybridization membrane indicates the patient's genotype.

Reverse dot blot analysis is simple and quick and does not require electrophoresis or Southern blotting. The technique is an excellent screening method and has sufficient discriminatory potential for many applications, but because relatively few alleles exist at each of the test loci, it generates a low LR and thus has a limited capability to distinguish individual genotypes at a high level of statistical significance. Consequently, the technique has been phased out in common laboratory usage in favor of methods based on the analysis of repetitive sequences.

Repetitive Sequence Analysis

As discussed in more detail in Chapter 1, VNTR loci have core repeats ranging from 14 to about 500 base pairs (bp) long, and different VNTR alleles contain two to several hundred tandem repeats of the core sequence. STR loci have core repeats from 1 to 13 bp long, and individual alleles usually have from 3 to 20 tandem core repeats (TCRs), although some have 100 or more TCRs. Because VNTRs and STRs are inherited in a mendelian fashion, and hundreds of VNTR and STR loci are present on every human chromosome, both types of repetitive sequence elements are useful for identity testing.

The amplicons generated by PCR of VNTR, often referred to as amplified fragment length polymorphisms, or AmpFLPs, are usually sufficiently different in size to be discriminated by direct staining after separation by simple gel electrophoresis. However, because STR alleles often differ in length by only a few bp, their electrophoretic separation requires a high-resolution methodology such as denaturing polyacrylamide gel electrophoresis or capillary electrophoresis. In practice, the number of repeats in an STR allele is easily determined by comparison with an allelic ladder that contains the majority of known alleles at the locus (26).

The use of STR loci versus VNTR loci for DNA typing has several advantages (27). First, because VNTR have a longer repeat unit, the different alleles have more variability in length, and, as discussed in Chapter 5, markedly different amplicon lengths can cause PCR amplification bias with preferential amplification of the shorter of allele. In the worst case scenario, biased amplification can result in undetected amplification of the larger allele, with resulting misinterpretations of the genotype (28,29). Second, testing of a partially degraded DNA sample is more likely to be successful using STRs because they are so short. This is an important technical consideration given that, in routine surgical pathology, many samples likely to be subjected to DNA typing are derived from formalin-fixed, paraffin-embedded (FFPE) tissue. Third, from a purely practical standpoint, because virtually all DNA-based forensic identity testing and paternity testing employs STRs, extensive technical resources are available to support STR-based testing in the clinical laboratory, including a large database of allele size distribution.

A set of 13 core STR loci (Table 23.3) was chosen by the Federal Bureau of Investigation of the United States for use in a national database of convicted felons known as the Combined DNA Index System or CODIS (8). When used together, the CODIS loci provide a test result with an extremely high LR, on average more than a trillion (30). Commercial kits for either monoplex or multiplex PCR amplification of CODIS loci have greatly simplified STR typing and made the method accessible to most molecular genetic laboratories (Table 23.2). Most commercial kits employ fluorophore-labeled primers, which not only increase the sensitivity of the technique but also make it quantitative (26,31). Multiplex STR is particularly useful for the analysis of DNA mixtures; the technique makes it possible to type minor components present at levels below 1% (32–34) and can even be applied to male-specific analysis of mixed specimens via the use of STR loci on the Y chromosome (35–37).

TABLE 23.3
THE CODIS STR LOCI[a]

Chromosome	Locus	Human Gene Name	Number of Repeats in Different Alleles[b]
2	TPOX	Thyroid peroxidase gene	5–14
3	D3S1358	NA[c]	8–20
4	FGA	Fibringen alpha-chain gene	12–51
5	D5S818	NA	7–16
5	CSF1PO	c-fms proto-oncogene (CSF1 receptor gene)	6–16
7	D7S820	NA	5–15
8	D8S1179	NA	7–19
11	TH01	Tyrosine hydroxylase gene	3–14
12	vWA	von Willebrand factor gene	10–25
13	D13S317	NA	5–16
16	D16S539	NA	5, 8–15
18	D18S51	NA	7–27
21	D21S11	NA	24–38

[a] For more information see www.cstl.nist.gov/biotech/strbase.
[b] Many of the CODIS loci also have variant alleles.
[c] Not applicable; not within the coding region of a gene.

TABLE 23.4
USES OF DNA TYPING METHODS IN IDENTITY TESTING

Medical uses
Typing for bone marrow or whole organ transplantation
Resolution of specimen labeling and identification issues
Identification of specimen contaminants
Distinguishing synchronous and metachronous tumors from tumor metastases
Evaluation of tumors in transplant recipients
Bone marrow engraftment analysis
Chimerism analysis
Diagnosis of hydatidiform moles

Identity determination
Forensic testing in criminal and civil cases
Postconviction exonerations
Paternity testing
Victim identification in mass disasters
Victim identification in war crimes
Family reunification

DNA databanks
Case to suspect matching
Case to case matching

Research
Anthropology
Plant forensics and breeding
Wildlife forensics and breeding

CLINICAL APPLICATIONS OF IDENTITY TESTING

Although DNA-based identity testing is most widely applied for forensic analysis, there are also numerous applications of the methodology in surgical pathology (Table 23.4).

Resolution of Specimen Identity Issues

One category of specimen identity issues is associated with deficiencies in specimen labeling, mismatches between the patient name on the container and the requisition slip, accessioning errors, and so on. Based on a College of American

Pathologists (CAP) Q-probes study, deficiencies of this type occur in about 6% of accessioned cases (38). Another category of specimen identity issues arises when a presumably extraneous tissue contaminant is present in a surgical or cytology specimen. A CAP Q-probes study designed to address this issue showed that presumed extraneous tissue is present in about 0.6% of slides evaluated prospectively and 2.9% of slides evaluated retrospectively with the specific intent to identify contaminants (39). Of note, approximately 30% of the contaminants encountered prospectively were abnormal or neoplastic, and about 10% presented some degree of diagnostic uncertainty (39).

Specimen Labeling and Accessioning Deficiencies

In some cases, identity must be determined based solely on the initial specimen because it would be difficult to obtain additional diagnostic tissue, and many different approaches to DNA-based testing have been shown to be ideally suited for resolution of specimen identification problems of this type. Allele-specific PCR based on HLA class II loci has been successfully applied to cases of presumed specimen mislabeling, but despite that fact that the method has advantages for typing partially degraded DNA derived from FFPE tissue (40,41), it has not been widely employed. The reverse dot blot approach has been used by many laboratories to resolve specimen identity issues (42–44), but because commercial dot blot kits are no longer marketed, the technique is no longer a viable option for routine clinical use. Instead, STR-based methods are employed by virtually all laboratories for specimen identity issues (45–48). The provenance of the tissue in question is quickly and easily determined by simply comparing its STR profile with the profile of a specimen of known origin, usually peripheral blood, a buccal swab, or even archival tissue. The number of loci used in the analysis can easily be adjusted to achieve the required LR.

Specimen Contamination

There is no doubt that immunohistochemical analysis of major blood group antigens is an extremely useful method for typing tissue contaminants (49,50). The method is simple and quick, does not require isolation of the putative contaminant by microdissection, and test interpretation is based on simple light microscopy. Nonetheless, blood group frequencies in some populations can limit the analysis by decreasing the likelihood that two unrelated specimens will be of discordant blood type (50).

DNA-based identity testing can also be used to demonstrate whether or not a suspect tissue fragment represents a contaminant, although for most DNA-based methods the potential contaminant must first be microdissected from the block before its relationship to the rest of the specimen can be determined. DNA-based methods that have been used successfully include allele-specific PCR (41,51), reverse dot blots (24,44), analysis of VNTR loci (52), and analysis of STR loci (45,48,53). Even FISH-based testing using probes for the X and Y chromosomes has been used to identify tissue contaminants (52), although this approach obviously has limited clinical utility because it provides useful information only in those cases in which the patient tissue and the contaminant are sex-mismatched. An example of the use of STR loci to resolve a specimen contamination issue that engenders diagnostic uncertainty is illustrated in Figure 23.1.

There are several important caveats to the use of DNA-based assays for evaluation of putative tissue contaminants. First, the chromosomal deletions that are a common feature of many types of dysplasia and malignancy can result in loss of heterozygosity (LOH) at test loci that complicates test interpretation. A difference in the DNA profile between two samples that is limited to allelic loss should therefore be interpreted with caution in order to avoid misinterpretation of loss of heterozygosity as evidence of genetic nonidentity, especially in those cases in which the suspect tissue fragment is neoplastic (48). Second, genetic duplication of a small chromosomal region, as well as improper segregation of an entire chromosome, can create a third allele at an STR locus (14). Although such occurrences are admittedly rare and are usually restricted to a single chromosome and a single STR locus, they can potentially complicate assignment of identity based on STR typing.

DISTINGUISHING SYNCHRONOUS AND METACHRONOUS TUMORS FROM TUMOR METASASES

Histopathologic features alone are not always sufficient to distinguish between tumor metastases and synchronous or metachronous tumors, but the difference can have profound implications for patient therapy and prognosis. DNA-based analysis in this setting is predicated on the fact that, according to the clonal model of carcinogenesis, all tumors arise from a single cell (54,55); a founder cell acquires a mutation that provides its progeny with a selective growth advantage, and from within this expanded population, another single cell acquires a second mutation that provides an additional growth advantage, and so on, until a fully malignant tumor emerges. Although the genetic instability that is a hallmark of most malignancies usually produces intratumoral heterogeneity, metastatic and recurrent tumors typically still have a genetic profile that is similar enough to the primary neoplasm to establish a relationship between the two (56–58).

Traditionally, the use of molecular analysis to establish a link between two tumors involved analysis of a panel of point mutations; larger scale structural changes such as translocations, insertions of viral genomes, or deletions; and patterns of X chromosome inactivation (59,60). In this type of analysis, for tumors that show an identical set of genetic features, the probability that the profile is due to random chance (estimated by the probability of the first genetic event occurring by random chance, multiplied by the probability of the second genetic event occurring by random chance, and so on) is used to determine the likelihood that the two tumors are of common origin (61–63). However, when the genetic profiles of two tumor specimens from this type of analysis are not identical, it is not always clear whether the result is evidence of a single tumor that has metastasized with genetic progression or is evidence of unrelated synchronous or metachronous tumors (62–67).

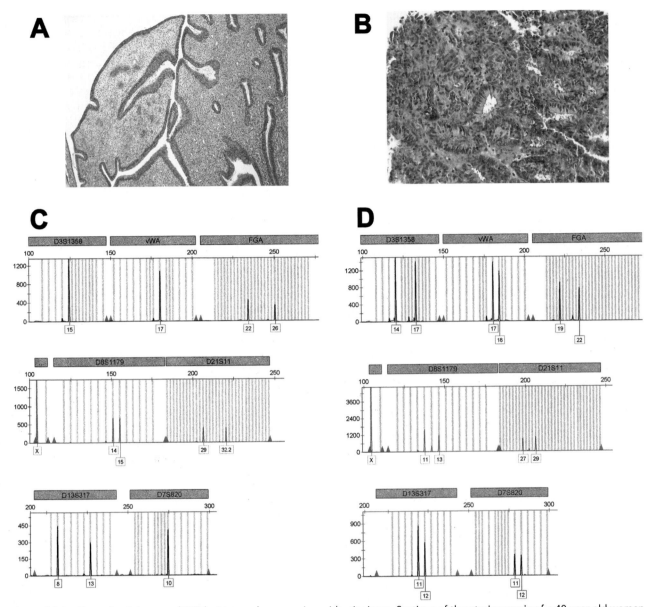

Figure 23.1 Example of the use of STR loci to resolve a specimen identity issue. Sections of the uterine cervix of a 40-year-old women with persistently abnormal pap smears showed unremarkable cervical mucosa (**A**, magnification 40×), but a detached fragment of an atypical glandular proliferation was also present (**B**, magnification 400×). DNA typing using a subset of the CODIS loci (Table 23.3) showed that the cervical mucosa (**C**) and atypical glandular fragment (**D**) had different genotypes, identifying the fragment as a contaminant. (See color insert.)

There is no standardized approach for dealing with problematic cases, although, in general, when the genetic profiles differ at only a few loci in a pattern that is consistent with genetic progression, and when the probability of the shared genetic events still supports a clonal relationship, the result is interpreted as evidence of a single tumor with metastasis (62,66,67). Nonetheless, the panel approach is hindered by low rates of single base pair changes and larger scale structural changes at the test loci, the extensive analysis required to establish the mutation rates of the various test loci in different tumor types, and the fact that evaluation of the pattern of X chromosome inactivation can be performed only on tumors arising in women.

Currently, the most common approach used to investigate the link between two neoplasms is LOH analysis. Even though there is overlap in the chromosomal regions characteristically deleted in various types of malignancies,

independent tumors typically show a unique pattern of chromosomal loss (68–70). Consequently, demonstration of a different profile of LOH using a panel of STRs provides evidence that two (or more) neoplasms in the same patient are most likely independently derived and therefore represent synchronous or metachronous tumors rather than tumor metastasis (64). The pattern of LOH at a panel of STRs also can be used to distinguish tumor recurrence or progression from second primary malignancies (56,71). A quantitative model has been developed that makes it possible to calculate the probability of the observed pattern of LOH in a pair of tumors, assuming either a common origin or an independent origin, from which it is possible to determine the likelihood ratio that the tumors have a common origin compared with an independent origin (72).

Genetic changes in STR alleles resulting from microsatellite instability (MSI) have also been used to investigate the relationship between different tumors in the same patient (73). As discussed in Chapter 2, MSI consists of random alterations in the length of repetitive DNA sequences that are usually the result of defects in mismatch repair genes, and the pattern of MSI in a primary tumor is generally retained in its metastases (64). PCR-based analysis of MSI at STRs, especially when coupled with PCR-based analysis of LOH at STRs, has proven to be a very useful method for distinguishing independent primary tumors from metastases in tumors of the lung (74,75), colon and rectum (76,77), stomach (78), endometrium and ovary (65,66,79), appendix (80), urinary bladder (67), and a variety of other sites (64,81–83).

EVALUATION OF NEOPLASMS IN ORGAN TRANSPLANT RECIPIENTS

Organ transplant recipients have a roughly 3- to 4-fold increased risk of developing some type of malignancy, although the risk is increased several hundred-fold for developing lymphoma, Kaposi's sarcoma, renal carcinoma, hepatobiliary carcinoma, anogenital carcinoma, and carcinoma of the skin and lip (84,85). However, not all of the malignancies that develop are of recipient origin. As initially recognized over 40 years ago, a subset of the tumors results from inadvertent transplantation of a malignancy from the donor to the graft recipient (86,87), as listed in Table 23.5. Although organs from donors with recognized neoplastic disease are no longer transplanted, a variety of malignancies continue to be transmitted to graft recipients from organ donors with unrecognized tumors (87–90).

In the first application of molecular genetic testing to evaluate the origin of a malignancy in a transplant recipient, RFLP analysis of several polymorphic loci on chromosome 7 and reverse dot blot analysis of an HLA locus were used to demonstrate that widespread melanoma in a renal transplant patient was of donor origin (91). More recently, PCR-based analysis of VNTR and STR loci has been used to clarify the origin of malignancies that developed in heart, kidney, and liver transplant recipients (92–94). Although the data seem to suggest that inadvertently transplanted malignancies occur at the highest rate after renal transplantation, this result is most likely due to the fact that a much higher number of kidney transplants have been performed than liver, heart, pancreas, or lung transplants.

However, documentation that a malignancy was inadvertently transplanted along with a donor organ does not automatically indicate that a histologically similar tumor in the recipient is of donor origin. In one interesting case, a renal transplant patient died of widely metastatic carcinoma 6 years after carcinoma of donor origin was identified in the failed allograft, but DNA evaluation demonstrated that the widespread metastatic carcinoma was nonetheless of recipient origin (95). Furthermore, inadvertent transmission of tumors does not occur only in transplant patients, but has also been shown to occur in other clinical settings. One such example is provided by a surgeon who presented with a sarcoma involving his hand at the site of an intraoperative injury he sustained some months earlier; genetic analysis of HLA genes and STR loci demonstrated that the surgeon's tumor had the same DNA profile as the malignant fibrous histiocytoma of the patient on whom he had been operating when he injured his hand (96).

From a technical perspective, interpretation of DNA typing carried out to evaluate tumors that arise in transplant recipients can be difficult because of the presence of chromosomal deletions and duplications, as discussed above. Similarly, MSI within a tumor of donor origin could produce an STR pattern that mimics the recipient's alleles at a specific locus (97), although testing of multiple loci would

---

TABLE 23.5

MALIGNANCIES TRANSMITTED BY ORGAN TRANSPLANTATION[a]

Cadaver donors
Malignant melanoma
Renal cell carcinoma
Lung carcinoma
Choriocarcinoma
Central nervous system tumors (including medulloblastoma and astrocytoma)
Hepatocellular carcinoma
Breast carcinoma
Colonic adenocarcinoma
Kaposi's sarcoma
Prostatic adenocarcinoma
Thyroid carcinoma
Lymphoma

Living related donors
Renal cell carcinoma

[a]Includes malignancies confined to the allograft, malignancies with local spread from the allograft, and malignancies with distant metastases.

readily exclude this source of error. Other factors that are unique to transplant recipients can cause additional problems. For example, even if a tumor is of donor origin, recipient inflammatory and vascular cells within the neoplasm can create a pattern of donor and recipient alleles that complicates identity determination (93,96). Similarly, the prolonged coexistence of both donor and recipient hematopoietic cells in the recipient following organ transplantation, a phenomenon known as microchimerism, can cause a complex pattern of donor and recipient alleles (98).

It is worth noting that inadvertently transplanted malignancies do not reflect the full spectrum of disease in organ transplant recipients for which DNA typing can be helpful for establishing the correct diagnosis. Some malignancies are not due to new or even transplanted neoplasms, but rather are recurrences of a tumor the recipient had before transplantation (99). And not all donor-derived neoplasms that arise in transplant recipients are malignant; for example, nephrogenic adenomas of the bladder in renal transplant recipients have been shown by interphase FISH to be derived from renal tubular cells of donor origin (100). Finally, medical rather than surgical disease can be a consequence of organ transplantation, as is demonstrated by the finding that hemolytic anemia in renal transplant recipients can result from the production of antibodies against recipient blood group antigens by biologically active "passenger" B-lymphocytes in the donor kidney (101–103).

BONE MARROW ENGRAFTMENT ANALYSIS

Even after successful engraftment of an allogeneic bone marrow transplant, a low percentage of hematopoetic cells of recipient origin persists in some patients, a phenomenon known as mixed chimerism. Mixed chimerism can be detected in bone marrow and peripheral blood (33,104) by a variety of molecular genetic methods, including conventional cytogenetics (105), FISH (105,106), RFLP analysis (107), PCR-based analysis of VNTRs and STRs (12,108,109), and assessment of SNPs (110). Laboratory detection and quantitation of the degree of mixed chimerism is referred to as bone marrow engraftment analysis.

Because PCR amplification of STR loci is rapid, quantitative, and informative in virtually all cases, it is the method of choice in most clinical laboratories that routinely perform bone marrow engraftment analysis (109). Before transplantation, both recipient and donor DNA are analyzed to determine the best loci for detection of recipient alleles within the donor allele background. Analysis of three or four STR loci is optimal for detection of mixed chimerism, for two reasons. First, loss of informative alleles as a result of chromosomal instability can be a source of error if testing is limited to only a single locus (12,13); second, the presence of stutter or shadow bands (resulting from polymerase slippage at repetitive regions [111], as discussed more fully in Chapter 5) can result in decreased test sensitivity by preventing detection of a low percentage of mixed chimerism if the informative allele colocalizes within the stutter bands. Because allogeneic bone marrow transplants are often between related individuals, identification of one informative locus, much less three or four, is sometimes difficult (112).

Although a level of mixed chimerism below 1% does not correlate with an increased risk of relapse in most studies (33,113,114), a higher percentage of mixed chimerism or an increasing level of mixed chimerism in patients monitored over time has been shown to correlate with an increased risk of relapse in some studies (32,115,116). Because there are a number of treatment strategies for patients who relapse after allogeneic bone marrow transplant, the use of bone marrow engraftment analysis to identify patients with developing relapse or at high risk of relapse provides an opportunity for early intervention that may be associated with better patient survival (117–120). However, some studies have failed to demonstrate an association between mixed chimerism and an increased rate of relapse (121–127). The contradictory results may be explained in part by variation in the patient populations under study and in part by differences in the sensitivity of the different DNA-based methods used to detect mixed chimerism. The lack of well-defined guidelines and assay performance standards, even among laboratories that use STRs for engraftment analysis, may also contribute to the conflicting results (112,128).

DEMONSTRATION OF NATURAL CHIMERISM

Although DNA-based identity testing of peripheral blood samples for mixed chimerism is most frequently performed in the context of bone marrow engraftment analysis, identity testing has also been used to document naturally occurring mixed chimerism in healthy individuals. For example, analysis of VNTR and STR loci has been used to demonstrate blood chimerism in twins (129,130), a finding that is consistent with prior studies that relied on RFLP analysis, blood group antigens, histocompatability antigens, or cytogenetic analysis (131–137). DNA typing has also been used to demonstrate long-term blood chimerism following solid organ transplantation resulting from passive transfer of donor hematopoietic cells along with the organ (138–140), and to demonstrate the persistence of fetal cells in maternal blood and tissues for decades, a situation known as fetal microchimerism (141,142).

The presence of natural chimerism in healthy individuals raises a couple of practical issues for clinical DNA-based identity testing. First, interpretation of a DNA profile should include an assessment of whether the test result could be caused by the phenomenon. Second, samples from nonhematopoietic tissues (such as hair-root or buccal swabs) likely constitute more reliable reference sources for testing somatic tissues; reference samples from blood should be reserved for testing of hematopoietic tissues (129,143).

Finally, for the sake of completeness, it must be noted that STR testing occasionally demonstrates a third allele in solid tissues in healthy individuals, albeit rarely (144). When the presence of a third allele is restricted to a single STR locus, the finding is usually attributed to duplication of the chromosomal region containing the STR locus or to improper segregation of the entire chromosome, rather than as evidence of chimerism.

IDENTITY TESTING
USING MITOCHONDRIAL DNA

Because most cells have at least several hundred mitochondria, each of which contains multiple copies of the mitochondrial genome, a cell typically has thousands of copies of each mitochondrial gene. As a result, identity testing based on mitochondrial DNA (mtDNA) has a higher sensitivity than testing based on nuclear DNA; mtDNA loci can often be amplified from samples that are so small or degraded that analysis of nuclear DNA is unsuccessful (8,145).

Although the mitochondrial genome is quite polymorphic, most of the variability among individuals is found in two hypervariable regions known as HV1 and HV2, each of which is several hundred bps long. Identity determination methods based on mtDNA target these hypervariable regions for PCR-based direct or indirect DNA sequence analysis (146–148) and, as with nuclear DNA typing, make use of population data to infer likelihood ratios when comparing mtDNA profiles (149). However, several features of mitochondrial genetics (Chapter 1) limit the utility of this approach. First, because mtDNA is maternally inherited, analysis can be used to assign a tissue sample only to a matrilineal family, not a specific individual. Transfer of paternal mtDNA into the fertilized ovum with subsequent recombination leading to hybrid mtDNA molecules has been described, but the effect appears to be minimal in the polymorphic regions of mtDNA most used in identity testing (150–152). Second, mtDNA has a much higher mutation rate than nuclear DNA, so a single individual often harbors different mtDNA sequences, a phenomenon known as heteroplasmy. Consequently, unknown and reference samples may contain sequence differences even when they originate from the same individual (153,154). Third, because all mtDNA polymorphisms are on the same fragment of DNA, variation at individual loci cannot be treated as independent events for calculation of statistical probabilities; relative to nuclear DNA, mtDNA polymorphisms therefore have a lower power of discrimination. Because of these limitations, use of mtDNA for identity determination is largely restricted to forensic settings in which only extremely limited material is available for analysis.

REFERENCES

1. Sensabaugh GF. Biochemical markers of individualaity. In: Saferstein R, ed. *Forensic Science Handbook.* Englewood Cliffs:Prentice-Hall, 1982:338–415.
2. Jeffreys AJ, Wilson V, Thein SL. Individual-specific 'fingerprints' of human DNA. *Nature* 1985;316:76–79.
3. Jeffreys A, Pena S. Brief introduction to human DNA fingerprinting. In: Pena S, et al., eds. *DNA Fingerprinting: State of the Science.* Basel: Birkhauser, Verlag; 1993:1–20.
4. Weedn VW. Forensic DNA tests. *Clin Lab Med* 1996;16:187–196.
5. Gill P, Jeffreys AJ, Werrett DJ. Forensic application of DNA "fingerprints". *Nature* 1985;318:577–579.
6. International Human Genome Sequencing Consortium. Initial sequencing and analysis of the human genome. *Nature* 2001;409:860–921.
7. Carey L, Mitnik L. Trends in DNA forensic analysis. *Electrophoresis* 2002;23:1386–1397.
8. Rudin N, Inman K, eds. *An Introduction to Forensic DNA Analysis,* 2nd ed. Boca Raton, FL: CRC Press Publishers; 2002.
9. Hirschhorn R. In vivo reversion to normal of inherited mutations in humans. *J Med Genet* 2003;40:721–728.
10. Erickson RP. Somatic gene mutation and human disease other than cancer. *Mutat Res* 2003;543:125–136.
11. Youssoufian H, Pyeritz RE. Mechanisms and consequences of somatic mosaicism in humans. *Nat Rev Genet* 2002;3:748–758.
12. Schichman SA, Lin P, Gilbrech LJ. Bone marrow transplant engraftment analysis with loss of an informative allele. *J Mol Diagn* 2002;4:230–232.
13. Zhou M, Sheldon S, Akel N, et al. Chromosomal aneuploidy in leukemic blast crisis: a potential source of error in interpretation of bone marrow engraftment analysis by VNTR amplification. *Mol Diagn* 1999;4:153–157.
14. Clayton TM, Whitaker JP, Sparkes R, et al. Analysis and interpretation of mixed forensic stains using DNA STR profiling. *Forensic Sci Int* 1998;91:55–70.
15. Budowle B, Moretti TR, Baumstark AL, et al. Population data on the thirteen CODIS core short tandem repeat loci in African Americans, U.S. Caucasians, Hispanics, Bahamians, Jamaicans, and Trinidadians. *J Forensic Sci* 1999;44:1277–1286.
16. Kupferschmid TD, Calicchio T, Budowle B. Maine Caucasian population DNA database using twelve short tandem repeat loci. *J Forensic Sci* 1999;44:392–395.
17. Martin P, Garcia O, Albarran C, et al. Spanish population data on the four STR loci D8S1179, D16S539, D18S51 and D21S11. *Int J Legal Med* 1999;112:340–341.
18. Allen RW, ed. *Standards for Parentage Testing Laboratories,* 3rd ed. Bethesda, MD: American Association of Blood Banks; 1998.
19. TWGDAM. Guidelines for a quality assurance program for DNA analysis. *Crime Lab Digest* 1991;18:44–75.
20. Wyman AR, White R. A highly polymorphic locus in human DNA. *Proc Natl Acad Sci USA* 1980;77:6754–6758.
21. Jeffreys AJ, Wilson V, Thein S. Hypervariable 'minisatellite' regions in human DNA. *Biotechnology* 1992;24:467–472.
22. Kan YW, Dozy AM. Polymorphism of DNA sequence adjacent to human beta-globin structural gene: relationship to sickle mutation. *Proc Natl Acad Sci USA* 1978;75:5631–5635.
23. Botstein D, White RL, Skolnick M, et al. Construction of a genetic linkage map in man using restriction fragment length polymorphisms. *Am J Hum Genet* 1980;32:314–331.
24. Tsongalis GJ, Wu AH, Silver H, et al. Applications of forensic identity testing in the clinical laboratory. *Am J Clin Pathol* 1999;112:S93–S103.
25. Baird ML. Use of the AmpliType PM + HLA DQA1 PCR amplification and typing kits for identity testing. *Methods Mol Biol* 1998;98:261–277.
26. Sprecher CJ, Puers C, Lins AM, et al. General approach to analysis of polymorphic short tandem repeat loci. *Biotechniques* 1996;20:266–276.
27. Butler JM. In: Butler JM, ed. *Forensic DNA Typing.* San Diego: Academic Press; 2001: 81–116.
28. Walsh PS, Erlich HA, Higuchi R. Preferential PCR amplification of alleles: mechanisms and solutions. *PCR Methods Appl* 1992;1:241–250.
29. Pai CY, Chou SL, Tang TK, et al. Prevention of false results from preferential PCR amplification of VNTR alleles. *J Formos Med Assoc* 1996;95:69–72.
30. Chakraborty R, Stivers DN, Su B, et al. The utility of short tandem repeat loci beyond human identification: implications for development of new DNA typing systems. *Electrophoresis* 1999;20:1682–1696.
31. Fregeau CJ, Fourney RM. DNA typing with fluorescently tagged short tandem repeats: a sensitive and accurate approach to human identification. *Biotechniques* 1993;15:100–119.
32. Bader P, Beck J, Frey A, et al. Serial and quantitative analysis of mixed hematopoietic chimerism by PCR in patients with acute leukemias allows the prediction of relapse after allogeneic BMT. *Bone Marrow Transplant* 1998;21:487–495.
33. Petit T, Raynal B, Socie G, et al. Highly sensitive polymerase chain reaction methods show the frequent survival of residual recipient multipotent progenitors after non-T-cell-depleted bone marrow transplantation. *Blood* 1994;84:3575–3583.
34. Thiede C, Florek M, Bornhauser M, et al. Rapid quantification of mixed chimerism using multiplex amplification of short tandem repeat markers and fluorescence detection. *Bone Marrow Transplant* 1999;23:1055–1060.
35. Hall A, Ballantyne J. The development of an 18-locus Y-STR system for forensic casework. *Anal Bioanal Chem* 2003;376:1234–1246.
36. Gill P, Brenner C, Brinkmann B, et al. DNA Commission of the International Society of Forensic Genetics: recommendations on forensic analysis using Y-chromosome STRs. *Forensic Sci Int* 2001;124:5–10.
37. Carracedo A, Beckmann A, Bengs A, et al. Results of a collaborative study of the EDNAP group regarding the reproducibility and robustness of the Y-chromosome STRs DYS19, DYS389 I and II, DYS390 and DYS393 in a PCR pentaplex format. *Forensic Sci Int* 2001;119:28–41.
38. Nakhleh RE, Zarbo RJ. Surgical pathology specimen identification and accessioning: A College of American Pathologists Q-Probes Study of 1,004,115 cases from 417 institutions. *Arch Pathol Lab Med* 1996;120:227–233.
39. Gephardt GN, Zarbo RJ. Extraneous tissue in surgical pathology: a College of American Pathologists Q-Probes study of 275 laboratories. *Arch Pathol Lab Med* 1996;120:1009–1014.
40. Bateman AC, Sage DA, Al-Talib RK, et al. Investigation of specimen mislabelling in paraffin-embedded tissue using a rapid, allele-specific, PCR-based HLA class II typing method. *Histopathology* 1996;28:169–174.
41. Bateman AC, Turner SJ, Theaker JM, et al. Polymerase chain reaction based human leucocyte antigen genotyping for the investigation of suspected gastrointestinal biopsy contamination. *Gut* 1999;45:259–263.
42. Shibata D, Namiki T, Higuchi R. Identification of a mislabeled fixed specimen by DNA analysis. *Am J Surg Pathol* 1990;14:1076–1078.
43. Giroti R, Kashyap VK. Detection of the source of mislabeled biopsy tissue paraffin block and histopathological section on glass slide. *Diagn Mol Pathol* 1998;7:331–334.
44. Shibata D. Identification of mismatched fixed specimens with a commercially available kit based on the polymerase chain reaction. *Am J Clin Pathol* 1993;100:666–670.
45. Kessis TD, Silberman MA, Sherman M, et al. Rapid identification of patient specimens with microsatellite DNA markers. *Mod Pathol* 1996;9:183–188.
46. Abeln ED, van Kemenade FD, van Krieken JH, et al. Rapid identification of mixed up bladder biopsy specimens using polymorphic microsatellite markers. *Diagn Mol Pathol* 1995;4:286–291.
47. Horn LC, Edelmann J, Hanel C, et al. Identity testing in cervical carcinoma in case of suspected mix-up. *Int J Gynecol Pathol* 2000;19:387–389.
48. O'Briain DS, Sheils O, McElwaine S, et al. Sorting out mix-ups: the provenance of tissue sections may be confirmed by PCR using microsatellite markers. *Am J Clin Pathol* 1996;106:758–764.
49. Ota M, Fukushima H, Akamatsu T, et al. Availability of immunostaining methods for identification of mixed-up tissue specimens. *Am J Clin Pathol* 1989;92:665–669.
50. Ritter JH, Sutton TD, Wick MR. Use of immunostains to ABH blood group antigens to resolve problems in identity of tissue specimens. *Arch Pathol Lab Med* 1994;118:293–297.

51. Bateman AC, Hemmatpour SK, Theaker JM, et al. Nested polymerase chain reaction-based HLA class II typing for the unique identification of formalin-fixed and paraffin-embedded tissue. *J Pathol* 1997;181:228–234.

52. Worsham MJ, Wolman SR, Zarbo RJ. Molecular approaches to identification of tissue contamination in surgical pathology sections. *J Mol Diagn* 2001;3:11–15.

53. Popiolek dA, Prinz MK, West AB. Multiplex DNA short tandem repeat analysis: a useful method for determining the provenance of minute fragments of formalin-fixed, paraffin-embedded tissue. *Am J Clin Pathol* 2003;120:746–751.

54. Nowell PC. The clonal evolution of tumor cell populations. *Science* 1976;194:23–28.

55. Fialkow PJ. Clonal origin of human tumors. *Biochim Biophys Acta* 1976;458:283–321.

56. Rolston R, Sasatomi E, Hunt J, et al. Distinguishing de novo second cancer formation from tumor recurrence: mutational fingerprinting by microdissection genotyping. *J Mol Diagn* 2001;3:129–132.

57. Lichy JH, Dalbegue F, Zavar M, et al. Genetic heterogeneity in ductal carcinoma of the breast. *Lab Invest* 2000;80:291–301.

58. Heinmoller E, Dietmaier W, Zirngibl H, et al. Molecular analysis of microdissected tumors and preneoplastic intraductal lesions in pancreatic carcinoma. *Am J Pathol* 2000;157:83–92.

59. Antonescu CR, Elahi A, Healey JH, et al. Monoclonality of multifocal myxoid liposarcoma: confirmation by analysis of *TLS-CHOP* or *EWS-CHOP* rearrangements. *Cancer Res* 2000;6:2788–2793.

60. Bagg A. Chronic myeloid leukemia: a minimalistic view of post-therapeutic monitoring. *J Mol Diagn* 2002;4:1–10.

61. Fujita M, Enomoto T, Wada H, et al. Molecular analysis of microdissected tumors and preneoplastic intraductal lesions in pancreatic carcinoma. *Am J Pathol* 2000;157:83–92.

62. Jacobs IJ, Kohler MF, Wiseman RW, et al. Clonal origin of epithelial ovarian carcinoma: analysis by loss of heterozygosity, *p53* mutation, and X-chromosome inactivation. *J Natl Cancer Inst* 1992;84:1793–1798.

63. Kuukasjarvi T, Karhu R, Tanner M, et al. Genetic heterogeneity and clonal evolution underlying development of asynchronous metastasis in human breast cancer. *Cancer Res* 1997;57:1597–1604.

64. Tang M, Pires Y, Schultz M, et al. Microsatellite analysis of synchronous and metachronous tumors: a tool for double primary tumor and metastasis assessment. *Diagn Mol Pathol* 2003;12:151–159.

65. Emmert-Buck MR, Chuaqui R, Zhuang Z, et al. Molecular analysis of synchronous uterine and ovarian endometrioid tumors. *Int J Gynecol Pathol* 1997;16:143–148.

66. Fujii H, Matsumoto T, Yoshida M, et al. Genetics of synchronous uterine and ovarian endometrioid carcinoma: combined analyses of loss of heterozygosity, *PTEN* mutation, and microsatellite instability. *Hum Pathol* 2002;33:421–428.

67. Diaz-Cano SJ, Blanes A, Rubio J, et al. Molecular evolution and intratumor heterogeneity by topographic compartments in muscle-invasive transitional cell carcinoma of the urinary bladder. *Lab Invest* 2000;80:279–289.

68. Vogelstein B, Fearon ER, Kern SE, et al. Allelotype of colorectal carcinomas. *Science* 1989;244:207–211.

69. Maitra A, Wistuba II, Washington C, et al. High-resolution chromosome 3p allelotyping of breast carcinomas and precursor lesions demonstrates frequent loss of heterozygosity and a discontinuous pattern of allele loss. *Am J Pathol* 2001;159:119–130.

70. Wistuba II, Tang M, Maitra A, et al. Genome-wide allelotyping analysis reveals multiple sites of allelic loss in gallbladder carcinoma. *Cancer Res* 2001;61:3795–3800.

71. Hunt JL, Tometsko M, LiVolsi VA, et al. Molecular evidence of anaplastic transformation in coexisting well-differentiated and anaplastic carcinomas of the thyroid. *Am J Surg Pathol* 2003;27:1559–1564.

72. Sieben NL, Kolkman-Uljee SM, Flanagan AM, et al. Molecular genetic evidence for monoclonal origin of bilateral ovarian serous borderline tumors. *Am J Pathol* 2003;162:1095–1101.

73. Mao L, Lee DJ, Tockman MS, et al. Microsatellite alterations as clonal markers for the detection of human cancer. *Proc Natl Acad Sci USA* 1994;91:9871–9875.

74. Matsuzoe D, Hideshima T, Ohshima K, et al. Discrimination of double primary lung cancer from intrapulmonary metastasis by *p53* gene mutation. *Br J Cancer* 1999;79:1549–1552.

75. Huang J, Behrens C, Wistuba I, et al. Molecular analysis of synchronous and metachronous tumors of the lung: impact on management and prognosis. *Ann Diagn Pathol* 2001;5:321–329.

76. Abe Y, Masuda H, Okubo R. Microsatellite instability of each tumor in sporadic synchronous multiple colorectal cancers. *Oncol Rep* 2001;8:299–304.

77. Krebs PA, Albuquerque A, Quezado M, et al. The use of microsatellite instability in the distinction between synchronous endometrial and colonic adenocarcinomas. *Int J Gynecol Pathol* 1999;18:320–324.

78. Ohtani H, Yashiro M, Onoda N, et al. Synchronous multiple primary gastrointestinal cancer exhibits frequent microsatellite instability. *Int J Cancer* 2000;86:678–683.

79. Lin WM, Forgacs E, Warshal DP, et al. Loss of heterozygosity and mutational analysis of the *PTEN/MMAC1* gene in synchronous endometrial and ovarian carcinomas. *Clin Cancer Res* 1998;4:2577–2583.

80. Szych C, Staebler A, Connolly DC, et al. Molecular genetic evidence supporting the clonality and appendiceal origin of pseudomyxoma peritonei in women. *Am J Pathol* 1999;154:1849–1855.

81. Takahashi T, Habuchi T, Kakehi Y, et al. Molecular diagnosis of metastatic origin in a patient with metachronous multiple cancers of the renal pelvis and bladder. *Urology* 2000;56:331.

82. Milchgrub S, Wistuba II, Kim BK, et al. Molecular identification of metastatic cancer to the skin using laser capture microdissection: a case report. *Cancer* 2000;88:749–754.

83. Kushima M, Fujii Hm, Murakami K, et al. Simultaneous squamous cell carcinomas of the uterine cervix and upper genital tract: loss of heterozygosity analysis demonstrates clonal neoplasms of cervical origin. *Int J Gynecol Pathol* 2001;20:353–358.

84. Penn I. Post-transplant malignancy: the role of immunosuppression. *Drug Saf* 2000;23:101–113.

85. Penn I. Cancers in renal transplant recipients. *Adv Ren Replace Ther* 2000;7:147–156.

86. Martin DG, Rubini M, Rosen VJ. Cadaveric renal homotransplantation with inadvertent transplantation of carcinoma. *JAMA* 1965;192:752–754.

87. Penn I. Transmission of cancer from organ donors. *Ann Transplant* 1997;2:7–12.

88. Conlon PJ, Smith SR. Transmission of cancer with cadaveric donor organs. *J Am Soc Nephrol* 1995;6:54–60.

89. Penn I. Donor transmitted disease: cancer. *Transplant Proc* 1991;23:2629–2631.

90. MacKie RM, Reid R, Junor B. Fatal melanoma transferred in a donated kidney 16 years after melanoma surgery [Letter]. *N Engl J Med* 2003;348:567–568.

91. Wilson LJ, Horvat RT, Tilzer L, et al. Identification of donor melanoma in a renal transplant recipient. *Diagn Mol Pathol* 1992;1:266–271.

92. Loh E, Couch FJ, Hendricksen C, et al. Development of donor-derived prostate cancer in a recipient following orthotopic heart transplantation. *JAMA* 1997;277:133–137.

93. Schmitt C, Cire K, Schattenkirchner S, et al. Highly sensitive DNA typing for detecting tumors transmitted by transplantation. *Transpl Int* 1998;11:382–386.

94. Stephens JK, Everson GT, Elliott CL, et al. Fatal transfer of malignant melanoma from multiorgan donor to four allograft recipients. *Transplantation* 2000;70:232–236.

95. Beckingham IJ, O'Rourke JS, Bishop MC, et al. The use of DNA typing to clarify the origin of metastatic carcinoma after renal transplantation: a clinical and medico-legal problem. *Transpl Int* 1994;7:379–381.

96. Gartner HV, Seidl C, Luckenbach C, et al. Genetic analysis of a sarcoma accidentally transplanted from a patient to a surgeon. *N Engl J Med* 1996;335:1494–1496.

97. Maehara Y, Oda S, Sugimachi K. The instability within: problems in current analyses of microsatellite instability. *Mutat Res* 2001;461:249–263.

98. Schlitt HJ, Hundrieser J, Hisananga M, et al. Patterns of donor-type microchimerism after heart transplantation. *Lancet* 1994;343:1469–1471.

99. Altimari A, Gruppioni E, Fiorentino M, et al. Genomic allelotyping for distinction of recurrent and de novo hepatocellular carcinoma after orthotopic liver transplantation. *Diagn Mol Pathol* 2005;14:34–38.

100. Mazal PR, Schaufler R, Altenhuber-Muller R, et al. Derivation of nephrogenic adenomas from renal tubular cells in kidney-transplant recipients. *N Engl J Med* 2002;347:653–659.

101. Borka P, Jakab J, Rajczy K, et al. Temporary donor-derived B-lymphocyte microchimerism leading to hemolysis in minor AB0-incompatible renal transplantation. *Transplant Proc* 2001;33:2287–2289.

102. Odabas AR, Tutucu KN, Turkmen A, et al. Severe alloimmune hemolytic anemia after renal transplantation. *Nephron* 2002;92:743–745.

103. Frohn C, Jabs WJ, Fricke L, et al. Hemolytic anemia after kidney transplantation: case report and differential diagnosis. *Ann Hematol* 2002;81:158–160.

104. Donckier V, Toungouz M, Goldman M. Transplantation tolerance and mixed chimerism: at the frontier of clinical application. *Transpl Int* 2001;14:1–5.

105. Diez-Martin JL, Llamas P, Gosalvez J, et al. Conventional cytogenetics and FISH evaluation of chimerism after sex-mismatched bone marrow transplantation (BMT) and donor leukocyte infusion (DLI). *Haematologica* 1998;83:408–415.

106. Durham D, Anders K, Fisher L, et al. Analysis of the origin of marrow cells in bone marrow transplant recipients using a Y-chromosome-specific in situ hybridization assay. *Blood* 1989;74:2220–2226.

107. Moses RD, Beschorner WE, Singer D, et al. Restriction fragment length polymorphism analysis with a cross-reactive HLA class II DR-beta gene probe for the detection of engraftment of MHC-mismatched marrow in the rhesus monkey. *Bone Marrow Transplant* 1989;4:475–481.

108. Leclair B, Fregeau CJ, Aye MT, et al. DNA typing for bone marrow engraftment follow-up after allogeneic transplant: a comparative study of current technologies. *Bone Marrow Transplant* 1995;16:43–55.

109. Van Deerlin VM, Leonard DG. Bone marrow engraftment analysis after allogeneic bone marrow transplantation. *Clin Lab Med* 2000;20:197–225.

110. Oliver DH, Thompson RE, Griffin CA, et al. Use of single nucleotide polymorphisms (SNP) and real-time polymerase chain reaction for bone marrow engraftment analysis. *J Mol Diagn* 2000;2:202–208.

111. Hauge XY, Litt M. A study of the origin of 'shadow bands' seen when typing dinucleotide repeat polymorphisms by the PCR. *Hum Mol Genet* 1993;2:411–415.

112. Schichman SA, Suess P, Vertino AM, et al. Comparison of short tandem repeat and variable number tandem repeat genetic markers for quantitative determination of allogeneic bone marrow transplant engraftment. *Bone Marrow Transplant* 2002;29:243–248.

113. Landman-Parker J, Socie G, Petit T, et al. Detection of recipient cells after non T-cell depleted bone marrow transplantation for leukemia by PCR amplification of minisatellites or of a Y chromosome marker has a different prognostic value. *Leukemia* 1994;8:1989–1994.

114. Mangioni S, Balduzzi A, Rivolta A, et al. Long-term persistence of hemopoietic chimerism following sex-mismatched bone marrow transplantation. *Bone Marrow Transplant* 1997;20:969–973.

115. Ramirez M, Diaz MA, Garcia-Sanchez F, et al. Chimerism after allogeneic hematopoietic cell transplantation in childhood acute lymphoblastic leukemia. *Bone Marrow Transplant* 1996;18:1161–1165.

116. Lawler M, Humphries P, McCann SR. Evaluation of mixed chimerism by in vitro amplification of dinucleotide repeat sequences using the polymerase chain reaction. *Blood* 1991;77:2504–2514.

117. Collins RH Jr, Shpilberg O, Drobyski WR, et al. Donor leukocyte infusions in 140 patients with relapsed malignancy after allogeneic bone marrow transplantation. *J Clin Oncol* 1997;15:433–444.

118. Kolb HJ, Mittermuller J, Clemm C, et al. Donor leukocyte transfusions for treatment of recurrent chronic myelogenous leukemia in marrow transplant patients. *Blood* 1990;76:2462–2465.

119. Kolb HJ, Schattenberg A, Goldman JM, et al. Graft-versus-leukemia effect of donor lymphocyte transfusions in marrow grafted patients. European Group for Blood and Marrow Transplantation Working Party Chronic Leukemia. *Blood* 1995;86:2041–2050.

120. Porter DL, Roth MS, McGarigle C, et al. Induction of graft-versus-host disease as immunotherapy for relapsed chronic myeloid leukemia. *N Engl J Med* 1994;330:100–106.

121. Molloy K, Goulden N, Lawler M, et al. Patterns of hematopoietic chimerism following bone marrow transplantation for childhood acute lymphoblastic leukemia from volunteer unrelated donors. *Blood* 1996;87:3027–3031.

122. Petz LD, Yam P, Wallace RB, et al. Mixed hematopoietic chimerism following bone marrow transplantation for hematologic malignancies. *Blood* 1987;70:1331–1337.

123. Roth MS, Antin JH, Bingham EL, et al. Use of polymerase chain reaction-detected sequence polymorphisms to document engraftment following allogeneic bone marrow transplantation. *Transplantation* 1990;49:714–720.

124. Suttorp M, Schmitz N, Dreger P, et al. Monitoring of chimerism after allogeneic bone marrow transplantation with unmanipulated marrow by use of DNA polymorphisms. *Leukemia* 1993;7:679–687.

125. van Leeuwen JE, van Tol MJ, Joosten AM, et al. Mixed T-lymphoid chimerism after allogeneic bone marrow transplantation for hematologic malignancies of children is not correlated with relapse. *Blood* 1993;82:1921–1928.

126. van Leeuwen JE, van Tol MJ, Joosten AM, et al. Persistence of host-type hematopoiesis after allogeneic bone marrow transplantation for leukemia is significantly related to the recipient's age and/or the conditioning regimen, but it is not associated with an increased risk of relapse. *Blood* 1994;83:3059–3067.

127. Schattenberg A, De Witte T, Salden M, et al. Mixed hematopoietic chimerism after allogeneic transplantation with lymphocyte-depleted bone marrow is not associated with a higher incidence of relapse. *Blood* 1989;73:1367–1372.

128. Antin JH, Childs R, Filipovich AH, et al. Establishment of complete and mixed donor chimerism after allogeneic lymphohematopoietic transplantation: recommendations from a workshop at the 2001 Tandem Meetings of the International Bone Marrow Transplant Registry and the American Society of Blood and Marrow Transplantation. *Biol Blood Marrow Transplant* 2001;7:473–485.

129. Rubocki RJ, McCue BJ, Duffy KJ, et al. Natural DNA mixtures generated in fraternal twins in utero. *J Forensic Sci* 2001;46:120–125.

130. Souter VL, Kapur RP, Nyholt DR, et al. A report of dizygous monochorionic twins. *N Engl J Med* 2003;349:154–158.

131. Hansen HE, Sondervang A. DNA profiles of chimeric twins, TS and MR using the single-locus-probe technique. *Hum Hered* 1993;43:98–102.

132. Pausch V, Bleier I, Dub E, et al. A further case of chimeric twins: genetic markers of the blood. *Vox Sang* 1979;36:85–92.

133. Bird GW, Wingham J, Nicholson GS, et al. Another example of haemopoietic (twin) chimaerism in a subject unaware of being a twin. *J Immunogenet* 1982;9:317–322.

134. Szymanski IO, Tilley CA, Crookston MC, et al. A further example of human blood group chimaerism. *J Med Genet* 1977;14:279–281.

135. Bird GW, Gibson M, Wingham J, et al. Another example of haemopoietic chimaerism in dizygotic twins. *Br J Haematol* 1980;46:439–445.

136. Angela E, Robinson E, North D. A case of twin chimerism. *J Med Genet* 1976;13:528–530.

137. Thomsen M, Hansen Hem, Dickmeiss E. MLC and CML studies in the family of a pair of HLA haploidentical chimeric twins. *Scand J Immunol* 1977;6:523–528.

138. Starzl T, Demetris AJ, Murase N, et al. Cell migration, chimerism, and graft acceptance. *Lancet* 1992;339:1579–1582.

139. Starzl T, Demetris AJ, Murase N, et al. Chimerism and donor-specific nonreactivity 27 to 29 years after kidney allotransplantation. *Transplantation* 1993;55:1272–1277.

140. Starzl T, Demetris AJ, Murase N, et al. Cell migration and chimerism after whole-organ transplantation: the basis of graft acceptance. *Hepatology* 1993;17:1127–1152.

141. Stevens AM, McDonnell WM, Mullarkey ME, et al. Liver biopsies from human females contain male hepatocytes in the absence of transplantation. *Lab Invest* 2004;84: 1603–1609.

142. Nelson JL. Microchimerism: incidental byproduct of pregnancy or active participant in human health? *Trends Mol Med* 2002;8:109–113.

143. Redline RW. Nonidentical twins with a single placenta: disproving dogma in perinatal pathology. *N Engl J Med* 2003;349:111–114.

144. Crouse CA, Rogers S, Amiott E, et al. Analysis and interpretation of short tandem repeat microvariants and three-banded allele patterns using multiple allele detection systems. *J Forensic Sci* 1999;44:87–94.

145. Andreasson H, Gyllensten U, Allen M. Real-time DNA quantification of nuclear and mitochondrial DNA in forensic analysis. *Biotechniques* 2002;33:402–411.

146. Butler JM, Levin BC. Forensic applications of mitochondrial DNA. *Trends Biotechnol* 1998;16:158–162.

147. Stewart JE, Aagaard PJ, Pokorak EG, et al. Evaluation of a multicapillary electrophoresis instrument for mitochondrial DNA typing. *J Forensic Sci* 2003;48:571–580.

148. de Souza Menezes J, de Almeida Drummond Franklin D, Seki H, et al. Single-strand conformation polymorphism of hyper-variable regions HV1 and HV2 of human mitochondrial DNA: detection by silver staining. *Forensic Sci Int* 2003;133:242–245.

149. Allard MW, Miller K, Wilson M, et al. Characterization of the Caucasian haplogroups present in the SWGDAM forensic mtDNA dataset for 1771 human control region sequences. Scientific Working Group on DNA Analysis Methods. *J Forensic Sci* 2002;47:1215–1223.

150. Eyre-Walker A, Smith NJ, Maynard-Smith J. How clonal are human mitochondria? *Proc R Soc Lond B Biol Sci* 1999;266:477–483.

151. Awadalla P, Eyre-Walker A, Maynard-Smith J. Linkage disequilibrium and recombination in hominid mitochondrial DNA. *Science* 1999;286:2524–2525.

152. Parsons TJ, Irwin JA. Questioning evidence for recombination in human mitochondrial DNA. *Science* 2000;288:1931.

153. Tully G, Bar W, Brinkmann B, et al. Considerations by the European DNA profiling (EDNAP) group on the working practices, nomenclature and interpretation of mitochondrial DNA profiles. *Forensic Sci Int* 2001;124:83–91.

154. Lutz S, Weisser HJ, Heizmann J, et al. Mitochondrial heteroplasmy among maternally related individuals. *Int J Legal Med* 2000;113:155–161.

The Future

24

TRENDS

Diagnosis

There is no doubt that molecular genetic analysis will play an increasing role in surgical pathology. The utility of many techniques, such as cytogenetics, polymerase chain reaction (PCR), and fluorescence in situ hybridization (FISH), has already been established. Other methods, such as gene expression profiling and proteomics, are currently primarily research tools but will likely find a niche in clinical laboratory testing in the future. Although it is impossible to predict the exact settings in which molecular testing will become a component of the pathologic evaluation of tissue specimens, several trends have emerged that will have a significant impact on the future of diagnostic genetic testing.

Analysis of Single Loci

Currently, most molecular tests performed in the context of diagnostic surgical pathology involve analysis of a single locus, whether by PCR to identify characteristic fusion transcripts, FISH to detect specific chromosomal aberrations, mutational analysis to detect precise sequence changes, in situ hybridization (ISH) to detect expression of individual genes, and so on. Despite the fact that analysis of single markers has established clinical value for many neoplasms, testing focused on individual loci often reflects an ignorance of other genes that have critical oncobiologic roles, which, if incorporated into the analysis, could increase the utility of the test result (1–4). Single genetic events are likely to be insufficient to account for all of the features of a neoplasm, and testing that involves a larger number of loci will likely provide more accurate diagnostic, prognostic, and therapeutic information (1,2). Analysis of additional loci will likely provide an explanation for many of the presumed false positive and false negative

results that are encountered when testing is limited to a single genetic region.

The fact that many of the molecular tests in routine use in diagnostic surgical pathology focus on single loci is a reflection of the immaturity of the field. Over a century of experience with light microscopy has shown that optimal pathologic evaluation of many neoplasms involves combined evaluation of the tumor's cytologic features, mitotic rate, architectural pattern, anatomic extent, and so on. Similarly, several decades of experience with immunohistochemistry has shown that a panel of immunostains often has greater diagnostic utility than a single immunostain. The fact that molecular testing currently relies on analysis of single genetic abnormalities is a reflection of our general ignorance of tumor biology rather than an optimized testing paradigm, and so it is to be expected that as our understanding of oncogenesis becomes more sophisticated, analysis of multiple loci will be used to provide more accurate information.

Microarray technology has made it possible to evaluate thousands of loci, if not tens of thousands, from individual tumor specimens. Although most microarray analysis in the context of surgical pathology has focused on global gene expression profiling, microarray methods for expression analysis targeted to specific cell-signaling pathways, metabolic pathways, or mutational patterns will likely emerge as other important approaches for the pathologic characterization of tumors (discussed more fully below).

Gene Expression Analysis

Even though gene expression profiling is still largely experimental, the use of the technique to clarify diagnostic groups, provide more accurate prognostic information, and predict response to specific therapeutic regimens indicates the enormous potential of the methodology. Once basic science studies have identified subsets of genes that show the greatest utility for testing of individual tumor

TABLE 24.1

POSSIBLE OBSTACLES TO CLINICAL APPLICATION OF ARRAY-BASED ANALYSIS

Technical issues
Cost of analysis
Lack of standardization between different array platforms
Requirement for fresh tissue
Tumor sample heterogeneity

Statistical issues
Lack of standard analysis between different studies
Selection bias

Epidemiologic issues
Tumor sample heterogeneity
Patient population heterogeneity
Selection bias

Experimental design issues
Cases for analysis usually selected based on conventional histopathologic evaluation
Lack of validation by independent case series
Lack of validation by prospective clinical trials
Overfitting artifacts

types, it can be anticipated that specialized microarrays (a colon cancer chip, a breast cancer chip, a non–small cell lung cancer chip, etc.) will be marketed for use in routine practice. However, there are several obstacles that may hinder the transition of gene expression analysis from basic science setting to clinical laboratories (Table 24.1).

Beyond purely technical, statistical, and epidemiologic issues (5–8), there are several significant experimental design issues that also need to be addressed. First, most microarray testing thus far has been performed on cases selected on the basis of conventional histopathologic evaluation. It is therefore not surprising when gene expression analysis produces results that show a high degree of correlation with histologic tumor type (2). Few studies have evaluated the role of microarray analysis that is not based on prior histopathologic evaluation, and it is rarely emphasized that tumor classification by light microscopy must precede microarray analysis in order to achieve the published results. These facts emphasize that traditional histopathologic evaluation and gene expression analysis are at present complementary, and suggest that claims that microarray analysis will revolutionize diagnosis are premature (9,10).

Second, the stringent rules used to formally assess the validity of novel therapeutic regimens in clinical trials are often not stringently applied to new diagnostic methods, and there is no regulatory oversight for validation of new diagnostic paradigms (reviewed in 11). Many issues (including analysis of complex patient populations, impact of tissue sample heterogeneity, possible selection bias) that are rigorously addressed in clinical studies of new diagnostic, prognostic, or therapeutic methods are often ignored in basic science reports (1,11).

Third, microarray analysis is particularly susceptible to overfitting artifacts. Overfitting occurs when a very large number of potential predictors is used to discriminate between a small number of outcome events (11). The magnitude of the problem is indicated by the informal rule applied in clinical epidemiology studies that there should be at least 10 events (tumor samples) for each variable (gene) in order to have confidence in the experiment results (12). Formal statistical analysis has demonstrated that, when the number of data points in a microarray experiment far exceeds the number of independent samples (e.g., 10 samples with disease, 10 samples without disease, and 6,000 data points for each sample), 98% of hypothetical models will fit with data sets that are randomly generated, even if confirmatory cross-validation analysis is performed (13). Validation of microarray results by an independent set of cases can minimize the problems generated by overfitting, but a recent survey has shown that only about 10% of microarray studies employ an independent set of cases to confirm the results (14).

The Tumor Microenvironment

It has recently become clear that the tumor microenvironment plays an important role in tumor development by a variety of different mechanisms. For example, lymphoma-specific chromosomal translocations in microvascular endothelial cells have been demonstrated in B-cell lymphoma (15). Altered patterns of gene expression in stromal fibroblasts that may promote neoplastic transformation through a paracrine mechanism have been described in the development of a number of carcinomas (16,17). Cytogenetic abnormalities in tumor-associated endothelial cells, as well as stromal exposure to carcinogens, have also been shown to correlate with carcinoma development (18,19). Although the role of the stroma in oncogenesis is only beginning to be understood, it is possible that molecular analysis of the tumor microenvironment may have diagnostic, prognostic, or therapeutic implications that are not yet recognized.

Phenotype-genotype Correlations

Just as a panel of a small number of immunohistochemical stains can be used to differentiate between two tumor types that are indistinguishable based on morphology, molecular tests can be used to distinguish tumors that have an identical morphologic and immunohistochemical appearance. However, it is probably naive to think that an increasingly detailed description of the DNA, RNA, protein, and metabolic features of neoplasms will entirely eliminate all diagnostic uncertainty. As we more completely understand the genetic and metabolic features of tumors in vitro, and concomitantly develop ever more complex models in silico, we simply move closer to the integration of all the genetic and metabolic information that already occurs within tumor cells in vivo. In the end, the heterogeneity of tumor phenotypes is simply a reflection of underlying genetic and metabolic heterogeneity; thus, an absolutely complete, absolutely accurate model of tumor biology will reflect this heterogeneity. A complete, accurate model will not only recapitulate the features of those tumors that easily fit into well-defined clinicopathologic groups, but will also faithfully reproduce the features of those tumors that do not match with precise diagnostic categories.

There is no doubt that specific patterns of mutation, gene expression, protein activation, and so on, have emerged (and will continue to emerge) that can be used as helpful, reliable guides for diagnosis. However, if an undifferentiated tumor harbors a set of mutations characteristic of a more well-defined tumor type, it suggests that there are unrecognized aspects of the genetic or metabolic profile of the undifferentiated tumor that have yet to be characterized. It is premature to assume that such differences are irrelevant.

Existing classification schemes are based on clinical data that correlate specific cytologic and morphologic features with outcome and response to treatment. For those tumors in which histopathologic evaluation and molecular analysis suggest different diagnoses, the hypothesis that the genetic diagnosis more accurately predicts clinical outcome must be proven by prospective clinical trials.

Prognosis

Although TNM stage is the most important prognostic indicator, and although complete excision with a negative margin also has a fundamental impact on survival, traditional histopathologic evaluation cannot be used to accurately predict which patients within TNM subgroups will suffer recurrences or die of their disease. Molecular testing therefore has the potential to provide information that can be used to more accurately stratify patients into prognostic categories.

However, a number of conceptual issues will need to be addressed before the role of molecular testing regarding prognosis is established (Table 24.2). First, the clinical relevance of staging information that is obtained only through extremely sensitive methods such as PCR will need to be established in randomized clinical trials (20–22). The demonstration that the presence of submicroscopic tumor in lymph nodes, peripheral blood, or bone marrow correlates with prognosis in retrospective studies does not imply that changes in treatment based on the presence on metastases will affect patient survival. Second, because retrospective studies are often compromised by unrecognized biases, a putative role of molecular tests for stratifying patients into different prognostic groups can be formally established only by prospective trials (23). For most putative prognostic markers, such trials have yet to be initiated, much less completed, and because prospective studies often take 5 to 10 years, meaningful integration of prognostic molecular testing into

---

TABLE 24.2

ISSUES CONFRONTING PROGNOSTIC MOLECULAR TESTING

- Does molecular analysis yield improved staging information compared with traditional staging methods?
- What is the clinical significance of submicroscopic metastasis (i.e., metastasis detected by molecular analysis but not traditional histopathologic evaluation)?
- What is the clinical significance of circulating DNA that harbors tumor specific mutations, compared with circulating tumor cells?
- Can quantitative PCR approaches overcome the specificity issues associated with illegitimate expression of marker loci?
- Can analysis of multiple loci overcome specificity issues associated with analysis of single loci?
- Can standardized markers and testing approaches be developed that make it possible to easily compare results from different institutions?
- How quickly will more cost-effective surrogate tests be developed to replace molecular tests?
- Will prospective trials confirm the results of retrospective studies?

Compiled from references 20 and 21.

routine clinical practice is a long-term process (20–23). Third, standardized testing protocols and standardized methods of statistical analyses must be developed so that the results from different institutions can be directly compared (22). Fourth, it will need to be established that molecular analysis provides information that cannot be obtained by more cost-effective surrogate markers (22).

Treatment

Molecular analysis will increasingly be used to stratify patients into more discrete therapeutic groups and to tailor therapy to individual patients. It is in this context that genetic analysis will likely come the closest to fulfilling the National Cancer Institute Director's Challenge for a molecular classification of cancer (24). In the future, pharmacogenetic testing to optimize treatment may become as integral a part of the pathologic evaluation of a malignancy as microscopic examination to assign a TNM stage and assess the adequacy of excision.

Pharmacogenetics

Pharmacogenetics is the study of the role of genetic variation to predict an individual patient's response to treatment with a specific drug (25). B0ecause genetic variation has been estimated to account for 20% to 95% of variability in drug disposition and effect (26), pharmacogenetics offers

the opportunity to not only increase the efficacy of therapy, but to also decrease harmful side effects (25,27–29).

In general, pharmacogenetic investigation falls into three categories. The first general category is the study of individual variation that influences drug disposition, including analysis of enzymes involved in drug metabolism, absorption, distribution, and excretion. The second category is analysis of inherited differences in the molecular targets of drugs. An increasingly important third category of investigation involves evaluation of acquired mutations that affect drug efficacy within individual tumors (29–31).

Although pharmacogenetics has traditionally involved correlation of specific alleles with drug response, in the future the field will doubtless expand to include genomics, proteomics, transcriptomics, metabolomics, and so on. Although each general approach has its own advantages and limitations (Table 24.3), all are subject to the same underlying set of challenges (27). First, the inherited component of drug response is usually polygenic, and so extensive genetic information from a large number of patients is required to identify all the polymorphisms associated with the drug's effect. Second, because the inherited component of drug response includes variations in drug disposition as well as the cellular target, detailed knowledge of the drug's metabolism as well as its mechanism of action is required if genomewide searches for associated polymorphisms are to be successful (5,6,25,27,32). Third, analysis depends on

---

TABLE 24.3

APPROACHES FOR MOLECULAR ANALYSIS OF PHARMACOGENETIC VARIATION

Approach	Advantages	Limitations
Sequence analysis	Provides information on the complete exonic sequence and splice junctions	Time consuming
		May detect irrelevant polymorphisms (i.e., low specificity)
Candidate polymorphism analysis	Quick and relatively inexpensive	Only helpful when tagged polymorphic loci are known
	Provides information regarding drug pharmacodynamics and pharmacokinetics	Requires extensive knowledge regarding what loci are important
	Hypothesis driven	
Expression profiling	Potentially provides information on genetic predispositions	Currently no database available
	May permit a direct assessment of drug effects	Data analysis is complex
Pathway approach	Accounts for associations between proteins in a metabolic pathway	Requires a detailed biochemical understanding of the pathway
	Provides information regarding drug metabolism and other biologic associations	Data analysis is complex
	Likely to explain interindividual variation in drug response	Requires large study sizes
	Hypothesis driven	
Genomics or proteomics	Provides a complete gene- or protein-expression profile (tumor or individual)	Optimal data management and data analysis techniques are not well defined
	Provides information on associations not previously suspected	Utility for prediction of toxicity is unknown
Compiled	Does not require a hypothesis	

Compiled from references 29 and 32.

objective quantification of drug responses and associated toxicities, which requires that patients are uniformly treated, systematically evaluated, and uniformly diagnosed (27). Fourth, pharmacogenetic relationships must be independently validated for different therapeutic indications of the same drug, as well as in different racial and ethic groups (27,33). And fifth, pharmacogenetic analysis must be performed on the patient's normal tissue as well as the tumor itself, because evaluation of normal tissue will not disclose mutations or epigenetic alterations in the neoplasm that independently affect the drug's disposition or its target.

Implications

The fact that pharmacogenetic testing will achieve a more significant role in the pathologic evaluation of tumors has a number of important implications for clinical trials. First, the presence of unrecognized molecular heterogeneity should be considered in trial design. Traditionally structured randomized clinical trials may not have enough statistical power to detect a therapeutic effect anticipated to occur in only a subset of patients (34,35). Second, the results from a clinical trial that involves one racial or ethnic group may not be predictive for patient groups of different race or ethnicity (33,36). Federal oversight of clinical trials in the United States has traditionally focused on ensuring enrollment of a diverse population of patients, so a radically different model of randomized clinical trials may be required (37). Third, pharmacogenetic analysis of tumors may become as important as, if not supplant, traditional eligibility criteria for clinical trials evaluating new therapeutic approaches (35).

Cost

It is unclear how molecular analysis used to tailor therapy to individual patients will affect future health care costs. Some have suggested that payers will have little enthusiasm for the analysis because of the cost of testing and because individualized therapy runs counter to adopted mechanisms of cost containment such as restricted drug formularies and therapeutic substitution (38). However, several studies have demonstrated that drug therapy tailored to an individual patient's genetic makeup actually reduces adverse drug reactions and thus can result in immediate cost savings (39,40).

EMERGING TECHNOLOGIES

DNA Sequence Analysis

Given that most tumors harbor mutations at many loci, DNA sequence analysis of a panel of genes may provide information that is more closely linked with diagnosis, prognosis, or therapeutic response. Advances in automation developed as part of the human genome project make it possible to realistically propose genomewide DNA sequence analysis as a component of the pathologic evaluation of individual tumors. Although possible from a technical viewpoint, the cost of such analysis is prohibitive and

so the approach is not yet feasible in routine practice. However, further advances in automation, coupled with a more complete understanding of the patterns of mutations that correlate with specific neoplasms, suggest that sequence analysis of a target set of genes may well become a routine component of the pathologic evaluation of tumor specimens.

Single Nucleotide Polymorphisms

Single-nucleotide polymorphisms (SNPs), discussed in more detail in Chapter 1, are common in the human genome. By some estimates, the human genome contains about 10 million SNPs that have frequencies higher than 1% (41,42). Once individual SNPs are linked with increased susceptibility to certain diseases, response to therapy, and so on, systematic analysis of SNPs may circumvent the need for more extensive DNA sequence analysis (27,34,43).

Systematic identification of SNPs that tag each of the common haplotypes of a genetic region is a very time consuming and expensive process (43). However, an international consortium recently identified a set of more than one million tagged SNPs that span the genome (42), a catalog that will be an important research tool. Nonetheless, it currently costs about U.S. $0.10 to evaluate one SNP in a patient sample (43), and so genomewide analysis still too expensive for clinical use, although increased automation and more refined SNP catalogs that decrease the cost of testing will likely make systematic analysis of SNPs an important clinical tool in the future.

Epigenetic Modifications

A technique that makes it possible to quantitatively detect the methylation status of every human gene individually has recently been deveoped (44). Given the effect that epigenetic changes have on gene expression, it is reasonable to anticipate that the pattern of methylation at defined sets of loci may eventually become a component of the pathologic evaluation of individual tumors. Paired genomewide DNA sequence or SNP testing may further enhance the diagnostic, prognostic, and therapeutic utility of genomewide methylation analysis.

Proteomics

In the same way that genomics refers to genomewide DNA sequence analysis and transcriptomics refers to global mRNA expression analysis, proteomics refers to analysis of the global pattern of protein expression. A number of different methods for high-sensitivity, high-throughput evaluation of protein expression profiles have been developed, methods that make it possible to compare changes in protein expression that correlate with specific mutations, epigenetic changes, transcriptional patterns, drug therapy and toxicity, and so on (45–49). Proteomic approaches that focus on overall patterns of expression have aleady been shown to provide novel methods for early diagnosis (50–52).

Although proteomics is itself a new method of analysis, it has already spawned a number of more advanced techniques that make possible even more detailed study of

TABLE 24.4

EMERGING CELLWIDE ANALYTIC TECHNOLOGIES

Technique	Use
Genomics	Genomewide analysis of DNA sequence and single nucleotide polymorphism variations
Pharmacogenetics	Characterization of genetic variation to predict individual patient response to drug therapy
Methylomics	Quantitative detection of the methylation status of every gene
Transcriptomics	Quantitative analysis of the level of transcription of every gene
Proteomics	Analysis of the global pattern of protein expression
Phosphoproteomics	Proteomic analysis targeted to proteins that undergo changes in phosphorylation during cell activation or signaling
Interactomics	Proteomic analysis of macromolecular networks
Metabolomics	Proteomic analysis of the entire range of cellular metabolic activities
Interferomics	Global analysis of the pattern of expression of small RNA molecules responsible for RNA interference

metabolic derangements in cells. For example, proteomics has been adapted to target proteins that undergo changes in phosphorylation during cellular activation or signaling, an approach known as phosphoproteomic analysis (53). Proteomics has also been adapted to study the global properties of macromolecular networks within cells (interactomics) and to evaluate the full range of cellular metabolic activities (metabolomics) (47,54,55). These various "omics" technologies are primarily research tools used in basic science laboratories, but there is little doubt that they will eventually find applications in the diagnostic, prognostic, or therapeutic evaluation of tumors (47,55) (Table 24.4).

RNA Interference

The recognition that several classes of short double-stranded or single-stranded RNA molecules have a profound role in the regulation of gene expression (see Chapter 1) indicates that altered RNA interference (RNAi) likely has a key role in the pathogenesis of many benign and malignant diseases. Reports that demonstrate that the profile of miRNAs (one class of small RNAs that mediate RNAi) is different in normal and neoplastic tissue (56), that alterations in miRNA are oncogenic (57,58), and that RNAi-based approaches can have therapeutic benefit (59–61) all suggest that analysis of specific small RNA molecules will likely have an important role in the pathologic evaluation of tumors, probably sooner rather than later.

It is likely that evaluation of genomewide patterns of RNAi will also prove useful for study of the role of small RNA molecules in the pathogenesis of disease. Analysis of

the genomewide pattern of RNAi will likely provide unrecognized links between DNA mutations, epigenetic modifications, and gene expression and so provide fundamental information needed to connect genomics, transcriptomics, and proteomics.

ETHICAL AND LEGAL ISSUES

The recent advances in genetic analysis have raised many ethical, legal, and social concerns, and several of these concerns directly affect pathologists. In a situation in which the diagnosis is certain but based on routine histopathologic examination alone, should a pathologist be held liable if additional confirmatory specialized testing is not performed (62)? What are the boundaries between standard ancillary tests in surgical pathology, genetic tests, and research tests (63–65)? Should informed consent for genetic testing differ from consent for conventional diagnostic and therapeutic tests? Faced with increased patient-driven demand for specialized testing, what is the appropriate venue for genetic testing; should patients have the option of direct access to genetic testing independent of any involvement by health care professionals (66)? When molecular analysis is performed, do physicians have a responsibility to disclose the test results, especially with regard to a duty to warn the patient's family members of a positive test result (63,67)? What are the obligations and liabilities of physicians regarding prophylactic therapy based solely on the results of genetic testing (68,69)? The importance of these issues is demonstrated by the fact that many of them concerns have already been the subject of litigation (63,69).

Broader social issues are also raised by molecular genetic testing in the context of surgical pathology. For example, do all patients have equal access to what are admittedly expensive tests (63,64)? Who should own or control the use of tissue specimens donated for research (70,71)? What are the boundaries between individual rights and legitimate public health interests for genetic tests or screening programs (67)?

Some of the most important ethical concerns surrounding genetic testing relate to the preservation of patient confidentiality to avoid discrimination in either employment or insurability. Fears that insurance companies will discriminate against individuals based on genetic test results may be based more on perception than fact (72,73), which is reassuring because much of the legislation thus far enacted does not reflect a sophisticated understanding of the process of medical underwriting in the insurance industry, but seems instead to have been generated primarily for political gain (65).

COST

Perhaps because the field of molecular genetic testing in diagnostic surgical pathology is still rather new, there is often a great deal of enthusiasm for analysis as an adjunct to traditional histopathologic evaluation simply because the testing can be done, with little critical evaluation of the associated cost. However, in the long run, the clinical utility of molecular analysis will not rest on its novelty factor. Cost issues will eventually play an important role in defining which molecular tests provide independent information that directly affects patient care and which tests simply increase laboratory costs.

There is no doubt that molecular genetic tests are expensive. Given that current reimbursement rates (at least in the United States) do not cover the cost of testing by even simple methods such as PCR, DNA sequence analysis, and membrane hybridization, it is difficult to imagine how laboratories will be able to afford to perform more complicated analysis such as gene expression profiling or proteomic analysis. Although technical improvements may eventually make these approaches more affordable, the cost of analysis by these advanced techniques currently excludes their application in routine clinical practice.

It is interesting to note that whereas rigorous cost-effectiveness analyses have been applied to pathologic evaluation of cytologic or surgical specimens (74–76), similar analyses are extremely rare for molecular genetic testing. Because managed care entities often evaluate whether or not they will pay for genetic tests based on cost-effectiveness analysis (77), such studies are critical if molecular analysis is to become an established component of surgical pathology. As noted above, genetic testing to tailor drug therapy to individual patients can result in immediate cost savings because it reduces adverse drug reactions; genetic testing for diagnosis (or for prognosis, or to direct therapy) is undoubtedly also cost effective because it not only establishes the optimal treatment, but also minimizes the costs and potentially harmful side effects of therapeutic regimens that are of no benefit.

Ethical Questions

Cost issues related to molecular testing include, indirectly, whether or not insurers will pay for treatments based on the result of molecular testing (78) and so raise several ethical questions. For example, if molecular testing makes it possible to distinguish between patients who are more or less likely to benefit from a therapy, will insurers refuse to pay for treatment of patients who are less likely to benefit? On what basis will medical insurers decide who is less likely to benefit? Will thresholds discriminate against patients of lower socioeconomic standing (who would be unable to pay for treatment if the insurance company refuses to pay) and patients of higher socioeconomic standing (who could afford treatment regardless of insurance coverage)?

IMPLICATIONS

The issues discussed previously emphasize several points that will most likely govern molecular genetic testing in the foreseeable future. First, from a purely practical perspective, the vast majority of cases can be diagnosed accurately and quickly by routine histopathologic evaluation (not to mention the fact that light microscopy is usually required to identify the specimens that should be referred for molecular genetic testing). Routine histopathologic diagnosis and molecular genetic analysis will continue to evolve to complement one another, rather than to compete with one another (79,80).

Second, even when a molecular test is devised that provides independent diagnostic, prognostic, or therapeutic information, the cost of genetic analysis will drive development of alternative approaches that will either replace the initial method or eliminate the need for molecular genetic analysis. Examples of this evolution in test methodology already exist and include immunohistochemical detection of chimeric proteins characteristic of specific tumor types as a replacement for detection of the underlying gene fusion by RT-PCR or FISH (Chapter 11) and solution-based detection of high-risk human papilloma virus (HPV) types as a replacement for ISH or PCR analysis of cervical biopsies (Chapter 16).

Third, many molecular tests are optimally performed on fresh tissue. Therefore, pathologists should not hesitate to freeze an aliquot of tumor from every case, if doing so will not compromise morphologic diagnosis, because the need for genetic testing cannot always be anticipated in advance. Pathologists should also submit an aliquot of tumor to their local tissue bank whenever possible, because fresh tissue is a such a valuable resource for translational research involving analysis of mutations that correlate with diagnosis, prognosis, or response to therapy; identification of tumor markers that can be used for screening or detection of early disease relapse; development of novel drug therapies; and so on (81,82).

Fourth, pathologists need to incorporate molecular genetic testing, in all its forms, into their individual and collective continuing medical education programs. Pathologists need to be prepared to advise their clinical colleagues on the settings in which molecular testing is appropriate and to ensure that the test results are correctly interpreted (63). The critical role of the laboratory physician in the broader context of genetic testing is highlighted by a recent study that showed that for almost one third of patients tested for *APC* gene mutations, the test results were incorrectly interpreted by the clinical physician who ordered the analysis (83).

REFERENCES

1. Rosai J. The continuing role of morphology in the molecular age. *Mod Pathol* 2001;14:258–260.
2. Oliveira AM, Fletcher JA. CHIPing soft tissue tumors: will the paradigms be changed? *Adv Anat Pathol* 2003;10:1–7.
3. Bongarzone I, Pierotti MA. The molecular basis of thyroid epithelial tumorigenesis. *Tumori* 2003;89:514–516.
4. Frayling IM. Methods of molecular analysis: mutation detection in solid tumours. *Mol Pathol* 2002;55:73–79.
5. Chicurel ME, Dalma-Weiszhausz DD. Microarrays in pharmacogenomics: advances and future promise. *Pharmacogenomics* 2002;3:589–601.
6. Ross JS, Linette GP, Stec J, et al. Breast cancer biomarkers and molecular medicine. II. *Expert Rev Mol Diagn* 2004;4:169–188.
7. Chicurel ME, Dalma-Weiszhausz DD. Oligonucleotide microarrays. In: Ladanyi M, Gerald W, eds. *Expression Profiling of Human Tumours: Diagnostic and Research Applications*. Totowa: Humana Press, Inc.; 2002:23–46.
8. Botstein D, Risch N. Discovering genotypes underlying human phenotypes: past successes for mendelian disease, future approaches for complex disease. *Nat Genet* 2003;33:228–237.
9. Hillan KJ, Quirke P. Preface to genomic pathology: a new frontier. *J Pathol* 2001;195:1–2.
10. He YD, Friend SH. Microarrays: the 21st century divining rod? *Nat Med* 2001;7:658–659.
11. Ransohoff DF. Rules of evidence for cancer molecular-marker discovery and validation. *Nat Rev Cancer* 2004;4:309–314.
12. Katz MH. Multivariable analysis: a primer for readers of medical research. *Ann Intern Med* 2003;138:644–650.
13. Simon R, Radmacher MD, Dobbin K, et al. Pitfalls in the use of DNA microarray data for diagnostic and prognostic classification. *J Natl Cancer Inst* 2003;95:14–18.
14. Ntzani EE, Ioannidis JP. Predictive ability of DNA microarrays for cancer outcomes and correlates: an empirical assessment. *Lancet* 2003;362:1439–1444.
15. Streubel B, Chott A, Huber D, et al. Lymphoma-specific genetic aberrations in microvascular endothelial cells in B-cell lymphomas. *N Engl J Med* 2004;351:250–259.
16. Allinen M, Beroukhim R, Cai L, et al. Molecular characterization of the tumor microenvironment in breast cancer. *Cancer Cell* 2004;6:17–32.
17. Bhowmick NA, Neilson EG, Moses HL. Stromal fibroblasts in cancer initiation and progression. *Nature* 2004;432:332–337.
18. Hida K, Hida Y, Amin DN, et al. Tumor-associated endothelial cells with cytogenetic abnormalities. *Cancer Res* 2004;64:8249–8255.
19. Maffini MV, Soto AM, Calabro JM, et al. The stroma as a crucial target in rat mammary gland carcinogenesis. *J Cell Sci* 2004;117:1495–1502.
20. Bustin S, Dorudi S. Molecular assessment of tumour stage and disease recurrence using PCR-based assays. *Mol Med Today* 1998;4:389–396.
21. Ross JS, Linette GP, Stec J, et al. Breast cancer biomarkers and molecular medicine. *Expert Rev Mol Diagn* 2003;3:573–585.
22. Oliveira AM, Fletcher CD. Molecular prognostication for soft tissue sarcomas: are we ready yet? *J Clin Oncol* 2004;22:4031–4034.
23. Hall PA, Going JJ. Predicting the future: a critical appraisal of cancer prognosis studies. *Histopathology* 1999;35:489–494.
24. http://www.cancerdiagnosis.nci.nih.gov/challenge/.
25. Weinshilbourn R. Inheritance and drug response. *N Engl J Med* 2003;348:529–537.
26. Kalow W, Tang BK, Endrenyi I. Hypothesis: comparisons of inter- and intra-individual variations can substitute for twin studies in drug research. *Pharmacogenetics* 1998;8:283–289.
27. Evans WE, McLeod HL. Pharmacogenomics: drug disposition, drug targets, and side effects. *N Engl J Med* 2003;348:538–549.
28. Ramaswamy S. Translating cancer genomics into clinical oncology. *N Engl J Med* 2004;350:1814–1816.
29. Ulrich CM, Robien K, McLeod HL. Cancer pharmacogenetics: polymorphisms, pathways and beyond. *Nat Rev Cancer* 2003;3:912–920.
30. Rosell R, Monzo M, O'Brate A, et al. Translational oncogenomics: toward rational therapeutic decision-making. *Curr Opin Oncol* 2002;14:171–179.
31. Workman P. The opportunities and challenges of personalized genome-based molecular therapies for cancer: targets, technologies, and molecular chaperones. *Cancer Chemother Pharmacol* 2003;52:45–56.
32. Schmitz G, Aslanidis C, Lackner KJ. Pharmacogenomics: implications for laboratory medicine. *Clin Chim Acta* 2001;308:43–53.
33. Tate SK, Goldstein DB. Will tomorrow's medicines work for everyone? *Nat Genet* 2004;36:34–42.
34. Johnson DH. Targeted therapy in non-small cell lung cancer: myth or reality. *Lung Cancer* 2003;41:3–8.
35. Betensky RA, Louis DN, Cairncross JG. Influence of unrecognized molecular heterogeneity on randomized clinical trials. *J Clin Oncol* 2002;20:2495–2499.
36. Service RF. Pharmacogenomics: going from genome to pill. *Science* 2005;308:1858–1860.
37. Noah L. The coming pharmacogenomics revolution: tailoring drugs to fit patients' genetic profiles. *Jurimetrics J* 2002;43:1–28.
38. Noah L. Pharmacogenetics [Letter]. *N Engl J Med* 2003;348:2042.
39. Phillips KA, Veenstra DL, Oren E, et al. Potential role of pharmacogenomics in reducing adverse drug reactions: a systematic review. *JAMA* 2001;286:2270–2279.
40. Roses AD. Genome-based pharmacogenetics and the pharmaceutical industry. *Nat Rev Drug Discov* 2002;1:541–549.
41. Gabriel SB, Schaffner SF, Nguyen H, et al. The structure of haplotype blocks in the human genome. *Science* 2002;296:2225–2229.
42. Altshuler D, Brooks LD, Chakravarti A, et al. for the International HapMap Consortium. A haplotype map of the human genome. *Nature* 2005;437:1299–1320.
43. Goldstein DB. Pharmacogenetics in the laboratory and the clinic. *N Engl J Med* 2003;348:553–556.
44. Lippman Z, Gendrel AV, Black M, et al. Role of transposable elements in heterochromatin and epigenetic control. *Nature* 2004;430:471–476.
45. Monteoliva L, Albar JP. Differential proteomics: an overview of gel and non-gel based approaches. *Brief Funct Genomic Proteomic* 2004;3:220–239.
46. Misek DE, Imafuku Y, Hanash SM. Application of proteomic technologies to tumor analysis. *Pharmacogenomics* 2004;5:1129–1137.
47. Stoughton RB, Friend SH. How molecular profiling could revolutionize drug discovery. *Nat Rev Drug Discov* 2005;4:345–350.
48. Merrick BA, Bruno ME. Genomic and proteomic profiling for biomarkers and signature profiles of toxicity. *Curr Opin Mol Ther* 2004;6:600–607.
49. Barry R, Soloviev M. Quantitative protein profiling using antibody arrays. *Proteomics* 2004;4:3717–3726.
50. Conrads TP, Zhou M, Petricoin EF 3rd, et al. Cancer diagnosis using proteomic patterns. *Expert Rev Mol Diagn* 2003;3:411–420.
51. Veenstra TD, Conrads TP. Serum protein fingerprinting. *Curr Opin Mol Ther* 2003;5:584–593.
52. Conrads TP, Hood BL, Issaq HJ, et al. Proteomic patterns as a diagnostic tool for early-stage cancer: a review of its progress to a clinically relevant tool. *Mol Diagn* 2004;8:77–85.
53. Espina V, Geho D, Mehta AI, et al. Pathology of the future: molecular profiling for targeted therapy. *Cancer Invest* 2005;23:36–46.
54. Vidal M. Interactome modeling. *FEBS Lett* 2005;579:1834–1838.
55. Bilello JA. The agony and ecstasy of "OMIC" technologies in drug development. *Curr Mol Med* 2005;5:39–52.
56. Lu J, Getz G, Miska EA, et al. MicroRNA expression profiles classify human cancers. *Nature* 2005;435:834–838.
57. He L, Thomson JM, Hemann MT, et al. A microRNA polycistron as a potential human oncogene. *Nature* 2005;435:828–833.
58. O'Donnell KA, Wentzel EA, Zeller KI, et al. c-*Myc*-regulated microRNAs modulate *E2F1* expression. *Nature* 2005;435:839–843.
59. Song E, Lee SK, Wang J, et al. RNA interference targeting Fas protects mice from fulminant hepatitis. *Nat Med* 2003;9:347–351.
60. Zhang W, Yang H, Kong X, et al. Inhibition of respiratory syncytial virus infection with intranasal siRNA nanoparticles targeting the viral NS1 gene. *Nat Med* 2005;11:56–62.
61. Bitko V, Musiyenko A, Shulyayeva O, et al. Inhibition of respiratory viruses by nasally administered siRNA. *Nat Med* 2005;11:50–55.
62. Dehner LP. On trial: a malignant small cell tumor in a child—four wrongs do not make a right. *Am J Clin Pathol* 1998;109:662–668.
63. Waldman L. The ethical, legal and psychosocial challenges of genetic testing: implications for primary medical care. *Mo Med* 2004;101:117–120.
64. Trent RJ, Yu B, Caramins M. Challenges for clinical genetic DNA testing. *Expert Rev Mol Diagn* 2004;4:201–208.
65. Rothstein MA, ed. *Genetics and life insurance: medical underwriting and social policy*. London: MIT Press; 2004.
66. Williams-Jones B. Where there's a web, there's a way: commercial genetic testing and the Internet. *Community Genet* 2003;6:46–57.
67. Hodge JG. Ethical issues concerning genetic testing and screening in public health. *Am J Med Genet C Semin Med Genet* 2004;125:66–70.
68. Palmer LI, Martin RC, Hein DW. Chemopreventive drug treatment in subjects with genetic predisposition to cancer: prescriber liability and healthcare disparities. *Pharmacogenomics* 2004;5:319–329.
69. Anderlik MR, Lisko EA. Medicolegal and ethical issues in genetic cancer syndromes. *Semin Surg Oncol* 2000;18:339–346.
70. Hakimian R, Korn D. Ownership and use of tissue specimens for research. *JAMA* 2004;292:2500–2505.
71. Ellis I, Mannion G, Warren-Jones A. Retained human tissues: a molecular genetics goldmine or modern grave robbing? A legal approach to obtaining and using stored human samples. *Med Law* 2003;22:357–372.
72. Stephenson J. Genetic test information fears unfounded. *JAMA* 1999;282:2197–2198.
73. Hall MA, Rich SS. Laws restricting health insurers' use of genetic information: impact on genetic discrimination. *Am J Hum Genet* 2000;66:293–307.
74. Mark DH. Visualizing cost-effectiveness analysis. *JAMA* 2002;287:2428–2429.
75. Esserman L, Weidner N. Is routine frozen section assessment feasible in the practice environment of the 1990s? *Cancer J Sci Am* 1997;3:266–267.
76. Raab SS. The cost-effectiveness of routine histologic examination. *Am J Clin Pathol* 1998;110:391–396.
77. Higashi MK, Veenstra DL. Managed care in the genomics era: assessing the cost effectiveness of genetic tests. *Am J Manag Care* 2003;9:493–500.
78. Service RF. Genetics and medicine: recruiting genes, proteins for a revolution in diagnostics. *Science* 2003;300:236–239.
79. Hill DA, O'Sullivan MJ, Zhu X, et al. Practical application of molecular genetic testing as an aid to the surgical pathologic diagnosis of sarcomas: a prospective study. *Am J Surg Pathol* 2002;26:965–977.
80. Ladanyi M, Bridge J. Contribution of molecular genetic data to the classification of sarcomas. *Hum Pathol* 2000;31:532–538.
81. Oosterhuis JW, Coebergh JW, van Veen EB. Tumour banks: well-guarded treasures in the interest of patients. *Nat Rev Cancer* 2003;3:73–77.
82. Teodorovic I, Therasse P, Spatz A, et al. Human tissue research: EORTC recommendations on its practical consequences. *Eur J Cancer* 2003;39:2256–2263.
83. Giardiello FM, Brensinger JD, Petersen GM, et al. The use and interpretation of commercial *APC* gene testing for familial adenomatous polyposis. *N Engl J Med* 1997;336:823–827.

Genetic Codes

1

THE NUCLEAR GENETIC CODE

First Position (5')	Second Position				Third Position (3')
	U	**C**	**A**	**G**	
U	UUU Phe UUC Phe UUA Leu UUG Leu	UCU Ser UCC Ser UCA Ser UCG Ser	UAU Tyr UAC Tyr UAA Stop UAG Stop	UGU Cys UGC Cys UGA Stop/Sec[1] UGG Trp	U C A G
C	CUU Leu CUC Leu CUA Leu CUG Leu	CCU Pro CCC Pro CCA Pro CCG Pro	CAU His CAC His CAA Gln CAG Gln	CGU Arg CGC Arg CGA Arg CGG Arg	U C A G
A	AUU Ile AUC Ile AUA Ile AUG Met	ACU Thr ACC Thr ACA Thr ACG Thr	AAU Asn AAC Asn AAA Lys AAG Lys	AGU Ser AGC Ser AGA Arg AGG Arg	U C A G
G	GUU Val GUC Val GUA Val GUG Val	GCU Ala GCC Ala GCA Ala GCG Ala	GAU Asp GAC Asp GAA Glu GAG Glu	GGU Gly GGC Gly GGA Gly GGG Gly	U C A G

1. The UGA codon has a dual role, serving as a STOP codon and as a Sec (selenocysteine) codon. For an in-frame UGA to dictate addition of Sec during protein synthesis, a Sec insertion sequence element must be present in the 3'-UTR of the mRNA (see reference 221 of Chapter 1).

THE MITOCHONDRIAL GENETIC CODE

First Position (5′)	Second Position				Third Position (3′)
	U	C	A	G	
U	UUU Phe	UCU Ser	UAU Tyr	UGU Cys	U
	UUC Phe	UCC Ser	UAC Tyr	UGC Cys	C
	UUA Leu	UCA Ser	UAA Stop	UGA Trp	A
	UUG Leu	UCG Ser	UAG Stop	UGG Trp	G
C	CUU Leu	CCU Pro	CAU His	CGU Arg	U
	CUC Leu	CCC Pro	CAC His	CGC Arg	C
	CUA Leu	CCA Pro	CAA Gln	CGA Arg	A
	CUG Leu	CCG Pro	CAG Gln	CGG Arg	G
A	AUU Ile	ACU Thr	AAU Asn	AGU Ser	U
	AUC Ile	ACC Thr	AAC Asn	AGC Ser	C
	AUA Met	ACA Thr	AAA Lys	AGA Stop	A
	AUG Met	ACG Thr	AAG Lys	AGG Stop	G
G	GUU Val	GCU Ala	GAU Asp	GGU Gly	U
	GUC Val	GCC Ala	GAC Asp	GGC Gly	C
	GUA Val	GCA Ala	GAA Glu	GGA Gly	A
	GUG Val	GCG Ala	GAG Glu	GGG Gly	G

Boxes indicate differences between the nuclear and mitochondrial genetic codes.

Amino acids

Amino Acid	3-Letter Abbreviation	1-Letter Abbreviation	Charge
Alanine	Ala	A	O
Arginine	Arg	R	+
Asparagine	Asn	N	O
Aspartic Acid	Asp	D	−
Cysteine	Cys	C	O
Glutamic Acid	Glu	E	−
Glutamine	Gln	Q	O
Glycine	Gly	G	O
Histidine	His	H	+
Isoleucine	Ile	I	O
Leucine	Leu	L	O
Lysine	Lys	K	+
Methionine	Met	M	O
Phenylalanine	Phe	F	O
Proline	Pro	P	O
Selenocysteine	Sec	U	O
Serine	Ser	S	O
Stop	X	X	
Threonine	Thr	T	O
Tryptophan	Trp	W	O
Tyrosine	Tyr	Y	O
Valine	Val	V	O

General Structure

$H_2N-\overset{\overset{H}{|}}{\underset{\underset{R}{|}}{C}}-COOH$

Charged Polar

Aspartic acid   Glutamic acid   Lysine   Arginine   Histidine

Acidic   *Basic*

Uncharged Polar

Asparagine   Glutamine   Serine   Threonine   Tyrosine   Cysteine   Selenocysteine

Amide Groups   *Hydroxyl Groups*   *Sulfhydryl Group*

Nonpolar

Glycine   Alanine   Valine   Leucine   Isoleucine   Proline

Methionine   Phenylalanine   Tryptophan

Summary of Recommended Nomenclature for Describing Mutations[1]

3

DESCRIPTION AT THE DNA LEVEL

- For genomic DNA and cDNA, the A of the ATG of the initiator Met codon is denoted nucleotide +1. There is no nucleotide zero. The nucleotide 5' to +1 is numbered −1. If there is more than one potential ATG, a reference consensus may be used. The numbering of nucleotides in the reference sequence in the databases should not be changed and will always be associated with the same (original) accession number.

- The use of lower case g for genomic or c for cDNA in front of the nucleotide number is recommended. To avoid confusion, a dot should separate these from the nucleotide number (g. or c. for genomic or cDNA, respectively). The accession number in primary sequence databases (Genbank, EMBL, DDJB) should also be included in the original publication/database submission.

- Nucleotide changes start with the nucleotide number and the change follows this number. 1997G>T denotes that at nucleotide 1997 of the reference sequence, G is replaced by a T.

- Deletions are designated by del after the nucleotide number. 1997delT denotes the deletion of T at nt 1997. 1997−1999del denotes the deletion of 3 nts. Alternatively, this mutation can be noted as 1997−1999delTTC. For deletions in short tandem repeats, the most 3' nt is arbitrarily assigned; e.g. a TG deletion in the sequence AATGTGTGCC is designated 1997−1998delTG or 1997−1998del (where 1997 is the first T before C).

- Insertions are designated by ins after the nucleotide interval number. 1997−1998insT denotes that T was inserted in the interval between nts 1997 and 1998. For insertions in short repeats, the most 3' nt interval is arbitrarily assigned; e.g. a TG insertion in the sequence AATGTGTGCC is designated 1997−1998insTG (where 1997 is the last G of the short TG repeat).

- Variability of short sequence repeats is designated as 1997(GT)6−22. In this case, 1997 is the first nucleotide of the dinucleotide GT, which is repeated 6 to 22 times in the population.

- A unique identifier for each mutation should be obtained. The OMIM unique identifier can be used (2), or database curators may assign such unique identifiers. Other existing databases, such as the HGMD (3,4), can also be used as a reference source for mutations that are already catalogued.

- Intron mutations when the full genomic sequence is not known can be designated by the intron (IVS) number, positive numbers starting from the G of the donor site invariant GT, negative numbers starting from the G of the acceptor site invariant AG. IVS4+1G > T denotes the G to T substitution at the nt + 1 of intron 4. IVS4−2A > C denotes the A to C substitution at nt −2 of intron 4. Alternatively the cDNA nucleotide numbering may be used to designate the location of the mutation in the adjacent intron. For example, c.1997+1G > T denotes the G to T substitution at nt +1 after nucleotide 1997 of the cDNA. Similarly, c.1997−2A > C denotes the A to C substitution at nt−2 upstream of nucleotide 1997 of the cDNA. When the full length genomic sequence is known, the mutation can also be simply designated by the nt number of the reference sequence.

- Two mutations in the same allele can be listed within brackets as follows: [1997G > T;2001A > C]. This will also allow the (i) designation of mutations that are only deleterious when they occur in the same allele with additional nucleotide substitutions; (ii) designation of haplotypes of different alleles.

DESCRIPTION AT THE PROTEIN LEVEL

- The codon for the initiator Methionine is codon 1.
- The single letter amino acid code is recommended. However, the three letter code is also acceptable.

- For amino acid nomenclature, the format is Y97S (Tyrosine at codon 97 substituted by Serine). The "wild type" amino acid is given before and the mutant amino acid after the codon number. Therefore there is no confusion as to the significance of G,C,T and A in the nomenclature.
- Stop codons are designated by X. For example R97X (Arginine codon 96 substituted by a termination codon).
- Deletions of amino acids are designated as: T97del denotes that the codon 97 for Threonine is deleted.
- Insertions of amino acids are designated as: T97−98ins denotes that a codon for Threonine is inserted at the interval between codons 97 and 98 of the reference sequence of the protein.
- The first report of a mutation in the literature should contain both a nucleotide and amino acid based name when appropriate.

COMPLEX MUTATIONS

- Recommendations for more complex mutations have been published (5) and can also be found online (6). Detailed description of such mutations and nomenclature proposals can usually be found in the original reference or by the unique identifier.

- Investigators that maintain mutation databases are encouraged to include a field of mutation consequence or mutation mechanism (if known) in their databases.

LACK OF CONSENSUS

The recommendations listed above do not always represent a full consensus, and updates and discussion of attentive nomenclature can be found online (6). For example,

- The "$\wedge$" sign may be used to determine the interval of an insertion rather than the "−" sign. For example, 1997$^{\wedge}$1998insG instead of 1997−1998insG.
- The designation of both deleterious mutations in the two alleles of a homozygote for a recessive disorder may be designated as [1997G > T + 2001A > G] to indicate the substitution in nucleotide 1997 of one allele and in nucleotide 2001 of the other allele of the same gene.
- Analogous to g. or c. for the genomic or cDNA numbering system, the p. symbol may be used to clearly distinguish the protein-based nomenclature.
- X may not be the best symbol for a termination codon.

REFERENCES

1. Used by permission of Antonarakis SE. Recommendations for a nomenclature system for human gene mutations. Nomenclature Working Group. *Hum Mutat* 1998;11:1–3. New York: Wiley.
2. http://www.ncbi.nlm.nih.gov/entrez/query.fcgi?db=OMIM.
3. http://archive.uwcm.ac.uk/uwcm/mg/hgmd0.html.
4. Stenson PD, Ball EV, Mort M, et al. Human Gene Mutation Database (HGMD): 2003 update. *Hum Mutat* 2003;21:577–581.
5. den Dunnen JT, Antonarakis SE. Mutation nomenclature extensions and suggestions to describe complex mutations: a discussion. *Hum Mutat* 2000;15(1):7–12.
6. http://www.dmd.nl/mutnomen.html.

Index